ESTHETICS *and* BIOMECHANICS *in* ORTHODONTICS

Second Edition

Ravindra Nanda, BDS, MDS, PhD
UConn Orthodontic Alumni Endowed Chair
Professor and Head
Department of Craniofacial Sciences
Chair, Division of Orthodontics
School of Dental Medicine
University of Connecticut
Farmington, Connecticut

ELSEVIER

ELSEVIER
SAUNDERS

3251 Riverport Lane
St. Louis, Missouri 63043

ESTHETICS AND BIOMECHANICS IN ORTHODONTICS ISBN: 978-1-4557-5085-6

Previous edition copyrighted 2005.

Library of Congress Cataloging-in-Publication Data

Esthetics and biomechanics in orthodontics / [edited by] Ravindra Nanda.—2nd edition.
p. ; cm.
Preceded by: Biomechanics and esthetic strategies in clinical orthodontics / Ravindra Nanda. c2005.
Includes bibliographical references and index.
ISBN 978-1-4557-5085-6 (hardcover : alk. paper)
I. Nanda, Ravindra, editor of compilation. II. Nanda, Ravindra. Biomechanics and esthetic strategies in clinical orthodontics. Preceded by (work):
[DNLM: 1. Malocclusion—therapy. 2. Biomechanics. 3. Esthetics, Dental. WU 440]
RK523
617.6'43—dc23

2013046414

Executive Content Strategist: Kathy Falk
Sr. Content Development Specialist: Courtney Sprehe
Publishing Services Manager: Deborah Vogel
Project Manager: Brandilyn Flagg
Designer: Ashley Miner

Last digit is the print number: 9 8 7 6 5 4 3 2 1

I dedicate this book, with love, to my cherished wife Catherine.
I truly appreciate all that you do for me.
It is because of you all things are possible.

CONTRIBUTORS

Mustafa Burhan Ateş, DDS, PhD
Assistant Professor
Department of Orthodontics
Faculty of Dentistry
Marmara University
Istanbul, Turkey

Zaher Aymach, DDS, PhD
Visiting Lecturer and Former Doctoral Resident
Division of Oral and Maxillofacial Surgery
Tohoku University
Sendai, Japan;
Post-Doctoral Fellowship–Trained
Department of Craniofacial Sciences
School of Dental Medicine
University of Connecticut
Farmington, Connecticut;
Post-Doctoral Resident
Department of Orthodontics
Howard University
College of Dentistry
Washington, DC

Bin Cai, DDS
Orthodontic Department
Guanghua School of Stomatology
Hospital of Stomatology
Sun Yat-sen University
Guangzhou, Guangdong, China

Taranpreet K. Chandhoke, DMD, PhD
Assistant Professor
Division of Orthodontics
Department of Craniofacial Sciences
School of Dental Medicine
University of Connecticut
Farmington, Connecticut

Aditya Chhibber, BDS, MDS
Division of Orthodontics
Department of Craniofacial Sciences
University of Connecticut Health Center
Farmington, Connecticut

R. Scott Conley, DMD
Robert W. Browne Professor of Dentistry
Clinical Associate Professor
Department of Orthodontics and Pediatric Dentistry
School of Dentistry
University of Michigan
Ann Arbor, Michigan

Tarisai C. Dandajena, DDS, MS, PhD
Assistant Professor of Orthodontics and Cell Biology
Department of Orthodontics and Department of Cell Biology
College of Dentistry and College of Medicine
University of Oklahoma Health Sciences Center
Oklahoma City, Oklahoma

Nejat Erverdi, DDS, PhD
Professor and Full-time University Staff
Marmara University
Istanbul, Turkey

Mithran S. Goonewardene, BDSc, MMedSc
Head and Program Director
Orthodontics Dental School
University of Western Australia
Nedlands, Western Australia

Urban Hägg, DDS, Odont Dr
Department of Orthodontics
Institute of Odontology
Faculty of Health Sciences
University of Copenhagen
Copenhagen, Denmark

Nandakumar Janakiraman, BDS, MDS
Division of Orthodontics
Department of Craniofacial Sciences
School of Dental Medicine
University of Connecticut
Farmington, Connecticut

Sunil Kapila, BDS, MS, PhD
Robert W. Browne Endowed Professor and Chair
Department of Orthodontics and Pediatric Dentistry
Graduate Orthodontics Program Director
University of Michigan
School of Dentistry
Ann Arbor, Michigan

Hiroshi Kawamura, DDS, PhD
Former Head and Chair
Division of Oral and Maxillofacial Surgery
Tohoku University
Sendai, Japan

Gregory J. King, DMD, DMSC
Professor Emeritus
Department of Orthodontics
University of Washington
Seattle, Washington

Vincent G. Kokich, DDS, MSD*
Professor
Department of Orthodontics
University of Washington
Seattle, Washington
Editor-in-Chief, *American Journal of Orthodontics and Dentofacial Orthopedics*

Vincent O. Kokich, DMD, MSD
Affiliate Assistant Professor
Department of Orthodontics
School of Dentistry
University of Washington
Seattle, Washington

Nazan Küçükkeleş, DDS, PhD
Department of Orthodontics
Faculty of Dentistry
Marmara University
Istanbul, Turkey

Harry L. Legan, DDS
Private Practice in Orthodontics
Nashville, TN and Laredo, Texas

Melih Motro, DDS, PhD
Department of Orthodontics
Faculty of Dentistry
Marmara University
Istanbul, Turkey

Padma Mukherjee, BDS, PhD
Assistant Professor
Predoctoral Program Director
Department of Orthodontics
Rutgers School of Dental Medicine
State University of New Jersey
Newark, New Jersey

Hiroshi Nagasaka, DDS, DDSc
Chief Surgeon
Division of Oral Surgery
Sendai Medical Center;
Former Lecturer
Division of Oral and Maxillofacial Surgery
Tohoku University
Sendai, Japan

Ram S. Nanda, BDS, DDS, MS, PhD
Professor and Chair Emeritus; Founder
Department of Orthodontics
University of Oklahoma
College of Dentistry
Oklahoma City, Oklahoma

Ravindra Nanda, BDS, MDS, PhD
UConn Orthodontic Alumni Endowed Chair
Professor and Head
Department of Craniofacial Sciences
Chair, Division of Orthodontics
School of Dental Medicine
University of Connecticut
Farmington, Connecticut

Şirin Nevzatoğlu, DDS, PhD
Assistant Professor
Department of Orthodontics
Faculty of Dentistry
Marmara University
Istanbul, Turkey

Peter W. Ngan, DMD
Certificates in Orthodontics and Pediatric Dentistry
Department of Orthodontics
School of Dentistry
West Virginia University
Morgantown, West Virginia

Marco Rosa, MD, DDS, D.Orthod
Assistant Professor
Postgraduate School in Orthodontics
Insubria University
Varese, Italy

*Deceased.

Bradley G. Shepherd, BDSc, MDSc
Private Practice in Prosthodontics
Perth, Australia

Junji Sugawara, DDS, DDSc
Visiting Professor
Division of Orthodontics
Department of Craniofacial Sciences
University of Connecticut Health Center
Farmington, Connecticut;
Visiting Professor
Division of Oral and Maxillofacial Surgery
Tohoku University;
Head, Orthodontic Section
SAS Orthodontic Center
Sendai, Japan

Jae-Hyun Sung, DDS, MSD, PhD
Professor Emeritus
Kyungpook National University
Daegu, South Korea

Madhur Upadhyay, BDS, MDS, MDentSc
Director (Orthodontic Fellowship Program)
Assistant Professor
Division of Orthodontics
Department of Craniofacial Sciences
School of Dental Medicine
University of Connecticut
Farmington, Connecticut

Flavio Andres Uribe, DDS, MDentSc
Associate Professor
Program Director
Division of Orthodontics
Department of Craniofacial Sciences
School of Dental Medicine
University of Connecticut
Farmington, Connecticut

Carlos Villegas, DDS
Sociedad Colombiana de Ortodoncia (SCO)
Asociación Colombiana de Cirugía Oral y Maxilofacial (ACCOMF)
World Federation of Orthodontists (WFO)
Asociación Latinoamericana de Cirugía Bucomaxilofacial (ALACIBU)
Medellín, Colombia

Benedict Wilmes, PhD
Department of Orthodontics
University of Duesseldorf
Duesseldorf, Germany

Ricky Wing Kit Wong, BDS, MOrth, PhD, MOrthRCS
Clinical Associate Professor
Orthodontics Unit of the Faculty of Dentistry
The University of Hong Kong
Pokfulam, Hong Kong

Sumit Yadav, BDS, MDS, PhD
Assistant Professor
Division of Orthodontics
Department of Craniofacial Sciences
School of Dental Medicine
University of Connecticut
Farmington, Connecticut

Satoshi Yamada, DDS, PhD
Orthodontist
SAS Orthodontic Center
Sendai, Japan

Hanife Nuray Yılmaz, DDS, PhD
Research Assistant in the Department of Orthodontics
Faculty of Dentistry
Marmara University
Istanbul,Turkey

Bjørn U. Zachrisson, DDS, MSD, PhD
Professor Emeritus
Department of Orthodontics
University of Oslo
Oslo, Norway

Xiao-Guang Zhao, BDS, MSD, PhD
Orthodontic Department
Guanghua School of Stomatology
Hospital of Stomatology
Sun Yat-sen University
Guangzhou, Guangdong, China

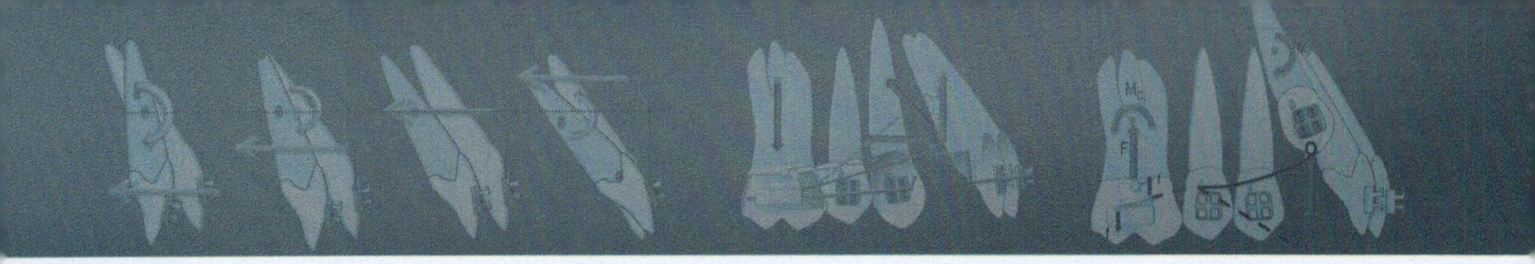

PREFACE

Esthetics and Biomechanics in Orthodontics combines two of the most important aspects of orthodontic treatment: *esthetics* and *biomechanics*. The basis of orthodontic treatment lies in the clinical application of biomechanic concepts, and understanding these concepts is imperative to achieving successful treatment outcomes. One of the key objectives of this book is to present how the esthetic objectives of orthodontic treatment can be successfully obtained with biomechanics-based orthodontic appliances. Some of the most eminent clinicians and scientists in the field of contemporary orthodontics have come together to provide you with state-of-the-art guidance on the how the principles of biomechanics can be applied to all orthodontic techniques to improve force delivery, prevent side effects, and achieve esthetically-pleasing, predictable results.

NEW TO THIS EDITION

13 NEW chapters

- Chapter 5: Biological Mechanisms in Orthodontic Tooth Movement
- Chapter 7: Biomechanics-Based Management of Impacted Canines
- Chapter 10: Molar and Incisor Positioning to Achieve Occlusal and Esthetic Objectives
- Chapter 13: Class II Correction with an Intermaxillary Fixed Noncompliance Device: Twin Force Bite Corrector
- Chapter 14: Treatment Strategies for Developing and Nondeveloping Class III Malocclusions
- Chapter 15 Clinical Practice Guidelines for Developing Class III Malocclusion
- Chapter 17: New Treatment Modalities for Class III Malocclusion
- Chapter 18: Achieving Optimal Esthetics with Palatal Mini-Implants: The Benefit Technique
- Chapter 19: Expanding the Limits for Esthetic Strategies by Skeletal Anchorage
- Chapter 21: Esthetics and New Approaches to Orthognathic Surgery
- Chapter 22: Surgery First: The Protocol of Innovative Surgical Orthodontics
- Chapter 24: Interdisciplinary Strategies for Treating Adult Patients
- Chapter 25: Missing Maxillary Lateral Incisors: New Procedures and Indications for Optimal Space Closure

KEY FEATURES

In addition to the thirteen new chapters, ***Esthetics and Biomechanics in Orthodontics*** includes:

- **Detailed case reports** representing key concepts to improve understanding all of the principles at play in the particular case
- High quality **photographs**, **radiographs**, and **line drawings** illustrating the various stages of treatment and biomechanical principles
- Chapters addressing **Individualized Orthodontic Diagnosis and Treatment Planning**, both fundamental components for successful treatment
- A **distinguished group of practitioners and scholars** from around the world bring their experience and expertise to each topic

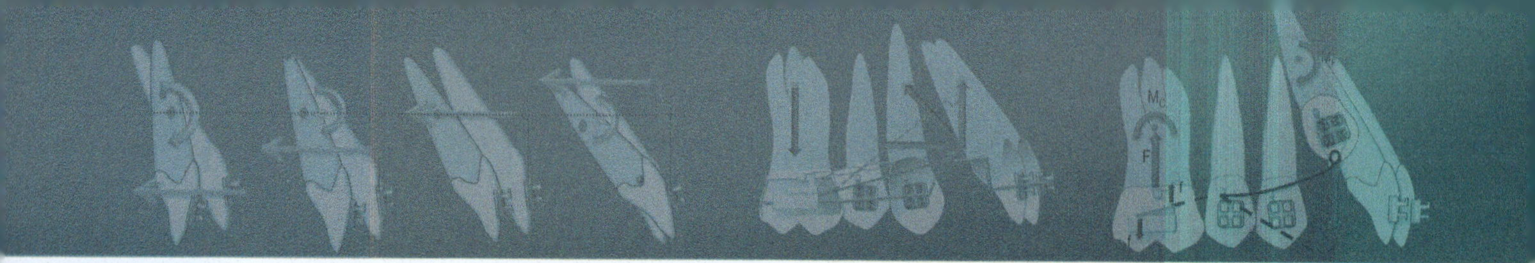

ACKNOWLEDGMENTS

My sincere thanks to all the contributors for agreeing to be part of this edition, and a special thanks to the new contributors who helped fill the gaps of the first edition.

Dr. Flavio Uribe deserves a special mention for helping me at each and every step. His work ethic and desire to innovate and share his innovations through his prolific writing is highly appreciated by all here at the University of Connecticut. The future of orthodontics is secure with researchers, clinicians, and mentors like him.

I also want to express my thanks to Madhur Upadhyay, Sumit Yadav, Preeti Chandhok, Amir Davoody, Jonny Feldman, and Nandakumar Janakiraman for their contributions at various stages. They helped to make this book possible.

My thanks also go to my two residents Thomas Dobie and Amir Assefnia for assisting with the design of cover of this edition and to Carlos Villegas for providing images of his patient.

A special thanks to Courtney Sprehe, my editor at Elsevier, for pushing me to complete this project. Her help at each and every step is much appreciated.

My special gratitude to late Vince Kokich for his legendary contributions to our profession and this book.

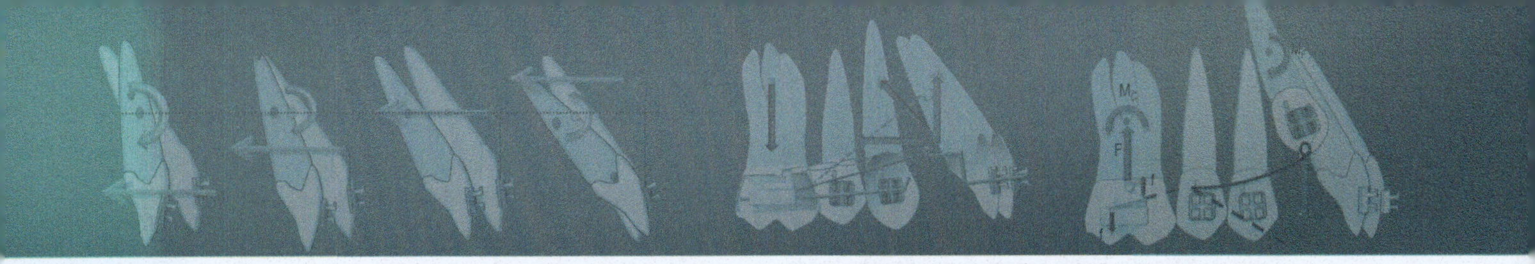

CONTENTS

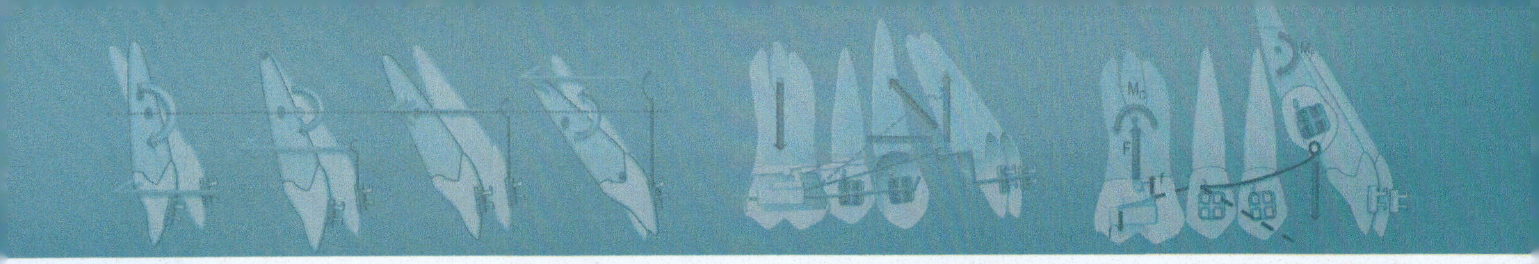

CHAPTER 1

Individualized Orthodontic Diagnosis

Flavio Andres Uribe, Taranpreet K. Chandhoke, and Ravindra Nanda

The term *diagnosis* is defined as the identification of a disease by careful investigation of its symptoms and history.[1] While not a true disease per se, malocclusions are the "disease" processes of orthodontics and the central focus of orthodontic diagnoses. Malocclusions can have esthetic and functional implications, and an accurate diagnosis is required to best understand their etiology and the treatment options for managing the abnormality. From an esthetic standpoint, there are psychological implications associated with malocclusions related to social acceptance and success.[2] From a functional standpoint, mastication, speech, and protection of the structures in the entire stomatognathic system can contribute to or be the result of the malocclusion that is present.

To define the abnormal or pathological characteristics of the malocclusion, there needs to be an appreciation of what is defined as "normal." This is a particular challenge because what is considered normal falls within a wide range. Variability is found throughout nature, so defining the limits of the normal range can be difficult. While esthetic perceptions vary through history and among individuals, races, and cultures, ideal occlusion and its functional implications are characterized by strict morphological features. Thus the definition of a normal occlusion involves both objective and subjective components.

Extensive research has determined the characteristics of normal functional occlusion. Concepts such as cusp-to-fossa or cusp-to-interproximal space occlusion, lateral and anterior guidance, and mutually protected occlusion are described comprehensively in other textbooks.[3] However, the criteria for ideal occlusal function are better defined in comparison to ideal esthetic values. Most of the occlusal concepts accepted today are derived from the assumed premise that good anatomy (i.e., good occlusal interdigitation) is analogous to proper function (Fig. 1-1).

From the esthetic standpoint, orthodontists base their judgment on cephalometric norms obtained many decades ago from population samples with vaguely defined parameters of esthetics. In general, these studies assumed that good occlusion was directly related to good facial esthetics. Although these measurements provide some objective guidelines that can be used to start defining how each patient differs from the norm, there are limitations to these analyses. Furthermore, it is not the absolute numeric amounts and their variation that dictate treatment but the accurate interpretation of these and all data obtained from the clinical examination and other patient records.

To accurately diagnose a malocclusion, orthodontics has adopted the problem-based approach originally developed in medicine.[4] Every factor that potentially contributes to the etiology, might contribute to the abnormality, or might influence treatment should be evaluated. Information is gathered through a medical and dental history, clinical examination, and records that include models, photographs, and radiographic imaging. A problem list is generated from the analysis of the database that contains a network of interrelated factors. The diagnosis is established after a continuous feedback between the problem recognition and the database. Ultimately, the diagnosis should provide some insight into the etiology of the malocclusion (Fig. 1-2).

The diagnosis and problem list is the framework that dictates the treatment objectives for the patient. Once formulated, the treatment plan is designed to address those objectives, from the mechanics to the sequence that will be used.

From the treatment objectives perspective, one or more treatment options can be developed to address each objective. Each treatment option will have advantages and disadvantages for the patient. During the process of obtaining informed consent from the patient, clear descriptions of the advantages, disadvantages, and risks of each treatment plan should be presented and the patient will ultimately determine the final treatment plan. The treatment plan then dictates the mechanics plan designed to achieve the desired goals with the greatest efficiency and fewest side effects.

This chapter discusses some of the objective measures that define the range of normality, both from an occlusal and a dentofacial standpoint. It is important to know that

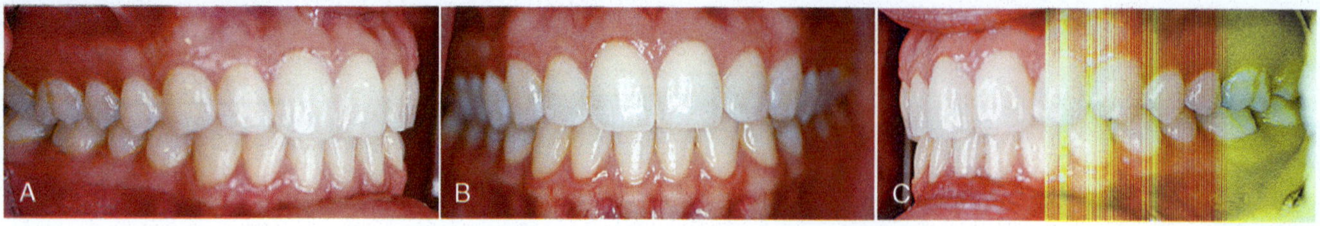

Figure 1-1 **A–C,** Frontal and lateral views of an ideal occlusion.

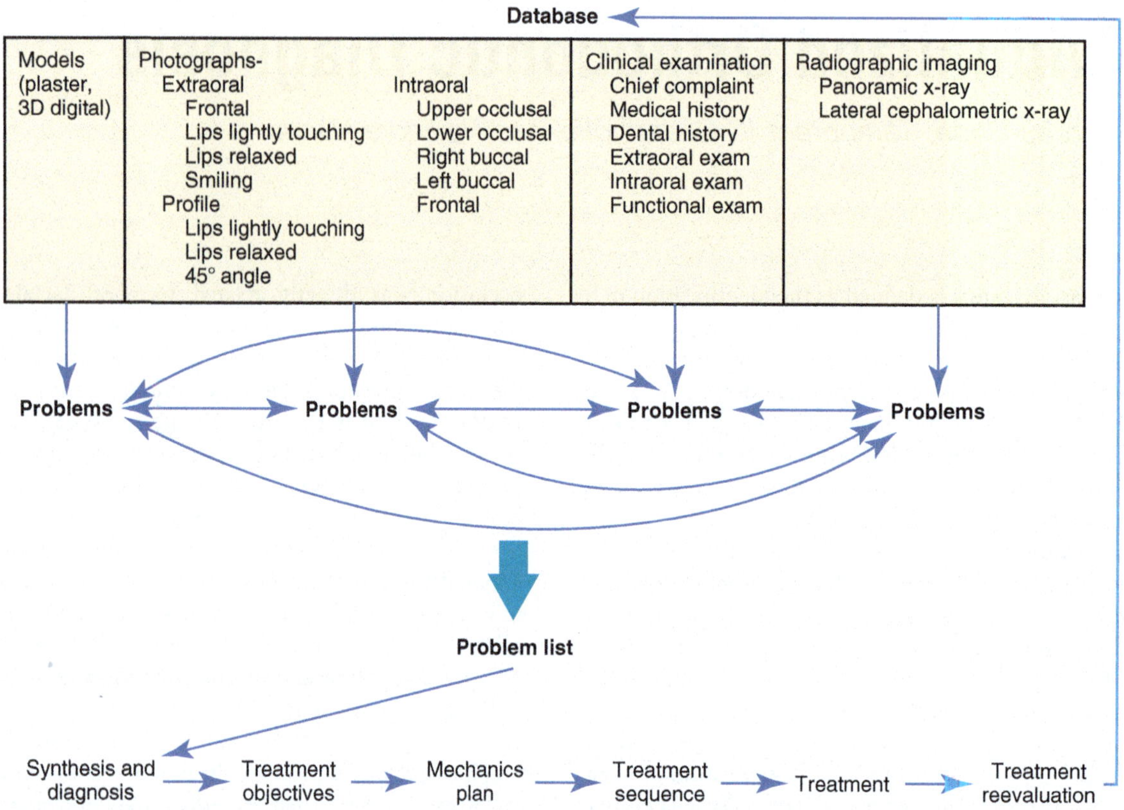

Figure 1-2 Steps in diagnosis and treatment planning.

although emphasis is placed on the entire dentofacial complex, there are limits to the amount of correction that can be achieved with orthodontic treatment.

The clinician has to work within certain constraints and understand the limitations of the various treatment options. For example, the soft tissue envelope allows for only a certain amount of correction. If major movements are needed, they may require other treatment options such as surgery or skeletal anchorage, which, although able to achieve a wider range of movements, are limited by the boundaries of the soft tissue envelope. The primary goal should be to achieve the best possible facial balance and functional occlusion.

Finally, while great care is taken in formulating a detailed treatment plan, it is important to realize that the diagnosis and treatment plan are dynamic processes. As the plan is executed, continuous monitoring and effective evaluation of the objectives are needed. Appropriate reassessment, adjustment, and corrective measures to the original plan are crucial if all specific goals and not only the occlusal goals are to be achieved.

As described above, very precise collection of data is needed to achieve a proper diagnosis. The database should include a thorough medical and dental history, a set of models, the necessary radiographs, and a clinical examination accompanied by extraoral and intraoral photographs.

CLINICAL EXAMINATION

Medical and Dental History

"What is the patient's chief complaint?" This question is the basis of the anamnesis. At a minimum, the treatment plan should aim to address this important fundamental component of the patient's initial screening. The clinician is responsible for accurately understanding and addressing the chief complaint. Some patients will have very specific goals for treatment while others will provide more generalized expectations. Clear communication is the key to understanding a patient's objectives. With young patients, it is usually the parents who voice their complaint about the child's teeth. Commonly, the child is lacking in motivation or is too shy

TABLE 1-1 Medical Conditions to be Considered in Orthodontic Treatment

Medical Condition	Implications	Action
Allergies	Allergic reaction	Determine material causing allergy and substitute a nonallergic material
Asthma	Root resorption	Monitor every 6 months for evidence of EARR
Coagulation disorders	Bleeding risk	Avoid treatment plans involving extractions if possible
Diabetes	Periodontal disease	Monitor adequate control of diabetes. Manage with a periodontist
Epilepsy	Gingival hypertrophy (medications)	Monitor excellent plaque control. Manage with a periodontist for possible surgical intervention during treatment
Heart valve conditions	Endocarditis	Premedication when fitting bands
High blood pressure patient taking calcium channel blockers	Gingival hyperplasia secondary to medications	Monitor oral hygiene. Complement brushing with chlorhexidine
HIV	Periodontal disease, opportunistic infections	Consult with physician about patient's general condition. Monitor oral hygiene and periodontal status
Leukemia	Mucositis, oral infections	Remove appliances until remission (consult physician)
Osteoporosis	Bisphosphonate-related ONJ, delayed tooth movement	Determine formulation of medication and explain potential limited outcomes of treatment to patient
Physical or mental handicap	Gingivitis, relapse (muscle hyperactivity or hypoactivity)	Electric toothbrushes may aid in oral hygiene. Consider mechanics plan in which manual dexterity is not needed (noncompliance mechanics)
Rheumatoid arthritis	TMJ degeneration	Monitor TMJ. Manage with an oral surgeon if severe arthritic degeneration
Transplant patient	Gingival hyperplasia related to immunosuppressant drugs	Monitor oral hygiene. Consider chemical complement to brushing such as chlorhexidine
Xerostomia (primary or secondary)	Caries	Monitor for loose appliances. Consider fluoride rinses as an oral hygiene supplement

EARR, External apical root resorption; *HIV*, human immunodeficiency virus; *ONJ*, osteonecrosis of the jaws; *TMJ*, temporomandibular joint.

to express himself or herself. The parents' concerns should be a major consideration but the child should also be involved through a set of simple questions that will guide the clinician in discovering the child's motivation for treatment, if any.

The medical history gives pertinent information about the physical well-being of the patient. Numerous medical conditions can affect treatment in one way or another (Table 1-1).[5] For example, a history of a cardiac malformation or anomaly may be an indication for premedication before certain orthodontic procedures.[6] A history of rheumatoid arthritis can have direct implications on the temporomandibular joint (TMJ) and thus on the occlusion. A patient with hemophilia may opt for a nonextraction treatment approach. All of these conditions may affect the delivery of treatment in the various phases: pre-treatment, treatment, and post-treatment.

Any metabolic disorder, such as diabetes, should be well-controlled before and during treatment, as healing is greatly hindered in uncontrolled types of diabetes.[7]

Another common medical condition of concern, especially in young patients, is asthma, not only because of the respiratory implications, but also because there is some evidence that patients with asthma who undergo orthodontic treatment have an increased incidence of root resorption.[8]

The above are some of the more common medical conditions, but it is important that all medical conditions be reviewed and further investigated (e.g., with a phone call to the patient's physician) if needed, as they may affect the treatment directly or indirectly. A more extensive review of these and other common medical disorders related to orthodontics can be found elsewhere.[5]

Another part of the medical history review specific to female patients is pregnancy. It is usually best to delay treatment until the pregnancy is over. The three basic reasons for postponing treatment are that radiographs usually are not recommended during pregnancy, there is an increased possibility of gingival hyperplasia due to hormonal influence, and in some instances the future mother's nutrition may be compromised as pain is elicited by tooth movement.

Other important information related to the medical history is the list of medications the patient may be taking and the existence of any allergies. Medications such as phenytoin (anticonvulsant), nifedipine (calcium channel blocker), and cyclosporine (immunosuppressive) need special attention, as they have the potential to cause a hyperplastic gingival response.[9] Some medications may also influence the progress of orthodontic treatment. Among these are oral bisphosphonates, which are used to treat osteoporosis in perimenopausal women through inhibition of osteoclastic activity, thereby reducing bone resorption. Proper osteoclastic activity is necessary to ensure physiological tooth movement. Local administration of bisphosphonates has been shown to significantly delay tooth movement and space closure in rats.[10,11] Studies have shown that patients taking bisphosphonates have increased treatment times, especially in extraction cases, and potentially compromised outcomes due to difficulty in achieving root parallelism and complete space closure.[12] There is an increased risk of osteonecrosis of the jaws (ONJ) with bisphosphonates, specifically with an intravenous formulation. However, this risk is significantly lower in patients taking oral bisphosphonates.

Potential allergies to the alloys used in orthodontics should also be identified. Hypersensitivity to nickel has been reported with a prevalence of up to 28%.[13] Allergies to other metals used in orthodontics, such as chromium and cobalt alloys, have also been reported.[14] It is important to know the nature of the reaction to each allergen. Allergies related to the airway are also a significant finding, as they impair normal nasal breathing thus potentially affecting the growth and development of the jaws.[15]

The use of tobacco should also be ascertained from the medical history. It is not uncommon to encounter adolescent and adult patients who smoke. Smoking can have an adverse effect on the periodontal condition of patients,[16] is a risk factor for periodontal disease, and has been shown to delay wound healing.[17] Health providers also have an important duty to dissuade teenagers and adults from tobacco use.

With more adult patients seeking orthodontic treatment, it is critical to determine whether these patients are periodontally stable for fixed treatment. Fixed appliance therapy will likely aggravate an underlying peridontal problem due to poor oral hygiene and activation of bone remodelling.[18] The orthodontist should take the necessary steps to minimize deleterious effects and also set realistic expectations for these patients. A full mouth series should be evaluated prior to the start of treatment and a focused clinical exam should be done to determine the periodontal status. Collaboration with a periodontist may be necessary to determine whether the patient is periodontally healthy for orthodontic treatment. If the patient has periodontitis, further periodontal therapy is indicated, which may involve a combination of therapies of scaling and root planing or open flap debridement depending on the severity of the disease.[19] It may also be indicated to increase the frequency of prophylaxis and monitoring by a general dentist or periodontist during fixed appliance treatment to ensure that the periodontal status remains stable.

Growth and Development

A specific section in the medical and dental interview should be dedicated to growth and development information. Most pediatricians keep a growth record of every child from birth (Fig. 1-3). A growth chart classifies the child under a height and weight percentile for comparison to the established norms for gender and chronological age. More importantly, the growth chart highlights any accelerations or peaks of growth that may have occurred. With this information, the objective is to evaluate the skeletal maturational level of the patient. The underlying rationale for this information is to properly time orthodontic treatment to the period that would be most efficient and effective.[20] This implies that treatment will rely not only on tooth movement, but also on modifying growth to achieve a wider range of movement, thereby correcting larger dentofacial discrepancies.

The pubertal growth spurt is associated with a differential maxillomandibular growth that involves a more anterior positioning of the mandible (Fig. 1-4). The timing of this spurt has been of interest to orthodontists. During this period the orthodontist should be able to influence growth of the mandible and the midface by mechanically affecting the environment. Experiments in animal models have shown the possibility of mandibular growth enhancement during this period.[21] Unfortunately, there is no clear evidence that this additional mandibular growth enhancement is predictably achievable in humans.[22] Although clinical studies have shown impressive results at the occlusal level, the results may be the sum of a combination of small orthopedic and dental movements.[23,24] Some of the orthopedic movements involve remodeling within the temporal bone that is difficult to quantify with traditional research methods.[25]

Chronological age, dental development, and eruption sequence are not good indicators of skeletal maturity. Biological indicators, such as menarche (females), voice change (males), hand-wrist ossification sequence, metacarpal ossification sequence, cervical vertebrae morphology, and statural growth curves, have been used to evaluate general skeletal craniofacial maturity.[20,26–28] Studies have shown a close correlation between peak height velocity and maximum acceleration in growth in the maxilla and mandible.[21,26,28,29]

Currently, there are no methods that can accurately predict the extent of craniofacial growth that a patient will ultimately achieve. This predictive inability becomes a problem in young patients with significant maxillomandibular discrepancies. For these patients a decision between a surgical approach or a growth modification approach is not simple. Moreover, these treatment strategies (surgery and growth modification) differ in timing, objectives, and often the direction of tooth movement. Some studies suggest that weak correlations can be drawn between final craniofacial form of growing children and their parents and other siblings.[30,31]

Although the absolute amount of growth cannot be predicted accurately, the direction of growth is more predictable. It has been shown that facial patterns are maintained.[32,33] Skieller et al. also published findings related to the morphology of the mandible in the prediction of growth patterns.[34] Some controversy relates to their findings, as their sample was made up of individuals with extreme patterns of vertical growth. Therefore the applicability of these predictive methods to individuals with less severe aberrations in their growth pattern might be limited.[35]

Finally, information regarding the timing of active growth cessation is important for young patients needing maxillofacial surgery. Radiographic films can be used to evaluate this feature. Use of cervical maturation indicators and hand-wrist films can provide further information on the stage of the patient's growth and is discussed later in the chapter. The best method to confirm that no further growth will occur in the craniofacial region is to take two sequential lateral head films with a 6- to 12-month interval; the superimposition of these radiographs should reveal no bony changes.[36]

Factors Influencing Craniofacial Growth

It is well known that many conditions affect the growth and development of the craniofacial complex. Knowing the

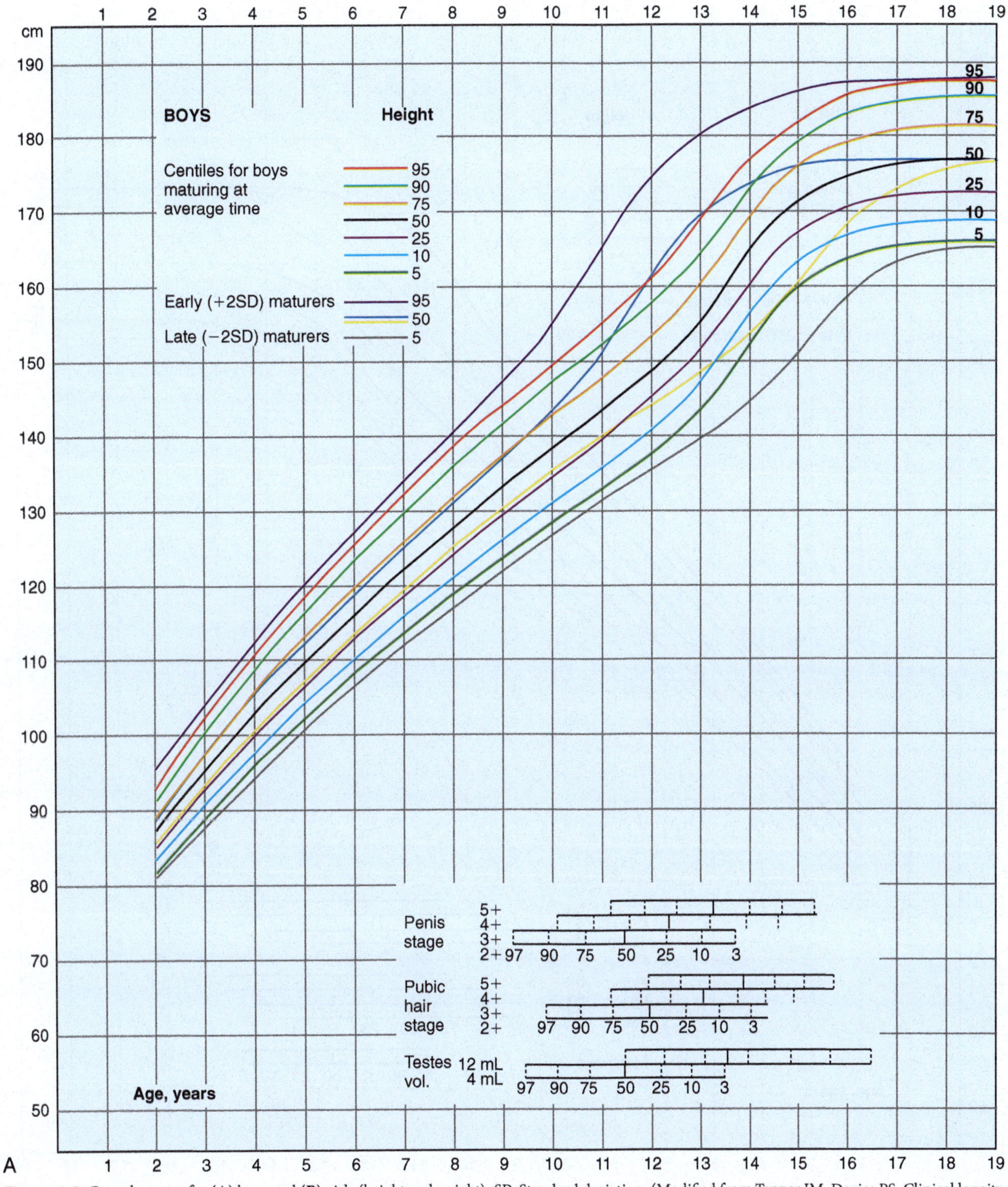

Figure 1-3 Growth curves for **(A)** boys and **(B)** girls (height and weight). *SD,* Standard deviation. (Modified from Tanner JM, Davies PS. Clinical longitudinal standards for height and height velocity for North American children. *J Pediatr.* 1985;107:317–329.)

Continued

etiology of the malocclusion is of prime importance for the diagnosis and eventual success of treatment. The etiology of the malocclusion is often multifactorial. In general, the etiologic factors can be categorized into genetic factors, environmental factors, or a combination of the two. Genetic information can be gathered from the interview with the guardian of the child patient or from the adult patient. This information is more important in patients where syndromes or extensive craniofacial deviations are present. Also, as mentioned, the parents' information may give some insight into the craniofacial form at the end of growth. The genetic component is also of further importance as it relates to

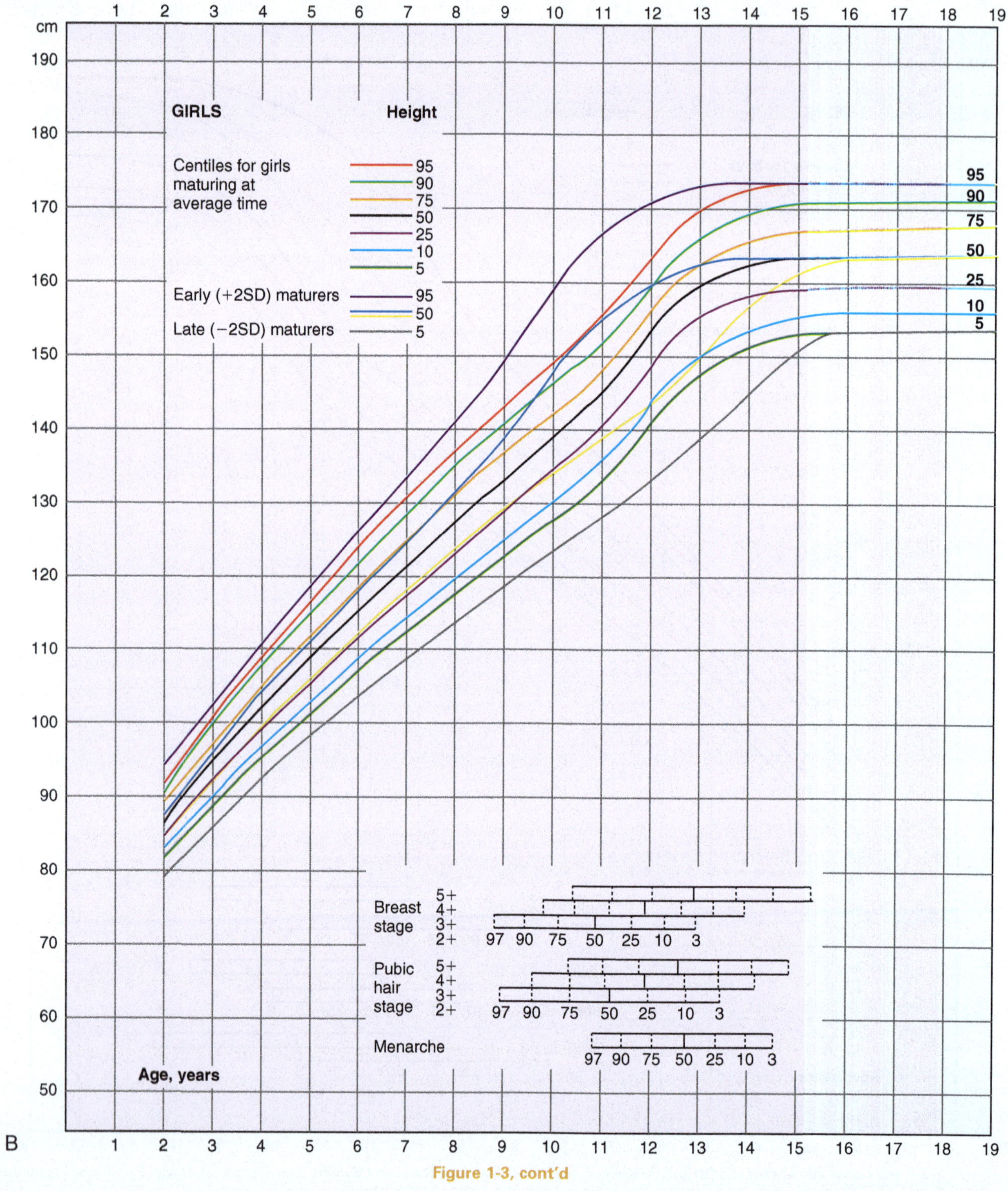

Figure 1-3, cont'd

abnormalities of tooth development and morphology, such as canine impaction, congenitally missing teeth, and abnormalities in tooth shape.[37,38]

Numerous environmental factors have been attributed to the etiology of malocclusions. The classic example is the habit of thumb-sucking. A long-term applied force (pressure) has been shown to affect skeletal hard tissues. The tissues of the musculature can apply constant low forces and result in adaption of the adjacent bony structures.[39] Muscular dysfunction by either hyperactivity or hypoactivity in certain disease processes also may affect the normal growth and development of the jaws.[40] If the forces exerted by the muscles are not in equilibrium, the net effect will be reflected in the hard tissues in the form of displacement and eventually conditions leading to malocclusion and maxillomandibular skeletal discrepancy.[41,42]

Frontal View

Traditionally, orthodontists have paid little attention to facial analysis from the frontal view and instead have focused mostly on anteroposterior changes (i.e., Angle classification). With the surge in three-dimensional (3D) imaging technology more information from the frontal view, especially relating to the soft tissue analysis, will be available in the future.[43]

When describing a patient from the frontal view, an overall assessment of the patient's symmetry is made. Attractiveness and pleasing facial esthetics have been linked to certain proportions and symmetry.[44,45] Minor asymmetries exist in all patients, even those who are visibly symmetrical, likely due to skeletal and soft tissue compensations during growth (Fig. 1-5).

Ideal facial proportions have been described since ancient times by Roman and Greek artists. Horizontal as well as vertical lines are used as reference planes to evaluate these proportions. The horizontal planes, such as the interpupillary, interauricular, alar base, and occlusal planes, should be parallel to each other and special attention should be paid to the presence of cants (Fig. 1-6). The proportions between these horizontal planes can also be evaluated on the profile view. From the frontal view the vertical reference lines are more important since it is only from this view that the transverse dimension can be evaluated (Fig. 1-7).

Midline

The frontal view is also helpful in the evaluation of the relationship between the facial and dental midlines. It is important to note that analysis of the facial midline can be difficult, especially in patients with deviated nasal septums (Fig. 1-8, A). Thus the commonly used technique of placing a piece of dental floss vertically through the facial midline to relate it to the dental midline can be deceiving. A better method is to assess the relationship between the Cupid's bow and the dental midline (Fig. 1-8, B).[46] Hence the dental midline can be related to an adjacent well-defined midsagittal anatomic structure. A more detailed analysis of the dental midline is included below since many other factors must be considered.

Finally, the chin is evaluated for any deviation in relation to the facial midline (Fig. 1-9, A). A view taken from above the patient (coronal) enhances the ability to detect any deviations (Fig. 1-9, B). Similarly, observing the patient from the lower (ventral) aspect of the mandible can complement this analysis (Fig. 1-9, C). This part of the clinical examination is very important, as a large chin deviation is an indication for further analysis, perhaps with additional radiographic imaging.

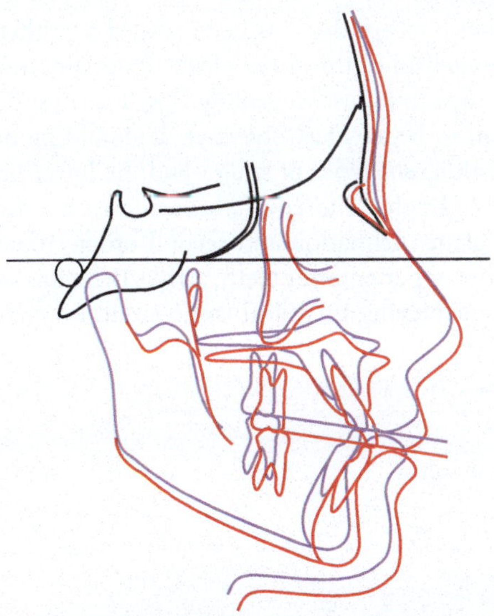

Figure 1-4 Differential growth of the mandible compared to the maxilla.

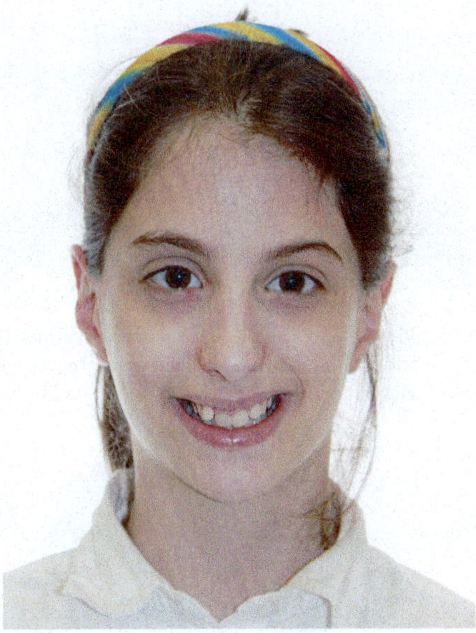

Figure 1-6 Maxillary cant evidenced at smile. More gingival display is appreciated in the upper right buccal segment than in the left buccal segment.

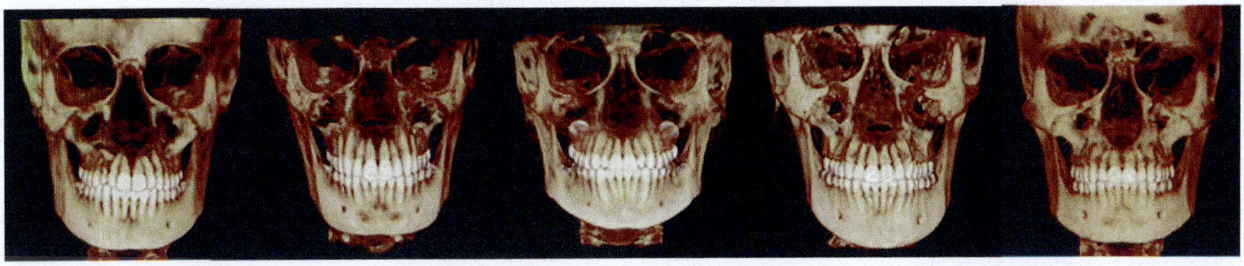

Figure 1-5 Cone beam computed tomography (CBCT) images from normal, Class I adolescent patients. Minor skeletal asymmetries are evident in these patients when examined in 3D.

Lips

A good analysis of the patient's lips is done at rest position or with the upper and lower lips lightly touching (Fig. 1-10, A). Indications of any muscle strain on lip closure should be noted (Fig. 1-10, B). Upper and lower lip lengths can be assessed in the frontal and profile views. Upper lip length when noted alone is not as important per se as its relationship to the upper incisors at rest and when smiling. The proper relationship between the upper lip and the amount of upper teeth exposure is a key factor in modern esthetic smile construction (Fig. 1-11). Full display of the upper incisor crown upon smiling has been linked to youthful smiles.[47] A differential diagnosis between a short or long lip and a maxillary vertical excess or deficiency is valuable in patients with an inadequate upper incisor display (Fig. 1-12).

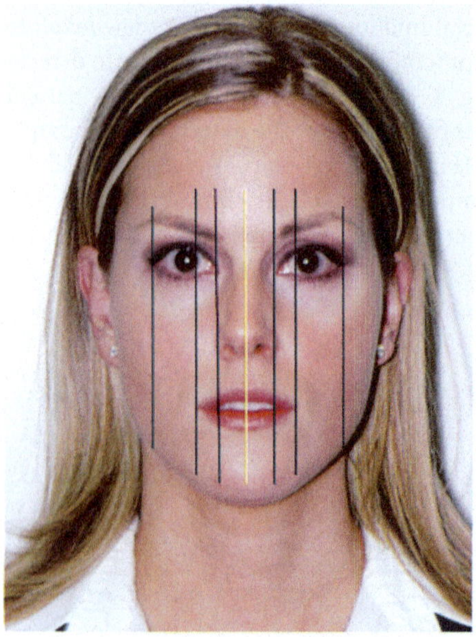

Figure 1-7 Vertical reference lines used to evaluate symmetry. The face is divided into six portions in the transverse analysis. The yellow line is an estimate of the facial midline.

Buccal Corridors and Smile Line

Other important relationships that can be evaluated only in the frontal view are the buccal corridors and the curvature of the smile line (relationship to lower lips). The buccal corridors and smile line concepts have been discussed extensively in the prosthetic literature.[48] The ideal esthetic parameter in smile design in the transverse dimension has been related to wide dental arches and narrow buccal corridors (Fig. 1-13). Some authors have described upper first molar display on a full smile as a feature of an attractive smile.[49] Although this does seem to be an attribute of beautiful smiles, its validity and applicability is doubtful. Anatomic structures limit the amount of transverse expansion needed to reduce the unattractive wide buccal corridors. The long-term periodontal health of teeth with expansion is not well understood. Computed tomography (CT) scans have shown that indiscriminate expansion of the maxillary arch results in buccal root dehiscences as these extend beyond the cortical plates.[50] Another important reason to avoid indiscriminate expansion relates to long-term stability.[51] Skeletal tissues (bones and teeth) are usually in equilibrium with the surrounding musculature; long-term stability might be compromised when teeth invade the neighboring muscle confinements.[41,42]

Another concept that has been related to esthetic smiles is the parallelism of the curve of the upper anterior teeth to the lower lip curvature on smiling (Fig. 1-14). Although this does seem to be an ideal objective, it should be noted that there are different types of smiles and the lower lip posture varies accordingly.[52] Moreover, this smile arc is a result of the occlusal plane inclination and second-order crown angulations in the upper anterior teeth.[53] Thus there are some limitations to achieving this ideal smile arc in every patient. A

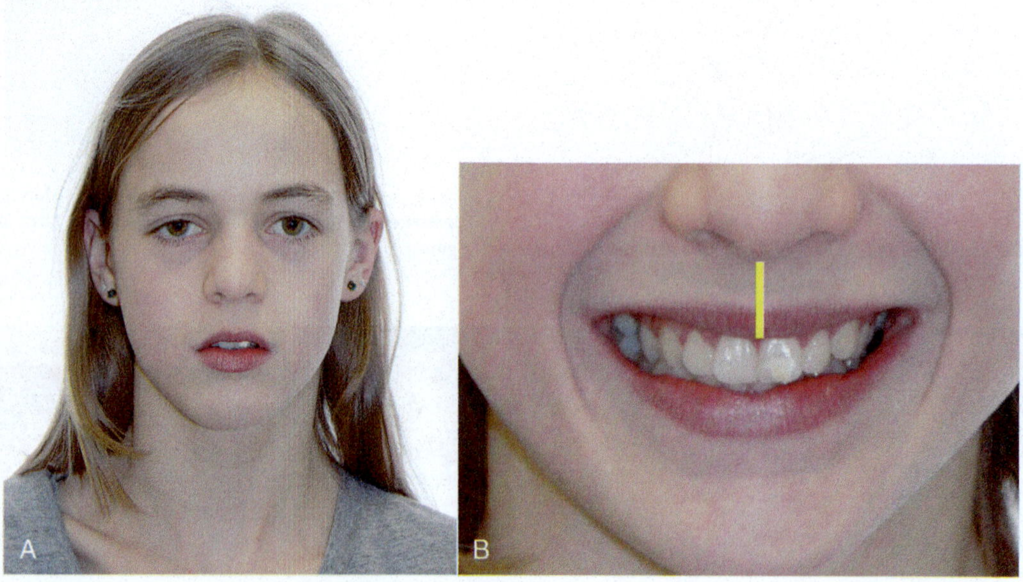

Figure 1-8 **A,** Patient exhibiting facial asymmetry, including a deviating chin and vertical discrepancy in the eyes. **B,** Same patient showing a coincident dental midline in relation to the philtrum.

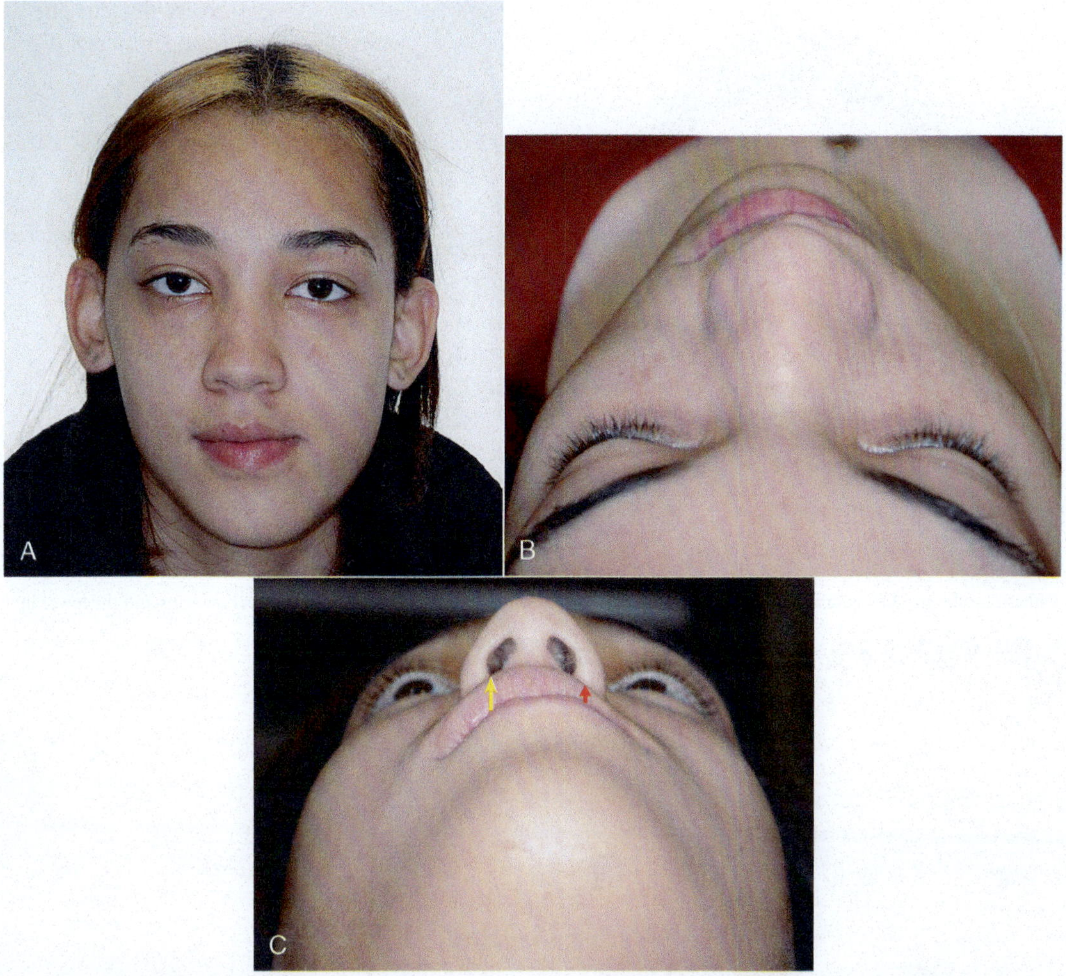

Figure 1-9 **A,** Patient with asymmetrical mandible. **B,** Coronal view to evaluate mandibular asymmetry during the clinical examination. **C,** Ventral view complements the assessment for mandibular asymmetry. In this patient the ventral view provides better information about the asymmetry. Arrows show the asymmetry between the left and right sides in the lip region.

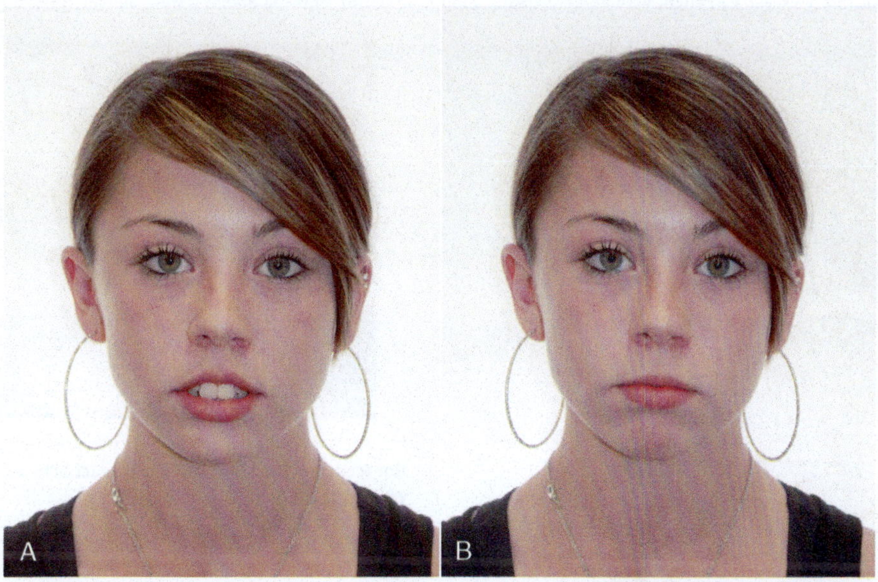

Figure 1-10 **A,** Patient showing incompetent lips at rest. **B,** Upon lip contact the mentalis strain is noted.

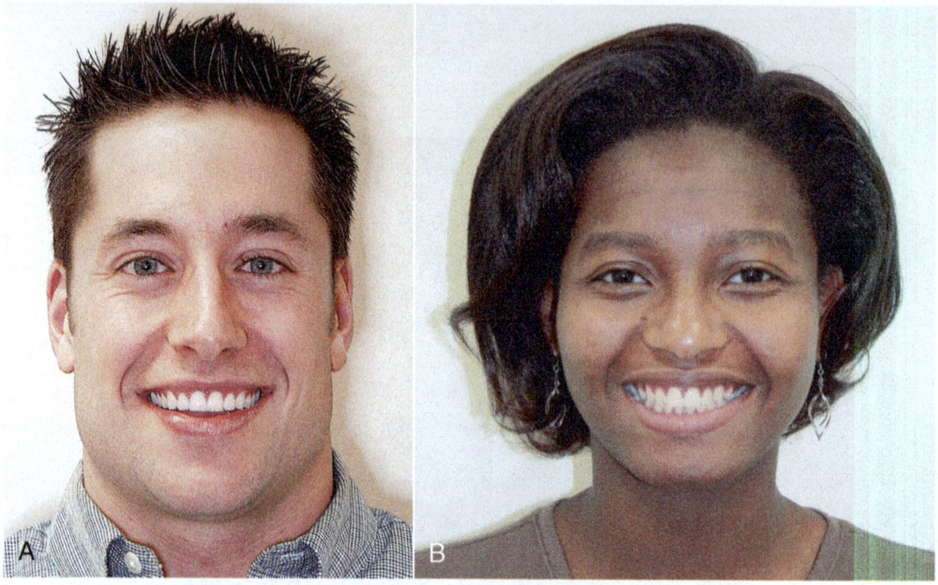

Figure 1-11 Esthetic smiles in (**A**) a man and (**B**) a woman. Note the relationship of the upper lip to the gingival margins and the lower lip to the smile arc.

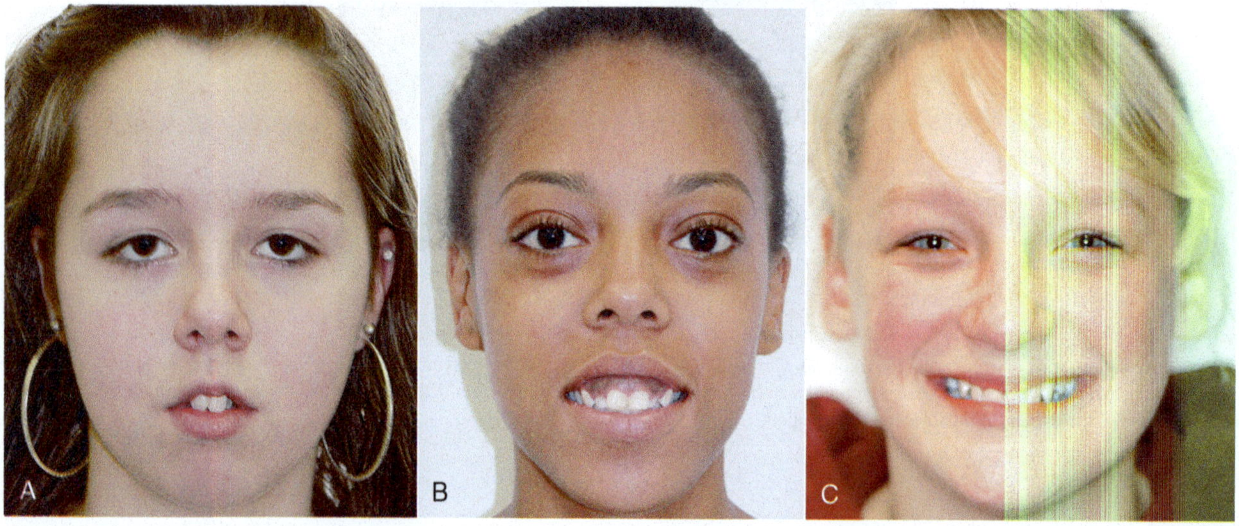

Figure 1-12 Differential diagnosis for incisor display. **A,** Patient with excessive incisor display due to a short upper lip. **B,** Patient with excessive maxillary display due to a vertical maxillary excess. **C,** Patient with an inadequate amount of incisor showing due to a short maxilla vertically.

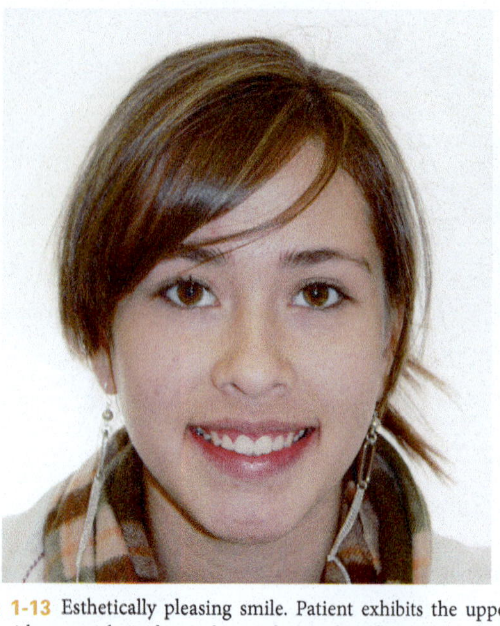

Figure 1-13 Esthetically pleasing smile. Patient exhibits the upper first molars with narrow buccal corridors and wide dental arches.

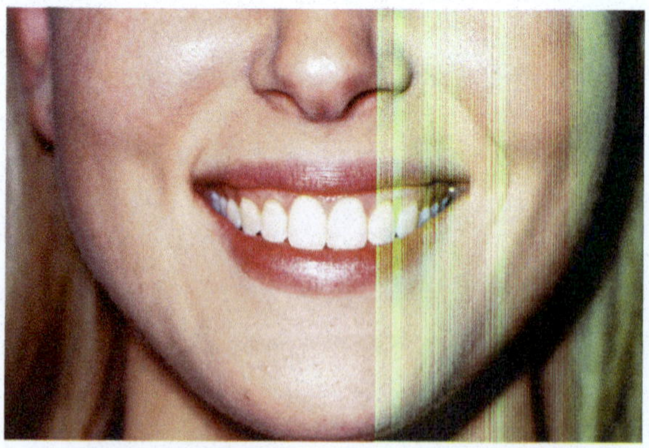

Figure 1-14 Ideal parallelism between the incisal edges of the upper anterior teeth and the lower lip. The contact between the incisors and the lip is very slight.

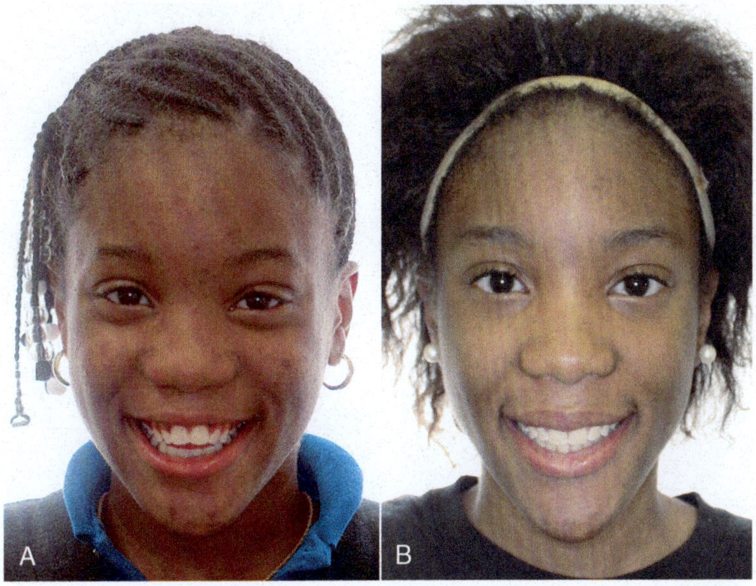

Figure 1-15 **A,** Reverse relationship between the upper incisors and the lower lips, which is frequently found in patients with a finger habit. **B,** Correction of the reverse relationship after treatment. A better esthetic relationship to the lower lip was achieved.

reasonable objective is to prevent a flat or reverse smile line (Fig. 1-15, A) and to obtain some degree of curvature that resembles the one found in the lower lip (Fig. 1-15, B).

Symmetry has always been linked to beauty. Not surprisingly, it has also been ascribed as one of the characteristics of a beautiful smile. This symmetry can be related to the size and shape of the teeth on both sides of each arch (see Fig. 1-11, A). Also, it is related to the relationship of the intraoral tissues to the lips on both the right and left sides. Therefore the same amount of gingival display should be seen upon smiling, on both sides of the arch. Reasons for any asymmetry include a cant in the maxillary skeletal base, different amounts of tooth eruption on the right and left sides, or asymmetrical smiles. It is estimated that 8.7% of normal adults have asymmetrical smiles (Fig. 1-16).[54]

The last feature related to symmetry in the smile is the dental midline. The ideal relationship of the dental midline to the facial midline was mentioned above. The upper dental midline has been considered more important than the lower dental midline in esthetic smile design. It has been shown that a discrepancy of <2 mm (to the right or left) between the upper dental midline and the facial midline is not readily perceived (Fig. 1-17, A).[55,56] However, any type of unparallel relationship between the interproximal contacts of the incisors related to the facial midline (incisal cant) is more easily perceived (Fig. 1-17, B).[57] Two further characteristics of an attractive smile are the gingival heights of the anterior teeth and the tooth shade. The gingival heights of the six upper anterior teeth are similar. The central incisors and the canines are at the same level, while the lateral incisors' free gingival level is approximately 0.5 mm incisal to the level of the canines and central incisors (Fig. 1-18). Moreover, the gingival heights of the premolars and molars should be approximately 1 and 1.5 mm less than the canines, respectively (Fig. 1-19).[58] The significance of tooth shade in the esthetic smile has been reviewed extensively in the prosthodontic literature.[49] Light shades have always been considered one of the most important characteristics of an esthetic smile. Therefore procedures such as tooth bleaching may be considered after orthodontic appliance removal. Tooth shade also becomes an important factor in patients where canine substitution for missing upper laterals is considered. Differences in the tone between the canines (dark yellow) and incisors may be an indication to opt to restore the laterals prosthetically instead of closing the edentulous space (canine substitution).

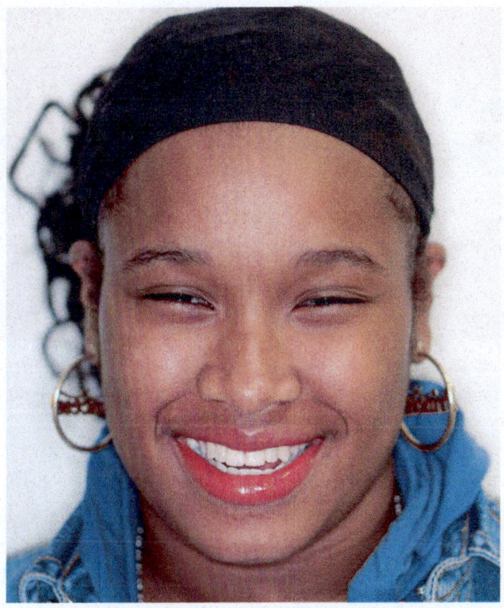

Figure 1-16 Asymmetrical smile with more tooth structure display on the right side. A reverse smile curve is also evident.

The last notable factor in the ideal smile is tooth shape. Incisors are the predominant teeth in the smile, especially the upper central incisor. The ideal proportion of this tooth

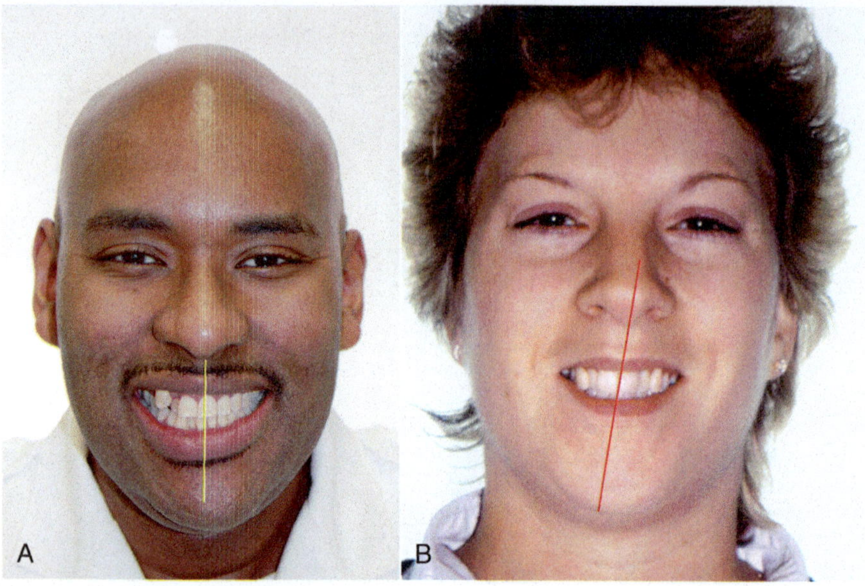

Figure 1-17 **A,** Patient with upper midline deviated approximately 2 mm to the right of the facial midline. **B,** Patient with upper midline deviated approximately 1 mm from the facial midline. The inclination of the line described by the interproximal contact area accentuates the midline discrepancy.

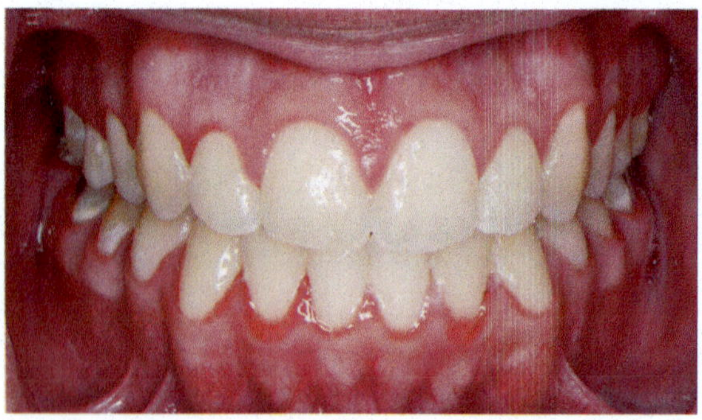

Figure 1-18 Proper gingival heights. The upper central incisors and canines have the same gingival height; the lateral incisors' gingiva is 1 mm below the canines and central incisors.

is found when the width approximates 75% to 80% of the height (Fig. 1-20).[59] Similarly, lateral incisor size is often small in the mesiodistal dimension and should be considered in determining final occlusion and overall treatment outcome. Tooth shape is discussed further later in the chapter.

Profile View

Orthodontists spend more time evaluating patients from the profile view. Most of the literature is based on analysis from lateral cephalometric films. The classification of malocclusions is also based on the anteroposterior dimension (i.e., Angle classification). Even though the vertical dimension can be analyzed from this view, interest in this dimension has lagged. Later chapters describe the importance of the vertical dimension in the treatment of various malocclusions by an application of sound biomechanical principles.

Anteroposterior Dimension

The anteroposterior dimension is the backbone of most contemporary orthodontic analyses. In this dimension the soft tissue convexity is initially assessed by observing the spatial relationship between the forehead, maxilla, and mandible. These are separate but interrelated anatomic structures with independent timings in development. Each structure provides feedback to the others to maintain a normal facial growth pattern.[60] Normally these three structures maintain a slight convexity that is reduced during puberty as a result of differential jaw growth.[33] During the pubertal growth spurt the mandible has a greater anterior displacement compared to the maxilla. It is important to note that at the end of growth there are also gender differences in the convexity of the profiles. On average the female profile is more convex due to a smaller chin projection.[61]

Once the magnitude of the facial profile convexity is assessed, the next step is to evaluate which of the three structures is contributing to the abnormality. With an increased angle of convexity or concavity, the question to be answered is which structure is causing the deformity (mandible or maxilla). It has been reported that the majority of skeletal convexities exhibit a deficient mandible.[62] On the other hand, studies show that approximately half of skeletal concavities present with a deficient maxilla.[63]

To evaluate maxillary and mandibular position during the clinical examination, an adequate reference plane must be determined. During the clinical examination the easiest assessment can be done using the natural head position. This can be achieved when the extraoral photographs are taken. More detailed analysis of the soft tissue spatial relationships in the anteroposterior dimensions is obtained from the lateral cephalograms.

Nose

Although the nose is outside the limits of what can be affected by orthodontic treatment, it is important for facial balance. More importantly, the apparent nose projection can

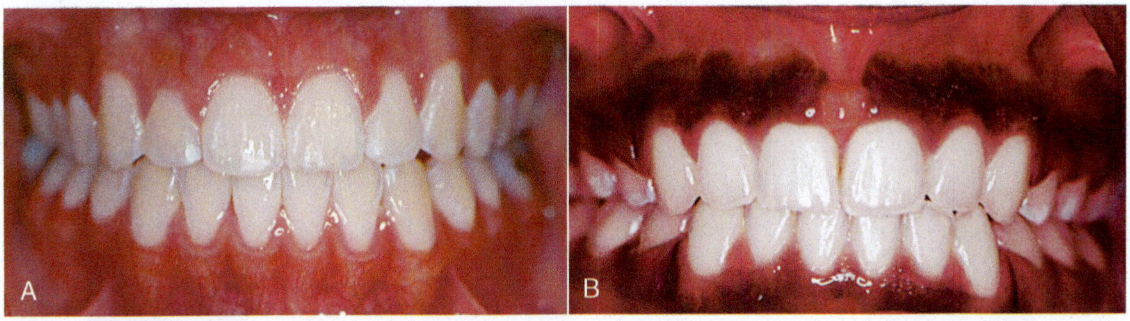

Figure 1-19 **A,** Gingival heights from the canines to the molars decrease gradually. **B,** Abrupt change in gingival heights between the canine and the second premolar. This situation is commonly seen in upper first premolar extraction.

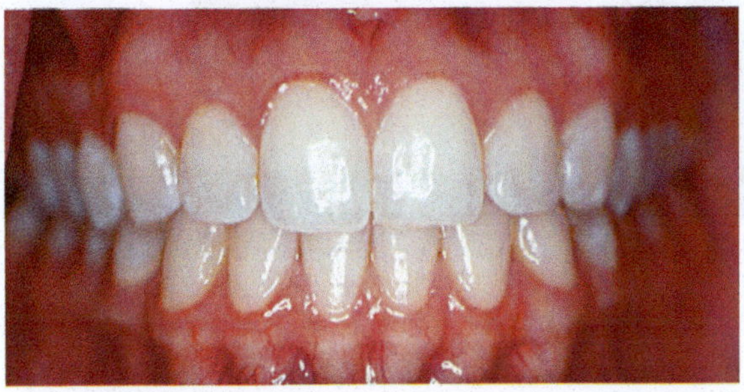

Figure 1-20 Proper tooth proportions and shape, especially on the upper central incisors, is a key element in an esthetic smile.

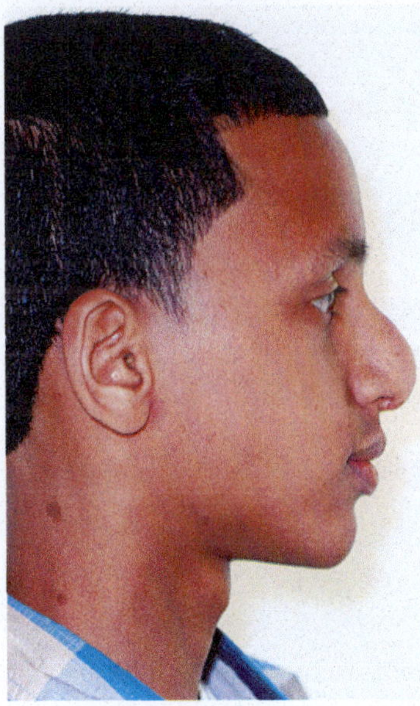

Figure 1-21 Patient with an abnormal nose contour.

be affected by the anteroposterior position of the lips. During the clinical examination, the length and height of the nose are evaluated. Any morphological variations in shape are noted (Fig. 1-21).

Lips

Lip response to orthodontic treatment is one of the most discussed topics in modern orthodontics. With the increased interest in esthetics, patients and practitioners are interested in not only the dental and skeletal changes, but also the response of the surrounding soft tissues to treatment. As teeth move, there is a direct effect on lip support. Although this is a subject of perpetual research, no good predictor of the precise lip response to orthodontic movement has been identified.[64] The only predictable variable is the direction of lip response. It has been established that if any lip changes occur, these will be in the direction of the upper anterior tooth movement.[65,66]

During clinical examination an overall assessment of the lips at rest is necessary. Special attention should be given to lip posture and tonicity. The influence of lip pressure in the etiology of certain types of malocclusions has been discussed in the literature.[67] To evaluate lip posture, the anteroposterior and vertical relationship of the lips (rest position) to the incisors is examined (Fig. 1-22).[68] In the anteroposterior dimension, a gap between the labial surface of the anterior teeth and the oral mucosa may be absent or present. In the vertical dimension, the lip line may be high (middle of the incisor root) or low. If the lips and the incisors contact each other, the exact location (incisal, middle, or apical third) of this junction is noted. The vertical and anteroposterior relationship of the lips to the incisors can aid in the prediction of upper lip movement in response to lingual incisor movement and the long-term stability of the incisors to labial movement as well.[69]

The relationship between the upper and lower lips is another important feature that must be evaluated. When the lips are at rest, the normal interlabial gap ranges from 1- to 3-mm. As the patient closes their lips, any strain on the perioral musculature, such as mentalis strain, may be indicative of an excessive interlabial gap. Another very important dimension to note is the amount of incisor display with the lips maintained at this rest position.

An excessive display of tooth or gum tissue may be the result of a single factor or a combination of factors, such as vertical maxillary excess, short upper lip, or supra-erupted upper incisors. From the profile view, a general indication of a short upper lip is evident when an obtuse angle is found between a line drawn from the commissure of the mouth to the labrale superioris and the horizontal reference plane (Fig. 1-23). In general, the lower lip is almost parallel to the horizontal plane; therefore these patients will present with an excessive interlabial gap.

Another important feature is lip thickness. It is well-known that lip thickness varies between different races.[70–72]

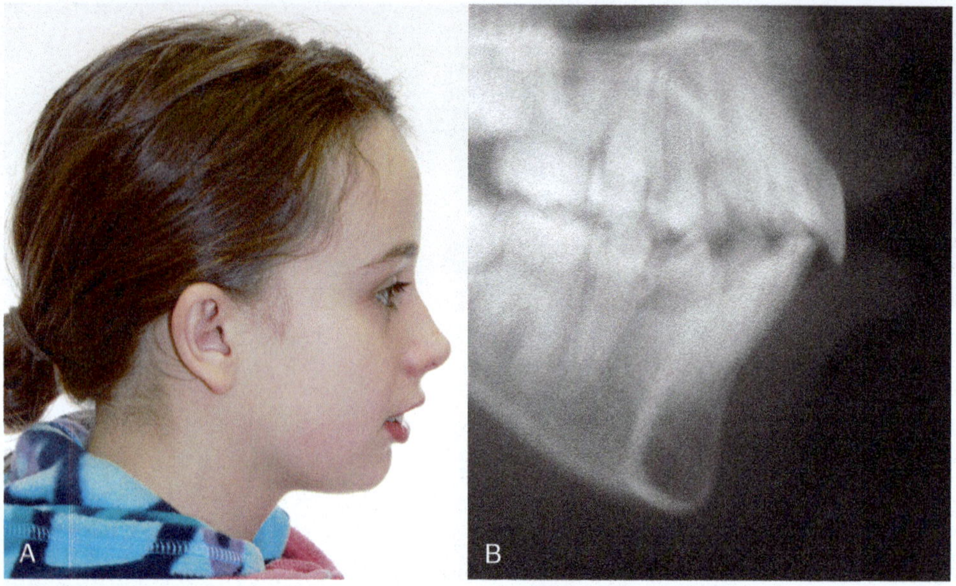

Figure 1-22 **A,** Patient with no contact between the crown of the upper incisors and the upper lip. The upper lip is not supported by the crowns of the upper central incisors. The effect on the upper lip after lingual tipping of the incisors would depend on the amount of movement of the coronal portion of the root. **B,** Lateral cephalometric film showing the vertical and anteroposterior relationship of the lip to the incisors. Intimate contact is noticed with the alveolar process of the anterior teeth in the maxilla.

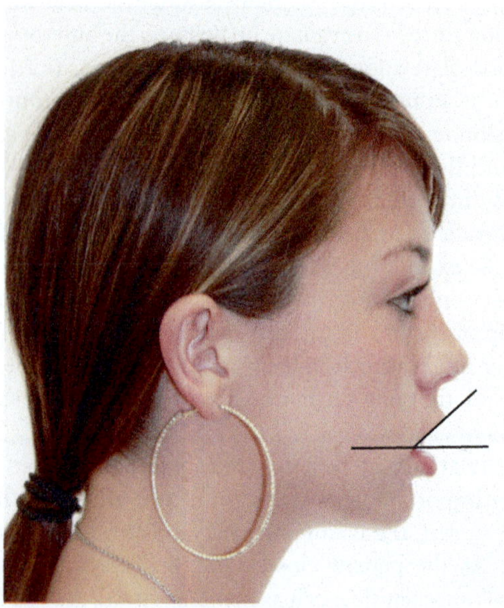

Figure 1-23 Large interlabial gap. There is a large angle between the horizontal plane and a line from the angle of the mouth to the labrale superioris.

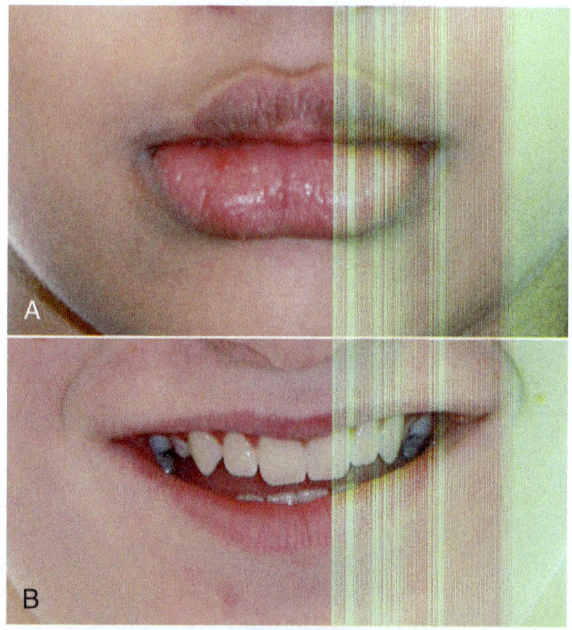

Figure 1-24 **A,** Patient with very thick lips. The response to incisor movement may be limited by the tissue mass. **B,** Patient with very thin lips that may be more susceptible to lip changes with tooth movement.

Moreover, the response to orthodontic tooth movement may be different between thin and thick lips. Some evidence suggests that thicker lips respond less and more variably to tooth movement than thinner lips (Fig. 1-24).[73]

The ideal anteroposterior position of the lips has been estimated by many studies using different reference lines. The definition of protrusive or retrusive lips varies with age, gender, and race. To define lip protrusion, different reference planes have been used. One of the most common reference planes used in clinical orthodontics is the E-line defined by Ricketts formed by a line passing from the tip of the nose to soft tissue pogonion (Pg').[74] The limitation of this reference line is that it is influenced by the anteroposterior position of the chin and nose. Any large deviation in the chin or nose position relative to the norm will give a false impression of lip position. To control for the nose variability, Burstone proposed the Sn–Pg' line extending from subnasale (Sn) to Pg' (Fig. 1-25).[75,76] Others have used different angles using the chin and lips as reference points and not incorporating the nose (Z angle, Steiner's S-line, and Holdaway angle).[77–79]

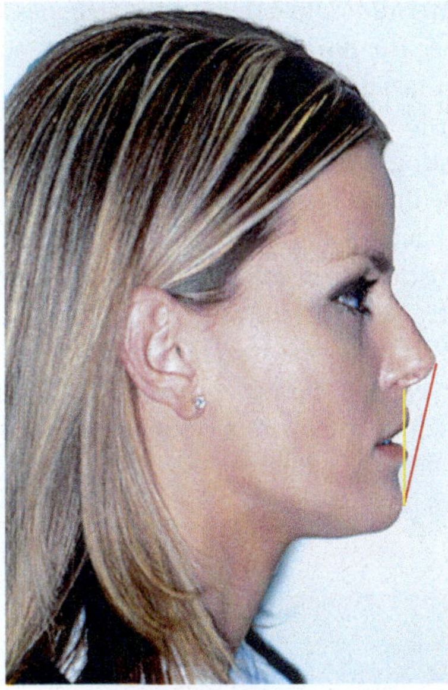

Figure 1-25 Relationship of the lips to two commonly used reference lines: E-line (influenced by the nose, red) and Sn–Pg' line (yellow).

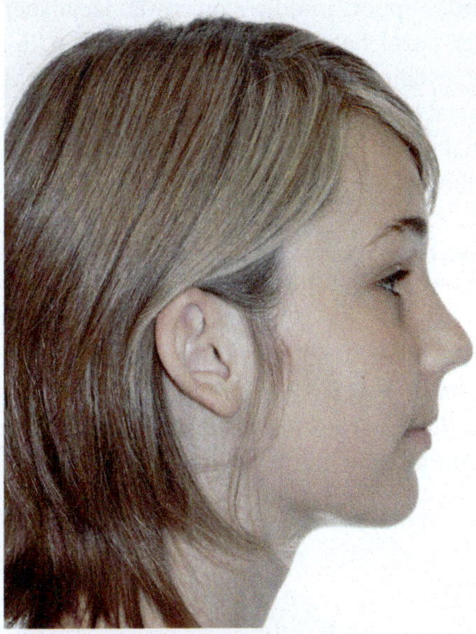

Figure 1-26 Obtuse nasolabial angle. The upturned nasal tip and retrusive lip contribute to the obtuse angle.

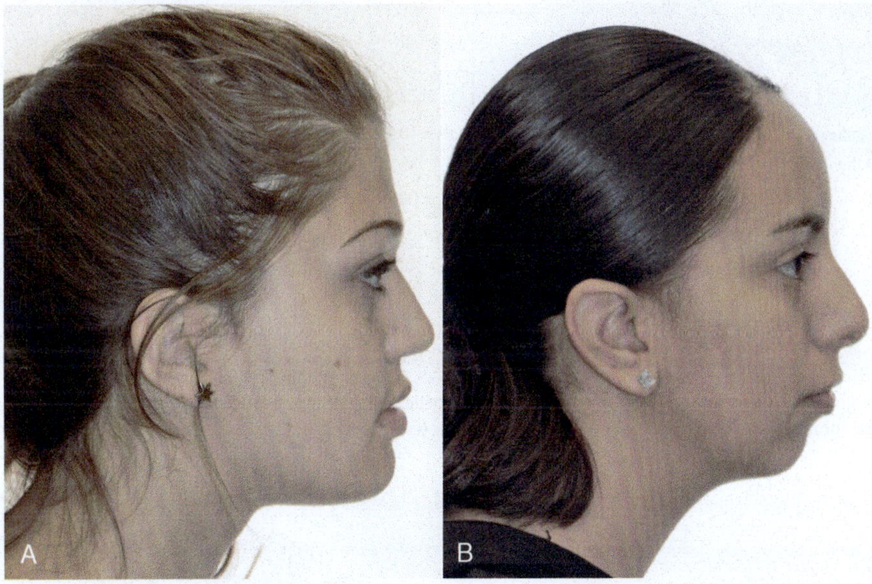

Figure 1-27 **A,** Parallel relationship of the chin–throat line to the horizontal plane. An adequate ratio between the lower facial height and throat depth is 1.2 : 1. **B,** Inadequate ratio between the lower facial height and throat depth (no throat depth) gives an unesthetic inclination of the chin–throat line.

The nasolabial angle is another important measurement related to lip protrusion. Although this angle is also influenced by the angulation of the nose (upturn or downturn of the nasal tip), it gives an indication of the upper lip inclination (Fig. 1-26).

Although numerically the soft tissue analysis can be better analyzed in a lateral cephalometric film, a general overview is achieved during the clinical examination. Using a combination of all these reference planes allows for a proper interpretation of the lip position.

Another important structure that is analyzed in the lateral view is chin projection. In adult patients, the ratio of the chin-to-throat depth length compared to the lower facial height is 1.2 : 1.[80] It seems that not only the length of this line but also the angulation to the true horizontal plane are important features in well-balanced faces. Normally, a parallel relation or slightly negative angle (throat point above the menton) is found in esthetically pleasing faces (Fig. 1-27, A). A deficient chin shows a reduction in the chin-to-throat depth length (Fig. 1-27, B).

Vertical Dimension

As stated above, the vertical dimension can be analyzed in both the frontal and the profile views. Both of these views can be related through the vertical dimension to provide a composite 3D analysis. The face can be divided into three equal thirds: upper, middle, and lower facial heights. The true upper facial height is seldom used, as it is measured from the trichion to the glabella. More commonly, the middle facial height is referred to as the upper facial height. The normal upper to lower facial height ratio is 1 : 1 (glabella [G] to subnasale [Sn] and Sn to soft tissue menton [Me']) (Fig. 1-28, A).

The lower facial third is very important since the effects of orthodontic treatment are most profound in this third. It is further subdivided into two proportional heights. One third of the lower facial height normally corresponds to Sn to St and two thirds from St to Me' (Fig. 1-28, B).

The vertical analysis is not limited to the anterior part of the face but also includes the posterior. The ratio between these two determines, to a degree, the steepness of the mandibular plane. The normal ratio of the lower facial height to the posterior facial height is 0.69.[81] An overall assessment of this relationship can be determined from the mandibular plane. Palpating and placing a flat object along the lower border of the mandible can give a general idea of the steepness of this plane.

In the vertical dimension from the profile view the face is generally categorized as convergent (short face) or divergent (long face). A short face is characterized by a flat mandibular plane angle with a similar posterior and anterior facial height, lip redundancy with a deep mentolabial sulcus, and short lower facial height (Fig. 1-29, A). At the other end of the spectrum, a long face is characterized by an increased

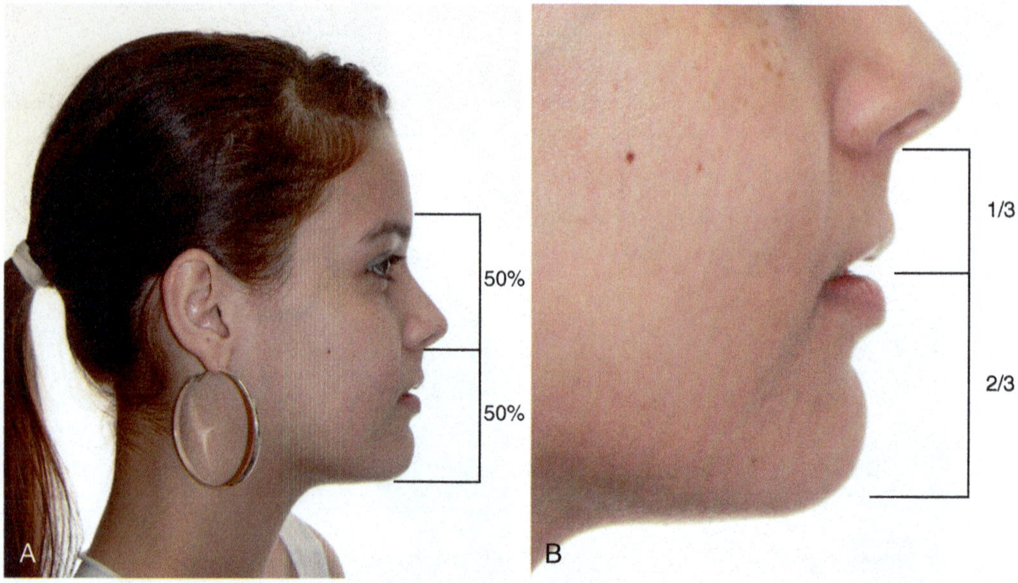

Figure 1-28 **A,** Facial heights divided into three equal thirds: trichion–glabella, glabella–subnasale, subnasale–menton. **B,** Lower facial height is further divided into unequal thirds: subnasale–stomion (one-third), stomiom–menton (two-thirds).

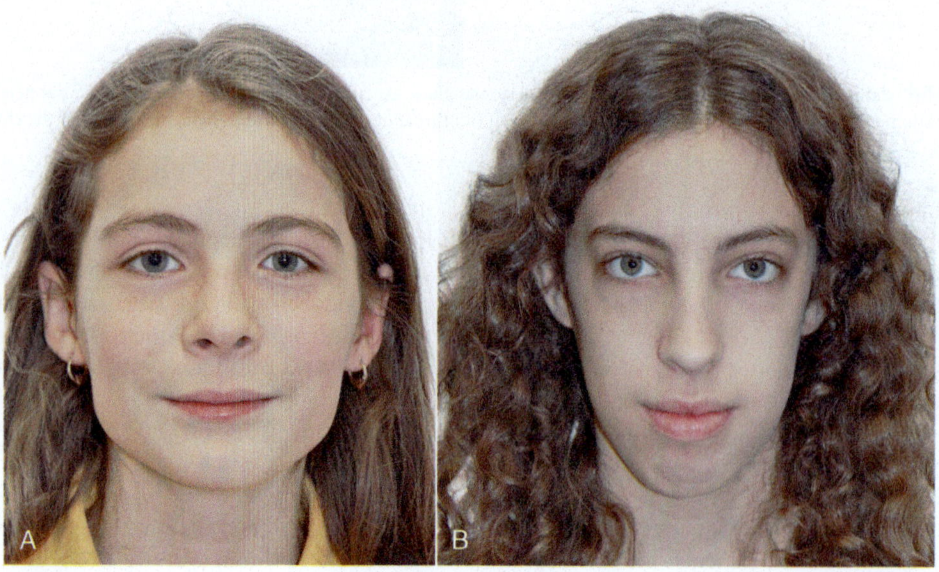

Figure 1-29 **A,** Short face (brachycephalic or euryprosopic). **B,** Long face (dolichocephalic or leptoprosopic).

anterior facial height relative to the posterior facial height, steep mandibular plane angle, possible lip incompetence with large interlabial gap, and shallow mentolabial sulcus (Fig. 1-29, B).

Most of the clinical analysis is static in nature; therefore during the examination it is important to pay close attention to the animation of the facial soft tissues. During this time an analysis of more natural lip function, including different smile heights, symmetry of the smile, and the amount of upper and lower incisor display during conversation, is more important than forced unnatural snapshots of animated features.

Photographs

Extraoral Photographs

Although the clinical examination provides an excellent opportunity for patient evaluation, it is important to document specific information (images, intraoral impressions). This information can be used later for data analysis (radiographs, photographs, and models), medicolegal reasons, and treatment progress and outcome evaluations.

Different photographic images from the profile and frontal views are recommended. Initially pictures of the patient with relaxed lips and lips lightly touching each other are taken from the frontal and profile views (Fig. 1-30, A–D). Frontal and profile view pictures are taken in the natural head position.

A 45 degree–angle image between the profile and frontal views provides information related to the amount of malar prominence and lower jaw shape (mandibular plane angle and gonial angle). This view usually confirms the findings of the analysis from the frontal and profile views (Fig. 1-30, E).

Finally, a frontal view photograph depicting a full smile should be taken. It is somewhat difficult to capture a natural, unposed smile. Usually this photograph does not reflect the full extent of the smile. Thus special attention is needed during the clinical examination to record important data such as the amount of tooth and gum display, the relationship of the upper teeth to the lower lip, and the width of buccal corridors (Fig. 1-30, F). During data analysis this information can be correlated to the still images. As an alternative, a video image of the different animated facial features has recently been suggested as part of the clinical record.[82]

Intraoral Photographs

A total of five views of the dentition and the occlusion are taken. These pictures include two buccal photos (left and right), two occlusal photos (upper and lower arch), and one frontal intraoral view. These photographs should be taken in maximum intercuspation (Fig. 1-31). Additionally, intraoral centric relation photographs are taken if a significant centric relation–centric occlusion (CR–CO) shift is present (mandibular shift).

Intraoral Examination

The intraoral examination for an orthodontic patient starts as does any other dental examination. First, an overall inspection of the oral mucosa in search of any pathological lesions is performed. Upon analyzing the soft tissue, special attention should be given to the gingival tissues. Periodontal status evaluation is of prime importance, especially in the adult, as discussed earlier in the chapter. It is not uncommon to find active periodontal disease in adults around the molar areas. A random probing should be done around the first and second molars and on some anterior teeth for every adult patient.

The quality of the attached gingiva is examined next. The thickness (gingivo-occlusal) and width of the attached gingiva are very important. Many times these are overlooked and recession may occur as the teeth are displaced labially out of their alveolar housing. It should be noted that recession also may be present before starting treatment (Fig. 1-32).

Continuing with the intraoral soft tissue analysis, the labial frenum attachment is evaluated. A high insertion into the attached gingiva might contribute to a persisting diastema (Fig. 1-33).[83] Moreover, high frenum attachments have also been linked to recession of the labial surface of the lower incisors.[84]

Oral Hygiene

Good oral hygiene is very important during orthodontic treatment and should be stressed from the start of treatment. It is well-established that orthodontic appliances hinder oral hygiene. Therefore careful evaluation of oral hygiene at the initial examination is needed and treatment should be delayed until good plaque control is achieved by the patient.

Tongue

Initially, the mucosa of the tongue should be screened for any signs of pathological lesions. A general evaluation of the shape and size of the tongue is performed and the tongue's relation to the lower dental arch should be noted. Evidence of indentations on the lateral borders of the tongue accompanied by generalized spacing between the teeth may suggest macroglossia.

The tongue is a powerful muscle that applies constant pressure to the lingual surfaces of the teeth, counteracting the lip pressure on the buccal surfaces.[37] Functional evaluation of the tongue during speech and swallowing could give some insight as to etiology of the malocclusion.

Finally, the lingual frenum is evaluated. Ankyloglossia or tongue-tie is found in some patients and may be a reason for impeded speech.[85]

Dentition

Before starting the dental examination, a thorough dental history should be taken. First, the patient is asked if he or she is under regular dental care. Although an affirmative answer does not mean that there is no active disease, it can be assumed that the patient or guardian has an interest in maintaining good oral health. A patient's oral hygiene habits (brushing frequency, use of floss, etc.) should be noted.

History of previous orthodontic treatment is also important. It might provide some insight into a patient's

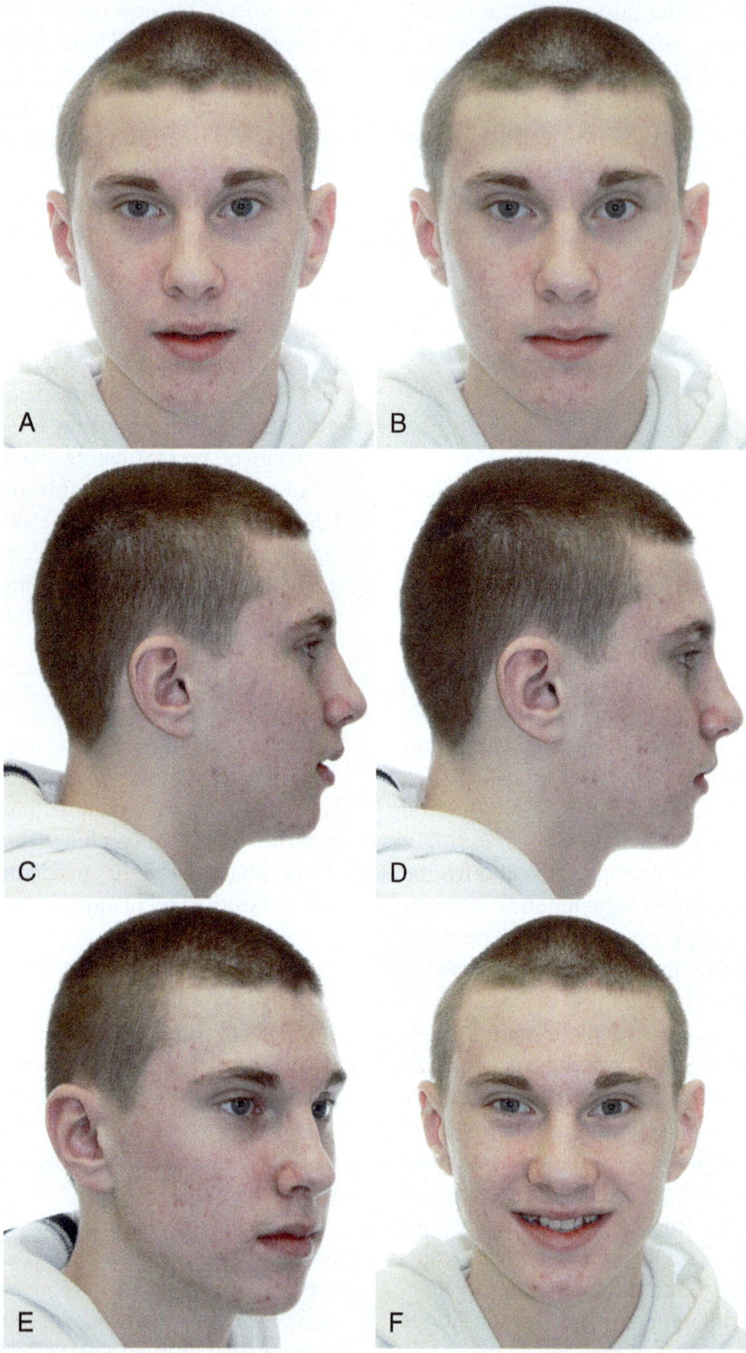

Figure 1-30 Extraoral photographs for the records. Frontal view (A) with lips at rest and (B) with lips lightly touching each other. Profile view (C) with lips at rest and (D) with lips lightly touching each other. E, Forty-five degree–angle photograph. Assessment of the cheek projection and mandibular plane angle is obtained from this view. F, Frontal view smiling photograph.

expectations, as well as relapse tendencies and sequelae (e.g., root resorption, decalcified lesions) after treatment. Additionally, the information can enable anticipation of complications that may have occurred with previous orthodontic therapy.

Within the dental history, the patient is questioned about previous trauma to the jaws or teeth. A history of trauma to the jaws may explain asymmetries, abnormal growth, or in some cases, TMJ symptoms. A history of trauma and the nature of the trauma (avulsion, luxation, fractures, etc.) to the teeth should be noted. Certain types of dentoalveolar trauma have been related to external root resorption and ankylosis.[86] Orthodontic movement can be a precipitating factor to this resorption in severely traumatized teeth (Fig. 1-34).[87]

Finally, any history of deleterious habits, such as thumb- or digit-sucking or a tongue posturing habit, might explain, in part, the etiology of the malocclusion. With regard to a

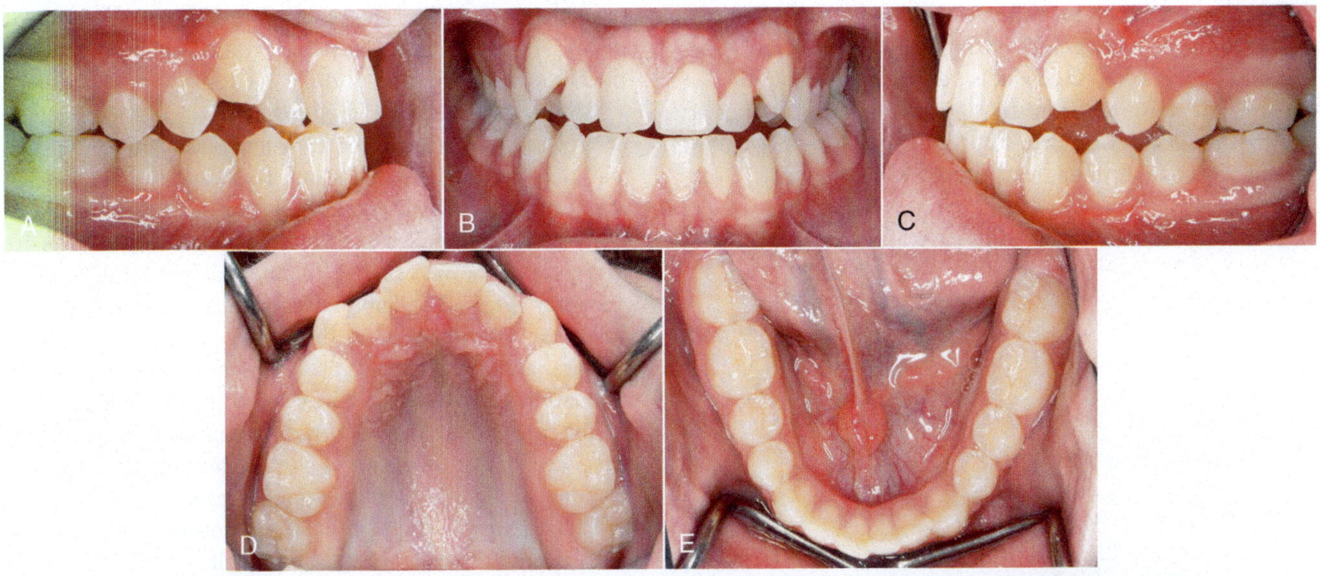

Figure 1-31 Intraoral records. **A,** Right buccal view. **B,** Frontal view. **C,** Left buccal view. **D,** Upper occlusal view. **E,** Lower occlusal view.

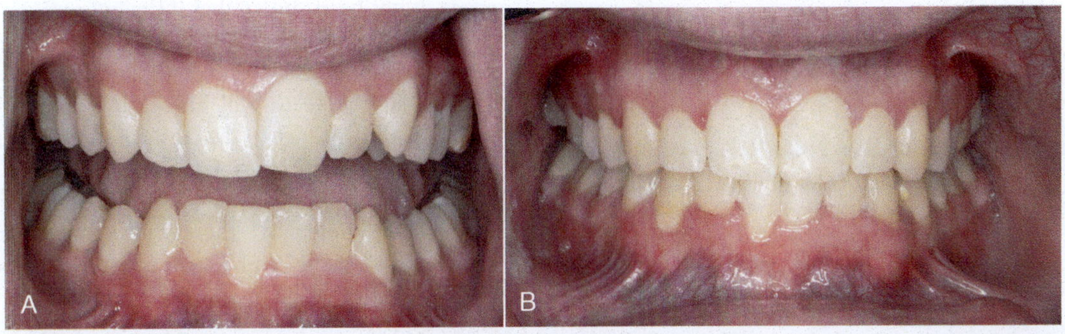

Figure 1-32 **A,** Preoperative photograph of the lower incisor gingival attachment. Incipient recession with a thin band of attached gingiva is seen. **B,** Postoperative photograph shows no attached gingiva in the lower right central incisor and slight progression of gingival recession. Grafting of this area is indicated.

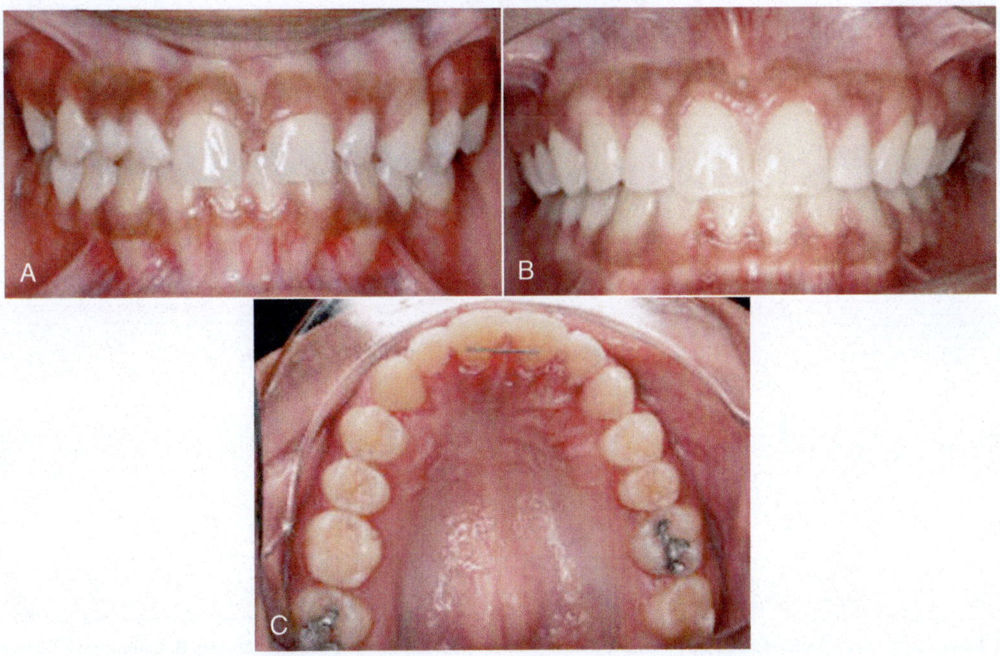

Figure 1-33 **A,** Thick band of labial frenum possibly contributing to the diastema. **B,** Diastema closure post-treatment with frenectomy complete. **C,** A bonded lingual retainer was placed between the incisors.

habit, it is important to find out if this is an active or past habit. In the case of an active habit, the frequency and time during the day when the habit is performed are noted.

The dental examination starts by counting the number of teeth. The specific aim is to inspect for any supernumerary or missing teeth. Primary teeth should be distinguished from permanent teeth and any tooth transpositions should be noted. The panoramic film is a useful aid for corroborating the clinical examination findings.

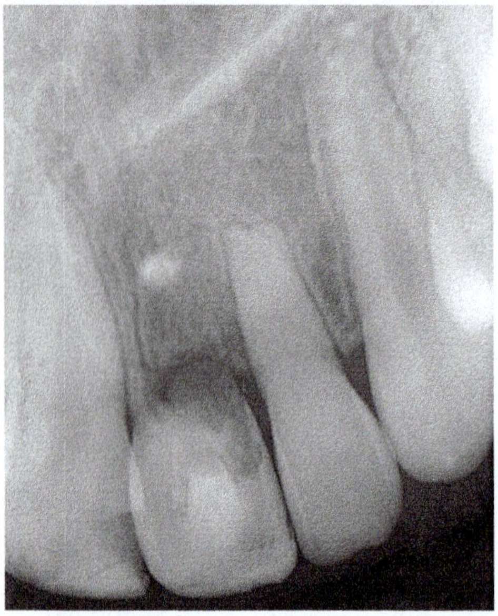

Figure 1-34 Radiograph of a patient with a history of severe trauma to the upper central incisor taken after orthodontic treatment. Note the calcification of the pulp chamber in the lateral incisor and the severe resorption of the root of the central incisor.

The size and shape of the teeth are critical for achieving an optimal esthetic outcome. Attention to morphological variation is especially important in the anterior segment. It is not unusual to find peg laterals, conical-shaped teeth, or other dental anomalies in this esthetic zone. Peg laterals are unsightly teeth that usually generate a Bolton tooth size discrepancy (Fig. 1-35). Subtle discrepancies in tooth size and shape are often noticed at the end of treatment when the occlusal and esthetic goals are not met. Therefore a careful evaluation of tooth size is needed from the beginning of treatment. Different restorative alternatives will dictate the specific distribution of spaces and positioning of the teeth to facilitate and enhance the restorative result.[88]

Open gingival embrasures, also known as "black triangles," are a common unesthetic finding in adults. These black spaces are closely related to tooth shape (Fig. 1-36) and are often a result of the papilla not filling the interproximal space. It has been shown that if the interproximal contact of two adjacent teeth is 5-mm or less from the crestal bone, a papilla will be present almost 100% of the time.[89] Thus triangular shaped teeth will have a low incisal contact that increases the distance to the crestal bone, resulting in a black triangle. At the initial examination the clinician should be aware that crowding between the upper incisors can displace the contact gingivally; therefore as proper alignment is achieved in the initial phases of treatment, the contact may

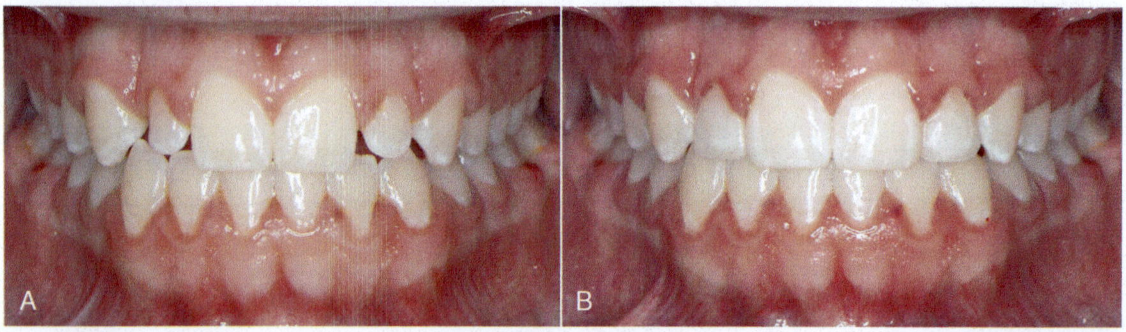

Figure 1-35 **A,** Morphology of the peg laterals creates wide unesthetic incisal embrasures. **B,** Restoration of these teeth is generally recommended in the last stages of treatment if composites are the selected restorative material.

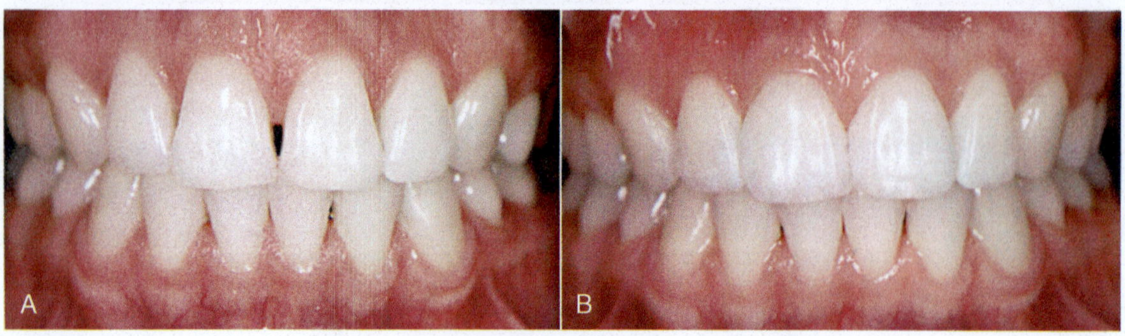

Figure 1-36 **A,** "Black triangle" as a result of the shape of the incisors. Contact between the incisors was too low. **B,** Good proportions between maximum height and width present in the incisal edge. Composite material was added to the mesial surfaces to alter the mesiodistal width in the middle and gingival thirds of the crowns.

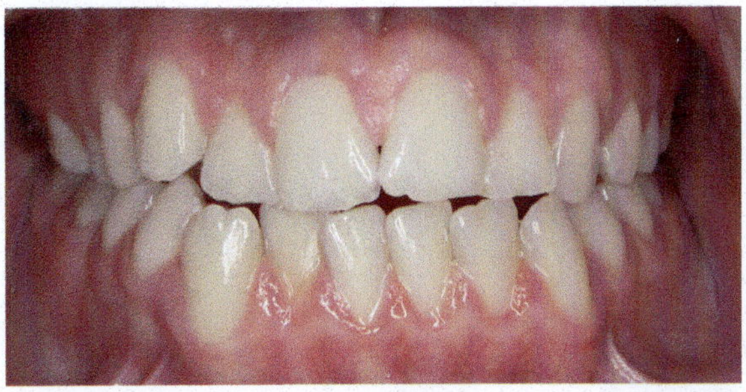

Figure 1-37 Abnormal morphology of the central and lateral incisors. The triangular shape can lead to "black triangles" interproximally once aligned.

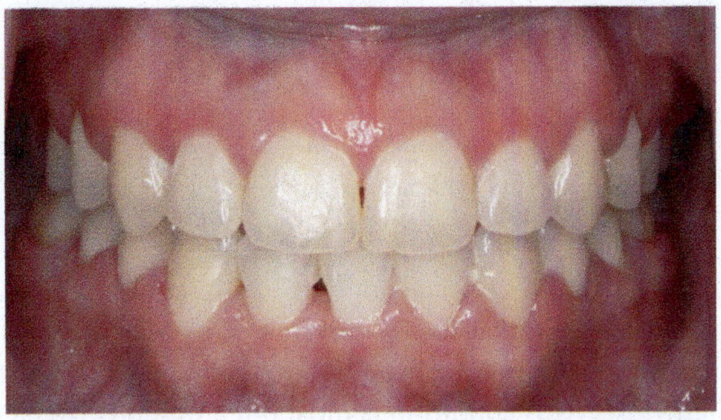

Figure 1-38 Post-treatment "black triangles" after the extraction of a lower incisor.

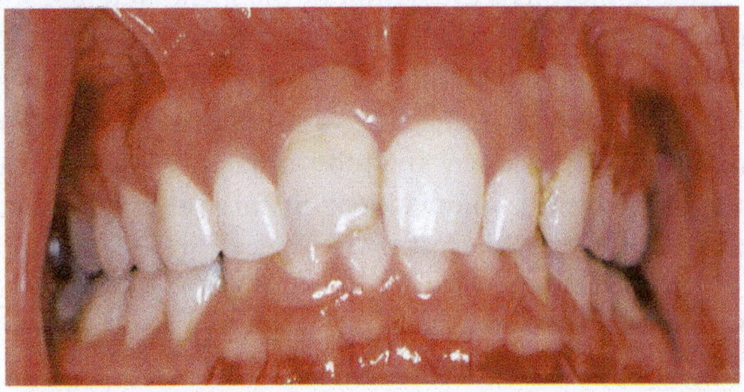

Figure 1-39 Abnormal morphology of the central incisors. The mesiodistal width is larger in the middle third compared to the incisal third, resulting in large incisal embrasures.

be displaced incisally, resulting in a black triangle (Fig. 1-37). The black triangle frequently found with the extraction of a lower incisor is often related to the bone recession that occurs after a tooth extraction (Fig. 1-38). Interproximal contact in the incisal third following lower incisor extraction also has been associated with these open gingival embrasures.[90]

Incisor crowns with a wider middle than incisal third also may result in excessive incisal embrasures (Fig. 1-39). Other abnormalities in tooth shape, such as irregularities in the borders of the incisors, may be related to a worn dentition or trauma to the incisors.

Tooth shape is related not only to the clinical crown but also to the root morphology and crown-to-root angulation. This is an important consideration in the straight-wire technique, as it is based on the coronal angulation to the occlusal plane in the three planes of space.[91] An acute angle between the root and the crown with a prescribed bracket may

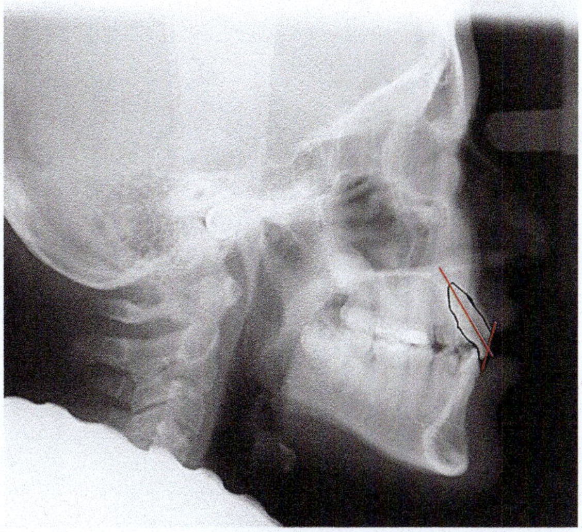

Figure 1-40 Acute crown–root angulation. Caution should be used during root correction of the incisors, as the lingual root portion may approximate the cortical plate of the palate.

position the root outside the cortical bone in the third order or displace the root against the tooth adjacent to it in the second order (Fig. 1-40).

Tooth shade is the final factor to be evaluated. It has been shown that patients prefer lighter shades. More importantly, any white or brown spots should be noted in the initial examination, to distinguish them from spots that can be caused by poor bacterial plaque control with fixed appliances.

The two most common dental diseases are caries and periodontal disease. Periodontal disease is more common in the adult population. Thus molars in all adult patients should be probed on all surfaces. Any additional probing will depend on the degree of periodontal involvement of the posterior teeth or will be based on the radiographic evidence obtained.

The deleterious effects of traumatic forces to teeth with periodontal disease have been well-reported (Fig. 1-41). Orthodontic forces have been shown to produce a similar breakdown effect on the tooth supporting structures in the presence of active periodontal disease. Therefore, as discussed earlier, prior to orthodontic treatment the clinician should ensure that no active disease is present and that suitable oral health conditions exist in the oral cavity.

Caries, the other common dental disease, is more prevalent in adolescents than in adults. Nevertheless, all patients should be screened for caries before and throughout orthodontic treatment. Any lesions present should be permanently restored and any pulpal involvement addressed before initiating treatment. It has been reported that infection within the confinement of the root canal can cause root resorption in response to an orthodontic force.[87] In addition, teeth with previous root canal treatment should be inspected for a good-quality seal and no signs of periapical pathology. Referring the patient to a general or pediatric dentist for cleaning and checkup before appliance placement is also recommended.

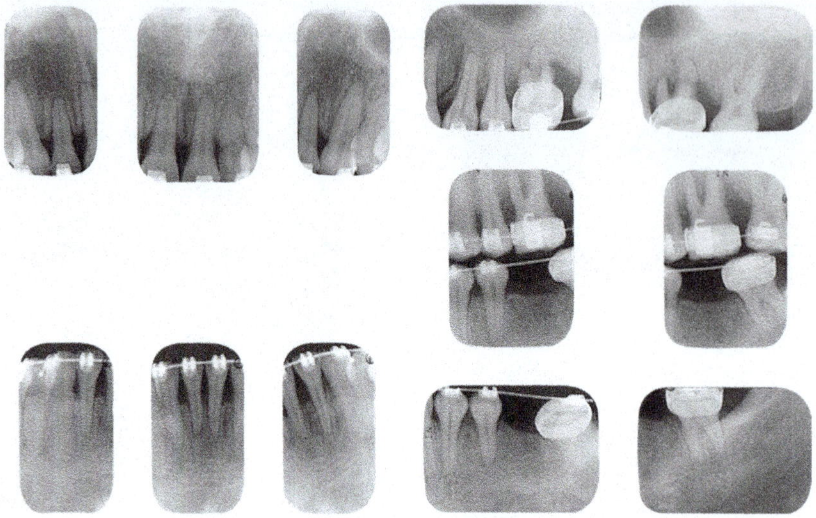

Figure 1-41 Patient with severe localized bone loss exacerbated by orthodontic appliances.

It is common for adults to present with missing teeth and heavily restored dentitions (i.e., crowns, bridges, and extensive amalgam or composite buildups). These patients should be checked for ill-fitting bridges and crowns. A good analysis of the tooth structure supporting the bridges should be done in collaboration with the restorative dentist. A multidisciplinary approach is needed in these cases to carefully plan the orthodontic movement that will facilitate ideal subsequent crown and bridge work. Furthermore, it should be anticipated that appliance insertion in heavily restored dentition is complicated. Banding and bonding procedures in these patients are difficult due to irregular tooth shapes and variable surface characteristics of the restorative materials. Hence appliance breakage during treatment is more common.

For the majority of patients, orthodontics is an elective procedure. Periodontal disease and caries affect many individuals seeking orthodontic treatment. Both dental diseases should be under control before orthodontic treatment is started. It should be stressed again that close communication with the general dentist is of key importance.

Tooth Eruption

As mentioned, there is great variation in the timing of eruption of different teeth among individuals. Delayed eruption of teeth is not a problem per se. However, an abnormal eruption sequence has been considered one of the factors involved in the etiology of malocclusion.[92] Other eruption disturbances, such as retained primary teeth, ankylosed teeth, and ectopic eruption, are important etiologic factors in malocclusion (Fig. 1-42). It has been reported that there is a correlation between the abnormal eruption sequence and direction, abnormal shape of teeth, and congenitally missing teeth.[37]

Dental Arches

During the intra-arch analysis, a general appreciation of the arch shape and an overall view of crowding or spacing are achieved. Intra-arch evaluation of the tooth relationships also includes marginal ridge discrepancies. Severe marginal ridge discrepancies between adjacent teeth may be indicative of ankylosis. This condition is most often found between the permanent first molars and the lower second primary molars (Fig. 1-43).

A more thorough evaluation of the intra-arch and inter-arch relationships can be achieved with the model analysis. Crowding, spacing, and problems with the angulations and orientation of teeth in the three dimensions of space can be analyzed more precisely in study models. Moreover, these models provide the unique possibility of analyzing the occlusion from the lingual aspect.

Extraoral Examination

Functional Analysis

One of the reasons that patients seek or are referred for orthodontic care is to achieve proper occlusal function. Therefore the orthodontist must have a good understanding of the critical concepts in occlusion and how they relate to other structures such as the TMJ.

Much has been discussed about which type of occlusion provides the best function.[93] In general, it is accepted that ideal occlusal function relates to a mutually protected occlusion.[93,94] This means that the posterior teeth protect the anterior teeth in maximum intercuspation by receiving the majority of the occlusal load and the anterior teeth protect the posterior teeth in the excursive movements. In lateral excursions, most clinicians agree that canine guidance is the ideal occlusal scheme. Yet group function on lateral movements can also be an acceptable occlusal scheme. Overall, balancing occlusal contacts is considered deleterious for occlusal function.

A good analysis of the different excursive movements is necessary in the initial clinical examination. The different excursive movements to be analyzed are anterior protrusive, lateral, and lateral protrusive movements. As mentioned above, any contacts between the posterior teeth during the

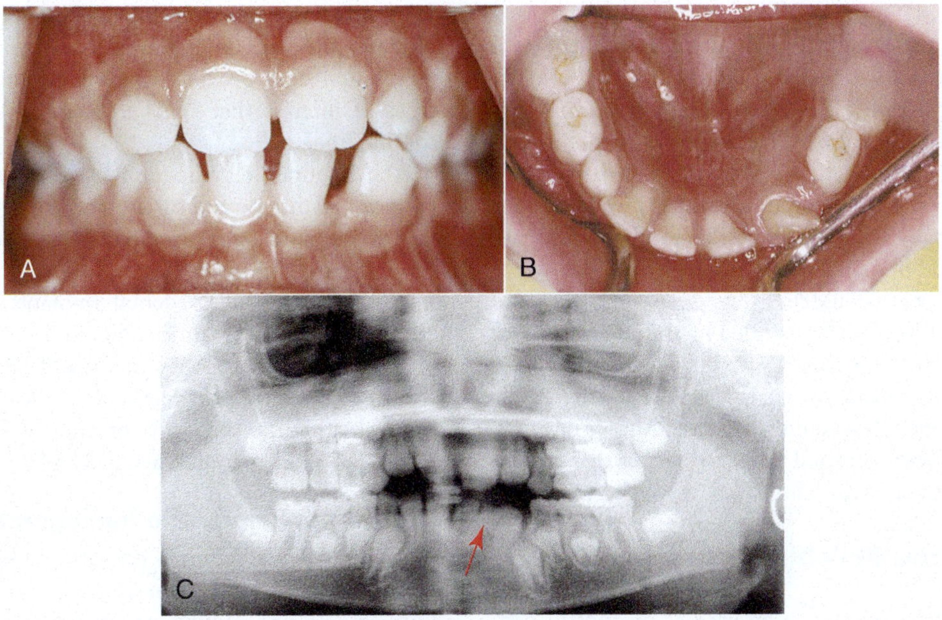

Figure 1-42 Ectopic eruption of lower left lateral incisor. **A,** Distal eruption of the lower lateral incisor exfoliated left primary canine instead of the lower lateral primary incisor. **B,** Space for the left permanent canine is greatly reduced. **C,** Panoramic radiograph shows that the primary left lateral incisor is still present *(arrow)* mesial to the lower left permanent lateral incisor. Eruption of the lower left permanent canine is hampered.

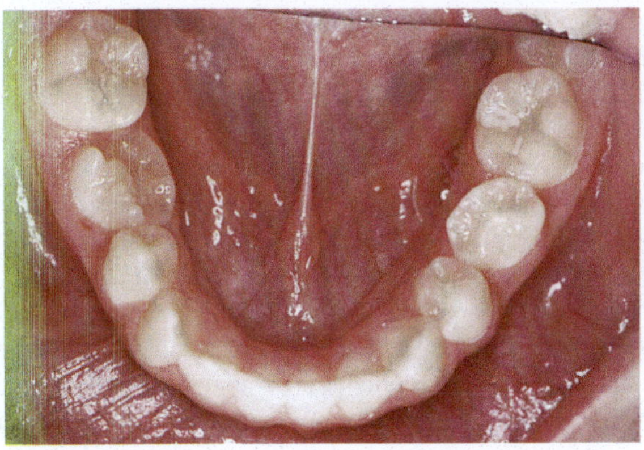

Figure 1-43 Thirteen-year-old patient with the lower right second primary molar submerged below the occlusal plane. This clinical finding is highly suggestive of ankylosis of this primary tooth.

anterior protrusive movement should be noted. In the lateral movements, attention should be given to any posterior contacts on the working side but most importantly on the balancing side. No anterior contacts should be present in lateral excursions. During all of these excursive movements, close attention should be paid to wear facets and how these relate interocclusally in the different end movements.

Temporomandibular Disorders

Temporomandibular disorders (TMD) encompass certain conditions in and around the TMJ. These disorders have been subdivided into internal derangements (within the articulation) and myofascial pain dysfunction (masticatory and cervical muscles).[95] Internal derangements are classified according to the relationship of the articular disc to the condyle during jaw opening. Four distinct stages of condyle-disc relationships have been found that denote progressive degeneration. The first stage starts with initial incoordination between the condyle and the disc during opening. The second and third stages are characterized by anterior displacement of the disc, which is not recaptured in the third stage. The fourth stage involves damage to the retrodiscal tissue.

The four major characteristics of myofascial pain dysfunction (MPD) are pain of unilateral origin, limited jaw opening, masticatory muscle tenderness, and no radiographic or clinical evidence of joint degeneration.[96] Each patient should be examined for the presence of any of these symptoms. The masticatory muscles and the temporomandibular articulation are palpated in search of any areas or trigger points that elicit pain.

In general, the TMJ examination should focus on evaluating jaw movements and areas of pain in and around the joint upon palpation or function. Mandibular movements should be painless and within a normal range (approximately 50-mm on maximum opening and 10-mm in lateral excursions).[94,97] The path followed during the opening movements of the mandible should be evaluated from the frontal view. This gives an indication of interferences, adhesions, or disc recapturing in the articulation. Although articular noises, such as clicking, popping, and crepitation, are important diagnostic findings, if any of these is the sole finding, it does not imply a diagnosis of TMD.[95]

In general, diagnosis and treatment of TMD is complex, as many other factors such as stress may be involved. In patients with a history of TMJ problems, a more advanced TMJ examination that may include the Helkimo index should be done.[98] Clinical examinations should be complemented with a very thorough medical and dental history that may include a psycho-stress analysis.[99]

CR–CO

A major area of controversy in orthodontics and dentistry overall is the relevance and importance of the centric relation.[100–103] Orthodontists should attempt to record the centric relation and detect whether any major shifts to the centric occlusion are present. It is normal to find a shift of approximately 1.5-mm in most individuals. The correlation between these small shifts and temporomandibular adverse effects is marginal but major shifts of 3- to 4-mm have been correlated with increased TMD.[104]

Some clinicians have recommended mounting every case in an articulator in order to treat an occlusion where CR–CO coincides. There is no evidence to support the need to mount every patient's models, less so if the potential source of error is considered in registering and transferring centric relation from the patient to an articulator.[105]

RADIOGRAPHIC RECORDS

Several radiographic images can be used as diagnostic aids for orthodontic therapy. The most commonly used images are the panoramic and lateral cephalometric radiographic films.

Before concentrating on any measurement analysis, a careful screening of each radiograph for any signs of pathology is indicated. Pathological images often pass undetected by clinicians, as attention usually centers on the orthodontic analysis instead of the anatomic structures. Interestingly, it was found that 6% of orthodontic patients show some kind of anomalous or pathological finding in orthodontic diagnostic radiographs (Fig. 1-44).[106,107]

Panoramic Radiograph

The panoramic radiograph provides a good general overview of the craniofacial anatomy, especially of the mandible, despite distortion of the image in some areas. Anatomy of the condyles should be examined carefully. Any asymmetry in length or width of the condyles, as well as in the shape of the articular surface, is noted. Ramus length and width symmetry should also be evaluated. Conditions such as hemimandibular hypoplasia or hyperplasia can be also detected in this radiograph.[108] The most important information available in this radiograph are the presence or absence of teeth, any variation in development or eruption timings, impaction of teeth, and variation in tooth anatomy.[109] The panoramic radiograph also provides general information on certain areas of interest that can be inspected closely with more specific imaging.

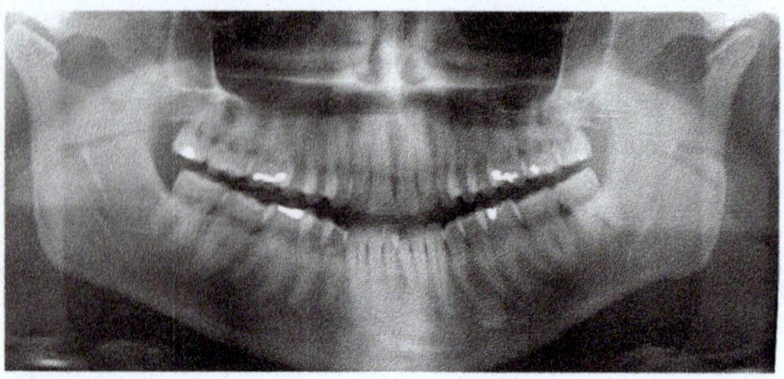

Figure 1-44 Condylar shape on panoramic radiograph is indicative of osteoarthritic changes. Note also the radiopaque structure between the root apices of the lower left premolars (compatible with idiopathic osteosclerosis).

The panoramic radiograph is also good for screening periodontal disease and caries. If an area looks suspicious for any of these diseases, a periapical or bitewing radiograph should be taken.

With the advent of dental implants and their use in anchorage, the panoramic radiograph is also an important tool for inspection of the quality and quantity (height and width) of bone for possible implant sites.[110] It is also useful for evaluating the proximity of implant sites to vital structures such as the mandibular canal and the maxillary sinuses.

Lateral Cephalometric Radiograph

The lateral cephalogram is one of the oldest and still most often used radiographic images in orthodontics. Its limitation, as with any radiograph, is that it displays only a 2D (vertical and anteroposterior) image of 3D structures. Most orthodontic research and growth and development data are based on information obtained from this radiograph. It has been used for evaluation of the hard tissue anatomy in the craniofacial structures, evaluation of growth, treatment planning, and treatment results.

Traditionally, angles and linear measurements have been used to evaluate the different anatomic structures in the craniofacial complex.[79,111] These measurements are compared to population means and the deviation from these norms is usually determined to be the problem. More recently, the development of numerous software programs enables an orthodontist to easily adopt his or her own relevant measurements from a plethora of cephalometric analyses. It should be emphasized that cephalometric analyses are only a diagnostic tool and are not diagnostic in themselves. Independent measures are meaningless if not interpreted properly; every deviation from the norm should be analyzed along with other measurements and within the whole context of the patient.

In the spatial analysis of an anatomic structure and its relation to others, three factors are important. The first is the size of the structure that can be measured, either in terms of height or width, and is usually defined by two points that determine a line. Second, the shape of the structure is usually defined by planes and angles and usually requires three or more points. Finally, the position of the structure is usually defined by angles and linear measurements to other reference structures.

The cephalometric analysis for orthognathic surgery (COGS) developed at the University of Connecticut has been divided into five major craniofacial components in an attempt to define their size, shape, and position.[75] These components are cranial base, maxilla, mandible, dentition, and soft tissue.

Before describing the specific spatial cephalometric analysis of these five components, a reference line or plane must be defined. This plane is important, as it will determine the orientation of the cranium in space. Many of the angular and linear measurements that analyze facial morphology relate back to this plane.

The Frankfurt horizontal (FH) plane was defined by anthropologists in the nineteenth century and was adopted in cephalometry as the horizontal reference line. Although still used, there are inherent problems with this reference line as both porion and orbitale are difficult landmarks to locate. It is especially difficult to visualize porion since it is a bilateral landmark and is often not well-defined on lateral head films. On the other hand, the sella-nasion (SN) line is composed of two easily visualized landmarks. At the University of Connecticut we have recommended an FH line located on average 7 degrees below the SN line.[112] This constructed FH reference line is more reproducible and thus allows better evaluation of treatment progress and outcome.

For an accurate interpretation of the different structures in space, a reference line that was based on a physiological posture instead of cranial anatomic landmarks has also been recommended. Studies have shown that variation in cranial base inclination may result in an unreliable impression of facial relationships.[113] A reference line that was made up of extracranial instead of intracranial points was recommended as being more reliable. This horizontal line should be parallel to the floor and represents the average head posture. The importance of this plane is that it not only reflects the normal position of the head in space, but also is a reproducible position not affected by intracranial landmarks. When a radiograph is taken in this natural head position (registered when a patient looks at a mirror in front of him or her at eye level), true vertical and horizontal reference lines can be traced.

Cranial Base

The cranial base, particularly the anterior portion, is an important structure in the cephalometric analysis. Since growth of the anterior cranial base is nearly completed early in life, it can be used as a reference for the other structures. The anterior cranial base is also used to superimpose successive cephalograms in order to evaluate the overall changes related to growth and treatment. By knowing the length of the cranial base, size correlations to the other structures (maxilla and mandible) can be estimated (Fig. 1-45).

The saddle angle formed by nasion (N) to sella (S) to articulare (Ar) (referred to as N–S–Ar) (see Fig. 1-45) and its influence on the craniofacial morphology has been evaluated in various studies. Its contribution to Class II and III malocclusions is somewhat controversial. It was proposed that an obtuse angle related to the former and an acute angle related to the latter[114] but recent studies have not found a strong correlation between the two.[115]

Maxilla

The second component of the cephalometric analysis is the maxilla. Initially, a general idea of its size is obtained by measuring the posterior border to the anterior border. This measurement is specifically defined as the distance from the anterior nasal spine to the posterior nasal spine (ANS–PNS). Thereafter the anteroposterior position is assessed. The distance from A point, which is related to a vertical reference line passing through N, provides good information relative to the position of the maxilla. It is important to remember that A point is affected by dentoalveolar movement. Another measurement used to assess the anteroposterior position of the maxilla is the perpendicular distance from PNS to a vertical line passing through pterygomaxillary fissure point (PTM) (Fig. 1-46).

To assess the vertical position of the maxilla, the distance from the ANS to the N is measured. This is known as the upper facial height and its absolute measurement is not as important as the relationship to the lower facial height

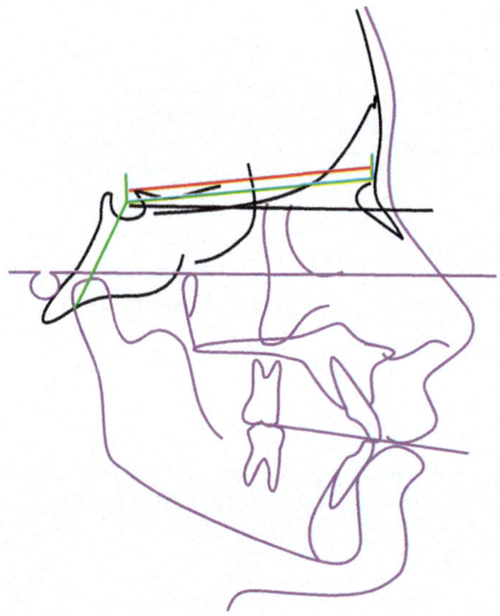

Figure 1-45 Measurements commonly used to evaluate the size and shape of the cranial base (first component in the cephalometric analysis).

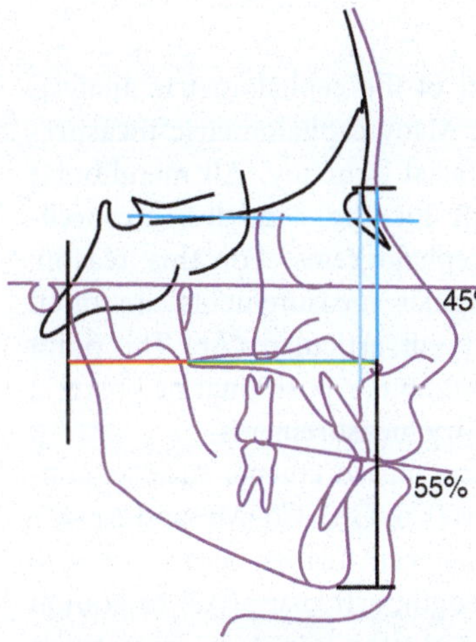

Figure 1-46 Commonly used measurements to evaluate size and position of the maxilla (second component). *ANS,* Anterior nasal spine; *FH,* Frankfurt horizontal; *PNS,* posterior nasal spine.

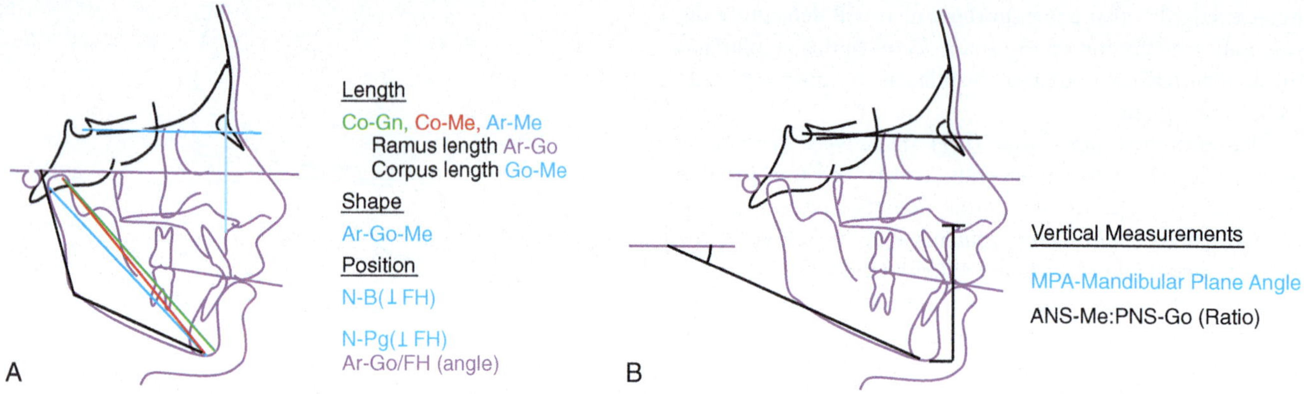

Figure 1-47 Measurements commonly used to evaluate size, shape, and position of the mandible (third component). **A,** Anteroposterior and **(B)** vertical images. *ANS,* Anterior nasal spine; *FH,* Frankfurt horizontal; *PNS,* posterior nasal spine.

(ANS–Me): 45% for the upper to 55% for the lower facial height (see Fig. 1-44).[112] Another important measurement indicating the vertical position or inclination of the maxilla is the angulation of the palatal plane (PNS–ANS) in relation to the horizontal line (see Fig. 1-44). Usually in skeletal open-bite patients this plane is tipped up anteriorly instead of being close to parallel, as is found in normal individuals.[116]

Mandible

The third major component of the cephalometric analysis is the mandibular position. Many cephalometric measurements relate to this craniofacial structure. All mandibular anatomic structures, except for the condyles, are well-visualized in the lateral cephalograms. For this reason, mandibular length and angular measurements are often taken from the constructed point, articulare (Ar). This point may be confounding, as mandibular positional or postural changes can give contradictory measurements.

To assess mandibular size, measurements such as condylion (Co) to gnathion (Gn) (Co–Gn), Co–Me, and Ar–Me are used (Fig. 1-47, A). These can further be divided into ramus height and corpus length: articulare (Ar) to gonion (Go) (Ar–Go) and gonion to menton (Go–Me), respectively (see Fig. 1-47, A). The anteroposterior position of the mandible is measured anteriorly by relating the distance of B point and the pogonion to a true vertical line (perpendicular to FH) passing through N (see Fig. 1-47, A). The difference between these two measurements gives an indication of the length of the hard tissue chin. Posteriorly, the anteroposterior position of the mandible can be evaluated from the angle formed by the ramus and the true horizontal (see Fig. 1-47, A). The shape of the mandible is defined by the gonial angle (Ar–Go–Me) (see Fig. 1-47, A).

The vertical anterior measurement of the mandible is calculated by quantifying the distance from ANS to Me (lower facial height). A ratio of the lower facial height to the posterior facial height (PNS–Go) can give an indication of the vertical pattern of the face (Fig. 1-47, B). These measurements can be correlated to the mandibular plane angle (true horizontal Go–Me, see Fig. 1-47, B). Traditionally, these angular measurements have been used to describe vertical

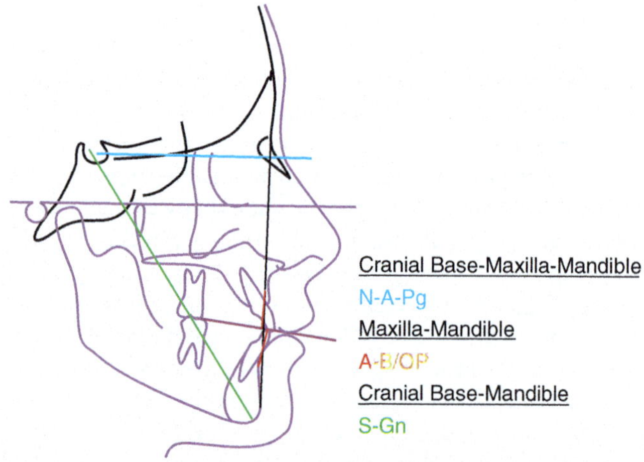

Figure 1-48 Cephalometric analysis between cranial base, maxilla, and mandible.

growth (high angle versus low angle) and facial patterns (long face versus short face).

Before starting the fourth major component (dental) of the cephalometric analysis, a set of measurements that relate the maxilla and mandible to each other and the cranial base needs to be mentioned. These measurements are A–B relative to the true horizontal and the occlusal plane and the angle of convexity (N–A–Pg) (Fig. 1-48). Lastly, the S–Gn line is an isolated measurement that correlates directly with direction (angle with respect to the true horizontal) and magnitude (absolute length) of mandibular growth and indirectly with the growth of the whole facial complex (see Fig. 1-48).

Dental Measurements

The spatial relationship of the teeth is described in terms of their horizontal and vertical position within the bones. One of the reference planes for the dental measurements is the occlusal plane, which on average has a downward inclination anteriorly of approximately 12 degrees related to the true horizontal or constructed FH plane.

Different types of occlusal planes have been described. Downs originally described the occlusal plane as a constructed line that bisects the upper and lower molars and the anterior teeth.[111] This plane does not take into consideration the axial inclinations of the posterior teeth. The inherent problem with this plane can be seen in patients who have no incisor overlap, such as in the case of an anterior open-bite.

A better method for defining this plane is the anatomic or functional occlusal plane. This occlusal plane follows the occlusal contacts of the posterior teeth and is extended anteriorly. It can be determined easily, as the longitudinal axis of the posterior teeth is almost perpendicular to this occlusal plane.

In the analysis of the dentition, the inclination of the upper incisors is evaluated in relation to the maxillary palatal plane and the true horizontal plane (Fig. 1-49). In the lower arch, the ideal relationship of the incisors to the mandibular plane has been considered to be an angle close to 90 degrees (see Fig. 1-49). The interincisal angle should confirm the findings of the upper and lower incisor inclination to the palatal and mandibular plane respectively (see Fig. 1-49).

Vertically, a measurement from ANS to 1 (ANS–upper incisor tip) determines the amount of eruption of the upper incisor. In the lower arch, the vertical height of the lower incisor is assessed by the measurement of Me to –1 (menton–lower incisor tip, see Fig. 1-49).

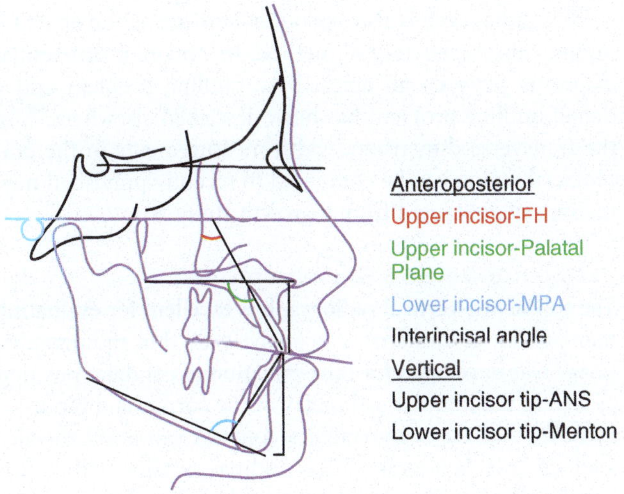

Figure 1-49 Measurements commonly used in the fourth component of the cephalometric analysis (dentition). *ANS*, Anterior nasal spine; *FH*, Frankfurt horizontal; *MPA*, mandibular plane angle.

Soft Tissue

Some of the reference lines used for cephalometric soft tissue analysis were introduced above in the description of the clinical examination. It is important to stress that these lines are only guidelines based on averages and that esthetics is highly subjective.

The soft tissue analysis should start by determining the general convexity of the profile (G–Sn–Pg; Fig. 1-50, A). Thereafter, the anteroposterior position of the maxilla and the mandible can be analyzed separately by drawing a line perpendicular to the horizontal reference line passing through the glabella, soft tissue nasion, subnasale, or any other anterior soft tissue landmark (depending on the analysis) and measuring the distance to the maxilla and the mandible (see Fig. 1-50, A). On average the mandible lies within this line (when a true vertical is drawn through the glabella) and the maxilla is 2- to 3-mm in front. It is important to determine the upper lip, lower lip, and soft tissue chin thickness since these elements might be compensating for a skeletal disharmony.

The next step in the soft tissue analysis is evaluation of the lips. In general, measurements of lip protrusion are made using Sn–Pg as the reference line (see Fig. 1-50, A). Other angles used to evaluate lip protrusion are the nasolabial angle for the upper lip and the mentolabial angle for the lower lip (see Fig. 1-50, A). To eliminate the influence of the nose when measuring upper lip inclination, an angle is measured between the true horizontal and a line is traced from Sn to the labrale superioris (Fig. 1-50, B). A similar measurement to evaluate lower lip inclination has been used by connecting a line from the depth of the mentolabial sulcus to the labrale inferioris and measuring the angle to FH (see Fig 1-50, B).

Growth Assessment

To complement the lip analysis, the curl of both lips is evaluated. This is an important esthetic feature. The depth of the

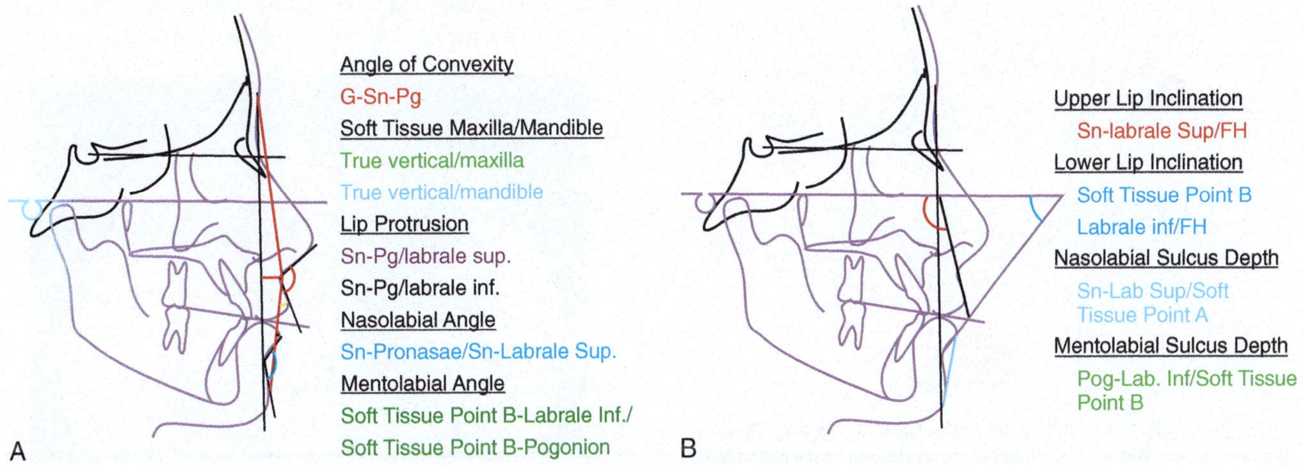

Figure 1-50 **A and B,** Soft tissue analysis (fifth component).

upper lip and the mentolabial sulcus is measured by drawing a line from the upper lip to Sn and the lower lip to Pg, respectively (see Fig. 1-50, B). Excessive depth in these measurements may indicate lip redundancy. Finally, a measurement of the chin to throat depth is important, especially in prospective surgery patients.

In general, when soft tissues are assessed, the tongue, soft tissue palate, and airway structures are often overlooked. It is important to evaluate the airway patency as well as the position of the hyoid bone. It has been reported that patients with obstructive sleep apnea have a low position of the hyoid bone.[117]

All cephalometric measurements and their deviations from the norms are only guides to describe the problems. An explanation for each deviation from the norm is examined in conjunction with the other measurements to obtain a cephalometric summary. Attention should be paid to contradictory measurements and an explanation for these should be sought. Cephalometric analysis is a tool and as such it is only one of the components in the database that needs to be complemented with the clinical examination, models, and other imaging.

Traditionally, hand-wrist radiographs have been used to evaluate skeletal maturity. The stage of ossification of the wrist and phalanges in the hand correlates to skeletal maturity (Fig. 1-51). However, efforts to correlate skeletal maturation to the cervical vertebrae have diminished the need for a hand-wrist radiograph. It has been shown that the peak of pubertal growth can be estimated adequately from a lateral cephalometric film.[118] Visual assessment of the lower border concavities and progressive elongation of the odontoid process (C2) and C3 and C4 vertebrae on the lateral cephalogram form the basis of this staging method. Based on this assessment, the patient can be placed in one of six cervical stage categories (CS1–CS6) and an estimation can be made on the growth stage of the patient relative to the peak in mandibular growth.[119]

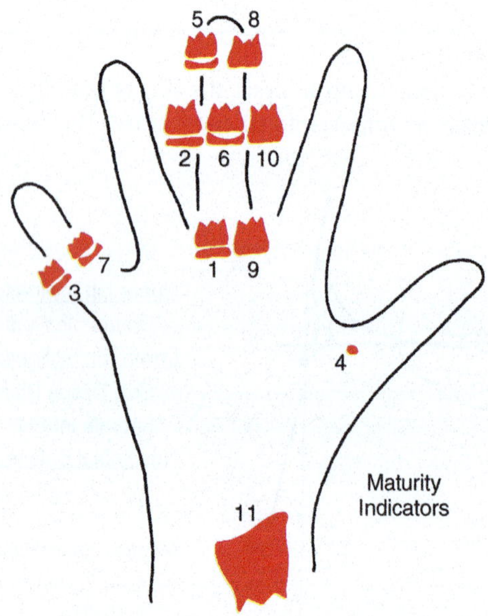

Figure 1-51 Hand-wrist radiograph with skeletal maturation indicators. (Redrawn from Fishman LS. Radiographic evaluation of skeletal maturation. *Angle Orthod.* 1982;52:88–112.)

Occlusal Radiograph

The occlusal radiograph has been used to locate supernumerary or impacted teeth. In conjunction with a panoramic radiograph, the occlusal x-ray has been reported to give a good indication of the location of the impacted or supernumerary tooth.[109] This radiograph is also indicated to evaluate the amount of suture distraction with rapid palatal expansion (Fig. 1-52).

Posteroanterior-Cephalometric Radiograph

The posteroanterior-cephalometric radiograph (posteroanterior cephalogram) is indicated in patients in whom a significant clinical asymmetry is noticed (Fig. 1-53). It can be used for both skeletal and dental base asymmetry detection. Mandibular ramus heights as well as corpus lengths can be evaluated. A large discrepancy between the lower borders of the mandible observed in a lateral cephalometric radiograph is highly indicative of a skeletal asymmetry that can be better evaluated with a posteroanterior cephalogram.

This radiograph is also a good tool for evaluation of dental midline discrepancies. A method to obtain a differential diagnosis between an apical base midline problem and a dental midline problem has been described elsewhere.[120] In the transverse dimension, width measurements in the craniofacial region can be compared to recently published normative data obtained from a growth study.[121]

Submento-Vertical Radiograph

The submento-vertical radiograph is excellent for evaluating mandibular asymmetry. An analysis of this radiographic image was developed for the evaluation of condylar position as well as mandibular symmetry of the corpus and ramus.[122] Symmetry of the zygomaxillary complex can also be evaluated on this radiograph. The findings obtained from this x-ray can be correlated to those found on the posteroanterior cephalogram for a 3D analysis of a skeletal asymmetry.

Cone Beam Computed Tomography

Cone beam computed tomography (CBCT) has gained popularity in recent years for imaging the craniofacial complex.

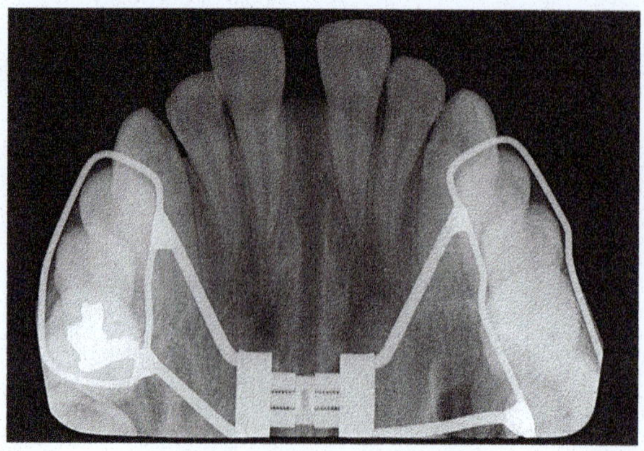

Figure 1-52 Occlusal radiograph depicting an open palatal suture.

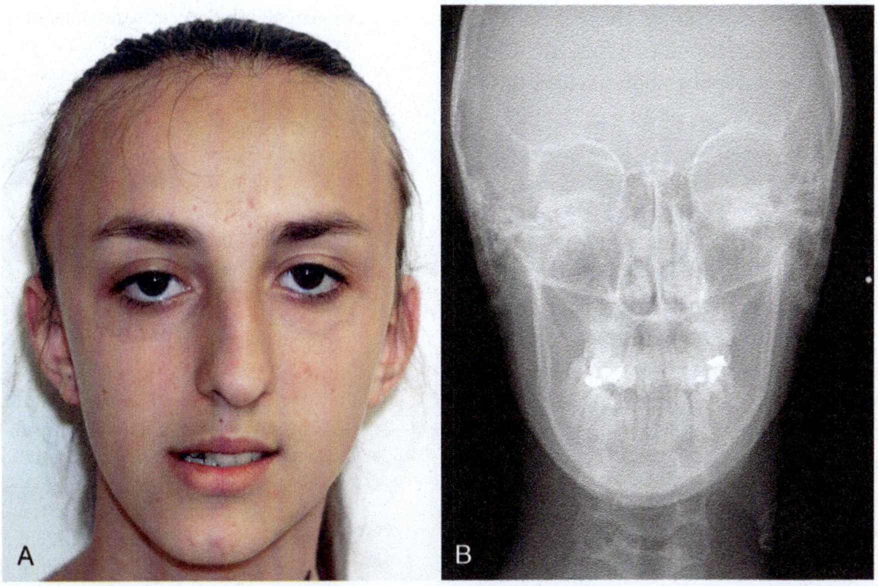

Figure 1-53 Significant mandibular asymmetry evident (**A**) in the clinical examination with the patient in centric occlusion and (**B**) on the posteroanterior cephalic radiograph in centric occlusion.

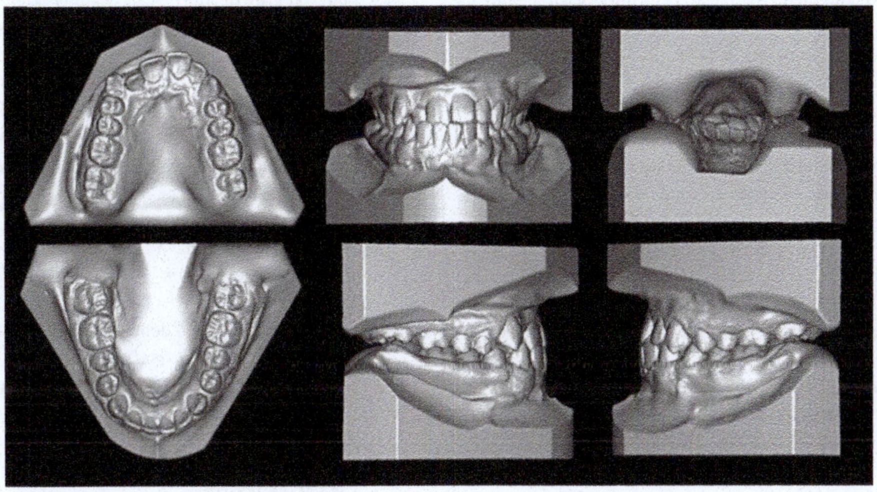

Figure 1-54 Composite montage of digital models in standard views (Orchestrate, Orthodontic Technologies, Rialto, CA.). Models can be manipulated in 3D and analyzed using digital software to make diagnostic measurements.

CBCT delivers a significantly lower dose of radiation compared to conventional CT methods and has distinct advantages over 2D images, including providing 1:1 orthogonal representations of structures. CBCT images can be used in lieu of other 2D images, such as panoramic radiographic projection and lateral cephalogram, with the software capable of generating these images from the 3D data. Caution should be exercised to minimize radiation doses to patients. Studies have shown great variability in the amount of radiation exposure between different CBCT machines and the control of the field of view and intensity can help to minimize these levels.[123-125] CBCT is a valuable tool for 3D surgical planning, which is discussed in Chapter 2. In addition, in cases with impacted teeth, CBCT images can provide a number of advantages over periapical and occlusal films for localization of these teeth, since they provide images free of distortion and overlapping structures.[124,126]

DIAGNOSTIC MODELS

One of the major advantages of models is the ability to inspect the malocclusion from the lingual aspect. Models also provide a more accurate and accessible way to evaluate arch shape, occlusion, and the 3D position of each tooth in space (first, second, and third order) and how it relates to the other teeth. Also, arch symmetry can be analyzed from the deviation of the teeth from the midsagittal suture.

Models also can be used for space analysis in the mixed dentition and as a template from which an occlusogram can be constructed. While traditionally stone models have been used, new technologies have further advanced the capabilities of digital 3D models. These models can be acquired through surface scanning of stone models or through the use of direct intraoral scanners, eliminating the need for an alginate impression (Fig. 1-54). A variety of software programs exist that are able to manipulate these models in all three dimensions and do a variety of analyses, including measuring Bolton discrepancies, space analysis, and doing occlusograms.[127]

SUMMARY

A synopsis of the most important components needed for the orthodontic diagnosis has been given. A detailed analysis of the clinical examination, radiographs, patient records, and additional imaging has been described. A good treatment outcome is heavily dependent on good data collection and analysis of the database. Ultimately, the diagnosis should answer the question "why?" so that later we can determine where we are going (objectives), how we are going to get there (treatment plan), and what techniques are going to be used (mechanics plan).

REFERENCES

1. Soanes C, Stevenson A., eds. *Concise Oxford English Dictionary*. 11th ed. Oxford, England: Oxford University Press; 2009.
2. Tobiasen JM. Social judgments of facial deformity. *Cleft Palate J*. 1987;24:323–327.
3. Ash M, Ramfjord SR. *Occlusion*. 4th ed. Philadelphia, PA: WB Saunders; 1995:472.
4. Barrows HS. *Practice-Based Learning*. Springfield, IL: Southern Illinois University School of Medicine; 1994:145.
5. Burden D, Mullally B, Sandler J. Orthodontic treatment of patients with medical disorders. *Eur J Orthod*. 2001;23:363–372.
6. Epstein JB. Infective endocarditis: dental implications and new guidelines for antibiotic prophylaxis. American Heart Association. *J Can Dent Assoc*. 1998;64:281–286, 289–292.
7. Devlin H, Garland H, Sloan P. Healing of tooth extraction sockets in experimental diabetes mellitus. *J Oral Maxillofac Surg*. 1996;54:1087–1091.
8. McNab S, Battistulla D, Taverne A, Symons AL. External apical root resorption of posterior teeth in asthmatics after orthodontic treatment. *Am J Orthod Dentofacial Orthop*. 1999;116:545–551.
9. Meraw SJ, Sheridan PJ. Medically induced gingival hyperplasia. *Mayo Clin Proc*. 1998;73:1196–1199.
10. Karras JC, Miller JR, Hodges JS, Beyer JP, Larson BE. Effect of alendronate on orthodontic tooth movement in rats. *Am J Orthod Dentofacial Orthop*. 2009;136(6):843–847.
11. Ortega AJ, Campbell PM, Hinton R, Naidu A, Buschang PH. Local application of zoledronate for maximum anchorage during space closure. *Am J Orthod Dentofacial Orthop*. 2012;142(6):780–791.
12. Lotwala RB, Greenlee GM, Ott SM, Hall SH, Huang GJ. Bisphosphonates as a risk factor for adverse orthodontic outcomes: a retrospective cohort study. *Am J Orthod Dentofacial Orthop*. 2012;142(5):625–634.e3.
13. Janson GR, Dainesi EA, Consolaro A, Woodside DG, de Freitas MR. Nickel hypersensitivity reaction before, during, and after orthodontic therapy. *Am J Orthod Dentofacial Orthop*. 1998;113(6):655–660.
14. Grimaudo NJ. Biocompatibility of nickel and cobalt dental alloys. *Gen Dent*. 2001;49(5):498–503; quiz 504–505.
15. Smith RM, Gonzalez C. The relationship between nasal obstruction and craniofacial growth. *Pediatr Clin North Am*. 1989;36(6):1423–1434.
16. Bergstrom J, Preber H. Tobacco use as a risk factor. *J Periodontol*. 1994;65(suppl 5):545–550.
17. Scabbia A, et al. Cigarette smoking negatively affects healing response following flap debridement surgery. *J Periodontol*. 2001;72(1):43–49.
18. Sanders, NL. Evidence-based care in orthodontics and periodontics: a review of the literature. *J Am Dent Assoc*. 1999;130(4):521–527.
19. Reichert C, et al. Interfaces between orthodontic and periodontal treatment: their current status. *J Orofac Orthop*. 2011;72(3):165–186.
20. Franchi L, Baccetti T, McNamara JA Jr. Mandibular growth as related to cervical vertebral maturation and body height. *Am J Orthod Dentofacial Orthop*. 2000;118(3):335–340.
21. Oudet C, Petrovic A, Stutzmann J. Time-dependent effects of a "functional"-type orthopedic appliance on the rat mandible growth. *Chronobiol Int*. 1984;1(1):51–57.
22. Chen JY, Will LA, Niederman R. Analysis of efficacy of functional appliances on mandibular growth. *Am J Orthod Dentofacial Orthop*. 2002;122(5):470–476.
23. Woodside, DG. Do functional appliances have an orthopedic effect? *Am J Orthod Dentofacial Orthop*. 1998;113(1):11–14.
24. Baccetti T, et al. Treatment timing for twin-block therapy. *Am J Orthod Dentofacial Orthop*. 2000;118(2):159–170.
25. Voudouris JC, et al. Condyle-fossa modifications and muscle interactions during herbst treatment, part 1. New technological methods. *Am J Orthod Dentofacial Orthop*. 2003;123(6):604–613.
26. Fishman LS. Radiographic evaluation of skeletal maturation: a clinically oriented method based on hand-wrist films. *Angle Orthod*. 1982;52(2):88–112.
27. Hagg U, Taranger J. Menarche and voice change as indicators of the pubertal growth spurt. *Acta Odontol Scand*. 1980;38(3):179–186.
28. Hagg U, Taranger J. Skeletal stages of the hand and wrist as indicators of the pubertal growth spurt. *Acta Odontol Scand*. 1980;38(3):187–200.
29. Silveira AM, et al. Facial growth during adolescence in early, average and late maturers. *Angle Orthod*. 1992;62(3):185–190.
30. Saunders SR, Popovich F, Thompson GW. A family study of craniofacial dimensions in the Burlington Growth Centre sample. *Am J Orthod*. 1980;78(4):394–403.
31. Suzuki A, Takahama Y. Parental data used to predict growth of craniofacial form. *Am J Orthod Dentofacial Orthop*. 1991;99(2):107–121.
32. Bishara SE. Facial and dental changes in adolescents and their clinical implications. *Angle Orthod*. 2000;70(6):471–483.
33. Nanda RS. The rate of growth of different facial components. *Am J Orthod*. 1955;41:658–673.
34. Skieller V, Bjork A, Linde-Hansen T. Prediction of mandibular growth rotation evaluated from a longitudinal implant sample. *Am J Orthod*. 1984;86(5):359–370.
35. Leslie LR, et al. Prediction of mandibular growth rotation: assessment of the Skieller, Bjork, and Linde-Hansen method. *Am J Orthod Dentofacial Orthop*. 1998;114(6):659–667.
36. Kokich VG. Managing complex orthodontic problems: the use of implants for anchorage. *Semin Orthod*. 1996;2(2):153–160.
37. Baccetti T. A controlled study of associated dental anomalies. *Angle Orthod*. 1998;68(3):267–274.
38. Peck S, Peck L, Kataja M. Concomitant occurrence of canine malposition and tooth agenesis: evidence of orofacial genetic fields. *Am J Orthod Dentofacial Orthop*. 2002;122(6):657–660.
39. Katz JL. The structure and biomechanics of bone. *Symp Soc Exp Biol*. 1980;34:137–168.
40. Kiliaridis S. Masticatory muscle influence on craniofacial growth. *Acta Odontol Scand*. 1995;53(3):196–202.
41. Proffit WR. Equilibrium theory revisited: factors influencing position of the teeth. *Angle Orthod*. 1978;48(3):175–186.
42. Weinstein S, et al. On an equilibrium theory of tooth position. *Angle Orthod*. 1963;33:1–26.
43. Mah J, Bumann A. Technology to create the three-dimensional patient record. *Semin Orthod*. 2001;7:251–257.
44. Scheib JE, Gangestad SW, Thornhill R. Facial attractiveness, symmetry and cues of good genes. *Proc R Soc Lond B Biol Sci*. 1999;266(1431):1913–1917.

45. Thornhill R, Gangestad SW. Facial attractiveness. *Trends Cogn Sci.* 1999;3(12):452–460.
46. Arnett GW, Bergman RT. Facial keys to orthodontic diagnosis and treatment planning: part I. *Am J Orthod Dentofacial Orthop.* 1993; 103(4):299–312.
47. Vig RG, Brundo GC. The kinetics of anterior tooth display. *J Prosthet Dent.* 1978;39(5):502–504.
48. Frush JO, Fisher RD. The dysesthetic interpretation in the dentogenic concept. *J Prosthet Dent.* 1958;8:55–58.
49. Dunn WJ, Murchison DF, Broome JC. Esthetics: patients' perceptions of dental attractiveness. *J Prosthodont.* 1996;5(3):166–171.
50. Fuhrmann RAW. Three-dimensional evaluation of periodontal remodeling during orthodontic treatment. *Semin Orthod.* 2002;8: 23–28.
51. Schiffman PH, Tuncay OC. Maxillary expansion: a meta analysis. *Clin Orthod Res.* 2001;4(2):86–96.
52. Sarver DM, Ackerman JL. Evaluation of facial soft tissues. In: Proffit WR, ed. *Contemporary Treatment of Facial Deformity.* St. Louis, MO: Mosby; 2003:92–126.
53. Burstone C. 2003. Personal communication.
54. Benson KJ, Laskin DM. Upper lip asymmetry in adults during smiling. *J Oral Maxillofac Surg.* 2001;59(4):396–398.
55. Beyer JW, Lindauer SJ. Evaluation of dental midline position. *Semin Orthod.* 1998;4(3):146–152.
56. Cardash HS, Ormanier Z, Laufer BZ. Observable deviation of the facial and anterior tooth midlines. *J Prosthet Dent.* 2003;89(3): 282–285.
57. Kokich VO Jr, Kiyak HA, Shapiro PA. Comparing the perception of dentists and lay people to altered dental esthetics. *J Esthet Dent.* 1999;11(6):311–324.
58. Caudill R, Chiche GJ. Establishing an esthetic gingival appearance. In: Chiche G, ed. *Esthetics of Anterior Fixed Prosthodontics.* Chicago, IL: Quintessence Publishing Co Inc; 1994:177–198.
59. Chiche G, Pinault A. Replacement of deficient crowns. In: Chiche G, ed. *Esthetics of Anterior Fixed Prosthodontics.* Chicago, IL: Quintessence Publishing Co Inc; 1994:53–73.
60. Petrovic A, Stutzmann J. [Growth hormone: mode of action on different varieties of cartilage (author's transl)]. *Pathol Biol* (Paris). 1980; 28(1):43–58.
61. Nanda RS, et al. Growth changes in the soft tissue facial profile. *Angle Orthod.* 1990;60(3):177–190.
62. McNamara JA Jr. Components of class II malocclusion in children 8–10 years of age. *Angle Orthod.* 1981;51(3):177–202.
63. Guyer EC, et al. Components of class III malocclusion in juveniles and adolescents. *Angle Orthod.* 1986;56(1):7–30.
64. Lai J, Ghosh J, Nanda R. Effects of orthodontic therapy on the facial profile in long and short vertical facial patterns. *Am J Orthod Dentofacial Orthop.* 2000;118(5):505–513.
65. Kocadereli IL. Changes in soft tissue profile after orthodontic treatment with and without extractions. *Am J Orthod Dentofacial Orthop.* 2002;122(1):67–72.
66. Rains M, Nanda R. Soft-tissue changes associated with maxillary incisor retraction. *Am J Orthod.* 1982;81(6):481–488.
67. Thuer U, Ingervall B. Pressure from the lips on the teeth and malocclusion. *Am J Orthod Dentofacial Orthop.* 1986;90(3):234–242.
68. Lapatki BG, et al. The importance of the level of the lip line and resting lip pressure in class II, division 2 malocclusion. *J Dent Res.* 2002; 81(5):323–328.
69. Burstone C. Arch form and dimension: anteroposterior positioning of the incisors. In: Burstone C, ed. *Problem Solving in Orthodontics: Goal-Oriented Treatment Strategies*, Chicago, IL: Quintessence Publishing Co, Inc; 2000:98–120.
70. Flynn TR, Ambrogio RI, Zeichner SJ. Cephalometric norms for orthognathic surgery in black American adults. *J Oral Maxillofac Surg.* 1989;47(1):30–39.
71. Lew KK, et al. Soft-tissue cephalometric norms in Chinese adults with esthetic facial profiles. *J Oral Maxillofac Surg.* 1992;50(11):1184–1189; discussion 1189–1190.
72. Rhine JS, Campbell HR. Thickness of facial tissues in American blacks. *J Forensic Sci.* 1980;25(4):847–858.
73. Oliver BM. The influence of lip thickness and strain on upper lip response to incisor retraction. *Am J Orthod.* 1982;82(2):141–149.
74. Ricketts R. Planning treatment on the basis of the facial pattern and an estimate of its growth. *Angle Orthod.* 1957;27:14–37.
75. Burstone C. The integumental profile. *Am J Orthod.* 1958;44:1–25.
76. Burstone CJ. Lip posture and its significance in treatment planning. *Am J Orthod.* 1967;53(4):262–284.
77. Holdaway R. A soft tissue cephalometric analysis and its use in orthodontic treatment planning: part I. *Am J Orthod.* 1983;84:1–28.
78. Merrifield L. The profile line as an aid in critically evaluating facial esthetics. *Am J Orthod.* 1966;52:804–822.
79. Steiner C. The use of cephalometrics as an aid to planning and assessing orthodontic treatment. *Am J Orthod.* 1960;46:721–735.
80. Legan H, Burstone CJ. Soft tissue cephalometric analysis for orthognathic surgery. *J Oral Surg.* 1980;38:744–751.
81. Horn A. Facial height index. *Am J Orthod.* 1992;102(2):180.
82. Sarver DM, Ackerman MB. Dynamic smile visualization and quantification: part 1. Evolution of the concept and dynamic records for smile capture. *Am J Orthod Dentofacial Orthop.* 2003;124(1):4–12.
83. Edwards J. The diastema, the frenum, the frenectomy: a clinical study. *Am J Orthod.* 1977;71:489–508.
84. Kopczyk R, Saxe SR. Clinical signs of gingival inadequacy: the tension test. *J Dent Child.* 1974;41:352–355.
85. Fletcher SG, Meldrum JR. Lingual function and relative length of the lingual frenulum. *J Speech Hear Res.* 1968;11(2):382–390.
86. Andreasen J, Andreasen FM. *Textbook and Color Atlas of Traumatic Injuries to the Teeth.* Copenhagen, Denmark: Munksgaard; 1994.
87. Hamilton RS, Gutmann JL. Endodontic-orthodontic relationships: a review of integrated treatment planning challenges. *Int Endod J.* 1999;32(5):343–360.
88. Kokich VG, Spear FM. Guidelines for managing the orthodontic-restorative patient. *Semin Orthod.* 1997;3(1):3–20.
89. Tarnow DP, Magner AW, Fletcher P. The effect of the distance from the contact point to the crest of bone on the presence or absence of the interproximal dental papilla. *J Periodontol.* 1992;63(12):995–996.
90. Uribe F, Holliday B, Nanda R. Incidence of open gingival embrasures after mandibular incisor extractions: a clinical photographic evaluation. *Am J Orthod Dentofacial Orthop.* 2011;139(1):49–54.
91. Andrews L. *Straight Wire: The Concept and Appliance.* San Diego, CA: K-W Publications; 1989.
92. Dale J, Dale HC. Interceptive guidance of occlusion with emphasis on diagnosis. In: Graber T, ed. *Orthodontics Current Principles and Techniques.* St. Louis, MO: Mosby; 2000:375–469.
93. Clark JR, Evans RD. Functional occlusion: I. A review. *J Orthod.* 2001;28(1):76–81.
94. Ash M, Ramfjord SP. *Occlusion.* Philadelphia, PA: WB Saunders; 1994.
95. Laskin DM. The clinical diagnosis of temporomandibular disorders in the orthodontic patient. *Semin Orthod.* 1995;1(4):197–206.
96. Greene C, Lerman MD, et al. The TMJ pain-dysfunction syndrome: heterogenicity of the patient population. *J Am Dent Assoc.* 1969;79: 1168–1172.
97. Cox S, Walker DM. Establishing a normal range for mouth opening: its use for oral submucous fibrosis. *Br J Oral Maxillofac Surg.* 1997; 35(1):40–42.
98. Helkimo M. Studies on function and dysfunction of the masticatory system. II. Index for anamnestic and clinical dysfunction and occlusal state. *Sven Tandlak Tidskr.* 1974;67:101–121.
99. Fricton JR. Management of masticatory myofascial pain. *Semin Orthod.* 1995;1(4):229–243.

100. Chhatwani B. More comments on Rinchuse Counterpoint. *Am J Orthod Dentofacial Orthop*. 1995;108(6):13A.
101. Hew SK. Comment on the Roth/Rinchuse responses. *Am J Orthod Dentofacial Orthop*. 1996;109(6):15A–16A.
102. Rinchuse DJ. A three-dimensional comparison of condylar change between centric relation and centric occlusion using the mandibular position indicator. *Am J Orthod Dentofacial Orthop*. 1995;107(3): 319–328.
103. Roth RH. Occlusion and condylar position. *Am J Orthod Dentofacial Orthop*. 1995;107(3):315–318.
104. McNamara JA Jr, Seligman DA, Okeson JP. Occlusion, orthodontic treatment, and temporomandibular disorders: a review. *J Orofac Pain*. 1995;9(1):73–90.
105. Clark JR, Hutchinson I, Sandy JR. Functional occlusion: II. The role of articulators in orthodontics. *J Orthod*. 2001;28(2):173–177.
106. Kuhlberg A, Norton LA. Finding pathology on cephalometric radiographs. In: Athanasious EA, ed. *Orthodontic Cephalometry*. London, England: Mosby-Wolfe; 1995:175–180.
107. Kuhlberg AJ, Norton LA. Pathologic findings in orthodontic radiographic images. *Am J Orthod Dentofacial Orthop*. 2003;123(2): 182–184.
108. Obwegeser HL, Makek MS. Hemimandibular hyperplasia–hemimandibular elongation. *J Maxillofac Surg*. 1986;14(4):183–208.
109. Jacobs SG. Radiographic localization of unerupted teeth: further findings about the vertical tube shift method and other localization techniques. *Am J Orthod Dentofacial Orthop*. 2000;118(4):439–447.
110. Tyndall D, Brooks S. Selection criteria for dental implant site imaging: A position paper of the American Academy of Oral and Maxillofacial Radiology. *Oral Surg Oral Med Oral Pathol Oral Radiol Endod*. 2000;89(5):630–637.
111. Downs W. Variations in facial relationships: their significance in treatment and prognosis. *Am J Orthod*. 1948;34:812.
112. Burstone CJ, et al. Cephalometrics for orthognathic surgery. *J Oral Surg*. 1978;36(4):269–277.
113. Moorrees C. Natural head position: the key to cephalometry. In: Jacobsen A, ed. *Radiographic Cephalometry*. Chicago, IL: Quintessence Publishing Co, Inc; 1995:175–184.
114. Bjork A. Cranial base development. *Am J Orthod*. 1955;41:198–225.
115. Dhopatkar A, Bhatia S, Rock P. An investigation into the relationship between the cranial base angle and malocclusion. *Angle Orthod*. 2002;72(5):456–463.
116. Cangialosi TJ. Skeletal morphologic features of anterior open bite. *Am J Orthod*. 1984;85(1):28–36.
117. Tangugsorn V, et al. Obstructive sleep apnea: a principal component analysis. *Int J Adult Orthodon Orthognath Surg*. 1999;14(3): 215–228.
118. Baccetti T, Franchi L, McNamara JA Jr. An improved version of the cervical vertebral maturation (CVM) method for the assessment of mandibular growth. *Angle Orthod*. 2002;72(4):316–323.
119. Baccetti T, Franchi L, McNamara JA Jr. The cervical vertebral maturation (CVM) method for the assessment of optimal treatment timing in dentofacial orthopedics. *Semin Orthod*. 2005;11(3):119–129.
120. Torres M. Treatment objectives and treatment planning. *Dent Clin North Am*. 1981;25(1):27–41.
121. Basyouni AA, Nanda SK. *An atlas of the transverse dimensions of the face*. Craniofacial Growth Series. Vol. 37. McNamara JA Jr, ed. Ann Arbor, MI: Center for Human Growth and Development, and Department of Orthodontics and Pediatric Dentistry, School of Dentistry, University of Michigan; 2001.
122. Forsberg CT, Burstone CJ, Hanley KJ. Diagnosis and treatment planning of skeletal asymmetry with the submental-vertical radiograph. *Am J Orthod*. 1984;85(3):224–237.
123. Ludlow JB, et al. Dosimetry of 3 CBCT devices for oral and maxillofacial radiology: CB Mercuray, NewTom 3G and i-CAT. *Dentomaxillofac Radiol*. 2006;35(4):219–226.
124. Guerrero ME, et al. The diagnostic efficacy of cone beam CT for impacted teeth and associated features: a systematic review. *J Oral Rehabil*. 2011;38(3):208–216.
125. Nervina JM. Cone beam computed tomography use in orthodontics. *Aust Dent J*. 2012;57(suppl 1):95–102.
126. Kapila S, Conley RS, Harrell WE Jr. The current status of cone beam computed tomography imaging in orthodontics. *Dentomaxillofac Radiol*. 2011;40(1):24–34.
127. Tomassetti JJ, et al. A comparison of 3 computerized Bolton tooth-size analyses with a commonly used method. *Angle Orthod*. 2001;71(5): 351–357.

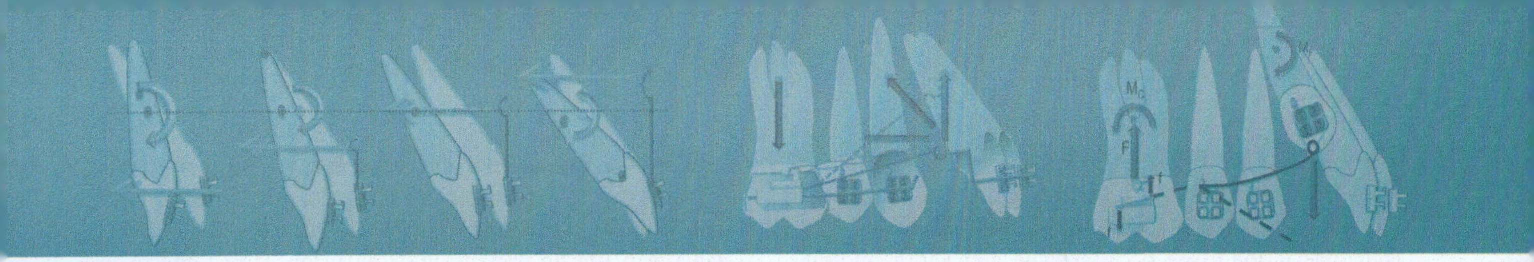

CHAPTER 2

Individualized Orthodontic Treatment Planning

Flavio Andres Uribe, Taranpreet K. Chandhoke, and Ravindra Nanda

A well-executed, individualized treatment plan is one of the most fundamental components of orthodontic treatment. Treatment planning begins with optimal diagnosis and sequential categorization of the identified problems in order of importance. From the problem list, specific treatment objectives are generated to address each identified problem. Greater priority is given to problems that appear to be more severe or for which earlier intervention is required. Also, a patient's chief complaint should be given high priority.

The treatment planning sequence should closely follow diagnostic findings (see Chapter 1) in the anteroposterior, transverse, and vertical dimensions. Although these dimensions have direct and indirect relationships to each other, each is analyzed separately in the problem list. In addition to problems in these three dimensions, any remarkable dental and medical findings and alignment issues are listed.

The most common medical and dental findings to be considered during orthodontic treatment are discussed in Chapter 1. The patient's medical history should be reviewed and any systemic disease or medical condition that may have an impact on the treatment plan should be included in the problem list. Not only may these conditions affect the course of orthodontic treatment, but orthodontic treatment may have detrimental effects on existing medical and dental problems and therefore these should be reviewed carefully. Furthermore, the effect of some medications on orthodontic treatment should be explored.[1,2]

Significant dental problems can have a direct impact on treatment planning. An example can be seen in a patient with extensive decay in the first molars. A decision between extracting or restoring these teeth has to be made not only from a purely orthodontic perspective, but also in conjunction with other factors, such as cost–benefit and long-term prognosis.

TREATMENT OBJECTIVES

The cornerstone of treatment planning is the treatment objectives. These can be visualized easily in three dimensions by means of a visualized treatment objective (VTO) and an occlusogram, which will be discussed later.[3]

Treatment objectives can be divided into general and specific treatment objectives. These categories are related but distinct as far as determination of treatment goals is concerned. General treatment objectives are those that can be applied to any orthodontic patient regardless of his or her malocclusion. These objectives include most of the characteristics of an ideal occlusion, such as Class I occlusion (canine), normal overjet and overbite, coincident midlines, slight curve of Spee, arch width coordination, and absence of crowding, spacing, rotations, and marginal ridge discrepancies.[4] These objectives do not provide the clinician with any specific information on how they are to be achieved. For example, an ideal overjet can be obtained in a Class II patient by retracting the upper incisors, flaring the lower incisors, or a combination of the two. Moreover, the nature of the incisor movement can be translation, controlled tipping, or uncontrolled tipping. If the specific objectives are not established, the clinician can choose any variety of methods, such as different appliances (Herbst, headgear, pendex, Twin Force bite corrector, elastics, bionator) or any therapy (extraction, nonextraction, surgery, implants) for Class II correction, since the only known objective is overjet reduction. A very wise phrase applies here: "If you don't know where you are going, it doesn't matter which road you take."[5]

To provide an individualized treatment plan, specific treatment objectives must be determined.[6] The general treatment objectives allow the orthodontist to communicate with the patient and guardian, while the specific treatment objectives act as a template (blueprint) for the desired treatment outcome.

Specific Treatment Objectives

Seven specific treatment objectives guide the clinician to achieve the desired outcome in the three planes of space: skeletofacial, soft tissue, occlusal plane, arch width, midlines, anteroposterior position of the incisors and molars, and vertical position of the incisors and molars.[4]

Skeletofacial Objectives

These objectives rely on understanding the growth status of the patient and often on the ability to predict the amount, direction, and rate of remaining growth. Due to the great variability in growth, it is difficult to define specific skeletofacial objectives. Perhaps this inability to accurately predict growth is the reason why many clinicians do not believe that specific objectives can be set in treatment planning for growing patients. This is not an issue in adult patients for whom skeletal objectives can be defined adequately, although for them a similar problem is encountered in determining the soft tissue objectives (see below).

Even though there is great variability in predicting growth, this objective is important and cannot be disregarded. A good approach is to underestimate future growth in skeletal Class II patients and overestimate growth in Class III patients. In this manner any additional growth (in a Class II patient) or limited growth (in a Class III patient) relative to the prediction would be favorable. Of course this is not always easy, especially in patients with moderate-to-severe dentofacial deformities, since growth can be the deciding factor between a surgical and nonsurgical approach to treatment.

Useful growth information is best obtained with a series of lateral cephalometric radiographs taken at 6-month to 1-year intervals. These radiographs provide important information since growth patterns are usually maintained in the majority of patients.[7] Unfortunately, serial cephalograms are often unavailable when a patient initially presents for treatment. Therefore an assessment of growth potential (amount of growth left in relation to puberty) and evaluation of craniofacial morphology (Bjork indicators)[8] may aid in the prediction.

It is important to note, however, that even if growth cannot be modified extensively at the level of the apical bases, significant skeletofacial changes can be achieved by affecting the dentoalveolar apparatus. This is especially evident in the vertical control of the molar, where favorable skeletofacial vertical and anteroposterior changes can be obtained with carefully selected mechanics.

In a nongrowing patient, surgery can substantially affect the skeletofacial objectives. As mentioned, the specific soft tissue component here directly relates to skeletal movements and can still be difficult to predict in these cases. However, pure skeletal changes, such as reducing mandibular prognathy in a Class III patient with a mandibular setback procedure, can be estimated and visualized with a VTO.

Soft Tissue Objectives

As mentioned above, soft tissue objectives are very much related to the skeletofacial objectives. The only aspect not covered in the skeletofacial objectives is the soft tissue changes due to dentoalveolar movement. The most remarkable changes in this area relate to the lips: reduction of interlabial gap and lip protrusion or retrusion. Direct effects on the soft tissue drape are seen with dentoalveolar movement in the vertical dimension at the molar level and in the anteroposterior dimension at the incisor level.

Anteroposterior incisor movement can result in changes at the lip level, at least to some degree.[9–11] Accurate prediction of soft tissue response to incisor movement is difficult. Therefore the soft tissue objectives should be set in terms of direction (more predictable) rather than magnitude of change.

Occlusal Plane Objectives

Occlusal plane objectives are often overlooked in treatment planning. Occlusal plane goals should be considered from a frontal and lateral perspective and in conjunction with skeletal and soft tissue objectives.[12] In the lateral view, anterior and posterior occlusal planes should be coincident. For example, in open-bite and deep overbite patients, the anterior and posterior occlusal planes are often at different levels. When determining specific objectives for a patient, it is a good idea to predetermine the level of the occlusal plane in order to apply proper mechanics during treatment. In deep bite patients it may be desirable to intrude anterior teeth to the level of the posterior teeth or vice versa. A straight wire ligated into all brackets has no ability to selectively intrude or extrude teeth. These mechanics are not optimal; the wire rather than the clinician ultimately controls the occlusal plane objectives. Similarly, in open-bite patients placement of a straight wire can have very undesirable results. The best option in this situation may be to treat the posterior and anterior segments separately.

Specific occlusal plane objectives in the frontal view should also be determined carefully. Often a cant in the anterior occlusal plane is associated with a midline deviation. This can be treated effectively by selective ligation of an intrusion arch or use of a cantilever to rotate the anterior teeth as a whole.[13]

Treatment objectives should outline not only the level of the occlusal plane, but also the cant. The term *level* refers to a parallel vertical movement, whereas the term *cant* refers to angular movement of the occlusal plane. A level change can be achieved, for example, by using an anterior bite plane, which allows eruption of posterior teeth. In addition, the application of box elastics to the posterior teeth aids in the occlusal plane leveling of the buccal segments by extrusion.[14] Indiscriminate use of Class II elastics for a prolonged period of time will invariably cant (steepen) the occlusal plane, whether or not this is a desired part of the treatment plan.

Arch Width Objectives

Arch width objectives relate mainly to the intercanine and inter-molar width. The lower intercanine width has been considered to be almost unalterable, as changes in this distance yield unstable results.[15] Any significant increase in the mandibular intercanine width may indicate a need for long-term fixed retention.[16] More leeway has been given to the alteration of the upper canine and molar width. Increasing the arch width depends largely on the occlusal and esthetic objectives.

For occlusal correction, a definitive indicator for expansion of the maxillary arch width occurs in a case with skeletal crossbite. However, from an esthetic perspective, some clinicians may expand the maxillary arch to fill the buccal corridors and approach treatment with a nonextraction, expansion treatment.

Midline Objectives

The midline is an important occlusal and esthetic objective. This topic is discussed extensively in this book. Needless to say, the facial and dental midlines should coincide. The planning of this objective becomes more elaborate when a surgical correction due to apical base midline problems is considered. In these patients the desired dental movement must be determined in conjunction with the apical base movement.[17] This is illustrated in Case 3 in this chapter, wherein an apical base discrepancy exists in the absence of a dental midline discrepancy. In this case, with the maxillary osteotomy performed, the maxilla is rotated such that the apical base deviation is corrected while the dental midline position is maintained.

Anteroposterior Objectives

Incisor Objectives. The incisor anteroposterior objectives should be planned with consideration given to the skeletofacial and soft tissue (lips) objectives.[18] The final anteroposterior position is decided after taking into consideration the nasolabial angle, facial convexity, size of nose, and ethnicity.[19] Anteroposterior objectives that cannot be obtained skeletally are obtained through dental compensations (camouflage). Usually the anteroposterior incisor objective is described in terms of the incisal edge (flare, maintain, or retract). The nature of the tooth movement should be described further (controlled tipping, uncontrolled tipping, or translation). If the incisal edge position is to be maintained, root correction (controlled root movement) is the other type of incisor movement in this plane.

The anteroposterior movement of the incisor depends largely on occlusion and esthetics. Arch crowding, protrusion, overbite, and overjet are some of the occlusal factors to consider. Esthetic considerations relate to lip changes (which vary greatly in magnitude) and third-order inclination of the upper incisors.[20] The final position of the upper incisors, due to their esthetic importance, must be decided during treatment planning.[21] This is especially the case in surgical patients, where the incisors are positioned ideally in space and the orthodontic and surgical movements are planned so that the incisor position is maintained. In adolescent patients the final upper incisor position also needs to be considered relative to the desired lower incisor position, the overjet, and the potential differential jaw growth.

Proper lower incisor inclination has been considered essential and tied to a cephalometric norm (90 to 95 degrees) by various techniques. Labial movement beyond this norm in patients with an ideal mandibular plane to the Frankfort horizontal plane (25 degrees) has been related to instability and gingival recession. Although evidence does not completely support the predisposition of recession after labial flaring,[22,23] this movement has traditionally been considered undesirable.[24] It may be necessary to evaluate that patient's oral hygiene, gingival biotype, and baseline recession prior to proceeding with a treatment plan that would further flare the lower incisors.[25]

Molar Objectives. The anteroposterior position of the molars greatly depends on the final position of the incisors. Once the incisor anteroposterior position is established, the molars will need to be protracted, maintained, or distalized, depending on the arch width and amount of crowding present. Incorporating growth into the planning of the anteroposterior molar position becomes somewhat challenging if growth modification is planned.

Vertical Incisor and Molar Objectives

As mentioned above, the final vertical position of the upper and lower incisors is influenced by the occlusion (overbite) and esthetics (incisor display). The vertical incisor position, together with the anteroposterior position, are good starting reference points for treatment planning. The vertical position of the incisors can be easily defined by boundaries determined by the incisor display and overbite.

The influence of the molar vertical position on the skeletofacial objectives makes these teeth a key factor in the vertical and anteroposterior dimensions. The molars can be held against growth (relative intrusion) or absolutely intruded with the use of implants. They can also be extruded for overbite correction, although the long-term stability of this type of extrusion in adults is questionable. Furthermore, extrusion of molars should be considered carefully due to the resultant clockwise rotation of the mandible, which may negate any positive changes that occur during adolescent mandibular growth.

DYNAMICS OF TREATMENT PLANNING

It must be emphasized that treatment plans and specific objectives are not static.[26] Due to the difficulty in accurate prediction of remaining growth, an undesirable outcome may be encountered during orthodontic treatment. Moreover, the biological response to the mechanical stimulus may also be unfavorable. It should be determined whether the undesirable outcome resulted from poor mechanics or unfavorable growth, or both. Ultimately, the treatment objectives should be adjusted after a reevaluation of the new clinical situation.

OCCLUSOGRAM, VISUALIZED TREATMENT OBJECTIVE, AND 3D VIRTUAL PLANNING

Two classic tools for visualizing the treatment plan are the occlusogram and the visualized treatment objective

(VTO). With the advent of computers, these two procedures have become less cumbersome to perform.[27] The occlusogram is a two-dimensional (2D) analysis of what would be considered a diagnostic wax setup.[28] Since it is done on either a piece of paper or a screen, it allows visualization of the original problem in comparison to the desired dental and skeletofacial corrections. Through the anteroposterior dimension, the occlusogram and VTO are related to each other, generating the three-dimensional (3D) visual goals of treatment.[29]

The advent of cone beam computed tomography (CBCT)-derived 3D planning extends the virtual planning capabilities for the clinician, providing an even more thorough analysis of the skeletal, dental, and soft tissue components to accurately determine the specific objectives of treatment. This is particularly valuable in surgical cases and in those that involve dentofacial deformities.[30–32] In addition, the digitally rendered 3D plan can be directly used for the fabrication of surgical splints without the use of conventional model surgery.

CASE REPORTS

Three cases are presented to illustrate different diagnosis and treatment planning strategies.

Text continued on p. 52

CASE REPORT 1

Patient Profile (Figs. 2-1 and 2-2)

- 17.10-year-old postpubertal female.
- Chief complaint: "My front teeth stick out and I want them straight."

Medical History

- History of smoking; patient reports smoking two cigarettes each day since the age of 10.
- No allergies; no medications.

Dental History

- Patient has received routine dental care.
- Presents in permanent dentition with second molar to second molar present in both arches.
- Minor occlusal restorations present on posterior teeth.
- History of supernumerary teeth resembling premolars present between maxillary first molar and second premolar.

Psychosocial Profile

Enthusiastic about receiving orthodontic treatment.

Cephalometric Summary (Fig. 2-3 and Tables 2-1 to 2-4)

Class II skeletal relationship with convex skeletal profile including:

- Retrognathic mandible
- Short mandibular body length
- Proclined maxillary and mandibular incisors
- Convex soft tissue profile
- Protrusive upper lip and retrusive lower lip

TABLE 2-1 Case 1: Cranial Base Analysis

Measurement	Value	Norm	SD	Dev Norm
Anterior CB [S-N] (mm)	65.1	69.6	3.0	−1.5*
Posterior CB [S-Ar] (mm)	34.6	38.0	4.0	−0.9
Saddle angle [SN-Ar] (degrees)	129.1	124.0	5.0	1.0*

CB, cranial base; *Dev Norm*, deviation norm; *SD*, standard deviation. * indicates number of SD from norm values.

TABLE 2-2 Case 1: Maxilla-Mandible to Cranial Base Analysis

Measurement	Value	Norm	SD	Dev Norm
SNA (degrees)	83.2	82.0	3.5	0.3
SNB (degrees)	74.8	80.9	3.4	−1.8*
ANB (degrees)	8.4	1.6	1.5	4.5****
N-A (HP) (mm)	0.1	−2.0	3.7	0.6
N-B (HP) (mm)	−12.7	−6.9	4.3	−1.4
N-Pg (HP) (mm)	−12.3	−6.5	5.1	−1.1
N-A-Pg (degrees)	14.8	5.6	3.0	3.1***
PNS-ANS (mm)	51.5	52.6	3.5	−0.3
Ar-PTM (mm)	36.1	32.8	1.9	1.7*
Y axis (mm)	114.5	128.5	6.0	−2.3
Y axis (degrees)	70.4	67.0	5.5	0.6
Ramus height [Ar-Go] (mm)	39.8	48.5	4.5	−1.9*
Corpus length [Go-Pg] (mm)	72.7	73.0	3.0	−0.1
MPA [MP-SN] (degrees)	33.3	33.0	6.0	0.1
Gonial angle [Ar-Go-Me] (degrees)	119.9	115.0	6.7	0.7
N-ANS (mm)	49.4	Ratio: 45.0 : 52.7		
ANS-Me (mm)	57.8	Norm: 45.0 : 55.0		

ANB, A point nasion B point; *ANS*, anterior nasal spine; *Dev Norm*, deviation norm; *HP*, horizontal plane; *MPA*, mandibular plane angle; *PNS*, posterior nasal spine; *PTM*, pterygomaxillary point; *SD*, standard deviation; *SNA*, sella-nasion A point; *SNB*, sella-nasion B point. * indicates number of SD from norm values.

TABLE 2-3 Case 1: Dentition

Measurement	Value	Norm	SD	Dev Norm
IMPA [L1-MP] (degrees)	107.9	95.0	7.0	1.8*
U1-Palatal plane (degrees)	115.7	110.0	5.0	1.1*
Inter-incisal angle [U1-L1] (degrees)	110.1	124.0	6.0	−2.3**
Wits [A-B/OP] (mm)	6.4	−1.0	1.0	7.4******

Dev Norm, Deviation norm; *IMPA*, incisor-mandibular plane angle; *SD*, standard deviation. * indicates number of SD from norm values.

CASE REPORT 1—cont'd

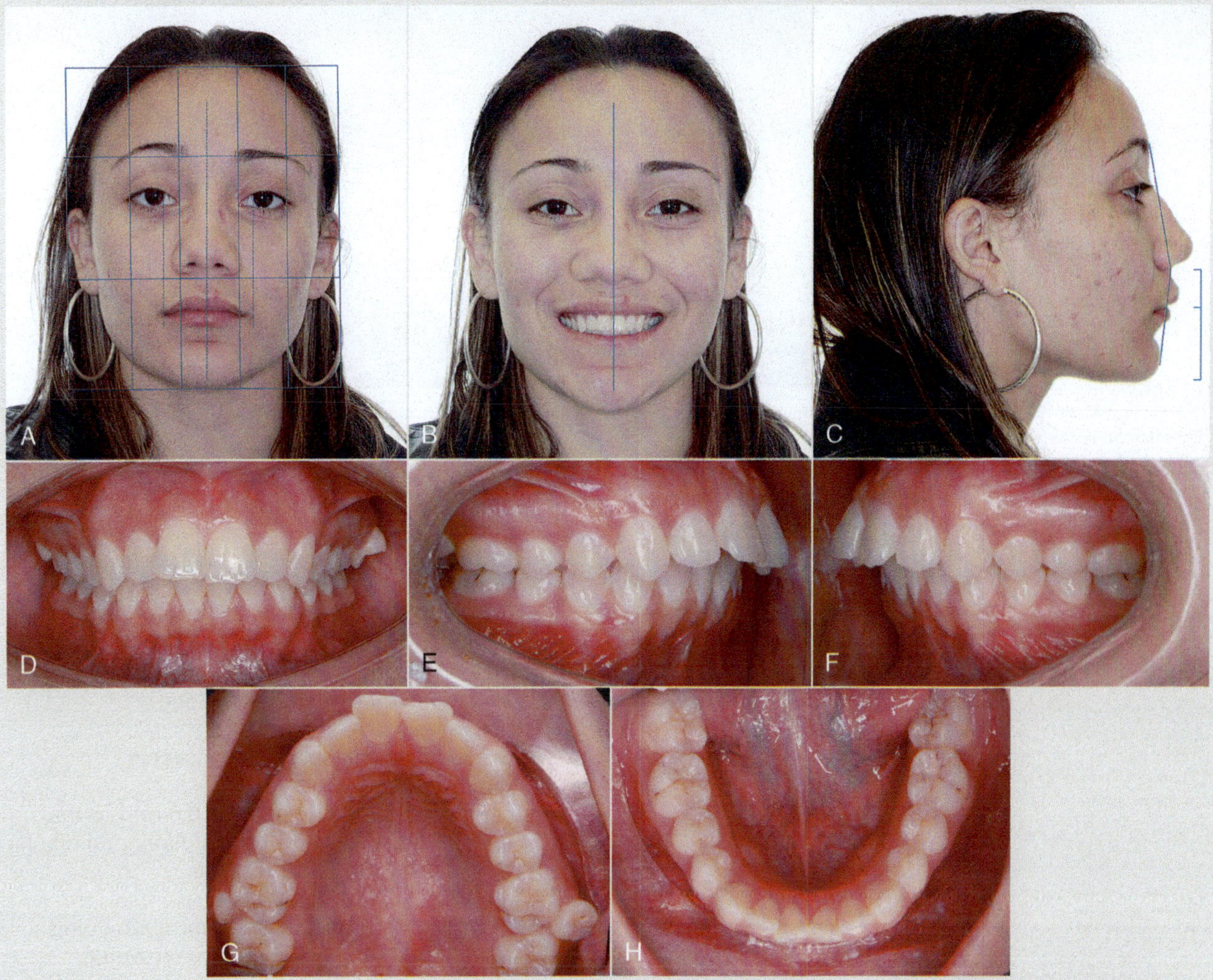

Figure 2-1 Case 1. **A,** Extraoral frontal view. Ovoid facial form; slight mentalis strain upon closure; no apparent pathology; interlabial gap 3.0 mm; 20% incisor display at rest clinically; midline—no major asymmetries; transverse fifths—normal intercommissural width at rest; vertical thirds—normal; mentolabial fold visible from this view. **B,** Extraoral smile. Incisor display on smile 90%; excessive mandibular incisor show; midlines: maxillary—0.5 mm right of facial, mandibular—on with facial; narrow smile. **C,** Extraoral profile. Convex soft tissue profile; protrusive upper lip; retrusive lower lip; lower facial height: throat depth within normal limits (WNL). **D,** Intraoral frontal view. Maxillary midline 0.5 mm to right of facial; mandibular midline on with facial; 40% overbite; good oral hygiene; slightly thin gingival biotype in lower incisor region. Intraoral right **(E)** and left **(F)** buccal views. Class II molar and canine (more severe on left); 7 mm overjet; protrusive maxillary and mandibular incisors. **G,** Intraoral maxillary occlusal view. 7-7 present with supernumerary teeth adjacent to molars; U-shaped arch; moderate crowding (5 mm); no caries present with some staining of pits and fissures. **H,** Intraoral mandibular occlusal view. 7-7 present; U-shaped arch; mild crowding (3 mm); small occlusal composites on lower 6s and staining of pits and fissures.

Overall Summary

- Convex and Class II skeletal and soft tissue profile.
- Supernumerary teeth in maxilla adjacent to first molars.
- Class II, Division 1 occlusion.
- 7-mm overjet; 40% overbite.

Problem List

1. Medical and dental findings of significance:
   - History of smoking
   - Supernumerary teeth adjacent to maxillary first molars
   - Impacted lower third molars
   - Small occlusal composite restorations on posterior dentition
   - Thin gingival biotype in lower incisor region
2. Anteroposterior:
   - Skeletal: Class II and convex skeletal profile due to retrognathic mandible
   - Dental: (1) Class II, Division 1 malocclusion (end-on on right, full-cusp on left); (2) severe Class II denture base discrepancy; (3) protrusive maxillary and mandibular incisors; (4) 7-mm overjet

Continued

CASE REPORT 1—cont'd

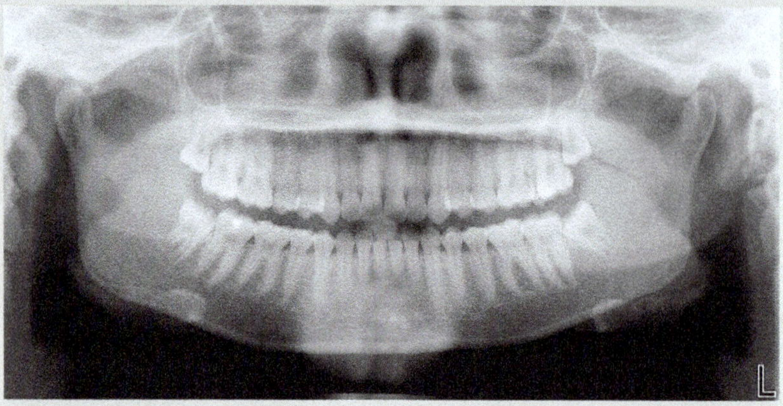

Figure 2-2 Case 1. Panoramic radiograph; erupting third molars, with lower left third molar inclined mesially and lower right third molar partially impacted on distal.

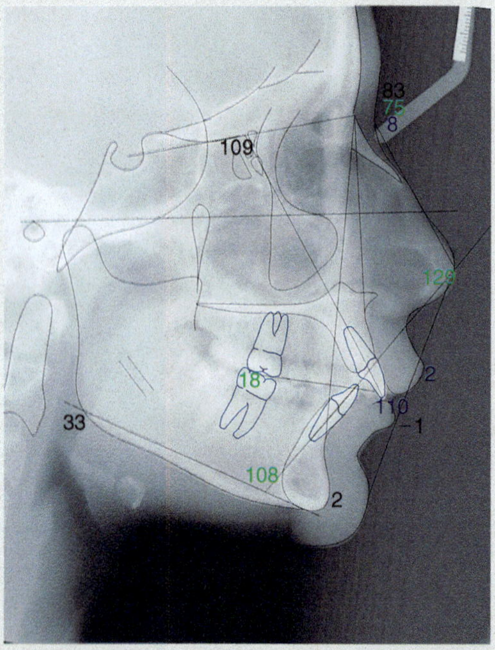

Figure 2-3 Case 1. A lateral cephalometric radiograph digital tracing.

TABLE 2-4 Case 1: Soft Tissue Analysis

Measurement	Value	Norm	SD	Dev Norm
ST convexity [G′-Sn-Pg′] (degrees)	20.7	12.0	4.0	2.2**
NLA [Col-Sn-UL] (degrees)	109.0	102.0	8.0	0.9
UL–SnPg′ (mm)	6.9	3.0	1.0	3.9***
LL–SnPg′ (mm)	2.5	2.0	1.0	−5.4*****

Dev Norm, Deviation norm; *LL*, lower lip; *NLA*, nasolabial angle; *SD*, standard deviation; *ST*, soft tissue; *UL*, upper lip. * indicates number of SD from norm values.

3. Vertical:
   - Skeletal: Slightly short ramus height, vertical thirds within normal limits
   - Dental: (1) 40% overbite; (2) 3-mm interlabial gap at rest, 20% incisor display at rest, 90% incisor display at smile; (3) Slightly accentuated lower curve of Spee
4. Transverse:
   - Skeletal: Normal skeletal transverse dimensions
   - Dental: (1) Maxillary midline 0.5-mm to the right of mandibular dental midline; mandibular midline on with facial midline.
5. Alignment:
   - Maxillary arch: moderate (5-mm) crowding
   - Mandibular arch: mild (3-mm) crowding

Treatment Objectives (Figs. 2-4 and 2-5)

1. Significant medical and dental objectives:
   - Educate patient on smoking cessation and provide options
   - Extract supernumerary teeth in maxillary arch and all four third molars
   - Continue to provide oral hygiene instructions and monitor
2. Skeletofacial: Reduce convexity of profile with camouflage treatment
3. Anteroposterior:
   - Incisors: (1) Retract the maxillary incisors; (2) maintain mandibular incisor position
   - Molars: (1) Maintain the maxillary molar position with maximum anchorage; (2) maintain mandibular molar position
4. Vertical:
   - Incisors: (1) Maintain maxillary incisor position; (2) maintain mandibular incisor position
   - Molars: (1) Maintain maxilla; (2) minor extrusion of mandibular molars for leveling of lower curve of Spee

CASE REPORT 1—cont'd

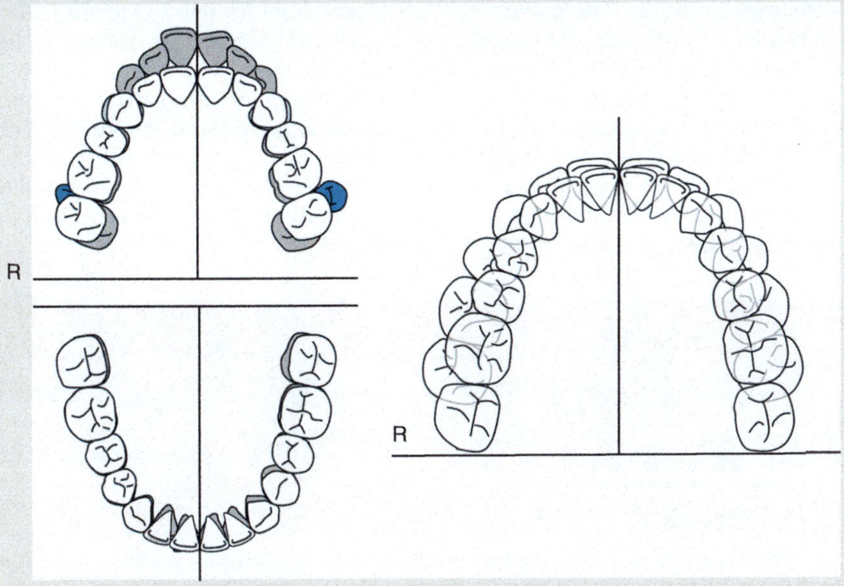

Figure 2-4 Case 1. Occlusogram. Pre-treatment tracing (gray) and post-treatment goal (white).

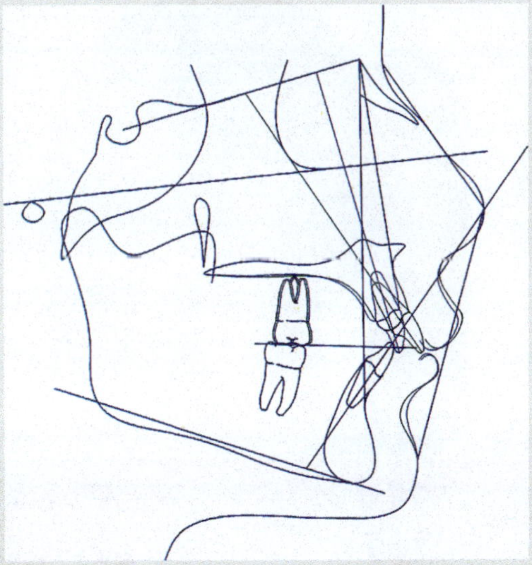

Figure 2-5 Case 1. Visualized treatment objective (VTO) using Dolphin® software (Chatsworth, CA.). Superimposed with pre-treatment tracing (black) and patient's VTO (blue).

5. Arch width/transverse: Maintain transverse dimensions
6. Midlines: Correct alignment of maxillary incisors to coincide midlines
7. Occlusal plane: Maintain natural occlusal plane
8. Soft tissue: Decrease convexity

General Treatment Plan (Table 2-5)

- Extract supernumerary teeth, third molars, and maxillary first premolars

TABLE 2-5 Case 1: Orthodontic Treatment Sequence

Maxilla	Mandible
Consultation and Place Separators; Refer for Extraction of Maxillary First Premolars, Supernumerary Teeth, and Third Molars	
Band first molars and bond remaining teeth	Band first molars and bond remaining teeth
Level and align	Level and align
Place infrazygomatic mini-implants (LOMAS*, 2 mm × 9 mm)	
En masse intrusion/retraction with 200-g Ni-Ti coil springs from mini-implants to soldered hooks on archwire (distal to lateral incisors) (Group A left, Group B right)	
Finish	Finish
Retention (circumferential Hawley retainer)	Retention (fixed lingual retainer)

Ni-Ti, Nickel-titanium.
*Mondeal Ortho, Mühlheim, Germany.

- Maximum direct anchorage in maxillary arch with infrazygomatic mini-implants for intrusion and retraction of maxillary incisors
- Finish Class II molar, Class I canine bilaterally

Treatment Progress

Patient was cooperative with oral hygiene and appliances throughout treatment and experiences no

Continued

CASE REPORT 1—cont'd

complications with the mini-implants. The patient was treated with 0.022-inch × 0.028-inch slot Carriere brackets with MBT prescription (Ortho Organizers Inc., Carlsbad, CA.). Once aligned, a 0.019-inch × 0.025-inch stainless steel wire was placed in the maxillary with soldered hooks between the maxillary lateral incisors and canines. Two infrazygomatic 2-mm × 9-mm mini-implants (LOMAS, Mondeal Ortho, Mühlheim, Germany) were placed with 200-g nickel-titanium (Ni-Ti) closed coil springs to the soldered hooks for en masse retraction of maxillary anterior teeth (Fig. 2-6). A canine Class I relationship was achieved within 8 months and the remaining space was closed in 4 months. The patient finished Class I canine, Class II molar and was given a circumferential wrap-around retainer for the maxillary arch and a lower fixed lingual retainer (Fig. 2-7).

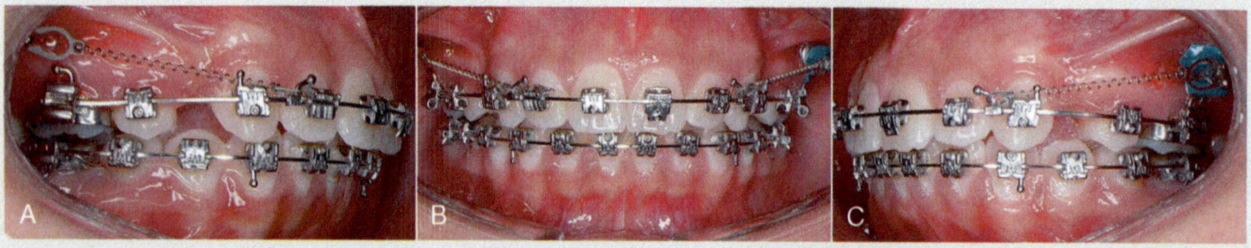

Figure 2-6 Case 1. Interim intraoral photographs after placement of infrazygomatic mini-implants and 200-g nickel-titanium (Ni-Ti) closed coil spring to soldered hooks to begin en masse retraction and intrusion. Right buccal (**A**), frontal (**B**), and left buccal (**C**) views.

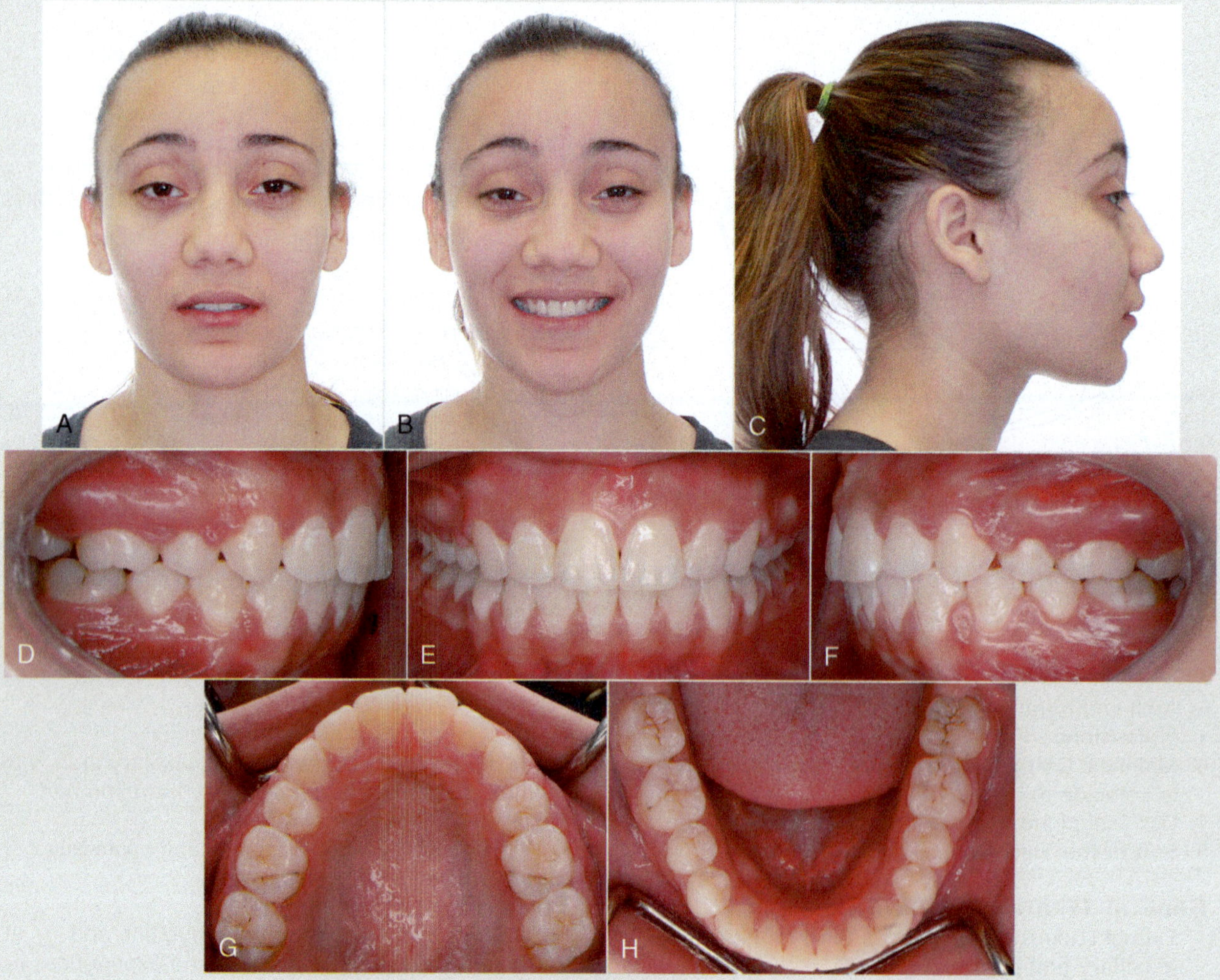

Figure 2-7 Case 1. Final records. **A,** Extraoral frontal view. **B,** Extraoral smile view. **C,** Extraoral lateral view. **D,** Intraoral right buccal view indicated Class II molar and Class I canine occlusion and ideal incisor relationship. **E,** Intraoral frontal view indicated improved overbite and overall improvement in esthetics. **F,** Intraoral left buccal view. Maxillary (**G**) and mandibular (**H**) occlusal views.

CASE REPORT 2

Overview

This case illustrates the complexity of managing impacted teeth from an orthodontic perspective. The fundamental component in developing a treatment plan in such cases is proper localization of the impacted teeth and determining the likelihood of aligning these teeth through a combined periodontal-orthodontic approach.

Radiographs are an important tool for determining whether a surgical approach is required and where to gain access to the impacted tooth. Numerous radiographic methods have been described in the literature using a combination of panoramic, periapical, and occlusal radiographs. Consecutive periapical x-rays with an incorporated mesial shift is widely used to determine the buccal or palatal position of impacted teeth by the application of Clark's SLOB (Same Lingual, Opposite Buccal) rule.[33] The primary limitation of traditional radiographs is that they are 2D representations and the localization of the impacted tooth can be challenging due to overlapping structures and distortion. Nearly 80% of clinicians need to use two or more supplemental radiographs to localize an impacted tooth.[34]

There are numerous benefits to using 3D imaging modalities with CBCT. Use of CBCT can be prescribed on a case-by-case basis; cases with impacted teeth are ideal for CBCT due to the orthogonal 1:1 representation and the ability to view the tooth successive slices, which eliminates the problem of overlapping adjacent teeth and other structures.[35,36] In addition, in cases where the impacted tooth is impinging on the adjacent tooth's root, root resorption can occur and be difficult to ascertain in both panoramic and intraoral images.[37,38] For these reasons, an accurate depiction of the true clinical position of the impacted teeth and potential compromise of adjacent teeth is greatly valuable and has a profound impact on the final treatment plan for the patient.

The small-volume CBCT has gained popularity, specifically since it further reduces the radiation dose from the traditional CBCT, focusing on only a small and focused field of view, such as 50-mm × 37-mm used in this case. Limiting this field of view to the area of interest can reduce the radiation dose to the patient but still provide the needed 3D information. A comparison of 14 CBCT devices showed significantly lower radiation exposure with small-volume CBCT compared to traditional full field of view CBCTs.[39] Based on that study, the Kodak 9000 3D CBCT (Kodak Dental Systems, Carestream Health, Rochester, NY.) used in this case had the lowest overall dose of radiation of the machines tested, with an effective dose of 19μSv in the anterior maxillary region. Conventional intraoral radiographs for detecting impacted canines include two periapicals or an occlusal x-ray, which have effective doses of 10μSv and 7μSv, respectively.[40,41]

Having 3D imaging of specific areas of interest aids the operator in exposing the correct part of the tooth and also in determining the placement of the bracket or gold chain. It also aids in developing the biomechanics plan to determine the most efficient way to orthodontically align these teeth.

Patient Profile (Figs. 2-8 and 2-9)

- 16.6-year-old, postpubertal female.
- Chief complaint: "Save my teeth. The bite is not good on the left."

Medical History

- Allergy to penicillin

Dental History

- Extensive dental care and routine oral hygiene visits
- Patient in mixed dentition:
  - Deciduous teeth present: Maxillary canines, second molars, left lateral incisor, and left first molar; mandibular second molars
  - Permanent teeth missing: Maxillary and mandibular second premolars and right maxillary and mandibular third molars and mandibular second molar
- Restorations present: Occlusal composite on mandibular deciduous second molars, root canal treatment and stainless steel crown on maxillary deciduous right second molar, and sealants on first molars

Psychosocial Profile

Patient is cooperative and enthusiastic to begin treatment. She is very self-conscious and concerned about her teeth.

Cephalometric Summary (Fig. 2-10 and Tables 2-6 to 2-9)

- Orthognathic, Class I skeletal and soft tissue profiles
- Mesofacial, with normal vertical thirds
- Upright upper incisors and retroclined lower incisors
- Normal nasolabial angle
- Retrusive lower lip

Overall Summary

- Class I skeletal and soft tissue profile
- Class I occlusion, 2-mm overjet
- Multiple impacted teeth in maxillary arch and retained deciduous teeth

Continued

CASE REPORT 2—cont'd

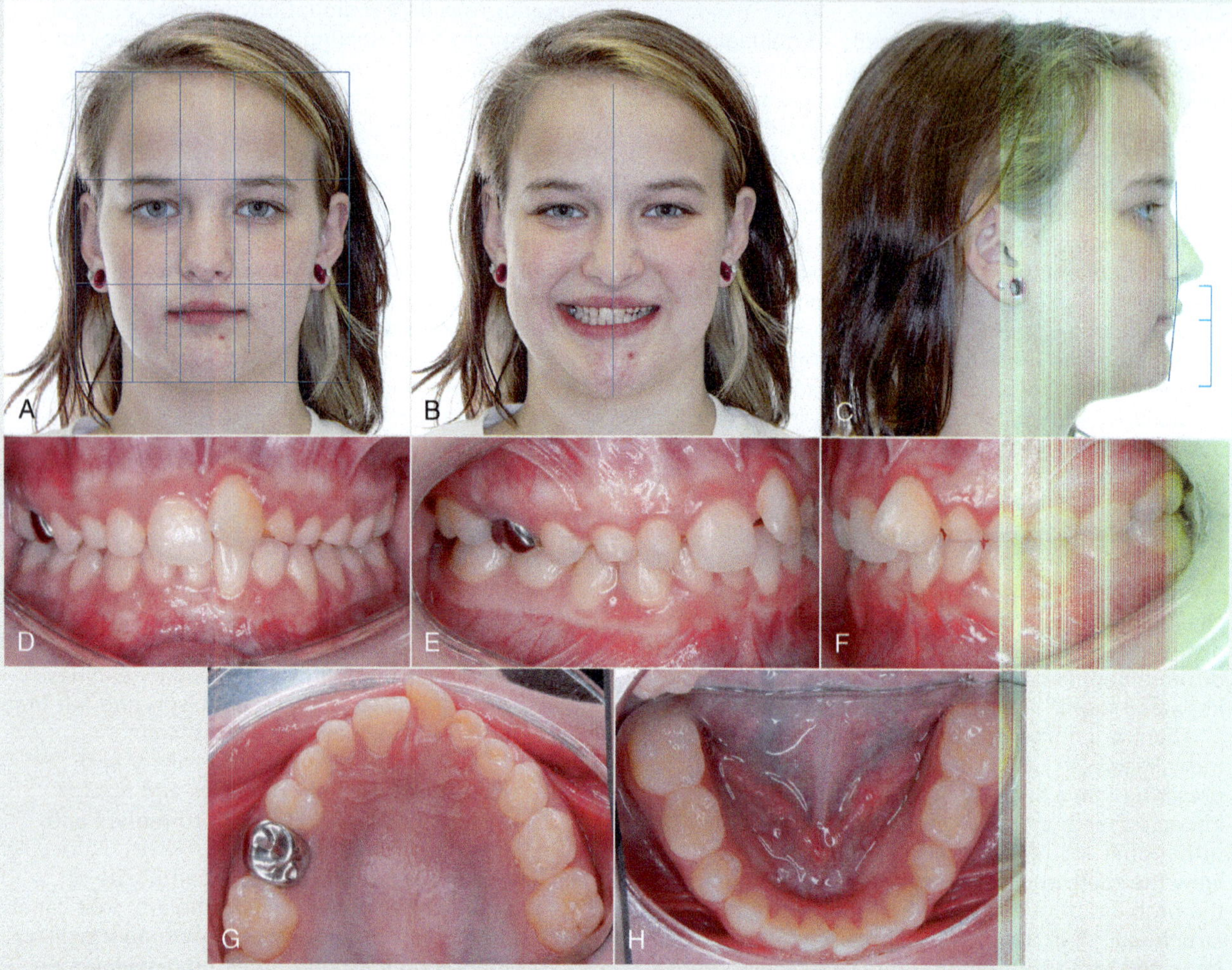

Figure 2-8 Case 2. **A,** Extraoral frontal view at rest. Ovoid facial form; vertical thirds normally proportioned; transverse fifths within normal range; nose and chin point on with facial midline; no maxillary incisor display at rest; no interlabial gap at rest. **B,** Extraoral smile. Maxillary incisor display on smile of 100%; 1–4 mm of gingival display upon smile; asymmetrical flat smile arc; upper and lower midlines coincident and on with facial midline on smile. **C,** Extraoral profile. Orthognathic facial profile with prominent chin button; retruded lower lip; nasolabial angle within normal range; slightly deep mentolabial fold; vertical thirds within normal proportions. **D–H,** Intraoral views. **D,** Intraoral frontal view. Maxillary and mandibular midlines coincident with facial midline; 70% overbite; fair oral hygiene; peg-shaped maxillary right lateral incisor; multiple deciduous teeth visible. **E and F,** Intraoral buccal views. Bilateral Class I relationship. **G,** Intraoral maxillary occlusal view. Retained deciduous teeth present: canines and second molars, left lateral incisor and left first molar; stainless steel crown on right deciduous second molar; sealants on first permanent molars and left deciduous second molar; U-shaped arch; adequate space for impacted teeth. **H,** Intraoral mandibular occlusal view. Retained deciduous second molars; mild crowding of 2 mm; U-shaped arch.

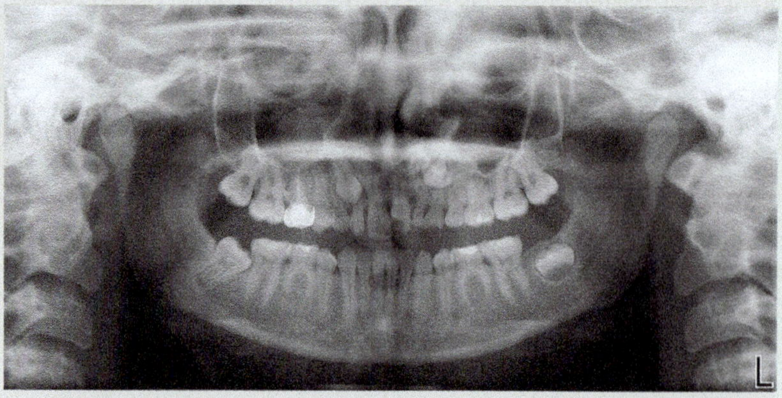

Figure 2-9 Case 2. Panoramic radiograph. Multiple impacted teeth visible in maxillary arch. Agenesis of second premolars in all quadrants. Developing third molars in maxillary and mandibular left quadrants. Agenesis of mandibular left second molar and mesial inclination of mandibular right second molar.

CASE REPORT 2—cont'd

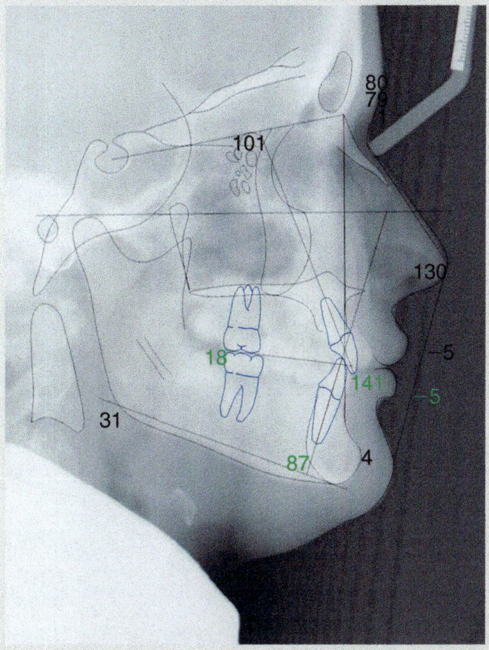

Figure 2-10 Case 2. Lateral cephalometric radiograph digital tracing.

TABLE 2-6 Case 2: Cranial Base Analysis

Measurement	Value	Norm	SD	Dev Norm
Anterior CB [S-N] (mm)	63.2	75.3	3.0	−4.0****
Posterior CB [S-Ar] (mm)	26.5	35.0	4.0	−2.1**
Saddle angle [SN Ar] (degrees)	123.4	124.0	5.0	−0.1

CB, cranial base; *Dev Norm,* deviation norm; *SD,* standard deviation. * indicates number of SD from norm values.

- Retained second primary molars in all four quadrants with agenesis of second premolars, mandibular left second molar and maxillary and mandibular right third molars

Interpretation of Small-Volume CBCT
(Fig. 2-11)

The small-volume CBCT was acquired at a voxel size of 76 μm, providing sufficient resolution to localize the unerupted teeth and adjacent structures. The images showed that the permanent left maxillary lateral incisor was horizontally impacted and was located lingual to the root of deciduous left lateral incisor and oriented in the buccolingual direction. Notable apical root resorption was detectable on the maxillary left deciduous canine and ectopic eruption of the maxillary left permanent canine. The maxillary left second premolar was also horizontally impacted in the buccolingual direction with notable apical root resorption on the maxillary left deciduous first molar.

TABLE 2-7 Case 2: Maxilla-Mandible to Cranial Base Analysis

Measurement	Value	Norm	SD	Dev Norm
SNA (degrees)	79.7	82.0	3.5	−0.7
SNB (degrees)	79.1	80.0	3.0	−0.3
ANB (degrees)	0.6	2.0	2.4	−0.6
N-A (HP) (mm)	−2.9	−2.0	3.7	−0.3
N-B (HP) (mm)	−5.3	−6.9	4.3	0.4
N-Pg (HP) (mm)	−1.6	−6.5	5.1	1.0*
N-A-Pg (degrees)	−5.5	2.6	5.1	−1.6*
PNS-ANS (mm)	46.7	52.6	3.5	−1.7*
Ar-PTM (mm)	25.7	32.8	1.9	−3.7***
Y axis (mm)	110.5	131.0	6.0	−3.4***
Y axis (degrees)	63.5	67.0	5.5	−0.6
Ramus height [Ar-Go] (mm)	42.2	46.8	2.5	−1.8*
Corpus length [Go-Pg] (mm)	63.8	83.5	5.0	−3.9***
MPA [MP-SN] (degrees)	30.7	33.0	6.0	−0.4
Gonial angle [Ar-Go-Gn] (degrees)	127.4	122.9	6.7	0.7
N-ANS (mm)	46.6	Ratio: 45.0 : 48.2		
ANS-Me (mm)	50.0	Norm: 45.0 : 55.0		

ANB, A point nasion B point; *ANS,* anterior nasal spine; *Dev Norm,* deviation norm; *HP,* horizontal plane; *MPA,* mandibular plane angle; *PNS,* posterior nasal spine; *PTM,* pterygomaxillary point; *SD,* standard deviation; *SNA,* sella-nasion A point; *SNB,* sella-nasion B point. * indicates number of SD from norm values.

TABLE 2-8 Case 2: Dentition

Measurement	Value	Norm	SD	Dev Norm
IMPA [L1-MP] (degrees)	87.5	95.0	7.0	−1.1*
U1-Palatal plane (degrees)	111.2	110.0	5.0	0.2
Inter-incisal angle [U1-L1] (degrees)	141.0	130.0	6.0	1.8*
Wits [A-B/OP] (mm)	−2.7	−1.0	1.0	−1.7*

Dev Norm, Deviation norm; *IMPA,* incisor-mandibular plane angle; *SD,* standard deviation. * indicates number of SD from norm values.

TABLE 2-9 Case 2: Soft Tissue Analysis

Measurement	Value	Norm	SD	Dev Norm
ST convexity [G′-Sn-Pg′] (degrees)	5.9	12.0	4.0	−1.5*
NLA [Col-Sn-UL] (degrees)	98.8	102.0	8.0	−0.4
UL–SnPg′ (mm)	3.1	3.0	1.0	0.1
LL–SnPg′ (mm)	0.3	2.0	1.0	−1.7*
Interlabial gap (mm)	0.7	2.0	2.0	−0.6

Dev Norm, Deviation norm; *LL,* lower lip; *NLA,* nasolabial angle; *SD,* standard deviation; *ST,* soft tissue; *UL,* upper lip. * indicates number of SD from norm values.

Continued

CASE REPORT 2—cont'd

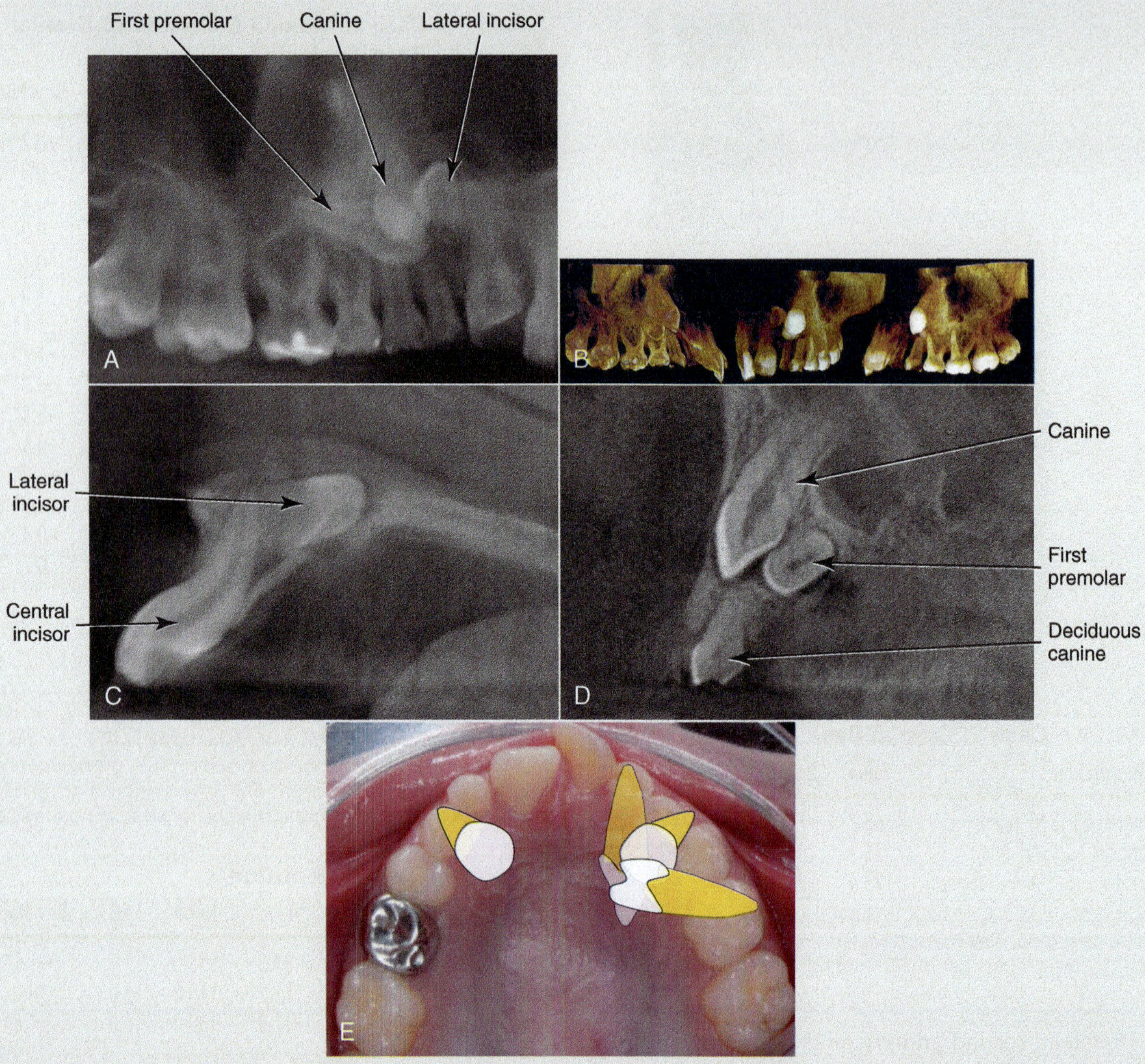

Figure 2-11 Case 2. Small-volume cone beam computed tomography (CBCT) of maxillary left quadrant. **A,** View from an oblique angle from the palatal aspect; the lateral incisor crown is pointing distal and horizontally impacted. The first premolar is also horizontally impacted, pointing toward the lateral incisor crown. **B,** Volume-rendered views from a direct palatal view (left panel), frontal view (center panel), and buccal view (right panel). Successive sagittal slices at the level of the left central incisor **(C)** indicating that the apex of the lateral incisor closely approximates the buccal cortex. At the level of the impacted canine **(D),** the horizontal impaction of the first premolar is evident, palatal to the canine. **E,** Schematic rendition of the impacted teeth from an occlusal clinical view.

Problem List

1. Medical and dental findings of significance:
   - See medical history above
   - Impacted maxillary permanent canines, right lateral incisor, and right first premolar
   - Presence of numerous deciduous teeth
   - Agenesis of second premolars and mandibular left second molar
   - Agenesis of right maxillary and mandibular third molars; evidence of third molar follicles in upper left and lower left quadrants
   - Peg-shaped upper right lateral incisor
   - Dilaceration of maxillary left central incisor
   - Mesial inclination of mandibular right second molar
   - Maxillary gingival height discrepancy and mild localized gingivitis in maxillary left quadrant
2. Alignment:
   - Maxillary arch: Adequate spacing; impacted maxillary canines, right lateral incisor and right first premolar

CASE REPORT 2—cont'd

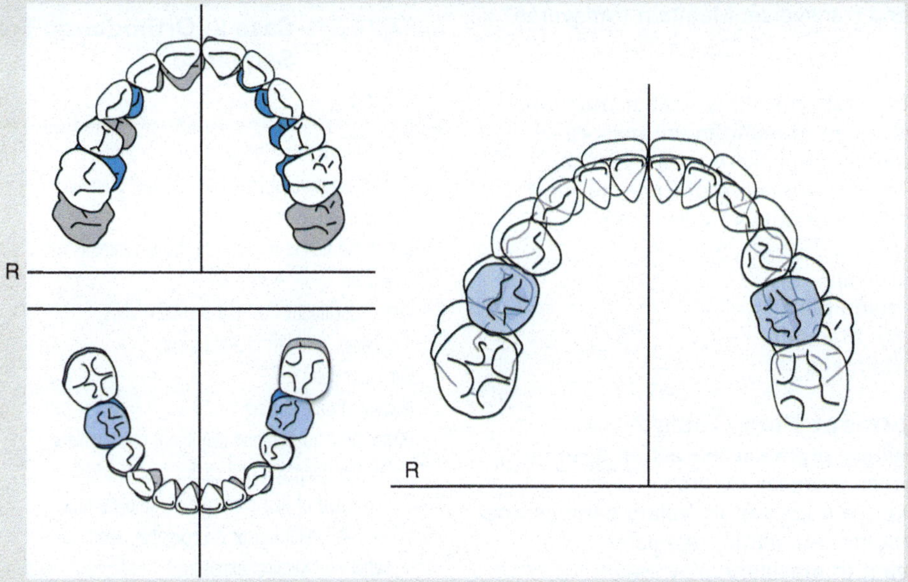

Figure 2-12 Case 2. Occlusogram. Pre-treatment teeth indicated by gray shading, with deciduous teeth in blue. Treatment goal indicated by white teeth.

- Mandibular arch: (1) Mild crowding (2 mm); (2) Bolton discrepancy (mandibular excess 1–2 mm).

3. Vertical:
   - Skeletal: Normal vertical thirds
   - Dental: (1) No incisor shown at rest; (2) 70% deep bite
4. Anteroposterior:
   - Skeletal: Within normal limits; orthognathic
   - Dental: (1) 2-mm overjet; (2) upright upper incisors, retroclined lower incisors
5. Transverse:
   - Skeletal: None
   - Dental: None

Treatment Objectives (Figs. 2-12 and 2-13)

1. Significant medical and dental objectives:
   - Improve oral hygiene
   - Continue to monitor eruption of the developing mandibular molars; upright mandibular right second molar to correct inclination
   - Extract deciduous maxillary canines, deciduous maxillary second molars, deciduous maxillary left lateral incisor, and deciduous maxillary left first molar
   - Maintain deciduous mandibular second molars with 1-mm interproximal reduction
   - Periodontal exposure of palatally impacted maxillary left lateral incisor and first premolar, with orthodontic traction to erupt
   - Monitor dilacerated maxillary left central incisor and refer to endodontist for evaluation.

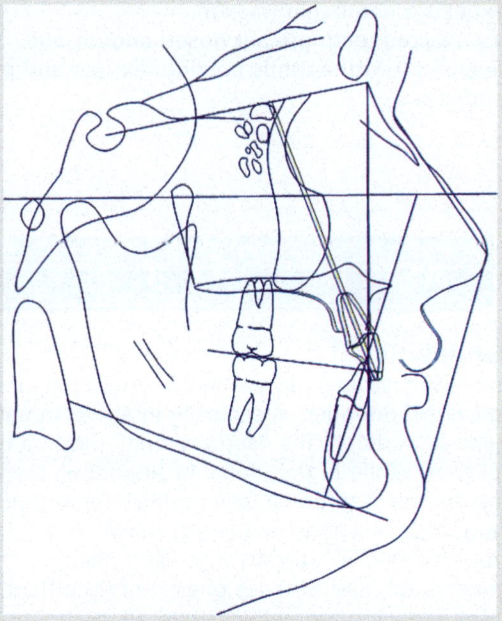

Figure 2-13 Case 2. Visualized treatment objective (VTO). Pre-treatment cephalometric tracing indicated in black with VTO in blue.

2. Skeletofacial: Maintain facial harmony.
3. Anteroposterior:
   - Incisors: (1) Maintain upper incisor position; (2) upright lower incisors
   - Molars: (1) Maxilla: Group C anchorage with 5-mm molar protraction; (2) mandible: Protract molars 2-mm. Finish with Class II molar relationship.

Continued

CASE REPORT 2—cont'd

4. Arch width and transverse: Maintain transverse dimension.
5. Vertical:
   - Incisors: Maintain maxillary incisor position; relative intrusion of mandibular incisors
   - Molars: Maintain maxillary molar vertical position; level lower curve of Spee through some extrusion of posterior dentition
6. Midlines:
   - Maintain maxilla
   - Maintain mandible
7. Occlusal plane: Maintain
8. Soft tissue: Maintain

General Treatment Plan (Table 2-10)

- Treat as maxillary premolar extraction case by closing E spaces in maxillary arch.
- Surgically expose impacted maxillary canines and left first premolar and extract respective deciduous teeth in maxillary arch. Begin orthodontic traction of impacted teeth. Once the left first premolar is partially aligned and the lateral incisor is accessible surgically, send for exposure and begin traction.
- If impacted teeth are ankylosed and do not respond to orthodontic traction, extract and place implants.

TABLE 2-10 Case 2: Orthodontic Treatment Sequence

Maxilla	Mandible
Refer patient to periodontist for consultation and exposure of impacted left first premolar and canines.	Maintain lower deciduous second molars and continue to monitor.
Determine timing of exposure for left lateral incisor.	
Extract deciduous first and second molars, canines, and left lateral incisor.	
Band 6s. Bond 7-7	Band 6s. Bond 7-7
Alignment and leveling.	Alignment and leveling
Orthodontic traction and alignment for maxillary left first premolar and canines; once initial alignment of first premolar is complete and the left lateral incisor is accessible, send patient for surgical exposure.	
Group A space closure	
Finish Class II molar and canine	Finish Class II molar and canine
Retention	Retention

CASE REPORT 3

Overview

This case illustrates the use of 3D virtual planning in surgical orthodontics, specifically in an asymmetrical patient. In addition, the "surgery first" method is employed. While in traditional orthognathic surgery cases there is a three-phase approach (presurgical orthodontics, surgery, and postsurgical orthodontics), the "surgery first" approach eliminates the first of these phases of treatment, thereby reducing the patient's overall treatment time. This method is detailed fully in Chapter 21.

Patient Profile (Figs. 2-14 and 2-15)

- 26.0-year-old adult Caucasian male.
- Chief complaint: "Correct my underbite and crooked smile."

Medical History

- Allergy to Percocet™
- History of surgery (rhinoplasty)

Dental History

- Patient has received routine dental care and reports prior history of orthodontic treatment.
- Presents in permanent dentition with second molar to second molar present in both arches.
- Large occlusal restoration on mandibular left first molar and maxillary second molars.
- Third molars previously extracted.

Psychosocial Profile

Highly enthusiastic and motivated patient with high esthetic expectations

Cephalometric Summary (Fig. 2-16 and Tables 2-11 to 2-14)

Class III skeletal relationship with concave skeletal profile including:

- Prognathic mandible relative to cranial base
- Compensated occlusion with proclined maxillary incisors and retroclined mandibular incisors

CASE REPORT 3—cont'd

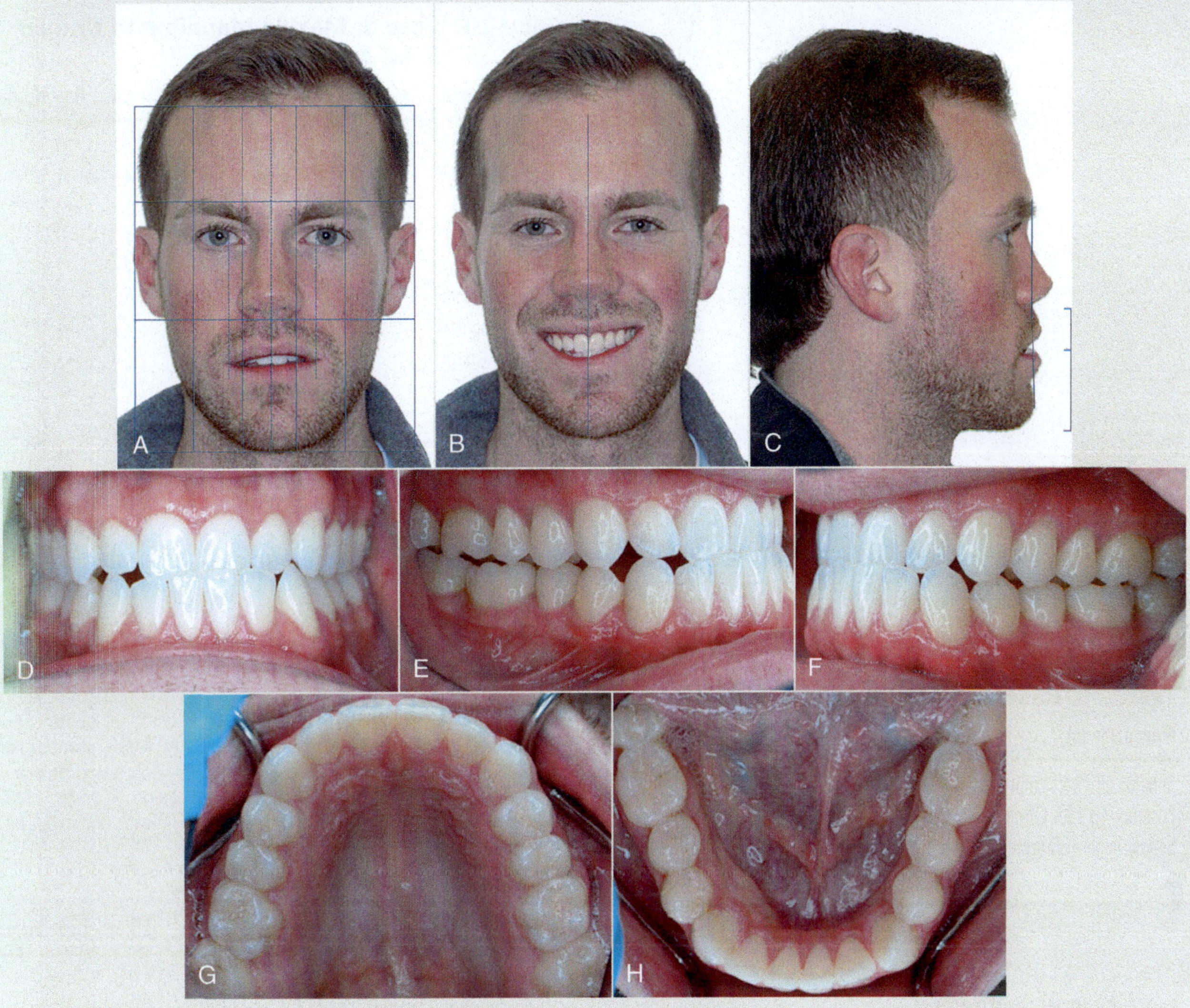

Figure 2-14 Case 3. **A,** Extraoral frontal view. Normofacial with ovoid facial form; chin point 7–8 mm to left of facial midline; maxillary dental midline on with facial midline; 7-mm interlabial gap at rest with 30% to 40% maxillary incisor display. **B,** Extraoral smile. 100% incisor display; maxillary cant evident with excessive gingival display in maxillary right quadrant; slight asymmetry of lips on animated smile. **C,** Extraoral profile. Concave soft tissue profile; nasolabial angle within normal limits; upper facial height to lower facial height 40:60; protrusive lower lip to Sn-Pg'. **D–H,** Intraoral views. **D,** Intraoral frontal view. Maxillary midline on with facial; mandibular midline 1–2 mm to left of facial; minimal overbite 10%; elongated lower incisors. **E and F,** Intraoral right and left buccal views. Class III malocclusion (full cusp on right, ¼ cusp on left); 1–2-mm negative overjet; compensated occlusion. **G,** Intraoral maxillary occlusal view. Second molar to second molar present; U-shaped arch; no crowding and healthy dentition. **H,** Intraoral mandibular occlusal view. Second molar to second molar present; U-shaped arch; minor spacing (~1 mm) distal to left lateral incisor.

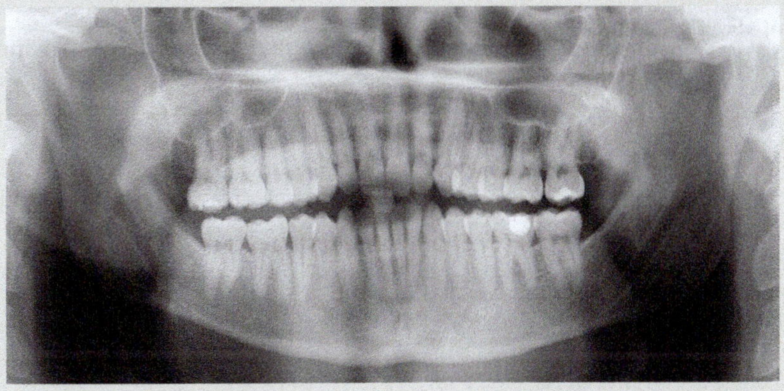

Figure 2-15 Case 3. Panoramic radiograph.

Continued

CASE REPORT 3—cont'd

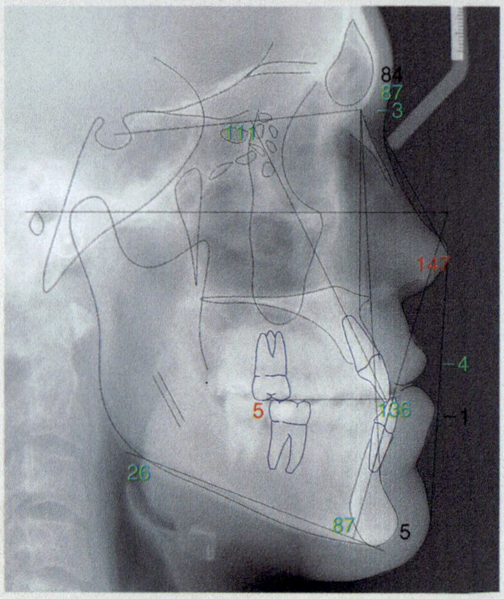

Figure 2-16 Case 3. Lateral cephalometric radiograph with digital tracing.

TABLE 2-11 Case 3: Cranial Base Analysis

Measurement	Value	Norm	SD	Dev Norm
Anterior CB [S-N] (mm)	72.2	77.3	3.0	−1.7*
Posterior CB [S-Ar] (mm)	35.4	37.0	4.0	−0.4
Saddle angle [SN-Ar] (degrees)	112.2	124.0	5.0	−2.4

CB, cranial base; *Dev Norm*, deviation norm; *SD*, standard deviation. * indicates number of SD from norm values.

- Class III Wits appraisal
- Concave soft tissue profile
- Protrusive lower lip

Overall Summary

- Concave, Class III skeletal and soft tissue profile
- Class III molar and canine occlusion with
  - 1–2-mm negative overjet
  - 10% overbite
- Maxillary cant with slightly excessive gingival display on the right on smile
- Chin point deviated 7–8 mm to left of facial midline
- Lower dental midline shifted to the left 1.5 mm

Problem List

1. Medical and dental findings of significance:
   - Incidental finding on CBCT: Lesion on the base of the skull (clivus) (Fig. 2-17)
     - Referred patient to medical radiologist for magnetic resonance imaging (MRI); lesion was 12.0 × 8.5 × 8.5 mm and determined to

TABLE 2-12 Case 3: Maxilla-Mandible to Cranial Base Analysis

Measurement	Value	Norm	SD	Dev Norm
SNA (degrees)	83.8	82.0	3.5	0.5
SNB (degrees)	87.4	80.9	3.4	1.9**
ANB (degrees)	−3.6	1.6	1.5	−3.5***
N-A (HP) (mm)	0.8	0.0	3.7	0.2
N-B (HP) (mm)	7.9	−5.3	6.7	2.0**
N-Pg (HP) (mm)	13.6	−4.3	8.5	2.1**
N-A-Pg (degrees)	−11.5	3.9	6.4	−2.4**
PNS-ANS (mm)	49.7	57.7	2.5	−3.2***
Ar-PTM (mm)	27.3	37.1	2.8	−3.5***
Y axis (mm)	145.3	140.0	6.0	0.9
Y axis (degrees)	60.5	67.0	5.5	−1.2*
Ramus height [Ar-Go] (mm)	54.4	53.0	4.5	0.3
Corpus length [Go-Pg] (mm)	75.7	73.0	3.0	0.9
MPA [MP-SN] (degrees)	20.6	18.6	5.0	0.4
Gonial angle [Ar-Go-Me] (degrees)	119.7	120.8	6.7	−0.2
N-ANS (mm)	53.0	Ratio: 45.0 : 60.0		
ANS-Me (mm)	69.6	Norm: 45.0 : 55.0		

ANB, A point nasion B point; *ANS*, anterior nasal spine; *Dev Norm*, deviation norm; *HP*, horizontal plane; *MPA*, mandibular plane angle; *PNS*, posterior nasal spine; *PTM*, pterygomaxillary point; *SD*, standard deviation; *SNA*, sella-nasion A point; *SNB*, sella-nasion B point. * indicates number of SD from norm values.

TABLE 2-13 Case 3: Dentition

Measurement	Value	Norm	SD	Dev Norm
IMPA [L1-MP] (degrees)	86.7	95.0	7.0	−1.2*
U1-Palatal plane (degrees)	116.4	110.0	5.0	1.3*
Inter-incisal angle [U1-L1] (degrees)	136.4	130.0	6.0	1.1*
Wits [A-B/OP] (mm)	−5.7	−1.0	1.0	−4.7****

Dev Norm, Deviation norm; *IMPA*, incisor-mandibular plane angle; *SD*, standard deviation. * indicates number of SD from norm values.

TABLE 2-14 Case 3: Soft Tissue Analysis

Measurement	Value	Norm	SD	Dev Norm
ST convexity [G′-Sn-Pg′] (degrees)	−5.1	12.0	4.0	−4.3****
NLA [Col-Sn-UL] (degrees)	102.0	102.0	8.0	0.0
UL–SnPg′ (mm)	4.8	3.0	1.0	1.8*
LL–SnPg′ (mm)	5.4	2.0	1.0	3.4***

Dev Norm, Deviation norm; *LL*, lower lip; *NLA*, nasolabial angle; *SD*, standard deviation; *ST*, soft tissue; *UL*, upper lip. * indicates number of SD from norm values.

CASE REPORT 3—cont'd

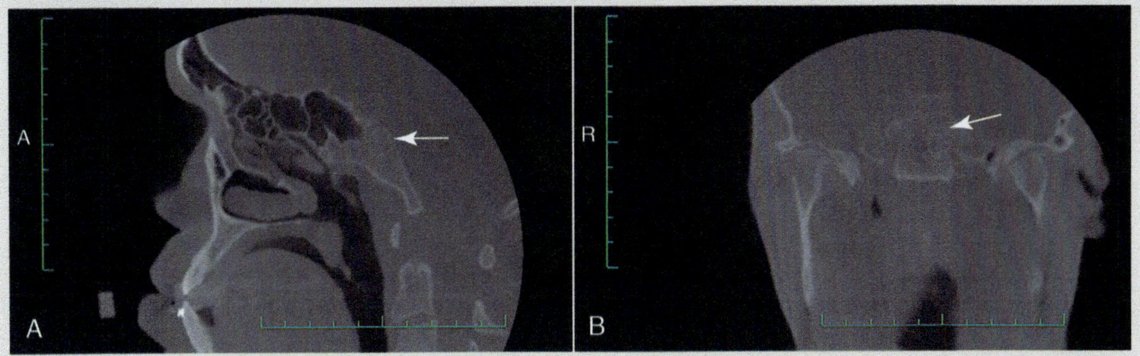

Figure 2-17 Case 3. Cone beam computed tomography (CBCT) images indicate lesion on base of the skull. Images acquired with Hitachi CB MercuRay CBCT scanner (Hitachi Medical Corp., Tokyo, Japan). **A,** Sagittal section with arrow pointing to lesion in the area of the clivus. **B,** Coronal section with arrow pointing to lesion.

TABLE 2-15 Case 3: Summarized Movements to Simulated Postsurgical Position by SimPlant® OMS*

Landmark	Definition	3D Movements		
		Anteroposterior	Transverse	Vertical
ANS	Anterior nasal spine	0.98 mm anterior	1.41 mm left	2.05 mm up
A	A point	0.97 mm anterior	1.18 mm left	2.06 mm up
ISU1	Midline of maxillary incisors	1.00 mm anterior	0.00 mm	2.00 mm up
UK9L	Maxillary left canine	1.78 mm anterior	0.37 mm left	1.14 mm up
U6L	Maxillary left first molar (mesiobuccal cusp)	2.04 mm anterior	1.05 mm left	0.87 mm up
UK9R	Maxillary right canine	0.26 mm anterior	0.32 mm left	2.83 mm up
U6R	Maxillary right first molar (mesiobuccal cusp)	0.02 mm anterior	1.01 mm left	3.12 mm up
ISL1	Midline of mandibular incisors	0.33 mm posterior	2.08 mm right	5.45 mm up
L6L	Mandibular left first molar (mesiobuccal cusp)	0.43 mm anterior	0.85 mm right	2.45 mm up
L6R	Mandibular right first molar (mesiobuccal cusp)	1.49 mm posterior	0.94 mm right	5.29 mm up
B	B point	0.69 mm anterior	2.78 mm right	5.15 mm up
Me	Menton	2.18 mm anterior	7.61 mm right	5.04 mm up

*Materialise, Leuven, Belgium.

be likely of chondroid origin and nonaggressive
- Recommended to recall for reevaluation with radiology in 6 months and clearance given to proceed with orthognathic surgery
- Allergy to Percocet™
- History of rhinoplasty and previous orthodontic treatment during adolescence

2. Anteroposterior:
   - Skeletal: Class III and concave skeletal profile due to prognathic mandible
   - Dental: (1) Class III malocclusion (full cusp on right, ¼ cusp on left); (2) severe Class III denture base discrepancy; (3) compensated incisors with proclined maxillary incisors and retroclined mandibular incisors; (4) 1–2-mm negative overjet
3. Vertical:
   - Skeletal: Maxillary cant present, indicated by excessive gingival display in maxillary right quadrant
   - Dental: (1) 10% overbite; (2) 7-mm interlabial gap at rest, 30% to 40% incisor display at rest, 100% incisor display visible on smile
4. Transverse:
   - Skeletal: Mandibular asymmetry, with chin point deviated to the left 3-mm relative to facial midline
   - Dental: (1) Maxillary midline 1 mm to the left of facial midline; mandibular midline 2-mm to the left of facial midline
5. Alignment:
   - Maxillary arch: No crowding or spacing
   - Mandibular arch: 1-mm spacing (distal to left lateral incisor)

Treatment Objectives (Figs. 2-18 and 2-19 and Table 2-15)

1. Significant medical and dental objectives:
   - Ensure that patient continues to be monitored by medical radiology for management of lesion on clivus

Continued

CASE REPORT 3—cont'd

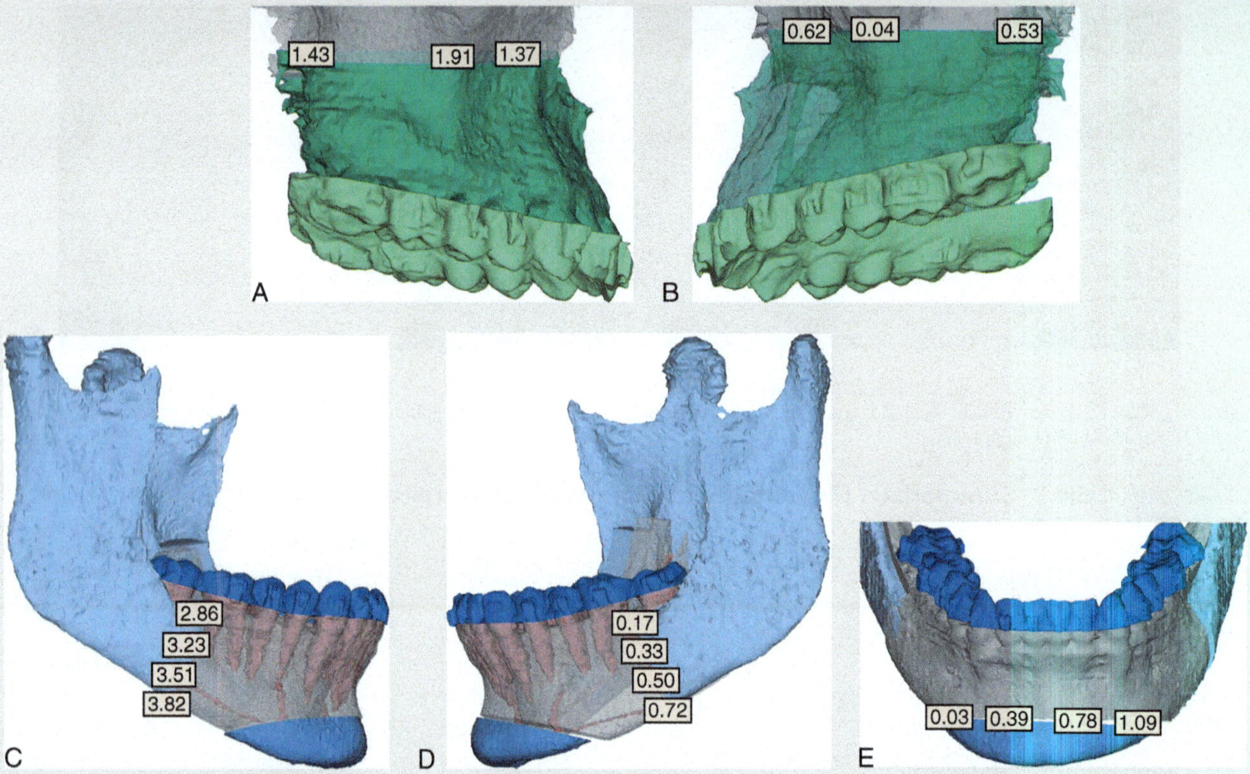

Figure 2-18 Case 3. Virtual 3D planning of surgical movements using Simplant OMS software (Materialise, Leuven, Belgium). **A and B,** Maxillary surgical movements from right and left views; Le Fort I osteotomy with asymmetrical impaction, indicating greater impaction on right. **C and D,** Mandibular surgical movements with right and left views; asymmetrical bilateral sagittal split osteotomies with greater setback on the right side. **E,** Lateral sliding genioplast for correction of chin point deviation with some vertical correction on left.

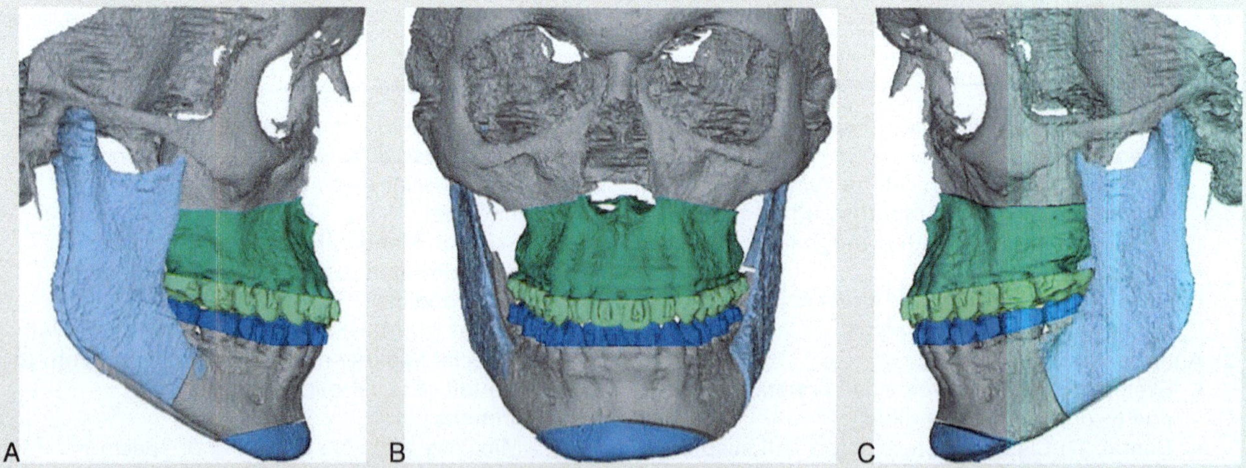

Figure 2-19 Case 3. Composite views of 3D surgical plan from (**A**) right, (**B**) front, and (**C**) left of patient.

CASE REPORT 3—cont'd

- Refer patient to oral and maxillofacial surgeon and ensure that patient is aware of the risks of surgical intervention
- Continue to provide oral hygiene instructions and monitor

2. Skeletofacial:
   - Surgical objectives:
   - Anteroposterior: Correct Class III and concave skeletal and soft tissue profile with bilateral sagittal split osteotomy (BSSO) and asymmetrical setback of the mandible (3-mm on right, 0.5-mm on left) and Le Fort I osteotomy
   - Vertical: Correct maxillary cant with asymmetrical maxillary osteotomy and impaction (3-mm on right, 1-mm on left)
   - Transverse: Correct lower midline deviation with asymmetrical BSSO setback (see above). Lateral sliding genioplasty to shift chin point 7–8 mm to right.
3. Anteroposterior:
   - Incisors: (1) Reduce maxillary incisor proclination; (2) procline lower incisors
   - Molars: Finish Class I molar and canine
4. Vertical:
   - Incisors: Maintain maxillary and mandibular vertical incisor position postsurgery
   - Molars: Maintain vertical molar position postsurgery
5. Arch width and transverse: Maintain transverse dimensions
6. Midlines: Maintain dental position postsurgery
7. Occlusal plane: Maintain occlusal plane
8. Soft tissue: Improve facial convexity

General Treatment Plan (Table 2-16)

- Orthodontic appliances placed 4 weeks prior to surgery.
- "Surgery first" approach (2 jaw): Le Fort I osteotomy (maxillary advancement, asymmetrical impaction), BSSO with asymmetrical mandibular setback and lateral sliding genioplasty. Immediate postsurgical occlusion will be overcorrected slightly to accommodate for dental decompensation during postsurgical orthodontics.
- Postsurgical orthodontics to finish Class I molar and canine with decompensation and final seating of occlusion.

Treatment Progress

The patient was bonded with 0.022-inch × 0.028-inch slot twin brackets with MBT prescription and 0.016-inch × 0.016-inch Ni-Ti maxillary and mandibular archwires with surgical hooks were placed in the operating room immediately prior to surgery. The computer-aided design (CAD)–generated surgical splints (Fig. 2-20) were removed immediately postsurgery. Two weeks after surgery the surgical hooks were removed, light Ni-Ti wires were placed, and the patient began wearing intermaxillary elastics. Orthodontic treatment lasted a total of 7 months Postoperative records show improvement in the facial profile overall and reduction in the asymmetry (Fig. 2-21). The patient was satisfied with the esthetic results and short treatment time.

TABLE 2-16 Case 3: Orthodontic-Surgical Treatment Sequence

Maxilla	Mandible
Refer Patient for Consultation with Oral Surgeon to Discuss Surgical Treatment Options and Risks	
Band first and second molars and bond remaining teeth 4 weeks prior to surgery	Band first and second molars and bond remaining teeth 4 weeks prior to surgery
CBCT for Simplant® OMS Virtual Planning and Generation of Surgical Splint	
Surgery: Le Fort I osteotomy with advancement and asymmetrical impaction	Surgery: BSSO with asymmetrical mandibular setback and lateral sliding genioplasty; bilateral skeletal anchorage plates placed for use in the event of potential relapse
Postsurgical Orthodontics	
Level and align Finish Class I molar and canine Retention (Essix retainer)	Level and align Finish Class I molar and canine Retention (Essix retainer)

BSSO, Bilateral sagittal split osteotomy; *CBCT*, cone beam computed tomography.

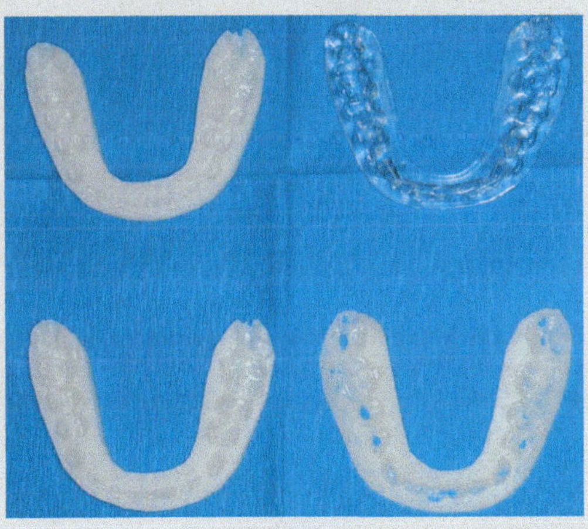

Figure 2-20 Case 3. Generation of intermediate and final surgical splints based on computer-generated 3D plan using computer-aided design (CAD) software and produced on a stereolithographic rapid prototyping machine (Medical Modeling, Golden, CO.).

Continued

CASE REPORT 3—cont'd

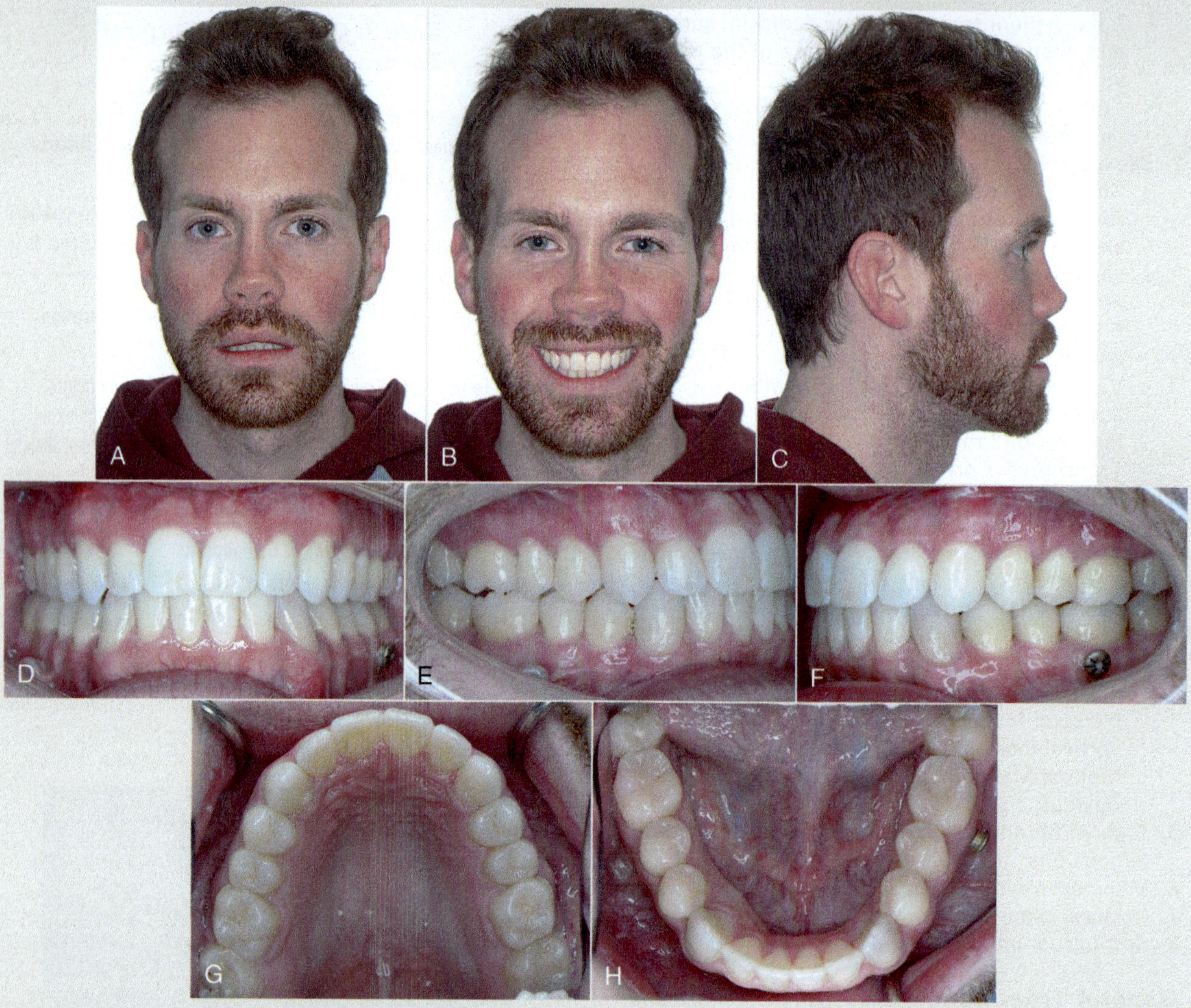

Figure 2-21 Case 3. Final records. **A,** Extraoral frontal view with improvement in asymmetry of chin. **B,** Extraoral smile with improvement in maxillary cant. **C,** Extraoral profile with notable improvement in facial proportions and convexity. **D,** Intraoral frontal photo with correction of anterior crossbite and more overbite. **E and F,** Right and left buccal view showing Class I molar and canine occlusion with ideal overjet and overbite. **G and H,** Maxillary and mandibular occlusal views showing improved alignment overall.

SUMMARY

This chapter described a systematic way to diagnose an orthodontic patient, devise a list of treatment objectives, and, based on that information, develop an individualized treatment plan. Specific treatment objectives provide the blueprint for the desired outcome. The importance of having specific objectives is highlighted when a decision is needed among the myriad of orthodontic appliances for correction of any malocclusion.

To obtain a consensus between the wishes of the patient and the clinician, more than one treatment plan is often developed. Different treatment plans give the patient options that may be helpful when difficult choices must be made due to issues related to finances, compliance, or other personal circumstances. Therefore, in instances where treatment plans are developed, the pros and cons of each option should be evaluated. An evaluation of the different options will help the clinician to successfully present the treatment plan to the patient as well as to obtain informed consent.

Once the treatment plan has been defined with specific goals, the appliance or group of appliances needed to achieve these goals is selected. Although the mechanics plan is done after the treatment objectives have been set, many seasoned clinicians tend to be biased by their own experience as to what can be achieved with the tools (appliances) they traditionally use. It is important to understand the biomechanics and potential side effects of all appliances chosen for treatment in order to achieve the desired treatment goals. A solid understanding of the effects of each appliance, when applied to specific populations, is essential as well. Knowledge of scientifically controlled trials that study various orthodontic appliances in different populations will help to achieve this goal.[42] Overall, it is important to remember that evidence-based orthodontics in conjunction with sound biomechanical knowledge allows the clinician to develop individualized mechanics with predictable results.

REFERENCES

1. Roberts WE, Hohlt WF, Baldwin JJ. Adjunctive orthodontic therapy in adults: biologic, medical, and treatment considerations. In: Bishara SE, ed. *Textbook of Orthodontics*. Philadelphia, PA: WB Saunders; 2001: 494–531.
2. van Venrooy JR, Proffit WR. Orthodontic care for medically compromised patients: possibilities and limitations. *J Am Dent Assoc*. 1985; 111(2):262–266.
3. Lindauer S. Orthodontic treatment planning. In Nanda R, ed. *Biomechanics in Clinical Orthodontics*. Philadelphia, PA: WB Saunders; 1997:23–47.
4. Kuhlberg AJ, Glynn E. Treatment planning considerations for adult patients. *Dent Clin North Am*. 1997;41(1):17–27.
5. Proffit WR, Sarver DM. Treatment planning: optimizing benefit to the patient. In: Proffit WR, Sarver DM, White RP, eds.*Contemporary Treatment of Dentofacial Deformity*. St. Louis, MO: Mosby; 2003:172–244.
6. Kuhlberg AJ. Steps in orthodontic treatment. In: Bishara SE, ed. *Textbook of Orthodontics*. Philadelphia, PA: WB Saunders; 2001:232–245.
7. Bishara SE. Facial and dental changes in adolescents and their clinical implications. *Angle Orthod*. 2000;70(6):471–483.
8. Bjork A. Prediction of mandibular growth rotation. *Am J Orthod*. 1969;55(6):585–599.
9. Burstone C. The integumental profile. *Am J Orthod*. 1958;44:1–25.
10. Kocadereli I. Changes in soft tissue profile after orthodontic treatment with and without extractions. *Am J Orthod Dentofacial Orthop*. 2002; 122(1):67–72.
11. Rains MD, Nanda R. Soft-tissue changes associated with maxillary incisor retraction. *Am J Orthod*. 1982;81(6):481–488.
12. Lamarque S. The importance of occlusal plane control during orthodontic mechanotherapy. *Am J Orthod Dentofacial Orthop*. 1995; 107(5):548–558.
13. Nanda R, Margolis MJ. Treatment strategies for midline discrepancies. *Semin Orthod*. 1996;2(2):84–89.
14. Nanda R. The differential diagnosis and treatment of excessive overbite. *Dent Clin North Am*. 1981;25(1):69–84.
15. Rossouw P, Preston CB, Lombard CJ, Truter JW. A longitudinal evaluation of the anterior border of the dentition. *Am J Orthod Dentofacial Orthop*. 1993;104(2):146–152.
16. Little RM. Stability and relapse of dental arch alignment. In: Burstone C, Nanda R, eds. *Retention and Stability in Orthodontics*. Philadelphia, PA: WB Saunders; 1993:97–106.
17. Torres M. Treatment objectives and treatment planning. *Dent Clin North Am*. 1981;25(1):27–41.
18. Sarver DM. The importance of incisor positioning in the esthetic smile: the smile arc. *Am J Orthod Dentofacial Orthop*. 2001;120(2):98–111.
19. Mejia-Maidl M, Evans CA. Soft tissue facial considerations and orthodontic treatment. *Semin Orthod*. 2000; 6(1): 3-20.
20. Peluso C, Kuhlberg A. *The axial inclination of central incisors and its effects on the perception of the facial profile*. Paper presented at: Annual American Dental Association Meeting, Scientific Program; 2002; Memphis, TN.
21. Arnett GW, Jelic JS, Kim J, et al. Soft tissue cephalometric analysis: diagnosis and treatment planning of dentofacial deformity. *Am J Orthod Dentofacial Orthop*. 1999;116(3):239–253.
22. Aziz T, Nassar U, Flores-Mir C. Prediction of lower incisor proclination during Xbow treatment based on initial cephalometric variables. *Angle Orthod*. 2012;82(3):472–479.
23. Vasconcelos G, Kjellsen K, Preus H, Vandevska-Radunovic V, Hansen BF. Prevalence and severity of vestibular recession in mandibular incisors after orthodontic treatment. *Angle Orthod*. 2012;82(1):42–47.
24. Allais D, Melsen B. Does labial movement of lower incisors influence the level of the gingival margin? A case-control study of adult orthodontic patients. *Eur J Orthod*. 2003;25(4):343–352.
25. Melsen B, Allais D. Factors of importance for the development of dehiscences during labial movement of mandibular incisors: a retrospective study of adult orthodontic patients. *Am J Orthod Dentofacial Orthop*. 2005;127(5):552–561; quiz 625.
26. Burzin J, Nanda R. The stability of deep bite correction. In: Burstone C, Nanda R, eds. *Retention and Stability*. Philadelphia, PA: WB Saunders; 1993:61–79.
27. Fiorelli G, Melsen B. The "3-D occlusogram" software. *Am J Orthod Dentofacial Orthop*. 1999;116(3):363–368.
28. Marcotte MR. The use of the occlusogram in planning orthodontic treatment. *Am J Orthod*. 1976;69(6):655–667.
29. Braun S. The extraction–nonextraction decision revisited. *Am J Orthod Dentofacial Orthop*. 1999;116(4):21A–22A.
30. Xia J, Ip HH, Samman N, et al. Computer-assisted three-dimensional surgical planning and simulation: 3D virtual osteotomy. *Int J Oral Maxillofac Surg*. 2000;29(1):11–17.
31. Swennen GR, Mollemans W, De Clercq C, et al. A cone-beam computed tomography triple scan procedure to obtain a three-dimensional augmented virtual skull model appropriate for orthognathic surgery planning. *J Craniofac Surg*. 2009;20(2):297–307.
32. Swennen GR, Mommaerts MY, Abeloos J, et al. A cone-beam CT based technique to augment the 3D virtual skull model with a detailed dental surface. *Int J Oral Maxillofac Surg*. 2009;38(1):48–57.
33. Jacobs SG. Radiographic localization of unerupted maxillary anterior teeth using the vertical tube shift technique: the history and application of the method with some case reports. *Am J Orthod Dentofacial Orthop*. 1999;116(4):415–423.
34. Southall PJ, Gravely JF. Vertical parallax radiology to localize an object in the anterior part of the maxilla. *Br J Orthod*. 1989;16(2):79–83.
35. Guerrero ME, Shahbazian M, Elsiena Bekkering G, Nackaerts O, Jacobs R, Horner K. The diagnostic efficacy of cone beam CT for impacted teeth and associated features: a systematic review. *J Oral Rehabil*. 2011; 38(3):208–216.
36. Kapila S, Conley RS, Harrell WE Jr. The current status of cone beam computed tomography imaging in orthodontics. *Dentomaxillofac Radiol*. 2011;40(1):24–34.
37. Ericson S, Kurol PJ. Resorption of incisors after ectopic eruption of maxillary canines: a CT study. *Angle Orthod*. 2000;70(6):415–423.
38. Ericson S, Kurol J. Incisor resorption caused by maxillary cuspids. a radiographic study. *Angle Orthod*. 1987;57(4):332–346.
39. Pauwels R, Beinsberger J, Collaert B, et al. Effective dose range for dental cone beam computed tomography scanners. *Eur J Radiol*. 2012; 81(2):267–271.
40. Patel S, Dawood A, Ford TP, Whaites E. The potential applications of cone beam computed tomography in the management of endodontic problems. *Int Endod J*. 2007;40(10):818–830.
41. Ngan DC, Kharbanda OP, Geenty JP, Darendeliler MA. Comparison of radiation levels from computed tomography and conventional dental radiographs. *Aust Orthod J*. 2003;19(2):67–75.
42. Huang GJ. Making the case for evidence-based orthodontics. *Am J Orthod Dentofacial Orthop*. 2004;125(4):405–406.

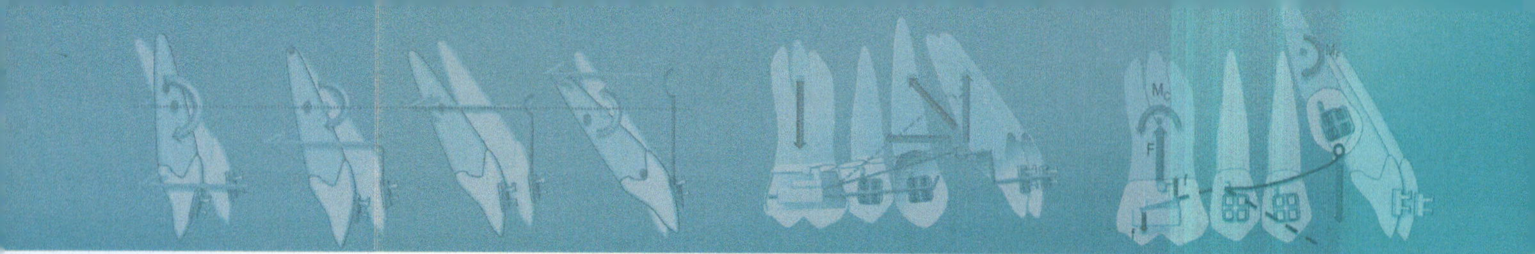

CHAPTER 3

Esthetics in Tooth Display and Smile Design

Bjørn U. Zachrisson

The orthodontic profession has always been in pursuit of the ideal dentition. At present, we are on the threshold of a paradigm shift that apparently will change the fundamental conceptual basis of orthodontics and the traditional emphasis in diagnosis and treatment planning.[1,2] The former emphasis on dental and skeletal components is still valid but greater attention than before is now required to the soft tissue aspects of orthodontics. In an effort to create natural esthetics, the orthodontist must give careful consideration to the patient in his or her entirety. Individual attributes of a tooth or segment of teeth may represent only part of the story, because teeth do not exist individually and separate from the patient to whom they belong. Combinations of tooth positions can create an effect that is greater than, equal to, or less than the sum of the parts.[3] The discipline of esthetics in orthodontics can be broken down into at least four parts: microesthetics (the elements that make teeth look like teeth), gingival esthetics, macroesthetics (the principles that apply when groupings of individual teeth are considered), and facial esthetics.[3] This chapter will focus on the principles of macroesthetics and facial esthetics in orthodontics and how to apply them clinically. The dynamic relationship between the teeth and the surrounding soft tissues during and after orthodontic corrections and the patient's facial characteristics will be emphasized. The display (amount and shape of crown structure that shows in various views and lip positions) will be related to age, sex, and facial characteristics. The purpose is to provide guidelines for orthodontists on how to analyze esthetic factors by viewing the patient from the front and to discuss some new concepts on how to achieve the desirable characteristics of tooth display in the vertical and transverse dimensions during normal social interaction.

EVALUATING ESTHETICS IN THE DENTIST'S CHAIR

Esthetics, which is derived from the Greek word for "perception," deals with beauty and the beautiful. It may be divided into two dimensions: objective (admirable) and subjective (enjoyable) beauty.[4] Objective beauty implies that the object possesses properties that make it unmistakably praiseworthy. Subjective beauty is value-laden and is related to the tastes of the person contemplating it. Contemporary techniques in orthodontics should lend objective esthetics to the entire orofacial complex, involving unity, form, structure, balance, color, function, and display of the dentition. In addition, the creation of subjective beauty according to an individual orthodontist's preferences may enhance the cosmetic value of the treatment rendered to each patient.

In discussing the principles of visual perception and its clinical application to dentofacial esthetics, Lombardi[5] remarked that detailed esthetic judgments can be made only by viewing patients from the front, in conversation, and observing facial expressions and smiling. The traditional dentist's view from above and behind the patient is skewed, differing markedly from the "true" perception of the patient in a mirror or by other persons during normal social interaction. For example, it is not possible to gain adequate information on such details as midline alignment (maxillary and mandibular relative to facial) and right-left symmetry of canine and premolar crown torque (Fig. 3-1, A) unless the patient is observed directly from the front (Fig. 3-1, B). A direct "eye-to-eye" view of the dentition can, in fact, be obtained when the patient is sitting in the dental chair[6]; the trick is to move the patient's head to the side of the headrest (see Fig. 3-1, B). With this method it is possible to analyze important esthetic factors during the treatment (Fig. 3-1, C and D), such as:

- Crown lengths of the upper and lower incisors
- Incisal edge contours (before and after recontouring)
- Position and symmetry of gingival margin levels on the upper and lower anterior teeth
- Axial inclinations of all anterior teeth
- Midlines (maxillary to mandibular and facial)
- Connector areas (the zone in which two adjacent teeth appear to touch)
- Symmetry and degree of crown torque of the canines and premolars
- Harmony of the front-to-back tooth display curve

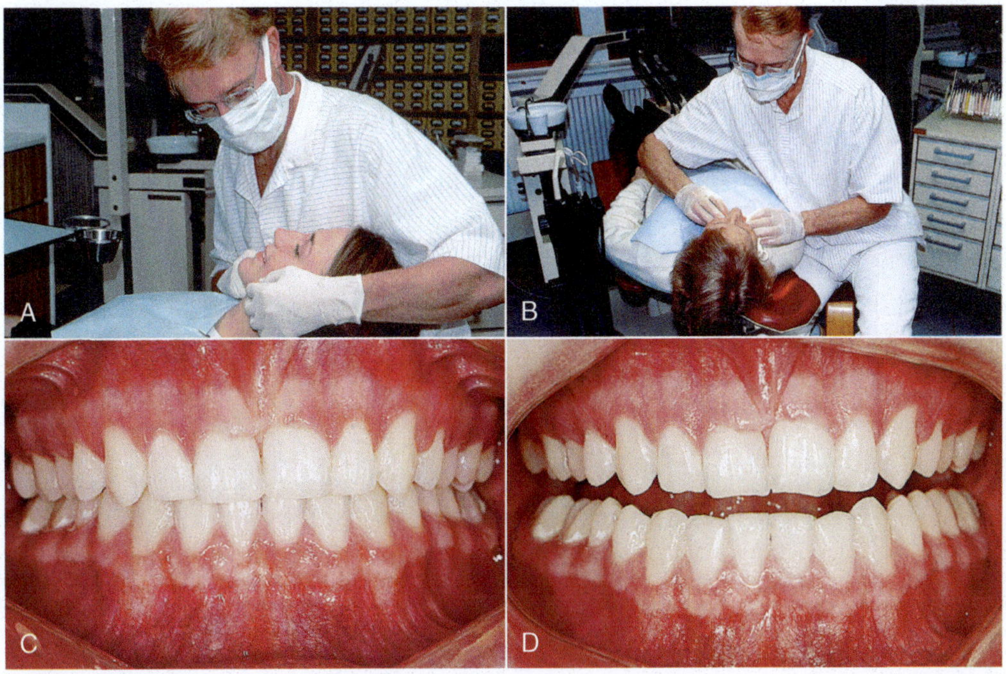

Figure 3-1 **A,** Unsuitable position for evaluating esthetics during treatment. Moving the patient's head to the side of the headrest (**B**) allows direct frontal view of dentition (**C**) and a realistic impression of esthetic features. **D,** The incisal edge contours can be examined on slight mouth opening.

It is important for a successful outcome that the clinician has learned to look at all of these aspects and has the ability to make the necessary corrections while the fixed appliances are still on, because "you can only change what you see."[7] After carefully studying the patient's dentition, the orthodontist can make the required finishing archwire bends and perform any other esthetic procedures needed. For analysis of tooth display when speaking and smiling and viewing the buccal corridors on smiling, a better impression is obtained when the patient is sitting up or standing in front of the dentist.[5,6]

STANDARDS OF NORMALITY

It is useful for esthetic oral rehabilitations to describe some average desirable characteristic features of smiles. These normative standards may serve as a guideline for enhancement of esthetics for the anterior component of the dentition.

Smile Type: Incisor and Gingival Display

Lip coverage of the maxillary incisors in full smiles is generally distinguished into three types: low, average, and high smiles.[8] The most frequent type[8,9] (found in about 70% of the young adult population) is the *average* smile that reveals 75% to 100% of the upper incisors. The *low* smile displays less than 75% of the maxillary incisors in a full smile and is found in about 20% of the population, whereas the *high* smile reveals the complete cervicoincisal length of the upper incisors and a contiguous band of gingiva and occurs in about 10% of the U.S. population.[8] A fourth type of lip line height may be defined as a "gummy" smile, which occurs when patients show more than 4-mm of gingiva on smiling (discussed later in the chapter).[10,11]

Upper lip coverage will always increase with age and therefore the percentage of high smiles may be greater among younger age groups[12,13] and smaller among older adults.[9,14] There is also a sexual dimorphism in that low smile lines are predominantly a male characteristic and high smiles are predominantly a female characteristic.[8]

It is noteworthy that some marginal gingival display in smiling is not as objectionable to laypersons as orthodontists may imagine.[10,13] We should therefore look on a moderately high smile type as an acceptable anatomic variation well within the usual range of lip-tooth-jaw relationships, especially among women.[12,13]

Smile Arc[15,16] (Smile Curve)

The relationship of the maxillary incisal curve to the inner contour of the lower lip can be divided into three types: parallel, straight, and reverse. In a survey of young adults in the Los Angeles area, Tjan et al.[8] found that a great majority (85%) had a maxillary incisal smile curve *parallel* to the inner contour of the lower lip, 14% showed a *straight* rather than a curved line, and only 1% had a *reverse* smile curve. Since parallelism is the normal finding in untreated persons, it is an optimal goal for objective beauty in esthetic oral rehabilitations,[17,18] including orthodontic (Figs. 3-2 and 3-3) and orthodontic-prosthetic treatments (Fig. 3-4). A straight or reverse smile curve may contribute to a less attractive facial appearance.[5,17] The reverse curve is frequently associated with marked abrasive wear of the upper incisors.

Number of Teeth Displayed in the Smile

The California survey[8] also revealed that in a typical or average smile in young adults, the six maxillary anterior

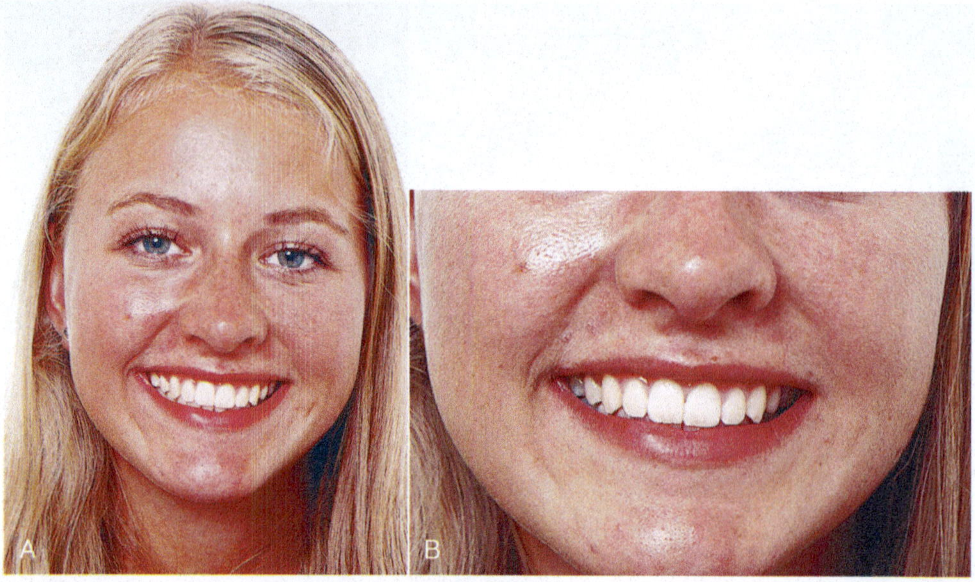

Figure 3-2 **A and B,** Esthetic smile curve (arc) with parallelism between maxillary teeth and inner contour of lower lip in four-premolar extraction case. Upright canine and premolar crowns contribute to fullness of smile.

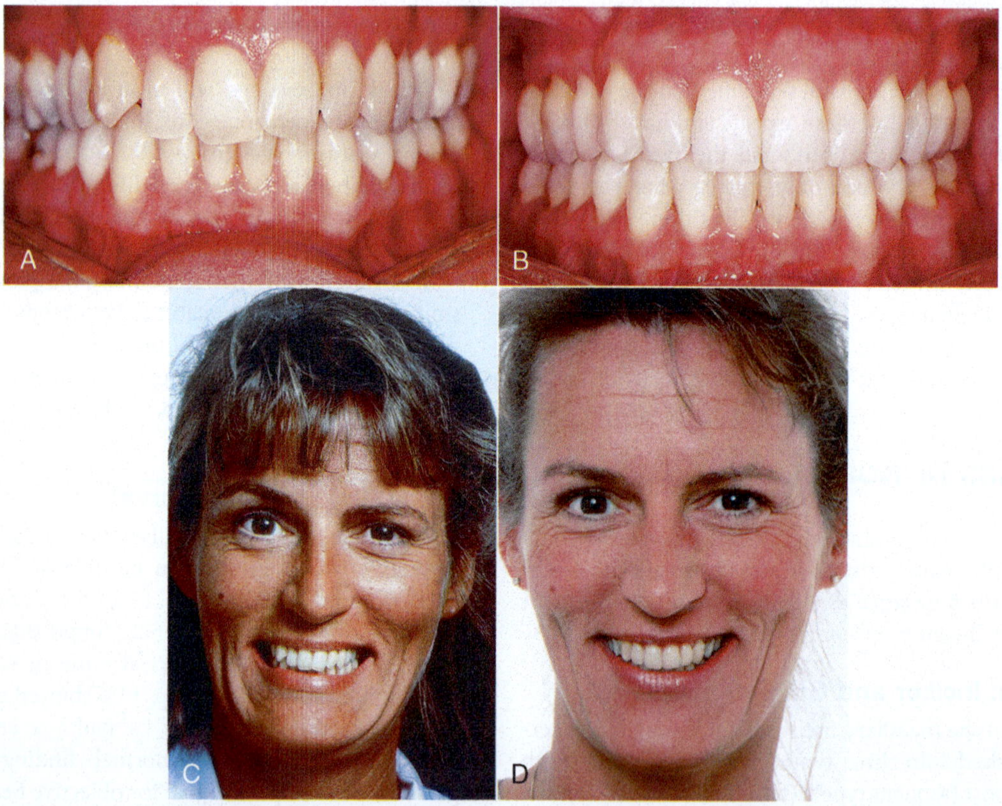

Figure 3-3 **A–D,** Improvement in parallelism between maxillary anterior tooth curve and lower lip contour with orthodontic treatment in adult female bimaxillary crowding case. Cant of maxillary central incisor midline is corrected.

teeth and the first or second premolars are displayed. The number of teeth displayed in the full smiles of 454 students was six anteriors only, 7%; six anteriors and first premolars, 48.5%; six anteriors and first and second premolars, 40.5%; and six anteriors, first and second premolars, and first molars, 4%.

VERTICAL POSITION OF THE INCISORS

Normal Age Changes in Lip-Incisor Relationship

Progressive changes with age on upper and lower lip positions are caused by the effects of gravity. Some normative

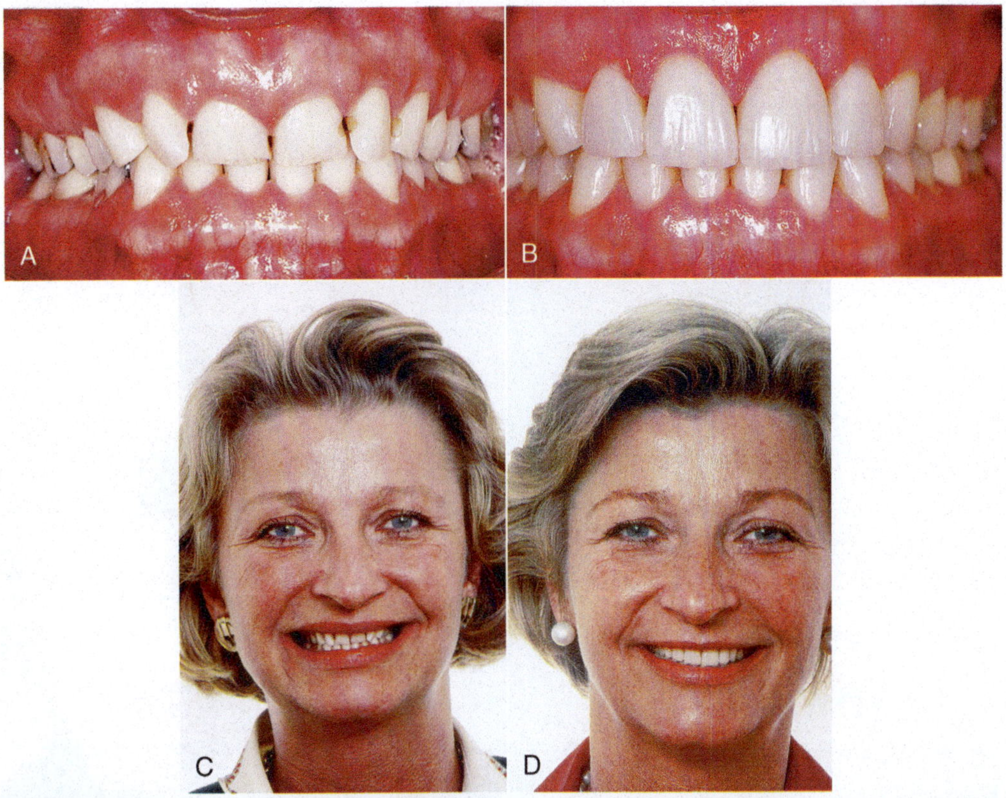

Figure 3-4 **A–D,** Orthodontic-prosthetic interdisciplinary approach to improve parallelism between maxillary incisor curve and lower lip contour in adult female Class II, Division 2 malocclusion with worn central incisors. Four porcelain laminate veneers (courtesy Dr. S. Toreskog, Göteborg, Sweden) were used to restore and elongate the maxillary incisors.

TABLE 3-1 Maxillary and Mandibular Incisor Display with Lips Gently Parted (in mm)

Age Group (Years)	Maxillary Central Incisor	Mandibular Central Incisor
Up to 30	3.5	0.5
30–40	1.5	1.0
40–50	1.0	2.0
50–60	0.5	2.5
Over 60	0.0	3.0

Modified from Vig RG, Brundo GC. The kinetics of anterior tooth display. *J Prosthet Dent.* 1978;39:502–504.

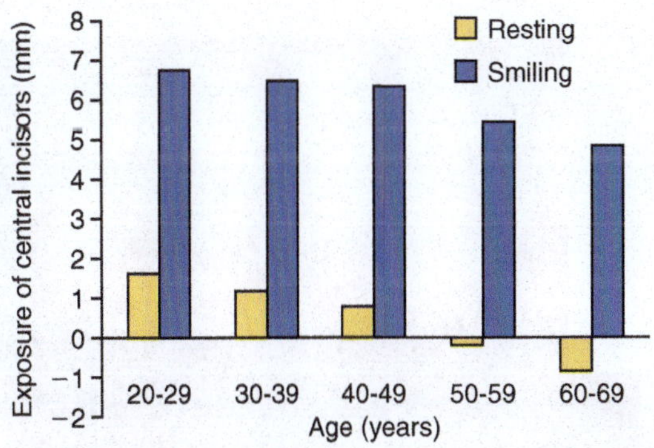

Figure 3-5 Comparison of maxillary incisor display by age with lips at rest and on smiling. (Reproduced with permission from Dong JK, Cho HW, Oh SC. The esthetics of the smile: a review of some recent studies. *Int J Prosthodont.* 1999;12:9–19.)

studies on the optimal vertical incisor positions in the faces of persons in different age groups are available. Peck et al.[13] showed that the normal display of maxillary incisors with relaxed lips at 15 years of age was 4.7-mm (standard deviation [SD] 2.0-mm) for boys and 5.3-mm (SD 1.8-mm) for girls. The sexual dimorphism is evident at all ages. For adults, Vig and Brundo[14] have provided normative mean values for different age groups (Table 3-1). Dong et al.[19] compared the age changes in maxillary and mandibular incisor display at rest and when smiling (Fig. 3-5) and confirmed the observations that the age changes with relaxed lips were dramatic (Fig. 3-6). Mandibular incisor display shows a corresponding increase with age. The amount of mandibular incisor display after age 60 is approximately equal to the amount of maxillary incisor display before age 30 (see Fig. 3-5 and Fig. 3-6, D).

There is a close correlation between the incisor exposure at rest and during normal speech.[20,21] The tooth display in speaking may be every bit as important as the tooth display in smiling to express personality and age. The most important information related to esthetics in treatment planning is obtained when the patient is observed during normal conversation. The tooth display on smiling will not provide the same information since when a person is smiling, the upper

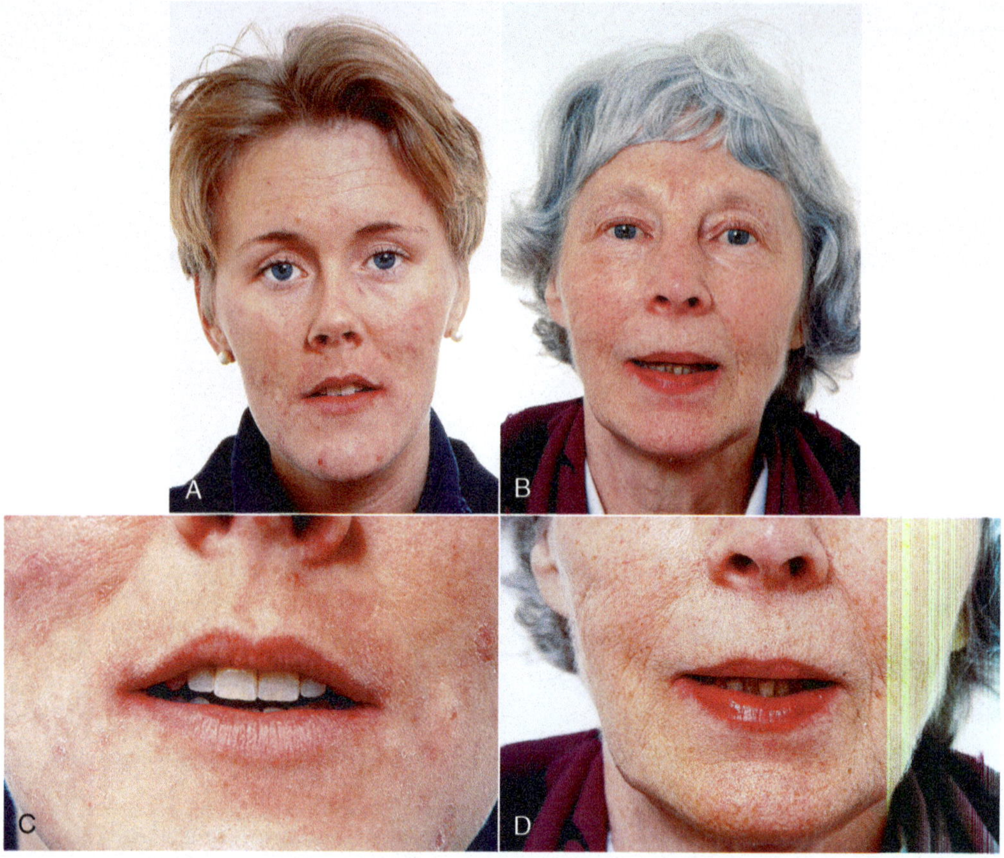

Figure 3-6 Age changes in vertical incisor display with relaxed lips, demonstrated by female patients aged 25 years (**A and C**) and 65 years (**B and D**). Note that the younger woman shows only maxillary incisors, whereas the older woman shows only mandibular incisors.

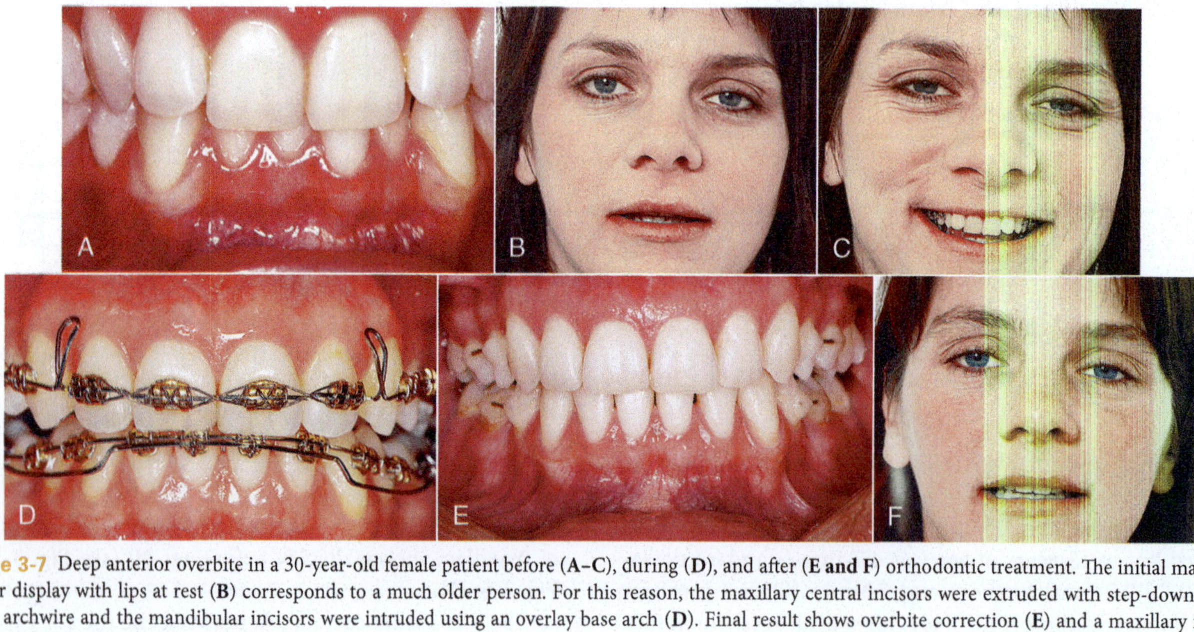

Figure 3-7 Deep anterior overbite in a 30-year-old female patient before (**A–C**), during (**D**), and after (**E and F**) orthodontic treatment. The initial maxillary incisor display with lips at rest (**B**) corresponds to a much older person. For this reason, the maxillary central incisors were extruded with step-down bends in the archwire and the mandibular incisors were intruded using an overlay base arch (**D**). Final result shows overbite correction (**E**) and a maxillary incisor display more relevant to the patient's age (**F**).

lip is raised actively by three different muscle groups.[22] For this reason, nearly everyone, irrespective of age, will display the maxillary incisors nicely in the full smile, even if only the mandibular incisors are visible during their speech. In other words, the age changes in incisor display are much more pronounced and apparent with the lips relaxed and when the patient is speaking than when he or she is smiling (Fig. 3-7).[15]

The sagging of the perioral soft tissue is partly due to the natural flattening, stretching, and decreasing elasticity of the

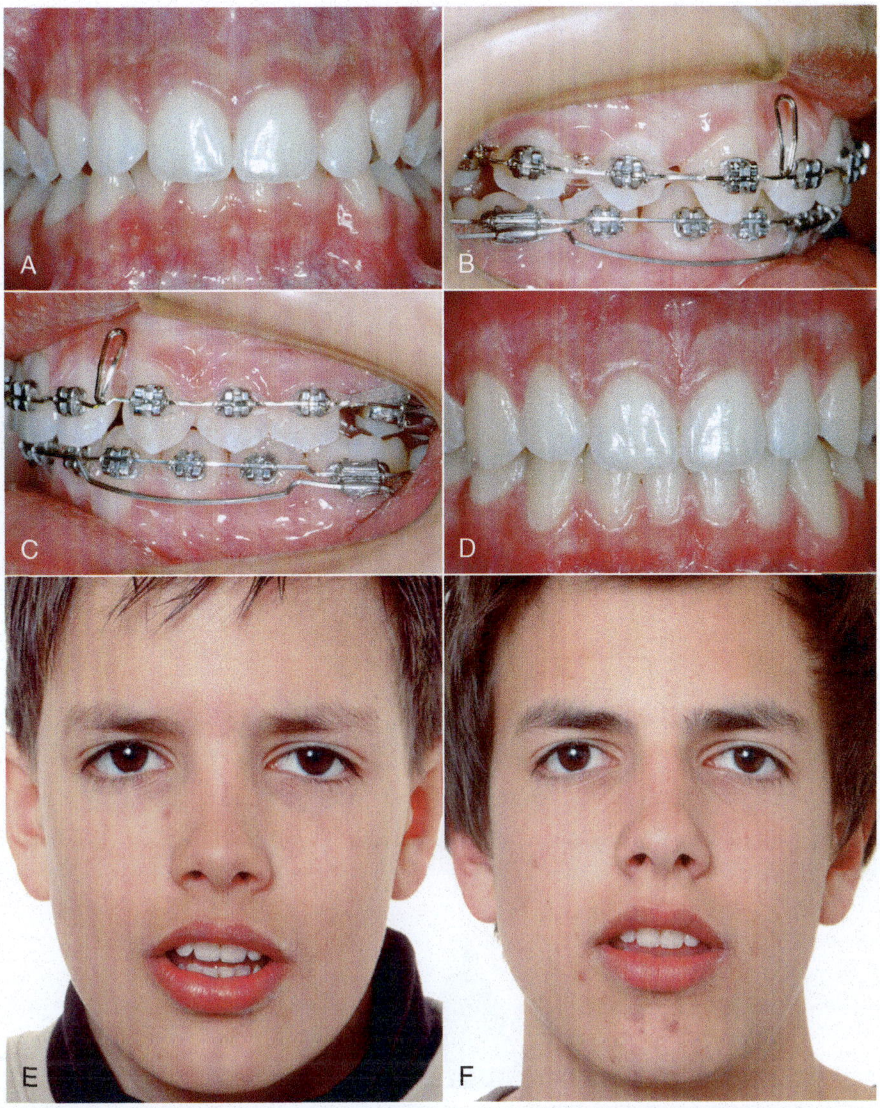

Figure 3-8 **A and E,** Young male patient with deep anterior overbite. **E,** Rest position photograph indicates that maxillary incisors should not be intruded. **B and C,** Mandibular incisor intrusion using 0.0175-inch × 0.025-inch CNA overlay arches from double tubes on the mandibular first molars. Final result demonstrates (**D**) overbite correction and (**F**) optimal maxillary incisor display with lips at rest.

skin.[23] The upper lip becomes longer and hides more and more of the maxillary incisors, while the drooping of the lower lip gradually exposes more of the mandibular incisors. As a consequence, show of maxillary incisors with relaxed lips signifies youth and beauty, whereas display of mandibular incisors is a characteristic of the elderly (see Fig. 3-6). The importance of the vertical dimension in tooth display has been demonstrated in prosthetic dentistry[13,14] and in orthognathic surgery involving maxillary repositioning.[24,25]

The guide for tooth position planning in orthodontic treatment should start with an appraisal of the position of the maxillary central incisal edge relative to the upper lip.[26,27]

This assessment is made with the patient's upper lip at rest, using a millimeter ruler or periodontal probe. This incisor position can be either acceptable or unacceptable, depending on the patient's age. The clinical guideline should be that the maxillary incisors should be moved in the vertical direction that improves their relationship to the resting lip position relative to the patient's age (Figs. 3-8 and 3-9; see Fig. 3-7). The relaxed lip position is the most reproducible functional position. It can and should be used as the guide,[26,27] whereas forced or posed smiles may vary considerably in the same patient and cannot be considered an accurate guide for incisor positioning.[27]

Spontaneous smiling records may also be recommended for diagnostic purposes. Because of the dynamic nature of spontaneous smiling, dynamic video recording of the spontaneous smile should be preferred.[9,20,21] Lip-tooth relationships follow a consistent pattern in natural rest position and during speech and spontaneous smiling.

Sex Differences

The sexual dimorphism in anterior tooth display implies that females have significantly more maxillary and less mandibular tooth exposure than males at all ages. In a group of adults, Vig and Brundo[14] found almost twice as much

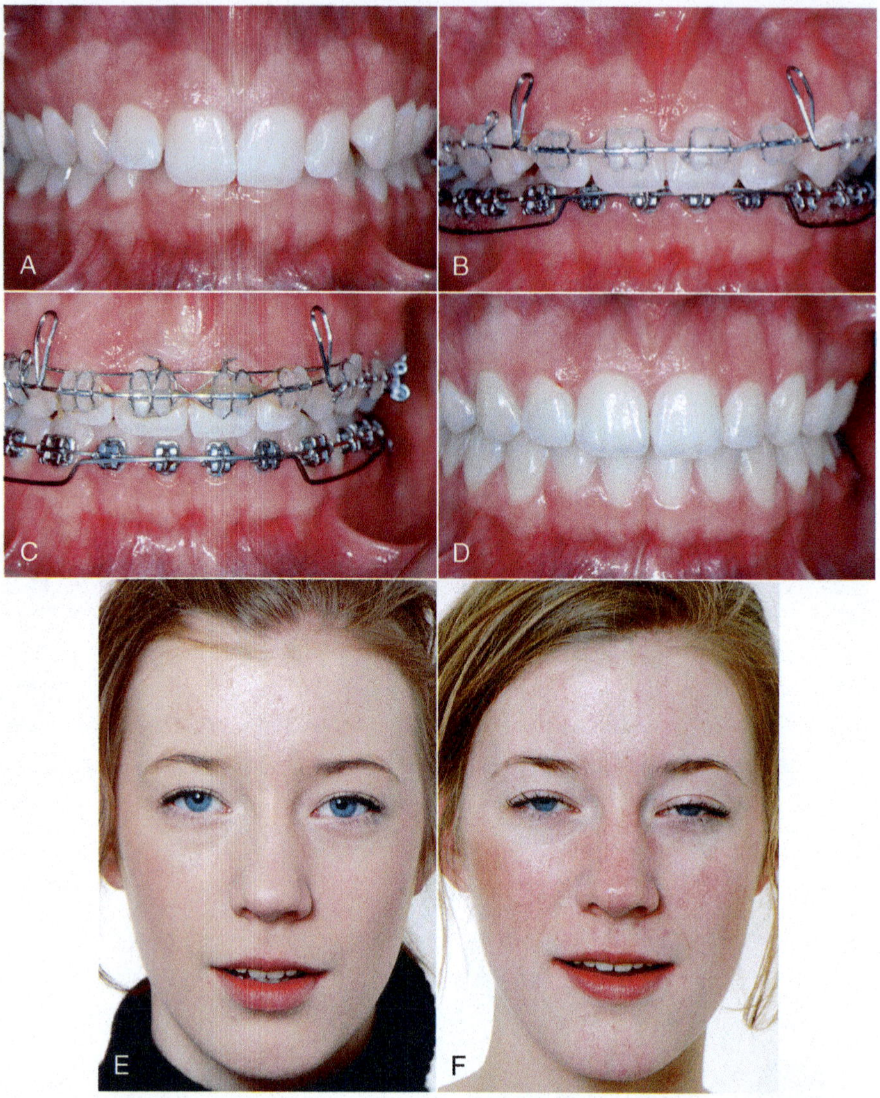

Figure 3-9 **A and E,** Eighteen-year-old female with Class II, Division 2 deep overbite malocclusion. **E,** The anterior overbite should not be treated with maxillary incisor intrusion, since the tooth display with lips at rest is good. **B-D,** The maxillary incisors were merely leveled and the deep bite correction was made with intrusion of the mandibular incisors. **C,** Von der Heydt torquing auxiliary was used to improve the maxillary incisor inclination. **F,** The incisor display with relaxed lips after treatment is unchanged.

maxillary anterior tooth display with the lips at rest in women (3.4-mm) as in men (1.9-mm). Men displayed much more of the mandibular incisors (1.2-mm compared to 0.5-mm).

Standardized Extraoral Records

A standardized procedure for recording the incisor display in (1) rest position (Fig. 3-10; see Figs. 3-4 to 3-9) and (2) a posed smile (see Figs. 3-2 to 3-4) both before and after orthodontic treatment is recommended and will help the clinician to avoid undesirable treatment effects on the maxillary incisor reveal. Each patient should be coached and asked to achieve the same lip position at least twice in succession before a photograph is taken. In rest position (instruct the patient to say "Emma" or "Mississippi"),[6,28] the teeth should be slightly apart and both the perioral soft tissue and the mandibular posture must be unstrained. In the posed smile (instruct the patient to bite together, smile, and say "Cheee …"),[6] the teeth should be lightly closed. As mentioned, the analysis of incisor display during spontaneous smiling should be made with video records.

CLINICAL IMPLICATIONS FOR DEEP OVERBITE CORRECTION

Average and Low Smile Types

The correction of deep anterior overbite can be made by various combinations of incisor intrusion and molar extrusion.[29,30] The treatment concepts for deep overbite cases have changed significantly during the past 10 to 15 years. This is due to the increasing attention now being paid to the esthetic importance of the vertical display of the *maxillary* incisors during normal speech and with relaxed lips.[6,7,26] While active intrusion of maxillary incisors with intrusion arches à la Burstone, utility arches à la Ricketts, overlay base-arches, and similar approaches has previously been considered a

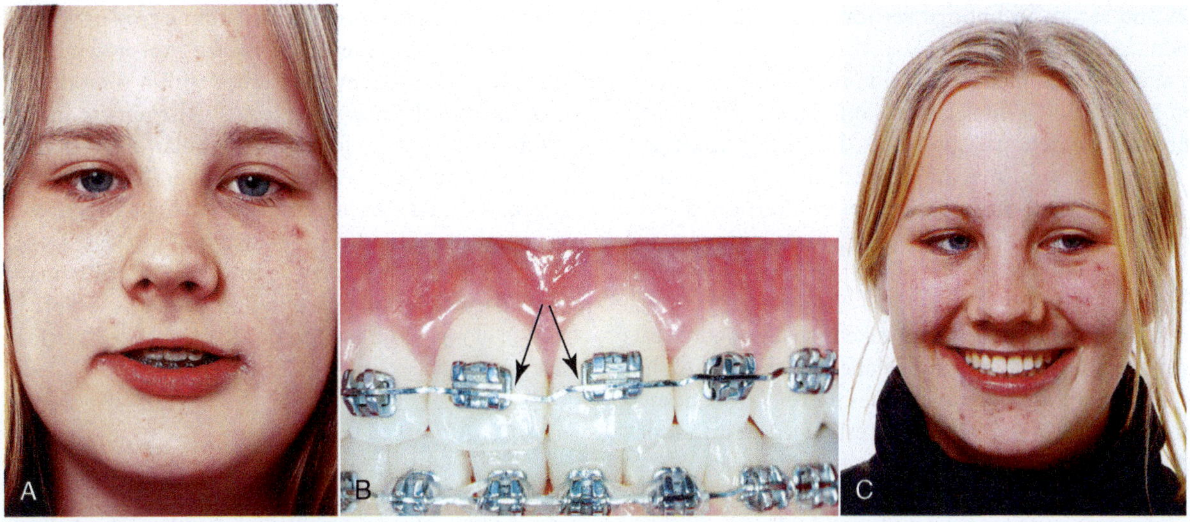

Figure 3-10 When smile curve is flattened during treatment (**A**), the central incisors may be extruded with step-down bends (*arrows* in **B**) to improve the curve and the parallelism to lower lip contour (**C**).

cornerstone of deep bite correction, the risk of too much intrusion (so-called "overintrusion") with such approaches is apparent.[28,30] Overintrusion may tend to hide the maxillary incisors behind the upper lip when the patient is speaking. Lindauer et al.[30] compared the outcomes from two common procedures used to reduce deep overbite: maxillary incisor intrusion using an intrusion arch and posterior eruption using an anterior biteplate. Both the intrusion arch and the biteplate procedures effectively reduced overbite significantly over a relatively short period of treatment. The intrusion arch patients displayed significant reductions in maxillary incisor display (mean change from 5.4- to 3.0-mm) accompanying documented incisor intrusion. This means that a maxillary intrusion arch will lead to a premature aged oral appearance. Such a mistake can go undetected by the orthodontist unless the upper central incisors show on speaking and smiling is recorded and analyzed properly. With increasing age of the patient and concomitant drooping of the upper lip, an unesthetic incisor display at adolescence will predictably worsen with time.[9,21]

In a child or adolescent patient, maxillary incisor intrusion beyond 4- to 5-mm below the upper lip at rest represents overintrusion of these teeth and unwanted aging of the patient. In a young adult between 20 and 30 years of age, there should be at least 3-mm of maxillary incisors showing. For an adult 30 to 40 years of age, approximately 1.5-mm of the maxillary incisors should show at rest position of the lips, and at age 40 to 50 years, about 1-mm should show. In patients more than 50 to 60 years of age, the maxillary incisors normally should not show at all when the lips are relaxed (see Fig. 3-6). According to Frush and Fisher,[31] an optimal incisor position for adults occurs when the maxillary lateral incisors show "when the patient is speaking seriously." The tips of the lateral incisors should show in varying degrees according to the sex and age requirements.

The tooth-to-lip position at rest should be monitored constantly throughout the orthodontic treatment. Since no orthodontist would wish to make his or her patients look older than they really are, it is important to carefully analyze each patient's tooth display on speaking before deciding whether maxillary intrusion mechanics should be used.[28] In some deep overbite cases, extrusion rather than intrusion of the maxillary incisors may be indicated (see Fig. 3-7) or a combination of orthodontics and prosthetic crown lengthening with porcelain laminate veneers will be the method of choice (see Fig. 3-4).

From an esthetic point of view, the best treatment strategy in the majority of deep overbite cases is to actively intrude the *mandibular* rather than the maxillary incisors. This is particularly true when the curve of Spee is marked and when the six mandibular anterior teeth are above the functional occlusal plane at the start of treatment. Mandibular incisor intrusion can be achieved with segmented intrusion arches, utility arches, overlay base-arches, etc. The rate of intrusion can be controlled by recording the position of the maxillary central incisal edges relative to fixed points on the mandibular appliances. Using overlay base-arches (see Figs. 3-7 to 3-9), the mandibular incisor intrusion usually occurs at a rate of 0.5-mm per month. It should be emphasized that it is not possible to effectively intrude mandibular incisors with one continuous archwire. Compared to a conventional continuous archwire, segmented mechanics (Burstone) will produce overbite correction by (1) more incisor intrusion and (2) less molar extrusion and subsequent posterior rotation of the mandible.[32,33]

Another situation that calls for the use of segmented archwires happens in children with reduced anterior overbite and maxillary canines erupting in a high position.[28] If a continuous leveling archwire is used, the intrusive counterforce on the incisors may overintrude them into functionally and esthetically unacceptable positions. In such instances, the first molars should be connected with a solid transpalatal bar to yield a reliable posterior anchorage unit and a cantilever wire from the extra molar tube used to bring down the canines and secure an optimal vertical incisor display after treatment.[7]

An alternative to incisor intrusion for deep overbite correction may be active molar extrusion. Such effects can be obtained with functional appliances, biteplates, headgears, etc.[34] Molar extrusion may be of merit in a growing child with normal or low-angle face type and vertical growth pattern[28] but it would be calamitous in a high-angle case and cannot be recommended in adults because of stability concerns.[34]

The second most common mistake in orthodontic treatment and finishing in the vertical plane is to create a straight smile line rather than an incisal smile curve.[15,28,35,36] Undesirable arc flattening is probably underestimated in orthodontics. Ackerman et al.[36,37] reported that as many as 32% of their patients got a flattening of the smile arc during orthodontic treatment. One reason why such changes may go unnoticed by orthodontists is that they are observed only when the patients are examined from the front.

It may seem difficult to achieve the desired parallelism between the maxillary incisors and the lower lip in smiling. In clinical practice, however, this appearance can readily be achieved if the maxillary central incisors are symmetrically positioned 0.5- to 1.5-mm longer than the lateral incisors[38] (see Fig. 3-10). If the lower lip shows a marked curvature in smiling, the distoincisal edges of the maxillary central incisors can be ground slightly with a diamond instrument, as this procedure will not affect the functional occlusion.[33]

It is particularly undesirable to combine maxillary incisor overintrusion with a straight rather than a curved arrangement of these teeth. This display gives the impression of a typical static denture that results in the so-called "denture mouth."[28,31]

High Smile Types: "Gummy" Smiles

As mentioned, a fourth category of smile line types is the "gummy" smile, defined as show of more than 4-mm of maxillary gingiva in full smiling.[11] This smile type has provoked considerable interest and concern among orthodontists. Its biological mechanism appears to involve the combined effects of anterior vertical excess, an increased muscular capacity to raise the upper lip in smiling, short upper lip, and associated factors such as excessive interlabial gap at rest and excessive overjet and overbite.[18,37]

A different treatment strategy may be needed for patients with high lip lines than for those with average or low smile types. Treatment alternatives include various combinations of orthodontic, periodontal, and surgical therapy. The differential diagnosis should take into consideration both the amount of maxillary incisor display at rest position of the lips and the amount of gingiva shown on smiling. If the maxillary incisor show at rest is optimal, active upper incisor intrusion should not be initiated. Instead, local gingivectomies or surgical crown lengthening with removal of crestal alveolar bone[39-41] should be done. Such procedures are particularly indicated in cases with altered passive eruption, excessive marginal gingivae, and short clinical crowns, since they will expose more of the anatomic crowns. When crestal alveolar bone is removed during surgical crown lengthening, the gingival margin will stabilize within 6 months at about 3-mm from the new bone level.[41] Attempts to inject botulinum toxin (Botox) for neuromuscular correction of excessively gummy smiles caused by hyperfunctional upper lip elevator muscles have been reported to be effective for about 6 months but the effect is transitory.[42]

Treatment of the most severe gummy smiles may require maxillary superior repositioning surgery (Le Fort I osteotomy), along with reduction of the associated vertical maxillary excess.[13]

MIDLINES

Dental to Facial Midline Positions

As mentioned, it is virtually impossible to check the relationship of the upper and lower midlines to the facial midline in the normal dentist-patient positions, since these allow only a view from the side (see Fig. 3-1). However, moving the patient's head to the side of the headrest will allow direct frontal observation.[6]

Midline Guides

The most practical guide to locate the midline of the face is to draw an imaginary vertical line that extends through soft tissue nasion and the midpoint of the Cupid's bow in the upper lip.[3,43]

A line between these landmarks not only locates the position of the facial midline but also determines the direction of the midline. Whenever possible, the maxillary dental midline should be coincident with the facial midline (Figs. 3-10 to 3-13). If this is not possible, the midline between the maxillary central incisors should be strictly vertical and parallel to the facial midline.[3,10,44,45]

Esthetically Acceptable Midline Deviations

Kokich Jr. et al.[10] reported an interesting interaction between maxillary central incisor midline deviation and crown angulation. As long as the dental midline was parallel to the facial midline, even a 4-mm maxillary midline deviation was not detected on photographs by dentists and laypersons. Similar findings from laypersons' perspectives were made by Springer et al.[46] However, all evaluators rated a 2-mm deviation in incisor angulation (canted midline) as noticeably unattractive. A significantly slanted dental midline is displeasing and will be noticed easily. These data demonstrate that a precise dental midline is not necessary for optimal esthetics as long as the incisal crown angulation is not canted (see Figs. 3-8 to 3-13). On the other hand, if the midaxis between the right and left maxillary central incisors is markedly canted, it will look unacceptably skewed even if the incisor contact point is located in the middle of the face.

While alignment of the maxillary and mandibular dental midlines is desirable in orthodontic treatment for occlusion reasons, the mandibular midline becomes a lesser issue in esthetics. The narrowness and uniform sizes of the

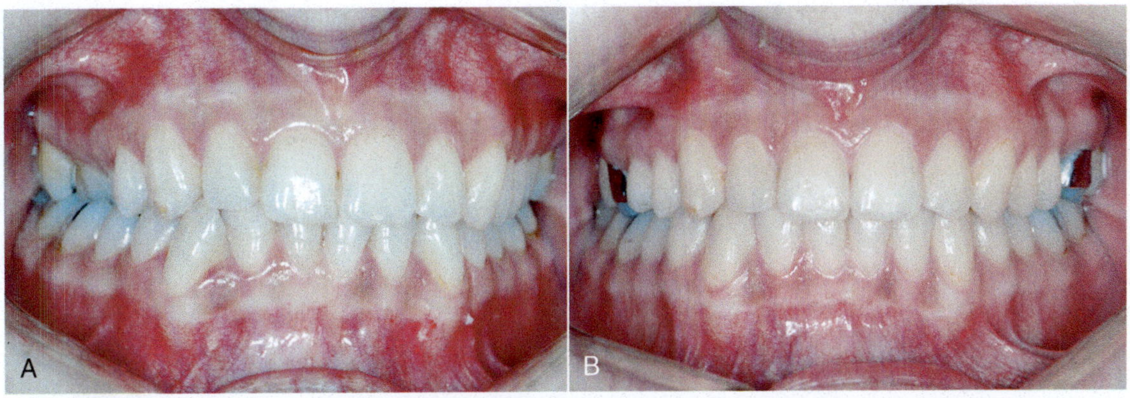

Figure 3-11 **A,** Adult female patient with rolled-in mandibular posterior teeth (particularly on the right side) and limited crossbite. Treatment included partial expansion in the maxillary right side. **B,** Uprighting of mandibular right canine, premolar, and molars was obtained by third-order bends in stainless steel archwire to provide desired lingual root torque. Note the symmetry of right and left sides after treatment.

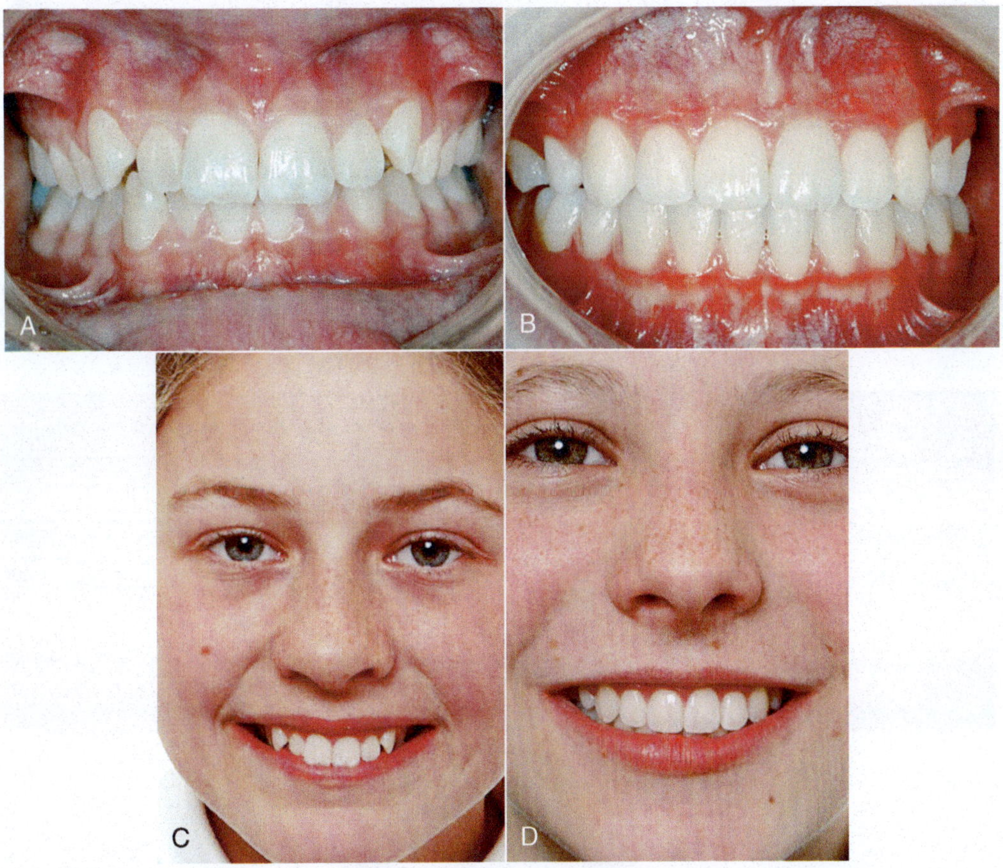

Figure 3-12 Maxillary premolar extraction case with full and radiant smile after orthodontic treatment. Note the lingually tilted maxillary premolars (**A**), canted midline, and extensive buccal corridors (**C**) at start. Maxillary and mandibular premolars and molars were uprighted. **B and D,** The dental midline coincides with the facial midline.

mandibular incisors make visualization of their midpoint more difficult.

Connector Area Versus Contact Point

Morley and Eubank[3] introduced the term *connector areas* as a useful tool and a visual goal to optimize smile esthetics in dental patients. The connector areas are larger, broader areas than the contact points between teeth and can be defined as the zone in which two adjacent teeth appear to touch. The most esthetic relationship between the maxillary anterior teeth is referred to as the 50-40-30 rule. This rule defines the ideal connector area between the two maxillary central incisors as 50% of their clinical crown length (Fig. 3-14; see Figs. 3-2, 3-12, and 3-13). The ideal connector area between a maxillary lateral incisor and a central incisor is 40% of the central incisor's clinical crown length, and between a lateral

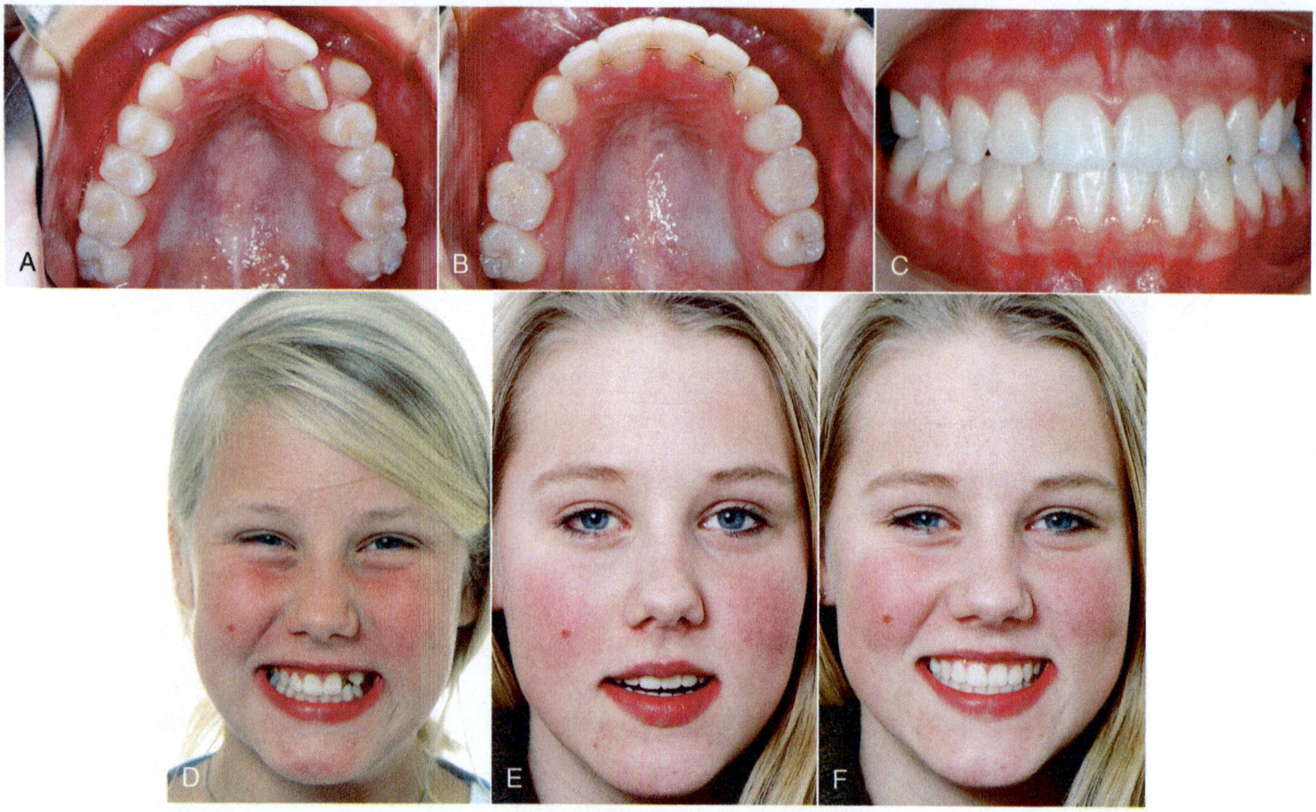

Figure 3-13 Desirable smile esthetics in young premolar extraction patient. **A and B,** Occlusal views before and after treatment. **D,** Facial view before treatment. **E,** Incisor display with relaxed lips is right for her age. **F,** The posed smile is full and attractive due to the upright canines and premolars and the dental midline is parallel to the facial midline. **C and F,** The connector area between the maxillary incisors and canines correspond to the 50-40-30 rule (see text).

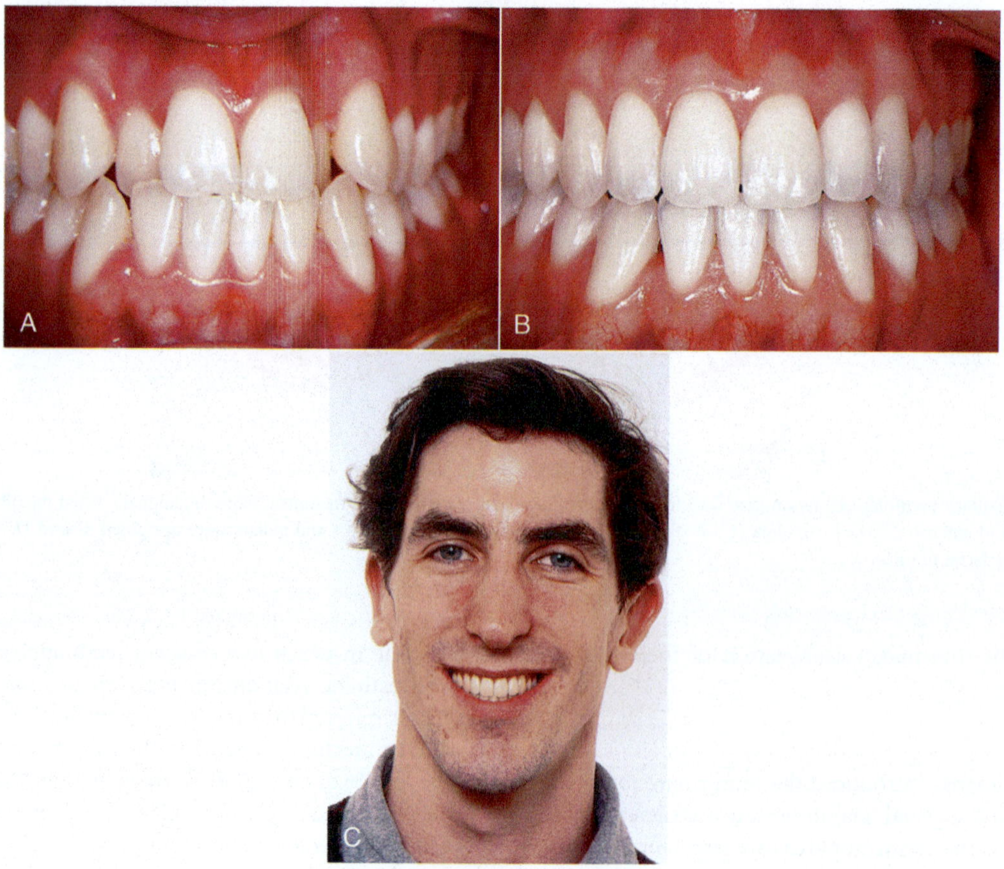

Figure 3-14 **A,** Nature's way of compensating for a small maxillary apical base is to tilt the maxillary posterior teeth (canines through molars) labially. This position was respected during the treatment, with outcome showing slight labial inclination of the crowns (**B**) to provide a full and pleasing smile (**C**).

incisor and a canine is 30% of the clinical crown length of the central incisors[3] (see Fig. 3-13).

The most important connector area is the one between the two maxillary central incisors. Since it should be quite long in orthodontically well-treated cases, it is clinically important to carefully check the clinical midaxis between the mesial surfaces of the central incisors before appliance removal. In cases of pre-treatment crowding it is almost always necessary to recontour these mesial surfaces by slight grinding (see Figs. 3-1, 3-3, 3-12, and 3-13). This will relocate the contact point in an apical direction to reduce or avoid interdental gingival recession[47] (dark triangles between the teeth due to loss of the gingival papillae) and result in an optimally long and vertical connector area (see Figs. 3-2 and 3-12 to 3-14). If the connector area is canted undesirably, it can be improved in the finishing stages of treatment using small artistic archwire bends. A prerequisite for detecting the need for such corrections is that the patient's dentition is studied from the front.

TRANSVERSE DIMENSION

Most orthodontists are familiar with the fact that too little lingual root torque of the maxillary central incisors during treatment will have a negative esthetic effect in most patients. Partly due to a different reflection of the incoming light, patients with optimal incisor crown inclination are considered to look more attractive than patients who finish orthodontic treatment with large interincisal angles. The current evidence regarding the most desirable esthetic labiolingual crown inclination of the maxillary canines, premolars, and molars is limited. Thus any discussion relative to what constitutes the most esthetic positions of the upper canines and posterior teeth in different patients will be subjective.

As discussed and illustrated elsewhere,[7,48,49] the fullness of the smile should be sought through adjustment of the clinical crown torque of the maxillary canines and premolars to their most esthetic appearance in different face types, rather than through nonextraction heroics or unnecessary lateral expansion and labial tipping of the maxillary dentition. Some important elements for the transverse dimension in orthodontics are:

- The labiolingual crown inclination of the terminal tooth in each quadrant that shows in smiling
- The crown inclination symmetry of contralateral teeth
- The harmony of the front-to-back tooth display curve
- The relationship between the size of the maxillary apical base and the labiolingual crown inclination of the maxillary teeth
- Occurrence of buccal corridors (negative space)

Terminal Tooth on Smiling

Generally speaking, about 90% of people show either the first or the second premolar as the last tooth when they are smiling.[8,16] To create the illusion of smile fullness, the last premolar displayed should be positioned relatively upright[42,43] (see Figs. 3-2, 3-10, and 3-11). It is particularly important to avoid a lingual inclination of the maxillary premolars in patients with a relatively small maxillary apical base (see Fig. 3-14) and in premolar extraction cases (Fig. 3-15; see Figs. 3-2, 3-12, 3-13).[48,49] When there is crown inclination asymmetry between the right and left last premolar on smiling, the smile invariably appears narrower on the side where the premolar has more tilt.[47]

The torque prescriptions for most preadjusted appliance systems tend to create too much lingual crown inclination of maxillary and mandibular canines and posterior teeth.[50] The view that the canines and premolars should have considerable lingual crown inclination (Fig. 3-16) in an optimally treated orthodontic case[51] irrespective of tooth size, jaw size, face type, and facial expressivity is disputed from an esthetic perspective.

The normative crown inclination values proposed by Andrews[51] (see Fig. 3-16) that have influenced available preadjusted appliance systems were based on careful study of 120 nonorthodontic patients with normal occlusion and teeth that were "straight and pleasing in appearance" and 1150 successfully treated orthodontic cases. Although this information has been of great value to our profession, study of already treated orthodontic cases may not be the optimal basis for optimal crown torque estimations from an esthetic perspective. Indeed, laypersons prefer straight upper canines and premolars according to an extensive computer-based survey based on slider technology on a large number of U.S. patients (n = 243).[52]

CROWN INCLINATION SYMMETRY ON CONTRALATERAL TEETH

Crown inclination symmetry of the contralateral teeth on the right and left sides of the maxilla and mandible will contribute to an optimally esthetic appearance (see Figs. 3-11 to 3-15). It is generally easier said than done to obtain bilateral crown inclination symmetry on canines and premolars (see Fig. 3-15). A prerequisite to detect asymmetries is to view the patient directly from the front at the start of orthodontic therapy so that the necessary correction bends can be made in the archwires.

Front-to-Back Progression

The front-to-back progression of the maxillary canine, premolars, and molars is a critical factor for the display of the dentition when the patient is speaking and smiling. The principles of gradation and smoothness must be observed, so the decrease in size and detail occurs gradually.[5] Lombardi[5] noted that the teeth should have a harmonious perspective from the dominant central incisors transitioning posteriorly, with each tooth in harmonious proportion to those adjacent. The apparent widths may or may not be in "golden proportion"[53,54] to one another. Analyzing students in California, Preston[54] found the golden proportion between the perceived width of the maxillary central and lateral incisors in only 17% of the cases and between any perceived lateral incisor and canine widths in none of the cases. He claimed

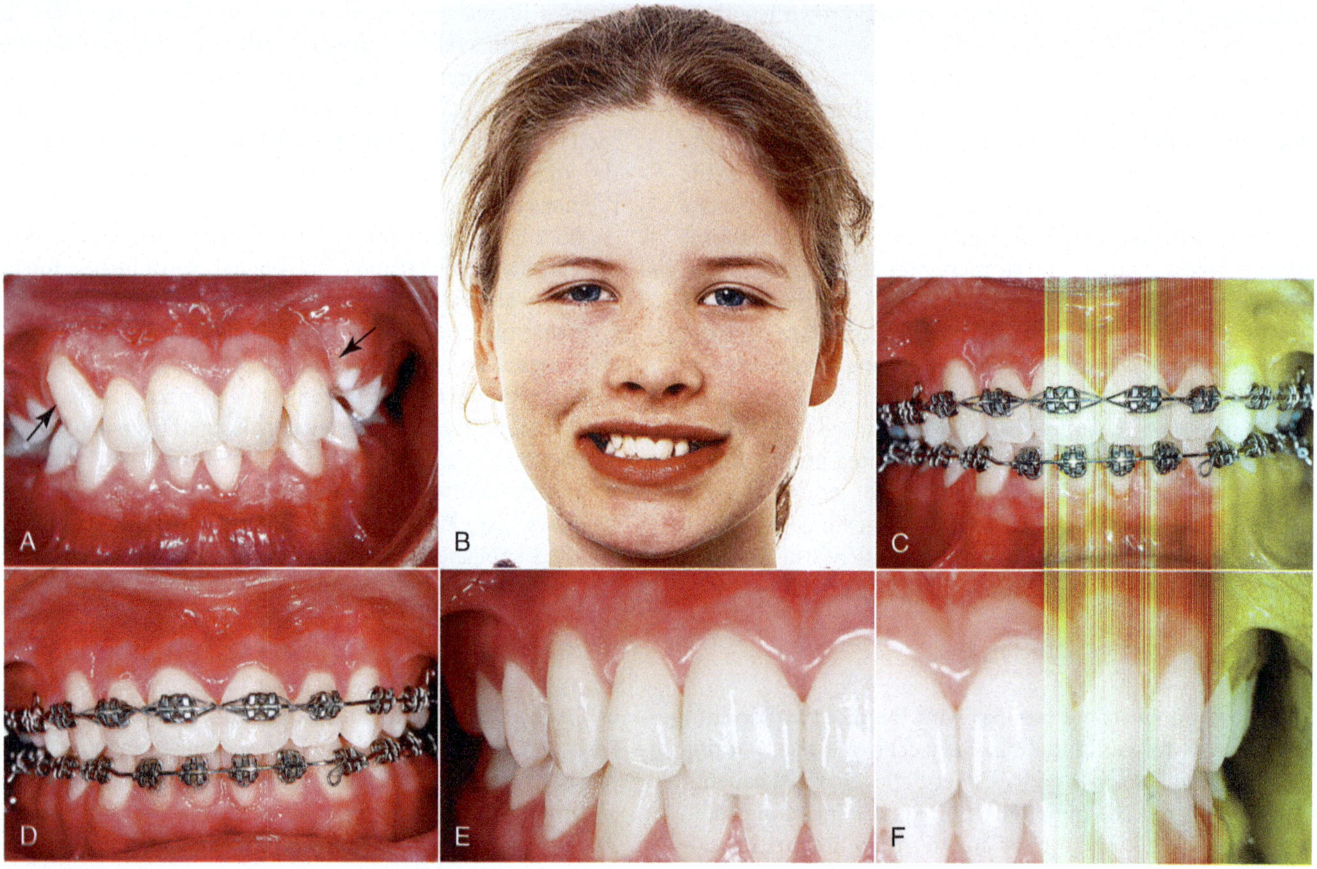

Figure 3-15 **A and B,** A markedly different clinical crown inclination between maxillary right and left canine *(arrows)* at start in young female patient. Due to the individualized torque with intentional lingual root torque bends in archwire, the right canine improved its inclination at 9 months (**C**) and 12 months (**E**) until it was upright and symmetrical with the left canine at the end of treatment (**D and F**). Also note the uprighted positions of maxillary and mandibular posterior teeth (**A, D, and F**).

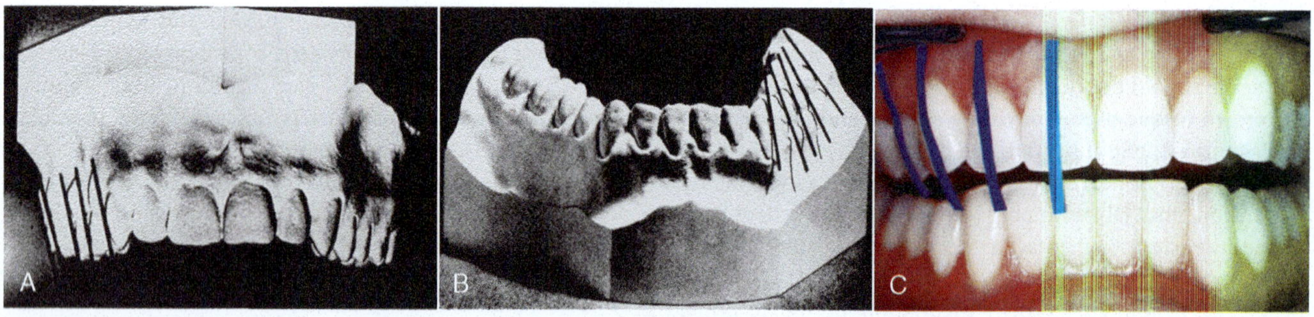

Figure 3-16 The optimal lingual crown inclination in normally occluded (**A**) upper and (**B**) lower posterior crowns according to Andrews.[51] **C,** Progressive medial tipping of the axial inclinations of the teeth according to Morley and Eubank.[3]

that there is nothing mystical or exclusively correct about the use of the golden proportion. Such use may well provide a pleasing outcome, as might many other approaches (see Figs. 3-10 to 3-15 and 3-18). From a clinical point of view, it may be more important to avoid any interruption of the harmony and gradual smoothness. This implies that canines and premolars with excessive lingual tipping (Figs. 3-17 and 3-18) or a premolar placed too far buccally[5] will lessen the harmony of the tooth display curve laterally and reduce the esthetic impression.

Apical Base Size and Crown Inclination Variations

Regarding jaw size, it appears to be a general rule for obtaining optimal esthetics that the smaller the maxillary apical base, the more labial tilt may be given to the canines and premolars to allow a broader smile (see Fig. 3-14). This will copy nature's way of compensating for different sizes of maxillae. For most patients, optimal esthetics will be achieved with upright canines or a very mild lingual crown inclination (see Figs. 3-2, 3-3, 3-9, 3-11 to 3-15, and 3-18). Too

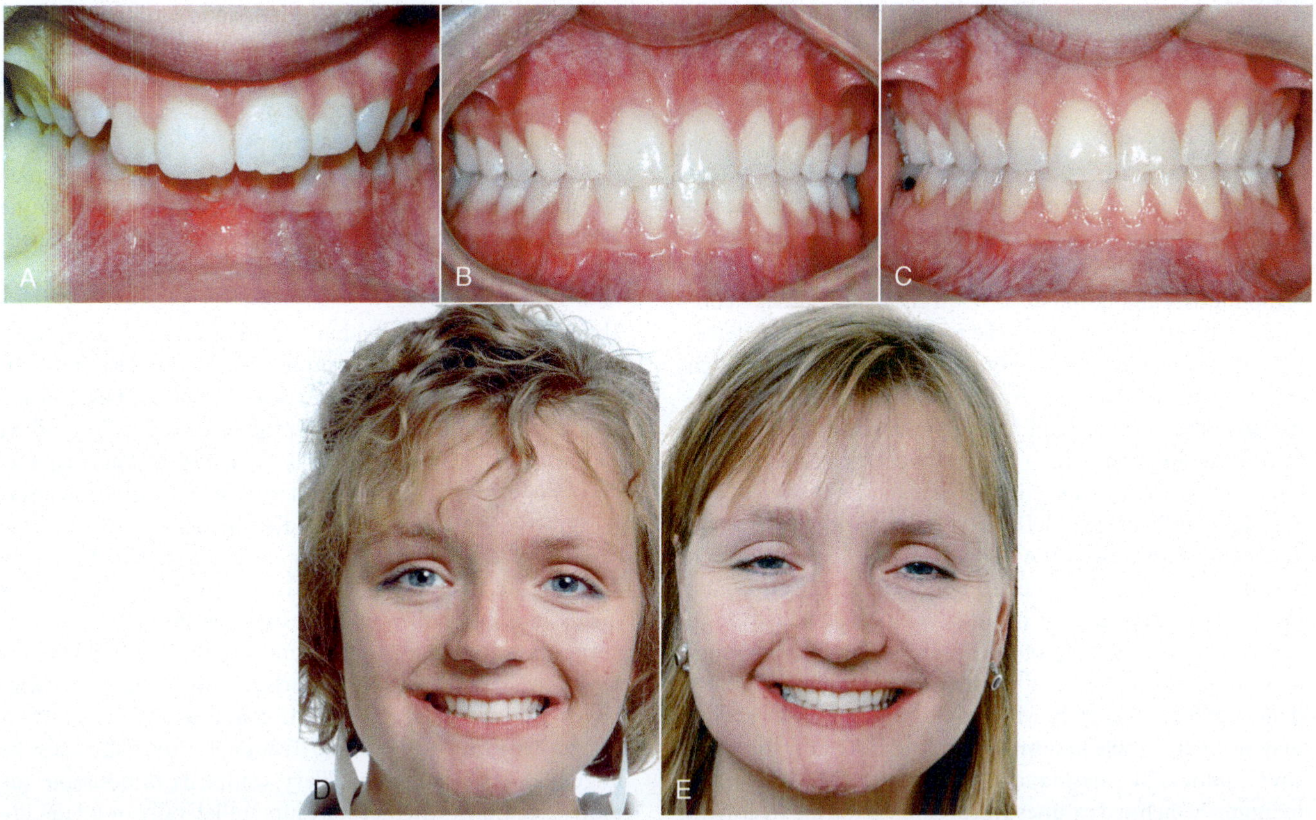

Figure 3-17 Undesirable smile esthetics in nonextraction Class II, Division 1 female patient. Marked lingual inclination of maxillary canines and premolars (**A**) remained undetected at the end of treatment (**B**) and 17 years later (**C**), providing a narrow smile with extensive buccal corridors throughout therapy and follow-up (**D and E**). Preadjusted appliance was used with negative torque values for canine and premolar brackets and no intentional third-order torquing bends.

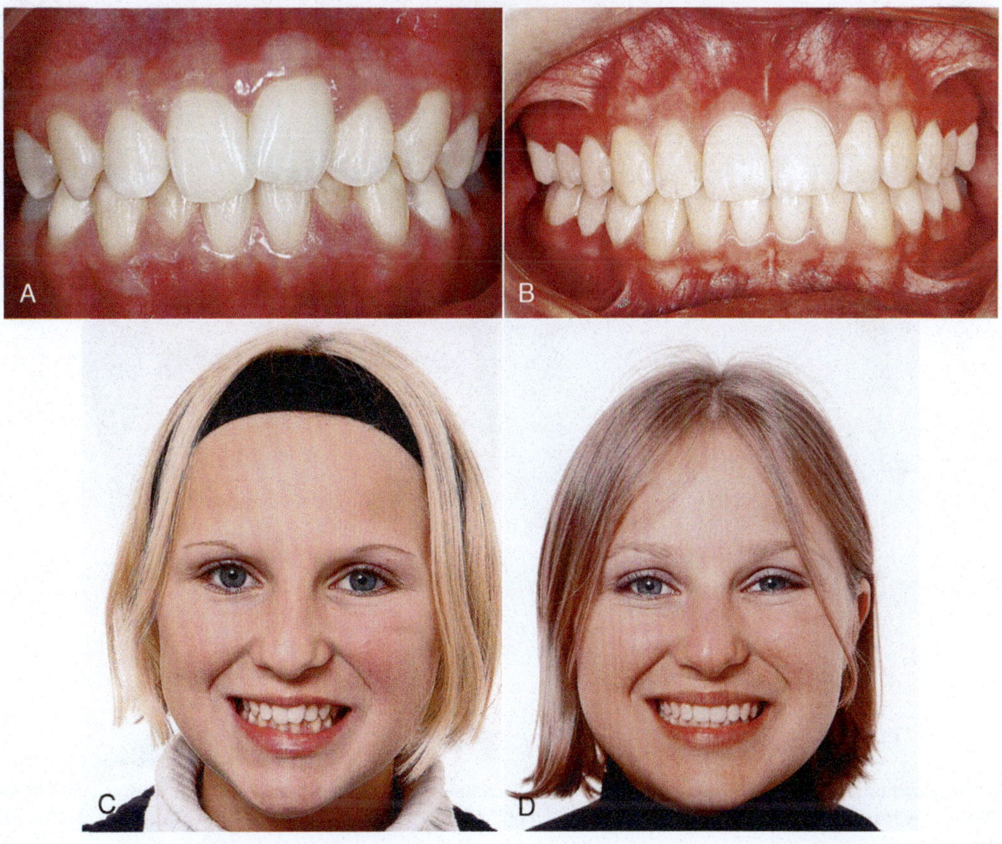

Figure 3-18 Adolescent female patient with mild bimaxillary crowding (**A**) treated without extraction and without lateral expansion and/or incisor proclination (**B**). Space along the dental arches was provided by stripping oval premolars and triangular incisors toward their ideal shapes. The improved fullness of the smile (compare **C and D**) is primarily due to intentional uprighting (lingual root torque placed in the archwires) of canines and posterior teeth.

much lingual crown inclination of the canines generally will disrupt the harmony of the front-to-back tooth display curve (see Fig. 3-17).

Buccal Corridors

Several studies have reported laypersons' perceptions of and reactions to the buccal corridors.[31,35,46,52,55] None found a specific relationship between this trait and smile esthetics. However, excessive buccal corridors are unesthetic to both orthodontists and laypersons.[46,55,56] Frush and Fischer[31] considered the buccal corridor to be a normal feature of a dentition that prevents the "sixty tooth smile" that is often characteristic of a denture. Apparently, the labiolingual inclination of the maxillary canine and premolars is as important as or more important than the presence or absence of dark buccal corridors for reflection of dental arch fullness (Figs. 3-19 and 3-20; see Fig. 3-18). It should be emphasized that dark shadows between the buccal surfaces of the dentition and the corners of the mouth are more apparent on frontal photographs than in real life, as they are generally due to inadequate flash lighting of the posterior areas of the mouth in routine photography.[36,37] If the pre-treatment maxillary dental arch is acceptable with regard to shape and width, it may seem preferable in terms of long-term stability to obtain smile fullness by intentionally adding buccal crown torque to lingually inclined canines and premolars during treatment (see Figs. 3-10 to 3-13 and 3-18). Maxillary lateral expansion is indicated whenever the maxillary and mandibular dental arches are notably constricted in the beginning, whether or not posterior crossbite is present. Excessive intentional lateral expansion of the dental arches is likely to introduce a disequilibrium and long-term relapse.[48,49]

The principles and considerations discussed above may be supplemented by a discussion of the optimal crown torque from an esthetic perspective for individual teeth, as follows.

Maxillary Canine

There is a very large individual variation in labiolingual inclination of the maxillary canines and premolars between patients. The patient in Figure 3-19, A and C, has a broad maxilla and marked lingual tipping of all teeth. In marked contrast, the patient in Figure 3-19, B and D, has a narrow maxillary apical base and a pronounced labial tilt of all clinical crowns. The crown torque discrepancies between these two patients demonstrate why it is unrealistic to try to produce the same orthodontic treatment result for both of them; it is also obvious that they cannot be treated to optimum esthetics using the same preadjusted bracket prescription system without marked third-order archwire bends. An individualized esthetic goal should be set for each patient before the orthodontic treatment is started. Excessive lingual tipping of the maxillary canine is undesirable for esthetic reasons, whether it occurs unilaterally or bilaterally (see Figs. 3-17 and 3-18).[52]

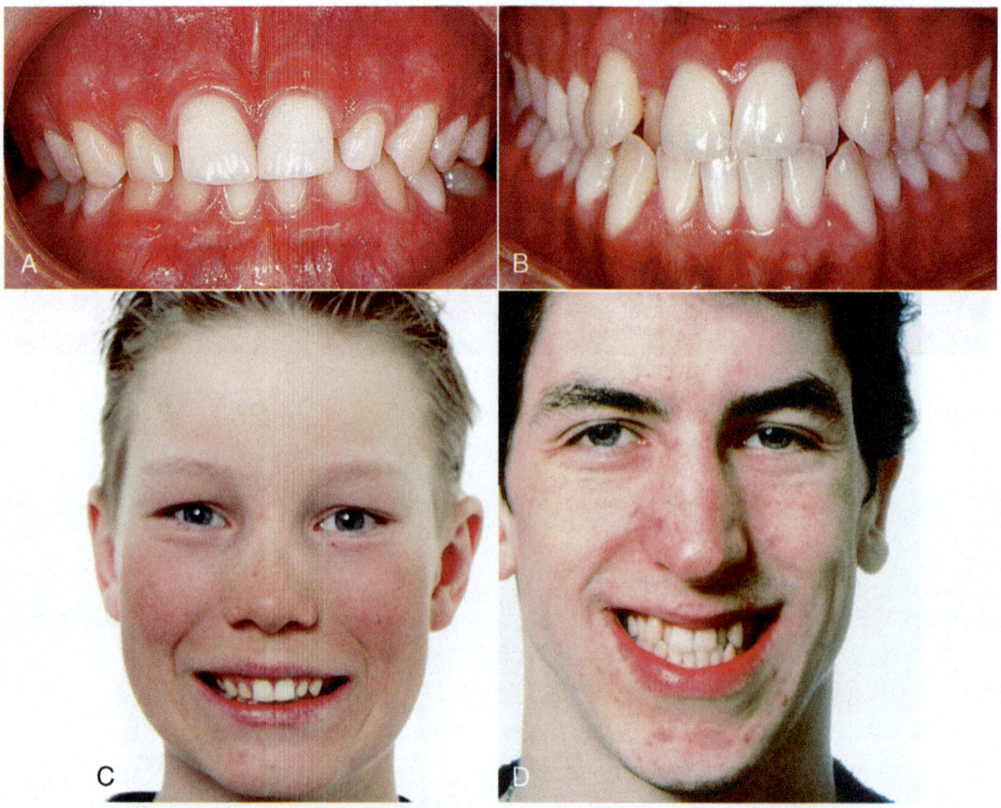

Figure 3-19 Two male patients demonstrate the wide range of individual variation in crown inclination of posterior teeth (canines through molars). **A and C,** The young boy has a large maxillary apical base with marked lingual tilt of the teeth. **B and D,** The older patient has a small maxilla, a large mandible, and labial tilt of the teeth.

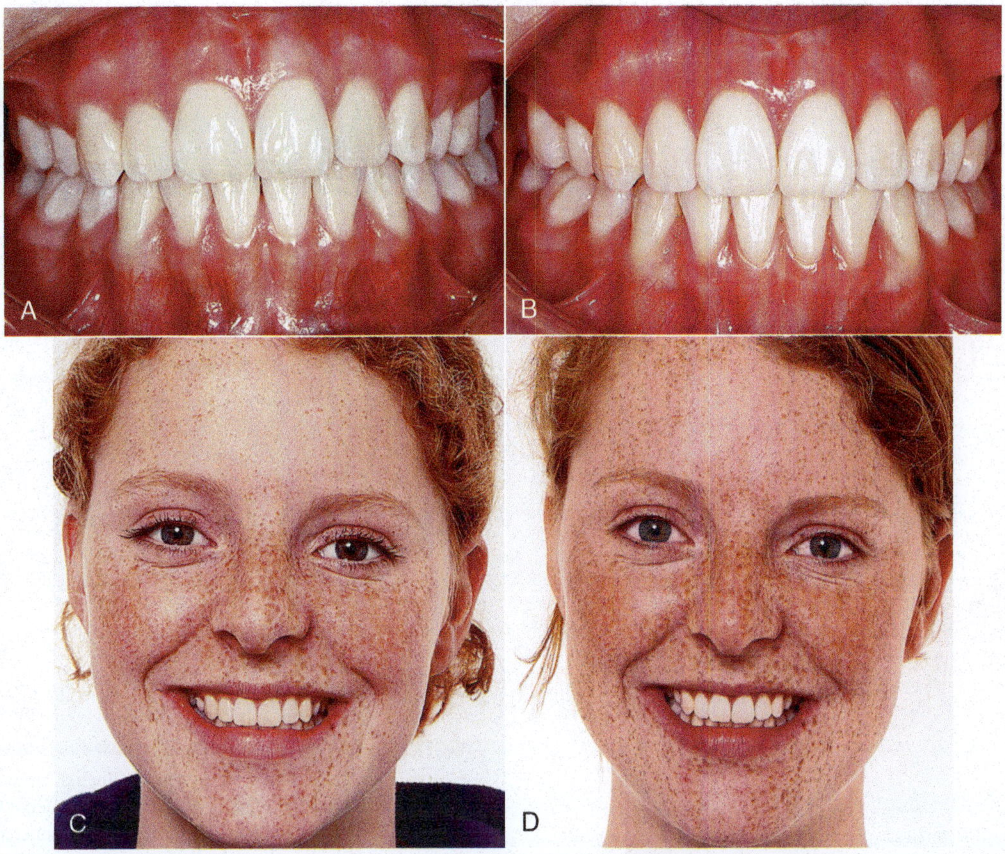

Figure 3-20 Importance of the premolar crown for fullness of the smile. A young female patient at the end of orthodontic treatment (**A and C**) and 5 years later (**B and D**). The post-treatment intraoral result may appear optimal according to the prevailing concepts (compare with Fig. 3-16, **A and C**). However, both smile photographs show that the lingually tilted premolars are almost hidden behind the upright canines. The smile is much narrower than for the patient with upright premolars in Figure 3-18, **D**.

It is surprisingly common that at the end of fixed appliance treatment, maxillary canine and premolar crowns are tipped lingually because the prescription in many modern brackets provides negative torque (lingual crown torque) for these teeth.[57,58] This affects smile esthetics negatively, especially in patients with narrow and tapered arch forms, by making the canines less prominent (see Fig. 3-17) and causing the first premolars to almost disappear on smile (see Fig. 3-20). To obtain a broader arch and more pleasing smile, the solution is not further lateral expansion across the premolars, but to use lingual root torque so that the crowns are uprighted. This gives the appearance of a broader smile without the risk of relapse that accompanies such expansion. Existing data confirm that the inclinations of these teeth remain as they were at the end of treatment.[58,59]

Uprighting the canines and premolars in this way does elongate their lingual cusps and potentially could lead to occlusal interferences that would be difficult for patients to tolerate. If this occurs (which is unlikely), reduction of the height of the lingual cusps is indicated.

To achieve symmetry of labiolingual crown inclination between the teeth on the right and left sides of the mouth, intentional individualization is needed (see Fig. 3-15). The easiest and most practical way to achieve symmetry is to carefully study each case from the front and make the necessary archwire bends early in treatment (see Fig. 3-15).

It is apparent from these and other cases that (1) the *preferred labiolingual crown inclination* of the maxillary canine *from an esthetic viewpoint* in a majority of cases *is relatively upright*[7,52] and (2) that *pre-treatment asymmetries in crown inclination between right and left canines will remain* after orthodontic therapy if no intentional measures are taken to correct them. Such adjustments may involve the use of individual archwire bends at different periods during treatment or possibly the use of custom brackets specifically engineered for the individual needs of each patient.

Maxillary First and Second Premolars

Premolars with an upright position will produce a broader smile than premolars that are tipped lingually. Particularly when orthodontic treatment has resulted in lingual tipping of the maxillary premolars behind upright canines, the smile becomes undesirably narrow in the posterior segments and does not reach an optimal fullness (see Fig. 3-20).

For this reason, the esthetically preferable first and second premolar crown torque for most patients is around 0 degrees.[7,52] For patients with a wide maxillary apical base, a few degrees of lingual crown torque may be desirable. For

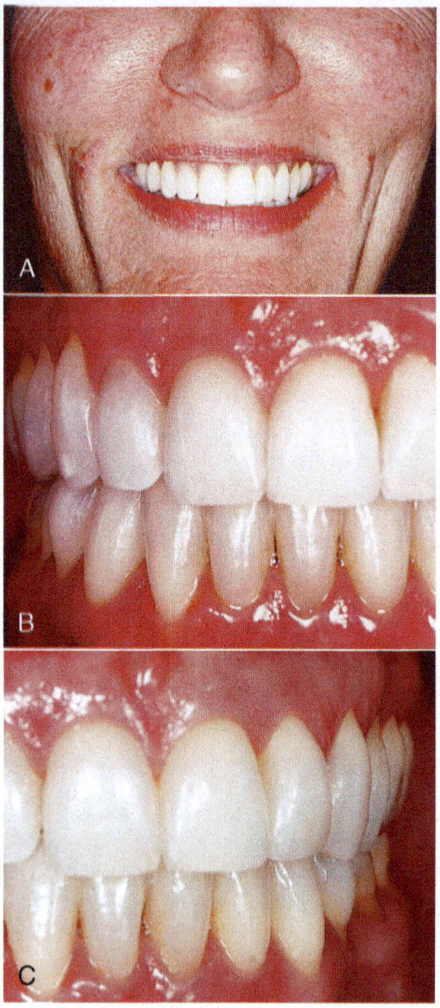

Figure 3-21 When the terminal teeth displayed in the smile are the maxillary first molars (**A**), their position should be upright to produce fullness of smile (**B and C**) (same patient as in Fig. 3-3).

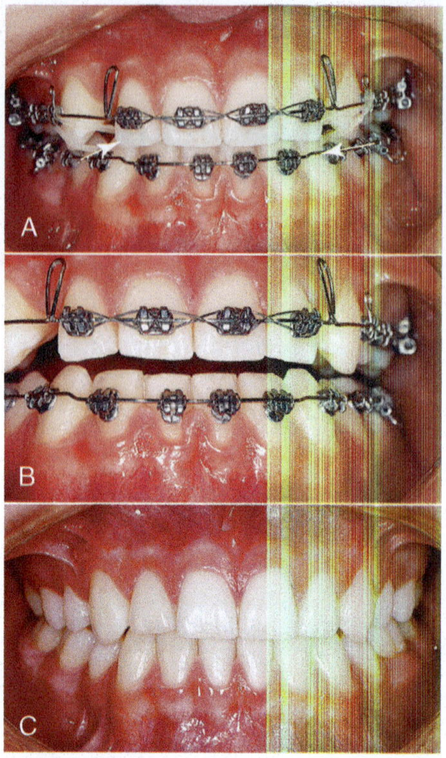

Figure 3-22 Unintentional excessive lingual tipping of mandibular canines (and premolars) during orthodontic treatment (**A and B**) is difficult and time consuming to correct and may remain undercorrected at the end of treatment (**C**). Note the right-left asymmetry of canine crown inclination throughout treatment.

patients with a small maxillary apical base, upright premolar crowns or even some labial crown inclination may produce a nice display of their dentitions (see Fig. 3-14).

Maxillary First Molar

Only a small percentage of a population show the maxillary first molars when smiling.[8] For these patients, the molars should be relatively straight to contribute to a full smile (Fig. 3-21).

Mandibular Canine

The optimal outcome of orthodontic treatment regarding the mandibular canines is to achieve (1) relatively upright positions when viewed from the front (see Figs. 3-11 and 3-21) and (2) bilateral crown inclination symmetry (see Figs. 3-9, 3-11, and 3-13). Upright rather than lingually tipped mandibular canines allow more labial crown torque of the maxillary canines, producing a broader smile. Many preadjusted prescription appliances place lingual crown torque in the mandibular canines, which appears undesirable both esthetically and functionally. Particularly when the mandibular canines are tipped lingually before orthodontic treatment is started, appliances with built-in lingual crown torque tend to produce an excessive lingual tipping of the canines (Fig. 3-22). The correction of such tipping toward the lingual is time-consuming and difficult and may remain unnoticed at the end of treatment (see Figs. 3-14 and 3-22). A mandibular canine torque prescription that induces some labial crown torque (lingual root torque) will counteract such side effects.

Mandibular Premolars and Molars

A common side effect of routine orthodontic treatment with both preadjusted and standard edgewise appliances is that the crowns of the mandibular posterior teeth tend to tip lingually.[50] This is undesirable not only from an esthetic point of view, but also for functional reasons. If the mandibular premolars and molars receive marked lingual crown torque, the lingual cusps of the maxillary posterior teeth may erupt into occlusion with their lingual cusps hanging down. This arrangement may cause balancing side interferences in side movements of the mandible. This side effect can be avoided by careful clinical observation and archwire bending and/or by using nontorqued attachments for the mandibular posterior teeth, including the second molars.

HOW TO ACHIEVE BOTH AN OPTIMAL SMILE AND DENTAL STABILITY

The available research evidence regarding long-term stability of orthodontic treatment results implies that the patient's pre-treatment mandibular intercanine width and mandibular arch form may be the optimal guide to future dental and arch form stability.[60–63]

If these measures are within a normal range, which implies that the intercanine width is around 25- to 26-mm, the mandibular incisors are in front of the A-pogonion line, and the arch form is symmetrical, with no need for transverse uprighting (buccal crown torque) of premolars and molars, then the mandible should be treated orthodontically without incisor proclination and lateral expansion (see Figs. 3-9, 3-12, 3-13, and 3-18). Mild to moderate dental crowding is managed by mesiodistal enamel reduction (stripping).

The maxillary dental arch is placed on top of and coordinated with the mandible. The original maxillary arch form is respected but frequently has to be rounded and slightly expanded posteriorly (see Fig. 3-13) to occlude properly with the mandibular teeth.[48,49] With this approach, smile fullness is sought not through lateral expansion or tipping of the maxillary dentition but rather through intentional adjustment of the labiolingual crown inclination of the maxillary canines and premolars to their most esthetic appearance (see Figs. 3-11 to 3-13).[48] Maxillary lateral expansion is indicated, however, whenever the maxillary and mandibular arches are notably constricted in the beginning, whether or not a posterior crossbite is present.

CLINICAL GUIDELINES

Vertical Dimension

The following guidelines are recommended to obtain an optimally esthetic tooth display in normal conversation and on smiling:

- Study the patient's dentition directly from the front to make a reliable esthetic evaluation. With the patient in the dental chair, move the patient's head to the side of the headrest, which allows an "eye-to-eye" perspective.
- Routinely take extraoral photographs with the lips at rest before and after treatment to record the maxillary incisor display. A short video that shows the patient speaking and smiling joyfully is helpful to record the spontaneous gingival display.
- Provide a curve of the maxillary incisors that is parallel to the inner contour of the lower lip on smiling. This is generally achieved by making the maxillary central incisors 0.5- to 1.5-mm longer than the lateral incisors.
- Avoid actively intruding the maxillary incisors when the pre-treatment vertical position is normal for the patient's age. Do not overintrude and hide the maxillary incisors behind the upper lip.
- Establish an age-appropriate vertical incisor display in rest position and normal conversation for each orthodontic patient.

Midlines

The following guidelines may be clinically useful for optimal smile design in orthodontic patients:

- A vertical line from nasion to the base of the philtrum may be the most practical guide to locate the facial midline.
- A precise dental midline coincident with the facial midline is not necessary for optimal esthetics.
- Moderate maxillary midline deviation is acceptable to most persons as long as the central incisor crown angulation is not significantly canted.
- Securing optimal connector areas between the maxillary anterior teeth according to the 50-40-30 rule is useful for esthetic smile design.
- The connector area between the two maxillary central incisors should be long (approximately half of their clinical crown lengths), vertical, and parallel to the facial midline.
- The mandibular midline is less important for esthetics.

Transverse Dimension

The most desirable and esthetic crown inclinations are not evidence-based but the following clinical recommendations are useful:

- Provide an individualized, esthetic, symmetrical labiolingual crown inclination of canines and premolars for each patient.
- Crown inclination asymmetries between contralateral canines and premolars in the right and left side of the mouth in the same patient are common. They must be (1) recognized early in treatment by studying the dentition from the front and (2) intentionally corrected by archwire torquing (or possibly by custom-made bracket torque prescriptions). Otherwise, the finished result will be asymmetrical with regard to clinical crown inclination.
- The terminal teeth shown on smiling should be straight to provide smile fullness. In about 90% of cases, the terminal teeth will be the maxillary first or second premolars.
- A smooth, gradual front-to-back tooth display curve laterally provides harmony and beauty to the treatment result. Any disruption will reduce the esthetic outcome.
- Avoid tipping the mandibular canines, premolars, and molars lingually during the orthodontic treatment.
- The secret to excellence in orthodontics is to learn to see important details in the dentition as they occur before, during, and after treatment.

SUMMARY

This chapter discussed some esthetic elements of tooth display and smile design associated with orthodontic treatment. Normative standards of the lip-incisor relationships were provided. The importance of an individual patient's display of the dentition during speech and on smiling was evaluated (1) in the vertical dimension, (2) with regard to midlines, and (3) in the transverse dimension. Multiple clinical guidelines were provided. Together, these clinical recommendations should be of value to improve the esthetic outcome of contemporary orthodontic treatment results.

REFERENCES

1. Ackerman JL, Proffit WR, Sarver DM. The emerging soft tissue paradigm in orthodontic diagnosis and treatment planning. *Clin Orth Res.* 1999;2:49–52.
2. Proffit WR. The soft tissue paradigm in orthodontic diagnosis and treatment planning: a new view for a new century. *J Esthet Dent.* 2000;12:46–49.
3. Morley J, Eubank J. Macroesthetic elements of smile design. *J Am Dent Assoc.* 2001;132:39–45.
4. Nash DA. Professional ethics and esthetic dentistry. *J Am Dent Assoc.* 1988;115:7E–9E.
5. Lombardi RE. The principles of visual perception and their clinical application to denture esthetics. *J Prosthet Dent.* 1973;29:358–382.
6. Zachrisson BU. Esthetic factors involved in anterior tooth display and the smile: vertical dimension. *J Clin Orthod.* 1998;32:432–445.
7. Zachrisson BU, Sinclair P. Master Clinician. Bjorn U. Zachrisson DDS, MSD, PHD. *J Clin Orthod.* 2012;41:531–557.
8. Tjan AHL, Miller GD, The JG. Some esthetic factors in a smile. *J Prosthet Dent.* 1984;51:24–28.
9. Desai S, Upadhyay M, Nanda R. Dynamic smile analysis: change with age. *Am J Orthod Dentofacial Orthop.* 2009;136:310.e1–310.e10.
10. Kokich VO Jr, Kiyak HA, Shapiro PA. Comparing the perception of dentists and lay people to altered dental esthetics. *J Esthet Dent.* 1999;11:311–324.
11. Van der Geld P, Oosterveld P, Schools J, Kuijpers-Jagtman AM. Smile line assessment comparing quantitative measurement and visual estimation. *Am J Orthod Dentofacial Orthop.* 2011;139:174–180.
12. Peck S, Peck L, Kataja M. Some vertical lineaments of lip position. *Am J Orthod Dentofacial Orthop.* 1992;101:519–524.
13. Peck S, Peck L, Kataja M. The gingival smile line. *Angle Orthod.* 1992;62:91–100.
14. Vig RG, Brundo GC. The kinetics of anterior tooth display. *J Prosthet Dent.* 1978;39:502–504.
15. Sarver DM. The importance of incisor positioning in the esthetic smile: the smile arc. *Am J Orthod Dentofacial Orthop.* 2001;120:98–111.
16. Sarver DM, Ackerman MB. Dynamic smile visualization and quantification: part 1. Evolution of the concept and dynamic records for smile capture. *Am J Orthod Dentofacial Orthop.* 2003;124:4–12.
17. Mack MR. Vertical dimension: a dynamic concept based on facial form and oropharyngeal function. *J Prosth Dent.* 1991;66:478–485.
18. Mack MR. Perspective of facial esthetics in dental treatment planning. *J Prosth Dent.* 1996;75:169–176.
19. Dong JK, Jin TH, Cho HW, Oh SC. The esthetics of the smile: a review of some recent studies. *Int J Prosthodont.* 1999;12:9–19.
20. Van der Geld P, Oosterveld P, Berge SJ, Kuijpers-Jagtman AM. Tooth display and lip position during spontaneous and posed smiling in adults. *Acta Odont Scand.* 2008;66:207–213.
21. Van der Geld P, Oosterveld P, Kuijpers-Jagtman AM. Age-related changes of the dental aesthetic zone at rest and during spontaneous smiling and speech. *Europ J Orthod.* 2008;30:366–373.
22. Rubin LR. The anatomy of a smile: its importance in the treatment of facial paralysis. *Plast Reconstr Surg.* 1974;53:384–387.
23. Peck S, Peck H. The aesthetically pleasing face: an orthodontic myth. *Trans Eur Orthod Soc.* 1971;47:175–185.
24. Rosen HM, Ackerman JL. Porous block hydroxyapatite in orthognathic surgery. *Angle Orthod.* 1991;61:185–191.
25. Turley PK. Orthodontic management of the short face patient. *Semin Orthod.* 1996;2:138–152.
26. Spear FM, Kokich VG, Mathews DP. Interdisciplinary management of anterior dental esthetics. *J Am Dent Assoc.* 2006;137:160–169.
27. Burstone CJ, Nanda R. JCO interviews Charles J. Burstone DDS, MS. part 1 facial esthetics. *J Clin Orthod.* 2007;41:79–87.
28. Zachrisson BU. Mechanical intrusion of maxillary incisors: a treatment strategy to be abandoned? *World J Orthod.* 2002;3:358–364.
29. Shroff B, Yoon WM, Lindauer SJ, Burstone CJ. Simultaneous intrusion and retraction using a three-piece base arch. *Angle Orthod.* 1997;67:455–462.
30. Lindauer SJ, Lewis SM, Shroff B. Overbite correction and smile aesthetics. *Semin Orthod.* 2005;11:62–66.
31. Frush JP, Fisher RD. The dynesthetic interpretation of the dentogenic concept. *J Prosthet Dent.* 1958;8:558–581.
32. Weiland FJ, Bantleon HP, Droschl H. Evaluation of continuous arch and segmented arch leveling techniques in adult patients: a clinical study. *Am J Orthod Dentofacial Orthop.* 1996;110:647–652.
33. AlQabandi A, Sadowsky C, Sellke T. A comparison of continuous archwire and utility archwires for leveling the curve of Spee. *World J Orthod.* 2002;3:159–165.
34. Simons ME, Joondeph DR. Change in overbite: a ten-year postretention study. *Am J Orthod.* 1973;64:349–367.
35. Hulsey CM. An esthetic evaluation of lip-teeth relationships present in the smile. *Am J Orthod.* 1970;57:132–144.
36. Ackerman JL, Ackerman MB, Brensinger CM, Landis JR. A morphometric analysis of the posed smile. *Clin Orth Res.* 1998;1:2–11.
37. Ackerman MB, Ackerman JL. Smile analysis and design in the digital era. *J Clin Orthod.* 2002;36:221–236.
38. Brisman AS. Esthetics: a comparison of dentists' and patient's concepts. *J Am Dent Assoc.* 1991;100:345–352.
39. Kokich VG. Esthetics: the orthodontic-periodontic-restorative connection. *Semin Orthod.* 1996;2:21–30.
40. Garber DA, Salama MA. The aesthetic smile: diagnosis and treatment. *Periodontol 2000.* 1996;11:18–28.
41. Brägger U, Lauchenauer D, Lang NP. Surgical lengthening of the clinical crown. *J Clin Periodontol.* 1992;19:58–63.
42. Polo M. Botulum toxin type A (Botox) for the neuromuscular correction of excessive gingival display on smiling (gummy smile). *Am J Orthod Dentofacial Orthop.* 2008;133:1955–2003.
43. Zachrisson BU. Dental to facial midline positions. *World J Orthod.* 2001;2:266–269.
44. Beyer JW, Lindauer SJ. Evaluation of dental midline position. *Semin Orthod.* 1998;4:146–152.
45. Johnston CD, Burden DJ, Stevenson MR. The influence of dental to facial midline discrepancies on dental attractiveness ratings. *Eur J Orthod.* 1999;21:517–522.
46. Springer NC, Chang C, Fields HW, et al. Smile esthetics from the layperson's perspective. *Am J Orthod Dentofacial Orthop.* 2011;139:e91–e101.
47. Tarnow DP, Magner AW, Fletcher P. The effect of the distance from the contact point to the crest of bone on the presence or absence of the interproximal dental papilla. *J Periodontol.* 1992;63:995–996.
48. Zachrisson BU. Making the premolar extraction smile full and radiant. *World J Orthod.* 2002;3:260–265.
49. Zachrisson BU. Maxillary expansion: long-term stability and smile esthetics. *World J Orthod.* 2001;2:266–272.
50. Ugur T, Yukay F. Normal faciolingual inclinations of tooth crowns compared with treatment groups of standard and pretorqued brackets. *Am J Orthod Dentofacial Orthop.* 1997;112:50–57.
51. Andrews LF. The six keys to normal occlusion. *Am J Orthod.* 1972;62:296–309.
52. Ker AJ, Chan R, Fields HW, Beck M, Rosenstiel S. Esthetics and smile characteristics from the layperson's perspective: a computer-based survey study. *J Am Dent Assoc.* 2008;139:1318–1327 (including online-only supplemental data).
53. Ricketts RE. The biologic significance of the divine proportion. *Am J Orthod.* 1982;81:351–370.
54. Preston JD. The golden proportion revisited. *J Esthet Dent.* 1993;5:247–251.
55. Martin AJ, Buschang PH, Boley JC, Taylor RW, McKinney TW. The impact of buccal corridors on smile attractiveness. *Europ J Orthod.* 2007;29:530–537.

56. Ioi H, Kang S, Shimomura T, et al. Effects of buccal corridors on smile esthetics in Japanese and Korean orthodontists and orthodontic patients. *Am J Orthod Dentofacial Orthop*. 2012;142:459–465.
57. Zachrisson BU. Facial esthetics: guide to tooth positioning and maxillary incisor display. *World J Orthod*. 2007;8:190–196.
58. Zachrisson BU. Proper quality orthodontics vs the new mechanical "systems." *World J Orthod*. 2007;8:412–419.
59. Zachrisson BU. Buccal uprighting of canines and premolars for improved smile esthetics and stability. *World J Orthod*. 2006;7:406–412.
60. Little RM, Wallen TR, Riedel RA. Stability and relapse of mandibular anterior alignment: first premolar extraction cases treated by traditional edgewise orthodontics. *Am J Orthod*. 1981;80:349–365.
61. Little RM, Riedel RA, Årtun J. An evaluation of changes in mandibular anterior alignment from 10 to 20 years postretention. *Am J Orthod Dentofacial Orthop*. 1988;93:423–428.
62. Felton JM, Sinclair PM, Jones DL, Alexander RG. A computerized analysis of the shape and stability of mandibular arch form. *Am J Orthod Dentofacial Orthop*. 1987;92:478–483.
63. Dyer KC, Vaden JL, Harris EF. Relapse revisited—again. *Am J Orthod Dentofacial Orthop*. 2012;142:221–227.

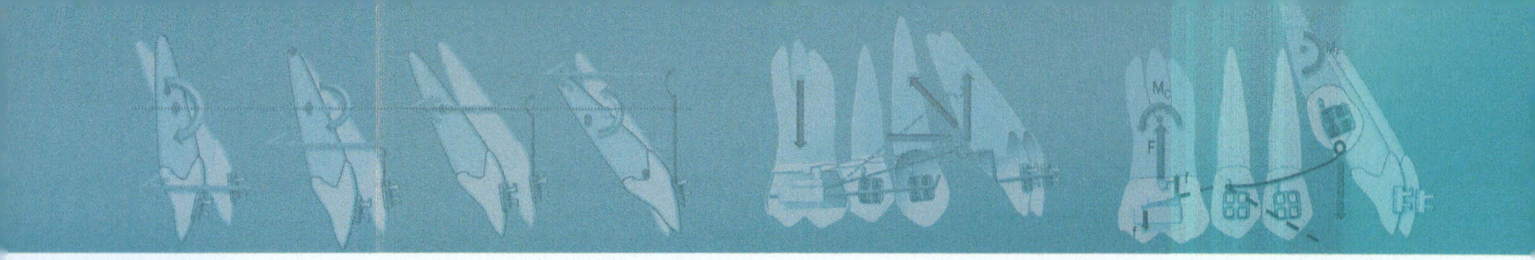

CHAPTER 4

Biomechanics in Orthodontics

Madhur Upadhyay and Ravindra Nanda

The physical concepts that form the foundation of orthodontic mechanics are the key to understanding how orthodontic appliances work and are critical in designing treatment methodologies and appliances. These physical concepts are not unique to orthodontics but are the elementary laws of mechanics in general. In this chapter we outline the ground rules and fundamentals that guide orthodontic tooth movement. All appliance systems reported in the past and all systems that will be reported in the future will use these principles of mechanics. However, let us start from the beginning: What does the word "mechanics" mean?

Mechanics can be defined as a branch of physics concerned with the mechanical aspects of any system. This can be divided into two categories: statics, the study of factors associated with nonmoving (rigid) systems, and dynamics, the study of factors associated with systems in motion, such as a moving car or a plane. When the knowledge and methods of mechanics are applied to the structure and function of living systems (biology)—for example, a tooth and its surrounding oral architecture—it is called biomechanics. It is our belief that the study of biomechanics of tooth movement can help researchers and clinicians to optimize their force systems applied on teeth to get better responses at the clinical, tissue, cellular, or molecular level of tooth movement.

APPROACHES TO STUDYING TOOTH MOVEMENT

Two approaches are used to study the biological and mechanical aspects of tooth movement: a quantitative approach and a qualitative approach. The quantitative approach involves describing movement of teeth or the associated skeletal structures in numerical terms. We all are familiar with terms such as 3-mm of canine retraction or 15 degrees of incisor flaring. Merely describing tooth movement quantitatively does not describe the complete nature of the movement. It is also important to understand the type or nature of tooth movement that has occurred. A qualitative approach describes movement in nonnumerical terms (i.e., without measuring or counting any parts of the performance). This approach is often followed at the clinical level or inferred from x-rays and/or stone models such as tipping and translation.

Both qualitative and quantitative analyses provide valuable information about a performance. However, a qualitative assessment is the predominant method used by orthodontists to analyze tooth movement. The impressions gained from a qualitative analysis may be substantiated with quantitative data and many hypotheses for research projects are formulated in such a manner.

BASIC MECHANICAL CONCEPTS

System and Frame of Reference

The concepts related to the movement of teeth to a large degree rest firmly on some fundamental principles of physical mechanics, which deals with analyzing the action of forces on bodies. A first step in examining any type of movement is to first identify the system. A system is a body or group of bodies or objects whose motion is to be examined; it might be a ball, a car, or a tooth. We also need to identify a frame of reference within which a system's movement takes place. This can be either the stationary environment or something that is also moving. Using a stationary frame of reference is least complicated. For example, the movement of teeth can be described in relation to the stable skeletal structures of the head and face, as is done quite routinely with cephalometric superimpositions. On the other hand, moving reference frames can also be used. An example would be intrusion of incisors (Fig. 4-1). Here, careful attention should be given to choosing the reference frame for measuring intrusion. Do you want to measure the movement of teeth relative to each other, to some other structure in the craniofacial complex, or to an outside external reference frame?

Establishing a Frame of Reference

The simplest and the most intuitive way of identifying direction of tooth movement is to create planes or axes of measurement according to the relationship of teeth to the ground.

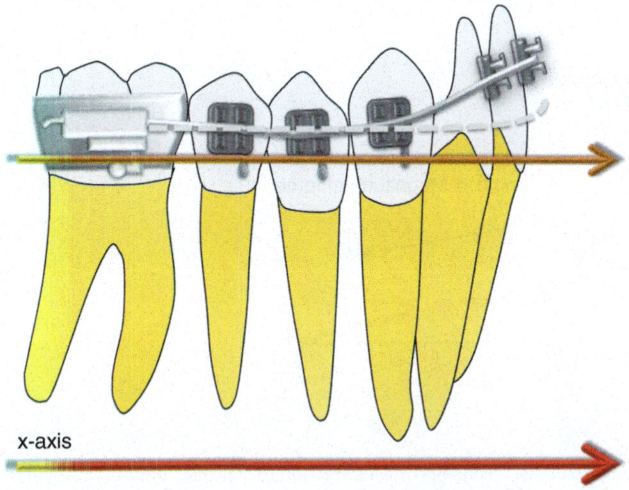

Figure 4-1 The amount of intrusion of the incisors can be measured using two different methods. Method 1: The reference frame chosen is the posterior teeth, indicated by the orange axis. During intrusion of the incisor the posterior teeth will not remain stationary and will show some movement (i.e., the reference frame itself will move). Therefore any measurement made on the incisor will provide information relative to the posterior teeth, not the "absolute" movement of incisors. Method 2: A reference frame outside the system is chosen, indicated by the red axis. This reference frame is not included in the system and is therefore free of any type of movement.

The axes or planes of measurement are then identified as spatial. Any plane or axis that is parallel to the ground is identified as a horizontal plane or axis. Any plane or axis that is perpendicular to the ground is identified as a vertical plane or axis. The two axes that are perpendicular to each other but parallel to the ground are designated as the x and y axes. The x axis is parallel to the ground and directed forward and backward relative to the object of measurement. Forward is designated as positive (+) and backward is designated as negative (–). The y axis is directed left and right relative to the object of measurement. The left direction is designated as positive and the right direction is designated as negative. The third axis, which is perpendicular to the other two, is vertical and is designated as the z axis. The upward direction is positive and the downward direction is negative. These three axes (x, y, and z) are used to describe the location of a tooth or a system under study and the direction of movement. The spatial axes do not change with the body or object changing orientations in space. They are fixed relative to the ground and the observer (Fig. 4-2).

Force

The role of force in everyday life is a familiar one. Indeed it seems almost superfluous to try to define such a self-evident concept as force. To put it in a simple way, force can be thought of as a measure of the push or pull on an object. However, from our perspective, such a simplistic definition is not good enough. The study of the mechanics of tooth movement demands a precise definition of force. So, what is force? A force is something that causes or tends to cause a change in motion or shape of an object or body. In other words, force causes an object to accelerate or decelerate. It is measured in Newtons (N) but in orthodontics force is nearly always measured in grams (g).

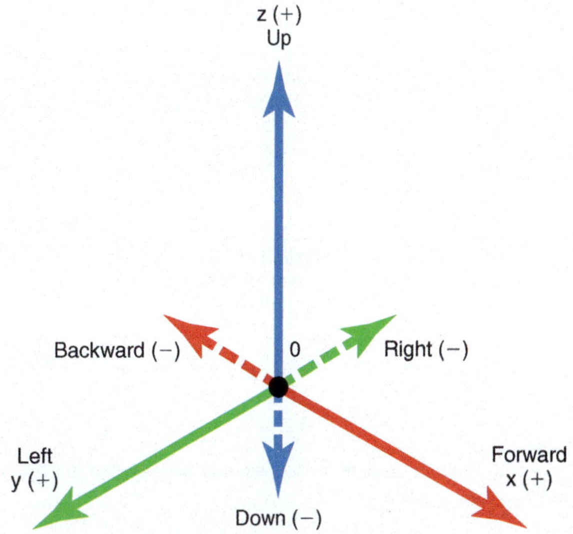

Figure 4-2 The three spatial axes used to orient any system in three-dimensional (3D) space.

$$1\ \text{N} = 101.9\ \text{g}\ (\approx 102\ \text{g})$$

Force has four unique properties, as shown in the graphic representation of a force acting at an angle to a central incisor in Figure 4-3:

- Magnitude: The "amount" of force being applied (e.g., 1 N, 2 N, 5N).
- Direction: The way the force is being applied or its orientation to the object (e.g., forward, upward, backward).
- Point of application: Where the force is applied on the body or system receiving it (e.g., in the center, at the bottom, at the top).
- Line of action of force: This is a straight line constructed in the same plane and in the direction of force extending through the point of application.

Force Diagrams and Vectors

Physical properties (such as distance, weight, temperature, and force) are treated mathematically as either scalars or vectors. Scalars, including temperature and weight, do not have a direction and are completely described by their magnitude. Vectors, on the other hand, have both magnitude and direction. Forces may be represented by vectors.

To move a tooth predictably, a force must be applied with an optimal magnitude, in the desired direction, and at the correct point on the tooth. Changing any of the four properties, discussed above, will affect the quality of tooth displacement. A force may be represented on paper by an arrow. Each of its four properties may be represented by the arrow whose length is drawn to a scale selected to represent the magnitude of the force—for example, 1-cm = 1 N or 2-cm = 2 N (Fig. 4-4). The arrow is drawn to point in the direction in which the force is applied and the tail of the arrow is placed at the point of force application. The line of action of

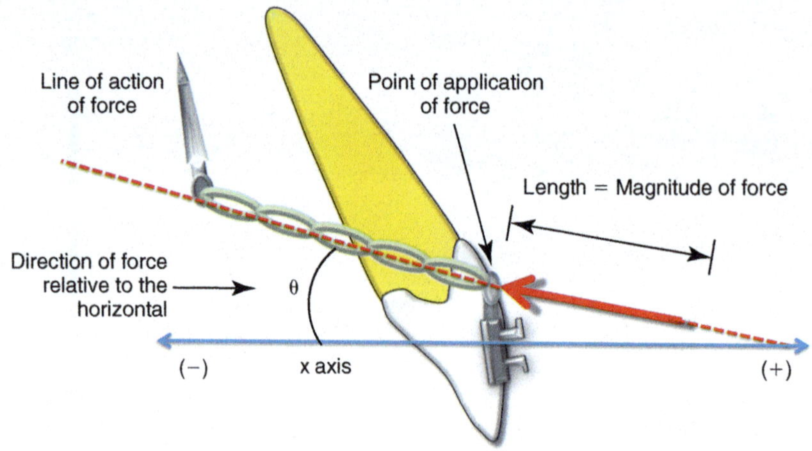

Figure 4-3 The four properties of an external force applied to a tooth illustrated by an elastic chain applying a retraction (distalizing) force on a maxillary incisor to a mini-implant.

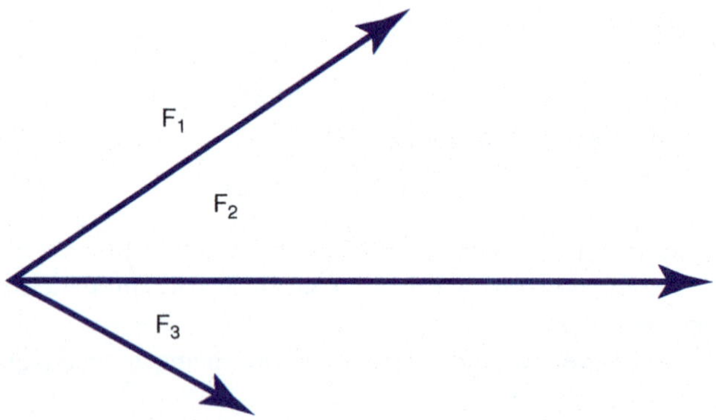

Figure 4-4 The length of the force vector describes the magnitude of the force vector. Example: $F_1 = 2$ N, $F_2 = 3$ N, $F_3 = 1$ N.

the force may be imagined as continuing indefinitely in both directions (head and tail ends), although the actual arrow, if drawn to scale, must remain a given length. A graphic representation of a force of 1 N acting at an angle of 30 degrees to a central incisor is shown in Figure 4-3.

Principle of Transmissibility

The principle of transmissibility is very important in vector mechanics, especially in understanding equilibrium and equivalent force systems, as we will see later. It implies that a force acting on a rigid body results in the same behavior regardless of the point of application of the force vector as long as the force is applied along the same line of action.

The Effect of Two or More Forces on a System: Vector Addition

Teeth are often acted upon by more than one force. The net effect or the resultant of multiple forces acting on a system, in this case teeth, can be determined by combining all of the force vectors. This process of combining all of the forces may be found by a geometric rule called vector addition, or vector composition. We place the vectors head to tail, maintaining their magnitudes and directions, and the resultant is the vector drawn from the tail of the first vector to the head of

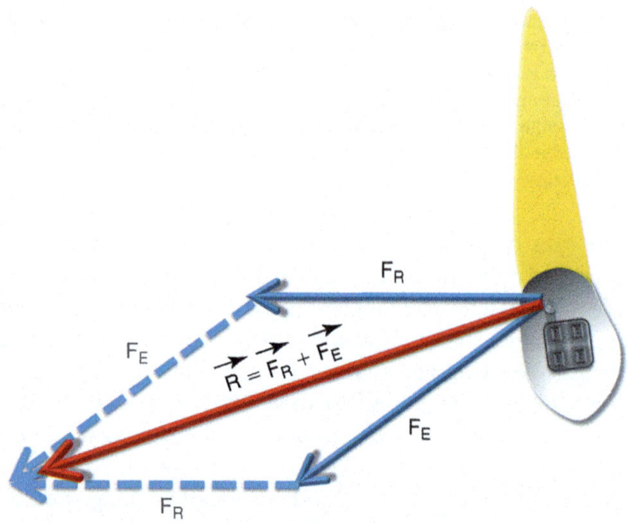

Figure 4-5 The law of vector addition by the parallelogram method. F_R can be thought of as a retractive force on the incisor and F_E as a force from a Class II elastic. The net effect of the two forces is represented by the resultant R.

the final vector. Vector addition can be accomplished graphically by drawing diagrams to scale and measuring or by using trigonometry.

Figure 4-5 shows how the two forces are visualized as two sides of a parallelogram and how the opposite sides are then drawn to form the whole parallelogram. The resultant force, R, is represented by the diagonal that is drawn from the corner of the parallelogram formed by the tails of the two force vectors.

The Directional Effects of Force: Vector Resolution

Often an occasion arises in which the observed movement of a system or a single force acting on a system will be analyzed in terms of identifying its component directions. In such cases the single vector quantity given is divided into two components: a horizontal component and a vertical component. The directions of these components are relative to some reference frame, such as the occlusal plane or the Frankfort horizontal (FH) plane, or to some axis in the system itself. The horizontal and vertical components are usually perpendicular to each other. Such a process may be thought of as the reverse of the process of vector composition. The operation is called vector resolution and is the method used to determine two component vectors that form the one vector given initially.

For example, a mini-implant as shown in Figure 4-6, A is being used for retraction of anterior teeth. It may be useful to resolve this force into the components that are parallel and perpendicular to the occlusal plane, in order to determine the magnitude of force in each of these directions. Resolution consists of three steps (see Fig. 4-6, B and C): (1) draw the vector given initially to a selected scale, (2) from the tail of the vector, draw lines representing the desired directions of the two perpendicular components, and (3) from the head of the vector, draw lines parallel to each of the two direction lines so that a rectangle is formed. Note that the new parallel lines constructed have the same magnitude and direction as the corresponding lines on the opposite side of the rectangle.

It is important to note that if it is desirable to estimate the magnitude of the components, simple trigonometric rules can be invoked to do so. In particular, the sine and cosine are very useful in finding the horizontal and vertical components of the force vector. In this case if, for example, the horizontal component of magnitude (F_H) makes an angle (θ) with the force (F), we can derive the components using the definitions of sine and cosine:

$$\text{Horizontal component } (F_H): F_H / F = \cos\theta;\ F_H = F\cos\theta$$

$$\text{Vertical component } (F_V): F_V / F = \sin\theta;\ F_V = F\sin\theta$$

With a little practice, it is easy to get the component directly as a product, skipping the step involving the proportion. Think of sin θ and cos θ as fractions that are used to calculate the sides of a right triangle when the hypotenuse is known. The side is always less than the hypotenuse and the sine and cosine are always less than 1. To get the side opposite the angle, simply multiply the hypotenuse by the sine of the angle. To get the side adjacent to the angle, multiply the hypotenuse by the cosine of the angle.

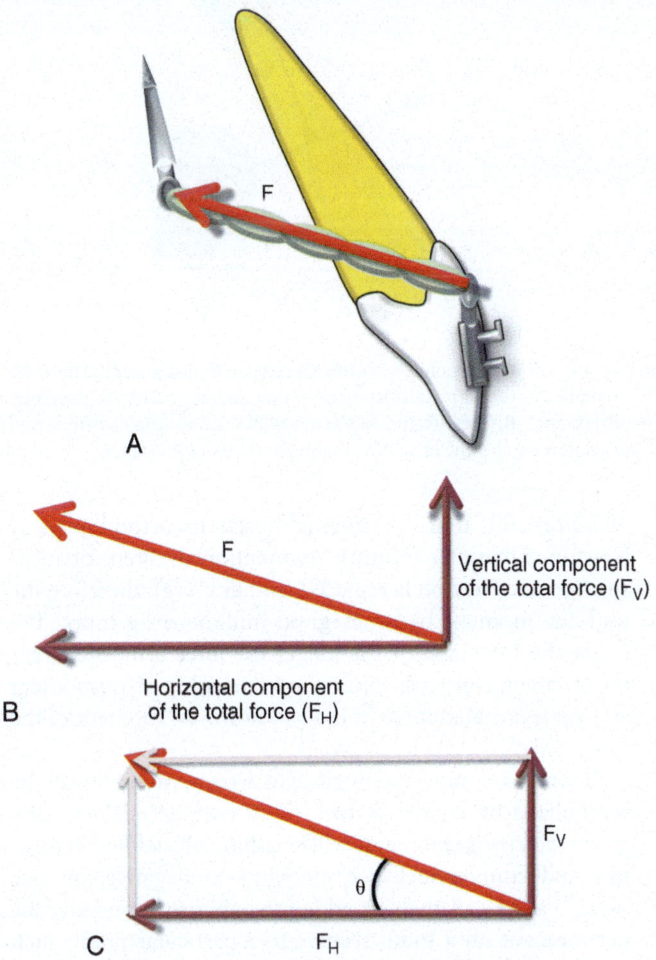

Figure 4-6 The process of vector resolution. F = force.

CENTER OF RESISTANCE, CENTER OF GRAVITY, AND CENTER OF MASS

Once a force is applied to a body, its nature of motion is regulated to a large extent by its center of mass. The center of mass of a body may be thought of as that point at which all of the body's mass seems to be concentrated (i.e., if a force is applied through this point, the system or body will move in a straight line). On similar lines recall that the earth exerts a force on each segment of a system in direct proportion to each segment's mass. The total effect of the force of gravity on a whole body, or system, is as if the force of gravity were concentrated at a single point called the center of gravity. Again, if a force is applied through this point, it will cause the body to move in a straight line without any rotation. The difference between the center of mass and the center of gravity is that the system in question in the latter is a "restrained system" (restrained by the force of gravity).

Teeth are part of a restrained system. Besides gravity they are more dominantly restrained by periodontal structures that are not uniform (involving the root but not the crown) around the tooth. Therefore the center of mass or the center of gravity will not yield a straight line motion if a force is applied through it because the surrounding structures and their composition alter this point. A new point analogous to the center of gravity is required to yield a straight line motion; this is called the center of resistance (C_{RES}) of the tooth (Fig. 4-7).

The center of resistance can also be defined by its relationship to the force: a force for which the line of action passes through the center of resistance producing a movement of pure translation. It must be noted that, for a given tooth, this movement may be mesiodistal or vestibulolingual, intrusive or extrusive. The position of the center of resistance is directly dependent on what may be called the "clinical root" of the tooth. This concept takes into account the root volume, including the periodontal bone (i.e., the distance between the alveolar crest and the apex), incrementing this value with the thickness (i.e., the surface) of the root.[1]

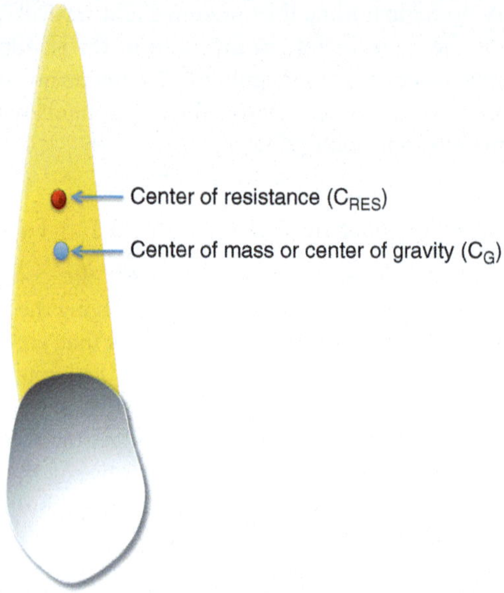

Figure 4-7 The C_{RES} of a tooth is usually located slightly apical to the C_G. The periodontal structures surrounding the tooth root cause this apical migration of the C_{RES}.

Thus the position of the center of resistance is also a function of the nature of the periodontal structures and the density of the alveolar bone and the elasticity of the desmodontal structures, which are strongly related to the patient's age.[2–4] These considerations implore us to speak of the "center of resistance associated with the tooth" rather than "the center of resistance of the tooth."

Moment (Torque)

When an external force acts on a body at its center of gravity (C_G) it causes that body to move in a linear path. This type of force, with its line of action through the C_G or C_{RES}, is called a centric force. On similar lines eccentric forces (off-center forces) act away from the C_{RES} of a body. What kind of effect will these forces have? Besides causing the body to move in a linear path, the eccentric force will have a turning effect on the body called torque; in other words, the force will also impart a "moment" on the body. The off-axis distance of the force's line of action is called the force arm (or sometimes the moment arm, lever arm, or torque arm). The greater this distance, the greater the torque produced by the force. The specifications of the force arm are critical. The force arm is the shortest distance from the axis of rotation to the line of action of force. Invariably the shortest distance is always the length of the line that is perpendicular (90 degrees) to the force's line of action ($d_\perp$). The symbol $\perp$ designates perpendicular. Force arm is critical in determining the amount of moment acting on the system.

The amount of moment (M) acting to rotate a system is found by multiplying the magnitude of the applied force (F) by the force arm distance ($d_\perp$):

$M = F\,(d_\perp)$, where F is measured in Newtons and $d_\perp$ is measured in millimeters (Fig. 4-8, A).

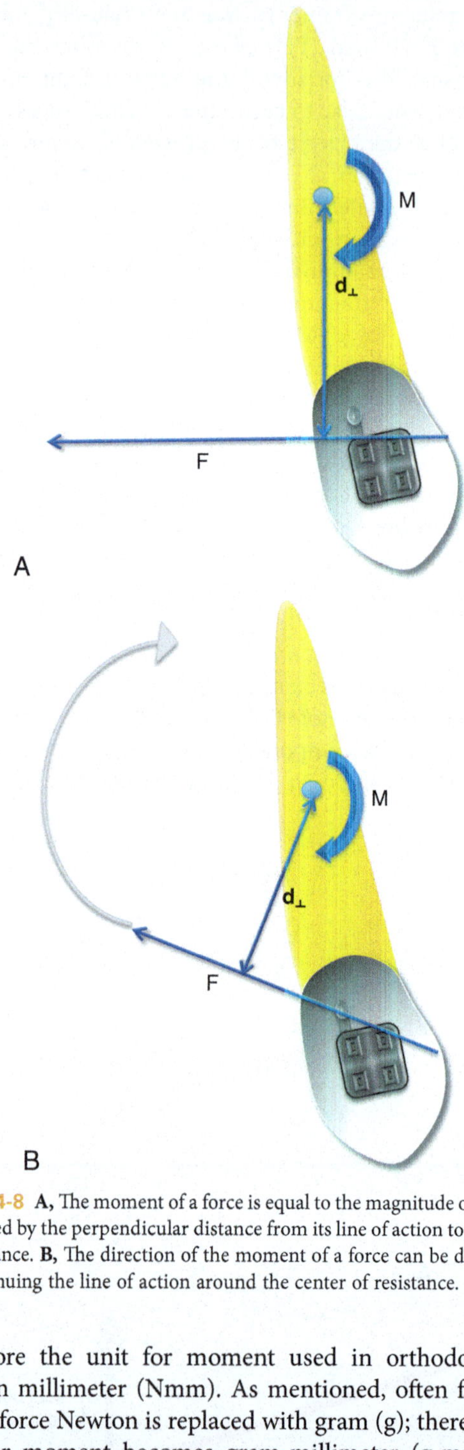

Figure 4-8 **A,** The moment of a force is equal to the magnitude of the force multiplied by the perpendicular distance from its line of action to the center of resistance. **B,** The direction of the moment of a force can be determined by continuing the line of action around the center of resistance.

Therefore the unit for moment used in orthodontics is Newton millimeter (Nmm). As mentioned, often for measuring force Newton is replaced with gram (g); therefore the unit for moment becomes gram-millimeter (g-mm). The larger the force and/or the longer the force arm, the larger the moment. Due to this intrinsic relationship of the moment and the associated force, it is also known as "moment of the force" (M_F).

If forces are indicated by straight arrows, moments can be symbolized by curved arrows. With two-dimensional diagrams, clockwise moments will be arbitrarily defined as positive and counterclockwise moments as negative, or vice versa. Values can then be added together to determine the net moment on a tooth relative to a particular point, such as the center of resistance. Point of application and line of

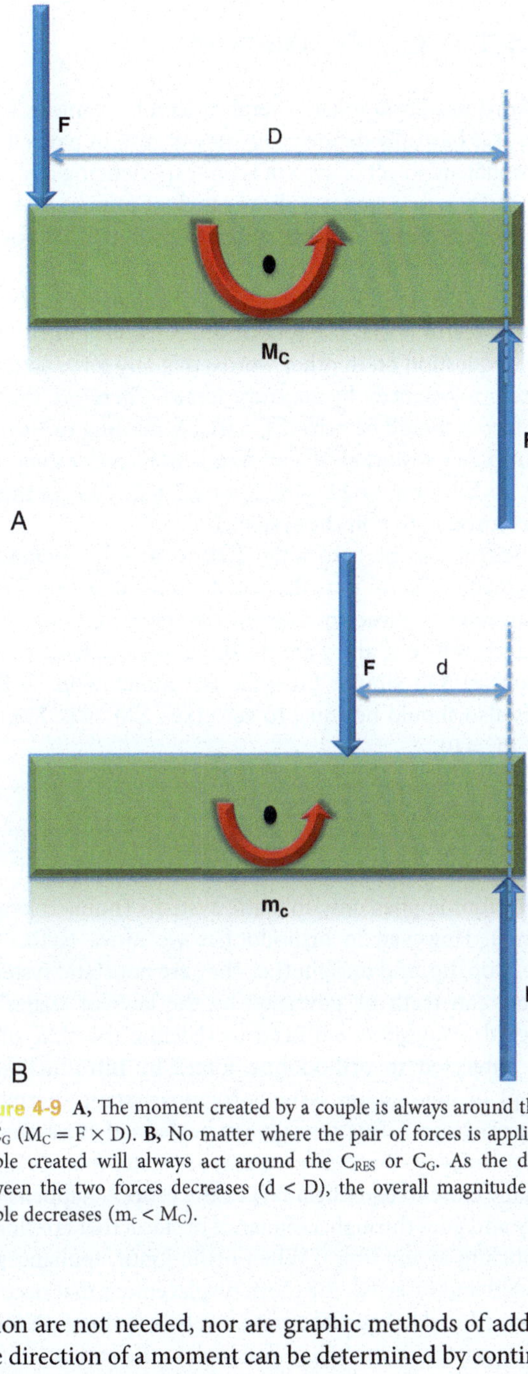

Figure 4-9 **A,** The moment created by a couple is always around the C_{RES} or C_G ($M_C = F \times D$). **B,** No matter where the pair of forces is applied, the couple created will always act around the C_{RES} or C_G. As the distance between the two forces decreases ($d < D$), the overall magnitude of the couple decreases ($m_c < M_C$).

action are not needed, nor are graphic methods of addition. The direction of a moment can be determined by continuing the line of action of the force around the center of resistance, as shown in Figure 4-8, B.

Couple (A Type of Moment)

A couple is a form of moment. It is created by a pair of forces that have equal magnitudes but opposite sense (direction) to one another with noncoincidental line of action (parallel forces). Because the forces have the same magnitude but are oppositely directed, the net potential of this special force system to translate the body upon which it acts is nil and there is only rotation.

A typical couple is shown in Figure 4-9. Although the couple's vector representation is shown midway between the two forces, the vector has no particular line-of-action

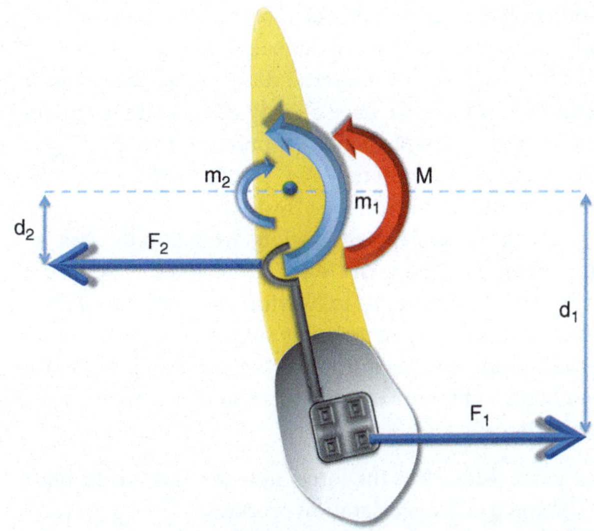

Figure 4-10 A couple created by two equal and opposite forces acting on a tooth. The total moment (M) is the vector addition of the two moments (m_1, m_2) generated by the two forces (F_1, F_2). Here, $m_1 = F_1 \times d_1$, $m_2 = F_2 \times d_2$. Because the two moments are in the opposite direction, one of the moments will be assigned a negative sign and the other a positive sign. The net moment (M) will be obtained by adding the two: $M = m_1 + (-m_2)$.

location and may be drawn through any point of the plane of the couple. Therefore a couple is also known as a "free vector." This freedom associated with the couple vector has far-reaching implications in clinical orthodontics and to certain force analysis procedures. As an example, no matter where a bracket is placed on a tooth, a couple applied at that bracket can only cause the tooth to feel a tendency to rotate around its center of resistance. This is also referred to as the moment of the couple (M_C).

The magnitude of the couple (M_C) is dependent on both force magnitude and distance between the two forces. The moment created by a couple is actually the sum of the moments created by each of the two forces. If the two forces of the couple act on opposite sides of the center of resistance, their effect to create a moment is additive. If they act on the same side of the center of resistance, they are subtractive (Fig. 4-10). Either way, no net force is felt by the tooth, only a tendency to undergo pure rotation.

EQUILIBRIUM AND NEWTON'S LAWS

No object is ever acted on by a single force. The essential factor causing acceleration is the net force, which is the resultant force or unbalanced force. For instance, if two equal and opposite forces act on a body, there is no net force to cause acceleration and the body's velocity remains constant. This condition of constant velocity or no velocity (rest) is called equilibrium. For example, the teeth in the mouth are at rest; they are not moving at all or rather they are at equilibrium (i.e., the sum of all forces acting on the teeth is zero). This brings us to a very important law in mechanics: Newton's First Law of Motion, often called the law of inertia. According to this law, a body or object remains at rest or, if in motion, remains in uniform motion with constant speed, unless it is acted on by a net unbalanced external force. This First Law is, of course, merely a statement of the quantitative definition of force we have already given and recognizes an essential property of matter. In practical use the First Law fully justifies the inherent rest position of a tooth or the inertia of the tooth, which is "rest."

To extend the laws of motion, we naturally seek a law describing what happens when a net force is applied to a body. And this brings us to Newton's Second Law of Motion, which states that if an object is subjected to an unbalanced system of forces, the object will be accelerated in the direction of the net force exerted. In its simplified version this can be written as:

$F = ma$, where F is the force, m is the mass of the body, and a is the acceleration produced

We can immediately see that the First Law is simply a special case of the Second Law (i.e., if the net force acting on a body is zero, then the acceleration is automatically zero).

Newton's Third Law of Motion (Action and Reaction) is directly related to what is done in day-to-day orthodontics. According to this law, forces always occur in pairs. Any time a wire puts a force on a bracket, the bracket puts the same force on the wire (Fig. 4-11). When swimming, a person interacts with the water, pushing the water backward while the water simultaneously pushes the person forward; both the person and the water push against each other. Facts such as these can be summarized as follows: Whenever one body exerts a force on a second body, the second body exerts a force on the first body; these forces are equal in magnitude and oppositely directed. Newton called these paired forces action and reaction. It is essential to understand that the two forces act on different bodies and hence cannot add up to zero.

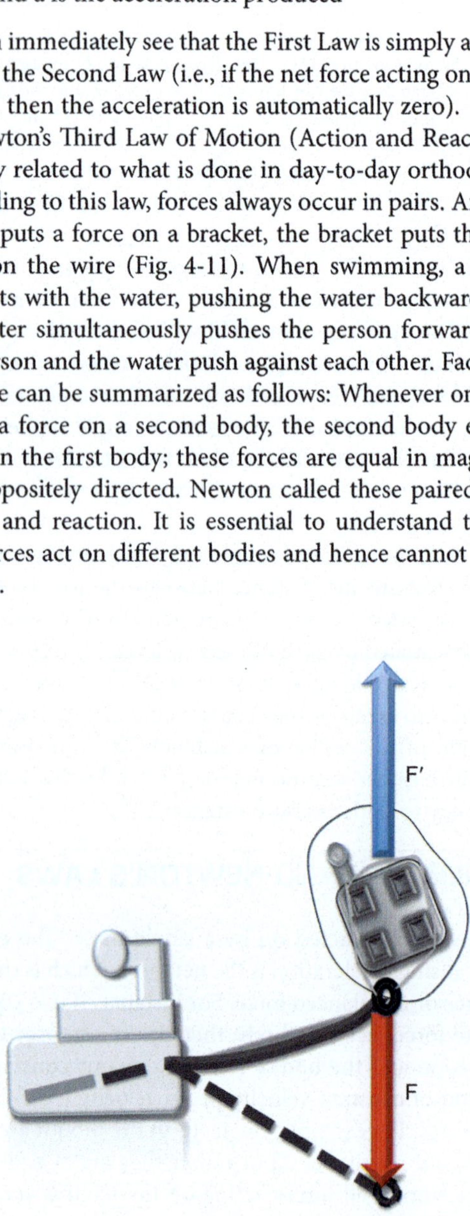

Figure 4-11 A cantilever spring exerting a force (F) on the bracket (*in red*). Per Newton's Third Law of Motion, the bracket will put an equal and opposite force (F′) on the cantilever wire (*in blue*).

CONCEPT OF EQUILIBRIUM

The word *equilibrium* has several different meanings but in statics it is basically defined as a state of rest; in particular, it means that an object or system is not experiencing any acceleration. Therefore statics is that branch of physics that deals with the mechanics of nonaccelerating objects or, for our convenience and understanding, "nonmoving" objects. Such a system is said to be in equilibrium. To achieve equilibrium, we must see to it that no unbalanced force is applied to the body in question or, in other words, that any force acting on a system is balanced by contrary forces. Therefore the sum of all forces should be zero ($\Sigma F = 0$). (According to Newton's Second Law of Motion, if a system is not accelerating, then $a = 0$, so $\Sigma F = ma$ or $\Sigma F = m(0)$ or $\Sigma F = 0$. That is, there is no net force acting on the system.)

A vector can be zero only if each of its perpendicular components is zero; thus the single vector equation $\Sigma F = 0$ is equivalent to three component equations: $\Sigma F_x = 0$, $\Sigma F_y = 0$, and $\Sigma F_z = 0$ (x, y, and z are the three spatial axes discussed previously). On similar lines the net moment in all three planes also should be equal to zero (i.e., $\Sigma M_x = 0$, $\Sigma M_y = 0$, and $\Sigma M_z = 0$).

EQUILIBRIUM IN ORTHODONTICS (THE QUASI-STATIC SYSTEM)

Equilibrium applies only to static systems (nonaccelerating systems). However, in orthodontics we move teeth. They move, stop, tip, and upright (i.e., they are not static systems). So how can teeth be governed by the laws of statics? To answer this question, we need to redefine the state of the teeth subjected to orthodontic forces by introducing the concept of quasi-static systems (or quasi-static thermodynamic processes). This concept can be defined as a system or process that goes through a sequence of states that are infinitesimally close to equilibrium (i.e., the process happens very slowly and goes through a sequence of states that are close to equilibrium at any time). When orthodontic appliances are activated and inserted, the tooth displacement that occurs is very small and takes place over a relatively long period of time. At any point in time, if you look in the patient's mouth you do not see any movement; however, after waiting for a sufficient period the movement can be appreciated. Therefore at any instant a force analysis may be carried out by invoking the laws of equilibrium without erring appreciably. In other words, the inertia of any appliance element or a tooth is negligibly smaller and may be neglected. For this reason, the physical laws of statics are considered adequate to describe the instantaneous force systems produced by orthodontic appliances. However, these laws cannot be used to describe how the force systems will change as the teeth move and an appliance deactivates and alters its configuration.

The solutions to problems in statics involving forces and moments call for ingenuity and common sense. There are no simple rules of procedure. The most common source of error

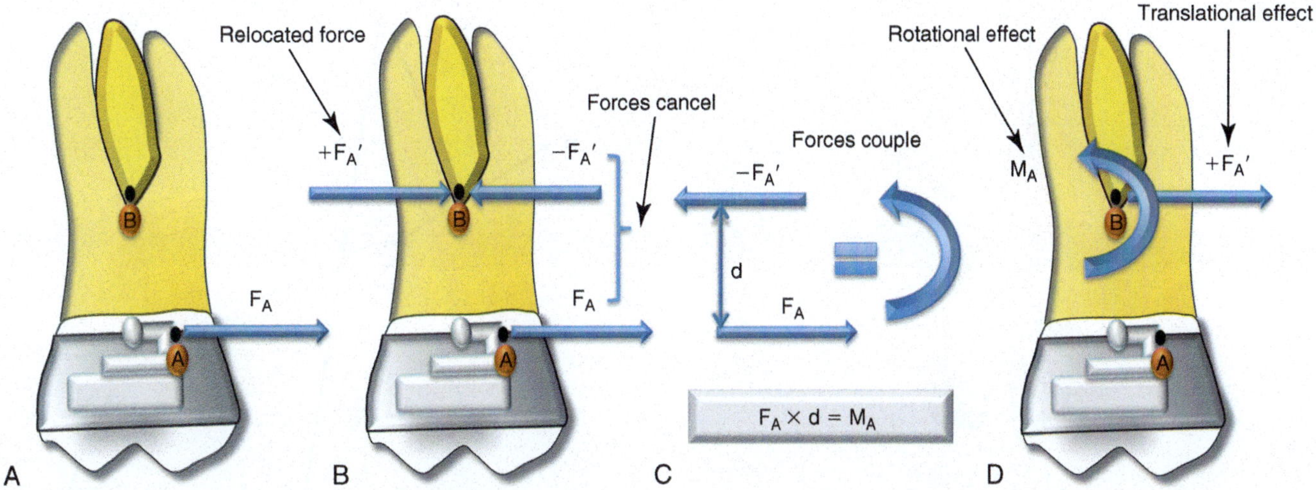

Figure 4-12 Creating equivalent force systems. The net effect of the force system depicted in **A** and **D** is the same. **B** and **C** show how to transform **A** to **B.**

is failure to identify the object whose equilibrium is being considered. You must learn to consider all forces acting on the body. Of course, Newton's Second and Third Laws of Motion are of great help in this regard. By using the Third Law, it is easy to figure out that if an appliance is exerting a force on a tooth, the tooth is exerting the same force on the appliance (see Fig. 4-11), and the same principle applies to all other teeth to which the appliance is connected. Because the appliance is not moving (static), the sum of all forces and moments produced by the appliance should be zero.

Principle of Equivalent Force Systems

The principle of equivalent force systems is an elegant way of redefining the forces and moments acting on a body. It helps to visualize not only the translatory movement of a tooth but also the rotation, tip, and torque experienced. An equivalent force system is a system of forces and/or moments that can be replaced with a different set of forces and/or moments and still achieve the same basic translational and rotational behavior. To understand the practical implication of this principle, let us discuss relocating a force system on a molar.

Application of Equivalent Force Systems: Moving the Force System to a Different Location

Figure 4-12 shows a force acting on the tooth at point A (F_A). Now suppose that you want to compute the effects of this force system at a different location, such as point B, which in this case is the C_{RES} of the molar (remember that the C_{RES} of the molar has been chosen arbitrarily; point B can be any other point on the molar). To determine the required translational effect, introduce two equal but opposite forces ($+F_A'$ and $-F_A'$) at point B. We can easily do this because such an introduction of forces will not affect the system in any way, as these forces are equal and opposite and therefore the resultant of these newly added forces is $F_A' + (-F_A') = 0$, or zero net translational effect. Make sure that the magnitude of these new forces is equal to F_A acting at point A. Now, by applying the law of vector addition the original force F_A plus the new negative force $-F_A'$ will cancel each other out. With this in mind, you can see that the only force that now remains on the molar is the newly relocated force F_A', which is now acting at point B. Congratulations! You have relocated the force.

Now that you have relocated the force, examine the two other forces on the molar: F_A acting at point A and $-F_A'$ acting at point B. These two forces are parallel, acting in opposite directions and separated by a distance (d). This setup is the very definition of a moment (couple), previously discussed. Remember that moments and couples cause rotation of a body; therefore the added rotational effect of this couple is what you must include when you move a force. Also, a couple is a free vector; therefore it applies the same rotational behavior regardless of where on the body it is acting. As a result, you can freely move the moment of the couple to point B on the molar as long as the magnitude and sense of the moment vector remain unchanged. The magnitude of this moment can be calculated by multiplying the force F_A or $-F_A'$ by d ($M_A = F_A \times d$). The point of application of a moment or couple doesn't matter when creating an equivalent force system. If you want to move a moment, just move it.

In summary, to relocate a force system you simply need to take the original force and apply it to the new location, plus compute the newly applied moment (which is the product of the force and the distance between the two points) and apply that at the new location maintaining its sense and direction.

There are two simple rules that allow the calculation of equivalent force systems. Two force systems are equivalent if (1) the sums of the forces in all three planes of space (x, y, and z) are equal and (2) the sums of moments about any point are identical.

CENTER OF ROTATION

Center of rotation is a fixed point around which a two-dimensional figure appears to be rotated as determined

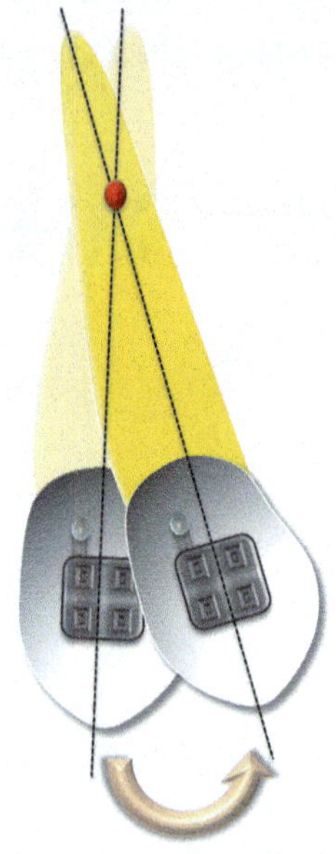

Figure 4-13 Center of rotation (*red dot*) of a tooth. Note that the center of rotation is the only point that has remained stationary.

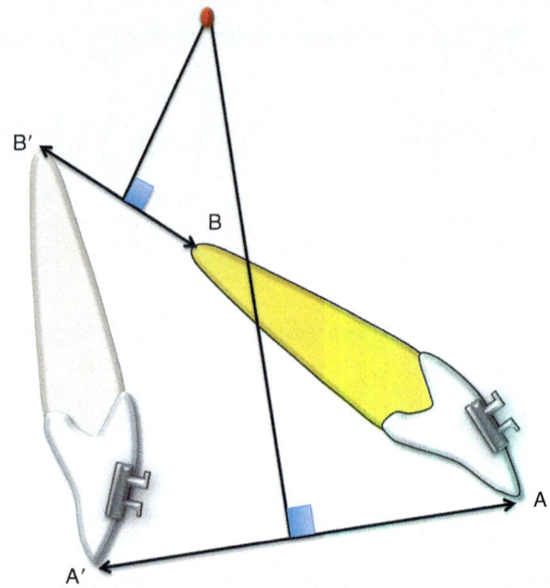

Figure 4-14 A and A′ represent the cusp tip before and after movement. A line has been drawn connecting these points. At the midpoint of this line a perpendicular has been constructed. The point at which this perpendicular intersects any other perpendicular constructed in a similar manner (here, the apex has been selected as the other point) is the center of rotation (*red dot*).

from its initial and final positions. (Note that a two-dimensional figure always rotates around a point while a three-dimensional figure rotates around an axis; that is, a two-dimensional object has a center of rotation while a three-dimensional object has an axis of rotation.) In other words, in rotation the only point that does not move is called the center of rotation (C_{ROT}) (Fig. 4-13). The rest of the plane rotates around this one fixed point.

Although a single center of rotation can be constructed for any starting and ending positions of a tooth, it does not follow that the single point actually acted as the center of rotation for the entire movement. The tooth might have arrived at its final position by following an irregular path, tipping first one way and then another. As a tooth moves, the forces on it continuously undergo slight changes, so that a changing center of rotation is the rule rather than the exception. In determining the relationship between a force system and the center of rotation of the resulting movement, all that can really be determined is an "instantaneous" center of rotation.[5]

Estimating the Center of Rotation

The C_{ROT} can be estimated easily as shown in Figure 4-14. Take any two points on the tooth and connect the before and after positions of each point with a line. The intersection of the perpendicular bisectors of these lines is the center of rotation.[6]

TYPES OF TOOTH MOVEMENT (Fig. 4-15)

As discussed in the preceding section, the center of rotation is the key to defining the nature of tooth movement. Controlling the C_{ROT} automatically gives precise control over the type (extent) of tooth movement. When a single force is applied on a tooth, the tooth will move in the direction of the force applied. Additionally, depending on the distance of the force from the C_{RES} the tooth will experience a moment (M_F) around the C_{RES}. This combination of a force and a moment will cause the tooth to rotate as it moves, placing its C_{ROT} slightly apical to the C_{RES}.[1,5,7] This type of tooth movement is called simple tipping or uncontrolled tipping. It is easy to visualize here that the crown and the root will move in opposite directions. Tipping can happen in many different ways depending on where the C_{ROT} is along the tooth. However, for ease of classification they can be categorized into two groups:

- Controlled tipping: During such movement the C_{ROT} is located at the root apex. The tooth moves similar to the pendulum on a clock, with its apex fixed at a particular point and the crown moving from one side to the other.
- Root movement: Here, the C_{ROT} is located at the crown tip while the root is free to move in the direction of the force. Traditionally, in the orthodontic literature, this is not characterized as a tipping movement but mechanically the movement is similar to controlled tipping.

Almost the entire universe of tooth movement consists of tipping the crown, the root (rare), or a combination (most common). However, there is one tooth movement that is extremely rare and very difficult to achieve in its strictest sense: translation, sometimes known as bodily movement. Here, both the crown and the root move in equal amounts and in the same direction with no rotation. In this case the C_{ROT} is nonexistent or, in mathematical terms, approaches infinity.

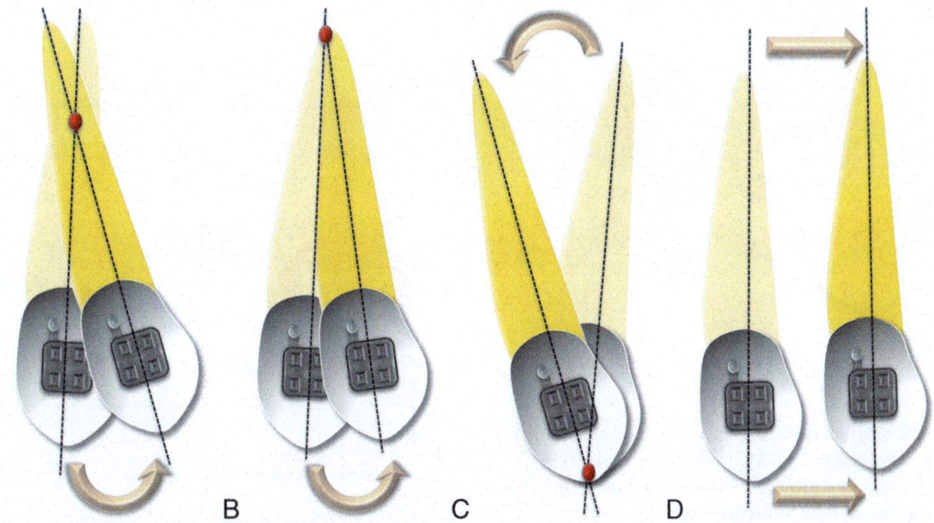

Figure 4-15 Types of tooth movement. **A,** Uncontrolled tipping. **B,** Controlled tipping. **C,** Root movement (torquing). **D,** Translation or bodily movement. The C_{ROT} in every case is depicted by a red dot. Note that during translation (**D**) the C_{ROT} is at infinity or, in other words, does not exist.

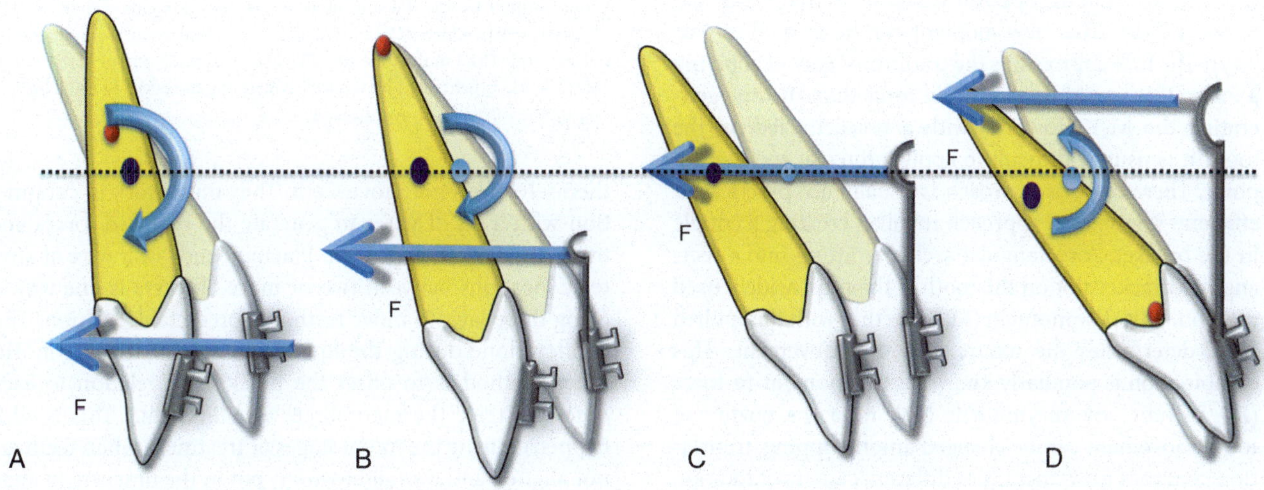

Figure 4-16 The application of a power arm to create different types of tooth movement. Note that the force has been kept constant through **A** to **D. A,** Uncontrolled tipping, no power arm. **B,** Controlled tipping produced by a power arm below the C_{RES} of the tooth. **C,** Translation, as the force is now being applied through the C_{RES} made possible by increasing the length of the power arm. **D,** Root movement with minimal crown movement; here, the power arm extends beyond the C_{RES}. (The red dot is the C_{ROT} and the blue dot is the C_{RES}.) Note how the M_F increases or decreases with an increase or decrease in the distance of force application from the C_{RES}.

Moment-to-Force (M/F) Ratios

Tipping (uncontrolled) is the most common tooth movement in everyday orthodontics but not always the preferred one. To modify this pattern of tooth movement and create a new one, the force system acting on the tooth needs to be altered. There are primarily two ways to accomplish this based on the mechanics involved:

1. Altering the point of force application (Fig. 4-16): A simple way of accomplishing this is to apply a force closer to the C_{RES} of the tooth. A rigid attachment, often called a power arm, can be attached to the bracket on the crown of the tooth. Then the force can be applied to this power arm. In this way the line of force can be moved to a different location, thereby altering its distance from the C_{RES}. This also causes a change in the moment of the force. For example, if the power arm can be made long and rigid to extend to the C_{RES} of the tooth, the moment arm (M_F) can be eliminated entirely, as the applied force will now pass through the C_{RES}. This method works beautifully when altering the tipping movement of the crown; however, for movements requiring higher levels of control, such as translation and root movement, this method poses certain problems. The "long" arms can be a source of irritation to the patient, by extending into the vestibule and/or impinging on the gingiva and cheeks. Additionally, the arms are sometimes not rigid enough and can undergo some degree of flexion under the applied force. (A clinical case showing translation with power arms has been described in Chapter 6.)
2. Altering the moment-to-force ratio (Fig. 4-17): An alternative method to alter the tooth movement is to play with the rotational component of the applied force (i.e., the

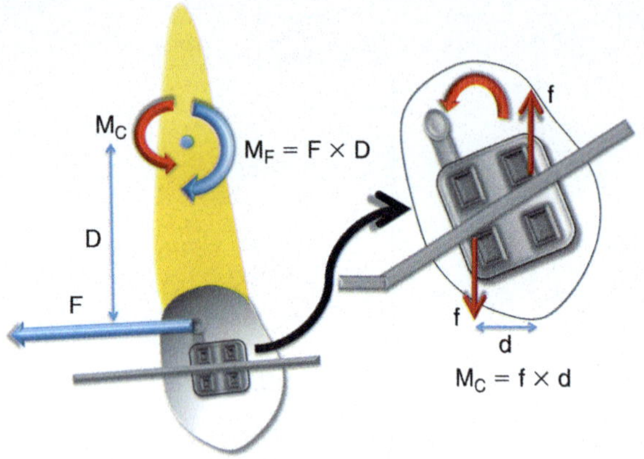

Figure 4-17 A schematic diagram depicting the generation of a moment due to a couple (M_C). It is the ratio of the M_C to the force applied (F) that determines the nature of tooth movement (M/F ratio). The higher the ratio, the greater will be the control over the tooth movement.

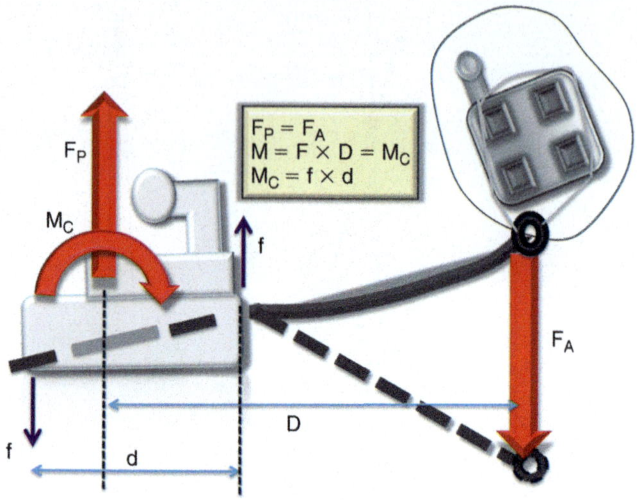

Figure 4-18 Schematic diagram illustrating a one-couple force system. The moment (M) generated by the system is the product of the force and the distance (D) separating the two forces, which causes the entire system to rotate. As with every rigid body system, this setup should be in equilibrium; in other words, the sum of all forces and moments should be zero. Therefore the two forces (F_P and F_A) should be equal. Also, the moment due to the couple (M_C) in the tube should be equal to the moment of the system (M). The M_C is generated by the wire contacting the edges of the tube generating the forces (f) shown in blue.

M_F). This is done by adding a counterbalancing moment (i.e., a moment in the opposite direction to that of the M_F) to the system. This new moment can be created in two ways. The first approach is the traditional way of applying a force (this would be a different force than the one generating the M_F). However, with a bracket fixed on the tooth it is usually difficult to apply a force at some other point. Therefore this approach is usually not practical or efficient. The second approach involves creating a couple in the bracket. A rectangular archwire fitting into a rectangular bracket slot on the tooth is the most widely used method. This new moment (M_C) together with the applied force determines the nature of tooth movement. This combination is popularly known as the moment-to-force (M_C/F) ratio. By varying this M/F ratio the quality of tooth movement can be changed among tipping, translation, and root movement (i.e., different centers of rotation along the long axis of the tooth are created by changing the magnitude of the couple and the applied force). In terms of the direction, the moment of the couple (M_C) is almost always going to be in the direction opposite the moment of the force (M_F) about the C_{RES}.

Note that in orthodontics moments are measured in gram-millimeters and forces are measured in grams, so that a ratio of the two has units of millimeters. This ratio is also indicative of the distance away from the bracket at which a single force will produce the same effect (i.e., through a power arm, as discussed above).

ORTHODONTIC FORCE SYSTEMS: APPLYING THE LAWS OF MECHANICS

From our discussion in the previous sections it is clear that orthodontic tooth movement follows certain principles of classical or Newtonian mechanics that need to be understood to carry out a particular type of tooth movement. Once you have mastered these fundamental laws, the next task it to put them into action. It is important to remember that the physical laws or the brackets on the patient's teeth by themselves will not move teeth. They must work in conjunction with a set of wires to generate the required forces and moments for moving teeth. Placing bends in a wire at strategic locations between two or more brackets is one way of using these laws to move teeth in a predictable fashion. This is often done during the finishing stages of treatment. The other method is to offset the brackets in relation to each other to create the same forces and moments. This is what happens during the initial stages of treatment when teeth are not aligned and a straight wire is put in the brackets to align them. Let's discuss these situations in detail.

Bends placed on a wire between two attachments or brackets or a straight wire linking maligned brackets or attachments can essentially create two kinds of force systems depending on how the wire is engaged in the brackets:

- One-couple force system
- Two-couple force system

One-Couple Force Systems

The orthodontic appliances capable of producing the most well-defined and dramatic tooth movements are often those that are the most simple biomechanically. These force systems are established between two attachments when a couple is created at one end of an attachment and a single force is created at the other. This usually involves a wire with a bend inserted in a bracket or tube while at the other end, instead of placing the wire in a bracket or tube slot, it is just tied to the attachment so that only one point of contact is created. This system therefore is also known as a one-bracket force system (Fig. 4-18). Due to the simple configuration of the action and reaction forces this system generates a statically determinate force system (i.e., all forces and moments created by such a system can be readily discerned, measured, and evaluated with remarkable precision). There are a number of clinical situations in which we make use of such a force system. Some of them have been discussed in Chapter 8.

A cantilever spring design is the essential component of all appliances using the one-couple force system. Figure 4-18 illustrates the mechanics involved when using a cantilever spring for canine extrusion. The mechanics shown apply to all one-couple force systems. Note that the spring is simply tied to an attachment or bracket and not inserted in the bracket slot so that there is only a single point of contact between the wire and the attachment, creating a single force with no couple as opposed to the two-point contact in the other attachment (tube). Such a quasi-static system (neither the wire nor the attachments are moving at a particular instant of time) will abide with the laws of equilibrium, as this is a "rigid system." Therefore the moment at the tube (M_C) should be opposed by another moment (M) in the opposite direction but one of equal magnitude. This M is produced by the equal and opposite forces (F_A and F_P) at the attachments. The forces again follow the law of equilibrium. (Note: The equal and opposite forces seen at the two attachments are not a consequence of Newton's Third Law of Motion.)

At the clinical level, the most consistent way to derive the force system produced by any orthodontic appliance is to remove the activated wire from its attachments and lay it passively over the attachment sites. The angle formed by the wire and the brackets will show the direction of the couple produced at the site of engagement, where the angle between the wire and bracket is largest.[8–10]

Two-Couple Force Systems

Two-couple force systems are established between two attachments when a wire is inserted in the bracket slots of two brackets or tubes. As the name suggests, these force systems involve forces and couples at both attachments when a straight wire is placed in a pair of nonaligned brackets or when a bend is placed between two aligned brackets. Therefore this force system is also known as a two-bracket force system. The dynamics of this two-bracket unit are fundamental in understanding the mechanical principles guiding the movement of teeth with sliding mechanics.

When compared to the force system described in the previous section (i.e., one-couple force systems) this constitutes a statically indeterminate force system (i.e., it is too complex to "precisely" determine all of the forces and moments involved at both attachments at a particular time). Inserting the wire into one attachment and using a force gauge to measure the force required to deflect the wire to the other bracket will not necessarily give an accurate assessment of the force produced by the wire. In this system, when the wire is placed over the slots of the two brackets where it will be inserted, the angle of entry of the wire at each bracket slot does show which bracket has the larger angle of entry and therefore the larger moment. This is important because, irrespective of the direction of the moment at the second bracket, the larger moment will dictate the direction of the associated net equilibrium of forces acting at each bracket.

As mentioned previously, the two-bracket force system can be described by two different approaches and has been described in detail in the orthodontic literature[11–13]: straight wire placed in angulated brackets (super-position method) and angulated (bent) wires in aligned brackets (subtraction method).

Straight Wire Placed in Angulated Brackets

This approach allows the orthodontist to use a straight wire in malaligned brackets. This triggers the activation of the force system. The force system can be accentuated by adding the proper bends whose force systems are summated to the straight-wire force system. This is known as the "superposition" method and is often used during the initial and leveling and aligning phases of orthodontic treatment or sometimes during finishing when bracket positions are changed for root correction.

The first step in understanding this method is to accurately define the system. Figure 4-19 shows the setup of such a system. The interbracket axis (D) connects the centers of the two attachments. This can also be called the "interbracket distance" or the x-x′ axis, as described in the beginning of this chapter. Both brackets make certain angles with this horizontal (x-x′) axis. The two attachment–wire segment can be fully defined if one knows θ_A, θ_B, and D. There are an infinite number of ways in which the brackets can be arranged relative to each other, in terms of both angulation and the distance. To make things easy, such a setup can be studies in six distinct geometries. Each geometry or arrangement of the brackets can be defined by the ratio of the bracket angulations relative to the x-x′ axis. Every geometry has its own unique set of force systems and is represented by a "class." Let us examine each class separately.

The reader will observe a gradual change in θ_A while θ_B is kept constant as we go through the various classes. Since,

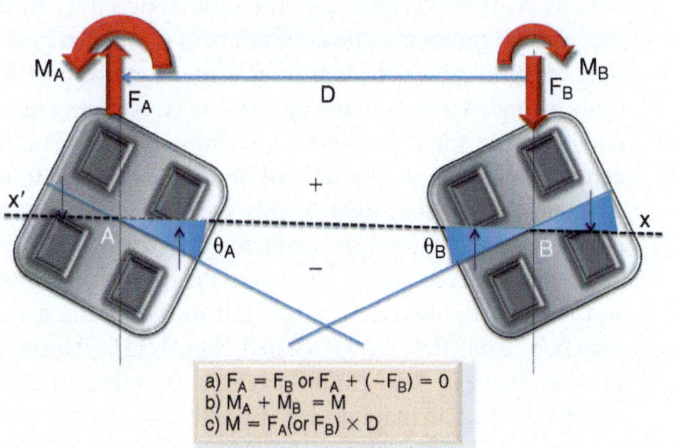

Figure 4-19 Wire-attachment geometry is defined by the interbracket distance (D) and the angles of the brackets at positions A and B relative to the horizontal reference frame (x-x′). The purple arrows show how the wire in the bracket creates the couples (M_A or M_B). Note: The equations mentioned in the box apply to all geometries (Classes I to VI) without exception.

by convention, θ_A is always either equal to or smaller than θ_B, the six classes can be used to describe any two-tooth segments, regardless of the teeth involved. A consistent sign convention is used to describe the angle of the brackets. The sign of the angle is the same sign as the moment required to place the wire into the bracket. At any point, if the axis of the bracket (blue line) goes below the x-x′ line, the sign convention for the angle created (for θ_A or θ_B) will be assigned a negative (−). All forces pointing downward and all moments in the counterclockwise direction are negative.

Class I: The two brackets here are angled the same amount and in the same direction with respect to the interbracket axis (D) (i.e., $\theta_A = \theta_B$ and $\theta_A/\theta_B = 1.0$) (Fig. 4-20). The two moments are equal; the ratio $M_A/M_B = 1$. Although the magnitude of the moments may vary, depending on the amount of activation and the interbracket distance, the ratio of M_A to M_B always remains +1 in Class I. In addition to the moment, two vertical forces are also produced: a negative force at position A and a positive force at position B. Force A equals force B as dictated by the laws of equilibrium.

Class II: The Class II geometry is characterized by θ_A having a magnitude of one-half of θ_B (Fig. 4-21). Two positive moments are created at the wire at positions A and B. The magnitude of the moment at A is 0.8 times the moment at B. A positive force is found at A and a negative force is found at B.

Class III: In Class III geometries the interbracket axis cuts across the two brackets; in other words, the angle made by bracket A with respect to the x-x′ axis or the wire is 0 degrees (Fig. 4-22). So, θ_A/θ_B is 0; thus a wire placed in the canine bracket (A) would cross the premolar bracket (B) at the center of the slot. Two positive moments are created at the wire at positions A and B. The magnitude of the moment at A is 0.5 times the moment at B. A positive force is found at A and a negative force is found at B.

Class IV: Here the bracket A is angled one-half of bracket B but in the opposite direction in relation to the x-x′ axis (i.e., $\theta_A = -0.5\theta_B$) (Fig. 4-23). The ratio between θ_A/θ_B is −0.5. In this geometry a positive moment is found at position B but no moment whatsoever is found at position A. Only a single force operates at position A, with an equal and opposite force at position B. Since no moment is acting in position A, the ratio of M_A/M_B is equal to 0. It is interesting to note that in this geometry the system almost behaves like a one-couple force system.

Class V: Bracket A is angled three-fourths of bracket B but in the opposite direction in relation to the interbracket axis (x-x′ axis) (i.e., $\theta_A = -0.75\theta_B$) (Fig. 4-24). The ratio between θ_A/θ_B is −0.75. In this example the moment at A is negative and its magnitude is two-fifths of the positive moment at B. The ratio of M_A/M_B is −0.4. Equal and opposite vertical forces act at positions A and B.

Class VI: In this class the bracket A is angled the same amount as bracket B but in the opposite direction so that the ratio of the angle (θ_A/θ_B) is −1.0 (Fig. 4-25). The force system acting on the wire is composed of equal and opposite moments (negative at A and positive at B) (i.e., M_A/M_B is −1.0). No vertical forces are present.

The six clinical classes actually represent a continuum of possible force systems that can place a wire between two brackets into equilibrium. The important thing here is to know the relative force system rather than the exact magnitude. For example, note how the magnitude of the vertical forces decreases as we go from Class I to II and so on until Class VI, where there are no vertical forces at all. In other words, we can say that as the ratio of θ_A/θ_B decreases the force magnitudes decrease. This can be easily figured out from the equations in Figure 4-19:

$$F_A \text{ or } F_B = M_A + M_B/D, \text{here} - F_A = F_B$$

Of more importance are the relative moments in each class and how the angulation of the brackets can change this. In a dynamic situation (i.e., at the clinical level), as the ratio of θ_A/θ_B changes from one class to the next, the force system on the wire, and hence on the teeth, will radically change.

Angulated (Bent) Wires in Aligned Brackets

Bending wires toward the end of orthodontic treatment is a common practice. It helps in giving final touches to a well-treated malocclusion. As with the superposition method, a gamut of possible locations and bend types can be placed. However, to understand the dynamics of such bends, they can be classified into the following categories based on the type of force system each can provide.

I. Step bends
II. Off-centered "V" bends
III. Centered "V" bends

In this approach it is important to first contour the wire passively between two brackets and then add the proper "V" or step bends. In other words, this approach first eliminates the force system produced by a straight wire in malaligned brackets and then creates the desired force system by adding bends in the wire. Therefore it is referred to as the subtraction method.

Each of these bends is distinct from the others in terms of the forces and moments produced at both ends.[12] It is important to remember that this method produces similar results to those of the superposition method described above and is also classified into various geometries. The various geometries can be categorized as follows:

I. Step bends. Step bends can replicate the Class I and II geometries described in the previous section. They require that two bends be placed on the wire anywhere along the interbracket distance.

Class I: A step in the wire between two brackets produces equal and opposite vertical forces and unidirectional couples whose moments are equal in magnitude (Fig. 4-26). Since the moments are in the same direction and of equal magnitude, the ratio is $M_A/M_B = 1$. This ratio defines the relative force system from a step in a wire that is identical to the Class I ratio found with a straight wire with parallel and stepped brackets (see Fig. 4-20). To create a Class I geometry with bends it

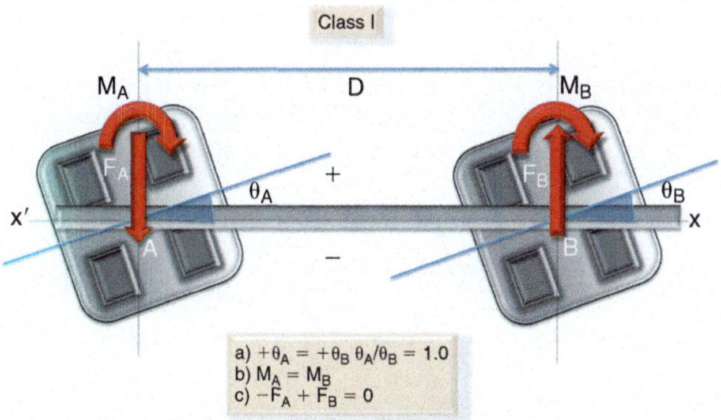

Figure 4-20 Class I geometry.

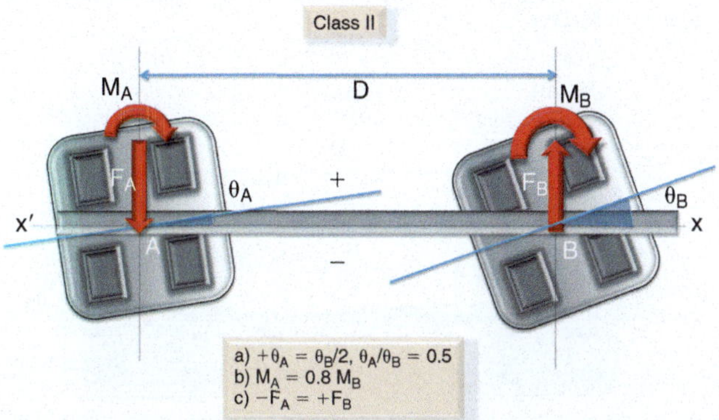

Figure 4-21 Class II geometry.

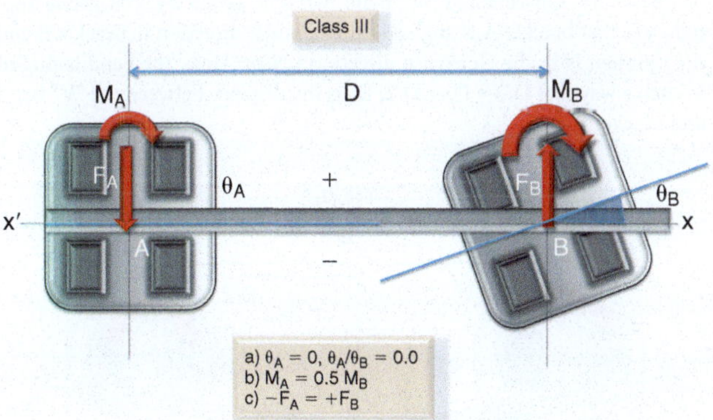

Figure 4-22 Class III geometry.

is important to remember that the wire segments going into the bracket slots should be parallel to each other (shown by blue lines in Fig. 4-26); in other words, the bend angulations should be similar and in the same direction (i.e., $\theta_A = \theta_B$ or $\theta_A/\theta_B = 1$).

For all practical purposes the shifting of the step mesiodistally does not alter the absolute or relative force system. Furthermore, the ratio $M_A/M_B = 1$ is independent of the interbracket distance. It also does not change with smaller or larger step bends.

Class II: The following geometry can be created when bend angulations are not equal to each other ($\theta_A \neq \theta_B$) and the wire segments going into the bracket slots if

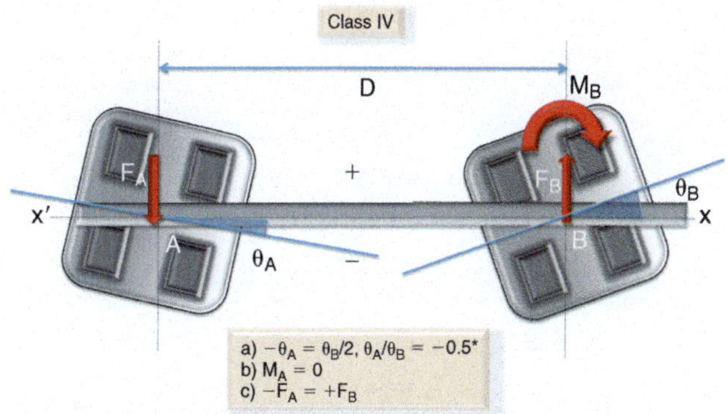

Figure 4-23 Class IV geometry. (*Negative sign indicates that bracket A is angled in the opposite direction to that of bracket B.) Note: There is no moment at bracket A.

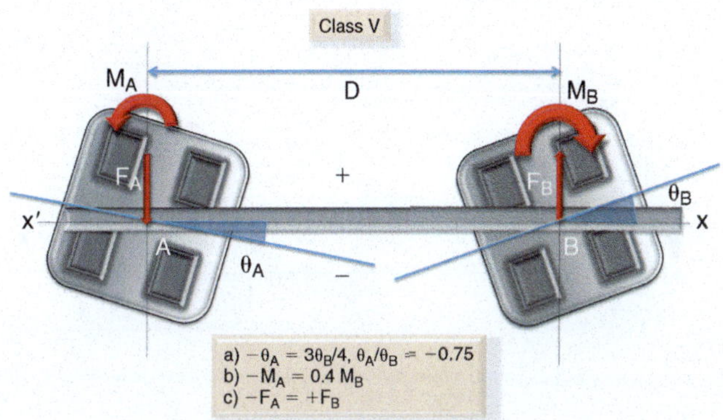

Figure 4-24 Class V geometry.

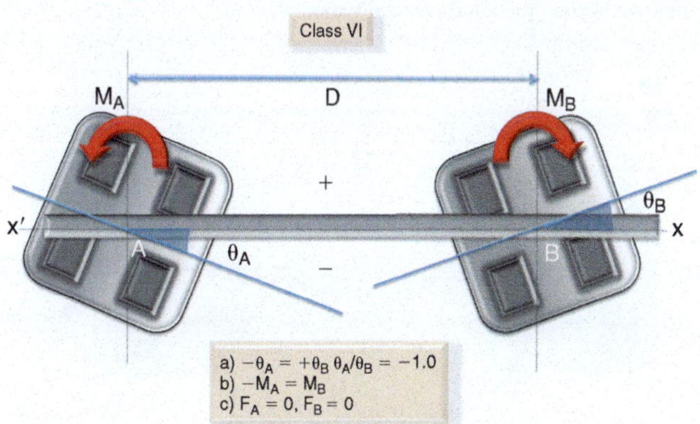

Figure 4-25 Class VI geometry. Note: The moments here are equal in magnitude but in the opposite direction. No vertical forces are created in this geometry.

extended with imaginary lines intersect beyond the interbracket span (Fig. 4-27).

II. Off-centered "V" bends. A "V" bend, as the name indicates, involves the placement of only one bend on the wire along the interbracket distance. Unlike a step bend, a "V" bend placed between two brackets radically alters the force system, depending on the mesiodistal placement of the bend. Therefore, based on the position of the bend, these bends can be arranged into the remaining geometries (Classes III to VI).

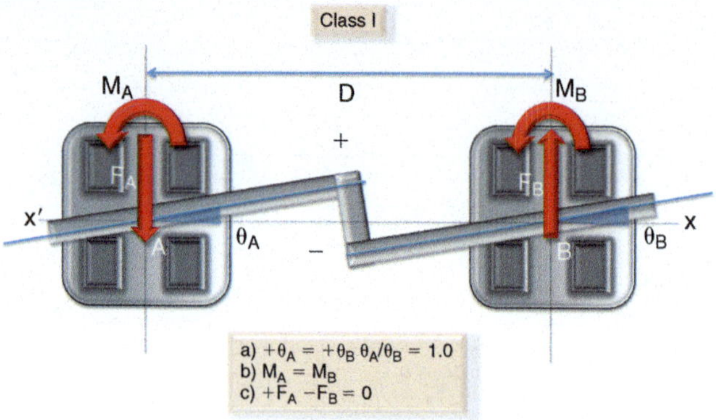

Figure 4-26 Step bends (bend angulations are made in such a way that the two blue lines are parallel to each other), Class I geometry. Note: It does not matter where the step bend is placed between the two brackets; the effect will be similar.

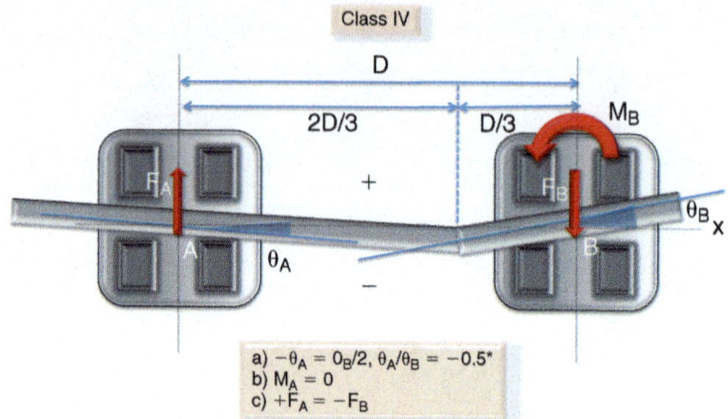

Figure 4-29 Off-centered "V" bend, Class IV geometry. (*Negative sign indicates that bracket A is angled in the opposite direction to bracket B.) Note: The bend is placed at one-third the interbracket distance. There is no moment at bracket A.

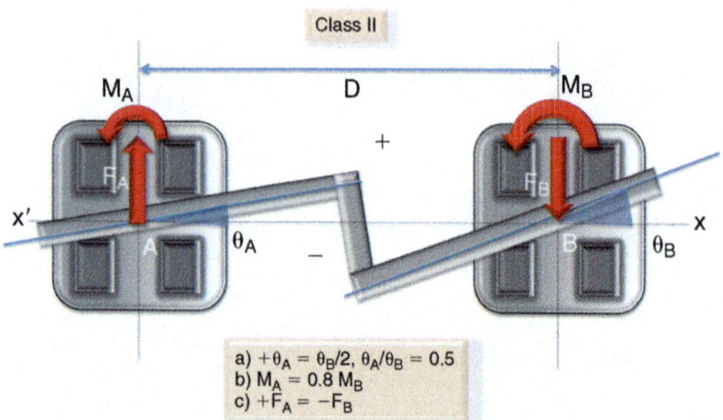

Figure 4-27 Step bends (bend angulations not at 90 degrees), Class II geometry. Note: The bends are placed in such a way that the two blue lines intersect beyond the interbracket distance.

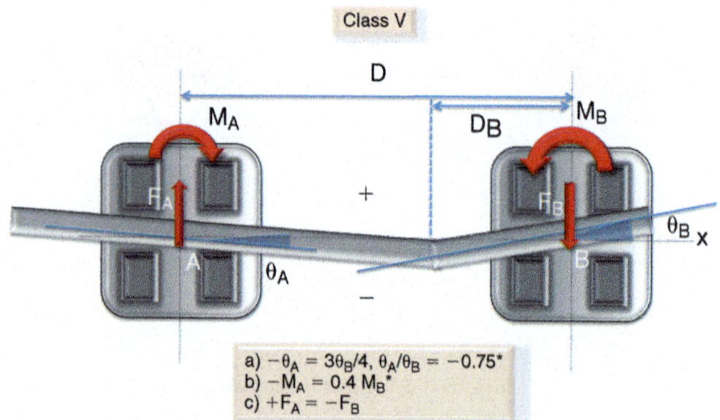

Figure 4-30 Off-centered "V" bend, Class V geometry. (*Negative sign indicates that bracket A is angled in the opposite direction to bracket B and the moment is in the clockwise direction.) Note: Here, the bend is placed in such a way that $D/3 < D_B < D/2$. D_B is the distance between the "V" bend and bracket B.

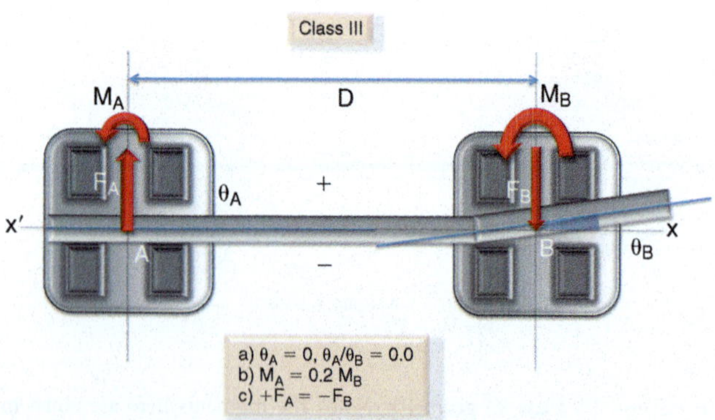

Figure 4-28 Off-centered "V" bend, Class III geometry. Note: The "V" bend is placed very close to one bracket.

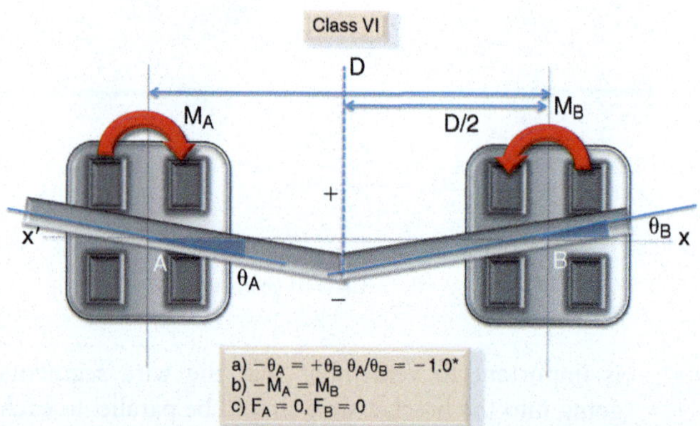

Figure 4-31 Centered "V" bend, Class VI geometry. (*Negative sign indicates that bracket A is angled in the opposite direction to bracket B and the moment is in the clockwise direction.) Note: Here, the bend is placed at half the interbracket distance. There are no vertical forces.

Class III: The "V" bend is placed very close to one of the brackets (Fig. 4-28). The bracket near the bend will have the bigger moment, while the moment at the other end will be much lower in magnitude but will have the same sense.

Class IV: The "V" bend is placed at one third the interbracket distance. No moment is found at the bracket further away from the bend (Fig. 4-29).

Class V: The bend is moved closer to the center of the interbracket distance (Fig. 4-30). From this point onward a moment is seen on the bracket further away from the bend but with an opposite sense.

III. Centered "V" bends.

Class VI: When the "V" bend is centered, equal and opposite moments are produced and hence there are no vertical forces (Fig. 4-31).

This analysis of the force systems leads to important clinical applications in the use of bends and bracket positioning and angulation in day-to-day orthodontics. It is important to emphasize again the need to appreciate the relative force system not the absolute force. In all of the bend geometries discussed, neither the height of the bend nor the interbracket distance changes the relative force system and obviously the absolute magnitude of the forces and moments will vary. This analysis also forms the basis for analyzing more intricate and complicated force systems that might be generated in an actual clinical situation.

SUMMARY

In this chapter we placed a strong emphasis on the fundamentals of the mechanical principles involved in tooth movement. Later in this book, we will see the clinical applications of these principles. It is our belief that by unraveling the basic mechanics of tooth movement and integrating them with newer advances we can make tooth movement more efficient with minimal side effects. Clinicians who understand the principles of tooth movement will have better control of their treatment mechanics and greater efficiency in tooth movement.

REFERENCES

1. Burstone CJ, Pryputniewicz RJ. Holographic determination of centers of rotation produced by orthodontic forces. *Am J Orthod.* 1980;77:396.
2. Davidian EJ. Use of a computer model to study the force distribution on the root of the maxillary central incisor. *Am J Orthod.* 1971;59:581–588.
3. Hay GE. The equilibrium of a thin compressible membrane. *Can J Res.* 1939;17:106–121.
4. Yettram AL, Wright KWJ, Houston WJB. Center of rotation of a maxillary central incisor under orthodontic loading. *Br J Orthod.* 1977; 4:23–27.
5. Christiansen RL, Burstone CJ. Centers of rotation within the periodontal space. *Am J Orthod.* 1969;55:351–369.
6. Smith RJ, Burstone CJ. Mechanics of tooth movement. *Am J Orthod.* 1984;85(4):294–307.
7. Pryputniewicz RJ, Burstone CJ. The effect of time and force magnitude on orthodontic tooth movement. *J Dent Res.* 1979;58(8):1754–1764.
8. Mulligan TF. *Common sense mechanics in everyday orthodontics.* Phoenix, AZ: CSM Publishing; 1998:1–17.
9. Isaacson RJ, Lindauer SJ, Rubenstein LK. Activating a 2 × 4 appliance. *Angle Orthod.* 1993;63:17–24.
10. Demange C. Equilibrium situations in bend force systems. *Am J Orthod Dentofacial Orthop.* 1990;98:333–339.
11. Koenig HA, Burstone CJ. Force systems from an ideal arch. *Am J Orthod.* 1974;65:270–289.
12. Burstone CJ, Koenig HA. Force systems from an ideal arch: large deflection considerations. *Angle Orthod.* 1989;59(1):11–16.
13. Koenig HA, Burstone CJ. Creative wire bending: the force system from step and V bend. *Am J Orthod Dentofacial Orthop.* 1988;93(1):59–67.

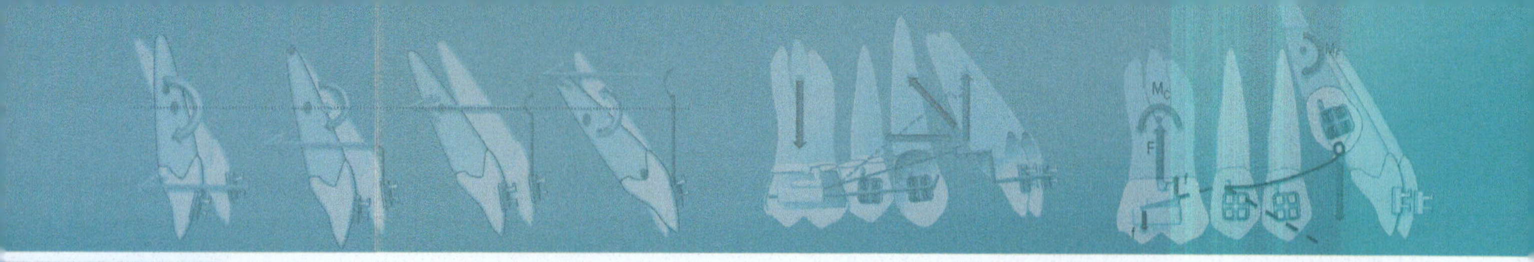

CHAPTER 5

Biological Mechanisms in Orthodontic Tooth Movement

Sunil Kapila and Gregory J. King

The goal of this chapter is to examine the relationships between orthodontic biomechanics and the underlying biological processes. The topics discussed include the factors affecting the rate of tooth movement, anchorage considerations, causes of relapse, and root resorption. All relevant biological principles underlying orthodontic tooth movement can be characterized as tissue remodeling. The process of orthodontic tooth movement is a resultant dynamic change in the shapes and composition of the investing bone and soft tissues. The dental and peridental tissues (dentin, cementum, periodontal ligament [PDL], and alveolar bone) all have active reparative mechanisms and will adapt under the normal forces of orthodontic appliances. At the most basic level, extrinsic forces set up localized areas of "pressure" and "tension" in the tissues adjacent to teeth and the subsequent responses satisfy the principles of Wolff's law of bone remodeling.[1]

When orthodontists use fixed appliances to apply force on teeth, predictable tooth movement is anticipated. This is accompanied by transiently increased tooth mobility and, occasionally, radiographic evidence of mild root resorption. Experienced clinicians also expect a certain amount of relapse to occur following orthodontic treatment. Other types of natural tooth migration commonly encountered are eruption of primary and succedaneous teeth as well as mesial or distal drifting of teeth. These physiological processes are not necessarily stimulated by biomechanical signals.

In rare instances teeth fail to erupt or move in response to forces (i.e., ankylosis). Each of these common clinical findings can be explained with a better understanding of the underlying biological principles that determine tooth movement.

TOOTH MOVEMENT

Clinical Responses

Kinetics of Orthodontic Tooth Movement

From a clinical perspective orthodontic tooth movement has three distinct phases: (1) displacement phase, (2) delay phase, and (3) acceleration and linear phase (Fig. 5-1).

Displacement Phase. The initial reaction of a tooth following force application is almost instantaneous (within a fraction of a second) and reflects the immediate movement of the tooth within the viscoelastic PDL cradle. These movements are generally predictable by biophysical principles and typically do not involve extensive amounts of tissue remodeling or deformation of the investing alveolar bone.[2] The fluid compartments within the PDL play an important role in the transmission and damping of forces acting on teeth.[3] The magnitude of the displacement response is also dependent on root length and alveolar bone height, which are factors that determine the location of a tooth's center of resistance and center of rotation (see Chapter 4).[4,5] For example, loss of alveolar bone results in a more apically positioned center of resistance, which affects the nature of both the initial displacement and net tooth movement (Fig. 5-2). Age is another factor affecting displacement. Young's modulus of the PDL has been shown to be greater in adults than in adolescents and this difference in biomechanical properties correlates to an equivalent or somewhat increased stress level in the PDL in adults. It is suggested that this might reduce the biological response of the PDL and thus delay tooth movement in adults.[6] The displacement capacity of a tooth can change even within the same individual; the elasticity of the PDL and alveolar bone has the potential to be substantially reduced at the end of tooth movement.[7]

Delay Phase. The second phase of the orthodontic tooth movement cycle is characterized by the absence of clinical movement and is generally referred to as the delay or latency phase. During this period there is no tooth movement but extensive remodeling occurs in all tooth-investing tissues. The absolute amount of force applied is not as relevant as the relative force applied per unit area. Depending on the localized compression of the PDL, there can be either (1) a partial occlusion of the blood vessels in the area or

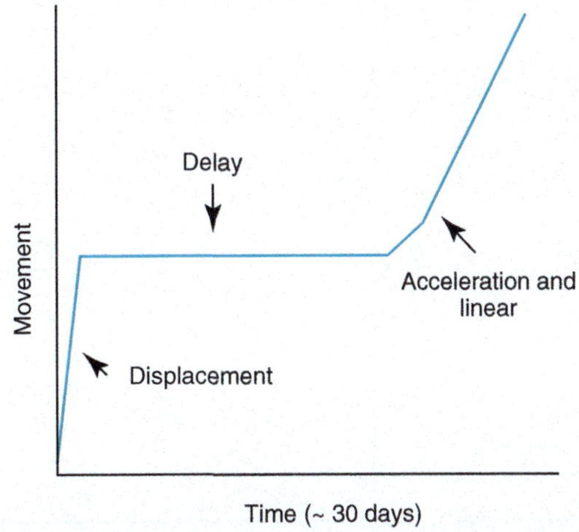

Figure 5-1 Phases of orthodontic tooth movement. The classic curve has three phases: an initial displacement that reflects the viscoelastic properties of the tooth supporting structures; a delay or lag period characterized by no movement; and a postlag phase with linear tooth movement. Minimal tooth movement occurs during the first two phases and most of the tooth movement occurs during the acceleration and linear phases, when alveolar bone remodeling occurs. The timeline is approximate, with considerable individual variation due to mechanical and biological differences.

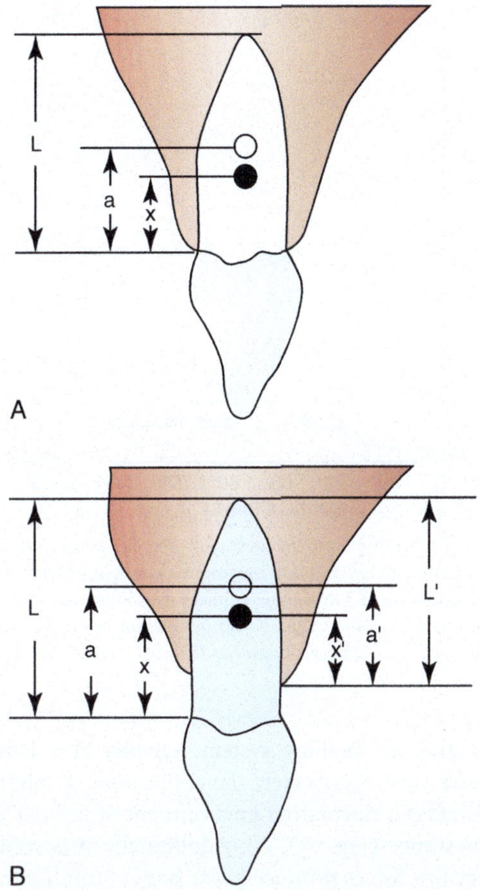

Figure 5-2 Degree of freedom within the viscoelastic periodontal ligament (PDL) apparatus (displacement) is affected by root lengths and alveolar bone heights. **A,** Varying root length (L) will cause shifts in the positions of the distance of the center of rotation (C_{ROT}) to the cervix (a) and the distance of the center of resistance (C_{RES}) to the cervix (x). **B,** Alveolar bone height changes can affect C_{ROT} and C_{RES}. (*a,* distance of the C_{ROT} to the cervix; *a′,* distance of the C_{ROT} to the alveolar crest; *L,* average root length; *L′,* varying alveolar bone heights; x, distance of the C_{RES} to the cervix; x′, distance of the C_{RES} to the alveolar crest.) Ultimately the patterns of tooth displacement will be determined by the change in the position of C_{RES} produced by changes in alveolar bone height or root length. (Modified with permission from Tanne K, Nagataki T, Inoue Y, Sakuda M, Burstone CJ. Patterns of initial tooth displacements associated with various root lengths and alveolar bone heights. *Am J Orthod Dentofacial Orthop.* 1991;100: 66–71.)

(2) an absolute occlusion of blood vessels when high excessive forces have been applied. In cases of partial blockage, the blood vessels delivering nutrients to the area have the capacity to adapt to the new environment and can undergo angiogenesis to bypass occluded areas. However, complete occlusion of vascular flow leads to temporary necrosis of the immediate area and follows a completely different pathway of tooth movement, which is slower to be initiated, starting after approximately 1 to 2 weeks. In either situation, structural and biochemical changes initiate a cascade of cellular mechanisms required for bone remodeling.

Aging has been shown to substantially affect the proliferative activity of the PDL cells and subsequent tooth movement, particularly during the delay phase.[8] However, some studies on molar movement in animal models have shown faster initial tooth movement in young subjects than in adults. Yet once tooth movement had reached the linear phase, the rate of tooth movement became equal in both groups. This indicates that the clinically observed increase in orthodontic treatment time for adults can be attributed primarily to the delay phase prior to the onset of tooth movement but the rate of migration is equally efficient once tooth movement has started.[9]

Acceleration and Linear Phase. The third phase of the orthodontic tooth movement cycle is characterized by rapid tooth displacement. Tooth movement is initiated in deference to the adaptation of the supporting PDL and alveolar bone changes. Studies on the bone-resorptive osteoclast response following orthodontic appliance activation indicate that when appliance reactivation occurs during the appearance of reactivation osteoclasts, a second cohort of osteoclasts can be recruited immediately. This causes immediate, significant tooth movement with no greater risk of root resorption.[10] The force magnitude directly affects the rate of tooth movement. High forces in excess of 100 g used in conventional orthodontic therapy to retract canine teeth have been shown to produce a lag phase of up to 21 days before tooth movement. Lower forces can induce tooth translation without a lag phase at rates that are still clinically significant.[11] The difference in rates of tooth movements can be explained by the different biological responses (frontal resorption versus undermining resorption) discussed later in the chapter. Equally as important as magnitude, however, is the timing of the force application. The force regimen has more influence on the rate of orthodontic tooth movement than the force magnitude.[12] Light continuous forces are much more conducive to orthodontic tooth movement

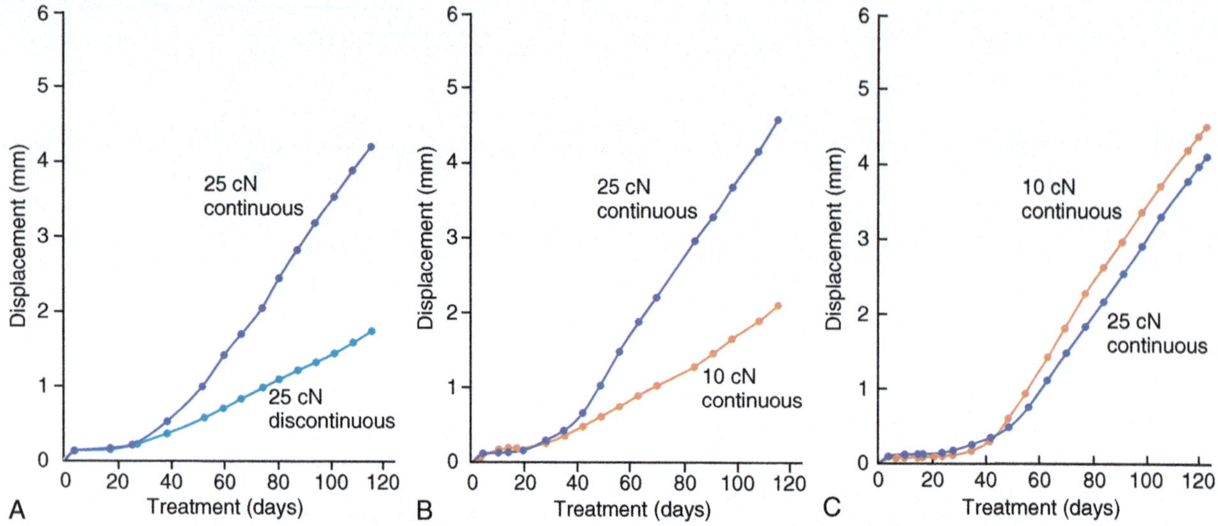

Figure 5-3 Time displacement curves for premolar tooth movement in a beagle dog experimental model demonstrating that (**A**) light continuous forces of 25 cN are more effective in tooth movement than light discontinuous forces and that (**B**) continuous forces of 25 cN produce greater movement than 10 cN in one animal, while (**C**) in another animal the two forces produce equal amounts of tooth movement, demonstrating individual variation and a plateau effect in the latter animal. (Reproduced with permission from van Leeuwen EJ, Maltha JC, Kuijpers-Jagtman AM. Tooth movement with light continuous and discontinuous forces in beagle dogs. *Eur J Oral Sci.* 1999;197:468–474.)

because the cell biology system remains in a constantly responsive state. Conversely the application of intermittent forces creates a fluctuating environment of cellular activity and quiescence (Fig. 5-3, A). Additionally, it is recognized that very low forces produce lower rates of tooth movement then higher forces (Fig. 5-3, B) up to a specific optimal threshold. Exceeding this optimal force does not result in substantially greater rates of tooth movement. This threshold may differ between individuals as demonstrated in experiments on beagle dogs where it was noted that 25 cN of force caused greater tooth movement than 10 cN of force in one animal but not in another (Fig. 5-3, B and C).

Ankylosis

In rare cases a tooth may not move at all, regardless of the amount of external force applied on it. A likely cause of this is a phenomenon known as "ankylosis" where the PDL fibers are conspicuously absent and therefore cannot serve as an intermediary between the root structure and the alveolar bone. The contact point is a direct fusion of the cementum layer to the cortical bone of the tooth socket. Apart from idiopathic ankylosis, the primary cause of ankylosis is extrinsic localized trauma.[13] In cases of severe dental trauma, such as avulsion or intrusion, there is injury to the periodontal membrane resulting in a direct fusion of the alveolar bone with the tooth. Consequences of this condition include progressive resorption of the root with replacement by bone (replacement resorption) and arrested growth of the alveolar process in growing patients. Individuals with congenitally missing succedaneous permanent teeth characteristically exhibit infraocclusion and overretention of ankylosed deciduous teeth.[14] Partial ankylosis can occur when only limited areas of the teeth are fused to the bone. If these localized regions of bone–tooth attachment can be overcome with sufficient force application, the remainder of the tooth that does have PDL support can proceed toward a normal pattern of tissue remodeling and tooth movement.

Principles of Anchorage in Orthodontics

The biomechanics of orthodontics are not always designed for the purpose of moving teeth. In certain cases the intent of the clinician may be to hold the position of certain teeth in the arch or to use groups of teeth comprising an "anchor unit" to serve as a foundation for pushing or pulling other teeth. Several types of anchorage are used in orthodontics: (1) extraoral anchorage appliances (e.g., headgear) where external skeletal structures are used, (2) intraoral osseointegrated implants and temporary anchorage devices (TADs) that are physically interlocked within the bone and therefore are very stable, and (3) dental anchorage, which is essentially the preparation and consolidation of teeth into units for use in pushing or pulling the rest of the dentition.

Dental anchorage is a term applied to the intentional minimization of migration of specific teeth through the supporting alveolar bone structure. The following section elaborates on dental anchorage since it is based on the premise of biological adaptation to orthodontic forces. Dental anchorage can be increased either by increasing the number of teeth consolidated into the anchor unit or by intentionally angulating specific teeth to better resist movement, or both. In general, teeth with greater root surface area tend to move less when used to move teeth with less root surface area. This occurs because the ability to resist movement is directly related to the periodontal fibers and bone surface area engaged in withstanding tooth movement. When forces are light and distributed over large surface areas, the compression on underlying periodontal structures leads to a partial vascular occlusion of the system and a transient ischemia.

Although limited, there is still oxygenation to the area, enabling the microsystem to adapt and recruit new blood vessels for initiation of frontal resorption to occur. Movement of teeth with frontal resorption occurs within 3 to 4 days. However, when hyalinization of bone occurs in areas of periodontal compression during force application, there is a significant retardation of tooth movement while undermining resorption occurs. In this case the resistance to tooth movement is due to complete vascular occlusion in the compression area causing localized necrosis of bone and undermining resorption. When this happens the teeth start moving only after 12 to 15 days of bone remodeling. Therefore anchorage preparation is affected by the magnitude of forces applied, the total root surface area of the teeth upon which the forces are applied, and the angulation of the teeth.

Increasing numbers of adults are seeking orthodontic treatment today and in these cases anchorage becomes a critical concern. Extraoral anchorage appliances are not usually a feasible alternative for these individuals. Therefore the clinician must maximize all available resources, such as the engagement and colligation of second molars (and third molars, if present) into the dental anchorage unit as well as the use of palatal anchorage devices such as the Nance acrylic button appliance. Also in multidisciplinary cases, implants and other fixed restorative devices can and should be incorporated into the treatment plan for use as anchorage units during orthodontics. Finally, the introduction of TADs has provided substantial advantages for anchorage preservation in adults and adolescents alike and has opened up novel approaches to orthodontic biomechanics in complex cases.[15]

Histological Responses

In general, teeth can move through their investing tissues with or without histological evidence of tissue injury. There is no evidence that the intra-alveolar phase of tooth movement during physiological eruption, drift, or relapse is mediated by pathological processes.[16–18] However, most studies of orthodontic tooth movement have described pathological processes at sites of compression, including vascular collapse, compensatory hyperemia, and tissue necrosis. Hyperemic changes are not restricted to the periodontal tissues adjacent to compression but have also been variously described in the adjacent marrow spaces and the dental pulp.

Tooth Movement Without Injury

The most obvious course of physiological tooth movement is the intra-alveolar eruption of teeth. As the crown of a tooth completes mineralization and begins its process of migration through the alveolar bone, it becomes enclosed in a crypt. This crypt is translated bodily by a combined effort of osteoclastic bone resorption along the path of eruption and osteoblastic bone formation on the path that the crown has already taken. The rate-limiting factor of the earliest (intraosseous) stage of tooth eruption is bone resorption and eruption can be accelerated or retarded by the local delivery of factors that alter the rate of osteoclastic activity.[19] Certain hormones, such as parathyroid hormone–related protein (PTHrP), have been shown to be crucial in the normal tooth eruption processes and cementogenesis.[20,21] Pathological systemic conditions with dysfunctional PTH/PTHrP or their cognate receptors can lead to the prevention of normal tooth eruption and inhibition of normal cementogenesis.

As teeth erupt into the oral cavity, and even throughout life, there is a natural tendency for them to continue moving along the path of least resistance until they encounter an obstacle of resistance. Usually this barrier comes in the form of interproximal contact from an adjacent tooth or occlusal contact from a tooth in the opposing arch. In the absence of this resistance there will be continued mesiodistal tipping or supraeruption, depending on the location of deficient contact. Studies have shown that mesial drifting of a tooth can have clinical significance on its morphological composition. In the process of mesial migration, tensional forces on the distal root surfaces may account for the increased cementum thickness on the distal surfaces of mesially drifted teeth.[22] As for supraeruption, in a mouse model where the opposing molar was extracted to induce occlusal hypofunction, histological staining showed that after 15 days of hypofunction the PDL was significantly narrowed and the fibrous nature was very disorganized for a minimum of 30 days and up to 3 months. There was concurrent deposition of disorganized woven bone at the top of the interradicular septa, at the bottom of the sockets, and along the modeling sides.[23] Thus it is evident that loading is an integral part of the maintenance of the supporting structures surrounding the tooth.

Tooth Movement with Injury

Necrotic lesions at compression sites in the PDL space have been described in the early literature documenting the histological changes accompanying orthodontic tooth movement.[24] These areas are referred to as "hyalinization zones" because of their similarity in appearance to hyaline cartilage. Modern morphological techniques have elucidated that these so-called "hyalinizations" are in fact areas of focal tissue necrosis.[25] As long as these lesions persist, orthodontic tooth movement does not occur. This period is coincident with the delay phase of the tooth movement cycle. Specialized phagocytic cells are recruited and migrate to the site to remove these necrotic lesions. These cells remove the injured tissue from the periphery, resulting in the resorption of not only the necrotic soft tissue lesion but also the adjacent alveolar bone and cementum.[26]

The tissue responses at sites of tension are consistent with those that have been described for other sites where soft tissue separates bone. In addition to the PDL, such sites can be found naturally in the craniofacial complex at sutures and artificially at sites of osteodistraction. Tensile forces are known to initiate an exuberant osteogenic response at these locations, with the first bone being deposited on the stretched soft tissue scaffold (Fig. 5-4). Through remodeling processes new compact bone is eventually deposited at these sites. This so-called consolidation process is slow to occur and therefore tends to lag behind the tissue removal activity that is simultaneously occurring at compression sites. The clinical result

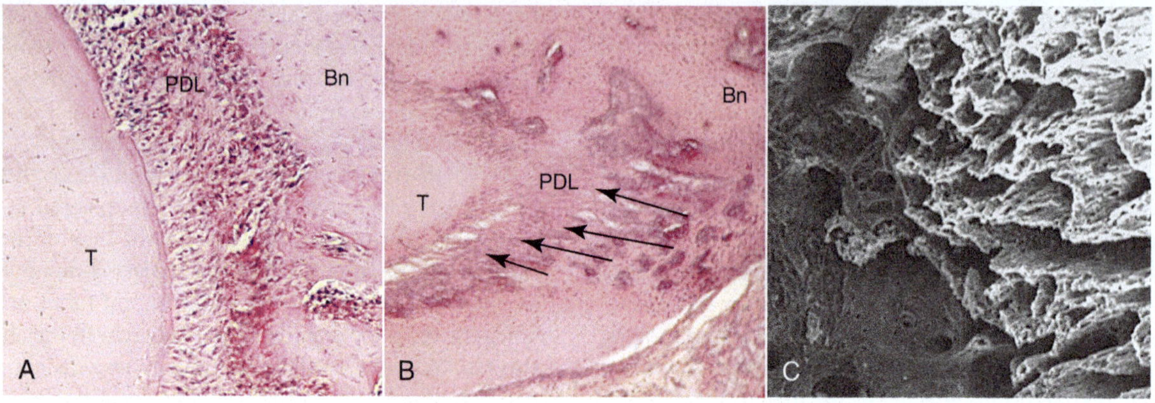

Figure 5-4 Morphological changes on the tension side during orthodontic tooth movement. **A,** Initial changes are characterized by stretching of the principal periodontal ligament (PDL) fibers, seen here as linear orientation of cell nuclei adjacent to the tooth. **B,** Later changes show deposition of bone on the stretched PDL fibers, oriented perpendicular to the tooth and socket wall *(arrows)*. *Bn,* Alveolar bone; *T,* tooth root. **C,** The three-dimensional organization of these initial bony spicules can be appreciated with a scanning electron micrograph of the alveolar bone on the socket wall after removal of the tooth and PDL. The micrograph is looking into the socket with the tension socket wall on the right.

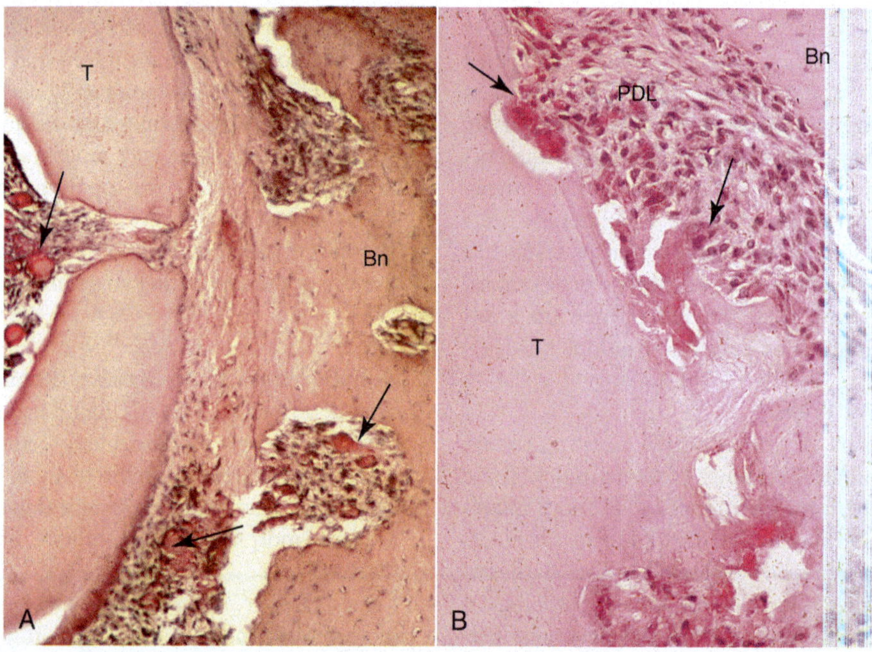

Figure 5-5 Morphological changes on the compression side showing tissue and cellular responses leading to root resorption during orthodontic tooth movement. **A,** Initial changes are characterized by focal areas of periodontal ligament (PDL) necrosis, so-called hyalinization, seen as the clear area in the PDL running vertically down the center of this micrograph. Areas of vascular congestion can be seen adjacent (pulp, PDL, and marrow spaces) to the necrotic PDL *(arrows)*. **B,** Later changes show removal of the necrotic PDL and adjacent tissues, including the root cementum and dentin from the periphery by osteoclasts, cementoclasts, and macrophages *(arrows)*. The remaining necrotic PDL is seen as the clear pink area in the lower middle of the micrograph. Vital adjacent PDL can be seen as the highly cellular areas above and below the necrosis. *Bn,* Alveolar bone; *T,* tooth root.

is the prevalence of increased mobility in teeth that are actively being treated orthodontically. This difference in timing between tissue removal and osteogenesis also accounts for the need to retain teeth that have recently been moved.

In addition to bone remodeling, histological evidence has shown that initial root resorption occurs in the peripheries of the necrotic PDL following orthodontic treatment (Fig. 5-5). This is a result of mononucleated nonclast macrophage-like and fibroblast-like cellular activity.[27,28] Minor resorptive lacunae created on the root surface by cementoclasts can be repaired gradually over time. However, heavy forces create extensive defects on the root surface, which exceed reparative capacity and lead to craterlike topography on the root surface and at the apex (Fig. 5-6).

Bone Turnover in Orthodontic Tooth Movement

Osteogenesis and Bone Modeling and Remodeling

Bone structure can be changed in three principle ways: (1) osteogenesis, (2) bone modeling, and (3) bone remodeling. Osteogenesis is when bone is formed on soft tissue and

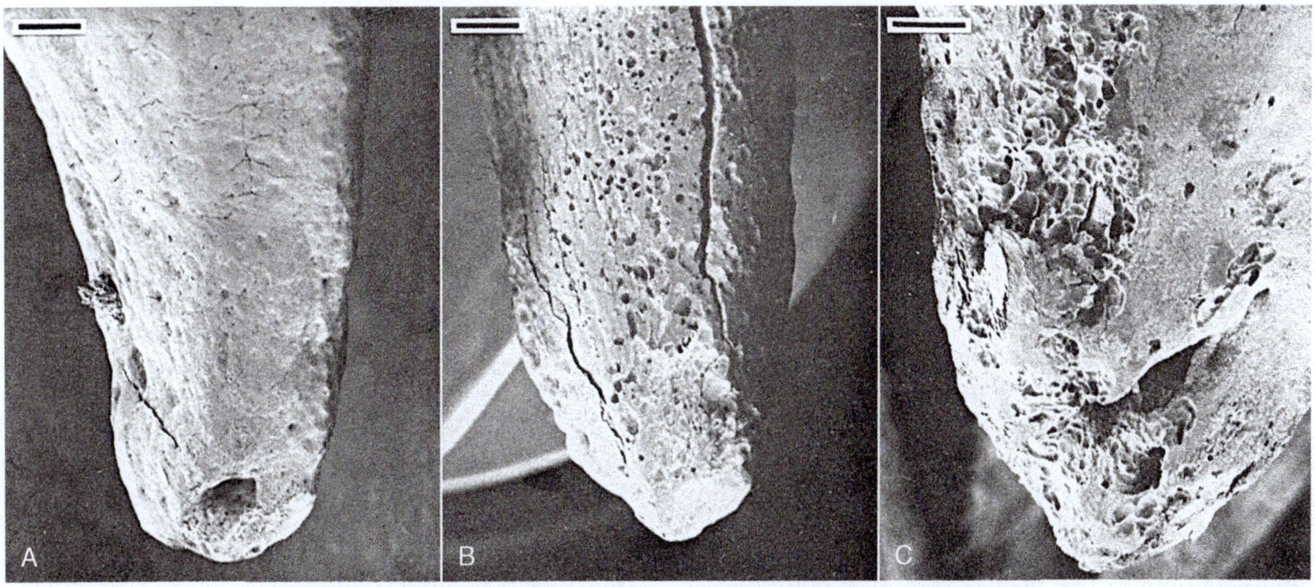

Figure 5-6 Tooth injury resulting in root resorption following bone remodeling. **A,** Apical third of the lingual root surface of the mandibular left bicuspid control tooth demonstrating the absence of resorption. **B,** Apical resorption and loss of root length association with a multitude of resorption pits over the lingual root surface as a result of 2 weeks' application of a continuous 10-g intrusive force. Many of the resorption loci have coalesced to form extensive invasive lesions. **C,** Lingual aspect of a maxillary right bicuspid showing early apical resorption caused by 14 days' intrusion with 50 g. Original magnifications for **A** and **B** are ×20 (bar = 300 mm) and for **C** is ×40 (bar = 200 mm). (Reproduced with permission from Harry MR, Sims MR. Root resorption in bicuspid intrusion: a scanning electron microscope study. *Angle Orthod.* 1982;52:235–258.)

generally occurs during embryonic development, the early stages of growth, and healing. There are two major subclassifications: intramembranous ossification and endochondral ossification, in which bone is formed on soft fibrous tissue and, usually, cartilage, respectively. Osteoblasts are a differentiation product from mesenchymal cells and act independently of osteoclasts, resulting in a large potential to create significant amounts of bone.

Modeling is characterized by bone formation on existing bone tissue over extended surface areas for significant periods of time. This type of bone turnover is prevalent during craniofacial growth and development and leads to change in shape of the structure or translation of the surface. For example, the mandibular alveolar process increases in length by resorptive modeling on the anterior surface of the ramus and by formative modeling on its posterior surface. From an orthodontics standpoint, modeling is important in normal growth of the craniofacial structure as well as changes in alveolar size and shape during tooth movement.

Remodeling is a reparative mechanism and involves a series of cellular events that occur cyclically throughout life (Fig. 5-7). It is the only physiological mechanism for maintaining and repairing the structural integrity of bone. The bone remodeling cycle begins with a period referred to as activation that is characterized by the recruitment and activation of osteoclasts at the site to be remodeled. This is followed by a resorptive phase when a "packet" of bone is removed. After a finite amount of time the resorptive process ceases. This phase is termed reversal. Reversal is followed by a formative phase characterized by the recruitment of bone formative cells to the site and the active repair of the defect created during the resorptive phase. Once the cycle is complete, the bone surface returns to a resting state. In healthy adults bone surfaces are primarily in a resting state, although a small fraction of the cell population can be seen to progress through the other phases. Remodeling is important in calcium homeostasis as well as in producing changes in bone matrices that modify the mechanical properties of the bone in response to altered loading. Remodeling and modeling of bone are differentiated by the fact that while

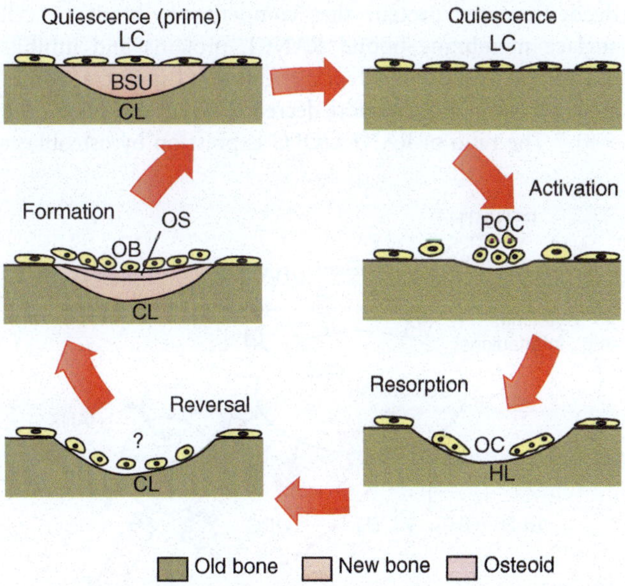

Figure 5-7 Cellular quiescence phase and five phases of cellular activity in remodeling of trabecular bone. *BSU,* Bone structural unit or newly formed bone structure; *CL,* closed lacunae; *HL,* Howship lacunae/resorption pit; *LC,* lining cells; *OB,* osteoblast; *OC,* osteoclasts; *OS,* osteoid; *POC,* osteoclast precursors.

osteoblast and osteoclast activities are found on the same site in remodeling, they occur on different sites in modeling, which enables morphological changes in the bone.

Cellular and Molecular Mechanisms of Bone Modeling and Remodeling

Skeletal integrity is the result of a dynamic interaction between bone-forming osteoblasts and bone-resorbing osteoclasts. The rate of remodeling is defined primarily by cells of the osteoblast lineage, which in addition to bone formation are also responsible for the activation and recruitment of osteoclast precursors.[29–31] The basis of communication between osteoblasts and osteoclasts was unclear until several groups independently identified the presence of an intermediary factor on the surface of osteoblasts that was responsible for the induction of osteoclastogenesis. This factor is a member of the tumor necrosis factor (TNF) superfamily and was termed receptor activator of nuclear factor κB ligand (RANKL).[32,33] Binding of RANKL to its cognate receptor, receptor activator of nuclear factor κB (RANK), expressed on the surface of osteoclast progenitor cells, induces osteoclastogenesis and activates osteoclasts (in the presence of macrophage colony-stimulating factor), resulting in increased bone resorption.[34,35] However, RANKL also has the potential to bind to osteoprotegerin (OPG), a soluble decoy receptor protein that competitively binds to cell surface membrane–bound RANKL proteins and inhibits RANKL activation of osteoclastogenesis. The interaction of RANKL with OPG therefore decreases bone resorption (Fig. 5-8).[36] The ratio of RANKL/OPG expression by osteoblasts is believed to be a key determinant of the rate of recruitment and activation of immature osteoclasts. In dentistry these genes have already been strongly implicated as the causative factors of alveolar bone changes. RANKL and OPG protein production has been detected in human periodontal cells.[37] Pathologically, lymphocytes and macrophages in periodontitis tissues show correlations with RANKL protein production and endothelial cells have associations with OPG production.[38] From an orthodontic perspective, it is very likely that pressure changes in the microenvironment of the tooth socket may cause up-regulation and down-regulation of the RANKL and OPG genes as a means of modulating protein production and ultimately bone remodeling.

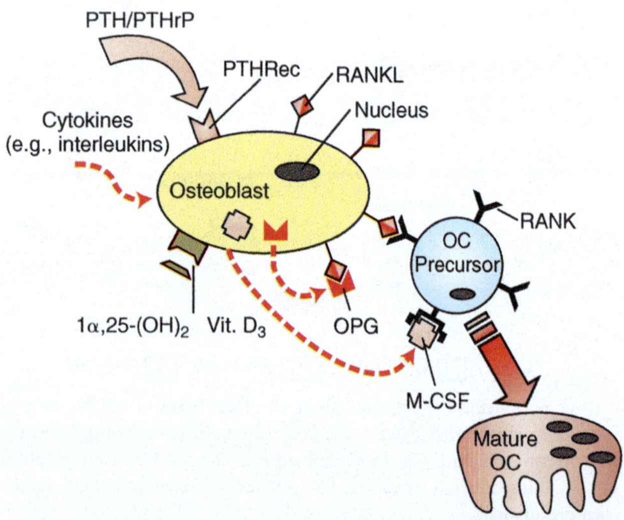

Figure 5-8 Regulation of osteoclastogenesis by osteoblasts. Receptor activator of nuclear factor κB ligand (RANKL) induces immature osteoclast (OC) precursors to differentiate into mature and functional osteoclasts, while osteoprotegerin (OPG) is a decoy receptor that acts as a competitive binding inhibitor of RANKL. Since RANKL is a cell surface–bound receptor protein, cell–cell interaction is required. Macrophage colony-stimulating factor (M-CSF) is also an essential co-factor. Vitamin D_3 and various cytokines have been demonstrated to have down-regulatory effects on OPG gene expression and up-regulatory effects on RANKL gene expression. *PTH*, Parathyroid hormone; *PTHRec*, PTH receptor; *PTHrP*, PTH-related protein.

Besides the prominent role of the RANKL/OPG ratio in the regulation of osteoclasts by osteoblasts, the rate of bone remodeling is controlled by other local and systemic mechanisms. Local, or paracrine, mechanisms involve numerous inflammatory cytokines (e.g., interleukins, TNFs, and growth factors) that have biological activities influencing individual phases of the cycle (Fig. 5-9).[39] In addition, there is evidence that alterations in the genetic expression of bioactive agents can occur directly on bone cells. Systemic control of bone remodeling occurs through several endocrine mechanisms, including the calciotropic hormones (e.g., parathyroid hormone [PTH] and 1α,25-$(OH)_2$ vitamin D_3) and the sex steroids (e.g., estrogen).[40–42] These factors act on osteoblasts as an intermediary to regulate osteoblast-osteoclast equilibrium and can either up-regulate or down-regulate a cascade of downstream signaling pathways that ultimately affect the expression of specific genes necessary to synthesize proteins involved in bone remodeling. For example, estrogen inhibits bone resorption, at least in part, by regulating the production of several cytokines, including interleukin-6 (IL-6), IL-1, RANKL, and OPG by cells of the osteoblastic lineage.[43] The potential implications and more recent findings on the applications of this knowledge to orthodontics are discussed at the end of the chapter.

The human bone remodeling cycle takes about 4 months and is characterized by a rapid period of resorption followed by a fairly slow period of formation. In a healthy adult bone resorption is coupled to formation so that there is no net loss or gain. However, in certain disease conditions this coupling can be lost, resulting in a net loss or gain of bone. Because it takes significantly more time to complete bone formation than it does to complete resorption, stimulation of large amounts of remodeling often leads to a net bone loss. This can be a temporary condition if the level of remodeling activity returns to normal, permitting formation to "catch up" with resorption as characterized by fracture healing. However, if high levels of bone remodeling persist, bone can be lost permanently, as in postmenopausal osteoporosis.

Conversely, increased bone density resulting in osteopetrosis is a clinical manifestation of certain syndromes, such as Albers-Schönberg disease and Paget disease, where there is an excessive hyperactivity of the osteoclasts resulting in a concurrent compensatory excessive deposition of bone. Rates of bone remodeling may be increased up to 20-fold,

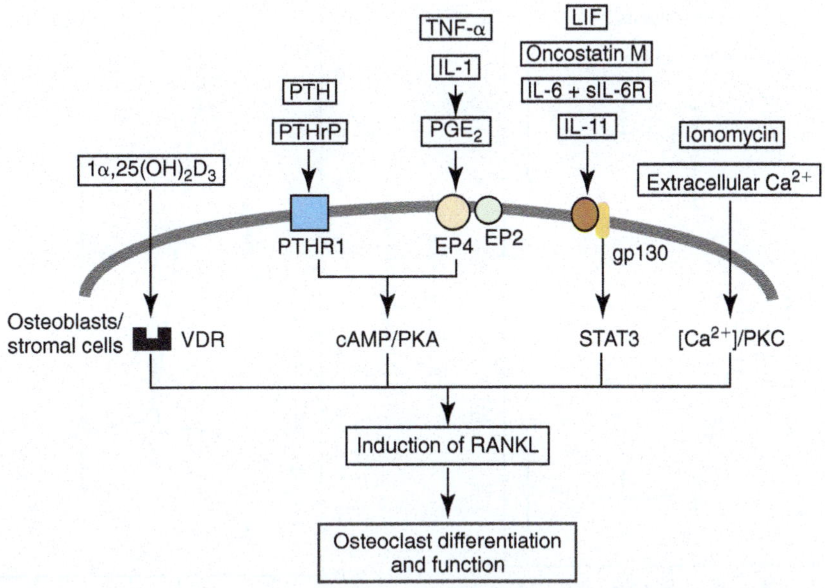

Figure 5-9 Paracrine and endocrine regulation of receptor activator of nuclear factor κB ligand (RANKL) in osteoblasts or stromal cells, which in turn induces osteoclastogenesis and results in the alteration of the osteoblast-osteoclast equilibrium. Hormones and cytokine factors: *1α,25(OH)$_2$D$_3$*; *1α*, vitamin D receptor; *PTH/PTHrP*, parathyroid hormone/PTH-related protein receptor; *PTHR1*, parathyroid hormone receptor type 1; *TNF-α*, tumor necrosis factor-α; *IL-1, IL-6, sIL-6R, IL-11*, interleukin-1, interleukin-6, soluble IL-6 receptor, interleukin-11; *PGE$_2$*, prostaglandin E$_2$; *LIF*, leukemia inhibitory factor. Pathways: *VDR*, Vitamin D receptor; *cAMP/PKA*, cyclic adenosine monophosphate/protein kinase A pathway; *STAT3*, signal transducer and activator of transcription 3 (important for the signal transduction of IL-6 and related cytokines); *[Ca^{2+}]/PKC*, calcium concentration/protein kinase C pathway. (Reproduced with permission from Takahashi N, Udagawa N, Takami M, Suda T. Cells of bone: osteoclast generation. In: Bilezikian JP, Raisz LG, Rodan GA, eds. *Principles of Bone Biology*. San Diego, CA: Academic Press; 2002:109–126.)

but this coupling is imperfect. Since the newly formed bone is laid down so quickly, it is irregular and chaotic, resulting in a composite mixture of lamellar and woven bone, which compromises the quality of the bone. The clinical consequences of this abnormal bone cell activity include diffuse sclerosis of the whole skeleton accompanied by pathological bone fragility and delayed physical development, profound intractable myelophthisic anemia, neurological deficits, and osteomyelitis, especially of the jaws and skull. Eruption and development of the dentition can be impeded and delayed due to the irregular bone remodeling adjacent to the tooth bud and crown.

BIOLOGICAL RESPONSES IN CLINICAL TREATMENT

In orthodontic tooth movement, sites of tension display osteogenesis over an extensive surface area, a framework consistent with modeling (Fig. 5-10, A). However, sites of compression undergo phases of a remodeling cycle (Fig. 5-10, B).[44] Since large amounts of remodeling are initiated at these sites, there is a net loss of alveolar bone over a short term, which subsequently returns to pre-treatment levels over the course of orthodontic treatment. This ultimately leads to the clinical characterization of teeth being actively moved (i.e., radiographic evidence of widening of the PDL and clinical evidence of increased tooth mobility). This, along with the persistence of stretched ligament and gingival fibers, leads to rapid relapse of orthodontically moved teeth and necessitates stabilization, at least until bone formation is able to return to pre-treatment levels.[45] Recent advances in the potential utility of biological mediators in enhancing anchorage[46] and post-treatment stability[47] are discussed later in the chapter.

There is a predictable relationship between mechanical strain and bone turnover. Increasing amounts of strain stimulate osteogenesis and conversely the lack of strain on bone (e.g., weightlessness during space flight) leads to osteopenia. Superficially this seems to contradict what happens in orthodontic tooth movement because sites of compression lose bone and sites of tension gain it. However, it is important to realize that the PDL is loaded in tension sites and unloaded in compression sites. The latter also exhibit evidence of tissue damage and infiltration of inflammatory cells releasing cytokines, which can also stimulate large amounts of bone resorption. Recent studies show that alveolar bone at sites distant from the tooth socket wall contribute to the bone remodeling response, and this is consistent with what would be predicted by the bone literature (i.e., bony trabeculae adjacent to compression sites are osteogenic and those next to tension sites are not).[48] Evidence also indicates that tissues are directly sensitive to deformations and strains in their immediate environment in addition to pressure or tension.[49]

Biological data are helpful in answering several clinically relevant questions in orthodontic tooth movement. How does bone density alter tooth movement? What is the relationship between force level and clinical response? How do intermittently applied forces compare to constant forces? What is the most effective rhythm for appliance reactivations? There is some controversy regarding the relationship

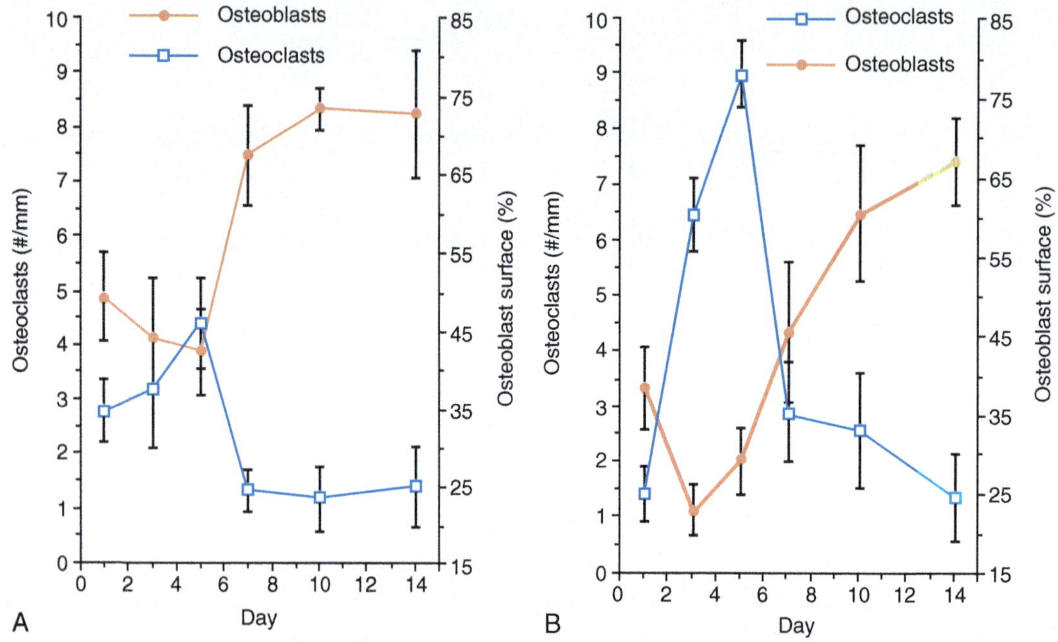

Figure 5-10 Cell dynamics associated with orthodontic tooth movement. **A,** Tension sites are characterized by an increase in osteoblasts and a reduction in resident osteoclasts in the latter part of the tooth movement. **B,** Compression sites are characterized by an influx of osteoclasts in the early part of the tooth movement followed by their reversal to baseline levels, followed by an increase in osteoblasts in the latter part of the tooth movement.

between alveolar bone density and orthodontic tooth movement. Moreover, the extent to which bone density affects root resorption is not fully understood. Some approaches to orthodontic treatment recommend taking advantage of the more dense cortical bone to enhance anchorage. This approach assumes that teeth would move more slowly through more dense alveolar bone. Although this appears to be a reasonable assumption, clinical studies have not been able to support the effectiveness of this approach. Some studies have found a relationship between root resorption and movement of teeth through dense cortical bone, while others have not. Orthodontic tooth movement in animal models has been shown to be accelerated when alveolar bone density is experimentally reduced, which also results in reduced risk of root resorption.[50] Today, bioactive agents show promise of being able to reduce localized bone density and the use of such agents in conjunction with conventional fixed appliances may provide more rapid tooth movement of individual teeth with less risk of root resorption.

The relationship between tooth movement and force magnitude is also controversial. Some data suggest that a force optimum exists, where there is a direct linear relationship at low force levels and an inverse one at high forces. Animal data have confirmed the direct linear relationship at low force levels but seem to suggest that there is a plateau at higher levels. Despite the persistence of biomechanical approaches to orthodontic treatment that assume the existence of an optimal force for orthodontic tooth movement, there is no direct evidence for it. Clinical studies aimed at addressing the concept are technically quite complex because of the difficulty of accurately measuring tooth movement and force magnitude and distribution in a clinical environment. As technology develops, intraoral biomechanical sensors with data storage capacities should become available. Highly sensitive methods for measuring orthodontic tooth movement in three dimensions using modern imaging instrumentation are also rapidly becoming a reality.[11,51] Together, these two advances should make clinical studies of this relationship feasible in the near future.

Orthodontists realize that the biomechanics can be quite complex. Most appliances can be considered to be slowly dissipating. The goal of constant force may not be routinely achieved even with the use of superelastic wires. Clinicians also commonly use appliances with interrupted and intermittent durations of force application. Superimposed on the mechanics are the usual forces associated with oral physiology (e.g., chewing, deglutition, and speech). Most studies have attempted to model this complex mechanical environment by asking simple questions or creating simplified models about its component parts.

What does it take to initiate orthodontic tooth movement? The bone literature suggests that significant amounts of osteogenesis can be stimulated by short exposures to dynamic strains.[52] Orthodontists expect to see tooth movement in response to less than constant force application (e.g., headgears and functional appliances). This is further supported by animal studies that have shown tooth movement with part-time exposure to mechanical signals.[53] A relevant question would be how long do the tissue changes stimulated during orthodontic tooth movement continue following appliance removal? Despite rapid relapse under these conditions, there is evidence that the cellular changes persist for a period of time, which would presumably be reflected in a more rapid response to a second appliance activation following a rest interval.[54] Some clinical studies have reported no difference in tooth movement when comparing constant and intermittent force protocols. Animal studies have suggested that the key factor may be the duration of force application, with forces for about one quarter of the time being effective, although other animals studies have shown that jiggling forces of extremely short duration can stimulate large numbers of osteoclasts and the tooth mobility characteristic of orthodontics.[55,56] This may be the case because intermittent protocols with short durations of force application provide long periods of time for significant amounts of relapse to occur.

Because most orthodontic appliances are slowly dissipating, clinical treatment can be viewed as a series of intermittent force applications. Experimental data from animal models suggest that reactivating an orthodontic appliance over longer intervals stimulates more efficient tooth movement than reactivations over short intervals.[10] Biochemical analysis of known markers of active bone metabolism have demonstrated that significant amounts of alveolar bone turnover continue for an indeterminate period following appliance decay.[57] Studies of tooth movement and tissue responses following reactivations indicate that linear tooth movement and rapid recruitment of osteoclasts can be achieved if reactivation is timed to coincide with the latter part of the bone remodeling cycle initiated by the first activation.[58] Clinical data on reactivation rhythm are extremely important to improving the efficiency and safety of treatment. Again, in the absence of sensitive means to monitor biomechanics and tooth movement in three dimensions, these experiments will be difficult to accomplish (Fig. 5-11).

Related to the concept of reactivation timing is how the circadian rhythm factors into the biology of tooth movement. Since there is a decreased metabolism at night during sleep, the question arises as to whether this becomes more favorable or less desirable for tooth movement. A research study was carried out on subjects divided into three groups: appliances were activated over 21 days either continuously throughout the experimental period, only during the light (0700 to 1900 hours) period, or only during the dark (1900 to 0700 hours) period.[59] Results demonstrated that the tooth movement in the whole-day and light-period groups was about twice that in the dark-period group. Histological

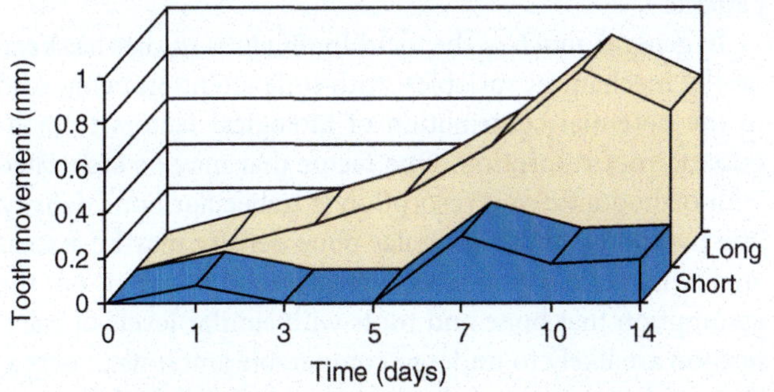

Figure 5-11 Orthodontic tooth movement curves following short (1 day) and long (10 days) interval reactivation schedules. Note the greater overall tooth movement without a delay period.

evaluation of the periodontal tissues confirmed that there was greater new bone formation on the tension side in the whole-day and light-period groups and more osteoclastic activity on the pressure side compared to the dark-period group. Overall, the light-period group exhibited decreased hyalinization of the PDL compared to the whole-day group. Therefore it is obvious that diurnal rhythms in bone metabolism and physiology have significant ramifications for orthodontic tooth movement.

The desirable goal of expediting tooth movement remains a perplexing and complex issue to resolve. Several historical approaches and some novel ones have recently been proposed to facilitate this goal. Prominent among these approaches are those dependent on physical or mechanical stimulation (vibrations, low-level laser, electrical current, and pulsed electromagnetic fields) and surgically facilitated orthodontic therapy (SFOT) (corticotomy, dentoalveolar distraction, periodontal distraction). Most of these have yet to be shown to expedite orthodontic tooth movement or, as in the case of corticotomies, appear to do so only transiently.[60,61] All of these approaches in principle attempt to modulate biological processes nonspecifically rather than to rationally use knowledge of bone biology to achieve the desired expedited tooth movement. Thus, for example, corticotomies result in short-term acceleration of tooth movement, which may be related to its modulation of a transient increase in RANKL[61] but has the caveat of significant patient morbidity and costs. In contrast, a more logical approach to achieving the goal of faster tooth movement would entail directly harnessing the biological regulation of bone turnover without large surgical procedures. Indeed, the local gene transfer of RANKL that results in a sustained overexpression of RANKL over time is accompanied by greater amounts and rates of tooth movement in experimental rats than in control rats or in rats subjected to corticotomies.[61,62] A consistent increase in RANKL expression and osteoclastogenesis occurs locally in the RANKL-vector injected side without either local inflammation at the injection site or systemic bony effects in the tibia. Thus local gene transfer or possibly local administration of pro-osteoclastic factors may prove to be a more attractive option than surgery or other options currently in use in enhancing tooth movement.

ROOT RESORPTION

Root resorption is a relatively common sequel of orthodontic treatment. Consequences range from slight tooth mobility resulting from mild amounts of root resorption to complete loss of teeth due to excessive root resorption. The type and magnitude of root resorption vary substantially from mild apical root blunting in a large number of cases, to lateral root resorption, to, infrequently but unfortunately, excessive root loss (Fig. 5-12). Because of the potential for significant clinical and legal implications of root resorption, assessment of the biological and mechanical basis of root resorption has been the subject of extensive research and discussion for almost a century. Yet because of the multiple factors contributing to

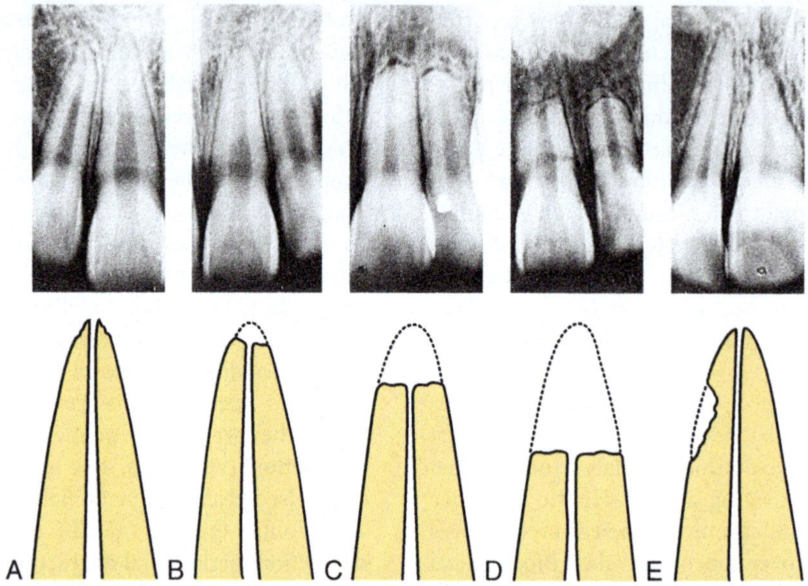

Figure 5-12 Types of root resorption observed in orthodontic patients. These are depicted radiographically (*upper panel*) and diagrammatically (*lower panel*) and range from **(A)** very mildly irregular apical root contours, to **(B)** mild apical root blunting, to **(C)** moderate apical root resorption, to **(D)** severe apical root resorption, to **(E)** lateral root resorption. (Modified from Goldson L, Malmgren O. Orthodontic treatment of traumatized teeth. In: Andreasen JO, ed. *Traumatic Injuries of the Teeth*. 2nd ed. Philadelphia, PA: WB Saunders; 1981:395.)

this process, the research findings are inconclusive and remain a highly debated topic in the literature.[63,64]

As early as 1914 clinical observers suggested a direct link between orthodontic treatment and root resorption.[65] In the late 1920s radiographic evidence demonstrating differences in root morphology before and after orthodontic treatment was presented.[66,67] Since then numerous potential causal relationships and contributory factors have been proposed and studied but definitive explanations of why root resorption occurs and what factors contribute to its occurrence have remained controversial. A comprehensive understanding of this problem has remained elusive because of the difficulty in comparing the results and conclusions of various studies that have used different experimental designs, patient populations, treatment mechanics, and analyses. Additionally, the variability in radiographic techniques and materials in different studies further contributes to the discrepant findings among studies. Finally, because of inherent differences in the characteristics of both the patient and the treatment, far too many potential etiologic factors have been considered in these studies, making it impossible to derive any meaningful conclusions. A better understanding of this important clinical problem requires controlled studies that are designed to examine the association between a limited set of variables and root resorption. The verification of the reliability of three-dimensional cone beam computed tomography (CBCT) relative to two-dimensional radiographs for assessing root resorption will be beneficial in better deciphering the variables associated with or contributing to root resorption.[68–72]

While the causative or contributory factors of orthodontic root resorption remain unknown, several studies have proposed a spectrum of factors that may predispose patients to root resorption. A hereditary component for orthodontic root resorption has been suggested by findings showing a significantly higher co-occurrence of root resorption among siblings than among nonsiblings (Fig. 5-13).[73] In the context of genetic predisposition to root resorption, findings also support the notion of an association, albeit small, between IL-1α, TNF-α, and osteopontin polymorphisms and root resorption.[74–76] Other studies have explored the relationship of force strength, as well as rate and direction of tooth movement, to root resorption with inconsistent findings.[77,78] A positive association between duration of treatment and root resorption has been demonstrated.[79,80] Root morphology, specifically abnormally shaped or dilacerated roots, also appears to influence the severity of root resorption.[81,82] Root resorption of varying degrees has been observed in the sagittal, transverse, and vertical planes of tooth movement.[83,84] Previous trauma to teeth treated orthodontically may also be a significant risk factor for root resorption.[85] However, because of the low incidence of trauma to teeth, this factor possibly accounts for root resorption in relatively few patients.

In general, much of the focus in previous studies has been on the mechanical variables, with little attention being paid to the potential contribution of biological factors to orthodontic root resorption. One factor that may be associated with orthodontic root resorption is trabecular bone density. The hypothesis that trabecular bone density may be associated with orthodontic root resorption is based on the assumption that bone and roots with similar levels of calcification are likely to undergo comparable amounts of degradation when exogenous forces are applied. While there is no conclusive evidence to support this hypothesis, some studies have provided indirect evidence for a potential association

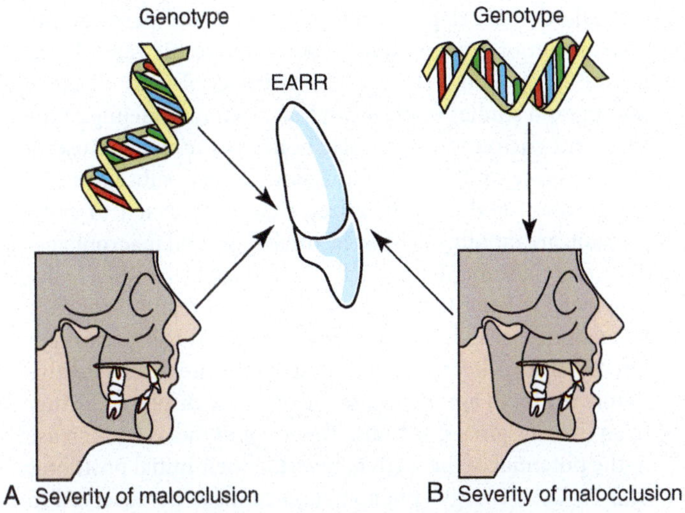

Figure 5-13 Competing models for the pathway through which an individual's genotype modulates the extent of external apical root resorption (EARR) experienced during the course of orthodontic treatment. **A,** The first paradigm suggests that the amount of EARR during treatment depends on an individual's genotype and, independently, on malocclusion. Genotype and malocclusion both have a modulating effect on the extent of EARR but they operate along separate biological and biomechanical pathways. With this model, a patient's genotype would have a direct effect on the extent of EARR and incorporating measures of severity of malocclusion into statistical design would not affect the estimate of heritability (h^2, the proportion of the total variance due to common genetic influences). **B,** The alternative paradigm is that genotype has an indirect effect acting through malocclusion. This model acknowledges that craniometric studies show that facial size and shape have moderately high genetic components. Because siblings share similar craniofacial relationships, the genetic influence on EARR would be modulated through malocclusion. With this model, inclusion of skeletodental covariates would alter h^2 estimates, although it is not clear a priori that estimates should necessarily increase or decrease. (Reproduced from Harris EF, Kineret SE, Tolley EA. A heritable component for external apical root resorption in patients treated orthodontically. *Am J Orthod Dentofacial Orthop.* 1997;111:301–309.)

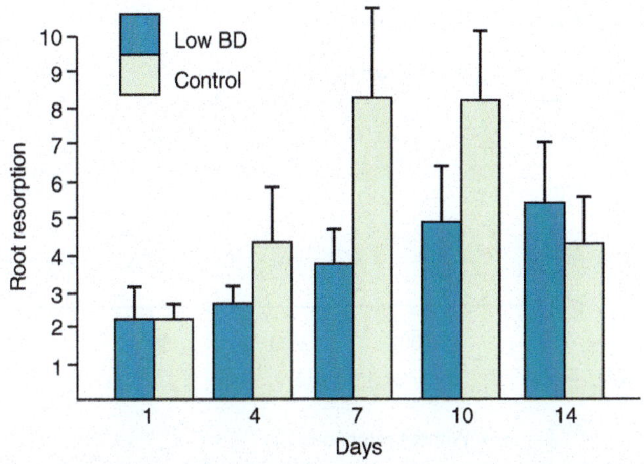

Figure 5-14 Root resorption comparison between normal (control) and low bone density (low BD). Note that there is less root resorption in the low-density group. (Reproduced from Harris EF, Kineret SE, Tolley EA. A heritable component for external apical root resorption in patients treated orthodontically. *Am J Orthod Dentofacial Orthop.* 1997;111:301–309.)

between bone density and root resorption. For example, it has been demonstrated that strong forces applied to teeth in less dense alveolar bone cause the same amount of root resorption seen in roots in dense alveolar bone subjected to much weaker forces.[78] Additionally, teeth being moved in close proximity to dense cortical bone undergo greater levels of root resorption than those in trabecular bone.[86] More appropriately, animal studies show that calcium-deficient rats exhibiting very low alveolar density have markedly low levels of root resorption following tooth movement (Fig. 5-14).[50] Similarly, studies on hypocalcemic rats have also demonstrated a proportional relationship between bone density and magnitude of root resorption.[87] These studies provide important insights into the potential association between bone density and root resorption but this association requires more definitive validation.

Finally, the contribution of biological mediators to orthodontic root resorption is coming under increasing scrutiny. In addition to the link between root resorption and gene polymorphisms for IL-1α, TNF-α, and osteopontin[74–76] that can generate varied gene products, some of which likely have greater predisposition to resorption, the RANK/RANKL/OPG pathway that is activated during orthodontic tooth movement may contribute to orthodontic root resorption.[88] When compressed in vitro, PDL cells from cases with severe external apical root resorption (EARR) produce higher levels of RANKL and lower amounts of OPG than cells from control subjects.[89,90] Also, RANKL immunoreactivity has been shown in tissues associated with root resorption as early as day 7 of tooth movement.[91] Finally, rats with higher pre-treatment levels of serum RANKL show more root resorption after tooth movement than rats with lower initial concentrations of RANKL,[92] suggesting that systemic levels of RANKL may be predictive of future root resorption. It is likely that findings such as these will lead to novel approaches to minimize orthodontic root resorption or to help identify patients who may be at a greater risk of root resorption, thereby enabling the clinician to proactively modify treatment objectives and plans.

ORTHODONTIC RELAPSE

Many biological and mechanical factors dictate the rate of tooth movement in orthodontics. Similarly this complex dynamic physiological environment also dictates the amount of relapse, which will occur following the completion of orthodontic treatment. Relapse can be defined as a natural tendency for a tooth or teeth to migrate back to their original pre-treatment position and angulation in the dental arch. In general, the amount of active tooth movement correlates strongly with the relapse potential (i.e., greater distances moved or greater rotations corrected result in a greater tendency for relapse).[93] Factors involved in clinical orthodontic relapse include force duration, distance of tooth movement, and mechanical management to minimize relapse occurrence. The role of gingival and transseptal fibers and the period of bone remodeling following orthodontic tooth

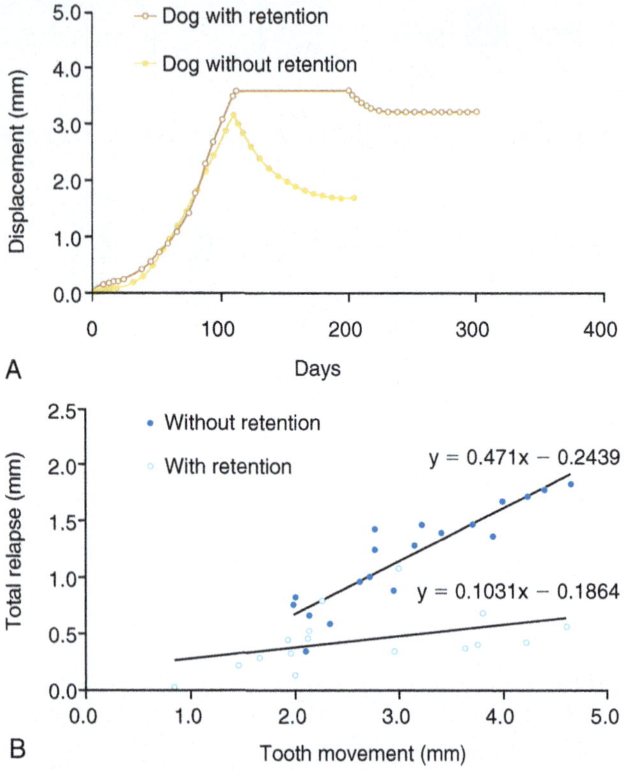

Figure 5-15 Retention enhances stability following orthodontic tooth movement and larger movements correlate with increased relapse, particularly in the absence of retention. **A,** Time–displacement curves of two dog premolars, one with retention and one without. **B,** Relationship between active tooth movement and the total amount of relapse with or without retention. The plots represent linear regression lines for the two different conditions. (Reproduced with permission from van Leeuwen EJ, Maltha JC, Kuijpers-Jagtman AM, van't Hof MA. The effect of retention on orthodontic relapse after the use of small continuous or discontinuous forces: an experimental study in beagle dogs. *Eur J Oral Sci.* 2003;111:111–116.)

movement also play significant roles in the ultimate magnitude of the relapse that occurs.

The potential for relapse is great during a critical period immediately after orthodontic treatment when the teeth and roots have been moved into the desired final position (Fig. 5-15). In the process of tooth movement, bone resorption occurs in areas of pressure and bone deposition occurs in areas of tension, as defined by Wolff's law.[1] The type of bone that is deposited in the area of tension is a rather soft, unorganized osteoid matrix. This bone is subsequently remodeled into organized lamellar bone architecture to provide a stronger alveolar support, a slow process that can take upward of 6 months.[54] At the same time, there are changes in the transseptal fibers attached to the roots of the teeth. The tensile forces cause transseptal fibers to adjust their length by rapid remodeling and this change continues to occur, as demonstrated by increased collagenous protein turnover within the middle third of the transseptal fibers following release of orthodontic force.[94] In all cases it is apparent that the retention mechanism used immediately after removal of the orthodontic appliances is a crucial component of the treatment plan.

Orthodontic relapse occurs when teeth are permitted to migrate out of position during postorthodontic remodeling of the supporting structures. Histological and electron micrograph studies have shown that rapid remodeling of the PDL and surrounding alveolar bones is the main cause of tooth relapse and that hyalinization formed subsequent to compression and/or mineralized tissues subjected to compression are rapidly resorbed by osteoclasts and macrophage-like and fibroblast-like cells.[18] Biological studies have provided evidence that teeth show a greater relapse tendency when continuous forces are used compared to intermittent forces.[95] This is because continuous forces are more effective in moving teeth and therefore the teeth are displaced farther from their original positions. The result of this is an increase in the potential of the teeth to revert to their initial positions. This "relapse energy" phenomenon can also be observed in situations where teeth require rotational correction.

As the tooth is rotated, the PDL is stretched (Fig. 5-16).[96] The greater the magnitude of rotation, the further these fibers become elongated. In its new milieu the PDL is able to reorganize and invest its fibrils in alveolar bone and cementum during the deposition of new bone and cementum. However, this process is slow and requires significant time.[97] Acceleration of this reorganization is facilitated by gingivectomy or circumferential supracrestal fiberotomy (CSF) aimed at surgically releasing the stretched free gingival fibers and allowing reattachment of these fibers in a less stressed or less stretched configuration.[98,99] Scanning electron microscopy and histological evaluation of postfiberotomy teeth confirm that there is an eventual reparative reattachment of the collagen fibers of the PDL (Figs. 5-17 and 5-18). Long-term evaluation at 4 to 6 years and 12 to 14 years after active treatment validates that CSF is effective in improving retention of tooth position.[45] This study also validated that there was neither a clinically significant increase in the periodontal sulcus depth nor a decrease in the labially attached gingiva of the CSF teeth observed at 1 and 6 months following the surgical procedure. However, recent biochemical studies propose that the rotational relapse of a tooth is not due to "stretched" collagen fibers but rather is a result of a change in the elastic properties of the whole gingival tissue.[100] Unlike bone and PDL, which regain their original structure after the removal of force, the gingival tissue does not regain its pre-treatment structure and it may be this tension that contributes to orthodontic relapse.[101]

Biological enhancement of bone maturation or diminishing its degradation by osteoclasts could provide a possible basis for enhancing post-treatment stability. Indeed a recent study[47] demonstrated that the local administration of the RANKL decoy ligand, OPG, inhibits postorthodontic relapse in an animal model of orthodontic tooth movement. Specifically, OPG injections significantly diminished postorthodontic relapse from 63% of total movement in vehicle control rats to as low as 24% in animals receiving OPG 24 days after appliance removal. Histologically the bone and periodontal tissue around teeth appeared normalized as early as 8 days after OPG administration, while the vehicle control group

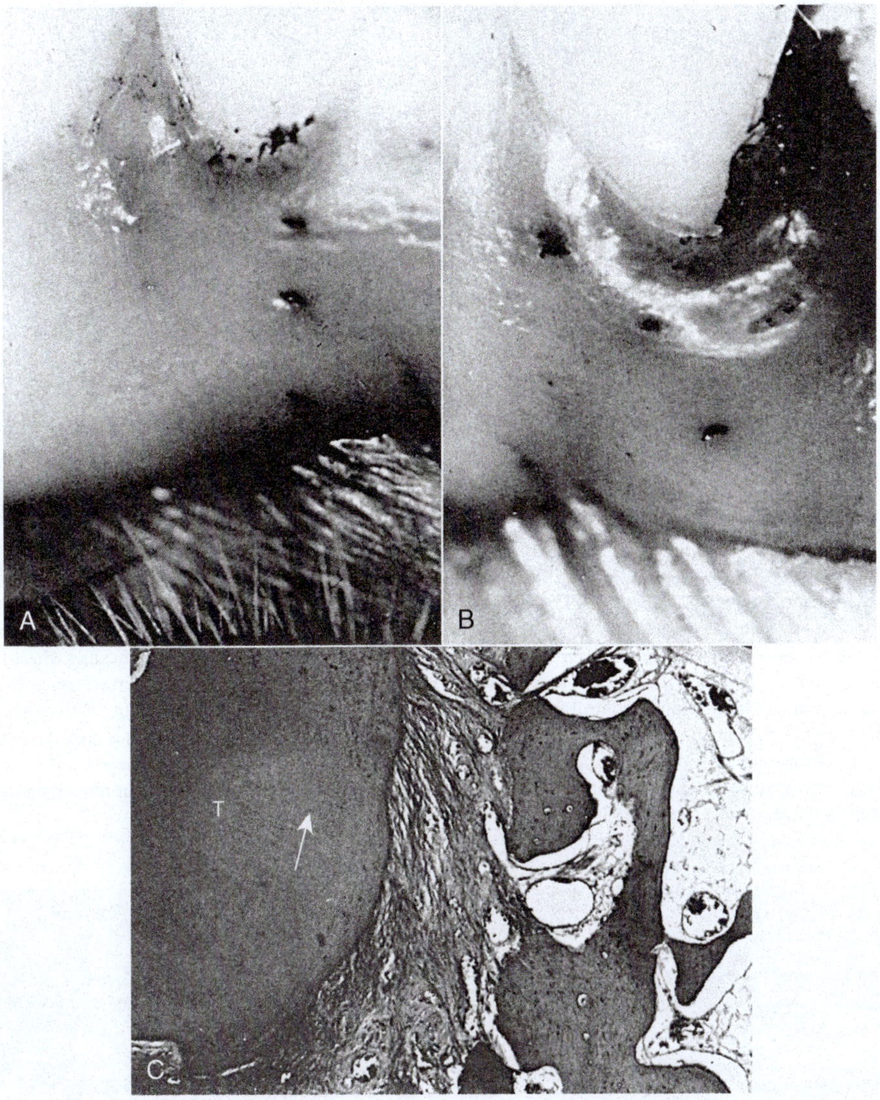

Figure 5-16 Stretching of periodontal ligament (PDL) and gingival tissue by orthodontic rotation of teeth. **A,** Tattoo marks on gingiva before rotation of the tooth. **B,** Tattoo marks on gingiva show deviation in direction of rotational movement of the tooth. **C,** PDL stretched and deviated (*arrow*) during rotation of the tooth (T). Magnification of original is ×64. (Reproduced from Edwards JG. A study of the periodontium during orthodontic rotation of teeth. *Am J Orthod.* 1968;54:441–461.)

showed only partial tissue recovery 24 days following tooth movement. Quantitative bone measures derived from micro-computed tomography had fully recovered to pre-tooth-movement values in OPG-treated animals, while these parameters had recovered only partially or had not recovered in the vehicle control rats 24 days after orthodontic treatment. The profound decrease in postorthodontic relapse by local OPG administration indicates that osteoclasts are critical to bone maturation following tooth movement and points to the potential pharmacological use of OPG or other RANKL inhibitors for orthodontic retention.

The factors noted above are considered intrinsic factors of orthodontic relapse related to the immediate supporting structures of PDL and alveolar bone surrounding the teeth. These relapse factors should be differentiated from extrinsic factors, such as continual craniofacial skeletal growth, external forces from facial muscles, and occlusal interdigitation. Despite the numerous studies over the years defining all of the variables and contributory factors related to orthodontic relapse, the degree of postretention anterior crowding is still both unpredictable and variable and no pre-treatment variables, from clinical findings, casts, or cephalometric radiographs before or after treatment, seem to be useful predictors.

FUTURE USES OF BIOLOGICAL PRINCIPLES IN ORTHODONTIC TREATMENT

In the future, the principles gleaned from molecular biology and tissue engineering are expected to become part of the therapeutic regimen used during orthodontic treatment. This paradigm of orthodontic treatment may involve the delivery of bioactive agents in combination with conventional biomechanics. Numerous agents that have activities

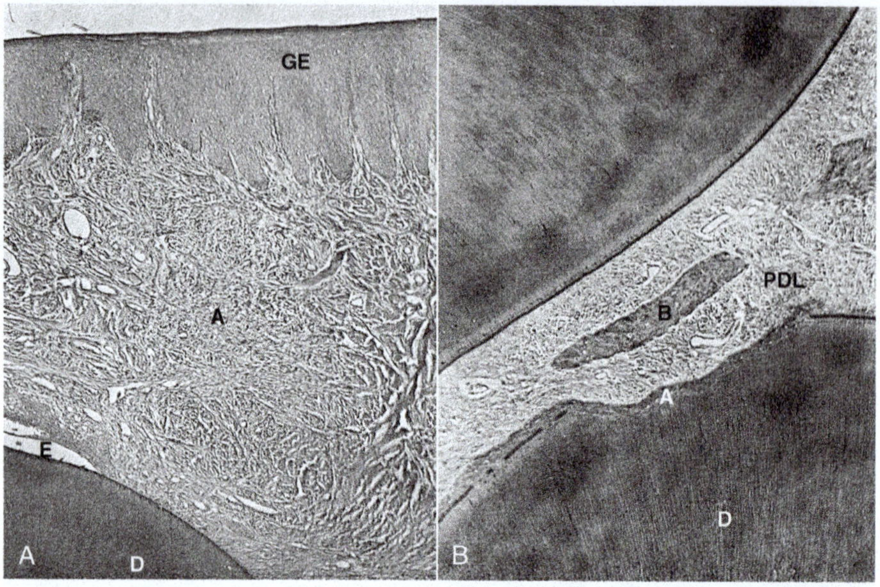

Figure 5-17 Histological changes of periodontal ligament (PDL) fiber adaptations in the presence and absence of surgical intervention. **A,** Shows the PDL arrangement of an incisor with total repair 42 days following surgical intervention. Overall, there is good orientation of the PDL ligaments as they slowly start to reattach and reorganize into the more familiar parallel collagen bundles. The supragingival tissue shows a zone of healing where the fibers are much sparser than the adjacent fiber bundles. Fiber organization outside the area of healing is very similar to the fiber arrangement observed in comparable areas of unrotated incisors. **B,** Histological section of a nonsurgical control incisor with a similar degree of tooth rotation as in **A.** PDL shows areas of compression and damage on the distolingual aspect and a widening on the mesiolabial aspect. Observation of the supragingival tissues displays a generalized discontinuity of the fiber pattern, areas of hemorrhage, and fiber disorganization. No evidence of any area of scarring or healing is observed. *A,* Area of resorption undergoing healing; *B,* bone; *D,* dentin; *GE,* gingival epithelium. (Modified from Brain WE. The effect of surgical transsection of free gingival fibers on the regression of orthodontically rotated teeth in the dog. *Am J Orthod.* 1969;55:50–70.)

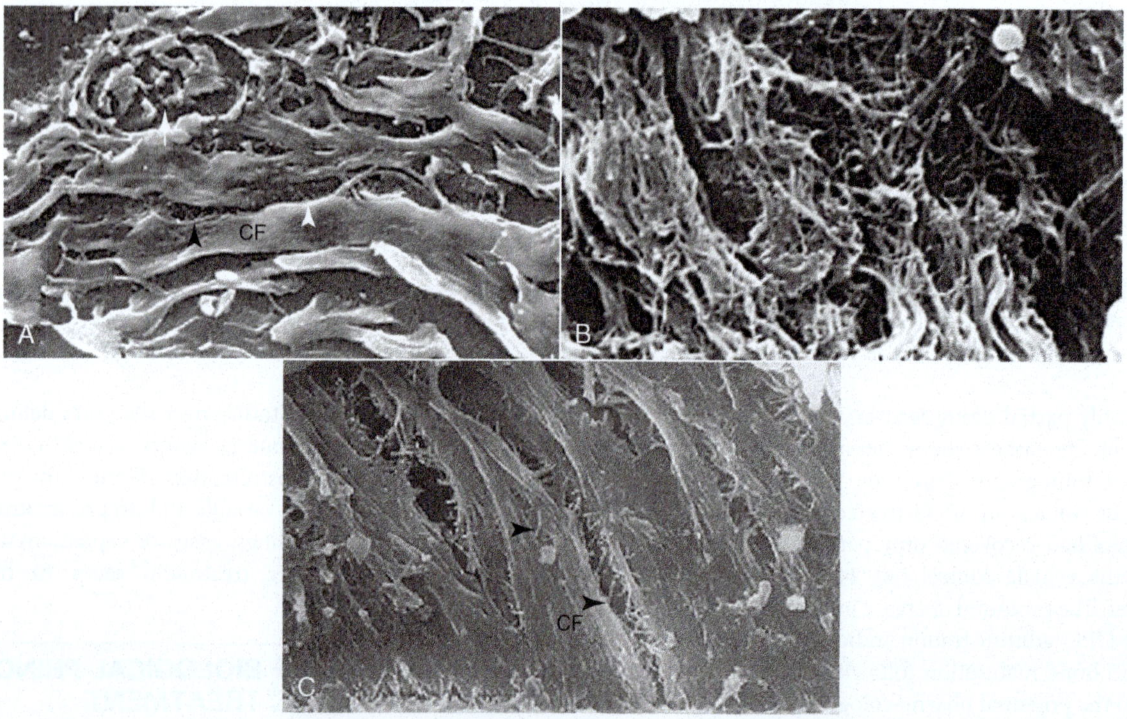

Figure 5-18 Teeth that have undergone surgical release of the gingival fibers demonstrate greater stability after orthodontic treatment. This is primarily due to the reattachment capability of the collagen fibers of the periodontal ligament (PDL). **A,** Observations with scanning electron microscopy (SEM) of supraalveolar fibers in palatal, buccal, and transseptal gingival areas reveal well-organized, parallel, and densely packed collagen fiber (CF) bundles with thin fibers connecting the large fiber bundles (*arrowheads*). **B,** SEM analysis of the different gingival regions after rotation and retention reveal disorganized, torn, and ripped collagen fibers. **C,** After gingival fiberotomy and release of retention the teeth remain stable in their rotated positions. SEM shows large, parallel, and densely packed collagen fibers. There is normalization of the longitudinally sectioned parallel and densely packed CF bundles interconnected with thinner fibers (*arrowheads*), resembling untreated controls. (Reproduced from Redlich M, Rahamin E, Gaft A, Shoshan S. The response of supraalveolar gingival collagen to orthodontic rotation movement in dogs. *Am J Orthod Dentofacial Orthop.* 1996;110:247–255.)

TABLE 5-1 Bioactive Agents That Have Been Shown to Enhance or Decrease Rates of Orthodontic Tooth Movement in Animal Models

Increase Tooth Movement Rate	Decrease Tooth Movement Rate
• Osteocalcin[104] • Nitric oxide[105] • Misoprostol[106] • Prostaglandin E2[107] • RANKL gene[61,62]	• Bisphosphonates[108] • Nitric oxide synthase inhibitor[109] • Echistatin[110] • MMP inhibitor[111] • Clodronate[112] • OPG gene[113] • OPG protein[46,47]

MMP, Matrix metalloproteinase; *OPG,* osteoprotegerin; *RANKL,* receptor activator of nuclear factor κB ligand.

that should be of significance in accelerating or preventing tooth movement already exist and indeed have been shown to modulate experimental tooth movement in animal models (Table 5-1). For example, localized application of calciotropic or osteoclastic agents has significant effects on local bone remodeling dynamics and may be used to facilitate tooth movement, such as retraction of canines into extraction spaces,[61,62] to impair tooth movement in cases with high anchorage needs,[46] or to enhance retention.[47] The increasing knowledge about the biological mechanisms in orthodontic tooth movement combined with smart local pharmaceutical delivery systems will facilitate the utility of these biomolecules in orthodontic therapy. Data on efficacy and safety, as well as means of delivery in the context of orthodontic treatment, will likely be forthcoming.

Advances in technological bioassays may also facilitate the biological diagnostics and monitoring of bone turnover and metabolism as well as markers of root resorption. Medical researchers have already attempted to establish relationships between molecular biochemical markers of bone remodeling (e.g., osteocalcin, alkaline phosphatase, and procollagen I) and the metabolic rate of bone turnover in clinical subjects.[102] However, the correlation and interpretation of results are complicated by numerous variables, such as age, pubertal stage, growth velocity, mineral accrual, hormonal regulation, nutritional status, and circadian variation. Yet the rapid progress in developing more sensitive and specific assays, as well as recent discoveries of more specific metabolic bone markers or bioactive agents associated with root resorption, is making this potential assessment of bone and root turnover a likely reality in the near future.[74-76,92,103]

REFERENCES

1. Wolff J. *The Law of Bone Remodeling* (trans.). Berlin, Germany: Springer-Verlag; 1986:1–22.
2. Dorow C, Krstin N, Sander FG. Experiments to determine the material properties of the periodontal ligament. *J Orofac Orthop.* 2002;63:94–104.
3. van Driel WD, van Leeuwen EJ, Von den Hoff JW, Maltha JC, Kuijpers-Jagtman AM. Time-dependent mechanical behaviour of the periodontal ligament. *Proc Inst Mech Eng H.* 2000;214:497–504.
4. Tanne K, Nagataki T, Inoue Y, Sakuda M, Burstone CJ. Patterns of initial tooth displacements associated with various root lengths and alveolar bone heights. *Am J Orthod Dentofacial Orthop.* 1991;100:66–71.
5. Yoshida N, Jost-Brinkmann PG, Koga Y, Mimaki N, Kobayashi K. Experimental evaluation of initial tooth displacement, center of resistance, and center of rotation under the influence of an orthodontic force. *Am J Orthod Dentofacial Orthop.* 2001;120:190–197.
6. Tanne K, Yoshida S, Kawata T, Sasaki A, Knox J, Jones ML. An evaluation of the biomechanic response of the tooth and periodontium to orthodontic forces in adolescent and adult subjects. *Br J Orthod.* 1998;25:109–115.
7. Tanne K, Inoue Y, Sakuda M. Biomechanic behavior of the periodontium before and after orthodontic tooth movement. *Angle Orthod.* 1995;65:123–128.
8. Kyomen S, Tanne K. Influences of aging changes in proliferative rate of PDL cells during experimental tooth movement in rats. *Angle Orthod.* 1997;67:67–72.
9. Ren Y, Maltha JC, van't Hof MA, Kuijpers-Jagtman AM. Age effect on orthodontic tooth movement in rats. *J Dent Res.* 2003;82:38–42.
10. King GJ, Archer L, Zhou D. Later orthodontic appliance reactivation stimulates immediate appearance of osteoclasts and linear tooth movement. *Am J Orthod Dentofacial Orthop.* 1998;114:692–697.
11. Iwasaki LR, Haack JE, Nickel JC, Morton J. Human tooth movement in response to continuous stress of low magnitude. *Am J Orthod Dentofacial Orthop.* 2000;117:175–183.
12. van Leeuwen EJ, Maltha JC, Kuijpers-Jagtman AM. Tooth movement with light continuous and discontinuous forces in beagle dogs. *Eur J Oral Sci.* 1999;107:468–474.
13. Andersson L, Malmgren B. The problem of dentoalveolar ankylosis and subsequent replacement resorption in the growing patient. *Aust Endod J.* 1999;25:57–61.
14. Kurol J. Infraocclusion of primary molars: an epidemiological, familial, longitudinal, clinical and histological study. *Swed Dent J.* 1984;21(suppl):1–67.
15. Nanda R. *Temporary Anchorage Devices in Orthodontics.* St. Louis, MO: Mosby Elsevier; 2009.
16. King GJ, Keeling SD, McCoy FA, Ward TH. Measuring dental drift and orthodontic tooth movement in response to various initial forces in adult rats. *Am J Orthod Dentofacial Orthop.* 1991;99:456–465.
17. Marks SC Jr, Schroeder HE. Tooth eruption: theories and facts. *Anat Rec.* 1996;245:374–393.
18. Yoshida Y, Sasaki T, Yokoya K, Hiraide T, Shibasaki Y. Cellular roles in relapse processes of experimentally-moved rat molars. *J Electron Microsc (Tokyo).* 1999;48:147–157.
19. Marks SC Jr. The basic and applied biology of tooth eruption. *Connect Tissue Res.* 1995;32:149–157.
20. Philbrick WM, Dreyer BE, Nakchbandi IA, Karaplis AC. Parathyroid hormone–related protein is required for tooth eruption. *Proc Natl Acad Sci USA.* 1998;95:11846–11851.
21. Ouyang H, McCauley LK, Berry JE, Saygin NE, Tokiyasu Y, Somerman MJ. Parathyroid hormone–related protein regulates extracellular matrix gene expression in cementoblasts and inhibits cementoblast-mediated mineralization in vitro. *J Bone Miner Res.* 2000;15:2140–2153.
22. Dastmalchi R, Polson A, Bouwsma O, Proskin H. Cementum thickness and mesial drift. *J Clin Periodontol.* 1990;17:709–713.
23. Levy GG, Mailland ML. Histologic study of the effects of occlusal hypofunction following antagonist tooth extraction in the rat. *J Periodontol.* 1980;51:393–399.
24. Rygh P. Ultrastructural changes in pressure zones of human periodontium incident to orthodontic tooth movement. *Acta Odontol Scand.* 1973;31:109–122.
25. Rygh P. Hyalinization of the periodontal ligament incident to orthodontic tooth movement. *Nor Tannlaegeforen Tid.* 1974;84:352–357.

26. Rygh P. Elimination of hyalinized periodontal tissues associated with orthodontic tooth movement. *Scand J Dent Res.* 1974;82:57–73.
27. Brudvik P, Rygh P. The initial phase of orthodontic root resorption incident to local compression of the periodontal ligament. *Eur J Orthod.* 1993;15:249–263.
28. Brudvik P, Rygh P. Non-clast cells start orthodontic root resorption in the periphery of hyalinized zones. *Eur J Orthod.* 1993;15:467–480.
29. Suda T, Takahashi N, Martin TJ. Modulation of osteoclast differentiation. *Endocrinol Rev.* 1992;13:66–80.
30. Takahashi N, Akatsu T, Udagawa N, et al. Osteoblastic cells are involved in osteoclast formation. *Endocrinology.* 1988;123:2600–2602.
31. Udagawa N, Takahashi N, Akatsu T, et al. Origin of osteoclasts: mature monocytes and macrophages are capable of differentiating into osteoclasts under a suitable microenvironment prepared by bone marrow-derived stromal cells. *Proc Natl Acad Sci USA.* 1990;87:7260–7264.
32. Anderson DM, Maraskovsky E, Billingsley WL, et al. A homologue of the TNF receptor and its ligand enhance T-cell growth and dendritic-cell function. *Nature.* 1997;390:175–179.
33. American Society for Bone and Mineral Research President's Committee on Nomenclature. Proposed standard nomenclature for new tumor necrosis factor family members involved in the regulation of bone resorption: American Society for Bone and Mineral Research President's Committee on Nomenclature. *J Bone Miner Res.* 2000;15:2293–2296.
34. Hsu H, Lacey DL, Dunstan CR, et al. Tumor necrosis factor receptor family member RANK mediates osteoclast differentiation and activation induced by osteoprotegerin ligand. *Proc Natl Acad Sci USA.* 1999;96:3540–3545.
35. Nakagawa N, Kinosaki M, Yamaguchi K, et al. RANK is the essential signaling receptor for osteoclast differentiation factor in osteoclastogenesis. *Biochem Biophys Res Commun.* 1998;253:395–400.
36. Simonet WS, Lacey DL, Dunstan CR, et al. Osteoprotegerin: a novel secreted protein involved in the regulation of bone density. *Cell.* 1997;89:309–319.
37. Hasegawa T, Yoshimura Y, Kikuiri T, et al. Expression of receptor activator of NF-kappa B ligand and osteoprotegerin in culture of human periodontal ligament cells. *J Periodontal Res.* 2002;37:405–411.
38. Crotti T, Smith MD, Hirsch R, et al. Receptor activator NF kappaB ligand (RANKL) and osteoprotegerin (OPG) protein expression in periodontitis. *J Periodontal Res.* 2003;38:380–387.
39. Takahashi N, Udagawa N, Takami M, Suda T. Cells of bone: osteoclast generation. In: Bilezikian JP, Raisz LG, Rodan GA, eds. *Principles of Bone Biology.* San Diego, CA: Academic Press; 2002:109–126.
40. Huang JC, Sakata T, Pfleger LL, et al. PTH differentially regulates expression of RANKL and OPG during osteoblast development. *J Bone Miner Res.* 2004;19:235–244.
41. Suda T, Ueno Y, Fujii K, Shinki T. Vitamin D and bone. *J Cell Biochem.* 2003;88:259–266.
42. Bord S, Ireland DC, Beavan SR, Compston JE. The effects of estrogen on osteoprotegerin, RANKL, and estrogen receptor expression in human osteoblasts. *Bone.* 2003;32:136–141.
43. Cheung J, Mak YT, Papaioannou S, Evans BA, Fogelman I, Hampson G. Interleukin-6 (IL-6), IL-1, receptor activator of nuclear factor kappaB ligand (RANKL) and osteoprotegerin production by human osteoblastic cells: comparison of the effects of 17-beta oestradiol and raloxifene. *J Endocrinol.* 2003;177:423–433.
44. King GJ, Keeling SD, Wronski TJ. Histomorphometric study of alveolar bone turnover in orthodontic tooth movement. *Bone.* 1991;12:401–409.
45. Edwards JG. A long-term prospective evaluation of the circumferential supracrestal fiberotomy in alleviating orthodontic relapse. *Am J Orthod Dentofacial Orthop.* 1988;93:380–387.
46. Dunn MD, Park CH, Kosteniuk PJ, Kapila S, Giannobile WV. Local delivery of osteoprotegerin inhibits mechanically mediated bone modeling in orthodontic tooth movement. *Bone.* 2007;41:446–455.
47. Hudson JB, Hatch N, Hayami T, et al. Local delivery of recombinant osteoprotegerin prevents post-orthodontic relapse. *Calcif Tissue Int.* 2012;90:330–342.
48. Verna C, Zaffe D, Siciliani G. Histomorphometric study of bone reactions during orthodontic tooth movement in rats. *Bone.* 1999;24:371–379.
49. Mundy GR. Cellular and molecular regulation of bone turnover. *Bone.* 1999;24(5 suppl):35S–38S.
50. Goldie RS, King GJ. Root resorption and tooth movement in orthodontically treated, calcium-deficient, and lactating rats. *Am J Orthod.* 1984;85:424–430.
51. Ashmore JL, Kurland BF, King GJ, Wheeler TT, Ghafari J, Ramsay DS. A 3-dimensional analysis of molar movement during headgear treatment. *Am J Orthod Dentofacial Orthop.* 2002;121:18–30.
52. Judex S, Boyd S, Qin YX, et al. Adaptations of trabecular bone to low magnitude vibrations result in more uniform stress and strain under load. *Ann Biomed Eng.* 2003;31:12–20.
53. Gibson JM, King GJ, Keeling SD. Long-term orthodontic tooth movement response to short-term force in the rat. *Angle Orthod.* 1992;62:211–216.
54. King GJ, Keeling SD. Orthodontic bone remodeling in relation to appliance decay. *Angle Orthod.* 1995;65:129–140.
55. Proffit WR, Sellers KT. The effect of intermittent forces on eruption of the rabbit incisor. *J Dent Res.* 1986;65:118–122.
56. Konoo T, Kim YJ, Gu GM, King GJ. Intermittent force in orthodontic tooth movement. *J Dent Res.* 2001;80:457–460.
57. King G, Latta L, Rutenberg J, Ossi A, Keeling S. Alveolar bone turnover and tooth movement in male rats after removal of orthodontic appliances. *Am J Orthod Dentofacial Orthop.* 1997;111:266–275.
58. Gu G, Lemery SA, King GJ. Effect of appliance reactivation after decay of initial activation on osteoclasts, tooth movement, and root resorption. *Angle Orthod.* 1999;69:515–522.
59. Miyoshi K, Igarashi K, Saeki S, Shinoda H, Mitani H. Tooth movement and changes in periodontal tissue in response to orthodontic force in rats vary depending on the time of day the force is applied. *Eur J Orthod.* 2001;23:329–338.
60. Long H, Pyakurela U, Wang Y, Liaoa L, Zhoua Y, Laic W. Interventions for accelerating orthodontic tooth movement: a systematic review. *Angle Orthod.* 2013;83:164–171.
61. Iglesias-Linares A, Moreno-Fernandez AM, Yañez-Vico R, Mendoza-Mendoza A, Gonzalez-Moles M, Solano-Reina E. The use of gene therapy vs corticotomy surgery in accelerating orthodontic tooth movement. *Orthod Craniofac Res.* 2011;14:138–148.
62. Kanzaki H, Chiba M, Arai K, et al. Local RANKL gene transfer to the periodontal tissue accelerates orthodontic tooth movement. *Gene Ther.* 2006;13(8):678–685.
63. Baumrind S, Korn EL, Boyd RL. Apical root resorption in orthodontically treated adults. *Am J Orthod Dentofacial Orthop.* 1996;110:311–320.
64. Goldson L, Henrikson CO. Root resorption during Begg treatment: a longitudinal roentgenologic study. *Am J Orthod.* 1975;68:55–66.
65. Ottolengui R. The physiological and pathological resorption of tooth roots. *Items Interest.* 1914:36:332–362.
66. Ketcham AH. A preliminary report of an investigation of apical root resorption of vital permanent teeth. *Int J Orthod.* 1927:13:97–127.
67. Ketcham AH. A progress report of an investigation of apical root resorption of vital permanent teeth. *Int J Orthod.* 1929;15:310–328.
68. Alqerban A, Jacobs R, Fieuws S. Comparison of two cone beam computed tomographic systems versus panoramic imaging for localization of impacted maxillary canines and detection of root resorption. *Eur J Orthod.* 2011;33:93–102.
69. Alqerban A, Jacobs R, Souza PC, et al. In-vitro comparison of two cone-beam computed tomography systems and panoramic imaging for detecting simulated canine impaction-induced external root resorption in maxillary lateral incisors. *Am J Orthod Dentofacial Orthop.* 2009;136:764-e1–764-e11.

70. Durack C, Patel S, Davies J, Wilson R, Mannocci F. Diagnostic accuracy of small volume cone beam computed tomography and intraoral periapical radiography for the detection of simulated external inflammatory root resorption. *Int Endod J*. 2011;44:136–147.
71. Ponder S, Benavides E, Kapila S, Hatch N. Quantification of external root resorption by low- vs. high-resolution cone beam computed tomography and periapical radiography: a volumetric and linear analysis. *Am J Orthod Dentofacial Orthop*. 2012;143:77–91.
72. Ren H, Chen J, Deng F, Zheng L, Liu X, Dong Y. Comparison of cone-beam computed tomography and periapical radiography for detecting simulated apical root resorption. *Angle Orthod*. 2013;83: 189–195.
73. Harris EF, Kineret SE, Tolley EA. A heritable component for external apical root resorption in patients treated orthodontically. *Am J Orthod Dentofacial Orthop*. 1997;111:301–309.
74. Al-Qawasmi RA, Hartsfield JK Jr, Everett ET, et al. Genetic predisposition to external apical root resorption. *Am J Orthod Dentofacial Orthop*. 2003;123:242–252.
75. Al-Qawasmi RA, Hartsfield JK Jr, Everett ET, et al. Genetic predisposition to external apical root resorption in orthodontic patients: linkage of chromosome-18 marker. *J Dent Res*. 2003;82:356–360.
76. Iglesias-Linares A, Yañez-Vico R, Moreno-Fernández A, et al. Osteopontin gene SNPs (rs9138, rs11730582) mediate susceptibility to external root resorption in orthodontic patients. *Oral Dis*. 2013. doi:10.1111/odi.12114.
77. McFadden WM, Engstrom C, Engstrom H, Anholm JM. A study of the relationship between incisor intrusion and root shortening. *Am J Orthod Dentofacial Orthop*. 1989;6:390–396.
78. Reitan K. Initial tissue behavior during apical root resorption. *Angle Orthod*. 1974;44:68–82.
79. Dermaut LR, De Munck A. Apical root resorption of upper incisors caused by intrusive tooth movement: a radiographic study. *Am J Orthod Dentofacial Orthop*. 1986;90:321–326.
80. Taithongchai R, Sookkorn K, Killiany DM. Facial and dentoalveolar structure and the prediction of apical root shortening. *Am J Orthod Dentofacial Orthop*. 1996;110:296–302.
81. Mirabella AD, Artun J. Risk factors for apical root resorption of maxillary anterior teeth in adult orthodontic patients. *Am J Orthod Dentofacial Orthop*. 1995;108:48–55.
82. Newman WG. Possible etiologic factors in external root resorption. *Am J Orthod*. 1975;67:522–539.
83. Harry MR, Sims MR. Root resorption in bicuspid intrusion: a scanning electron microscope study. *Angle Orthod*. 1982;52:235–258.
84. Wainwright WM. Faciolingual tooth movement: its influence on the root and cortical plate. *Am J Orthod*. 1973;64:278–302.
85. Linge L, Linge BO. Patient characteristics and treatment variables associated with apical root resorption during orthodontic treatment. *Am J Orthod Dentofacial Orthop*. 1991;99:35–43.
86. Horiuchi A, Hotokezaka H, Kobayashi K. Correlation between cortical plate proximity and apical root resorption. *Am J Orthod Dentofacial Orthop*. 1998;114:311–318.
87. Engstrom C, Granstrom G, Thilander B. Effect of orthodontic force on periodontal tissue metabolism: a histologic and biochemical study in normal and hypocalcemic young rats. *Am J Orthod Dentofacial Orthop*. 1988;93:486–495.
88. Tyrovola JB, Spyropoulos MN, Makou M, Perrea D. Root resorption and the OPG/RANKL/RANK system: a mini review. *J Oral Sci*. 2008;50:367–376.
89. Nishijima Y, Yamaguchi M, Kojima T, Aihara N, Nakajima R, Kasai K. Levels of RANKL and OPG in gingival crevicular fluid during orthodontic tooth movement and effect of compression force on releases from periodontal ligament cells in vitro. *Orthod Craniofac Res*. 2006;9:63–70.
90. Yamaguchi M, Aihara N, Kojima T, Kasai K. RANKL increase in compressed periodontal ligament cells from root resorption. *J Dent Res*. 2006;85:751–756.
91. Nakano Y, Yamaguchi M, Fujita S, Asano M, Saito K, Kasai K. Expressions of RANKL/RANK and M-CSF/c-fms in root resorption lacunae in rat molar by heavy orthodontic force. *Eur J Orthod*. 2011;33: 335–343.
92. Tyrovola JB, Perrea D, Halazonetis DJ, Dontas I, Vlachos IS, Makou M. Relation of soluble RANKL and osteoprotegerin levels in blood and gingival crevicular fluid to the degree of root resorption after orthodontic tooth movement. *J Oral Sci*. 2010;52:299–311.
93. Reitan K. Principles of retention and avoidance of posttreatment relapse. *Am J Orthod*. 1969;55:776–790.
94. Row KL, Johnson RB. Distribution of 3H-proline within transseptal fibers of the rat following release of orthodontic forces. *Am J Anat*. 1990;189:179–188.
95. van Leeuwen EJ, Maltha JC, Kuijpers-Jagtman AM, van't Hof MA. The effect of retention on orthodontic relapse after the use of small continuous or discontinuous forces: an experimental study in beagle dogs. *Eur J Oral Sci*. 2003;111:111–116.
96. Edwards JG. A study of the periodontium during orthodontic rotation of teeth. *Am J Orthod*. 1968;54:441–461.
97. Reitan K. Tissue rearrangement during retention of orthodontically rotated teeth. *Angle Orthod*. 1959;29:105–113.
98. Boese LR. Increased stability of orthodontically rotated teeth following gingivectomy in *Macaca nemestrina*. *Am J Orthod*. 1969;56:273–290.
99. Brain WE. The effect of surgical transsection of free gingival fibers on the regression of orthodontically rotated teeth in the dog. *Am J Orthod*. 1969;55:50–70.
100. Redlich M, Rahamim E, Gaft A, Shoshan S. The response of supraalveolar gingival collagen to orthodontic rotation movement in dogs. *Am J Orthod Dentofacial Orthop*. 1996;110:247–255.
101. Redlich M, Shoshan S, Palmon A. Gingival response to orthodontic force. *Am J Orthod Dentofacial Orthop*. 1999;116:152–158.
102. Szulc P, Seeman E, Delmas PD. Biochemical measurements of bone turnover in children and adolescents. *Osteoporos Int*. 2000;11: 281–294.
103. Woitge HW, Seibel MJ. Biochemical markers to survey bone turnover. *Rheum Dis Clin North Am*. 2001;27:49–80.
104. Hashimoto F, Kobayashi Y, Mataki S, Kobayashi K, Kato Y, Sakai H. Administration of osteocalcin accelerates orthodontic tooth movement induced by a closed coil spring in rats. *Eur J Orthod*. 2001;23:535–545.
105. Shirazi M, Nilforoushan D, Alghasi H, Dehpour A-R. The role of nitric oxide in orthodontic tooth movement in rats. *Angle Orthod*. 2002;72: 211–215.
106. Sekhavat AR, Mousavizadeh K, Pakshir HR, Aslani FS. Effect of misoprostol, a prostaglandin E_1 analog, on orthodontic tooth movement in rats. *Am J Orthod Dentofacial Orthop*. 2002;122:542–547.
107. Seifi M, Eslami B, Saffar AS. The effect of prostaglandin E_2 and calcium gluconate on orthodontic tooth movement and root resorption in rats. *Eur J Orthod*. 2003;25:199–204.
108. Igarashi K, Mitani H, Adachi H, Shinoda H. Anchorage and retentive effects of a bisphosphonate (AHBuBP) on tooth movements in rats. *Am J Orthod Dentofacial Orthop*. 1994;106:279–289.
109. Hayashi K, Igarashi K, Miyoshi K, Shinoda H, Mitani H. Involvement of nitric oxide in orthodontic tooth movement in rats. *Am J Orthod Dentofacial Orthop*. 2002;122:306–309.
110. Dolce C, Vakani A, Archer L, Morris-Wiman JA, Holliday LS. Effects of echistatin and an RGD peptide on orthodontic tooth movement. *J Dent Res*. 2003;82:682–686.
111. Holliday LS, Vakani A, Archer L, Dolce C. Effects of matrix metalloproteinase inhibitors on bone resorption and orthodontic tooth movement. *J Dent Res*. 2003;82:687–691.
112. Liu L, Igarashi K, Haruyama N, Saeki S, Shinoda H, Mitani H. Effects of local administration of clodronate on orthodontic tooth movement and root resorption in rats. *Eur J Orthod*. 2004;26:469–473.
113. Kanzaki H, Chiba M, Takahashi I, Haruyama N, Nishimura M, Mitani H. Local OPG gene transfer to periodontal tissue inhibits orthodontic tooth movement. *J Dent Res*. 2004;83:920–925.

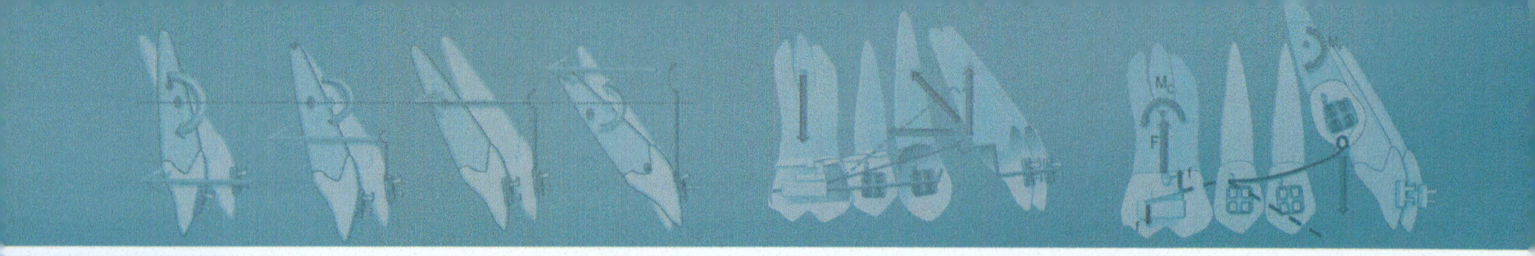

CHAPTER 6

Biomechanical Basis of Extraction Space Closure

Madhur Upadhyay, Sumit Yadav, and Ravindra Nanda

Tooth movement to close space is one of the most desired goals of orthodontic treatment. For years, orthodontists have searched for an efficient force system that can work quickly, accurately, and effectively to close extraction spaces. Orthodontic tooth movement is the result of the controlled application of mechanical forces to the teeth and periodontium. The stimulus provided by activated orthodontic appliances provides the necessary mechanical force to elicit a biological response. This perturbation temporarily disrupts the physiological equilibrium of the dentofacial complex and causes tooth movement in the direction of the net force, resulting in the closure of space.

To carry out such movements, orthodontic tools should be chosen on the basis of the biological responses of the periodontium surrounding the teeth (not yet an exact science) and their biomechanical properties as well as the appliances being used to move them (a much more exact science), rather than on the basis of anecdotal reports of success (since failures are rarely described). Therefore in this chapter we refrain from showing many clinical cases (which many orthodontists have in plenty) and instead describe the science behind orthodontic space closure.

FUNDAMENTALS OF SPACE CLOSURE

Before embarking on the details of the mechanics involved in space closure it is important to comprehensively analyze the basic tenets of the approach to this orthodontic problem.

The Basics

In space closure the objective is simple: to bring together opposing teeth or segments of teeth by applying a force between them. This force is usually applied on the bracket attached to the crown of the teeth (Fig. 6-1) and is occlusal and buccal to the center of resistance (C_{RES}) of the units experiencing the force. This generates moments (moment due to force, or M_F), which cause tipping and rotation of the teeth in the direction of the applied force. The clinical observation of the amount of tipping and rotation will depend on the amount of space closure. A greater amount of space closure will yield greater degrees of side effects. The amount of space requiring correction can vary depending on the severity. Less than 2-mm of spacing can be categorized as minor, greater than 2-mm but less than 4-mm is moderate, while anything greater than 4-mm is severe. Large spaces need good anchorage control over the desired tooth movement (i.e., effectively managing the unwanted moments [causing tipping and rotation] created during space closure).

With efficient mechanical appliances and sound application of the fundamentals learned in Chapter 4, almost any desired tooth movement can be obtained. In a nutshell, the nature of tooth movement can be controlled by applying a counteracting moment (M_C) to the M_F. In Figure 6-1, the tipping showed can be controlled by this M_C. The easiest way to generate this M_C is to place a straight wire in the tipped brackets (Fig. 6-2). This ratio of moment to force (M_C/F ratio) at the orthodontic bracket can bring about various types of tooth movement. However, the type of tooth movement seen during space closure also depends on the tooth and the objectives of the overall treatment. For example, canines and molars usually need to be translated while the anterior teeth or incisors can do well with simple tipping. Root movement is frequently required for final alignment of the roots, especially during finishing. All these movements require different M_C/F ratios as we will see in the next section.

Moment to Force (M/F) Ratio

The M/F ratio is a good way to describe or predict the quality of tooth movement. In the literature it has been stated that an M/F ratio of 5 : 1 is required for tipping, of 7 : 1 is required for controlled tipping, of 10 : 1 is required for translation, and of 12 : 1 is required for root correction. However, these ratios cannot be applied universally for all teeth and in all situations. For example, for translation the ratio of 10 : 1 applies for a single rooted tooth where the distance of the bracket or the point of force application is 10-mm from the C_{RES} of the

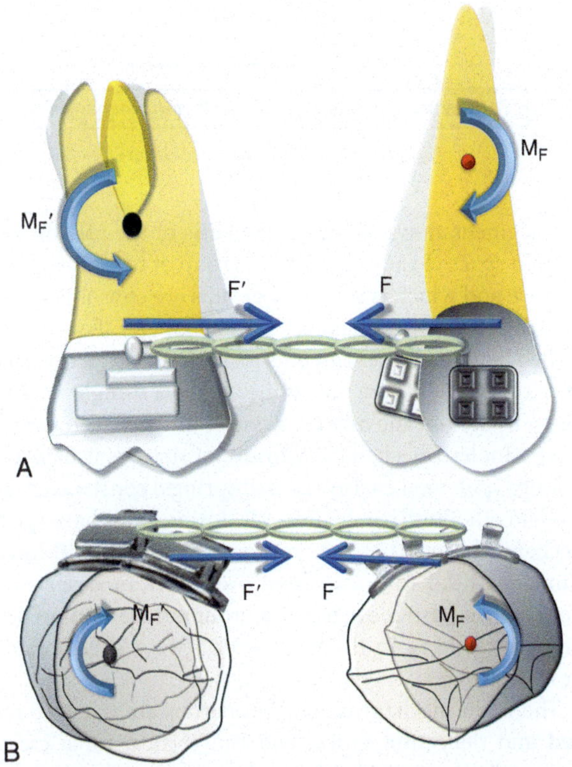

Figure 6-1 Basic dynamics of space closure. **A,** The magnitude of force for both teeth is equal (F = F′) but the moment due to force (M_F) is not necessarily equal ($M_F \neq M_F'$). For the definition of M_F, see Chapter 4. **B,** Occlusal perspective of the same. Tipping will occur in all planes of space.

tooth and the amount of force applied is 100 g. A more general way of defining M/F ratio for tooth movement should follow a qualitative approach, not a quantitative approach. High, moderate, and low M/F ratios can do this aptly.

As seen in Chapter 4 and in Figure 6-1, a single force applied at the bracket of a tooth will produce uncontrolled tipping with the center of rotation (C_{ROT}) slightly apical to the C_{RES}. Now if a counterbalancing moment (M_C) is applied and is high enough, it can perhaps negate the M_F. (Note: In Figure 6-2, the M_C is generated when the opposite ends and corners of the bracket contact the wire placed in the slot.) This will result in translation. A further increase will cause root movement into the space. At these relatively high M/F ratios, stresses reportedly distribute more evenly through the entire root with minimal changes in the mechanical properties during activation; this reduces injuries to teeth and surrounding tissues. A moderate M_C will only partially oppose the M_F, leading to controlled tipping with the apex remaining stationary. It is apparent from this discussion that regulating the M_C/F (or M_C/M_F) ratio is key in producing different types of tooth movement for space closure.

However, it is important to mention that the nature of tooth movement can also be regulated by varying the point of force application (see Chapter 4 for a detailed discussion on this).

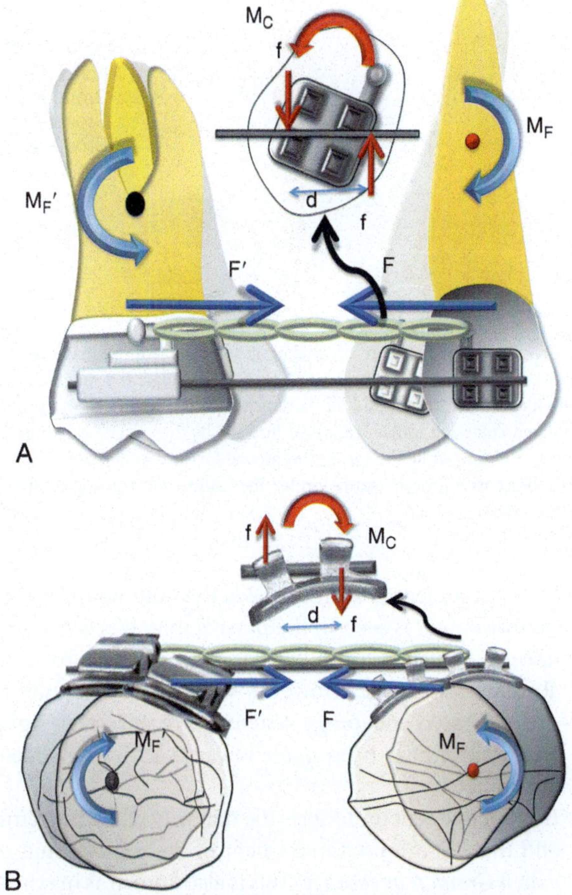

Figure 6-2 Mechanics of uprighting a tipped tooth. **A,** A simple way to generate a counteracting moment (M_C) is to place a straight wire in tipped brackets. The interaction of the M_C and moment due to force (M_F), or the moment to force (M/F) ratio, dictates the nature of tooth movement. Note that M_F = F × distance from the center of resistance (C_{RES}), while M_C = F × d (distance between the two couple forces). **B,** Occlusal perspective of the same. Uprighting will occur due to the wire-bracket interaction. Thus the quality of tooth movement is an interplay of moment due to a couple (in red) and the force (in blue).

Anchorage

As discussed, space closure involves the gradual closure of space between two teeth or two segments of teeth when one or both move toward each other. Depending on the needs of the patient, one set of teeth or one tooth can be classified as the active unit while the other is classified as the passive or reactive unit. These two units have completely different roles during tooth movement. The active unit undergoes the majority of the movement while the passive unit resists any kind of movement and provides the resistance necessary to facilitate the movement of the active unit, thereby serving as an anchorage. Therefore *anchorage* can be defined as the resistance offered by the passive unit toward any type of unwanted movement when the active unit is undergoing the desired movement. The set of teeth that offers this anchorage or resistance is also called the "anchorage unit." The anchorage setup for different situations can be broadly classified into four types (Fig. 6-3):

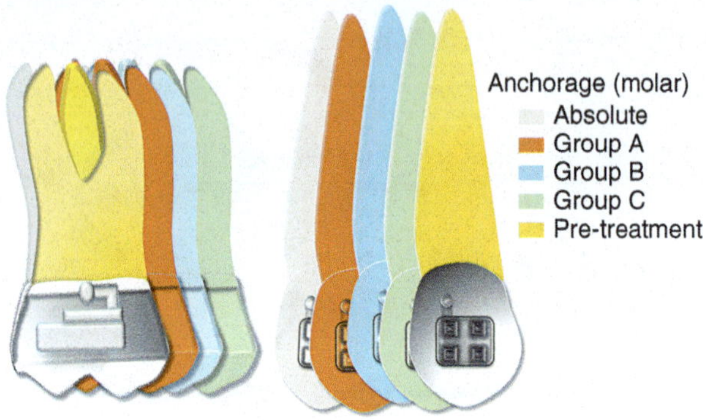

Figure 6-3 Classification of anchorage (for an approximate space of 8 mm). Each increment represents 2 mm. To calculate the movement of a particular shaded tooth, add all increments preceding it. For example, for the green color the molar has move forward by 2 (orange) + 2 (blue) + 2 (green) = 6 mm, while the canine has moved forward only 2 mm. Therefore this represents a group C situation for the canine and a group A situation for the molar.

1. If all movement is seen in the active unit and absolutely no movement is seen in the passive unit, it is called *absolute anchorage*. Clinically, it is very difficult to obtain absolute anchorage. However, with the development of skeletal based anchorage systems in recent years, significant strides have been made towards achieving absolute anchorage.
2. If the active unit undergoes the majority of the movement and there is minimal movement of the passive unit, it is called *Group A anchorage*. This is also known as maximum or high anchorage.
3. If the movement is shared equally among the active and passive units, it is called *Group B anchorage*. This is also known as moderate or medium anchorage.
4. If the majority of movement is seen in the passive unit, it is called *Group C anchorage*. This is also known as low or minimal anchorage. Needless to say, when there is Group C anchorage for a particular set of teeth, it means there is Group A anchorage for the other set. Thus in many ways the term *Group C anchorage* is redundant.

One of the easiest ways to generate Group A anchorage is by creating a high M/F ratio. In rare situations anchorage might even go beyond absolute anchorage and you might notice a net "anchorage gain." For example, during en masse retraction of the anterior teeth, the incisors and the molar both can move distally. This sometimes occurs when skeletal anchorage is used to reinforce anchorage.

METHODS OF SPACE CLOSURE

Space closure can be accomplished by adopting friction-based mechanics, often called "sliding mechanics," or without friction, also known as "segmental mechanics" (Fig. 6-4).

Segmental Mechanics

The basic premise of this concept is that all teeth in the upper or lower arch are not connected to each other by a continuous wire but are divided into discrete groups or segments.

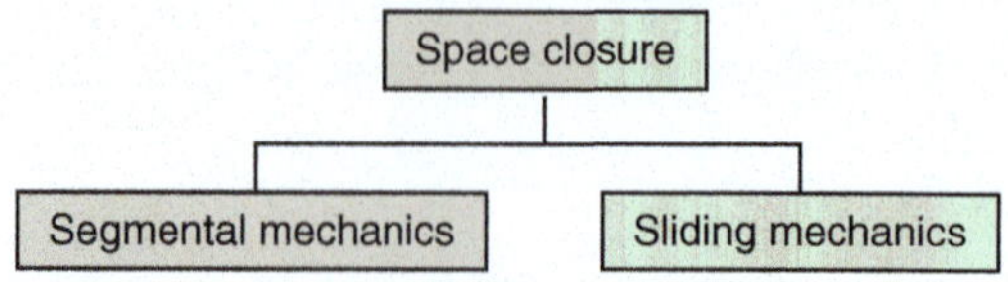

Figure 6-4 Methods for space closure.

This segmentation is done on the basis of the role the teeth serve in space closure (i.e., which group of teeth is supposed to move and which is not). The groups are consolidated into segments: active and passive (for anchorage). Force is then applied between these segments to close the extraction space. Since the segments are not connected by a straight wire (i.e., the teeth are not moving on a wire), this is also referred to as "frictionless mechanics." Closure of space is usually done by loops (potential energy–loaded springs) constructed from regular orthodontic archwires. All closing loops have specific mechanical properties (i.e., response to mechanical forces). Clinicians need to know these properties in order to use them optimally to move teeth or groups of teeth in predetermined directions. In the next section we will elaborate on these properties.

The main mechanical loop properties are the M/F ratio, load and deflection ratios, and the vertical force created. Among these, the M/F ratio can be considered the most significant because it is related to the type of tooth movement.

Concept of Differential Moments

Typically, for severe space closure scenarios a high M/F ratio loop is desirable, while minor spaces can be dealt with loops expressing a low M/F ratio. This is because with more space, teeth have a tendency to show more tipping. Therefore a high M/F ratio will ensure that they remain upright through the space closure.

For example, during incisor retraction the high M/F ratio for the posterior teeth will encourage anchorage preservation as it resists any tipping into the extraction space. In fact, a large posterior moment can cause distal crown movement, thereby opening up more extraction space. On the other hand, the low M/F ratio for the incisors encourages tipping. Simply described, methods using differential M/F ratios may be represented mathematically by the inequality $M_{Cp}/F \neq M_{Ca}/F$ and $M_{Cp}/F \gg M_{Ca}/F$ (here, *a* indicates anterior and *p* indicates posterior).

The application of such unequal moments must also comply with the laws of equilibrium discussed in Chapter 4. Because the moments created at each end of the loop or spring are unequal, the total force system must have additional effects. Vertical forces (intrusive and extrusive) are therefore also acting on the two segments. The magnitude of the vertical force depends on the difference between the two moments and the distance between the two segments.

In contemporary orthodontics, many closing loop shapes are being used, such as vertical or teardrop loops, T-loops, L-loops, Gjessing springs, and others.[1–6] These loop types can be further modified by adding a coil, altering the height, tipping the vertical legs (to increase the M_C), and so on.

Optimizing Loops for Space Closure: How Loop Design Affects the M/F Ratios

Researchers and clinicians have tried to design and refine loop geometry to obtain the highest M/F ratios possible, with the primary objective of reinforcing anchorage. Mechanical properties of closing loops depend on many factors, such as loop height, width, shape, and position; wire material; cross-sectional dimensions; and so on.[4,5,7–9] Let's look into some of these factors in detail.

Loop Height

Loop height, in particular, affects the M/F ratio considerably. As the loop height increases, the M/F ratio increases. Unfortunately, no loop can reach a M/F ratio greater than its height. Burstone and Koenig[7] reported that a 6-mm-high vertical loop had a M/F ratio of approximately 2 whereas a 10-mm-high vertical loop had a M/F ratio of about 4 for a 7-mm horizontal loop length. For a T-loop, as the gingival horizontal length increases, the M/F ratio increases as well to an upper limit and then levels off. Loop length and coil (helix) have only minor effects on the M/F ratio. There is a limit to which the height of a loop can be extended as it starts creating both bending difficulties and inconvenience to the patient when inserted in the mouth.

Loop Shape

The shape of a loop is another important factor to adjust the mechanical properties. The M/F ratio generated by T-loops is higher than that of vertical loops with the same loop height.[7,9] A so-called Opus loop introduced by Siatkowski[4,5] has an L shape with a helix in the apical portion of the L to increase the M/F ratio. Siatkowski reported that the Opus 70 loop, with the vertical legs tipped 70 degrees backward, had a M/F ratio as high as 8.7 mm, which is much higher than can be obtained by vertical loops or T-loops with similar dimensions. However, L-loops with similar dimensions as the Opus loop have given the highest M/F ratios to date (Fig. 6-5).[10]

Loop Placement

The final position of a loop between the active and passive units can significantly modify the M/F ratio.[8,11,12] In fact, this is the primary mechanism by which differential moments are created for space closure. This is known as "off-centered positioning of the loop." Higher moment is produced at the bracket closer to the loop. This principle is directly borrowed from the V-bend principles discussed in Chapter 4. Off-centered V-bends produce a greater moment on the closest tooth. As the loop is activated by horizontal activation (discussed below), the two legs of the loop form an angle with each other (Fig. 6-6). This angle can be further accentuated by placing bends in the loop, thereby increasing the differences in the M/F ratios between the two segments of teeth.

Let us now examine how loop placement and the preactivation bends are clinically used to control space closure. Two clinical situations are presented: canine retraction and incisors retraction.

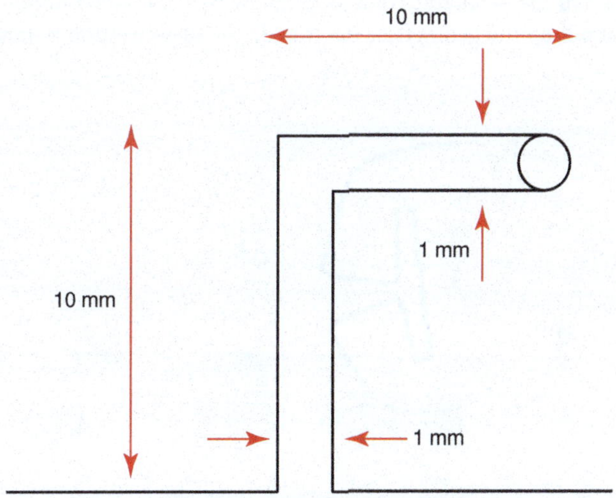

Figure 6-5 An L-loop with a helix.

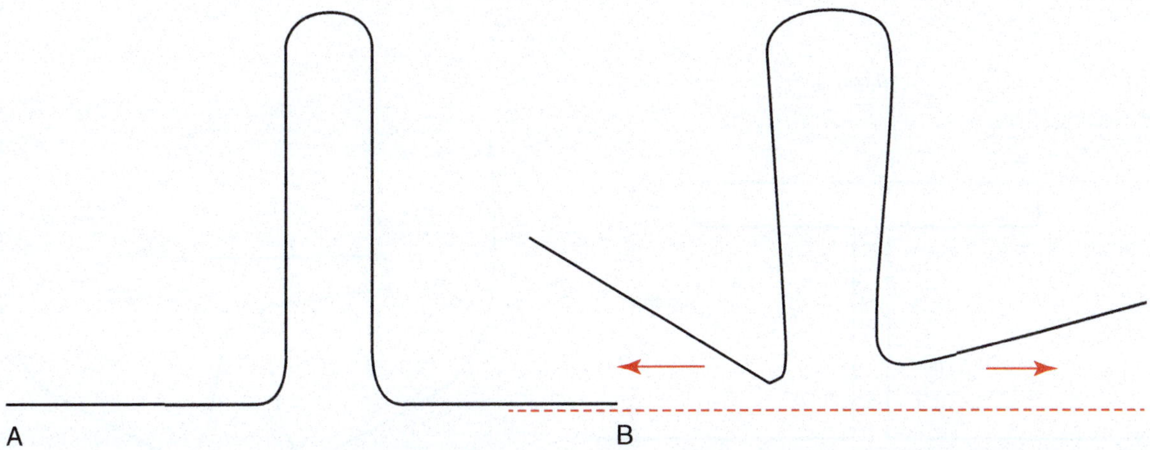

Figure 6-6 **A,** A typical vertical loop. **B,** After horizontal activation the two legs are at an angle to each other. This angulation creates a moment opposite in direction to that created by the moment due to a force (M_F).

Segmental Mechanics for Space Closure

Canine Retraction

Canine retraction is the movement of the canine in a distal direction from a position close to the lateral incisors to a position next to the premolar along the gentle curvature of the arch.

Setup. Let us consider that there is an anteroposterior space of approximately 8-mm to be closed distal to the canine. Before space closure can be initiated with a loop, it is important to ensure that the teeth or segments of teeth to be incorporated for tooth movement or anchorage are adequately aligned so that a 0.021-inch × 0.025-inch stainless steel wire (in a 0.022-inch slot bracket) can be used to hold them as separate units. The only link between the two units should be the loop.

Preactivation of the Loop (Figs. 6-7 and 6-8). Before the loop can be inserted into the extraction space, certain "preactivation bends" must be placed so that the loop gives a V- or U-shaped outline overall. Remember from Chapter 4 that the mechanics of a loop can be worked out by understanding the geometries described. The preactivation bends are also known as the alpha bend (anterior curvature) and beta bend (posterior curvature). The bends are necessary to create the moment (M_C) that will counteract the moment generated by the force (M_F). The greater the degree of bend, the higher the M_C generated. Also, higher moment is created on the tooth closer to the loop (see discussion of off-centered "V" bends in Chapter 4).

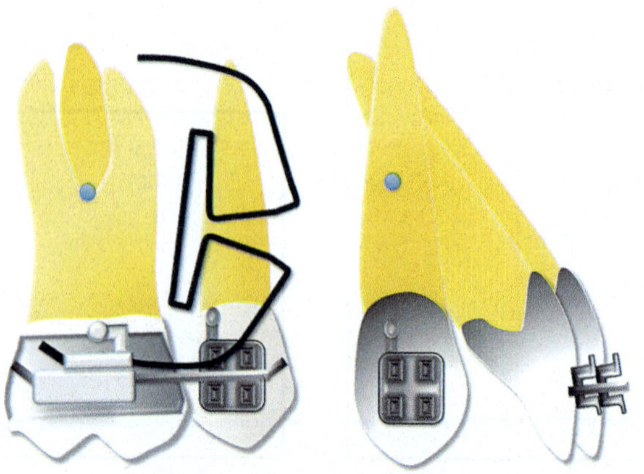

Figure 6-7 The setup for segmental retraction of the canine: 0.021-inch × 0.025-inch stainless steel wires as stabilizing units. Inserting the loop with preactivation bends.

Activation of the Loop. The final activation of the loop is done only when it is placed in the bracket slots. The wire is pulled distally through the posterior tube and cinched. The amount of distal pull is guided by the amount of space to be closed. For an 8-mm extraction space, ideally 8-mm of activation is good. This activation step is necessary to generate the required force and M_F for space closure.

Once the loop has been activated and placed at the desired location, tooth movement is initiated by "deactivation" of the loop. Space closure with loops progresses via three distinct phases, which can be delineated comprehensively at both the theoretical and the clinical level. The quality and nature of tooth movement is primarily determined by the interaction of the M_F and M_C generated as the teeth move toward each other.

Phase I (Tipping). In the initial phases of retraction the spring is fully activated and therefore the force is high, resulting in a high moment ($M_F = F \times d$, where d is the distance between the point of application of force and the C_{RES} of the canine). This condition results in a M_C/M_F ratio <1, placing the C_{ROT} of the canine close to the apex. The canine therefore shows considerable crown movement with minimal root movement (Fig. 6-9, A). This phase represents a classical example of "differential moments," described earlier in the chapter. Due to the nature of movement of the canine versus the molar (crown tipping of canine versus root tipping of molar) the anchorage demand on the molars is minimal, or in other words the chance of "anchor loss" is minimal. Hence, the anchorage demand from the molar is less. It is important to remember that if the operator does not place enough preactivation bends on the loop, this phase might show uncontrolled tipping of the canine with rapid dumping of the canine.

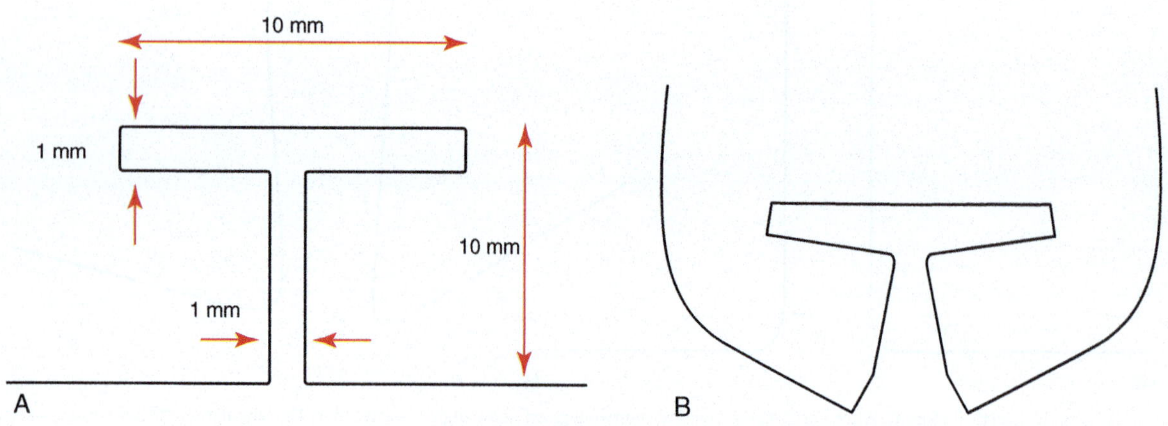

Figure 6-8 **A,** T-loop. **B,** With preactivation bends.

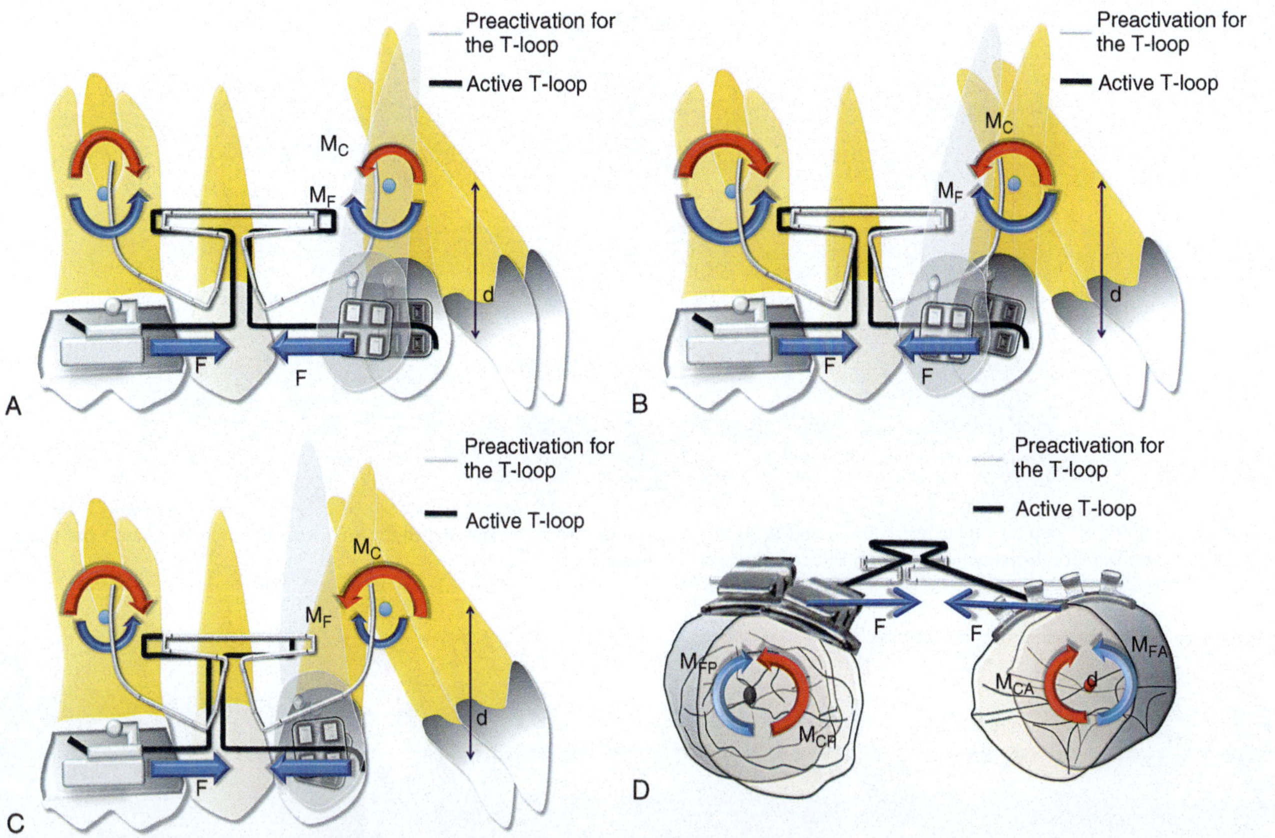

Figure 6-9 Space closure with loops. **A,** Phase I of loop deactivation (simple tipping). As $M_F \ggg M_C$, there is minimal root movement with more crown movement. $M_F = F \times d$. Note: The stabilizing wires for the passive segments are not shown. **B,** Phase II of loop deactivation (translation). As $M_F = M_C$, there is equal crown and root movement. Therefore the canine is undergoing bodily movement. (Remember that such a situation rarely exists where the moments are perfectly balanced.) **C,** Phase III of loop deactivation (root movement). As $M_C \ggg M_F$, there is minimal crown movement and more root movement. **D,** Occlusal perspective of the same. The V-bend placed in the T-loop will generate the counteracting moment or moment due to a couple (M_C) to oppose the rotation of the molar and canine. To have no rotation during retraction, $M_F = M_C$.

Phase II (Translation). As the canine is distalized and the distance between the two attachments decreases, the force levels drop. This causes a reduction in the M_F as well. At some point, $M_C = M_F$ ($M_C/M_F = 1$). Such a situation will place the C_{ROT} at infinity. At this stage the canine is translating as the moments are cancelled out (Fig. 6-9, B). Here, both the molar and the canine tend to translate. However, it is important to remember that this will not happen at the same time for the two teeth as the M_F values are different for the canine and molar. Also, the probability of anchor loss in this phase is high, because there is no net moment on the molar to reinforce anchorage and there is greater anchorage demand on the molar due to canine translation.

Phase III (Root Movement). The force levels continue to drop and so does the M_F but the M_C drop is not that significant (as it depends on the elasticity of the wire). Therefore, at this stage the M_C/M_F ratio is >1, thereby reversing the net moment (Fig. 6-9, C). This results in more root movement than crown movement, paving the way for root correction (as in phase I the canine had tipped). The canine therefore is undergoing root tipping or root uprighting while the molar shows predominantly crown tipping. Therefore this phase is vulnerable to showing some molar mesial movement (anchor loss). Anchorage reinforcement may be needed.

Note that for ease of understanding, the vertical forces generated due to the unequal moments have not been shown in Figure 6-9. Also, all phases will be similar to the one described above from an occlusal perspective as well (Fig. 6-9, D).

It is important to remember that the M_C/M_F ratio is responsible for optimizing the quality of canine movement while the force is responsible for the actual distal movement. Once the canine has undergone all of these phases of movement, complete deactivation of the loop has occurred. It now needs to be reactivated and then the canine will undergo the same kind of movement described above. Depending on the initial position of the canine a clinician might not want the canine to go through all three phases of distalization. For example, in crowded arches the canine is often mesially tipped and a simple uprighting of the canine is more than enough to close the extraction space (Fig. 6-10). Therefore, the spring can be removed once it has completed phase I.

Incisor Retraction

Retraction of incisors will proceed in a similar way as that described above. However, from an anchorage perspective it places less demand on the posterior teeth or the anchor units. This can be largely attributed to the nature of movement desired for the incisors. Usually the incisors have to

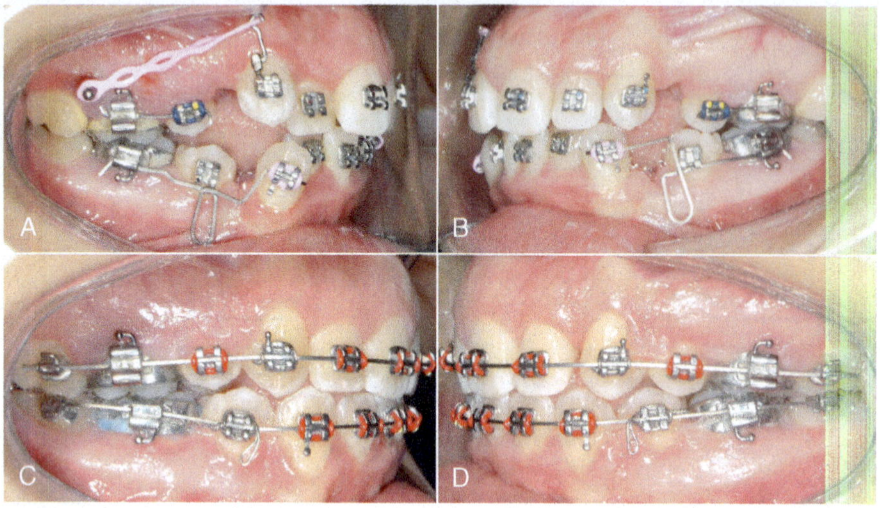

Figure 6-10 A reverse loop for canine retraction. **A and B,** As the lower canines were mesially tipped the loop was only used for phase I and phase II of retraction. **C and D,** Once the retraction was complete, continuous wires were placed.

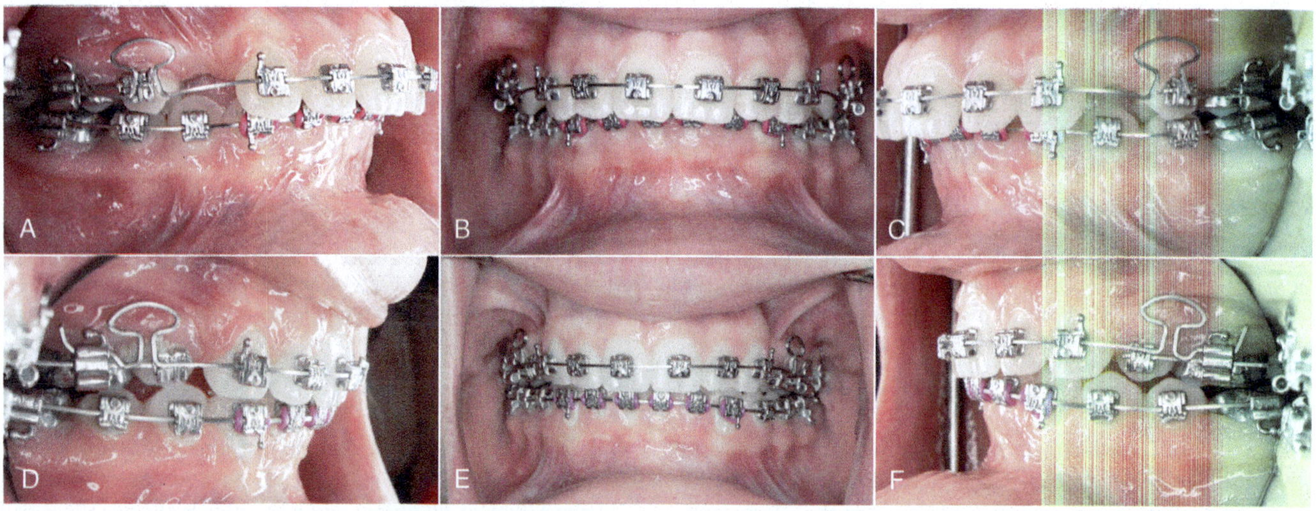

Figure 6-11 A mushroom loop for en masse retraction of the incisor and canine. Note the offset placement of the loop to preserve anchorage of the posterior segment. **A–C,** At the beginning of retraction. **D–F,** After space closure.

undergo only tipping for extraction space closure, with minimal translation and in only rare circumstances root uprighting. In terms of mechanics it means placing a high moment (M_C) on the posterior/anchor unit while considerably less moment is needed for the incisors. Therefore phase I is generally more than sufficient to complete the space closure process when incisors are being retracted. In terms of loop mechanics, more moment (M_C) must be created for the posterior unit ($M_{Cp} \ggg M_{Ca}$). This can easily be done by using any of the techniques described previously but the most common and easiest approach is the offset placement of the loop (Figs. 6-11 and 6-12). In this case the offset will be closer to the posterior segment. The moments and the forces created will follow the same rules as the V-bends discussed in Chapter 4.

From a theoretical standpoint segmental mechanics is arguably the most efficient way to move teeth. However, due to its overreliance on the operator's skills in terms of loop

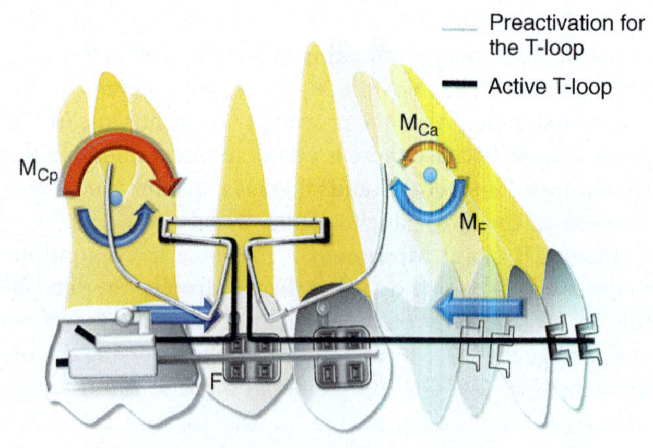

Figure 6-12 Mechanics of incisor retraction (simple tipping). As $M_F \ggg M_C$, there is minimal root movement and more crown movement. Note that the loop is placed toward the posterior segment to create a greater moment ($M_{Cp} \ggg M_{Ca}$) on it than on the anterior teeth.

fabrication, positioning, preactivation bends, activation, etc., segmental mechanics is highly technique sensitive. The clinician should be extremely careful in using this technique. On the other hand, sliding mechanics is less sensitive to technique but follows the same principles described above for space closure.

Sliding Mechanics

Ever since the Andrews straight-wire appliance[13] was introduced there has been a gradual but paradigm shift from closing loop mechanics to sliding mechanics. The objective is simple: to create a force system that can work efficiently and shorten the orthodontic treatment period. Sliding mechanics contributes to achieving more control during space closure (i.e., fewer side effects such as tipping and rotation), improving patient comfort, and preventing excessive force application.

By definition, in sliding mechanics force is applied between two teeth or segments of teeth such that they move or slide on a straight wire inserted in the respective brackets of the two segments so that a significant amount of friction is generated between the wire and the bracket surfaces. With the closing loop mechanics, activated loop create force only at the bracket level, and control is created by generating moments (via preactivation bends) whereas in sliding mechanics, retraction forces can be transferred to any height level on a power arm to move the teeth in a preprogrammed direction (e.g., controlled tipping, translation).

Two methods have been used for extraction space closure. The first method is two-step retraction, which involves canine retraction followed by incisor retraction. The second method is "en masse" retraction of the six anterior teeth.

Canine Retraction

A continuous archwire engages the brackets affixed to the facial surfaces of the teeth. In particular, the wire within the bracket attached to the canine crown and supported at neighboring posterior and perhaps anterior dental sites is intended to guide the tooth during its distal displacement.

To begin, let us assume that the teeth have been leveled and aligned to a degree that the archwire chosen for retraction sits passively through the bracket slots. Typically, for canine retraction the method used to provide the distal force (F) is a spring or an elastomeric element (module, chain, O-ring, or tied thread). Orthodontic tooth movement occurs as a result of mechanical force exerted on the crown and maintained there over some finite period of time. It is important to mention that this distal driving force will typically decrease with time if an elastomeric element is involved.

For the ease of understanding the details involved in this seemingly continuous and smooth process, we have divided it into four distinct phases as we did for segmental mechanics in the previous section. The beginning and end of each phase are defined by four instantaneous views of the mechanics involved. Each phase represents a characteristic movement pattern distinct from the other three. Each part of Figure 6-13 represents an instant of time during the retraction process. The force system shown is exerted on (not by) the canine; accordingly, the symbols for the delivered force and the couple partially represent their displacement potentials.

Phase I. This is the initiation of canine retraction. A single force (F) is applied on the canine bracket in a distal direction (Fig. 6-13, A). This force produces a moment (M_F) acting at the C_{RES} of the canine, causing it to tip as it is being distalized. Since there is some degree of play between the archwire and the bracket slot, the tooth is free to tip in the mesiodistal direction in an uncontrolled manner, creating a C_{ROT} slightly apical to the C_{RES} (from Chapter 4). This can also be referred to as the "unsteady state" of canine retraction, as it is undergoing uncontrolled tipping.

Phase II. The canine is now tipped to the extent that the aforementioned clearance (or play) between the bracket slot and the wire has been eliminated (Fig. 6-13, B). The sketch in Figure 6-13, B depicts the canine somewhat later in time relative to Figure 6-13, A. Archwire–bracket slot contact now exists. This two-point contact by the archwire exerts a pair of parallel, equal in magnitude, noncollinear forces to form the M_C. (The two forces will be of the same magnitude if the wire, because of its occluso-apical location and that of the bracket, generates no net potential to extrude or intrude the tooth.)

This M_C opposes the M_F, resulting in less tipping of the canine when compared to phase I. As the wire further deflects, M_C continues to increase and the C_{ROT} moves to the apex of the canine, creating controlled tipping of the canine. This can also be called the "controlled state" of canine retraction. With a preangulated bracket slot the initial clearance can be zero with some local second-order rotation required to engage the wire in the slot. If this is the case, M_C exists from the start of the retraction process. Also note that, as M_C appears, some frictional resistance to these sliding mechanics arises but is assumed to be small. The magnitude of M_C is, principally, directly related to the local bending of the guiding archwire at the canine bracket site and therefore is intricately associated with the wire properties, such as stiffness and resiliency. The size of M_C also, to a much lesser extent, is associated with the location of the canine bracket relative to support sites mesial and distal to it.

Phase III. As distal crown tipping continues, the magnitude of M_C increases directly with the local wire bending deformation. (Presumably the archwire maintains its elasticity throughout the retraction process.) With the accompanying distal displacement of the crown and relaxation of the driving component (elastomeric) of the appliance, F decreases in magnitude. The possibility then arises that the couple to force (M_C/F) ratio may be reduced to nearly equal the distance between the crown center (where the bracket is placed) and the C_{RES} of the canine. In other words, here $M_C = M_F$. Therefore the net moment acting on the canine has decreased to zero, signifying that the C_{ROT} has migrated

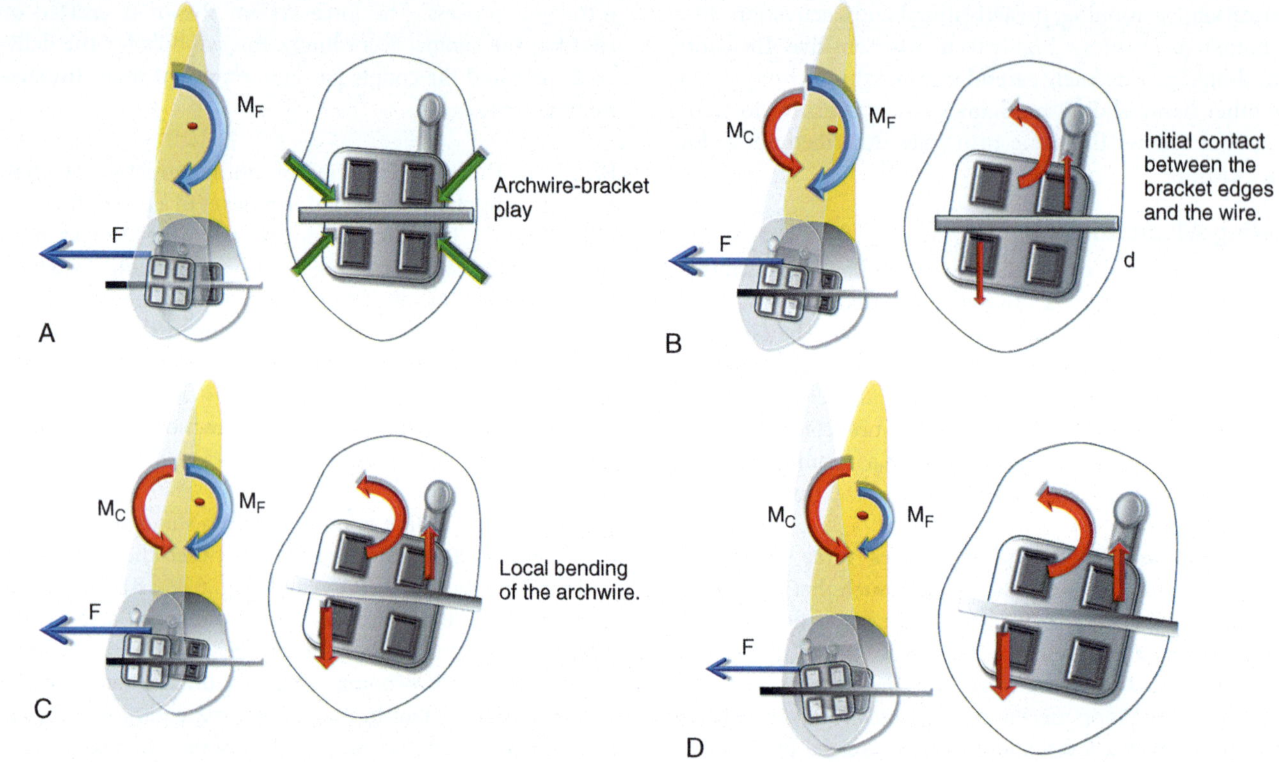

Figure 6-13 Mechanics of canine retraction with sliding mechanics. **A,** Phase I (the unsteady state/uncontrolled tipping). The archwire-bracket play allows for uncontrolled tipping of the canine. Note: Due to the play, no M_C is generated. **B,** Phase II (the controlled state/controlled tipping). The archwire-bracket play no longer exists. There are signs of initial contact between the archwire and the bracket edges giving rise to M_C. Here, $M_F \ggg M_C$. **C,** Phase III (the steady state/translation). The contact between the archwire and the bracket edges has increased, leading to an increase in the M_C. Simultaneously there can be a decrease in the force levels, causing a decrease in M_F. Here $M_F = M_C$. **D,** Phase IV (the restorative state/translation). There is a pronounced decrease in the force levels, causing a decrease in M_F. Here, $M_F \ll M_C$.

apically and the tipping displacement has potentially transformed into bodily movement. This mechanical configuration is shown in Figure 6-13, C. This situation can be attained either by a reduction in M_F or by an increase in M_C. It is important to remember that the relative values matter more than the absolute values. If this delicate balance of forces and moments is maintained, the canine will continue translating. This phase is also called the "steady state." However, this phase is at best only a theoretical possibility and for all practical reasons is impossible to attain.

Phase IV. For the canine distalization to enter this phase it must be assumed that the distal driving force is undergoing a constant decay through the retraction process. As discussed, the bodily displacement format may exist only momentarily. As the F decreases, so does the M_F; however, because of the angulated bracket and the local bending of the archwire, the M_C does not decrease as readily as the M_F. Therefore in this phase $M_C \gg M_F$ and the M_C/F ratio is greater than in the previous phase (Fig. 6-13, D). This results in restoration of the axial inclination of the canine (uprighting or root correction). This can be called the "restorative state" of canine retraction and can be clinically referred to as the second-order torquing of the canine. A tremendous amount of frictional force is generated at the wire-bracket interface, resulting in the relocation of the C_{ROT} gingival to the C_{RES} anywhere between the bracket and the C_{RES}. Remember that if the distal force does not show decay, this phase is never reached; instead, the canine might be relegated to just the first two phases (i.e., tipping only).

In a similar evaluation form, the occlusal view, the bracket is labial to the C_{RES} and hence a distal force will again create a M_F that will rotate the canine distally inward. This will be phase I (the unsteady state). Until the point play exists between the wire and the bracket from an occlusal view, the canine is free to rotate. During phase II (the controlled state) the archwire begins to deflect as the diagonally opposite ends of the bracket contact the archwire. A M_C is generated, which minimizes the M_F. In phase III (the steady state) the moments are equally balanced and there is no change in the position of the canine from an occlusal perspective. In phase IV (the restorative state) the rotated canine starts derotating because M_C exceeds M_F in magnitude.

Force Transmitted to the Anchor Teeth

The setup for canine retraction described above is a "friction-based" system in which the canine, through the application of a force, is made to slide distally guided by a continuous archwire that connects the incisors to the molars. The canine is the link between the posterior teeth (premolars and

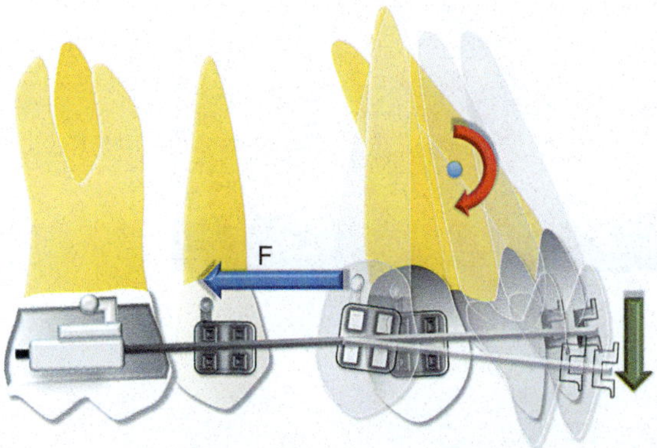

Figure 6-14 Incisor extrusion during canine retraction. Note the deflection of the archwire.

molars) and anterior teeth (incisors). Therefore it is not difficult to imagine that any change in its position might have a direct effect on the incisors and the molars. Let us consider carefully what those side effects might be.

Effect of Canine Retraction on the Incisors. An implicit advantage of canine retraction on a continuous arch system lies in limiting the possibility of unpredicted canine movement (e.g., flaring or rotation). Despite the advantages of sliding mechanics, canine retraction does present its own set of problems. When pure forces generated from springs or elastics are induced at the canine, especially when an archwire with a low load-deflection rate is being used or the force levels are too high, the wire tends to deform with undesirable side effects on other teeth (Fig. 6-14). Due to the tipping of the canine described in phases I to III, a constant stress is created on the wire, resulting in its elastic deflection. This deflection of the wire creates an extrusive force on the incisors and a moment that tends to cause lingual tipping. This tendency for archwire deflection can be reduced by using higher stiffness archwires and/or lighter forces for retraction. Auxiliary archwires, such as an overlay intrusion arch or cantilever springs, can also help to minimize the assumed deflection of the archwire.

Effect of Canine Retraction on the Molars. According to Newton's Third Law of Motion, the retraction force on the canine should exert the same force on the molar. This force will create a moment on the molar, causing it to tip mesially. The molar will then undergo all four phases of mesialization as described for the canine. However, the degree of movement may vary depending on the surrounding bone, tooth characteristics, number of additional teeth ligated to the molar, etc. An important side effect seen quite often clinically, especially when heavier forces are used, is the presence of a lateral open bite due to simultaneous tipping of the canine and molar crowns with no root correction. This can largely be attributed to the increased levels of retraction forces preventing the tooth from entering into phase III or phase IV of sliding movement.

Incisor Retraction

During space closure the incisors also follow the same phases of retraction as the canine. The dominant phases in incisor retraction are phases I and II (i.e., tipping).

Although clinically incisor retraction is similar to canine retraction, at the mechanical level there are a few differences. When tipped back, the bracket of a canine undergoes a second-order interaction with the archwire; in contrast, due to its position an incisor bracket has a third-order interaction. This third-order interaction lends itself to a greater degree of play compared to the second-order interaction of the canine. Therefore the dominant phases in incisor retraction are phases I and II (i.e., tipping), as the greater degree of play allows for more tipping. The questions that arise in such a situation are: What if we do not want this tipping? Or what if we are looking for more control on incisor retraction from the initiation of retraction? To achieve these goals we want to introduce an M_C in the first phase of retraction.

Some common ways of doing this are:

1. Bending the wire (V-bend, as discussed in Chapter 4)
2. Placing a curve in the main archwire
3. Torquing the archwire (twisting the wire)
4. Increasing the stiffness and size of the archwire

Another method of minimizing the tipping movement of the incisors and canine is by decreasing the M_F produced without compromising the magnitude of force. This can be achieved by changing the point of force application relative to the C_{RES} of the teeth. This can be easily achieved by using a "power arm" (Fig. 6-15). The effects of such mechanics on the incisor tooth are described in detail in Chapter 4.

MINI-IMPLANT–DRIVEN MECHANICS OF TOOTH MOVEMENT

Why Do We Need Mini-Implants for Space Closure?

The extraction of premolars and anterior teeth retraction is generally indicated when there is obvious protrusion of teeth and there is a strong esthetic need. While retracting anterior teeth in a full cusp Class II malocclusion or in a Class I bialveolar dental protrusion case, anchorage control assumes profound importance because maintaining the posterior segment in place becomes very critical. A loss in molar anchorage can not only compromise correction of the anteroposterior discrepancy, but also affect the overall vertical dimension of the face. The application of mini-implant–supported anchorage can circumvent the anchorage issues in such situations, maintaining a Class II molar relationship while establishing a Class I canine relationship for esthetics and functional guidance.

Where to Use Mini-Implants

Mini-implants (MIs) serve as anchorage units in situations where there is a need for absolute anchorage.[14-18] They are used to generate a constant and predictable force system, so that accurate and precise movement of the active units can

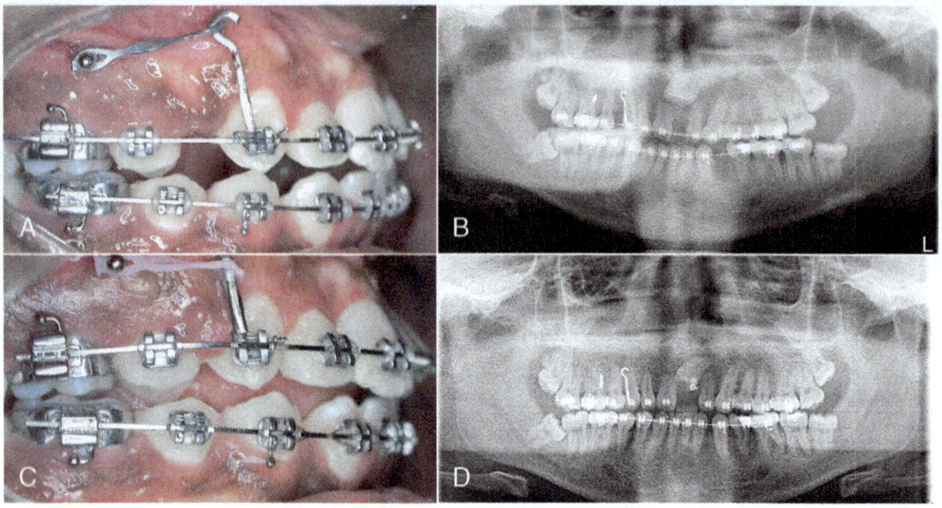

Figure 6-15 Canine distalization using a "power arm." **A and B,** Initiation of retraction. Note that the length of the power arm is approximately close to the C_{RES} of the canine. **C and D,** After completion of distalization. No tipping has occurred.

be achieved without the concern about the possibility of anchor loss. In other words, MIs help in eliminating the element of unpredictability that is associated with the traditional anchorage units (usually the posterior teeth), thereby making the orthodontist completely in charge of the tooth movement desired.

Basic Principles of Mini-Implant Use

To maximize the potential of MIs, it is crucial to understand the underlying mechanics behind the force application from an MI to the active unit or teeth. This section details the fundamental biomechanical principles involved in the usage of such devices and their practical applications.

Here is a simple example to elucidate the need to understand the mechanics involved with MIs. When using conventional mechanics, force application is usually parallel to the occlusal plane and hence we are required to deal with the force only in one plane. However, because MIs are usually placed apical to the occlusal plane into the bone between the roots of teeth, force applied is always at an angle (Fig. 6-16). (Note: The preferred location for MI placement is between the roots of the second premolars and first molars close to the mucogingival junction. Care should be taken that the MIs are not inserted too far apically in the movable mucosa, since this can lead to implant failure due to persistent inflammation around the MI site.) This angulated force lends itself to be broken into two components (by the law of vector resolution, discussed in Chapter 4): a horizontal retractive force (r) and a vertical intrusive force (i). The force applied with MIs in such a setup is also closer to the C_{RES} of the anterior unit. Therefore, the M_F with MIs is significantly less than with conventional mechanics. Clinically it means there is less tendency for the teeth to tip.

In addition, with conventional mechanics the molars or posterior segments usually serve as the anchor unit, with the rest of the arch serving as the active unit. The force system is therefore differentially expressed in the active unit and the anchorage or passive unit within the same arch. In contrast, when MIs are incorporated as the third counterpart, selective movement of the anterior and posterior segments is possible. Precise planning for the amount of the desired tooth movement is thus a prerequisite before active treatment can be initiated.

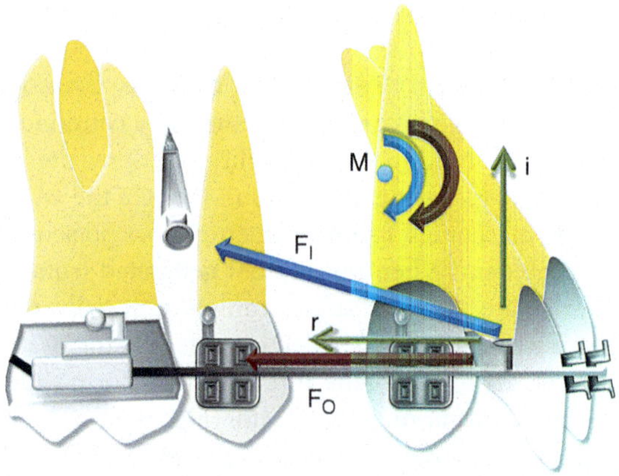

Figure 6-16 The vector of force varies between conventional mechanics (F_O) and implant-based mechanics (F_I) for space closure. Biomechanical design of the force system involved during en masse retraction of the anterior teeth with implants. Here, $F \gg r > i$, where F is total force, i is intrusive component, and r is retractive component. Also, the moment created by the implant is significantly less than that created by conventional mechanics. (Force application with implants is closer to the C_{RES} and $M = F \times$ distance to the C_{RES}.)

Mechanics of Space Closure with Mini-Implants

According to Figure 6-16 (a pictorial description of the initial force system for en masse retraction), the force (F) exerted by the nickel-titanium (Ni-Ti) coil springs (bilaterally) has two distinct components: a larger and predominantly retractive force (r) and a smaller intrusive force (i), causing en masse retraction and some intrusion of the anterior teeth. Additionally, there is a clockwise moment (M) on the anterior segment as the total force passes below the estimated C_{RES} of the anterior teeth. This moment causes the anterior teeth to tip. The degree of tipping will be regulated by the thickness and stiffness of the archwire. For example, a 0.017-inch × 0.025-inch stainless steel archwire has approximately 12 to 14 degrees of play in a 0.022-inch slot, assuming that the wire is completely passive when retraction starts, while a 0.016-inch × 0.022-inch stainless steel archwire has 16 to 18 degrees of play (Fig. 6-17). Therefore the latter will show greater amounts of tipping and a prolonged phase I and phase II of retraction compared to the former. A clinician should judiciously select the archwire for space closure.

For example, if the anterior teeth are flared at the beginning, more tipping is required; hence a thicker wire will be of limited use, as the effective play will be less. If instead the teeth are upright and there is a need for more control on the incisors, a thicker wire should be the choice (Fig. 6-18). As discussed, another method of obtaining control over the incisors during space closure is the use of power arms. This can be employed with implants as well (Fig. 6-19). For a complete list of approximate play for different archwire sizes, refer to Table 6-1.

Once the anterior teeth have tipped by the amount of play available between the bracket slot and the wire (clearance),

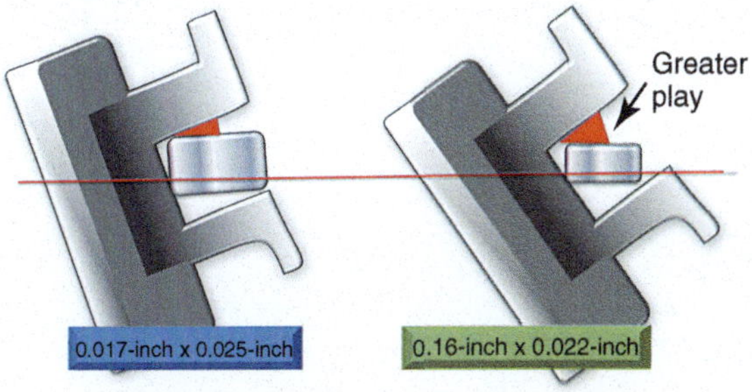

Figure 6-17 The amount of play between the bracket and archwire depends on the size of the archwire.

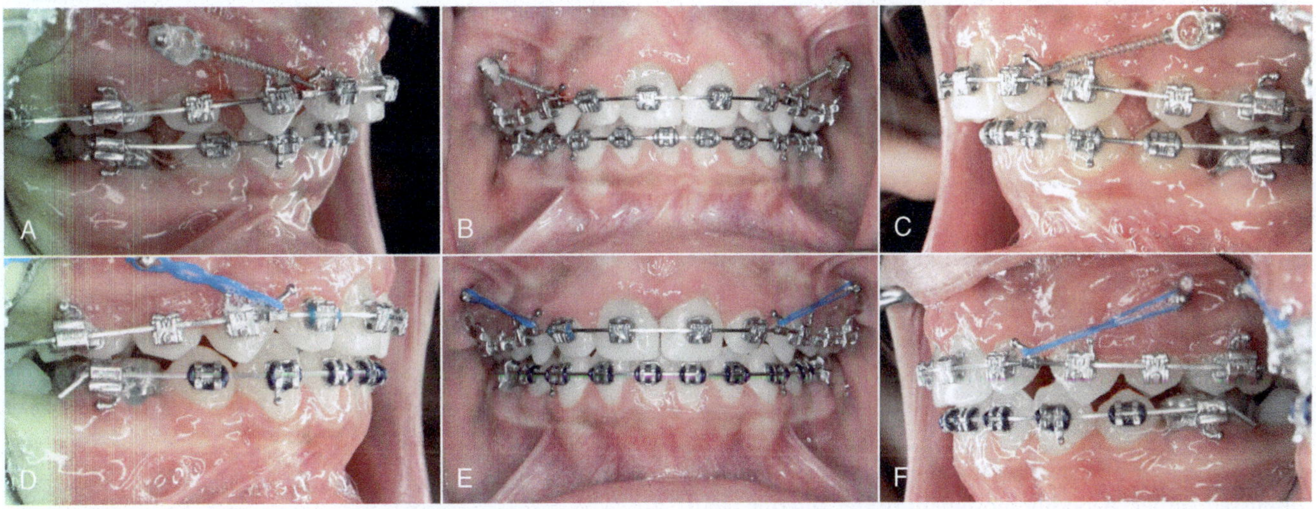

Figure 6-18 En masse space closure with mini-implant–supported anchorage. **A–C,** The incisors were upright at the beginning of space closure, so a 0.019-inch × 0.025-inch stainless steel archwire was used. **D–F,** After space closure. The axial inclination of the incisors was maintained to a large extent.

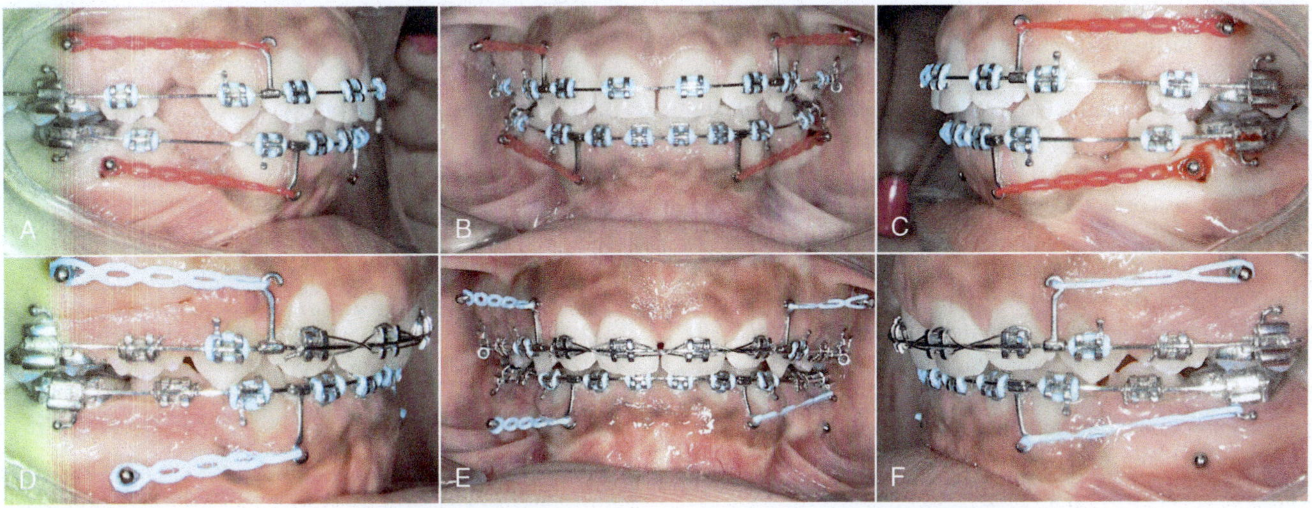

Figure 6-19 Mini-implants with power arms for space closure. **A–C,** Before. **D–F,** After.

TABLE 6-1 Amount of Wire Bracket Play in the Third Order for Different Archwire Sizes

Archwire Size (inches) (for stainless steel)	Amount of Play (degrees)
0.016 × 0.022	16–18
0.017 × 0.025	13–14
0.019 × 0.025	6–8
0.021 × 0.025	2–3

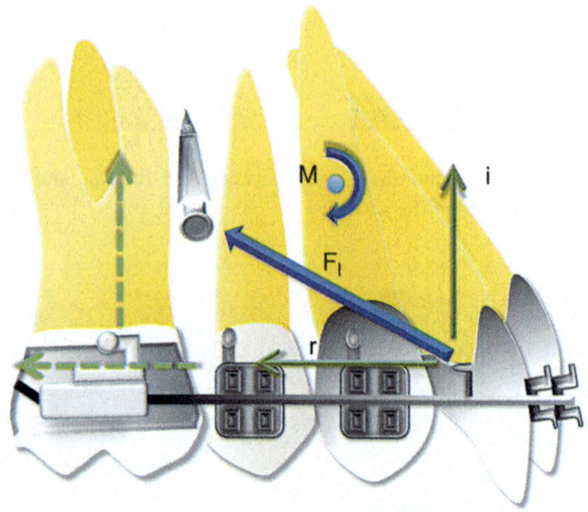

Figure 6-20 Biomechanical design for the force system involved after space closure. Retraction of the upper anterior teeth is still in progress. Note the increase in the angulation of the total force relative to the occlusal plane. (Here, $F_I \gg r \approx i$.) Such a mechanical configuration has important implications for vertical control and Class II correction.

no further tipping occurs, as the brackets lock onto the wire in that position and a counteracting M_C is generated, as discussed earlier. A bodily movement of the anterior teeth can be expected if the retractive force is continued but biological limitations can also play a decisive role.

After the extraction spaces are closed, contact between the canine and the second premolar is established. From this point on, further continuation of the retraction results in transmission of the total force to the posterior segments through the interdental contacts, producing a distal and intrusive force on the posterior teeth and a moment (M) on the entire arch (Fig. 6-20). These mechanics has often been employed to correct Class II molar relationships without extractions.

The biomechanics involved during en masse retraction with MI-assisted anchorage has other advantages that are quite distinct from other conventional methods, especially in high-angle patients. One such advantage, which is quite obvious, is the fact that there is no possibility of molar mesialization or anchorage loss in such a setup, since no retractive force is being applied from the molars. Therefore it is an effective way of compensating for a Class II malocclusion with large overjet.

SUMMARY

Space closure is the most critical aspect of orthodontics, especially in cases undergoing extraction. This chapter covers only the essential fundamentals of space closure, providing a stepping stone for further advanced reading in this area. A more detailed description involving the role of friction and archwire properties is beyond the scope of this book. Nonetheless, understanding the forces and moments involved during this procedure and their customized application for individual cases and situations can significantly enhance the outcome of treated cases.

REFERENCES

1. Gjessing P. A universal retraction spring. *J Clin Orthod.* 1994;28:222–242.
2. Hoenigl KD, Freudenthaler J, Marcotte MR, Bantleon HP. The centered T-loop: a new way of preactivation. *Am J Orthod Dentofacial Orthop.* 1995;108:149–153.
3. Martins RP, Buschang PH, Gandini LG Jr. Group A T-loop for differential moment mechanics: an implant study. *Am J Orthod Dentofacial Orthop.* 2009;135:182–189.
4. Siatkowski RE. Continuous arch wire closing loop design, optimization, and verification: part I. *Am J Orthod Dentofacial Orthop.* 1997;112:393–402.
5. Siatkowski RE. Continuous arch wire closing loop design, optimization, and verification: part II. *Am J Orthod Dentofacial Orthop.* 1997;112:487–495.
6. Coimbra ME, Penedo ND, de Gouvea JP, Elias CN, de Souza Araujo MT, Coelho PG. Mechanical testing and finite element analysis of orthodontic teardrop loop. *Am J Orthod Dentofacial Orthop.* 2008;133:188.e9–e13.
7. Burstone CJ, Koenig HA. Optimizing anterior and canine retraction. *Am J Orthod.* 1976;70:1–19.
8. Faulkner MG, Fuchshuber P, Haberstock D, Mioduchowski A. A parametric study of the force/moment systems produced by T-loop retraction springs. *J Biomech.* 1989;22:637–647.
9. Safavi MR, Geramy A, Khezri AK. M/F ratios of four different closing loops: 3D analysis using the finite element method (FEM). *Aust Orthod J.* 2006;22:121–126.
10. Techalertpaisarn P, Versluis A. Mechanical properties of Opus closing loops, L-loops, and T-loops investigated with finite element analysis. *Am J Orthod Dentofacial Orthop.* 2013;143:675–683.
11. Kuhlberg AJ, Burstone CJ. T-loop position and anchorage control. *Am J Orthod Dentofacial Orthop.* 1997;112:12–18.
12. Firouz T, Kuhlberg AJ, Nanda R. Efficacy of extraction space closure by precalibrated T-springs. *Inf Ortho Kiefer.* 1998;30:663–674.
13. Andrews LF. *Straight Wire: The Concept and Appliance.* San Diego, CA: L.A. Wells Company; 1989.
14. Upadhyay M, Yadav S, Nagaraj K, Uribe F, Nanda R. Mini-implants vs fixed functional appliances for treatment of young adult Class II female patients: a prospective clinical trial. *Angle Orthod.* 2012;82(2):294–303.
15. Upadhyay M, Yadav S, Nanda R. Vertical dimension control during en masse retraction with mini-implant anchorage. *Am J Orthod Dentofacial Orthop.* 2010;138:96–108.
16. Upadhyay M, Yadav S, Nagaraj K, Patil S. Treatment effects of mini-implant for "en masse" retraction of anterior teeth in bialveolar dental protrusion cases: a randomized controlled trial. *Am J Orthod Dentofacial Orthop.* 2008;134:18–29.
17. Upadhyay M, Yadav S, Nagaraj K, Nanda R. Dentoskeletal and soft tissue effects of mini-implants in Class II Div 1 patients. *Angle Orthod.* 2009;79:240–247.
18. Upadhyay M, Yadav S, Patil S. Mini-implant anchorage for en masse retraction of maxillary anterior teeth: a clinical-cephalometric study. *Am J Orthod Dentofacial Orthop.* 2008;134:803–810.

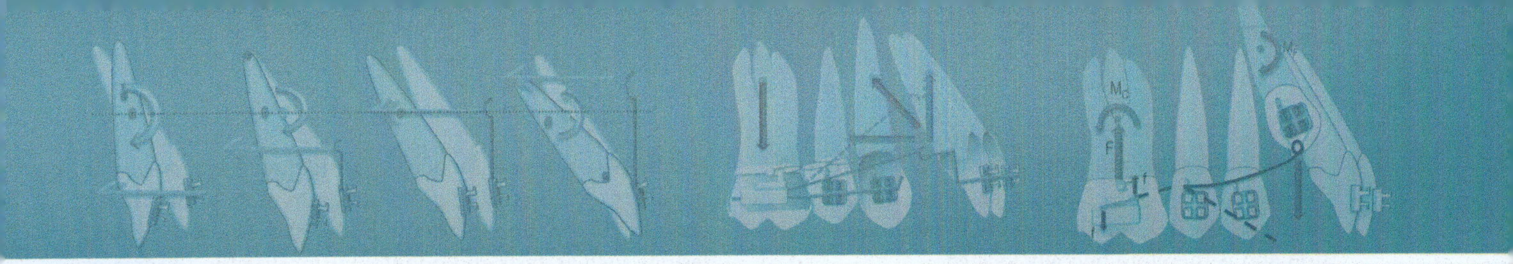

CHAPTER 7

Biomechanics-Based Management of Impacted Canines

Sumit Yadav and Ravindra Nanda

Maxillary canines are important both esthetically and functionally and are the second most commonly impacted teeth after the third molars.[1–6] The frequency of unerupted maxillary canines is approximately 0.8% to 2% in the general population, with ethnic variations.[4] The incidence of canine impaction is twice as common in females as in males and the teeth are palatally impacted in 85% of these patients and buccally impacted in 15%.[6] Patients with impacted maxillary canines are perceived to be more difficult and time consuming to treat than those with a routine malocclusion.

Position of the impacted canines and treatment mechanics are the two major factors affecting total treatment time and the final position of the canines in the oral cavity.[7,8] With new technologies such as cone beam computed tomography (CBCT), the impacted canine can be precisely located in three dimensions.[7] An optimal force system is then needed for the treatment and this system is defined as that which results in a greater biological response with minimal tissue damage, resulting in rapid tooth movement with few or no deleterious effects.[9]

Traditional force systems are attenuated as a result of deactivation during tooth movement or because of the physical properties of the force delivery system.[10] Appliance design has been focused on improving force delivery. Although an ideal spring that can deliver a continuous force day after day is only a theoretical possibility, various inter-arch and intra-arch mechanics have been devised for the successful management of impacted canines. Oppenhuizen[11] and Jacoby[12] devised an extrusion spring for palatally impacted canines using prefabricated 0.018-inch stainless steel archwires. Bowman and Carano[13] devised new directional force springs called Kilroy I and Kilroy II, used for palatally and buccally impacted canines, respectively. Haydar et al.[14] used microscrews with either an elastic traction or a ligature wire for management of the impacted tooth. Vardimon et al. recommended the use of magnets to treat impacted canines on the basis of a less invasive surgical procedure, effective forces at short distances, and controlled spatial guidance.[14a]

However, none of these authors have discussed the mechanics involved with the use of their appliances. The use of improper mechanics (direction and magnitude of force applied, direction and magnitude of reactionary force) when treating impacted and ectopically erupted canines increases the chance of root resorption of the adjacent teeth. A knowledge of mechanics is essential for effective treatment and an important step toward evidence-based treatment.[10,15]

DIAGNOSIS OF CANINE IMPACTION

The diagnosis of canine impaction is based on both clinical and radiographic examinations.

Clinical Examination

The following clinical signs along with radiographic diagnosis might be indicative of impacted canines:

1. Delayed eruption or migration of the permanent maxillary lateral incisors
2. Delayed eruption of the permanent canine (beyond 14 to 15 years of age)
3. Prolonged retention of the deciduous canine (beyond 14 to 15 years of age)
4. Absence of normal canine bulge
5. Presence of palatal bulge

Radiographic Diagnosis

Numerous radiographic methods have been proposed for the accurate localization of the impacted canines:

1. Periapical films: A single periapical film provides the orthodontist with a two-dimensional representation of the impacted canines and surrounding dentition.[16] To evaluate the position of the canine buccolingually, a second periapical film should be obtained by one of the following methods:
   - Clark's rule (or same lingual opposite buccal [SLOB] rule): Two periapical films are taken of the same area, with the horizontal angulation of the cone changed when the second film is taken. If the impacted canine

moves in the same direction as the cone, it is lingually positioned. If the impacted canine moves in the opposite direction, it is situated closer to the source of radiation and is therefore buccally located.

- Buccal object rule: The basic premise of this technique deals with the foreshortening and elongation of the images on the films. If the vertical angulation of the cone is changed by approximately 20 degrees in two successive periapical films, the buccal object will move in the direction opposite to the source of radiation. On the other hand, the lingual object will move in the same direction as the source of radiation.

2. Occlusal films: These serve as an adjunct along with the periapicals in determining the buccolingual position of the impacted canine.[16]
3. CBCT: CBCT can exactly locate the position of impacted canines in three dimensions of space. This three-dimensional imaging technique can also assess any damage to the roots of adjacent teeth and the quantity and quality of bone surrounding each tooth.[17,18]

SURGICAL EXPOSURE

Some research and much debate have surrounded the merits of open versus closed eruption techniques. There appear to be subtle differences between the two eruption techniques in relation to treatment duration and deleterious effects on the periodontal tissue. Two schools of thought exist regarding the eruption techniques; however, the choice between using an open or a closed eruption technique is typically based on individual preference. A simple palatal impaction (cusp tip of the canine at the same level of the cement-enamel junction of lateral incisor or central incisor) usually requires open surgical exposure whereas closed surgical exposure is usually favored when the tooth is more deeply embedded in the bone since open surgical exposure may necessitate excessive removal of the surrounding bone. Individual palatally impacted canines may lead to autonomous eruption after open surgical exposure; however, the orthodontic literature lacks sufficient clinical evidence as to which palatally impacted canine will respond favorably to which eruption technique.[19–21] Closed eruption technique has been much criticized regarding the direction of tooth eruption (direction of force) and its deleterious effects (root resorption of lateral incisor). However, with the advent of three-dimensional radiography (CBCT), the exact location of the impacted tooth can be identified and an optimal force system can be applied, which may result in rapid tooth movement with minimal deleterious effect on the impacted and the adjacent tooth.[20,21]

ETIOLOGY

The etiology of impacted canines is obscure and multifactorial. However, primary etiologic causes of maxillary canine impactions include (1) arch length deficiency (buccal canine impactions), (2) disturbances in tooth eruption sequence (hormonal or disease induced), (3) trauma to the maxilla or maxillary dentition, (4) prolonged retention of deciduous canine, (5) rotation of tooth buds, and (6) pathological lesions such as cysts and odontomas localized in the area of permanent canines and lateral incisors. It is hypothesized that palatally impacted canines are associated with a hypoplastic or missing lateral incisor (guidance theory) or with aplasia of the premolars or third molars (genetic theory). Palatally impacted canines are often present with adequate arch space whereas buccally impacted canines are thought to be associated with dental arch deficiencies.

Guidance Theory

The permanent maxillary canine lacks the guiding force during the process of eruption into the oral cavity because of extra space in the apical part of the maxilla resulting from a hypoplastic or missing lateral incisor. This theory purports that impacted canines are frequently found in persons with peg-shaped or missing maxillary lateral incisors. Even if these impactions are genetically determined, guidance theory states that the palatal canine impaction usually occurs as a result of local environmental disturbances.

Genetic Theory

According to genetic theory, the eruption anomaly of the maxillary permanent canine is the result of a developmental disturbance of the dental lamina. Evidence for this theory is found in familial and bilateral occurrences, sex differences, and the increased incidence of other dental issues such as ectopic eruption of the first molars and infraocclusion of the primary molars.[22–25] Research has even shown that palatally impacted canines usually coexist with either hypodontia or agenesis of the third molars.[26] Transcription factors such as *MSX1* and *PAX9*, which have been correlated with agenesis of molars, might be involved in palatal canine impactions.[27] Baccetti showed that unilateral palatally impacted canines correlated significantly ($p < 0.05$) with aplasia of maxillary lateral incisors whereas bilateral palatally impacted canines have significant correlation ($p < 0.05$) with agenesis of third molars, supporting the genetic etiology of palatal canine displacement.[28]

BIOMECHANICAL CONSIDERATIONS

Cantilever springs with a single force direction and point of force application are commonly used for the management of impacted and ectopically erupted canines (Fig. 7-1). Cantilever springs produce force on the impacted and ectopically placed canines in all three spatial planes, depending on the position of the canines (see Fig. 7-1; Fig. 7-2). The major force directed on the impacted and ectopically placed canine is vertical (extrusive force) and labial/lingual. In horizontal canine impactions, a pure couple force system with high moment-to-force ratio is advantageous to upright the impacted canine before pulling it out in the oral cavity. Cantilever-based appliances or springs (one-couple force systems) are designed to have a low load deflection rate. The

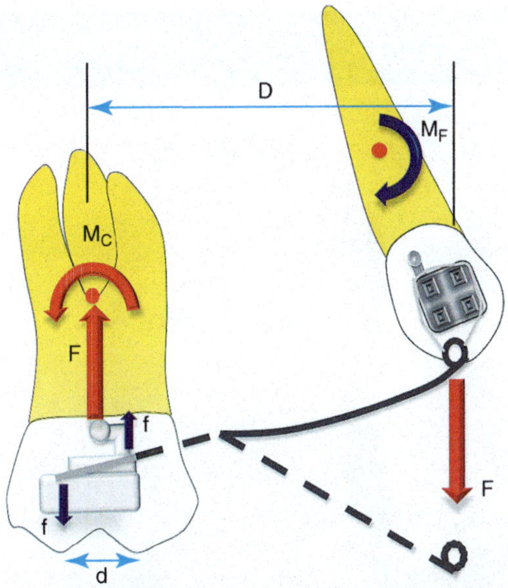

Figure 7-1 Anteroposterior view: A cantilever spring design for extrusion of a canine (a one-couple force system). The dotted line indicates the passive state of the spring while the solid design shows that it is in the activated state; in other words, from this point on the spring will gradually undergo deactivation. The force (F) exerted on the canine and molar per Newton's Third Law of Motion is equal and opposite. Once activated, the spring generates a couple in the auxiliary tube (M_C), where $M_C = F \times D$. D is the distance between the center of resistance (C_{RES}) of the molar and the point of application of the force on the canine. M_C can also be calculated by the product of the force of the couple (f) and the length of the auxiliary tube (d); that is, $M_C = f \times d$. Because the force does not pass through the C_{RES} of the canine, it generates a moment due to force (M_F). On the molar, as the force is assumed to pass through the C_{RES}, no moment due to force is generated. Note: Always differentiate between a moment due to a force and a moment due to a couple.

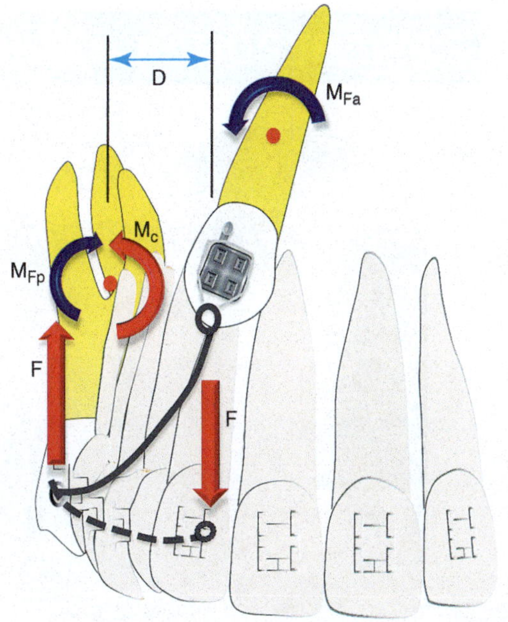

Figure 7-2 Transverse view: A cantilever spring design for extrusion of a canine (a one-couple force system). M_{Fp}: Since the force is buccal to the center of resistance (C_{RES}) of the molar, a moment due to the applied force is generated. Likewise, a moment is generated on the canine (M_{Fa}). Here, the net moment acting on the molar (M) can be obtained by subtracting the moment due to the force from the moment due to the couple (M_C). Therefore, $M = M_C - M_{Fp}$.

force systems delivered by these appliances (springs) tend to stay optimal and consistent in their magnitude, which prevents them from having any deleterious effects on the surrounding periodontium through the entire range of tooth movement. Additionally, an acceptable magnitude of force is maintained in the appliance during treatment to avoid frequent reactivations. A single force is exerted on the canine for eruption and alignment. The reactionary force and the moment are dissipated on the molar (see Figs. 7-1 and 7-2), which can be controlled by using a palatal arch and/or ligating the molar to the rest of the arch. Any spring that allows a modification of the force system during the period of getting an impacted canine out in the oral cavity and aligned in the arch is advantageous as long as clinicians are aware of structural mechanics and spring geometry.

Text continued on p. 132

CASE REPORT 1

A 13-year-old postpubertal girl presented with a chief complaint of crooked anterior teeth. Extraoral examination revealed a dolichofacial growth pattern with a straight soft tissue profile and an obtuse nasolabial angle. Intraoral examination showed that she had a bilateral Class I molar relationship and palatally impacted maxillary canines (Fig. 7-3). After leveling and aligning, a 0.032-inch CNA (Connecticut new arch form, Ortho Organizers, Carlsbad, CA.) transpalatal arch and a 0.019-inch × 0.025-inch CNA archwire were placed in the maxillary arch. Cantilever springs (0.017-inch × 0.025-inch CNA wire) applying 80 g of force (occlusal/extrusive) were placed bilaterally from the auxiliary tube of the molar bracket (Fig. 7-4). Springs were activated at each visit and after 5 months maxillary canines erupted in the oral cavity. At this point, the direction of the force was changed from occlusal to bucco-occlusal and force was reduced to 30 g. After 12 months of cantilever mechanics, the crowns of both maxillary canines were in the arch (see Fig. 7-4). Finishing and detailing were accomplished with a 0.017-inch × 0.025-inch CNA archwire. Total treatment time was 18 months (Fig. 7-5).

Continued

CASE REPORT 1—cont'd

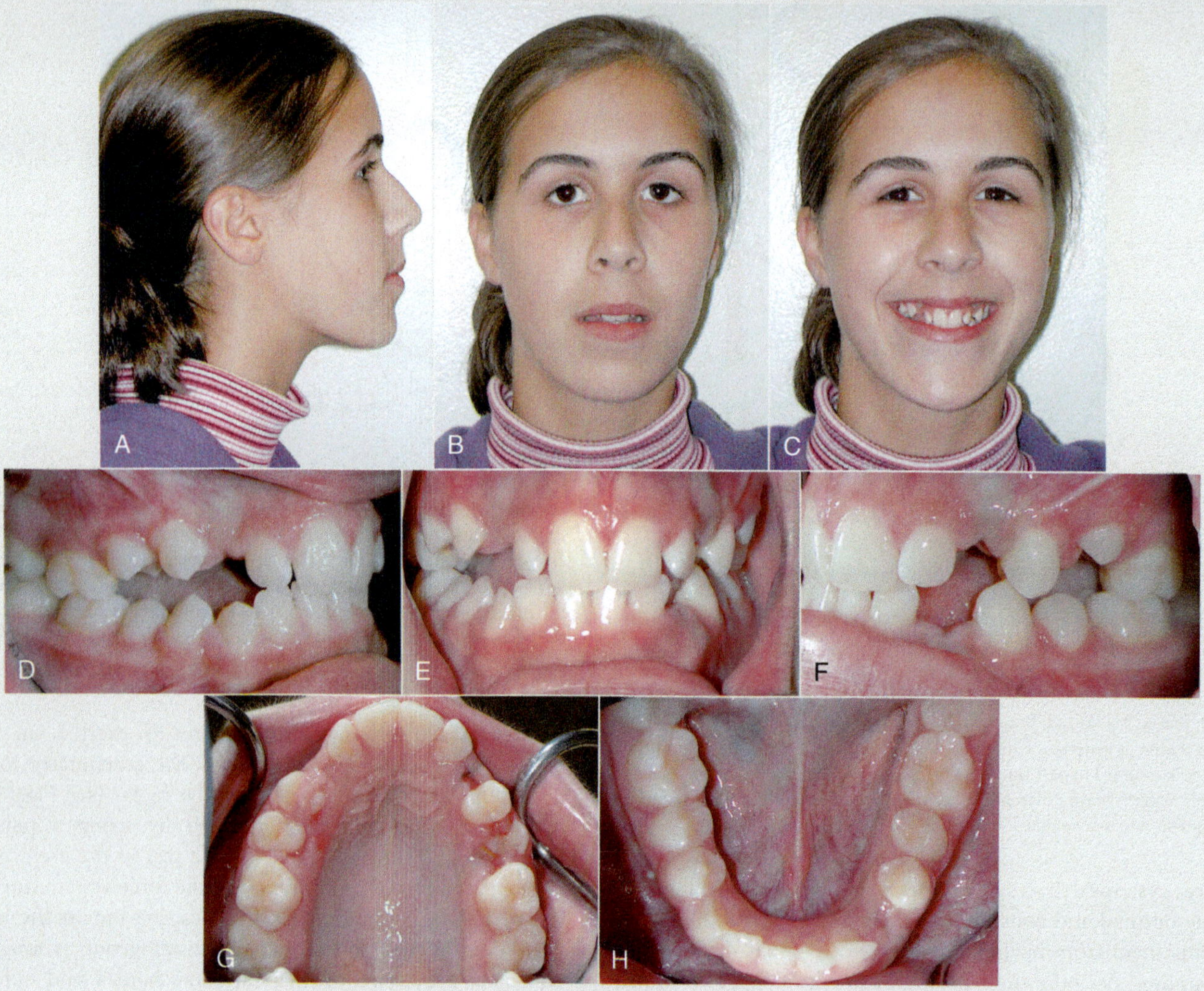

Figure 7-3 **A–C,** Pre-treatment facial views. **D–H,** Pre-treatment intraoral views.

CASE REPORT 1—cont'd

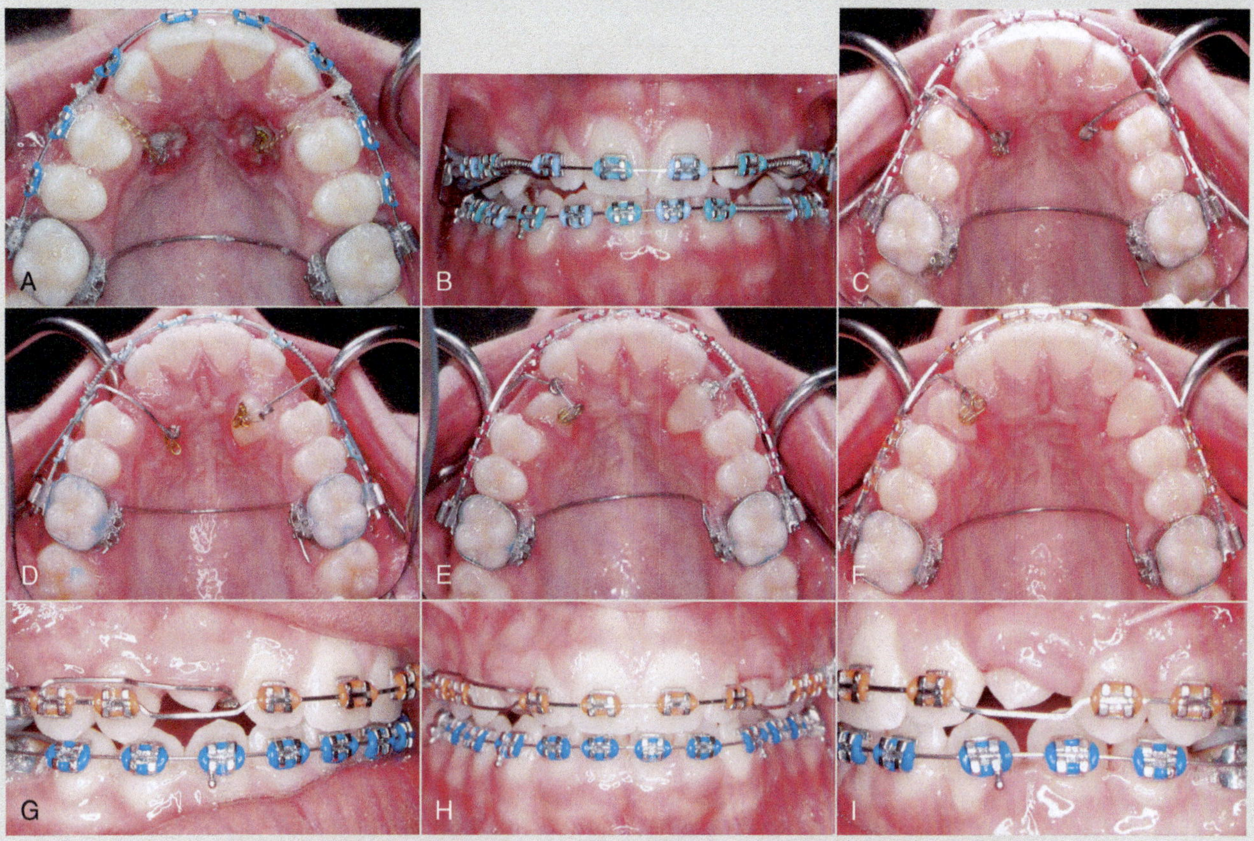

Figure 7-4 **A-F,** Mid-treatment intraoral (occlusal) views. **G–I,** Mid-treatment intraoral views.

Continued

CASE REPORT 1—cont'd

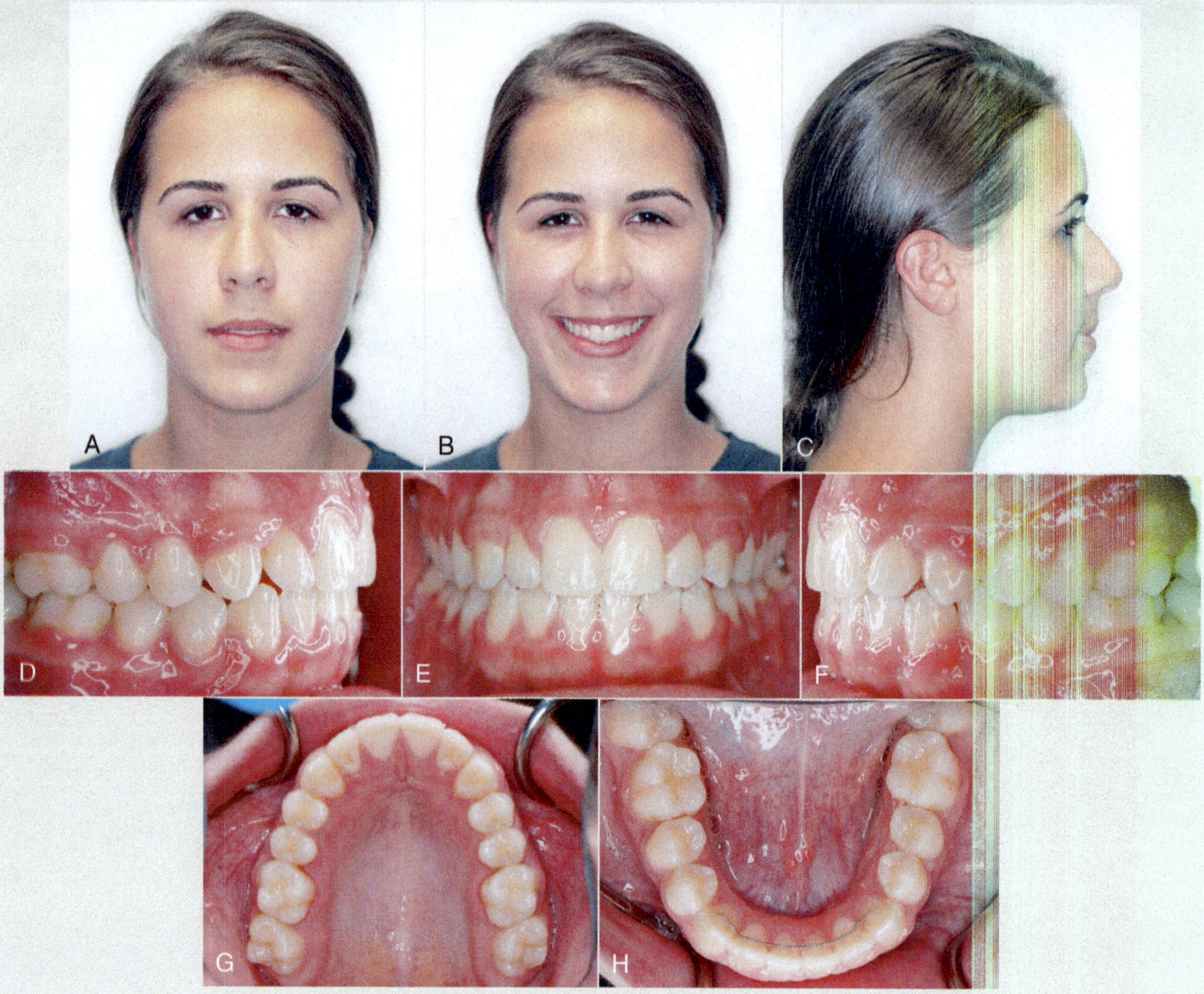

Figure 7-5 **A–C,** Post-treatment facial views. **D–H,** Post-treatment intraoral views.

CASE REPORT 2

An 11.7-year-old postpubertal girl was referred by her general dentist regarding a missing right maxillary canine. Extraoral examination revealed a dolichofacial growth pattern with a straight soft tissue profile (Fig. 7-6, A–C). Intraoral examination showed that she had a Class I molar relationship and a palatally impacted right maxillary canine (Fig. 7-6, D–H). After initial leveling and aligning, a 0.032-inch CNA transpalatal arch and a 0.019-inch × 0.025-inch CNA archwire were placed in the upper arch. A cantilever spring (0.017-inch × 0.025-inch CNA) was placed from the right auxiliary tube of the molar bracket (Fig. 7-7). Seventy-five grams of bucco-occlusal force were applied and after 6 months the canine erupted into the arch. Finishing and detailing were accomplished with a 0.017-inch × 0.025-inch CNA and a 0.017-inch × 0.025-inch braided stainless steel archwire. Total treatment time was 16 months (Fig. 7-8).

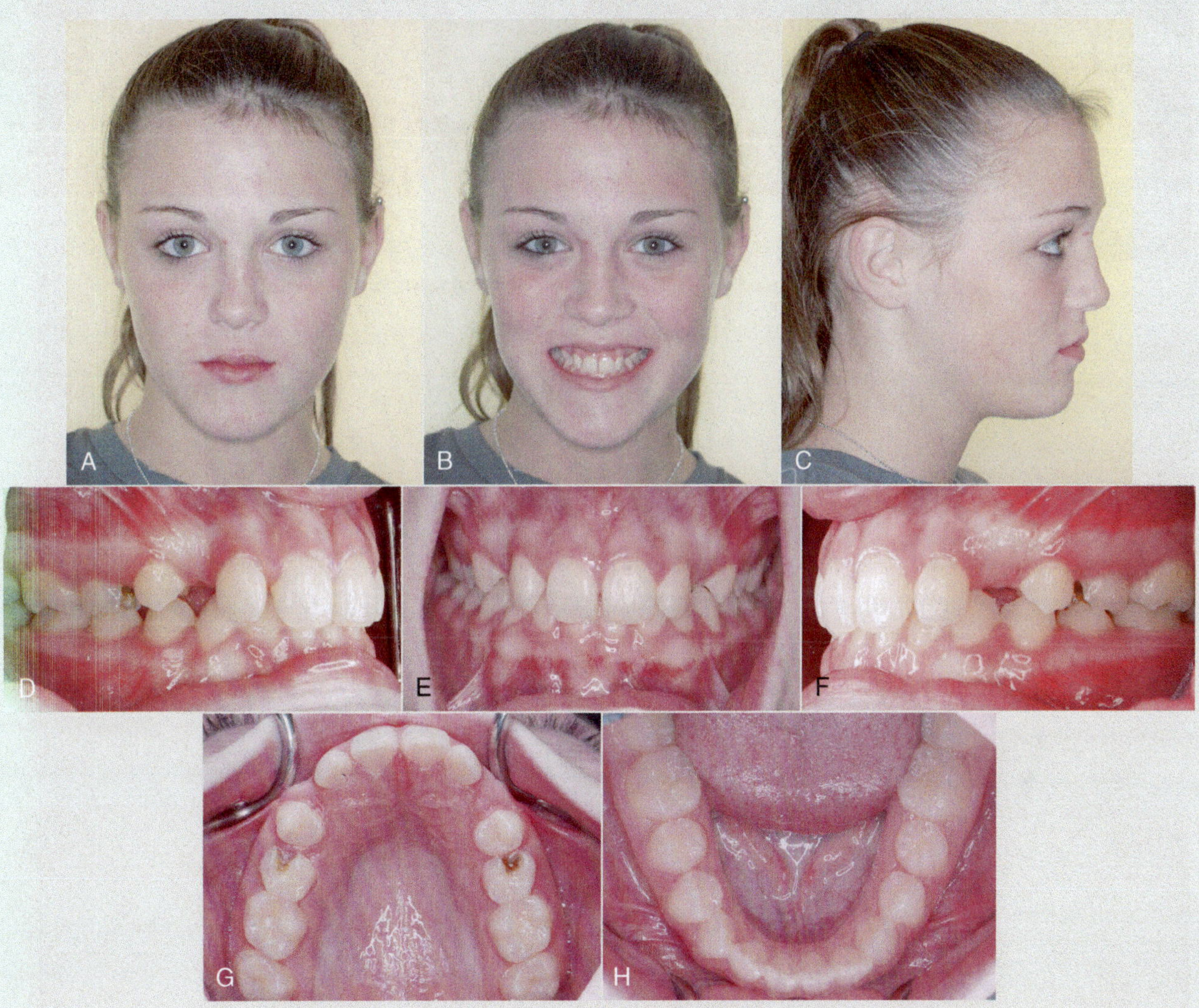

Figure 7-6 **A–C,** Pre-treatment facial views. **D–H,** Pre-treatment intraoral views.

Continued

CASE REPORT 2—cont'd

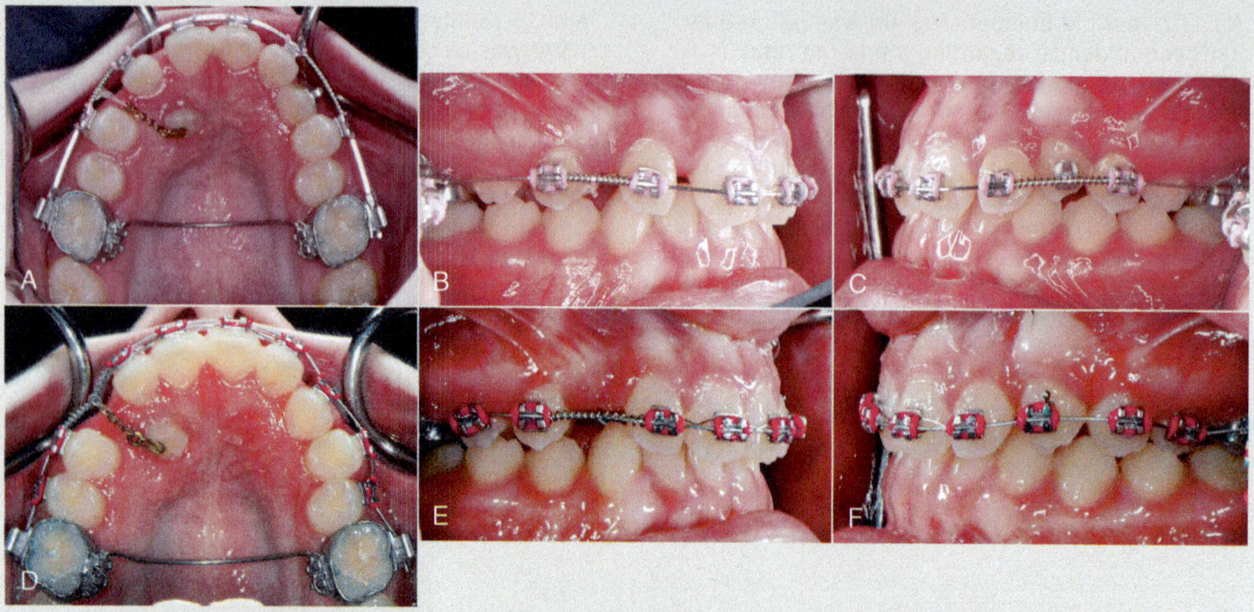

Figure 7-7 **A–F,** Mid-treatment intraoral views.

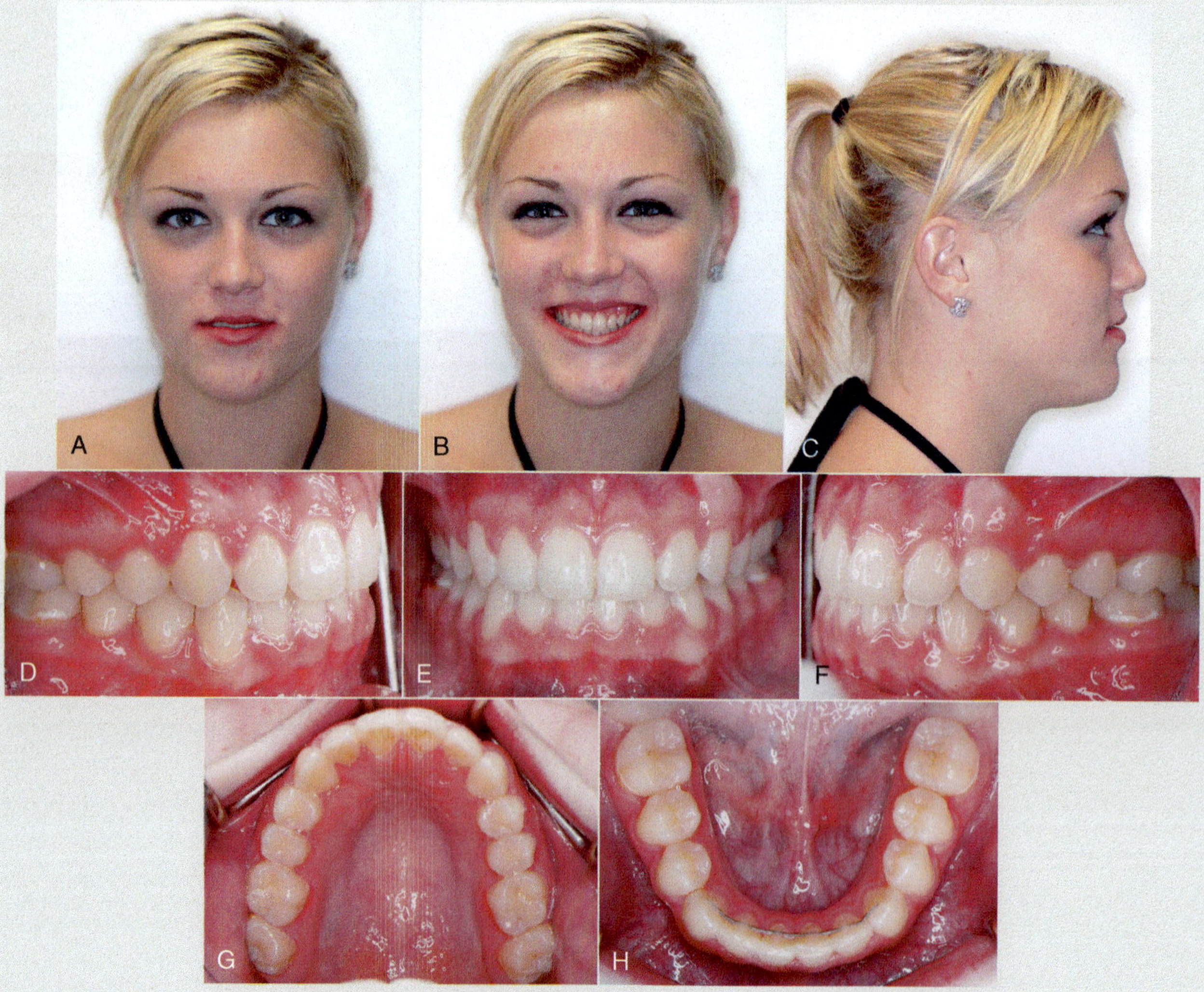

Figure 7-8 **A–C,** Post-treatment facial views. **D–H,** Post-treatment intraoral views.

CASE REPORT 3

A 12-year-old postpubertal girl presented with a chief complaint of irregularly placed upper front teeth. Extraoral examination revealed a brachyfacial growth pattern with a convex soft tissue profile and obtuse nasolabial angle (Fig. 7-9, A–C). Intraoral examination showed that she had a bilateral Class I molar relationship and highly placed maxillary canines in the buccal vestibule (Fig. 7-9, D–H). The deciduous maxillary left canine was overretained and the patient had a crossbite tendency due to a narrow transverse maxillary dimension (see Fig. 7-9, D–H). The deciduous left maxillary canine was extracted and a hyrax expander was placed to correct the transverse discrepancy (Fig. 7-10, A–E). Cantilevers (0.017-inch × 0.025-inch CNA) were placed bilaterally from the auxiliary tube of the molar bracket to bring the highly placed canines into the arch (see Fig. 7-10, A–E). Further alignment of the canines was done using a 0.016-inch nickel-titanium (Ni-Ti) wire piggybacked over a stiffer 0.017-inch × 0.025-inch CNA base archwire (Fig. 7-10, F–K). Finishing and detailing were accomplished with a 0.017-inch × 0.025-inch CNA and a 0.016-inch × 0.022-inch braided stainless steel archwire. Total treatment time was 15 months (Fig. 7-11).

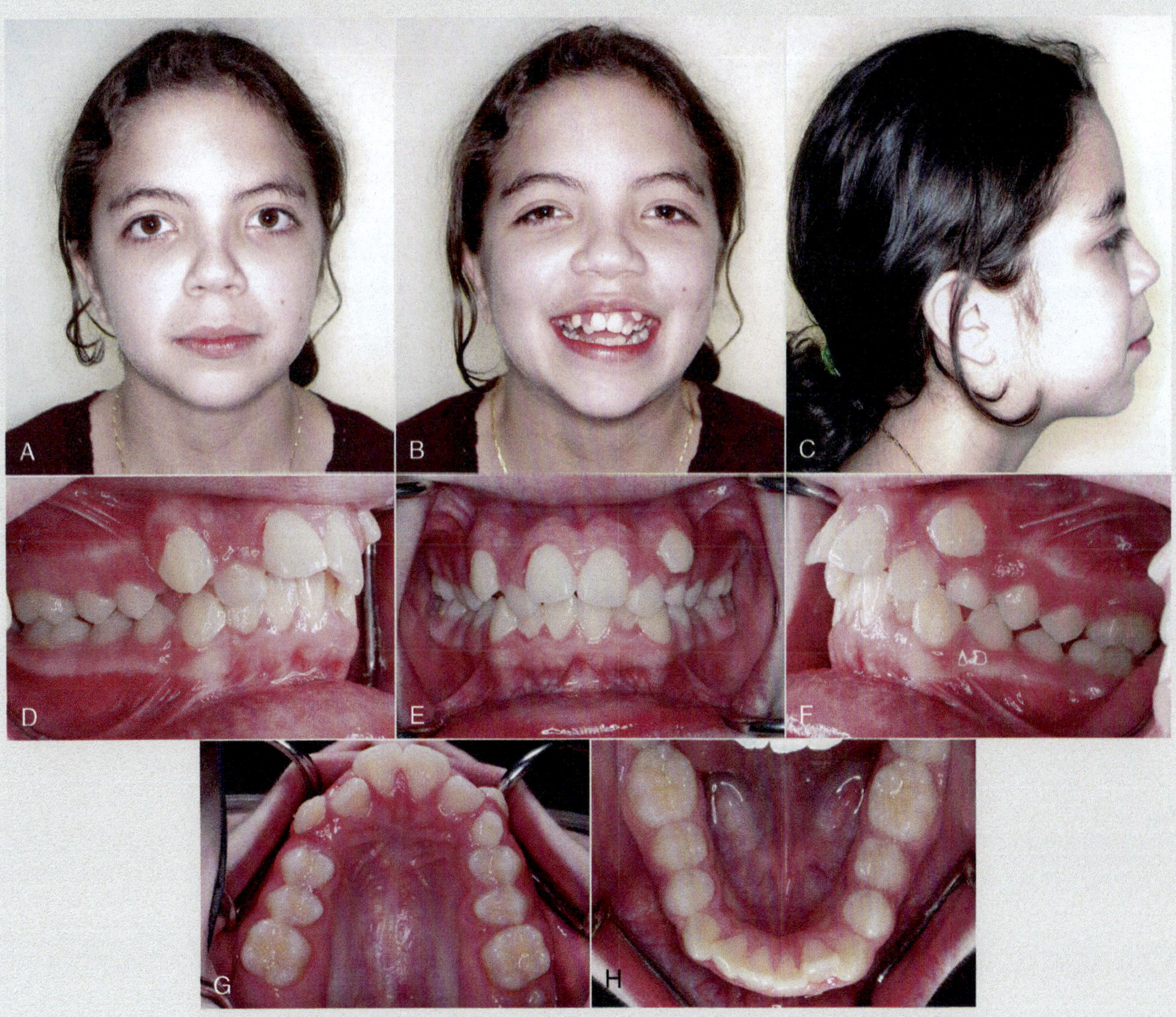

Figure 7-9 **A–C,** Pre-treatment facial views. **D–H,** Pre-treatment intraoral views.

Continued

CASE REPORT 3—cont'd

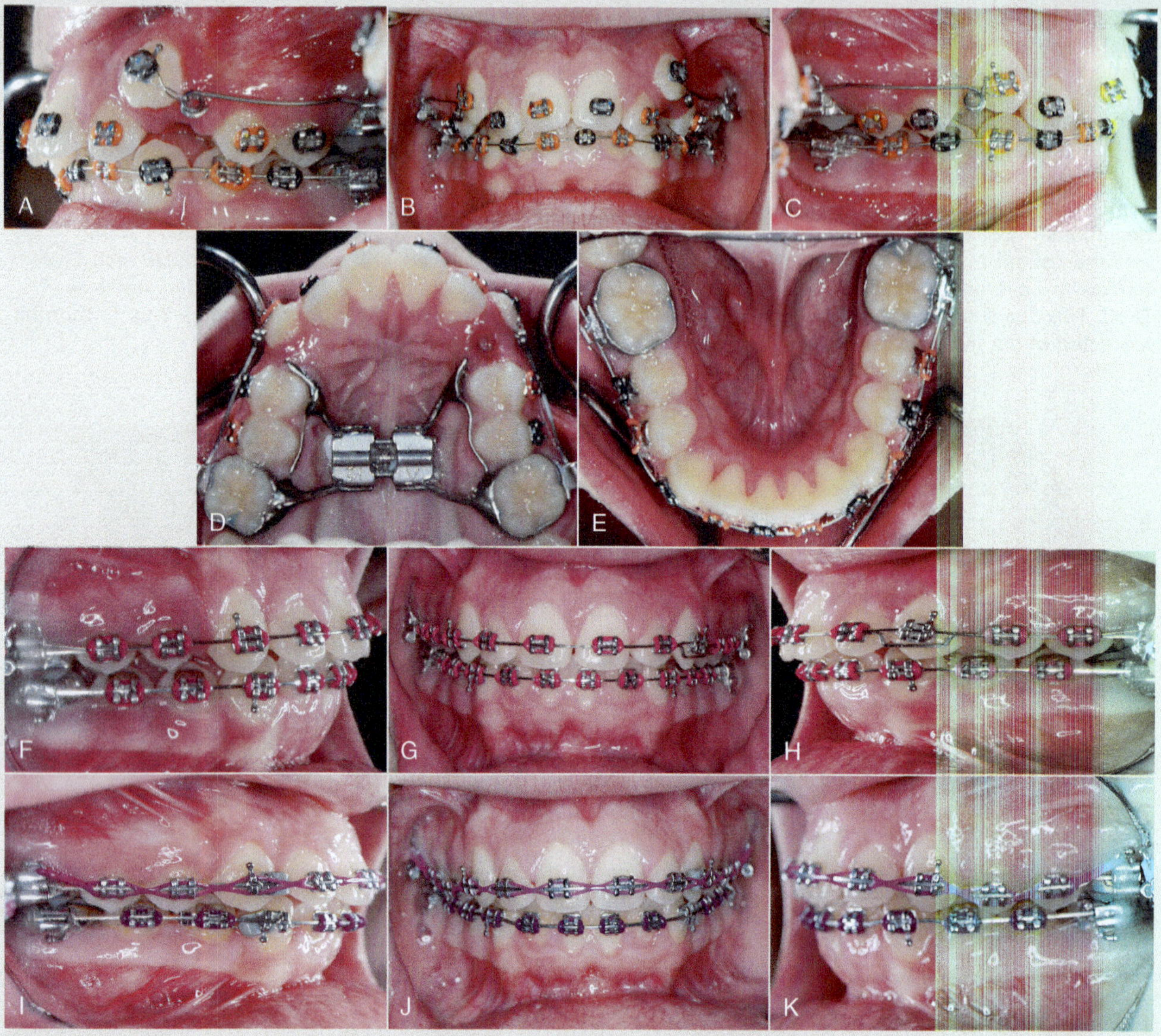

Figure 7-10 **A–K,** Mid-treatment intraoral views.

CASE REPORT 3—cont'd

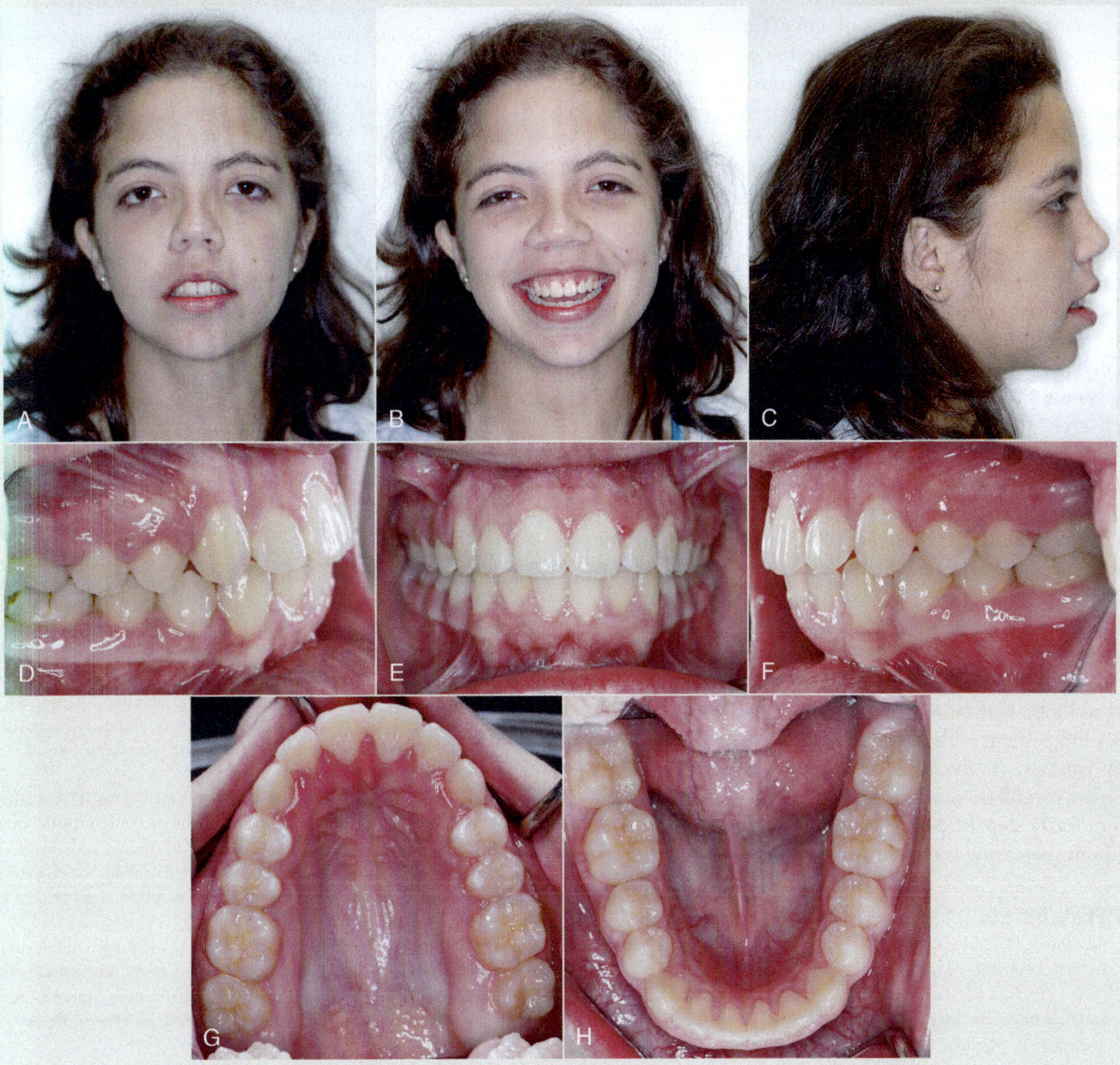

Figure 7-11 **A–C,** Post-treatment facial views. **D–H,** Post-treatment intraoral views.

The therapeutic approach to impacted and ectopically placed canines is interdisciplinary. Although many factors account for the final outcome, the three-dimensional force system acting on the canines is perhaps the single most important factor. Correction of impacted and ectopically placed canines usually requires eruption of the canines into the oral cavity and a buccolingual movement to get the canines into the arch. The single force system (cantilever mechanics) has been used effectively to bring about controlled three-dimensional movement in both impacted and ectopically placed canines in the direction predetermined by the treatment goals. The force required to get the canines (impacted or displaced) into the arch is relatively low. However, to prevent the undesirable tipping of the maxillary first molar, a transpalatal bar (0.032-inch round CNA wire) was used in all three case reports (in the third case an inactivated hyrax was used as the transpalatal bar). Furthermore, the cantilever springs were made from a 0.017-inch × 0.025-inch archwire, which has a low load deflection rate, thus reducing the frequency of reactivation. In all of the case reports, patients were treated with a closed-eruption surgical exposure technique and the canines were brought into the arch through attached mucosa, which resulted in an adequate zone of attached keratinized gingiva, good bone support, and no excessive periodontal probing depths.

SUMMARY

Orthodontic and esthetic outcomes are frequently compromised in patients with impacted or ectopically placed maxillary canines. In the three case reports presented in this chapter, careful treatment planning and meticulous mechanics at each step helped us to achieve the desired results without increasing the treatment time significantly.

REFERENCES

1. Bishara SE. Clinical management of impacted maxillary canines. *Semin Orthod.* 1998;4:87–98.
2. Peck S, Peck L, Kataja M. The palatally displaced canine as a dental anomaly of genetic origin. *Angle Orthod.* 1994;64:249–256.
3. Thilander B, Myrberg N. The prevalence of malocclusion in Swedish schoolchildren. *Scand J Dent Res.* 1973;81:12–21.
4. Ericson S, Kurol J. Radiographic assessment of maxillary canine eruption in children with clinical signs of eruption disturbance. *Eur J Orthod.* 1986;8:133–140.
5. Bedoya MM, Park JH. A review of the diagnosis and management of impacted maxillary canines. *J Am Dent Assoc.* 2009;140:1485–1493.
6. Cooke J, Wang HL. Canine impactions: incidence and management. *Int J Periodontics Restorative Dent.* 2006;26:483–491.
7. van Vlijmen OJ, Kuijpers MA, Berge SJ, et al. Evidence supporting the use of cone-beam computed tomography in orthodontics. *J Am Dent Assoc.* 2012;143:241–252.
8. Holberg C, Steinhauser S, Geis P, Rudzki-Janson I. Cone-beam computed tomography in orthodontics: benefits and limitations. *J Orofac Orthop.* 2005;66:434–444.
9. Burstone CJ, Tanne K. Biomechanical basis of tooth movement [in Japanese]. *Nihon Kyosei Shika Gakkai Zasshi.* 1986;45:541–551.
10. Yadav S, Chen J, Upadhyay M, Jiang F, Roberts WE. Comparison of the force systems of 3 appliances on palatally impacted canines. *Am J Orthod Dentofacial Orthop.* 2011;139:206–213.
11. Oppenhuizen G. An extrusion spring for palatally impacted cuspids. *J Clin Orthod.* 2003;37:434–436.
12. Jacoby H. The "ballista spring" system for impacted teeth. *Am J Orthod.* 1979;75:143–151.
13. Bowman SJ, Carano A. The Kilroy spring for impacted teeth. *J Clin Orthod.* 2003;37:683–688.
14. Haydar SG, Uckan S, Sesen C. A method for eruption of impacted teeth. *J Clin Orthod.* 2003;37:430–433.
14a. Vardimon AD, Graber TM, Drescher D, Bourauel C. Rare earth magnets and impaction. *Am J Orthod Dentofacial Orthop.* 1991;100(6):494–512.
15. Yadav S, Chen J, Upadhyay M, Roberts E, Nanda R. Three-dimensional quantification of the force system involved in a palatally impacted canine using a cantilever spring design. *Orthodontics (Chic.).* 2012;13: 22–33.
16. Sajnani AK, King NM. Diagnosis and localization of impacted maxillary canines: comparison of methods. *J Investig Clin Dent.* 2012;4:252–256.
17. Alqerban A, Jacobs R, Fieuws S, Willems G. Comparison of two cone beam computed tomographic systems versus panoramic imaging for localization of impacted maxillary canines and detection of root resorption. *Eur J Orthod.* 2011;33:93–102.
18. Botticelli S, Verna C, Cattaneo PM, Heidmann J, Melsen B. Two- versus three-dimensional imaging in subjects with unerupted maxillary canines. *Eur J Orthod.* 2011;33:344–349.
19. Parkin NA, Deery C, Smith AM, Tinsley D, Sandler J, Benson PE. No difference in surgical outcomes between open and closed exposure of palatally displaced maxillary canines. *J Oral Maxillofac Surg.* 2012;70: 2026–2034.
20. Parkin N, Benson PE, Thind B, Shah A. Open versus closed surgical exposure of canine teeth that are displaced in the roof of the mouth. *Cochrane Database Syst Rev.* 2008;(4):CD006966.
21. Mathews DP, Kokich VG. Palatally impacted canines: the case for pre-orthodontic uncovering and autonomous eruption. *Am J Orthod Dentofacial Orthop.* 2013;143:450–458.
22. Peck S, Peck L, Kataja M. Site-specificity of tooth agenesis in subjects with maxillary canine malpositions. *Angle Orthod.* 1996;66:473–476.
23. Peck S, Peck L, Kataja M. Concomitant occurrence of canine malposition and tooth agenesis: evidence of orofacial genetic fields. *Am J Orthod Dentofacial Orthop.* 2002;122:657–660.
24. Peck S, Peck L. Palatal displacement of canine is genetic and related to congenital absence of teeth. *J Dent Res.* 1997;76:728–729.
25. Pirinen S, Arte S, Apajalahti S. Palatal displacement of canine is genetic and related to congenital absence of teeth. *J Dent Res.* 1996;75:1742–1746.
26. Becker A. Palatal displacement of canine is genetic and related to congenital absence of teeth. *J Dent Res.* 1997;76:1526.
27. Litsas G, Acar A. A review of early displaced maxillary canines: etiology, diagnosis and interceptive treatment. *Open Dent J.* 2011;5:39–47.
28. Baccetti T. A controlled study of associated dental anomalies. *Angle Orthod.* 1998;68:267–274.

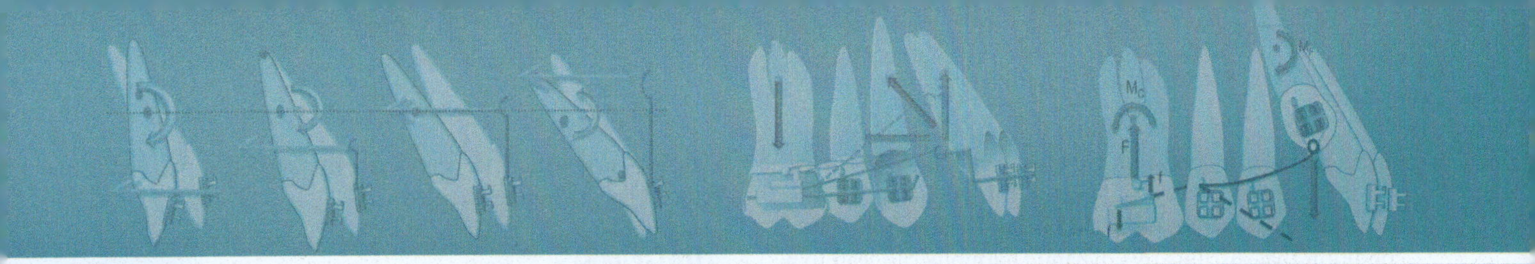

CHAPTER 8

Management of Deep Overbite Malocclusion

Madhur Upadhyay and Ravindra Nanda

Deep overbite is perhaps the most common malocclusion and is also the most difficult to treat successfully. Excessive incisal overlap, which varies widely from patient to patient, is one of the primary manifestations of dental malocclusion.[1] Before embarking on a detailed discussion of deep bite malocclusion it is imperative to understand the concept of overbite. One of the earliest definitions of overbite was put forward by Strang,[2] who defined it as "the overlapping of the upper anterior teeth over the lowers in the vertical plane." However, since the crown length of the upper and lower incisors varies significantly in individuals, a notation of overbite as a percentage is more descriptive and desirable. Therefore the same definition when put in terms of percentage defines overbite as "the amount and percentage of overlap of the lower incisors by the upper incisors."

The ideal overbite in a normal occlusion may range between 2- and 4-mm or more appropriately between 5% and 25% (overlap of the mandibular incisors by the maxillary incisors) (Fig. 8-1). According to Nanda,[3] even a range of 25% to 40% without any associated functional problems during various movements of the temporomandibular joint (TMJ) may be considered normal. However, overlaps greater than 40% should be considered "excessive" (deep bite), as they have the potential to cause deleterious effects on the overall dental health of the surrounding periodontal structures and the TMJ. At 5 to 6 years of age the percentage of overbite varies between 36.5% and 39.2%.[4] Between 9 and 12 years of age the overbite usually increases, whereas in the period between 12 years and adulthood it decreases.[5] Thereafter it remains largely unchanged, varying between 37.9% and 40.7% unless affected by other factors such as abrasion or loss of teeth, causing reduced vertical dimension. Severe deep bites (overbites >5-mm) are found in nearly 20% of children and 13% of adults, representing about 95.2% of vertical occlusal problems.

One of the most severe forms of excessive overbite is the *cover bite*[6] (Fig. 8-2), which is most often associated with the Class II, Division 2 malocclusion. This condition was first recorded in 1912 in the German literature as *Deckbiss*.[7] It is characterized by complete covering or concealment of the mandibular incisors' crowns due to excessive overbite and retroclination of the maxillary incisors. Another term that has been used previously to denote a severe form of deep bite is the *closed bite*[8] (Fig. 8-3). This is mostly seen in adults and very rarely in young children and is characterized by excessive overbite resulting from loss of posterior teeth.

ETIOLOGY

A deep bite malocclusion overlies a multitude of hidden skeletal or dental discrepancies. Accordingly, a deep bite should not be approached as a disease entity; instead, it is considered a clinical manifestation of an underlying skeletal or dental discrepancy.

From a developmental standpoint, skeletal or dental overbite is caused by either genetic or environmental factors, or a combination of both. Skeletal deep bites usually have a horizontal growth pattern and are characterized by (1) growth discrepancy of the maxillary and mandibular jawbones, (2) convergent rotation of the jaw bases, and/or (3) deficient mandibular ramus height. In such situations the anterior facial height is often short, particularly the lower facial third. On the other hand, dental deep bites show either supraocclusion (overeruption) of the incisors[2,9] or infraocclusion (undereruption) of the molars,[2,5,9,10] or a combination of the two. Other factors that can affect this condition include alteration in the tooth morphologies, premature loss of permanent teeth resulting in lingual collapse of the maxillary or mandibular anterior teeth, mesiodistal width of anterior teeth, and age-related natural deepening of the bite.

Deep bites primarily caused by environmental factors can also be classified as "acquired deep bites." It is a well-known fact that there is a dynamic equilibrium of forces between the structures around the teeth, namely, the tongue, the buccinator, the mentalis and the orbicularis oris muscles, and the occlusal forces that assist in the balanced development and maintenance of the occlusion. Any environmental condition that disrupts this dynamic harmony can lead to a malocclusion. Some examples are:

1. A lateral tongue thrust or abnormal tongue posture causing infraocclusion of the posterior teeth
2. Wearing away of the occlusal surface or tooth abrasion
3. Anterior tipping of the posterior teeth into extraction sites
4. Prolonged thumb-sucking

Hence deep bite etiology must be considered in detail in order to formulate a comprehensive diagnosis and treatment plan for each patient so that optimal skeletal, dental, and esthetic results can be attained.

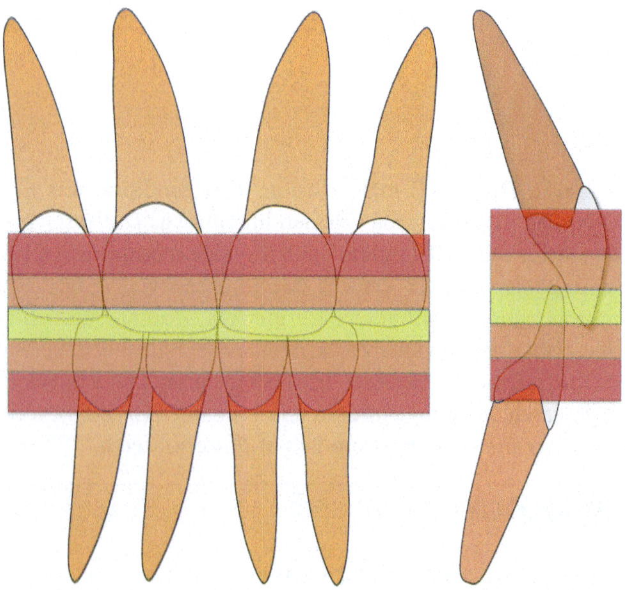

Figure 8-1 Zones of overbite: 5% to 25% is normal (*yellow*), 25% to 40% is increased overbite (*orange*), and >40% excessive (deep) overbite (*red*).

DIAGNOSIS

A deep overbite can be corrected either by extrusion of posterior teeth or by inhibition and genuine intrusion of anterior teeth, or by a combination of the two (Fig. 8-4). The choice of treatment is based in part on the etiology of deep bite, the amount of growth anticipated, the vertical dimension, the relationship of the teeth to the adjoining soft tissue structures, and the desired position of the occlusal plane.

Growth Considerations

It is widely accepted that correction of deep bite is both easier to accomplish and more stable when it is performed on growing patients than when it is attempted on those with no appreciable growth remaining.[11,12] Since growth tends to increase the vertical distance between the maxillae and the mandible, it is probably useful to treat such patients in a period of active mandibular growth. During the growth period, tooth eruption can be stimulated in the posterior segments and inhibited in the anterior because condylar growth allows for dentoalveolar growth. However, in adults such a movement is counteracted by the posterior occlusion, especially in a patient with a hypodivergent skeletal pattern. The stability of such a tooth movement, if performed, is highly questionable, as it leads to alterations in muscle physiology, thereby increasing the chances of relapse. In such malocclusions and others in which growth stimulation is no longer possible, fixed or removable mechanical appliances are needed to achieve optimal treatment results. In some patients a surgical procedure may be required. For example, in patients with vertical maxillary excess, a Le Fort I osteotomy with maxillary impaction might be required to

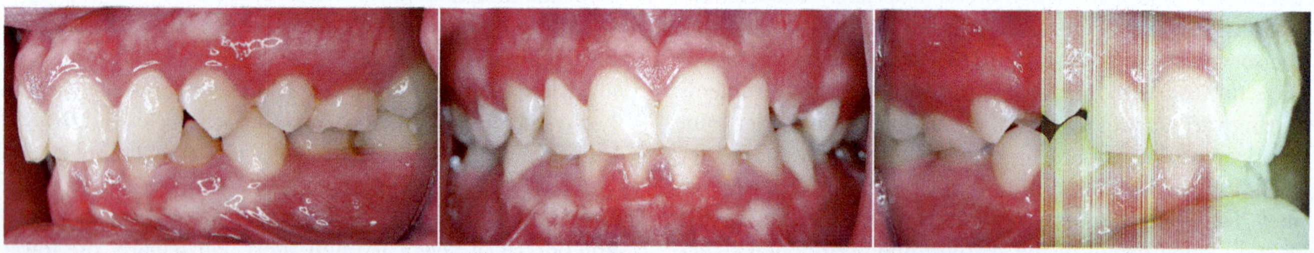

Figure 8-2 Example of cover bite malocclusion. Note that the lower incisors are completely concealed by the upper incisors.

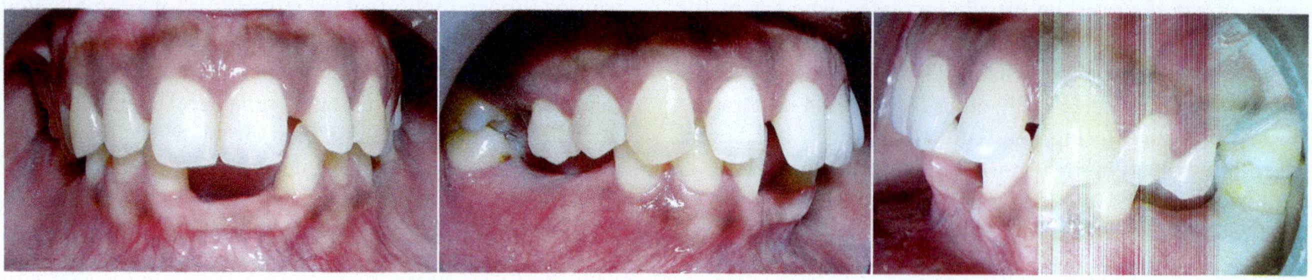

Figure 8-3 Example of closed bite.

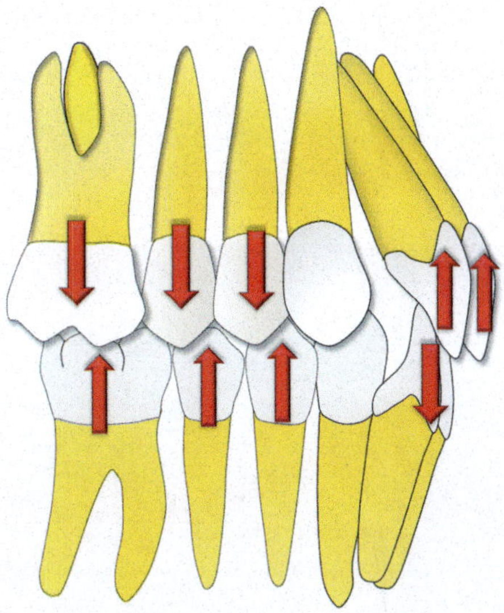

Figure 8-4 Deep bite malocclusion can be treated by either intrusion of incisors or extrusion of posterior teeth.

achieve optimum dentofacial esthetics. A detailed discussion of this subject is beyond the scope of this chapter and can be found elsewhere.[13]

Assessment of the Vertical Dimension

Schudy[14] advocated correction of deep bite with eruption of premolars and molars as the treatment of choice, while others[3,15] have preferred intrusion of incisors to treat the majority of their patients. Instead of following anecdotal information it is important to carefully consider the influence of extrusive or intrusive mechanics on the vertical facial height of a patient, as this in turn may affect the anterior-posterior relationship of the maxilla and mandible.

In general, eruptive mechanics should not encroach on the freeway[8] or interocclusal space, which is defined as the distance between the occlusal or incisal surfaces of the maxillary and mandibular teeth when the mandible is in the physiological rest position. The average is between 2- and 4-mm. When there is a larger than normal free space, greater opportunities exist for correction by guiding vertical alveolar development. For example, in a Class II, Division 2 patient with a hypodivergent facial pattern, redundant lips, and a flat mandibular plane angle, the deep bite can be corrected and facial esthetics improved by increasing the lower facial height or facial convexity. However, in most other Class II malocclusions it is not always desirable to increase the vertical dimension, since doing so would tend to accentuate the point A–point B discrepancy and increase an abnormally large lower face.

Soft Tissue Evaluation

In the present era, "soft tissue relationships" form an important diagnostic tool for deep bite correction. The clinician should always consider the maxillary incisor position relative to the lip position to determine whether to maintain, intrude, or extrude the maxillary incisors relative to the upper lip. With increased emphasis on smile esthetics and smile design, the use of dynamic smile analysis is gaining precedence over static photographs in diagnosing malocclusions and formulating appropriate treatment plans for their correction.[16]

Incisal exposure should be considered in three different clinical situations during initial examination: in relaxed lip position, while smiling, and during speech. In a relaxed lip position, 2- to 4-mm of incisor exposure, which includes the incisal edges, is considered acceptable. When smiling, the average incisor exposure is almost two-thirds that of the upper incisor, according to Maulik and Nanda.[16] They also reported that in most pleasing smiles the upper lip in males does not show any gingiva; however, females can have 1- to 2-mm of gingival exposure. If this condition is met and a deep bite is still present, the treatment plan should focus on either posterior extrusion (if the vertical parameters permit) or lower incisor intrusion (Fig. 8-5). In contrast, an occlusal plane "significantly" below the ideal might show excessive gingiva, which might then require selective intrusion of the upper incisors (Fig. 8-6). Incisor exposure during speech may give additional information, as different facial muscles are involved.

Another important factor to consider is the "interlabial gap." In patients exhibiting a large interlabial gap it might not be desirable to perform posterior extrusive mechanics, as this might further worsen the esthetics of the patient by increasing the interlabial gap. In fact, an increase in the interlabial gap may cause several other problems, such as inability to close the lips without strain and associated functional problems. Similarly, in individuals with redundant upper and lower lips or no interlabial gap but who show excessive overbite, posterior extrusive mechanics may be desirable.

Flaring (proclining) the incisors is yet another option that primarily camouflages deep bites. It is especially useful in patients who have retroclined incisors to begin with (e.g., Class II, Division 2 cases). However, rapid labial tipping of mandibular incisors must be avoided to minimize risk of root resorption, gingival recession, and bone dehiscence, especially on a narrow symphysis with questionable labiolingual width of the alveolar bone.[17] Another contraindication can be undesirable facial esthetics.

TREATMENT

Treatment mechanics for deep bite correction depend on a number of etiologic variables and the associated treatment plan. Nevertheless, as already mentioned, there are three ways to treat deep bite malocclusions: intrusion of the upper and lower incisors, extrusion of the upper and lower posterior teeth, or a combination of the two.

Intrusion of the Upper and Lower Incisors

Incisor intrusion is generally indicated in a patient with a vertical maxillary excess, a large interlabial gap, a long lower facial height, or a steep mandibular plane. Some of the appliances that can achieve "true incisor intrusion"[18] are discussed below.

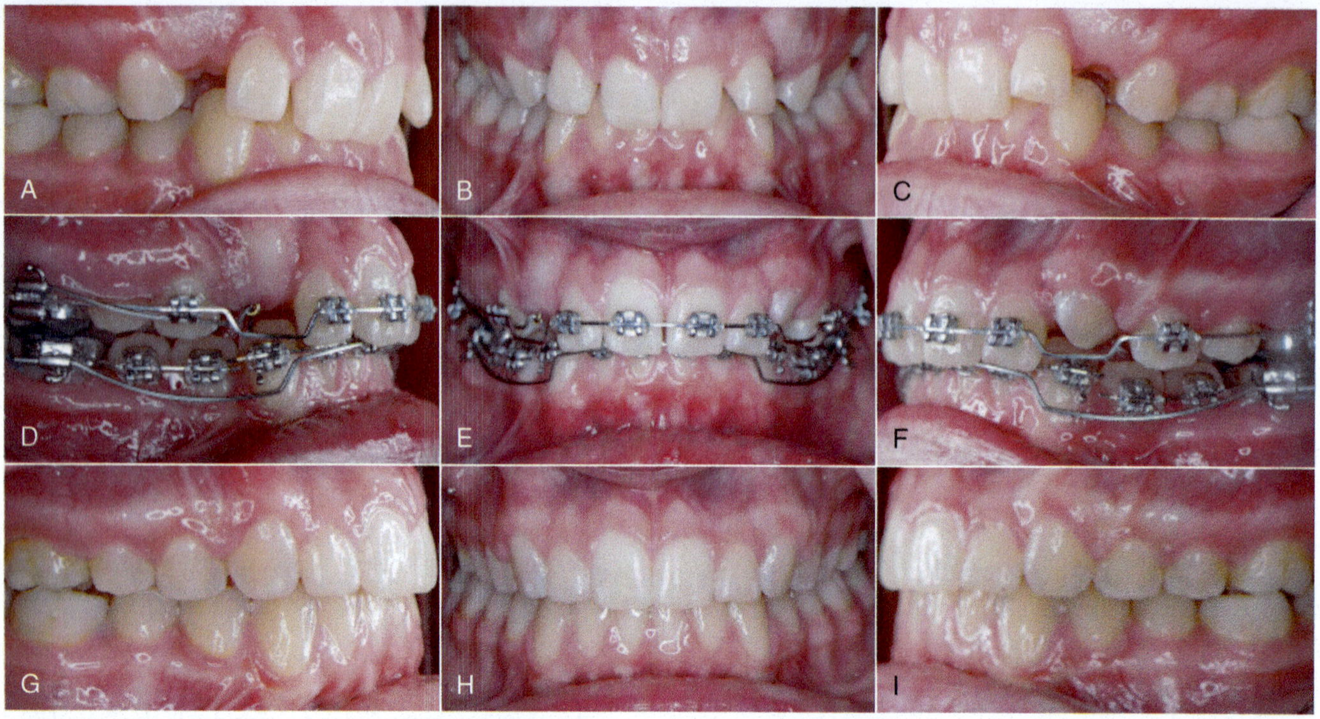

Figure 8-5 **A–C,** This adolescent female patient had the chief complaint of excessive overbite. On careful analysis it was observed that her upper incisor exposure was adequate both at rest and during smiling. **D–F,** The decision was made to intrude the lower incisors only so the deep bite malocclusion could be resolved without significantly affecting the patient's smile esthetics. Segmental intrusion of the lower incisors was carried out with an overlay intrusion arch. **G–I,** Treatment results.

Intrusion Arch

An intrusion arch can be made from 0.016-inch × 0.022-inch or 0.017-inch × 0.025-inch CNA (Connecticut Nickel Titanium Archwires). Alternatively, preformed intrusion archwires—the Connecticut Intrusion Arch (CTA)[19] (Ultimate Wireforms, Bristol, CT.) fabricated from a nickel-titanium (Ni-Ti) alloy that provides the advantages of shape memory, springback, and light continuous force distribution—can also be used (Fig. 8-7, A). The appliance setup includes two passive posterior (stabilizing) units and one active anterior unit (the intrusion arch). The passive units consist of stiff or rigid segmented wires (0.017-inch × 0.025-inch stainless steel or higher dimension wires) in the molars and premolars bilaterally. Inclusion of as many teeth as possible in the posterior segment minimizes side effects. The anterior segment, which includes either two or four incisors, is constructed with similar wires. Remember that the higher the dimension of the stainless steel wires, the more predictable the tooth movement is.

The intrusion arch is activated by placing a 30-degree gingival bend 2- to 3-mm mesial to the molar tubes so that the wire lies passively in the vestibular sulcus. Activation is accomplished by bringing it occlusal and tying it to the anterior segment as a point contact, as opposed to placing it directly into the bracket slots as is done with the utility arch.[20,21] The intrusion arch uses a one-couple force system, which makes the appliance statically determinant (i.e., the various forces and moments in this setup can be quantified to an appreciable degree of accuracy). The intrusion arch can also be tied back or cinched to prevent flaring of the incisors if the intrusive force is being applied anterior to the center of resistance (C_{RES}) of the incisors. The reciprocal action of the intrusion arch on the molars or the buccal segments is the extrusion and/or distal tip back of the crowns and the mesial movement of the roots (Fig. 8-7, B). This can be very helpful in a Class II, Division 1 patient who requires correction of the molar relation to a Class I. In such patients a buccal segment is often not needed, as it may prevent distal tip back of molars. However, in Class I malocclusions with deep bite, a tip back may cause steepening of the occlusal plane. Increasing the number of teeth in the anchor unit is one way to minimize such side effects. Another method is to use relatively low forces to the order of 40 g for the upper four incisors and 30 g for the lower incisors. As a general guideline, 10 to 15 g of force per incisor is acceptable to prevent posterior side effects.[22] Recent evidence has shown that the intrusive forces can be made so light that reactive forces on the anchor teeth remain well below the force levels needed for extrusion and tipping.[22] Therefore the use of a headgear to prevent side effects is completely avoidable. Additionally, low forces help to minimize root resorption. On average, after the initial activation period of 3 to 4 weeks the base arch should intrude 0.4- to 0.6-mm per month.[23]

Another useful clinical application of intrusion arch, besides its other uses,[19] is in preventing the side effects associated with canine retraction. A popular method of canine retraction is "frictional mechanics" employing a continuous arch system. The obvious advantages of this system (compared to frictionless mechanics) are reduced possibility of unpredicted canine movement (e.g., rotation, flaring, and extrusion of the canine) and minimal wire bending. However, when an archwire with a low load-deflection rate is used it tends to deform, leading to undesirable side effects on the anterior teeth in the form of extrusion of the incisors or deepening of the bite.[24] This type of deep bite can also be termed "iatrogenic deep bite," which in the present context means deep bite induced inadvertently by the clinician (Fig. 8-8). With larger or rigid archwires the system might develop excessive friction leading to delayed tooth movement, anchorage loss, or maybe even cessation of canine retraction. Therefore the use of a 0.016-inch × 0.022-inch CTA as an overlay archwire to optimize the biomechanical system for canine retraction, as shown in Figure 8-9, is recommended.

The counterclockwise moment (if tied anterior to the C_{RES} of the anterior teeth) and the intrusive force on the incisors ensure the stability of the incisors by counteracting the iatrogenic forces generated by canine retraction. Additionally, molar anchorage is reinforced due to a tip-back moment on the posterior segment.

Utility Arch

The utility arch (Fig. 8-10) is similar in design to the CTA. It is stepped down at the molars, passes through the buccal vestibule, and is stepped up at the incisors to avoid distortion from occlusal forces. The difference is that for intrusion the utility arch is tied into the incisor brackets, which create a two-couple force system the moment of which tends to tip the incisor crowns facially and the molar distally. Although

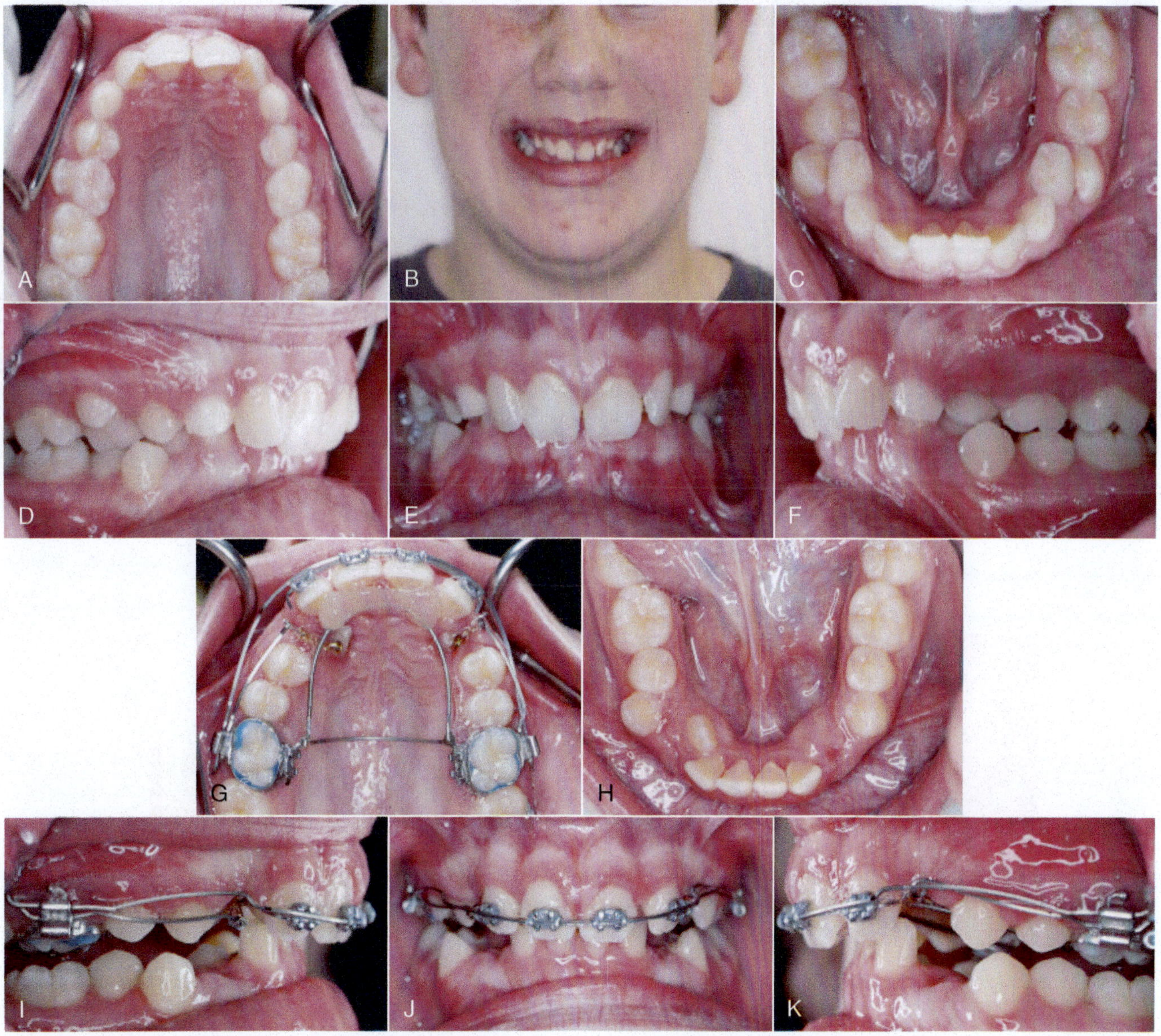

Figure 8-6 **A–F,** Pretreatment photographs. **G–P,** Extremely light forces delivered through a Connecticut Intrusion Arch (CTA) were used to selectively intrude only the upper central incisors. **Q–V,** Treatment results show a significant improvement in the gingival exposure and the smile as well as the correction of the deep overbite.

Continued

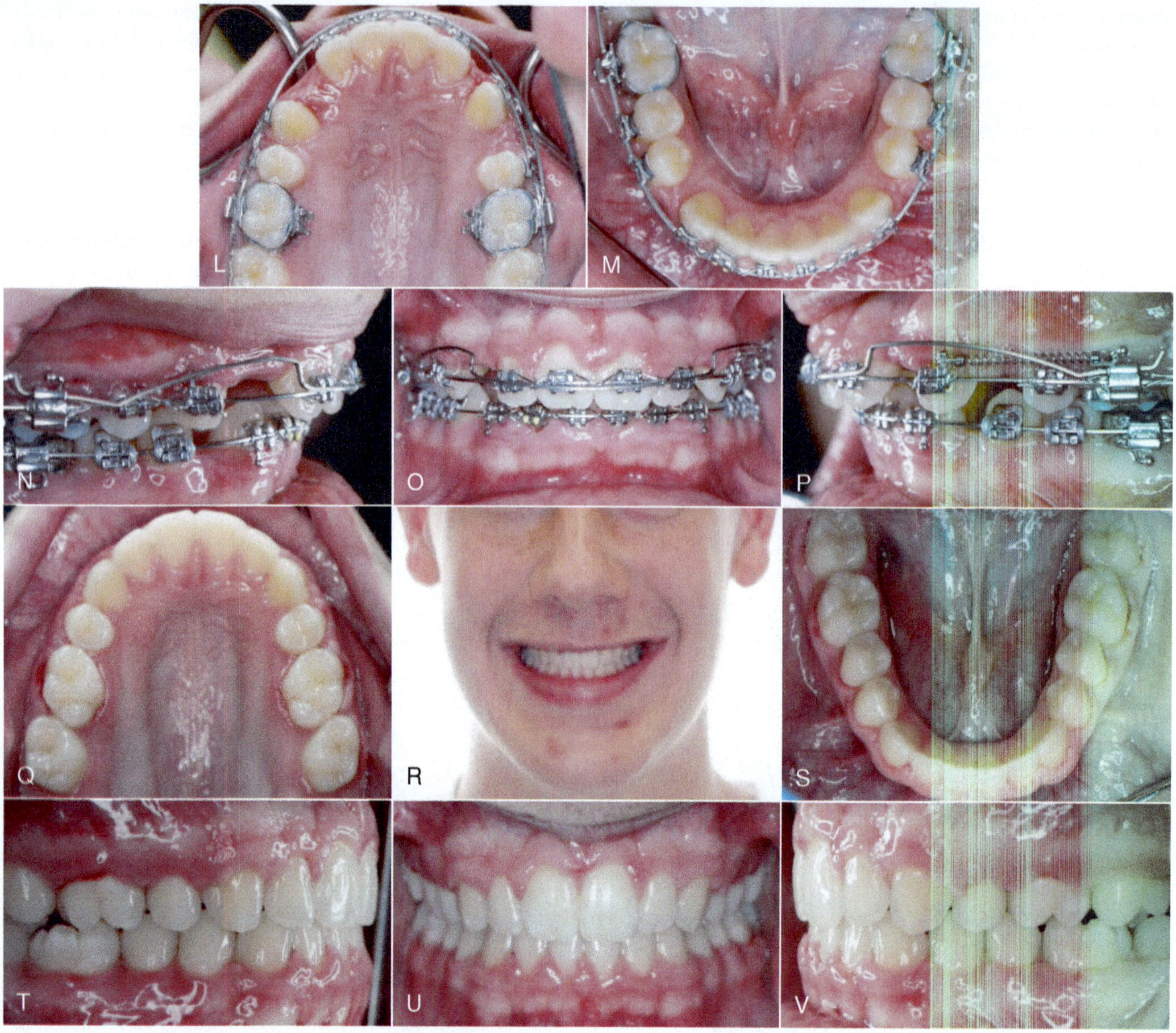

Figure 8-6, cont'd

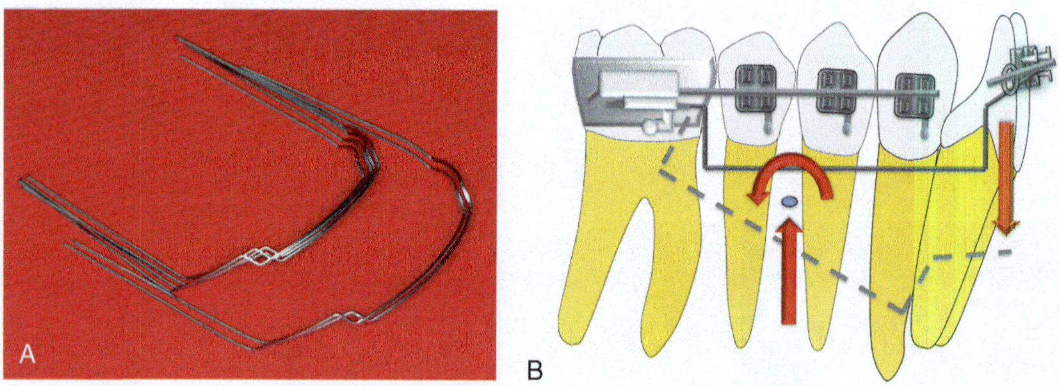

Figure 8-7 **A,** Preformed upper and lower Connecticut Intrusion Archwire (CTA) made from nickel-titanium (Ni-Ti) alloy. **B,** The biomechanical design of lower incisor intrusion with the CTA.

the facial tipping of incisors can be avoided by cinching or tying back the intrusion utility arch, any force that tends to bring the anchor teeth mesially is undesirable. Incorporating a "twist" or "torque bend" in the incisor segment is another way of controlling the tendency of the teeth to tip facially; however, this will increase the intrusive force on the incisor segment and the extrusive force on the molar. It is well known that heavier forces do not increase the amount or rate of intrusion.[25,26] Another problem is that, unlike the CTA, this being a two-couple system means that it is impossible to accurately determine the magnitude of the reactive forces (statically indeterminate), which makes it rather impossible to adjust the archwire to prevent side effects. Therefore in our clinical practice we prefer to use the CTA. Also, considerable chair time is saved as the CTA involves no wire bending and needs minimal adjustment.

Three-Piece Intrusion Arch

Labial tipping of incisors gives the clinical impression of deep bite correction because it influences the vertical incisal edge position. Similarly, during extensive retraction of incisors development of a deep bite (iatrogenic) is common due to uprighting of the incisors (Fig. 8-11). It is therefore important to control the labio-lingual inclination of the anterior teeth as they are intruded and retracted, especially if they are flared to begin with.

A three-piece intrusion arch[27] uses segmental mechanics to simultaneously intrude and retract incisor teeth in a

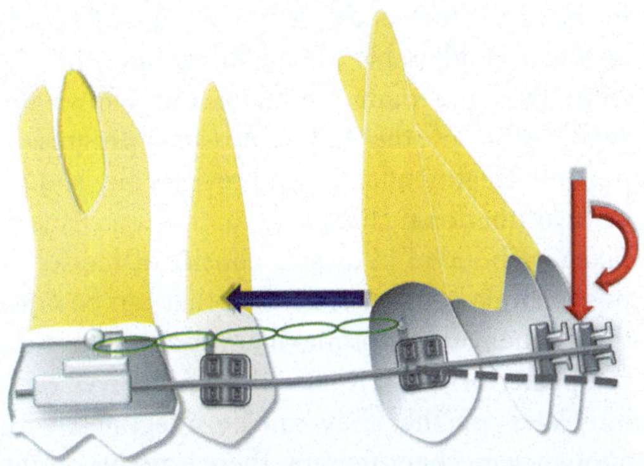

Figure 8-8 Development of deep bite (iatrogenic) during canine retraction (sliding mechanics) due to occlusal deflection of the archwire.

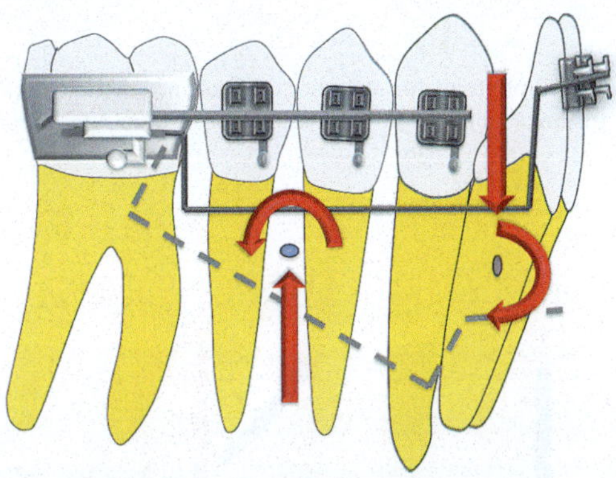

Figure 8-10 Biomechanical design of lower incisor intrusion with the Ricketts utility arch.

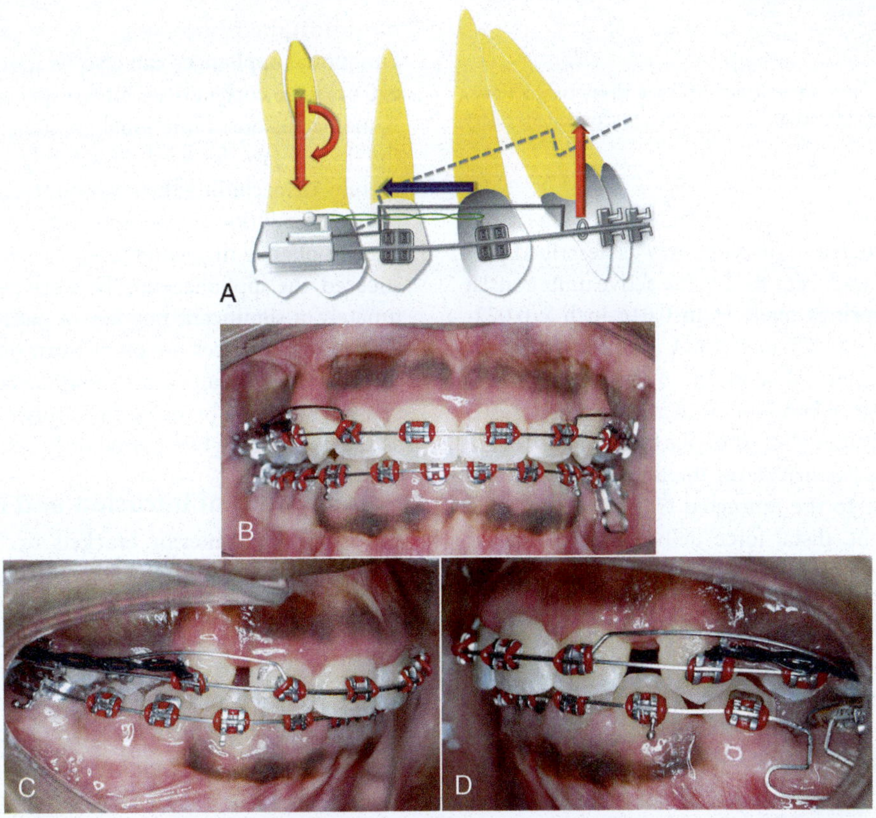

Figure 8-9 A, Application of Connecticut Intrusion Archwire (CTA) to prevent deepening of the bite and simultaneously to augment anchorage during canine retraction. B–D, Clinical views demonstrating the application described in A.

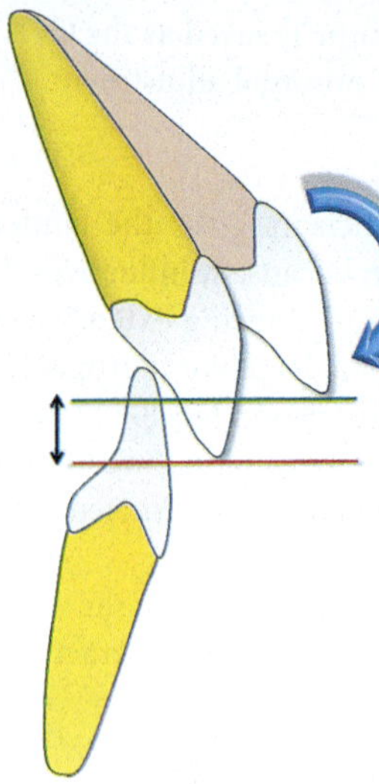

Figure 8-11 Uprighting (or retraction) of proclined incisors during orthodontic treatment might lead to development of deep bite (iatrogenic in nature).

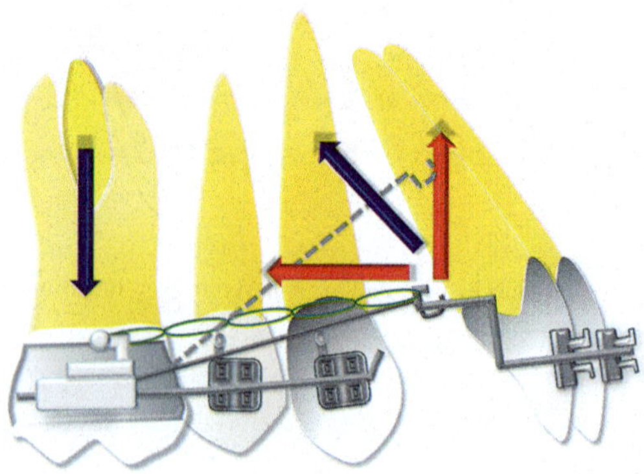

Figure 8-12 A sketch of the biomechanics involved when using a three-piece intrusion arch for simultaneous intrusion and retraction of maxillary incisors.

highly predictive manner. The passive units, with some modifications, are constructed in the same way as described previously for intrusion arch (Fig. 8-12). The active units consist of two segmented springs made from 0.016-inch × 0.022-inch or 0.017-inch × 0.025-inch CNA wires activated by placing a 30-degree gingival bend 2 to 3 mm mesial to the molar tubes. The gingival bend can be increased or decreased based on the desired amount of intrusive force. The wires are hooked to the distal extensions on the anterior segmented wire at a point close to the estimated C_{RES} of the incisors. Application of a light, distal force delivered by a Class I elastic or a power chain to the anterior segment helps to alter the direction of the intrusive force on the anterior segment, so that the forces are directed in an upward and backward direction through the C_{RES} of the anterior teeth or as required in a particular case (Fig. 8-13).

Extrusion of Upper and Lower Posterior Teeth

Biteplates

Currently, biteplates are the most popular appliances to correct deep bites by molar extrusion (Fig. 8-14). These appliances load the incisors for an intrusive effect but leave the posterior teeth free to erupt, thereby leveling the curve of Spee primarily by posterior extrusion, as the intrusive effect on the incisors at best is minimal. Sleichter[28] studied the vertical changes of molars and incisors with biteplate treatment. He found that alveolar height in the molar region increased while there was minimal change in the incisal area.

Two types of biteplates can be used: removable or fixed.

- Removable biteplates consist of an acrylic platform anchored to the maxillary dentition with arrowhead, Adams, or crib clasps. Anteriorly there is a labial bow, which helps to stabilize the biteplate and contact the teeth at the incisal one-third. By acting as a premature incisal stop, usually within the confines of the interocclusal space (freeway space), the block forces the posterior teeth from occlusal contact and allows them to erupt. It is advisable not to disocclude the posterior teeth by more than 2-mm, as this allows for close supervision of the follow-up and progress of the patient's treatment and also prevents any sudden TMJ or myofunctional change.
- Fixed or bonded biteplates consist of blocks of composite or glass ionomer cement that can be bonded on the lingual surface of maxillary incisors to disocclude the posterior teeth. Their advantages over removable biteplates are that they can be integrated with fixed appliance mechanotherapy, there is no need for patient cooperation, and the appliance itself is considerably less bulky.

Functional Appliances

Functional appliances can also be used to achieve posterior extrusion to correct deep bites, especially in low angle Class II malocclusions. Functional appliances help in positioning the lower jaw forward to an edge-to-edge relationship, thereby disoccluding the posterior teeth, which are then free to erupt. Eruption can be augmented by using elastics during fixed appliance mechanotherapy. However, for treatment to succeed, the appliance must be worn nearly full-time. Unfortunately, a significant number of patients do not cooperate fully and appliances are often worn only part-time and lost or broken while out of the mouth. Many of these problems can be overcome by using fixed functional appliances, such as the Twin Force bite corrector (Fig. 8-15).

Combination of Intrusion and Extrusion

By positioning anterior brackets occlusally and posterior brackets gingivally or by using reverse curve archwires, simultaneous intrusion of anterior teeth and extrusion of posterior teeth can be attained (Fig. 8-16). However, there is no definite control over such mechanics. Changes in the axial inclination of the buccal teeth and flaring of incisors due to an intrusive force anterior to the C_{RES} are some of the drawbacks that need to be addressed. Also, since extrusion is more easily accomplished than intrusion a reverse curve of Spee wire will extrude posterior teeth while obtaining minimal, if any, anterior intrusion.[29]

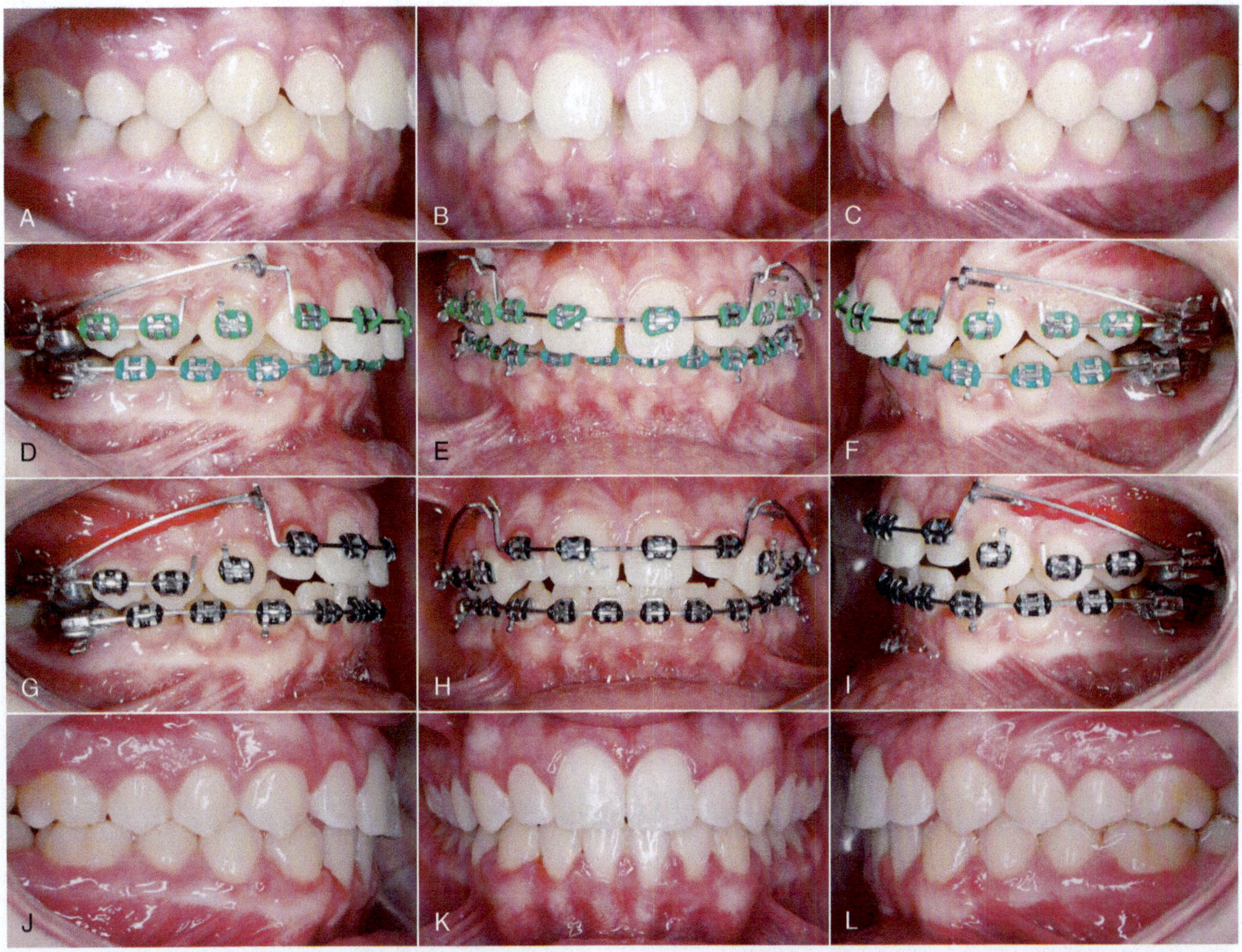

Figure 8-13 Adult patient showing a severe deep bite due to supraeruption of the incisors. **A–C,** Pre-treatment intraoral views. **D–I,** Three-piece intrusion arches were placed in both the upper and the lower arches for deep bite correction. **J–L,** Optimum overbite and overjet were established at the end of treatment.

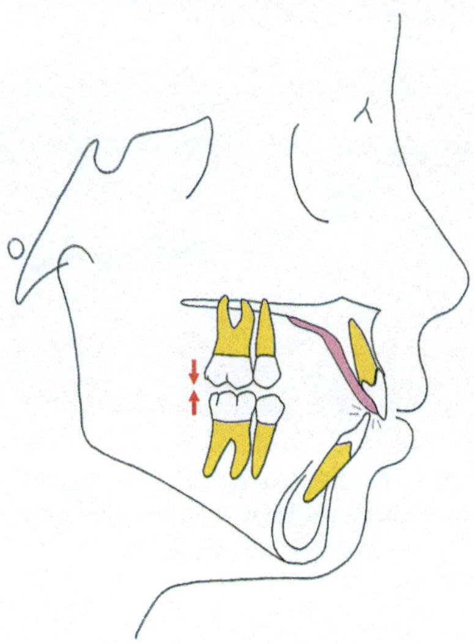

Figure 8-14 Mechanism of action of an anterior biteplate.

IMPLANTS FOR DEEP BITE CORRECTION

Anchorage control, especially in the vertical dimension, is of paramount importance if bite opening must be achieved by genuine intrusion of the anterior teeth. Additionally, if intrusion of all six anterior teeth (including the canines) is desired (instead of only four incisors), as in a "cover bite" malocclusion, extraoral appliances become a prerequisite in order to withstand the additional burden of anchorage. According to Burstone,[15] it is not possible to intrude all six anterior teeth at one time without producing undesirable axial inclination change in the posterior segment. An additional 20 to 30 g of force would be required on each side to intrude the canine, taking into account the root size and the dense surrounding bone. Although efficient, extraoral appliances require extensive patient cooperation. Recently it has also been shown that the chances of root resorption are greater with these appliances, possibly due to the "jiggling effect."[30] Esthetics and social issues are also of concern. In the past decade, skeletal anchorage systems such as mini-plates, palatal implants, mini-implants, and screws have revolutionized orthodontic

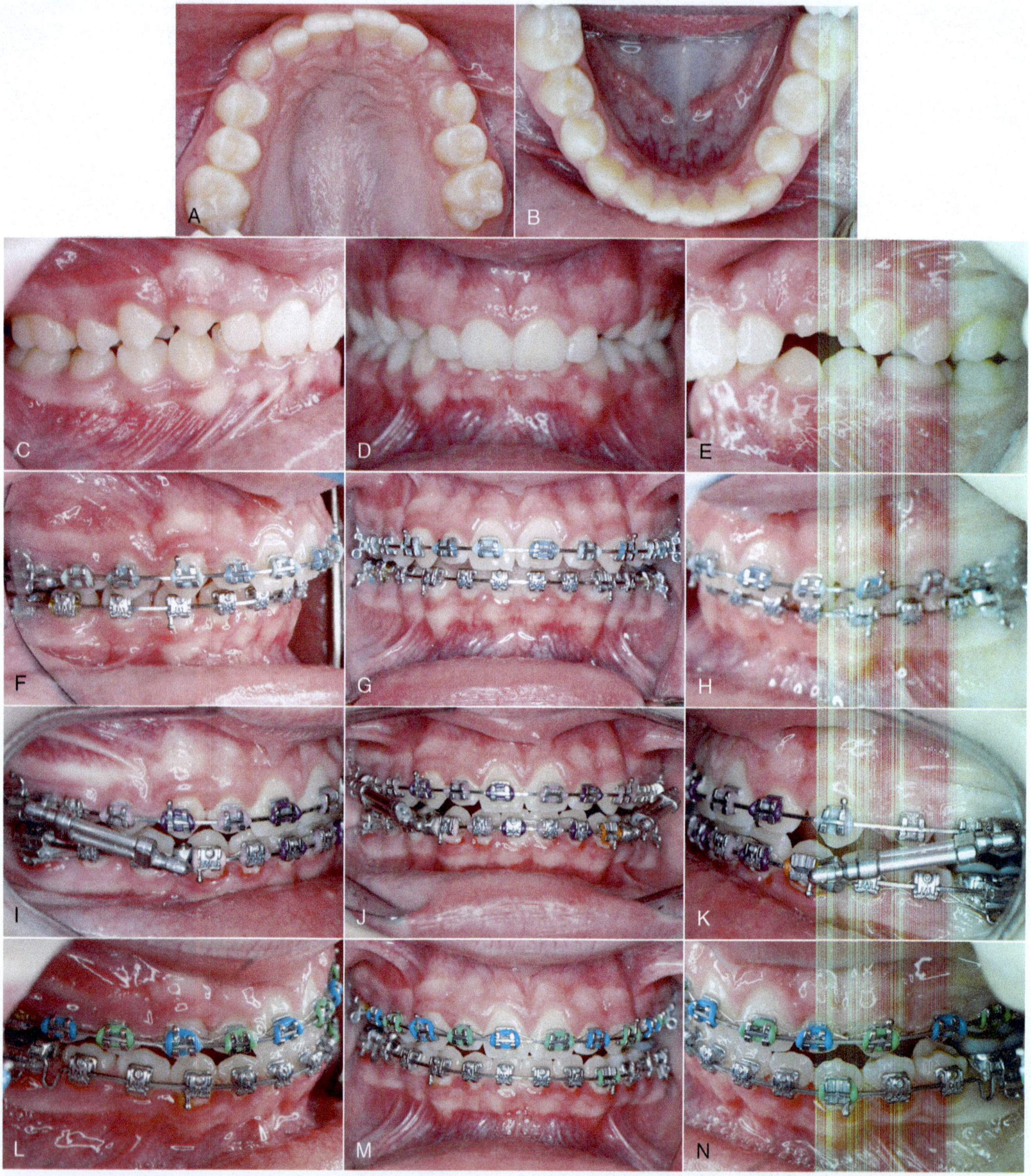

Figure 8-15 **A–E,** Pre-treatment clinical views of a Class II, Division 1 patient with severe deep bite. **F–N,** Patient was treated with a Twin Force bite corrector (fixed functional appliance). Note how the anterior positioning of the mandibular teeth in an edge-to-edge relationship with the maxillary incisors disoccludes the posterior teeth, which are then free to erupt. Alternatively, elastics can be used to augment their eruption.

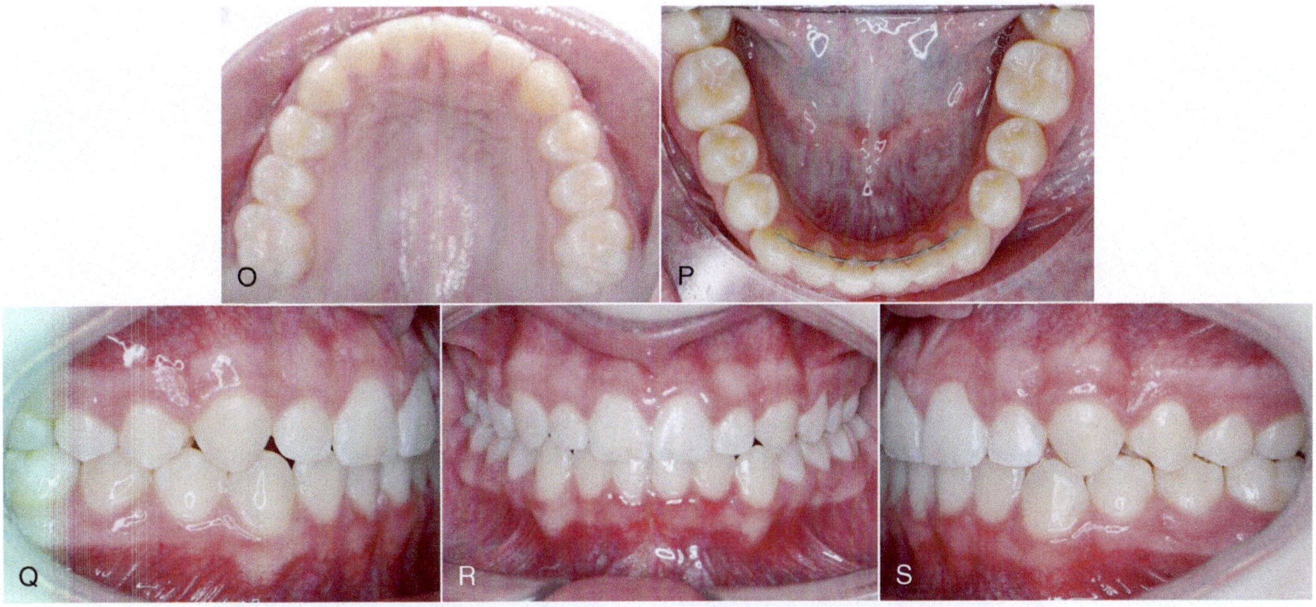

Figure 8-15, cont'd **O–S,** Results of treatment.

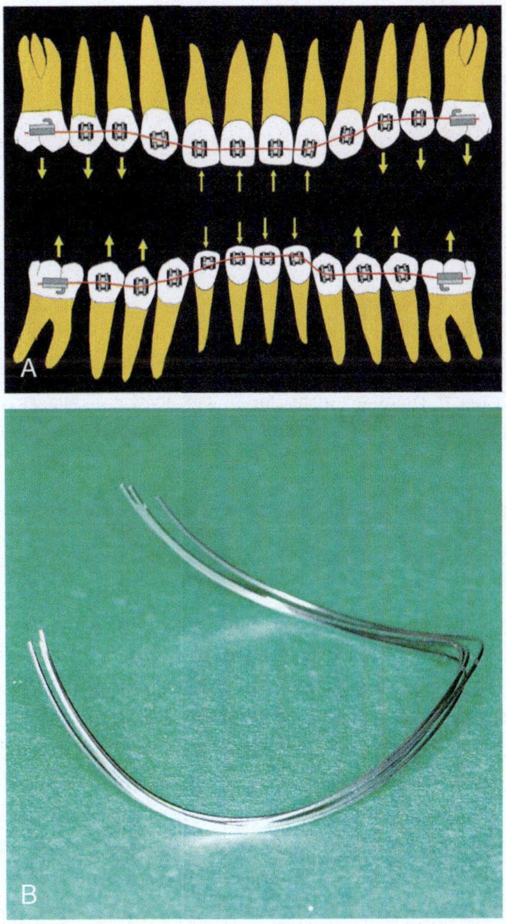

Figure 8-16 **A,** Simultaneous intrusion of anterior teeth and extrusion of posterior teeth can be accomplished by occlusal positioning of the anterior brackets relative to the posterior. **B,** Using reverse curve archwires will produce a similar effect.

anchorage and biomechanics by making anchorage more stable.[31–35] Mini-implants can be used effectively for en masse intrusion of anterior teeth[36] (Fig. 8-17).

Availability of sufficient interdental bone, less soft tissue irritation, and a larger anterior segment (if all six anterior teeth are included) that requires greater control are some of the factors that must be considered when placing mini-implants for intrusion of anterior teeth. We have found the interdental bone between the roots of the canine and lateral incisors, bilaterally, as an appropriate location for placement of mini-implants. The selection of the point of application of the intrusive force with respect to the C_{RES} of the anterior segment is also an important consideration in the placement of the implants, so that the nature of the tooth movement that will occur can be predicted more accurately. The C_{RES} of the six anterior teeth has been estimated to be halfway between the C_{RES} of the four incisors and canines.[36] True intrusion without axial inclination change can be obtained only by directing the intrusive force through the C_{RES} of the anterior teeth. In the patient described in Figure 8-17, a light distal force (r) was delivered by an elastic chain to the anterior segment to alter the direction of the intrusive force (i) so that true intrusion of the anterior teeth could be achieved along their long axes (Fig. 8-18). The distal force used was of very low magnitude, primarily to redirect the line action of the intrusive force.

RETENTION AND STABILITY

As discussed, correction of deep bite malocclusion can be attained by a variety of methods with fairly predictable results. However, the real challenge is maintaining the overbite over an appreciable period. The results of most studies concerning the stability of overbite correction suggest a decrease in the overbite during treatment followed by an

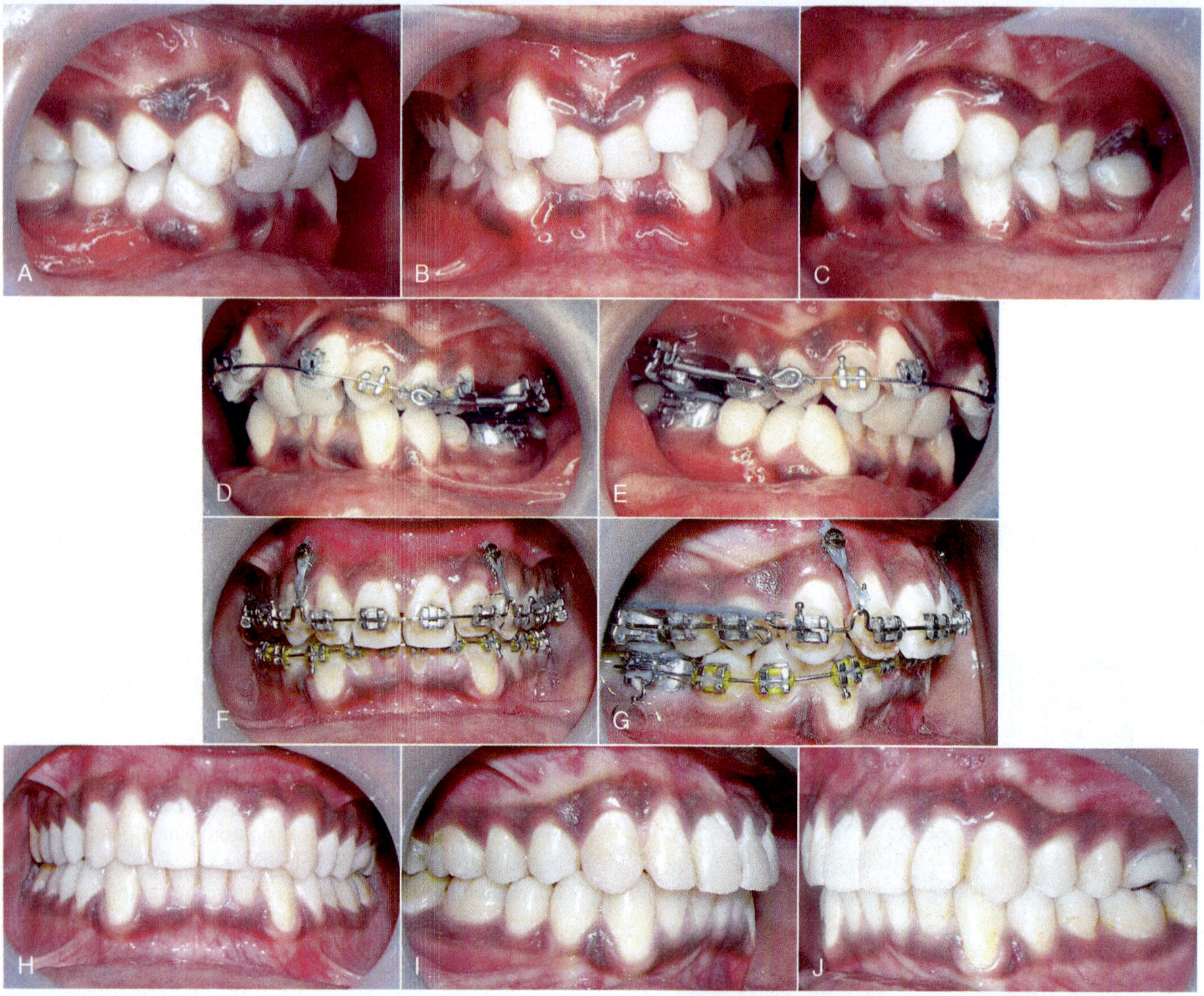

Figure 8-17 **A–C,** Sixteen-year-old postpubertal male patient presenting with a severe Class II, Division 2 malocclusion with 100% deep bite. **D and E,** In the first phase of treatment a Jones jig molar distalization appliance was used to distalize the maxillary molars by more than 6 mm, to achieve a Class I molar relation. **F and G,** In the second phase of treatment mini-implants were inserted between the roots of the maxillary lateral incisor and canine to intrude all maxillary anterior teeth en masse in a single step. More than 4-mm of intrusion was achieved without any posterior teeth extrusion. The implants remained stable throughout treatment. In the mandibular arch the incisors were proclined to alleviate the severe crowding. **H–J,** Good overjet and overbite were achieved after completion of active orthodontic treatment.

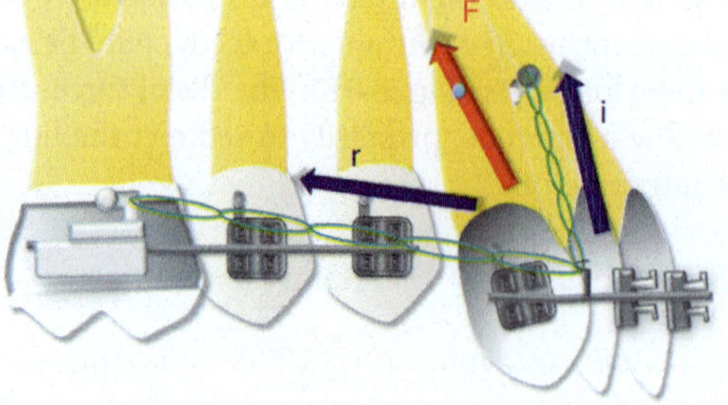

Figure 8-18 Biomechanical design for the en masse intrusion of the maxillary anterior teeth, where *i* is intrusive force, *r* is distal force, *F* is resultant force, and C_{RES} is center of resistance of the anterior teeth.

increase in the overbite after appliance removal, although at the clinical level this increase might not be significant.[37] The following are some factors that must be kept in mind when planning retention for deep overbite correction:

1. Age: Deep bite correction is usually achieved by the simultaneous intrusion of incisors and extrusion of the posterior teeth. Growing patients benefit the most with this approach because active vertical growth during deep bite correction ensures greater stability. Because growth tends to increase the vertical distance between the jaw bases, performing treatment during this period is most advantageous.
2. Facial type: Certain facial types have a greater potential for permanent correction than others. Hyperdivergent facial types usually exhibit a more favorable reaction to overbite correction when compared to

hypodivergent facial types. This can be attributed to the growth rate in the vertical direction, which is highest and lasts the longest in high angle patients.

3. Molar extrusion and incisor intrusion: The stability of molar extrusion in growing patients has been examined in previous studies, which suggest that this is a fairly stable procedure if the interocclusal space is not violated. Any eruptive movement beyond the interocclusal space might not be stable due to strong posterior occlusion or muscle stretching, especially in low angle individuals. For the same reason, in adults incisor intrusion is regarded as more stable. Other factors that can lead to relapse of incisor intrusion include continued lower incisor eruption, canting of the occlusal plane, incomplete leveling of the curve of Spee, and forward rotation of the mandible.
4. Inter-incisal angle: Riedel[38] has suggested that a large inter-incisal angle at the end of treatment is associated with relapse of deep overbite. This might be because a large inter-incisal angle tends to force the crowns of the mandibular incisors lingually and the apex of the maxillary incisors labially.[12] A study by Burzin and Nanda[37] showed that the axial inclination of the incisors did not change significantly during a 2-year post-treatment observation period. They suggested that ideal axial inclination of the incisors at the end of treatment could be a factor in overbite stability. Therefore maintaining optimum inter-incisal angle, incisal stops, and guidance between the maxillary and mandibular incisors is essential for maintaining overbite correction. The inter-incisal angle can be higher for dolichofacial patterns and less for brachyfacial patterns; however, in general an angle of 125 to 135 degrees ensures good stability for deep bite correction.

SUMMARY

Deep overbite is a common component of malocclusion in adults and children. Although a number of treatment modalities were discussed in this chapter, the importance of accurate diagnosis, which entails the precise estimation of the etiologic factors, cannot be undermined because effective treatment of deep bite and its retention in the long-term critically depend on it. Esthetic considerations such as maxillary incisor to lip relationship and gingival exposure on smiling are also important diagnostic features that must be considered in the treatment plan.

REFERENCES

1. Goldstein MS, Stanton FL. Various types of occlusion and amounts of overbite in normal and abnormal occlusion between two and twelve years. *Int J Orthod Oral Surg*. 1936;22:549–569.
2. Strang RHW. *A Textbook of Orthodontia*. Philadelphia, PA: Lea & Febiger; 1950.
3. Nanda R. The differential diagnosis and treatment of excessive overbite. *Dent Clin North Am*. 1981;25:69–84.
4. Dermaut LR, Pauw GD. Biomechanical aspects of Class II mechanics with special emphasis on deep bite correction as a part of the treatment goal. In: Nanda R, ed. *Biomechanics in Clinical Orthodontics*. Philadelphia, PA; WB Saunders; 1997:86–89.
5. Flemming HB. Investigation of the vertical overbite during the eruption of the permanent dentition. *Angle Orthod*. 1961;31:53–62.
6. Peck S, Peck L, Kataja M. Class II Div 2 malocclusion: a heritable pattern of small teeth in well-developed jaws. *Angle Orthod*. 1998;68:9–17.
7. Mayrhofer B. *Lehrbuch der Zahnkrankheiten*. Jena, Germany: Gustav Fischer Verlag; 1912:60–62.
8. Moyers RE. *Handbook of Orthodontics*. 4th ed. Chicago, IL: Year Book Medical Publishers; 1998:422–424.
9. Prakash P, Margolis HI. Dento-cranofacial relations in varying degrees of overbite. *Am J Orthod*. 1952;38:657–673.
10. Wylie WL. The relationship between ramus height, dental height and overbite. *Am J Orthod Oral Surg*. 1946;32:57–67.
11. Bell W, Jacobs J, Legan H. Treatment of Class II deep bite by orthodontic and surgical means. *Am J Orthod*. 1984;85:1–19.
12. Simons M, Joondeph D. Change in overbite: a ten-year post-retention study. *Am J Orthod*. 1973;64:349–367.
13. Proffit WR, White RP, Sarver DM. Long face problems. In: Proffit WR, White RP Jr, Sarver DM, eds. *Contemporary Treatment of Dentofacial Deformity*. St. Louis, MO: Mosby; 2003:464–506.
14. Schudy FF. The control of vertical overbite in clinical orthodontics. *Angle Orthod*. 1968;38:19–38.
15. Burstone CR. Deep overbite correction by intrusion. *Am J Orthod*. 1977;72:1–22.
16. Maulik C, Nanda R. Dynamic smile analysis in young adults. *Am J Orthod Dentofacial Orthop*. 2007;132:307–315.
17. Wehrbein H, Bauer W, Diedrich P. Mandibular incisors, alveolar bone, and symphysis after orthodontic treatment: a retrospective study. *Am J Orthod Dentofacial Orthop*. 1996;110:239–246.
18. Ng J, Major PW, Heo G, Flore-Mir C. True incisor intrusion attained during orthodontic treatment: a systematic review and meta-analysis. *Am J Orthod Dentofacial Orthop*. 2005;128:212–219.
19. Nanda R, Marzban R, Kulhberg A. The Connecticut intrusion arch. *J Clin Orthod*. 1998;32:708–715.
20. Ricketts RM. Bioprogressive therapy as an answer to orthodontic needs: part I. *Am J Orthod*. 1976;70:241–268.
21. Ricketts RM. Bioprogressive therapy as an answer to orthodontic needs: part II. *Am J Orthod*. 1976;70:359–397.
22. Steevenbergen EV, Burstone CJ, Prahl-Andersen B, Aartman IHA. The influence of force magnitude on intrusion of the maxillary segment. *Angle Orthod*. 2005;75:723–729.
23. Faber ZT. *The Relationship of Tooth Movement to Measured Force Systems: A Prospective Analysis of the Treatment Effects of Orthodontic Intrusion Arches* [master's thesis]. Storrs, CT: Division of Orthodontics, University of Connecticut; 1994.
24. Nanda RS, Ghosh J. Biomechanical considerations ion sliding mechanics. In: Nanda R, ed. *Biomechanics in Clinical Orthodontics*. Philadelphia, PA: WB Saunders; 1997:188–217.
25. Dellinger EL. A histologic and cephalometric investigation of premolar intrusion in the *Macaca speciosa* monkey. *Am J Orthod*. 1967;53:325–355.
26. Reitan K. Initial tissue behavior during apical root resorption. *Angle Orthod*. 1974;44:68–82.
27. Shroff B, Nanda R. Biomechanics of class II correction. In: Nanda R, ed. *Biomechanics in Clinical Orthodontics*. Philadelphia, PA: WB Saunders; 1997:143–155.
28. Sleichter CG. Effects of maxillary bite plane therapy in orthodontics. *Am J Orthod*. 1954;40:850–870.
29. Woods MG. The mechanics of lower incisor intrusion: experiments in non-growing baboons. *Am J Orthod*. 1988;93:186–195.
30. Deguchi T, Murakami T, Kuroda S, Yabuuchi T, Kamioka H, Yamamoto TT. Comparison of the intrusion effects on the maxillary incisors between implant anchorage and J-hook headgear. *Am J Orthod Dentofacial Orthop*. 2008;133:654–660.

31. Nanda R, Uribe FA. *Temporary Anchorage Devices in Orthodontics.* St. Louis, MO: Mosby Elsevier; 2009.
32. Upadhyay M, Yadav S, Nagaraj K, Patil S. Treatment effects of mini-implants for en-masse retraction of anterior teeth in bialveolar dental protrusion patients: a randomized controlled trial. *Am J Orthod Dentofacial Orthop.* 2008;134:18–29.e1.
33. Nagaraj K, Upadhyay M, Yadav S. Mini-implant anchorage for a skeletal class II malocclusion with missing mandibular incisors: a case report. *World J Orthod.* 2008;9(2):155–166.
34. Upadhyay M, Yadav S. Mini-implants for retraction, intrusion and protraction in a Class II division 1 patient. *J Orthod.* 2007;34(3):158–167.
35. Upadhyay M, Nagaraj K, Yadav S, Saxena R. Mini-implants for en masse intrusion of maxillary anterior teeth in a severe Class II division 2 malocclusion. *J Orthod.* 2008;35:79–89.
36. Melsen B, Fotish V, Burstone CJ. Vertical force considerations in differential space closure. *J Clin Orthod.* 1990;24:678–683.
37. Burzin J, Nanda R. The stability of deep overbite correction. In: Nanda R, Burstone CJ, eds. *Retention and Stability in Orthodontics.* Philadelphia, PA: WB Saunders; 1993:61–79.
38. Riedel RA. A review of the retention problem. *Angle Orthod.* 1960; 30:179–194.

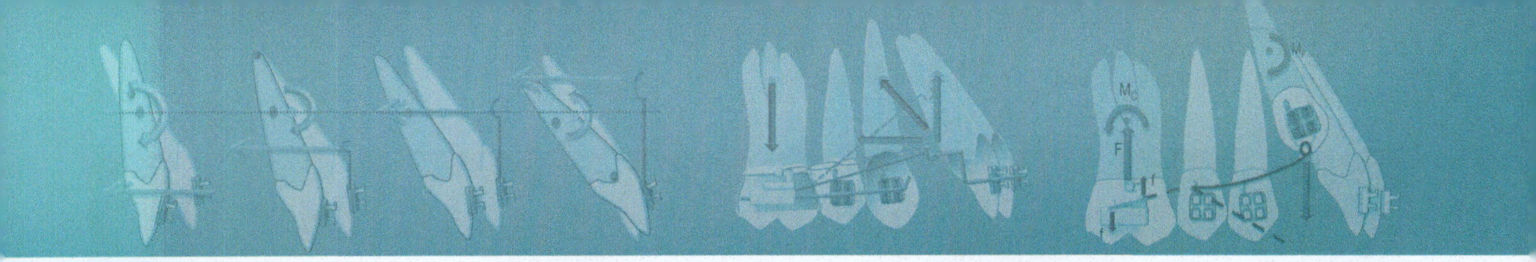

CHAPTER 9

Management of Open-Bite Malocclusion

Flavio Andres Uribe, Nandakumar Janakiraman, and Ravindra Nanda

Achieving an ideal treatment outcome depends on an accurate diagnosis in three dimensions, a good understanding of the interaction between the neuromuscular components of the orofacial region and the craniofacial skeleton, and the ability to provide individualized treatment mechanics.[1] Early research in the 1950s and 1960s clearly showed the mutual dependence in three dimensions of the dentofacial complex.[2] Despite the interest in three-dimensional (3D) diagnosis and treatment planning in orthodontics, the most widely used classification, introduced by Edward Angle, describes the malocclusion only in the anteroposterior dimension,[2] providing little information about the vertical or transverse facial and dental relationships.

The importance of the vertical dimension of the face was first recognized by Downs and later discussed by Wylie and Johnson.[3] Sassouni and Nanda[2] comprehensively described the skeletal characteristics caused by dimensional and positional imbalances in both vertical and anteroposterior dimensions. Their classification of the facial types included an assessment of vertical disproportions. The terms *skeletal deep bite* and *skeletal open bite* were used to describe the two extremes observed in this dimension.[2,4]

Sassouni[4] further investigated the vertical dimension of the dentofacial complex and found that disproportions in this dimension can be a cause for anteroposterior dysplasia. He further stated that addressing the vertical component of the malocclusion would bring about the desired outcome in the anteroposterior dimension.

During the same period, Schudy introduced the concept of facial divergence as the proportion of facial height to facial depth. He surmised that the ratio of depth to height affects not only the facial type but also the overbite. Hyperdivergent and hypodivergent facial types were described as the two extremes of facial divergence.[5] Later, Nanda showed that these vertical patterns are established early in life, even before the eruption of permanent teeth.[6]

Various terms used to describe increased vertical facial dimension have been used interchangeably, describing angles, growth tendencies, and occlusal traits and even implying etiology. The following terms are used most commonly to describe an increased vertical facial pattern: *dolichofacial, leptoprosopic, hyperdivergent, skeletal open bite, high angle, backward rotator, adenoid faces, long face syndrome*, and *vertical maxillary excess*. Although the relationship is not necessarily direct, an increased vertical facial pattern has been associated with an anterior open-bite malocclusion.

Open bite has been defined as an occlusal characteristic in which upper and lower teeth are not in contact and vertical overlap does not exist. The term was first introduced by Caravelli as early as 1842.[7] Although this type of malocclusion can occur unilaterally or bilaterally in the buccal segments, it most often occurs in the anterior segment. The anterior open-bite malocclusion is most obvious when a clearance is apparent between the upper and lower incisors from the frontal view. Of course, clinical diagnosis of an anterior open bite then becomes somewhat subjective because the diagnosis depends on the horizontal plane of assessment (Fig. 9-1).

This chapter describes the characteristics of anterior open bite, its etiology and differential diagnosis, contemporary and evidence-based treatment approaches in growing and nongrowing patients, treatment alternatives and retention protocols for successful management, and increased predictability of stability in the long-term.

CHARACTERISTICS OF ANTERIOR OPEN BITE

Björk[8] described the skeletal and dental characteristics common in patients with anterior open bite. He discussed the morphological characteristics associated with downward and backward mandibular rotation during growth. These characteristics include distal condylar inclination, short ramus, antegonial notching, obtuse gonial angle, excessive maxillary height, straight mandibular canal, thin and long symphysis, long anterior facial height, short posterior facial height, steep mandibular plane, divergent occlusal planes, acute intermolar and interincisal angulation, anteriorly tipped-up palatal plane, and extruded molars. Among all of these characteristics, the steepness of the mandibular plane

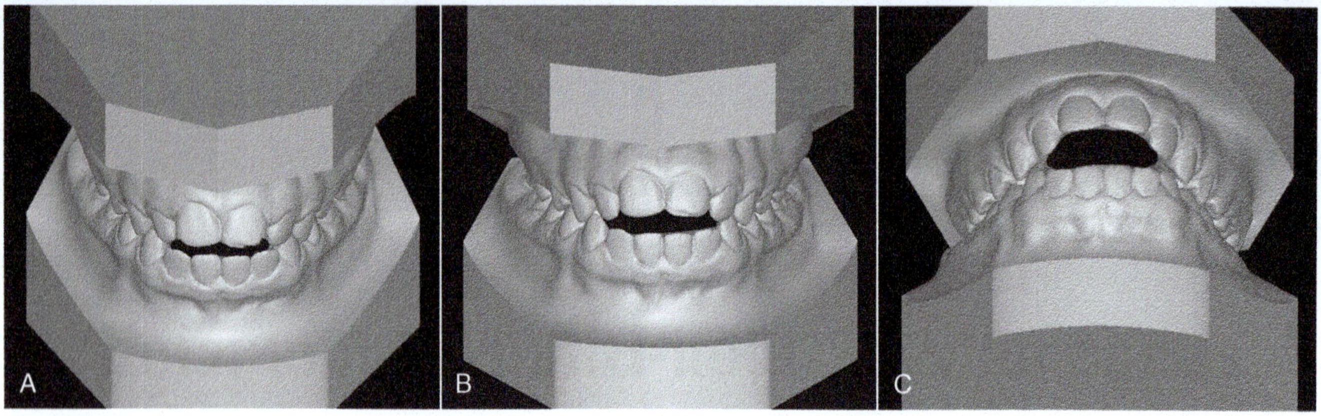

Figure 9-1 Evaluation of an anterior open bite from different planes. **A,** Minimal amount of anterior open bite is evident from the uppermost view angle. **B,** Increased open bite compared to **A.** Plane of assessment is almost perpendicular to the occlusal plane. **C,** The lowermost view angle reflects an extensive open bite, one that does not appear as extensive from the top view. The apparent magnitude of the open bite depends on the steepness of the occlusal plane and/or the plane of evaluation.

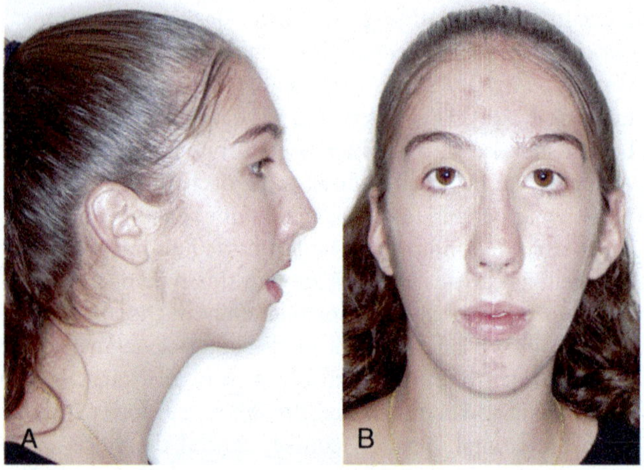

Figure 9-2 A large interlabial gap (>3 mm) is the most significant soft tissue characteristic of a skeletal open bite. **A,** Profile view. **B,** Frontal view with lips closed, showing the mentalis strain resulting from a large interlabial gap.

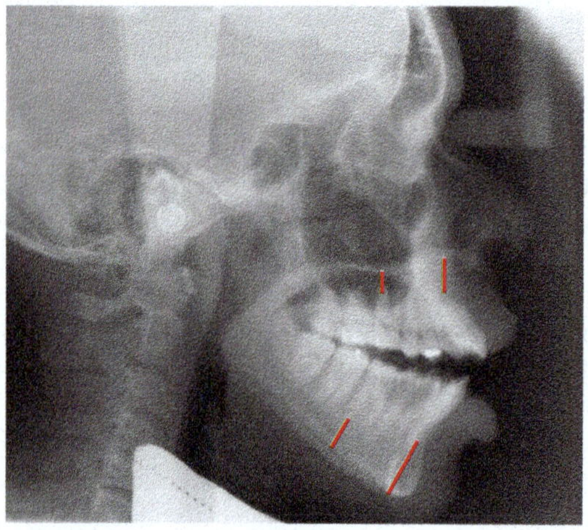

Figure 9-3 Excessive vertical height of the buccal segments is a common characteristic of skeletal anterior open-bite patients.

has been considered the key skeletal finding and thus the term *high-angle patients*.

Most soft tissue characteristics parallel those of the hard tissues: long lower facial height, steep mandibular plane, and short posterior facial height. In addition, a large interlabial gap is most evident on clinical examination of patients with a skeletal open bite[9–11] (Fig. 9-2).

Although all of the skeletal characteristics just mentioned are associated with an anterior open bite, in one study[12] only 13% of patients who had a cephalometric criterion for open-bite tendency had a vertical space between the incisors perpendicular to the occlusal plane. In many instances the skeletal open bite is camouflaged by overeruption of the anterior teeth. This issue makes classification of an open bite as either skeletal or dentoalveolar difficult. Often this malocclusion is the result of a combination of both factors.

Studies[10,11,13] have indicated that skeletal open bites are often related to excessive vertical growth of the dentoalveolar complex, especially in the region of the posterior maxillary molar (Fig. 9-3). Conversely, dental anterior open bites are primarily due to reduced incisor dentoalveolar vertical height[14] (Fig. 9-4). The difference between these two types of open bites is also reflected in the occlusal planes. The skeletal type of malocclusion generally has occlusal contacts only at the molar level, with both occlusal planes diverging anteriorly,[15] whereas the occlusal planes in the dentoalveolar open bite usually diverge from the first premolar forward (Fig. 9-5).

ETIOLOGY

The causes of open-bite malocclusions are often related to the environment. Among the environmental factors, the concept of form following function has been singled out as a primary cause. An example is the role of the muscular posture affecting, directly or indirectly, the development of skeletal and dental open bites.

Airway and Craniofacial Pattern

Airway maintenance is an important factor in determining the posture of various orofacial musculatures. Nasopharyngeal obstruction induced experimentally in primates[16,17]

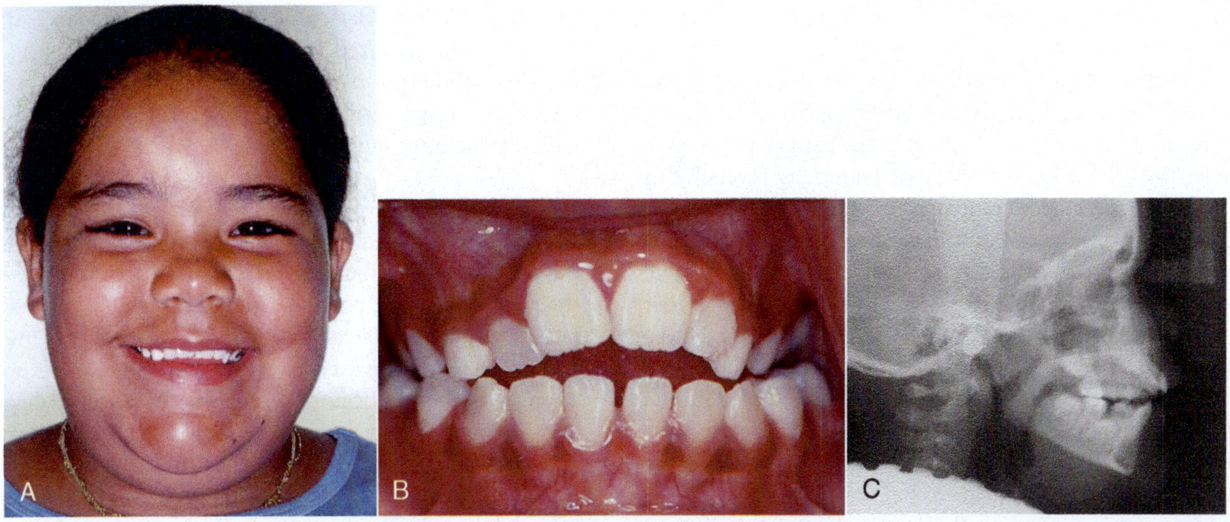

Figure 9-4 Reduced anterior dentoalveolar height characterizes a dental anterior open bite. **A,** Reduced incisal display as a result of restricted eruption of the maxillary incisors from a thumb-sucking habit. **B,** Anterior open bite from the finger habit. **C,** Reduced distance from the apex of the maxillary central incisors to the palatal plane.

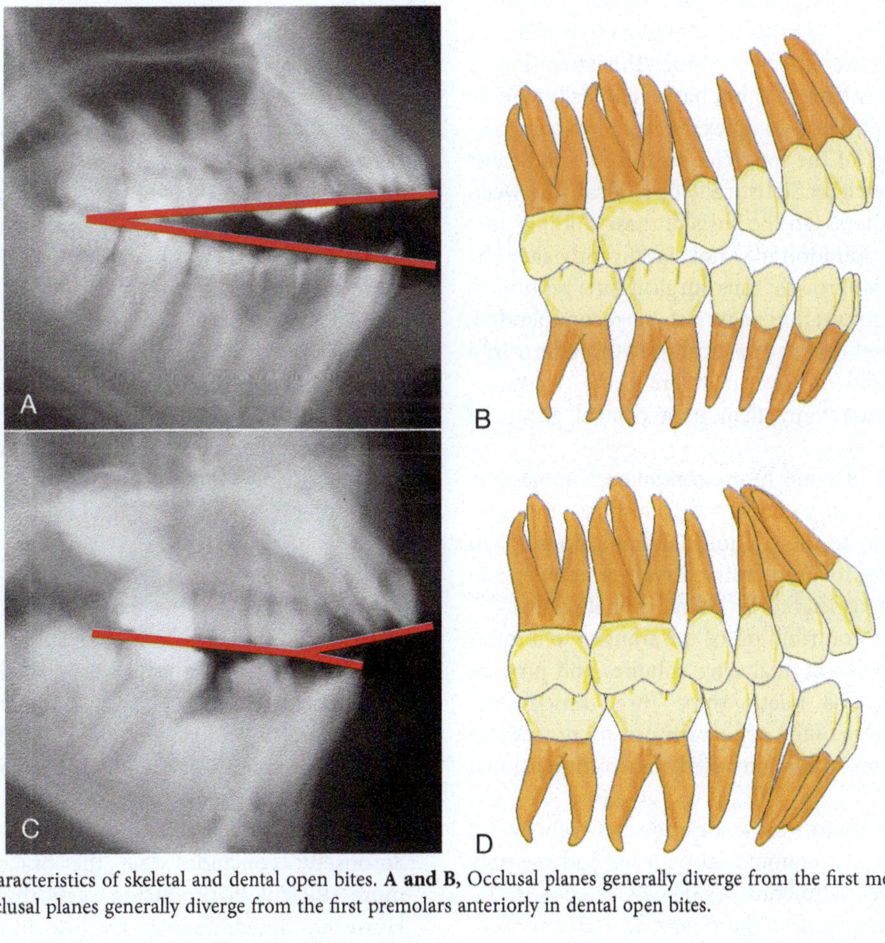

Figure 9-5 Occlusal characteristics of skeletal and dental open bites. **A and B,** Occlusal planes generally diverge from the first molar anteriorly in skeletal open bites. **C and D,** Occlusal planes generally diverge from the first premolars anteriorly in dental open bites.

contributed to a lower position of the tongue and mandible, with the lips separated to maintain airway patency. This positional change led to increased anterior facial height, steeper mandibular plane, and larger gonial angle. Of note, the responses of the primates varied greatly. When extrapolating these findings to humans, clinicians should be aware of the individual variations in response to similar stimuli when assessing the contribution of mouth breathing to craniofacial deformity.[16,17] Additionally, the experimental animal model does not translate well to humans because complete nasal obstruction is uncommon; the usual mode of respiration is oronasal.[18]

The association between mouth breathing and the vertical pattern of facial growth is rather weak. With the evidence available, predicting which children are at risk, at what age the growth pattern will change due to nasal obstruction, how much nasal obstruction must occur to alter the growth pattern, and finally if the acquired pattern is reversible is difficult.[18] Fields et al.[19] compared the mode of breathing in adolescents with normal and hyperdivergent vertical facial patterns. In patients with the hyperdivergent pattern, tidal volume and minimum nasal cross-sectional area were similar to those of patients with normal facial patterns but nasal respiration was significantly reduced. The authors concluded that the mode of breathing could be behaviorally determined rather than being anatomically dependent. Hence the relationship between nasopharyngeal obstruction and long face syndrome in children appears to be multifactorial.

Shanker et al.[20] conducted a longitudinal assessment of the interrelationships between the upper respiratory parameters (nasal resistance, breathing mode) and dentofacial morphology in 8- to 12-year-old children. The results indicated that the pattern of respiration was neither constantly oral nor constantly nasal and that the children often switched from one pattern to the other over time. This alteration in breathing pattern over time may not have a clinically significant effect on the dentofacial complex. Further, in a comparison of the indicators of the long face pattern, no indicator differed significantly either statistically or clinically between nasal and oral breathers. On the basis of these findings, the transient mode of respiration may not significantly alter the pattern of craniofacial growth; thus surgical intervention to alter the mode of respiration may not be recommended. Souki et al.[21] reported that the vertical growth pattern in a group of mouth breathers was no different after tonsillectomy and/or adenoidectomy than in a control group of mouth breathers.

With the advent of cone beam computed tomography (CBCT), research is being conducted to evaluate the relationship of the airway to the craniofacial dimensions.[22,23] In the past, these studies focused on the airway relationship in the two dimensions registered by lateral cephalograms.[24–26] With a 3D view, the contribution of the transverse dimension and the possibility of analyzing volumes will provide better evidence of this relationship. Three-dimensional CBCT-based evaluation of the upper airway is more accurate and more reliable than evaluation based on two-dimensional (2D) images.[27]

CBCT data may indicate an association between size of the airway and different craniofacial patterns and possibly relate the 3D anatomy to function. Using CBCT, Alves et al.[28] found that the dimensions of the pharyngeal airway were greater in nasal breathers than in mouth breathers. However, a consideration of variables that might affect the findings of these studies is important. The variables include positioning of patients during image acquisition, impact of the respiratory phase, airway patency, head posture, mandibular morphology, and the position of the tongue and hyoid bone. Hence standardization of CBCT settings and definition of the anatomic boundaries of the airway are necessary.[23,27] Because a standardized protocol for airway imaging is not available, making a reasoned judgment of the validity and reliability of upper airway models based on three-dimensional CBCT imaging is often difficult.[29]

Muscle and Its Contribution to Facial Pattern

A generally accepted notion is that hyperdivergent patients have weaker mandibular muscles and a weaker bite force than hypodivergent patients do. However, this relationship between the dentofacial complex (form) and jaw muscles (function) is still a matter of controversy. Whether or not the strength of the masticatory muscles is the primary determinant of the dentofacial complex is still not clear.[30] The influence of muscles of mastication on the orofacial region is difficult to understand but can be at least theoretically determined by analyzing its geometric properties (size of the muscle, orientation of the muscle, and mechanical advantage), intrinsic properties (muscle fiber size and distribution), and muscle recruitment patterns.[31]

Muscle Size

The total force exerted by a muscle is directly related to its cross-sectional area of muscle fibers, which can be measured by using computed tomography (CT) and magnetic resonance imaging (MRI). The cross-sectional area can give some insight into the strength of the masticatory muscle in the various facial types. The size of masseter and medial pterygoid muscles was larger by 50% in brachyfacial subjects than in dolicofacial subjects. The size difference was about 30% larger in brachyfacial subjects for the temporalis muscles and about 6% larger for the anterior digastric muscle. Among the masticatory muscles, the cross-sectional area of the masseter is highly sensitive to the variation in long face subjects. The difference in size indicates a different loading pattern during function in hyperdivergent and hypodivergent patients.[31]

Muscle Orientation

When analyzed in the sagittal plane, the masseter was obliquely oriented in long face subjects and vertically oriented in short face subjects. Because of the difference in the spatial orientation of the masseter and medial pterygoid muscles in the two groups, the vertical force component of the muscles was 3% and 2% higher in short face subjects than in long face subjects respectively. Due to this difference in orientation of masseter and medial pterygoid muscles, Spronsen[31] concludes that the brachyfacial subjects are more efficient in producing vertically directed bite forces. However, the differences in bite force between the two groups were quite small, even though they were statistically significant.[31]

The moment arm in the masticatory muscular force system is the perpendicular distance from the summit of the mandibular condyle to the line of action of the force. Small differences in values in the moment arm of the masseter and medial pterygoid muscles were observed in subjects with normal, hypodivergent, and hyperdivergent facial patterns. The moment arm at the region of the lower first molar was 8% smaller in the short face group than in the long face group. This difference is due to the morphology of the mandible and the spatial orientation of the masticatory muscles to the morphology between the short face and long face subjects. Because of the smaller moment arm and the associated biomechanical advantage, slightly larger bite forces were produced in brachyfacial subjects when compared with dolicofacial subjects.[31]

The maximum biting force was 155 N in long face subjects and 356 N in normal face subjects.[32] In other studies[33] bite force was 380 N in long face subjects and 720 N in short face subjects. However, the bite forces in children with hyperdivergent and normal facial patterns are similar,[34] although the forces differ significantly in adults of both groups. Explaining why the maximum bite forces are lower in long face groups than in other groups is difficult. Can this difference in bite forces be due to differences in the composition of muscle fiber? Rowlerson et al.[35] found that subjects with open bites had a higher percentage of type I fibers (slow contracting and fatigue resistant) in masseter muscle than did deep bite subjects. In contrast, compared with open-bite subjects, deep bite subjects had more type II fibers (fast contracting and relatively fatigable). A correlation exists between the vertical growth pattern and particular muscle fibers but further studies are necessary to evaluate the cause and effect relationship between the type of muscle fiber and vertical growth pattern of the face.

Based on the above findings, Van Spronsen[31] concludes that the influences of muscle orientation, moment arms, and biomechanical advantage on the open-bite malocclusion are generally weak. The influence of maximum bite forces in determining craniofacial morphology is controversial, because electromyographic studies have shown that maximum bite forces are produced for only 6 minutes per day.[36] The influence of the bite force of jaw muscle due to shorter duration of action on the developing craniofacial complex may be negligible or small.[37] Furthermore, Ueda et al.[38] reported that 90% of masticatory muscle activity is of low amplitude and may be related to long face morphology.

Finally, the vertical growth pattern is established early in life[39,40]; the craniofacial morphology is visible even before the development of weak musculature. Therefore the strength of association between the long face and weak musculature is rather weak and questionable. A hyperdivergent growth pattern, which is under a strong genetic influence, might result in a dentofacial morphology with weak musculature. These environmental interactions (weak musculature and others) on the genetically determined craniofacial structures could possibly determine the final expression of long face morphology.[31]

Role of the Tongue in Anterior Open Bite

Another major etiologic factor that reportedly contributes to open bites is an imbalance between the tongue and the perioral musculature.[41] Various habits, such as tongue thrusting and thumb- and finger-sucking, and anatomic conditions, such as macroglossia, have been reported as causative factors. These factors contribute to the development of an open-bite malocclusion by adversely affecting the development of the anterior dentoalveolar complex and inhibiting the normal eruption of teeth.[42] The force of the tongue or finger against the lingual surface of the incisors also causes concurrent flaring of the upper anterior teeth.[43]

Clinicians should carefully consider the role that the tongue plays in the etiology of open bite. Both the function and the anatomy of the tongue must be evaluated. From an anatomic point of view, a large tongue (macroglossia) can be responsible for splaying the anterior teeth and thus cause an open bite. Unfortunately, macroglossia is difficult to diagnose because no simple method is available to measure the volume of the tongue.[44] Certain features noted during clinical examination that indicate macroglossia include spacing and flaring of the anterior teeth, indentations on the lateral borders of the tongue, and lateral extension of the tongue onto the occlusal surface of the lower teeth[45] (Fig. 9-6).

From a functional point of view, deviant patterns of swallowing or tongue thrusting may contribute to the development of anterior open bite. However, some researchers claim that tongue thrusting appears to be a compensatory or adaptive behavior to the altered craniofacial skeleton. Swallowing, chewing, and speaking have little impact on the morphology of the dentition but the consequences of postural aberrations leading to changes in the resting pressure and posture of the tongue are marked.[46] Some clinicians have proposed that the

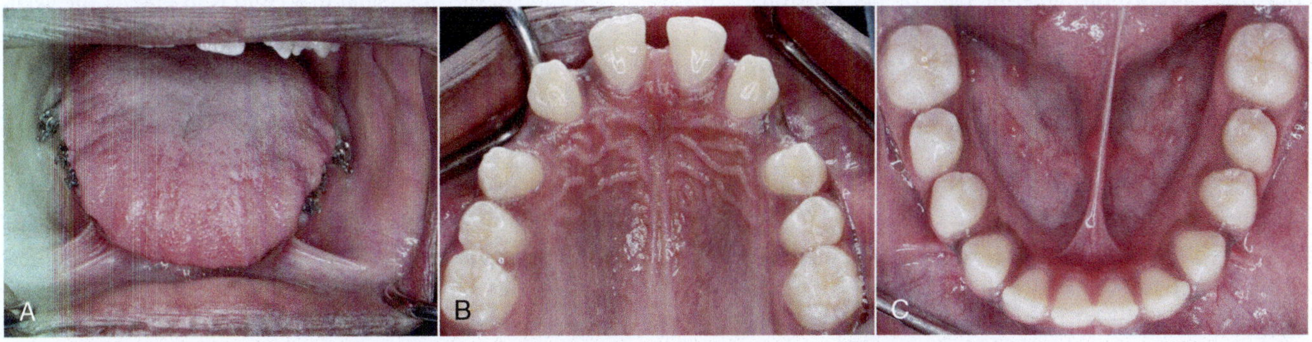

Figure 9-6 Patient with a large tongue. **A,** Intraoral clinical exam shows indentations on the lateral borders of the tongue and coverage of the occlusal surfaces of all lower teeth. **B and C,** Upper and lower arches depict generalized spacing.

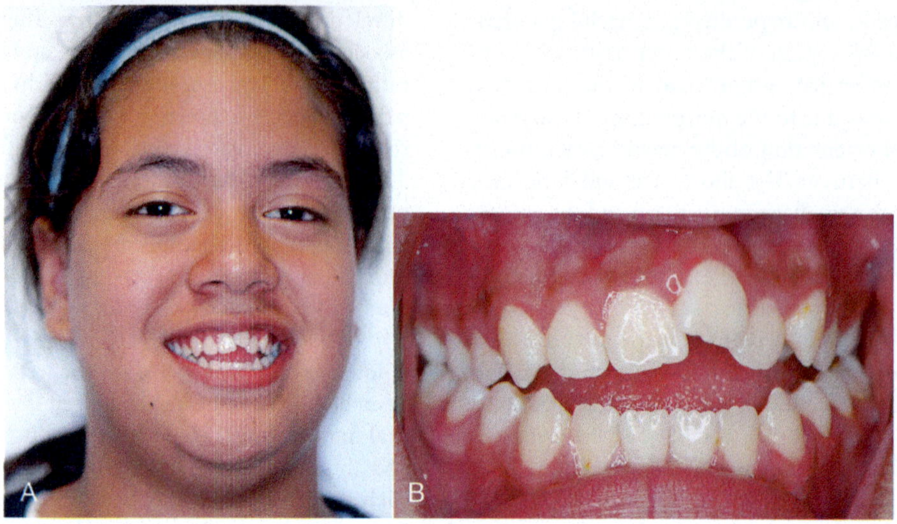

Figure 9-7 Anterior open bite exacerbated by an ankylosed maxillary left central incisor due to previous trauma. **A,** Smile view showing the reduced smile display in the ankylosed incisor. **B,** Frontal intraoral view showing the significant anterior open bite as a result of the ankylosed incisor.

resting posture of the tongue is a more significant factor contributing to the open bite, compared to any of the temporal active functional muscular activity.

Several techniques, such as cineradiography, videofluoroscopy, ultrasonography, and, more recently, kinetic MRI, have been used to evaluate tongue movements during deglutition.[47] Akin et al.[47] used cine MRI to compare tongue movements during swallowing between subjects with anterior open bite and control subjects. The images were obtained during stage 1 (loss of contact of the dorsal tongue with the soft palate), stage 2 (passage of the bolus head across the posterior/inferior margin of the ramus of the mandible), and stage 3 (passage of the bolus head through the opening of the esophagus). Significant differences were found between stages 2 and 3, the pharyngeal and esophageal stages, which are involuntary. The posture of the tip of the tongue was more anterior during all stages in the open-bite subjects than in the control subjects. These results indicate that, during swallowing, the tip of the tongue is thrust forward in open-bite subjects to maintain the anterior oral seal. During normal swallowing the position of the posterior dorsum of the tongue was significantly elevated in stages 2 and 3, a change that might be a normal movement for propulsion of a food bolus and protection of the airway. However, in the open-bite group, the anterior part of the dorsum of the tongue is lowered and its middle part is elevated. As a compensatory mechanism to avoid aspiration during swallowing, the rear part of the tongue has minimal or no movement and marked movements occur in the anterior and middle parts of the tongue.

Thumb-Sucking

Prolonged thumb-sucking is another common environmental factor often associated with anterior open bite. Children who suck their thumbs have a higher prevalence of anterior open bite than do control subjects of a similar age group.[48] Additionally, finger-sucking and a hyperdivergent facial pattern are significant risk factors not only for development but also for increased severity of an open bite.[49]

Trauma

Skeletofacial and dentoalveolar trauma are also etiologic factors of anterior open bite. Skeletal trauma involving the condyles can cause severe anterior open bites.[50] Arrested condylar growth or ankylosis of the condyle results in altered vertical growth of the mandible, clinically manifested as an anterior open bite. Trauma to the dentition, particularly the incisors, can result in localized anterior open bite if the damaged teeth become ankylosed before the patient finishes growing[51] (Fig. 9-7).

Finally, anterior open bites may develop in patients with degenerative diseases involving the condyles. Idiopathic condylar resorption[52] and juvenile rheumatoid arthritis[53] are two pathological conditions that involve condylar resorption.

Genetics

The genetic component of an open bite is related primarily to the patient's inherent growth potential. Traits such as anterior facial heights are, to a large degree, inherited.[54] Obtaining a thorough family history will help in predicting a patient's growth potential.

Although the main goal in a child is to predict the vertical skeletal relationships at the end of growth, growth patterns are established early in life and maintained in most people.[55,56] Therefore a skeletal open-bite pattern could be evident in the early mixed dentition. Numerous cephalometric planes have been used independently and combined to detect the early skeletal open-bite pattern. The overbite depth indicator index of the primary dentition might be useful for predicting a skeletal open-bite tendency in adolescence.[57] This index is a composite of cephalometric measurements involving the mandibular and palatal plane angles in relation to the A-B line and the Frankfort horizontal plane, respectively.

The Björk indicators are another useful method to help predict vertical growth patterns. However, these indicators are based on patients with extreme variations in vertical facial growth; thus they may be of limited value in patients with less severe open-bite skeletal patterns.[58,59]

The genetic component is an important contributing factor to open-bite malocclusion. Control of the vertical growth pattern by orthodontic means alone is difficult. However, changes in the dentoalveolar complex may directly affect the most representative skeletal features of an anterior open bite. For example, controlling the vertical eruption of the molars allows the mandible to rotate in a counterclockwise direction, reducing the excessive vertical skeletofacial pattern.

TREATMENT STRATEGIES

As described in Chapter 1, treatment strategies should address the cause of the malocclusion. Environmental factors that contribute to a patient's malocclusion, such as thumb-sucking or finger-sucking, should be identified during the clinical examination and then eliminated. The treatment of excess in the vertical dimension often mimics that of the treatment of anterior open bite. The different approaches can be separated according to the age of the patient. In growing patients, the focus of the approach is controlling the eruption of the molars, thereby affecting the skeleton. The same focus will also be beneficial if the patient has an anterior open bite. In adults, the excess vertical length has traditionally been treated with surgery, especially if the hyperdivergent features are associated with a marked dentofacial deformity that affects esthetics. These features are maxillary excess, increased mandibular plane angle, excessive gingival display, retrognathic mandible, long lower facial height, and excessive interlabial gap. Recently, these patients have been treated by using temporary anchorage devices (TADs). However, this approach is most often attempted only when the vertical excess is associated with an anterior open bite.

Treatment of Thumb-Sucking or Finger-Sucking

Children often have a habit of sucking on a finger or a thumb. Many children stop this habit on their own; others need assistance. Children should be encouraged by their parents to stop the sucking habit before the age of 4 years. Before this age, most adverse dental and skeletal effects caused by the habit usually return to the original state, creating a favorable environment for the eruption of permanent teeth.[42] Communication and positive reinforcement by the parents may help to modify any undesirable behaviors but unless a child is willing to stop the habit, these attempts may be unsuccessful.[60]

To help a child stop the habit, parents should note the time of the day at which the behavior occurs and then try to intervene. For example, if a child sucks a thumb or finger during sleep, mechanically obstructing the hand with a sleeping gown may be helpful.[61] If initial attempts are unsuccessful, an intraoral appliance that acts as a mechanical obstruction and reminder can be used.

Different intraoral appliances are available for behavior modification. These appliances consist of a stiff archwire with a series of loops that sit closely to the anterior part of the palate and attach to two upper molar bands. The loops act as a mechanical obstruction and a reminder of the habit. Usually, after 3 months spontaneous correction of any dentoalveolar or eruption problem occurs without use of any other appliance (Fig. 9-8).

Treatment of Tongue Thrusting

Patients with tongue thrusting can be treated effectively in the same manner as that used for patients who suck on a thumb or finger (Fig. 9-9), although different appliances, such as the habit appliance with lingual spurs or cribs (Fig. 9-10), have been suggested. In one study,[62] immediately after crib placement the tip of the tongue was positioned posteriorly during all stages of deglutition. Additionally, the anterior and middle parts of the dorsum of the tongue were at a lower position, reflecting a compensatory functional change for bolus propulsion and airway protection. However, no significant change occurred in the posterior part of the dorsum. Taslan et al.[63] reported a decrease in resting tongue pressure and swallowing pressure from 21 g/cm^2 to 13 g/cm^2 and 216 g/cm^2 to 143 g/cm^2, respectively, after 10 months of tongue crib therapy in patients with anterior open bite. This decrease in tongue pressure at rest and swallowing pressure after crib therapy was suggestive of tongue adaptation in response to the altered environmental changes. This altered tongue posture aided in the correction of an anterior open bite through an increase in overbite of 3.6-mm. The increase in overbite was attained by lingual inclination of the maxillary and mandibular incisors by 4 degrees each and by extrusion of 1.4-mm and 1-mm, respectively.[64]

Other devices to retrain the tongue posture, known as myofunctional appliances, are also effective in treating tongue thrusts. Myofunctional therapy aids in muscle retraining by using a series of tongue exercises to correct the deleterious resting and functional postures[65] and corrects the tendency for hyperdivergent growth. Types of functional appliances include the Frankel functional regulator, bionators, activators, and twin blocks.

In a longitudinal study,[66] considerable decreases in mandibular plane angle, palatal plane to mandibular plane angle, and gonial angle occurred in a group of patients treated with functional regulators. Compared with findings in the control group, the ratio of the upper to the lower anterior facial height and the ratio of the anterior to the posterior facial height changed to normal values in the treatment group. Improvement in skeletal open bite was due to lengthening of the ramus and favorable compensatory growth at the condyles. The functional regulator did not remove the wedge by intruding the molars. The authors[66] hypothesize that the forward rotation of the mandible is due to postural balance between the forward and backward rotating muscles brought about by lip seal exercises. Of note, the goal of most

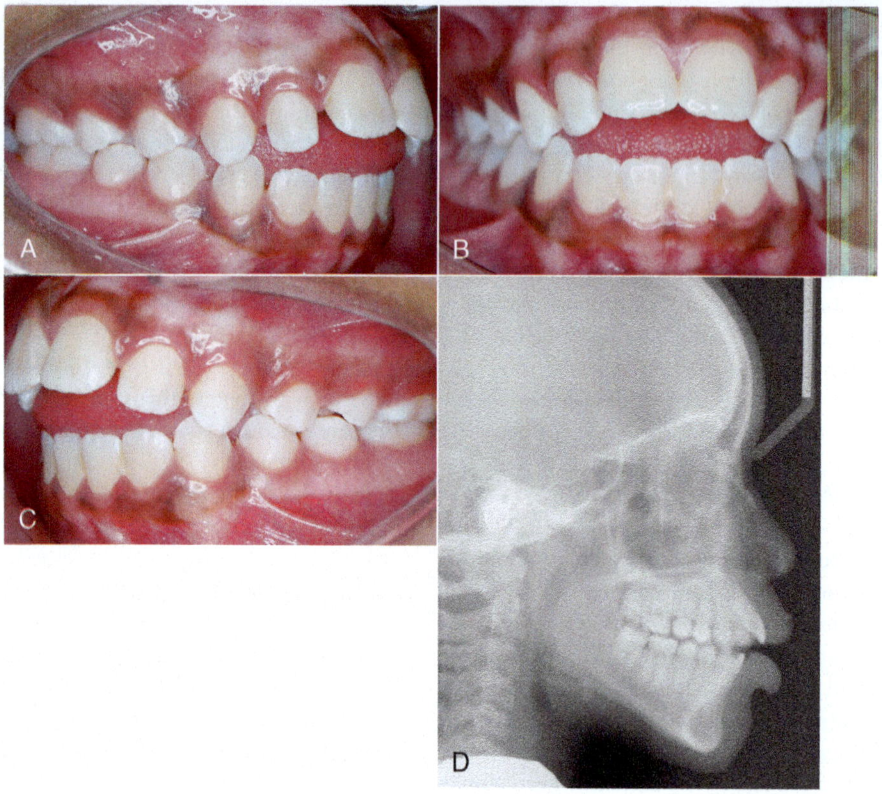

Figure 9-8 **A–C,** Patient with a finger-sucking habit resulting in an anterior open bite mesial to the first premolars. **D,** Lateral cephalogram showing characteristics of a dental open bite.

treatment strategies for patients with hyperdivergent facial patterns is to intrude the molars. On the contrary, correction with the functional regulator was primarily achieved by changing the existing deviant functional pattern of muscular environment.

Treatment of Macroglossia

If macroglossia is diagnosed, surgical resection may be performed to reduce the volume of the tongue. The open bite can then be corrected by retraction of the anterior teeth. After treatment, stability most likely will be enhanced, because the reduced tongue volume will better match the reduced arch length obtained after retraction of the incisors (Fig. 9-11). Although this procedure may help in the reduction and stability of anterior open-bite correction, the morbidity of the procedure, with potential sequelae in taste, sensation, and motor dysfunction, explains why this approach is not often chosen.[45,67]

Treatment of Airway Obstruction

Procedures that promote better breathing through the nose (turbinate surgery, adenoid and tonsil removal, allergy treatment) may help to reestablish normal growth patterns.[68] However, the growth direction of the mandible among patients varies greatly after any of these procedures.[69] This variability makes the decision to intervene with a resective surgical procedure difficult. Therefore the diagnosis of upper airway obstruction and the decision for surgical intervention should always be made by an appropriate team of specialists.

Correction of Open Bite by Incisor Extrusion

Extrusion of the upper and lower incisors is a common orthodontic treatment for anterior open bites. This treatment is appropriate if the patient has an open bite with a normal skeletal pattern but may also be used in patients with vertical dysplasias who have deficient incisor display at rest and when they smile. However, most patients with long face morphology and anterior open bite have posterior as well as anterior vertical maxillary excess (Fig. 9-12). Thus correction of the malocclusion in these patients by extrusion of the upper incisors may result in an excessive display of the incisors and gingival tissues, compromising not only the esthetic results but also the long-term stability of the outcome. Nonetheless, the short-term occlusal results are usually satisfactory.

Here the compliant and noncompliant are treatment methods. Vertical elastics are the most common method used for incisor extrusion in compliant patients. Extrusion arches are used in noncompliant patients.

Extrusion Arches

Extrusion arches are efficient tools used to correct upper and lower occlusal planes that diverge anterior to the first premolars. These archwires are indicated (1) when spontaneous correction of an anterior open bite does not occur after

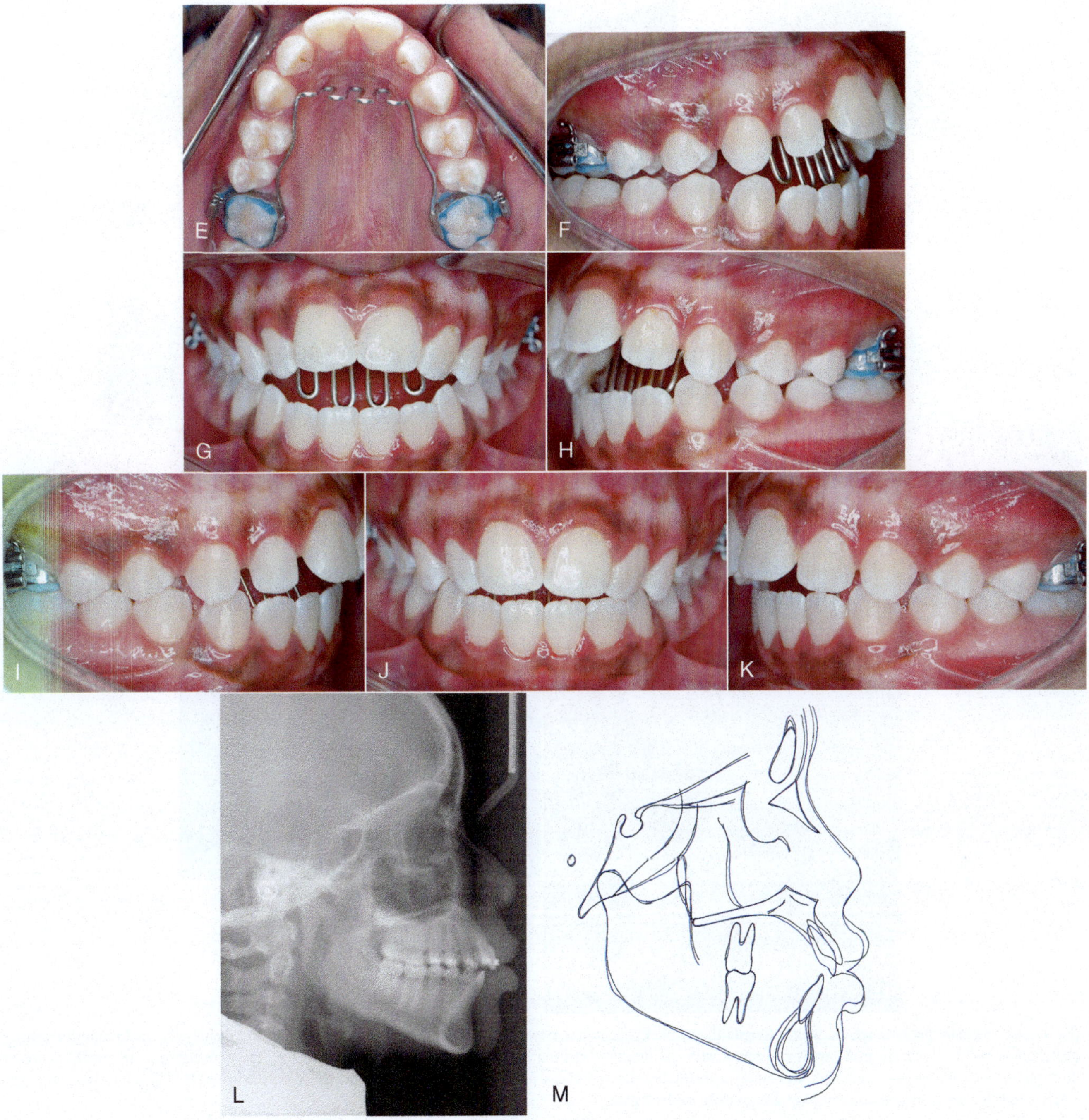

Figure 9-8, cont'd **E–H,** Habit appliance with loops acting as a mechanical obstruction in close approximation to the anterior portion of the palate. **I–K,** Spontaneous correction of the anterior open bite after habit appliance delivery. **L,** Lateral cephalogram showing the open-bite closure. **M,** Superimposition reflecting the incisor extrusion that results with spontaneous closure of an anterior open bite with the habit appliance.

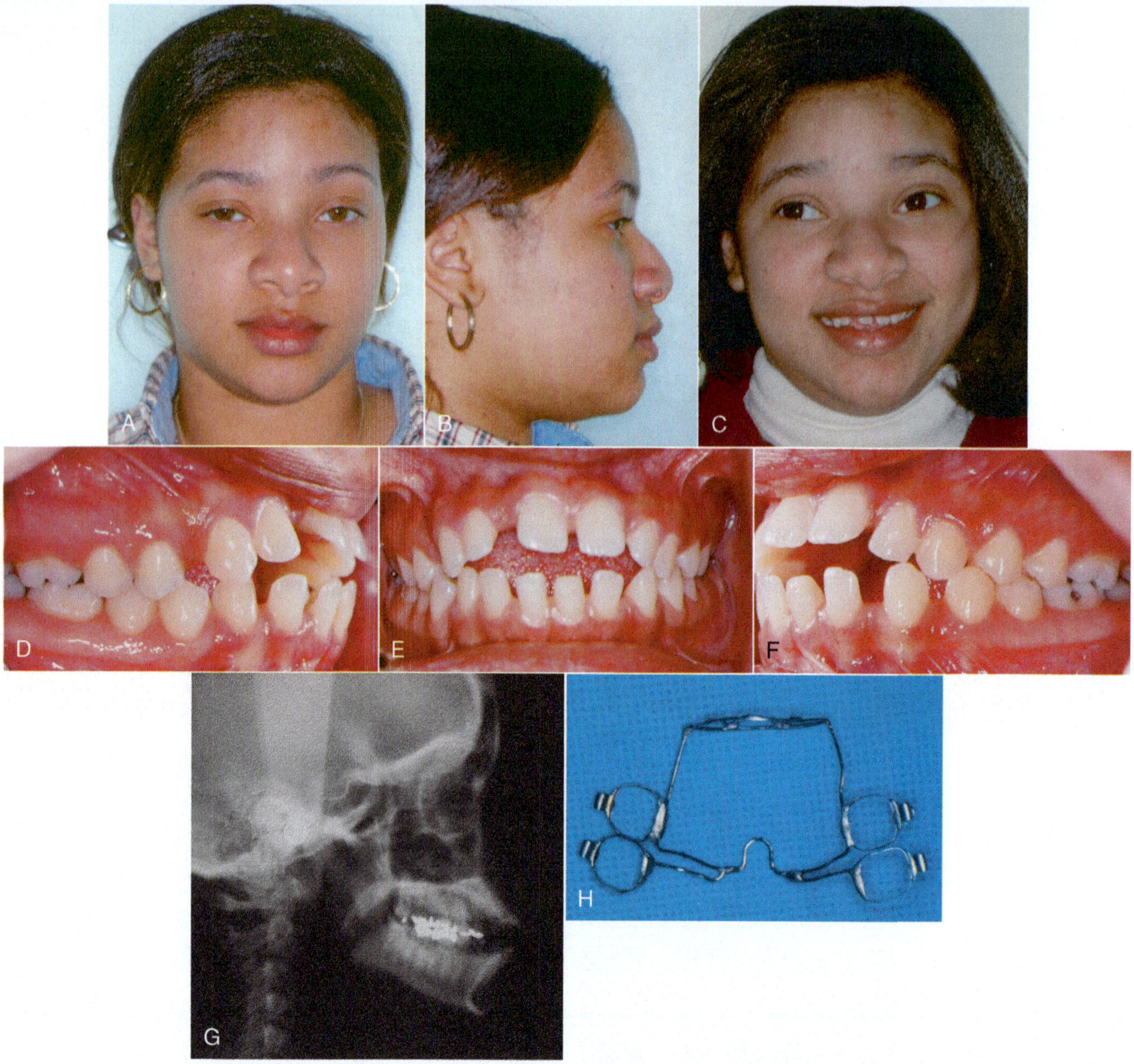

Figure 9-9 Female patient, age 18, with a tongue thrust. **A–C,** Extraoral views. On smile, only 50% of the incisors are displayed and an anterior tongue posture is evident. A reverse smile arc is consistent with the tongue thrusting habit. **D–F,** Intraoral views show a 3-mm anterior open bite with divergent occlusal planes from the first premolars. **G,** Lateral cephalogram shows a dental anterior open bite with dentoalveolar protrusion. **H,** Habit appliance with first and second molar bands and anterior loop design close to the palate.

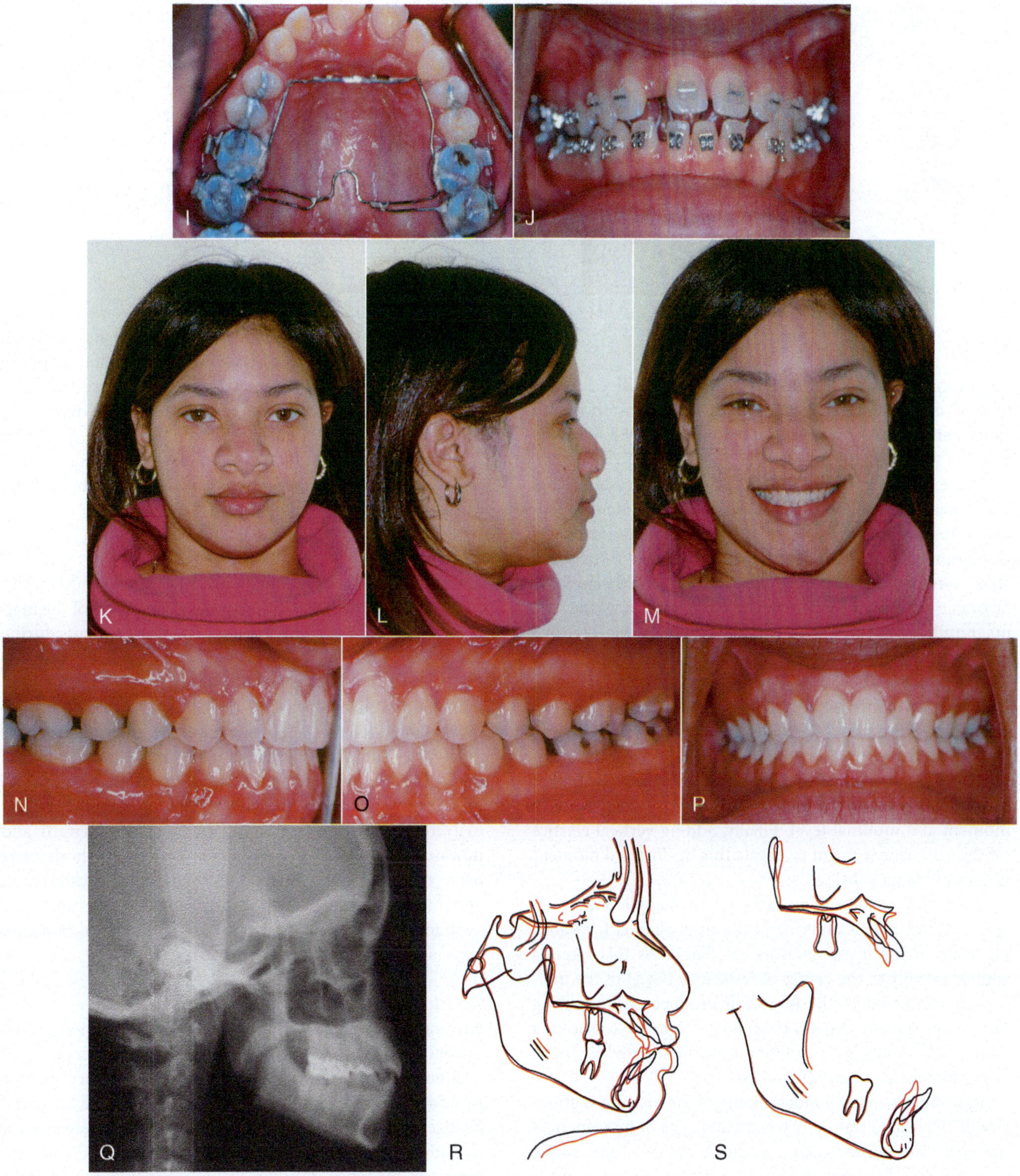

Figure 9-9, cont'd **I,** Intraoral view of the cemented habit appliance. **J,** Brackets are placed after 6 months of exclusive treatment with the habit appliance. Fifty percent of the negative open bite self-corrected. **K–M,** Extraoral views after treatment. A positive smile arc was obtained, with approximately 90% incisor show on smile. **N–P,** Adequate overbite was achieved with a good Class I relationship. **Q,** Final lateral cephalogram shows the overbite correction. **R,** General superimposition shows no maxillary or mandibular growth. Controlled lingual tipping of the upper and lower incisors reduced the dentoalveolar protrusion and anterior open bite. **S,** Regional maxillary and mandibular superimpositions show the same dental movements described previously (pre-treatment age, 18.8 years; post-treatment age, 21.5 years).

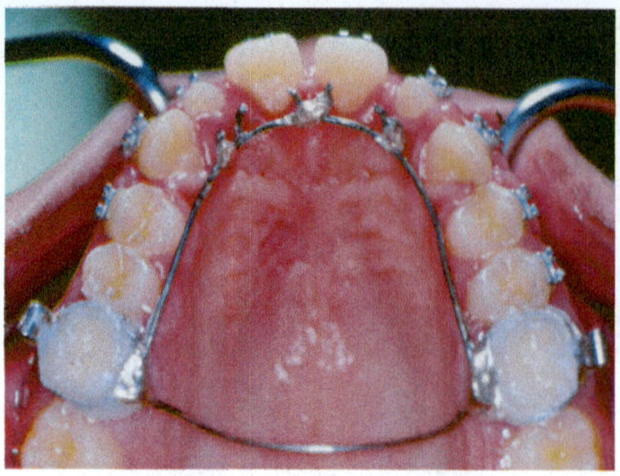

Figure 9-10 Habit-breaking appliance with lingual spurs.

tongue crib therapy, (2) when a constant extrusive force is desired in the anterior teeth with minimal posterior side effects, and (3) in noncompliant patients who will not wear anterior vertical elastics.

The extrusion arch is a one-couple force system (Fig. 9-13) that applies a single extrusive force to the anterior teeth and a tip-forward moment and intrusive force to the posterior segment. Often the tip-forward moment is undesirable.[70] On the other hand, the intrusive force on the molar is favorable in patients with anterior open bites; however, the magnitude of this force, which is the same as the extrusive force on the anterior teeth, most likely would not result in molar intrusion.

Different options are available to negate the tip-forward side effect. First, a buccal stiff sectional wire from the upper first molar to the first premolar is added. Second, the magnitude of the extrusive force should be kept low (extrusion of the incisors requires light forces) to maintain the posterior moment at a minimal level. Finally, adding vertical elastics off the posterior segment to negate this tip-forward moment is helpful[71] (Fig. 9-14).

The extrusive force of an extrusion arch applied to divergent occlusal planes anterior to the premolars is favorable, especially if the upper incisors are flared. As this force is applied labially to the center of resistance (C_{RES}) of the incisors, the moment of the force will produce an uprighting movement (crown lingual) (Fig. 9-15). Figure 9-16 shows a patient with anterior open bite that was corrected by using upper and lower extrusion arches.

In some instances, lingual tipping of the incisors is undesirable. Instead, a translatory extrusion type of movement is the goal. The same mechanics can be applied (one-couple force system); however, the force on the anterior segment is placed close to the canine in an anteroposterior direction by means of a three-piece extrusion arch (Fig. 9-17).

Vertical Elastics

Traditionally, vertical elastics have been used for closure of an open bite. Inter-arch mechanics with vertical elastics are indicated in patients with anterior open bites in which the occlusal planes diverge anteriorly. Vertical elastics from the lower incisors to the upper incisors result in a consistent force system of equal and opposite forces (Fig. 9-18). Reduction of the overbite by extrusion of the incisors is the result.

Although vertical elastics are a common method for incisor extrusion, certain problems are inherent with this type of treatment. First, response varies greatly among patients because of poor control of the force magnitude and degrees in compliance. Second, specific goals defined in the treatment plan (occlusal plane, position of incisors) cannot be achieved predictably because good mechanical control is difficult to achieve with indiscriminate use of elastics.

Multiloop Edgewise Archwire

The appliance known as the multiloop edgewise archwire (MEAW) relies on a combination of compliant and noncompliant mechanics in which archwires with specific shapes in conjunction with vertical elastics are used to correct an anterior open bite. Most of the reduction in the overbite is achieved by extrusion of the anterior teeth with negligible molar intrusion.[72] Additionally, the inter-molar angle is partially corrected, a change that may aid in stability after treatment.

Treatment in Growing Patients

The prevalence of open bite is two to three times higher in children than in adults.[73] Spontaneous correction of the malocclusion occurs in more than two-thirds of patients during the mixed dentition period.[74] Early treatment options are available for open bites that do not self-correct.[7] However, managing skeletal open-bite malocclusions and the long-term stability of the outcome depend on the orthodontist's ability to address the cause and to alleviate the 3D problems in skeletal, dental, and soft tissues. The primary aim is to inhibit the vertical development or intrusion of buccal dentoalveolar segments and to aid in favorable forward and upward rotation of the mandible. Various methods have been used to manage hyperdivergent facial patterns in growing patients: habit-breaking appliances, functional appliances, headgear, posterior bite blocks, vertical-pull chin cups, and clenching exercises.

Headgear

Extraoral maxillary traction appliances are commonly used to control the vertical dimension. Occipital and vertical-pull headgears have an intrusive force on the maxillary molars. In addition to the intrusive component of force, occipital headgears also have a distal force. This force system is ideal in patients with a Class II hyperdivergent growth pattern. However, evidence indicates little therapeutic benefit from use of a high-pull headgear, because an increase in the angle of the mandibular plane can occur.[75] Although control of the eruption of maxillary molars is effective, compensatory overeruption of the mandibular molars often occurs as well.[76]

Orthodontists generally avoid using cervical-pull headgear in patients with hyperdivergent facial patterns because molar extrusion can occur, leading to clockwise rotation of the mandible. However, contrary to this popular notion,

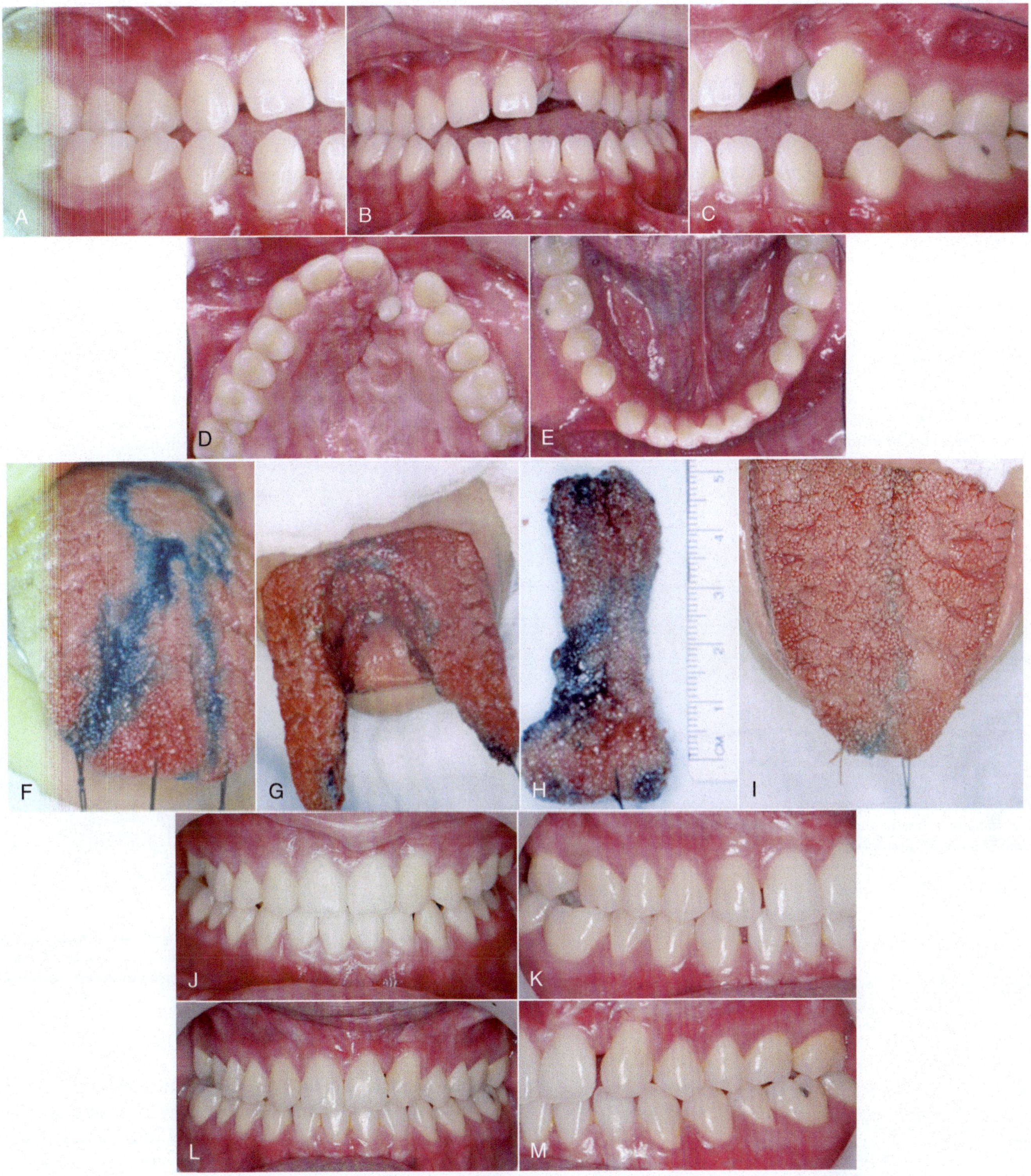

Figure 9-11 **A–E,** Intraoral views of a patient with a unilateral left cleft lip and palate. Significant spacing is observed in the lower arch due to a large tongue. **F,** Keyhole-design glossectomy. **G–I,** Lateral borders of the tongue to be approximated after tissue mass reduction. **J,** Anterior open-bite closure after surgical orthodontic treatment. **K–M,** Intraoral views illustrating 9-year stable result.

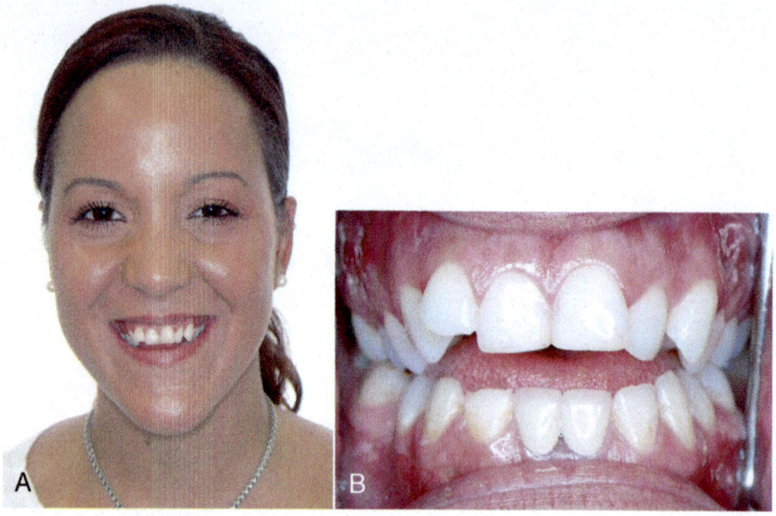

Figure 9-12 **A,** A Patient with posterior vertical maxillary excess and anterior open bite with slightly increased incisor display at smile. **B,** Correction of the anterior open bite by extrusion of the anterior teeth will accentuate the anterior vertical maxillary excess in detriment of facial esthetics.

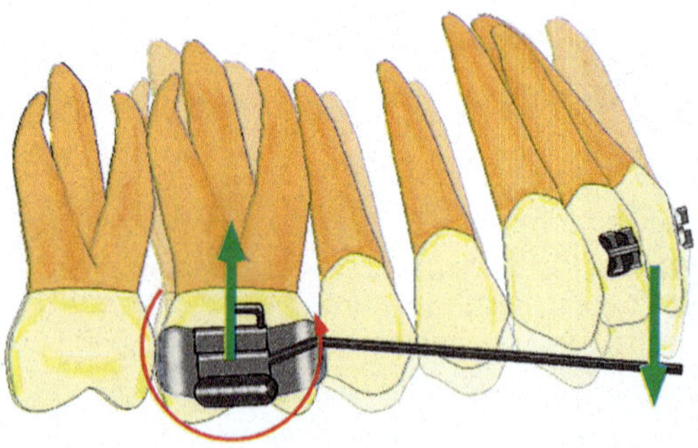

Figure 9-13 Extrusion arch force system. A one-couple force system with an anterior extrusive and a posterior intrusive force. The couple on the molar produces a tip-forward moment.

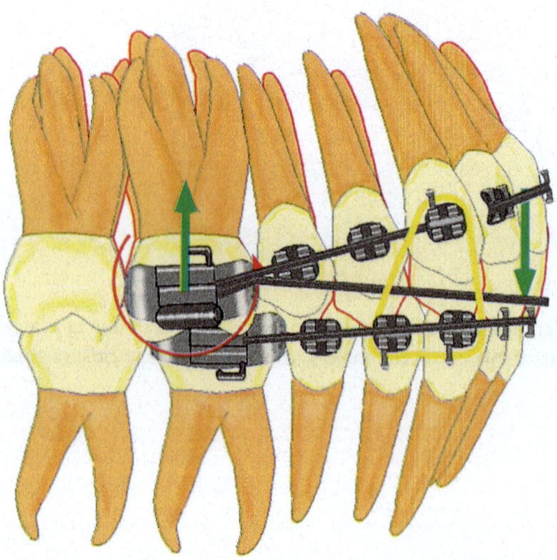

Figure 9-14 Vertical elastic added to the upper buccal segment to negate the tip-forward tendency produced by the one-couple force system in the extrusion arch.

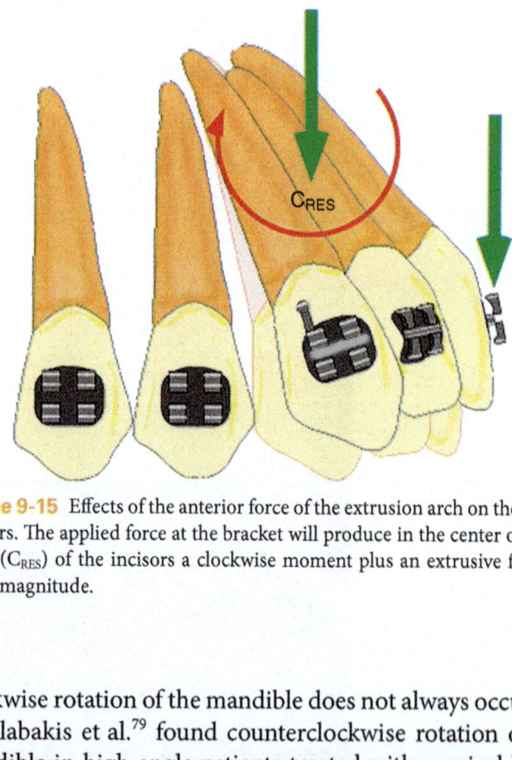

Figure 9-15 Effects of the anterior force of the extrusion arch on the upper incisors. The applied force at the bracket will produce in the center of resistance (C_{RES}) of the incisors a clockwise moment plus an extrusive force of equal magnitude.

clockwise rotation of the mandible does not always occur.[77,78] Haralabakis et al.[79] found counterclockwise rotation of the mandible in high angle patients treated with cervical headgear. Additionally, in another study[80] changes in vertical dimension in dolicofacial patients did not differ significantly between patients treated with cervical headgear and those treated with occipital headgear.

Posterior Bite Blocks

Passive acrylic bite blocks are functional appliances that open the mandible beyond the interocclusal distance by 3- to 4-mm and maintain the pressure applied by the masticatory muscles on the posterior teeth.[81] On the other hand, spring-loaded bite blocks[82] and magnetic bite blocks (active

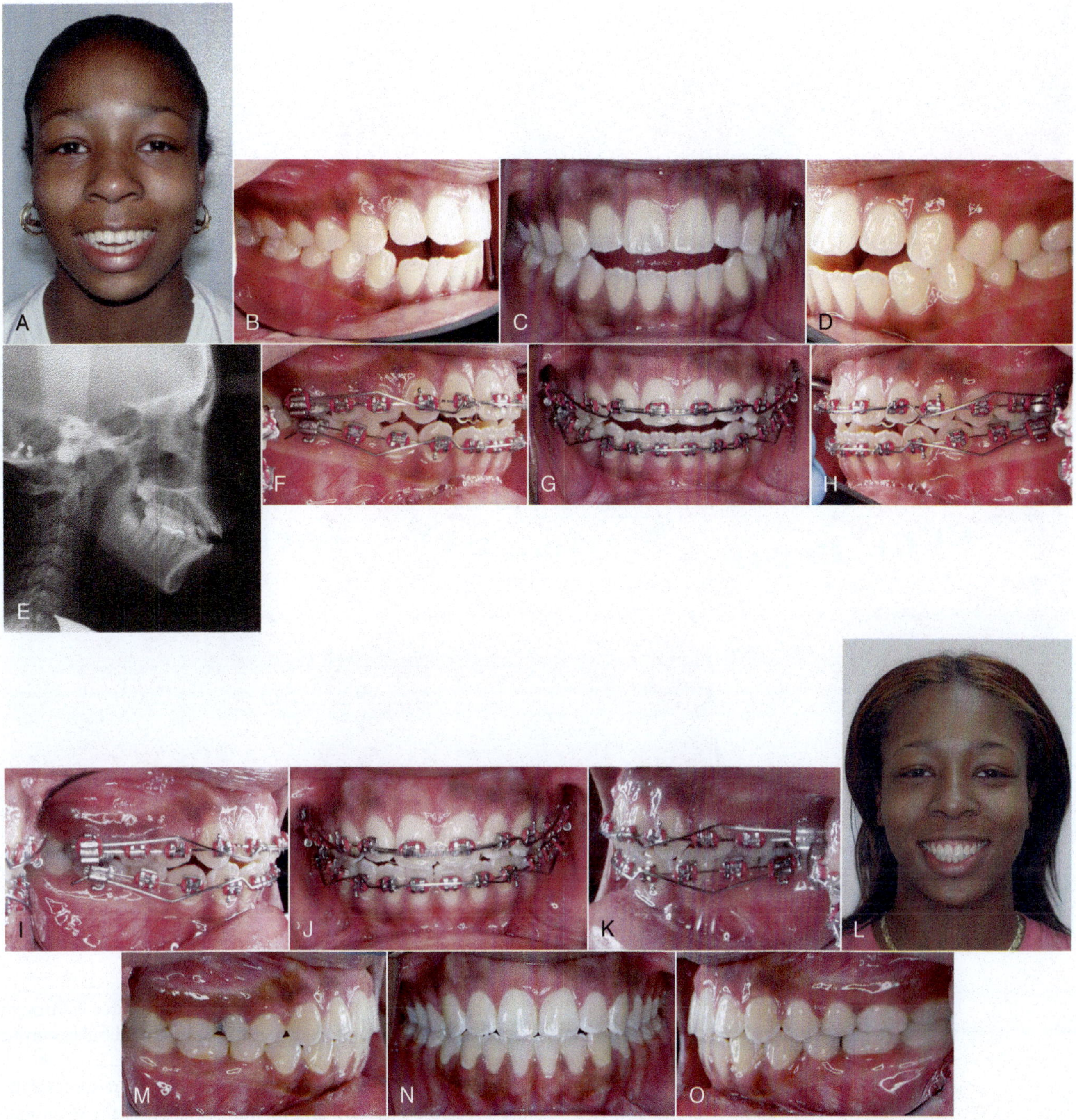

Figure 9-16 Treatment of a patient with extrusion arches on the upper and lower dentition. **A,** Frontal view on smile showing approximately 90% of incisor display. **B–D,** Preoperative intraoral photos showing a 3-mm anterior open bite and occlusal plane diverging anteriorly from the first premolars. **E,** Lateral cephalogram showing undererupted maxillary incisors. **F–H,** Upper extrusion arch with buccal segments to prevent molar tip forward. Lower extrusion arch tied to the lateral incisors with a continuous nickel-titanium (Ni-Ti) 0.016-inch wire. **I–K,** Good anterior open-bite correction with maintenance of the vertical relationship on the buccal segments. **L–O,** Final records showing the improved smile arc and good occlusion with positive overbite.

vertical correctors)[83] provide continuous vertical force on the occlusal surfaces of posterior teeth within the neuromuscular system. In experimental studies[84] in animals, an alteration in vertical dimension led to structural adaptations in the craniofacial complex. Although these appliances were effective in reducing the vertical dimension in growing patients, absolute intrusion of posterior teeth was minimal (0.5-mm).[82]

Vertical-Pull Chin Cup

Vertical-pull chin cups (VPCCs) have been used to control the increase in anterior facial height during the time of mixed and early permanent dentition.[85–87] VPCCs have been used in conjunction with fixed appliances, functional appliances, posterior bite blocks, and removable appliances (Fig. 9-19). The magnitude of force applied is 400 g per side and, according to recommendations, the VPCC should be worn

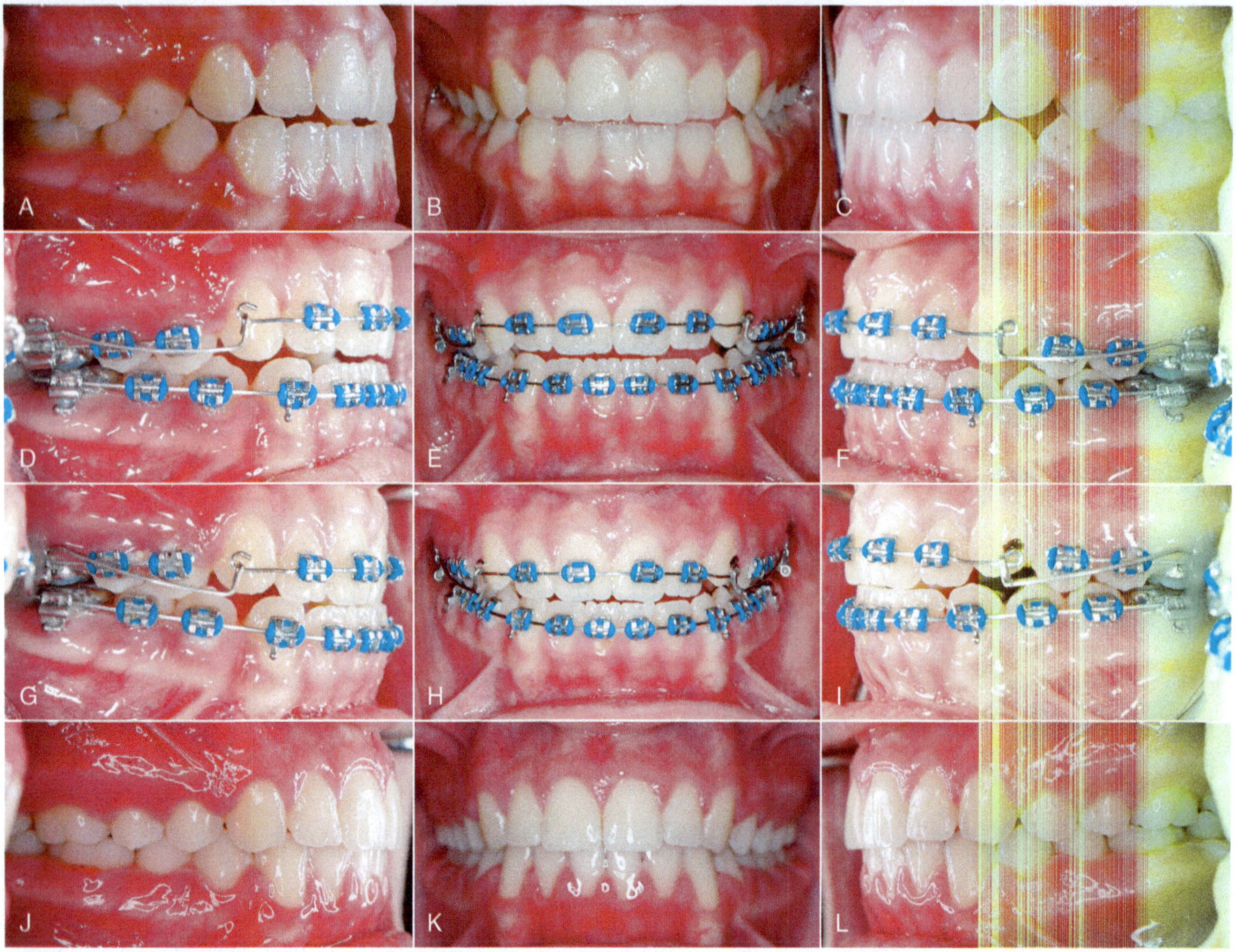

Figure 9-17 Three-piece extrusion arch. **A–C,** Intraoral records showing an anterior open bite with upright incisors. **D–F,** Three-piece extrusion arch delivered to extrude the incisors and slightly correct the incisor inclination by delivering a force posterior to the center of resistance. **G-I,** Incisor extrusion evident by referencing the movement to the adjacent canines. **J-L,** Intraoral final records showing good buccal occlusion, adequate overbite, and good incisor maxillary inclination.

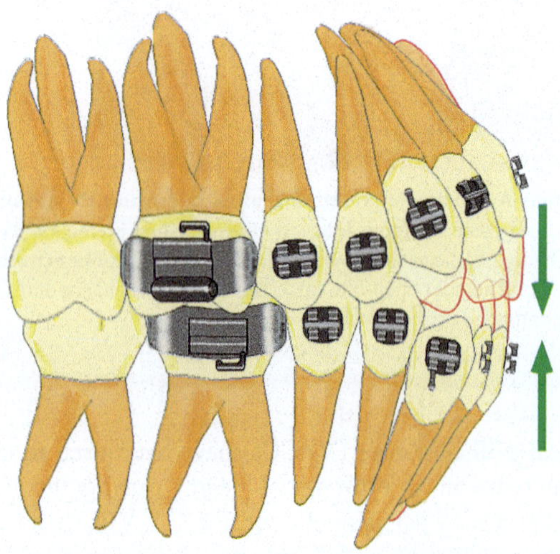

Figure 9-18 Force system of anterior vertical elastics (equal and opposite forces), which is favorable in anterior open bite with divergent occlusal planes anterior to the first premolars and reduced incisor display.

up to 12 hours per day. The direction of the force is through the anterior and inferior region of the mandibular corpus and 3 cm from the outer canthus of the eye. Iscan et al.[88] reported that skeletal and dental open bites were successfully corrected by upward and forward rotation of the mandible, significant eruption of the mandibular incisors, and inhibition of eruption in the mandibular posterior dentoalveolar region.

Masticatory Muscle Exercises

Isometric masticatory muscle exercise has been recommended as an adjunctive to orthodontic treatment[89,90] or alone in patients with hyperdivergent facial patterns. Isometric clenching exercises increase the contractile forces of the elevator muscles of the mandible. Masticatory exercises can produce favorable skeletal and occlusal changes in growing children. Significant reductions in anterior facial height, gonial angle, and counterclockwise rotation of the mandible have been reported.[91,92] Clenching exercises on a soft bite

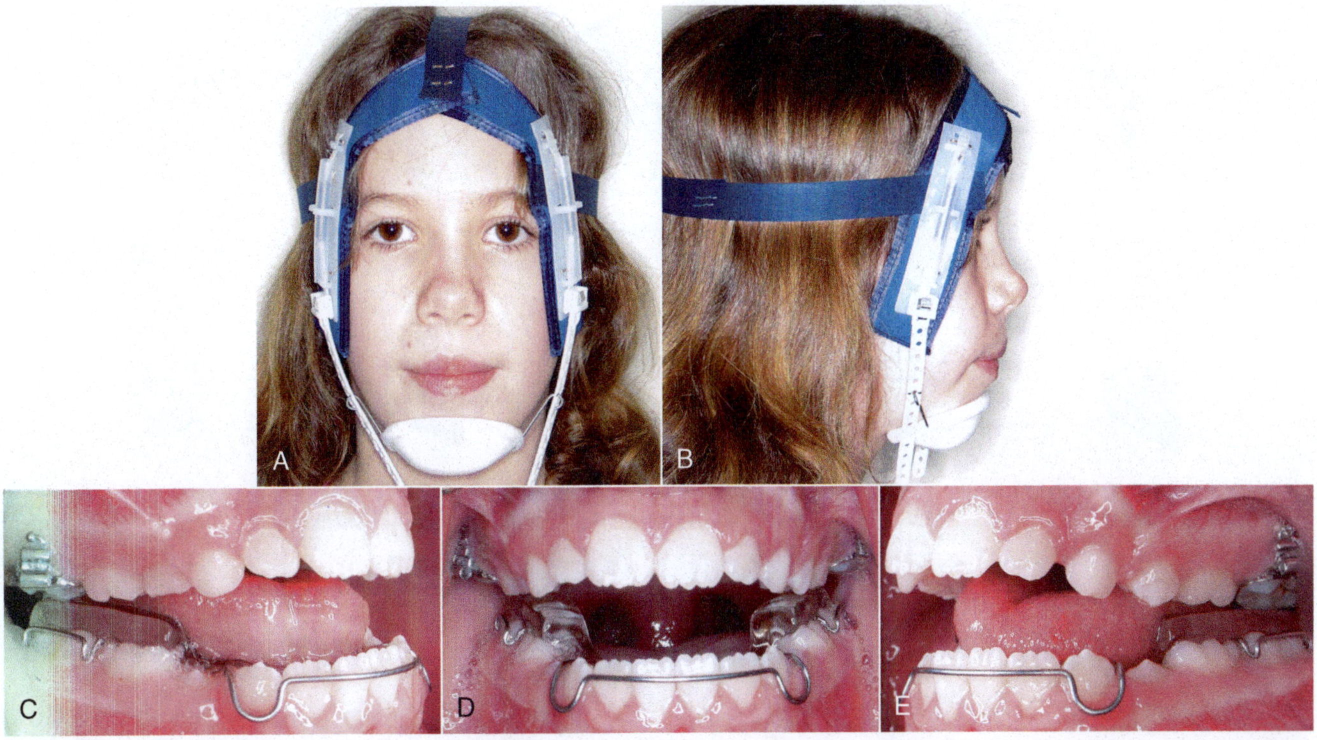

Figure 9-19 Vertical-pull chin cup **(A and B)** with removable occlusal splint **(C-E)** on the lower arch to control the eruption of the molars in a growing patient. (From Nanda R, Kapila S: *Current Therapy in Orthodontics*, St. Louis: Mosby, 2010.)

block[93,94] and chewing exercises with a hard gum[91,95] or tough pine tree resin[92] are the common methods of masticatory muscle exercises. A minimum of 45 to 150 minutes per day for 12 to 30 months of exercise appears to be necessary to produce clinically significant morphological changes in the dentofacial complex.[89]

Transpalatal Arch

The tongue affects the dentoalveolar complex during mastication, swallowing, and speech and at rest. Harnessing the forces generated by the musculature of the tongue on the palatal arch during swallowing can prevent the vertical development of the maxillary molars.[96] During deglutition, mean tongue pressure ranges from 37 to 709 g/cm^2.[97] Chiba et al.[97] measured the tongue pressure exerted on the palatal bar by altering the anteroposterior and vertical position of the transpalatal arch. Increased levels of pressure were recorded when the loop of palatal arch was 6-mm from the roof of the palate and anteroposteriorly between the second molars. DeBerardinis et al.[96] retrospectively analyzed the vertical holding appliance, which is a transpalatal arch with an acrylic pad. Compared with control subjects, for the duration of treatment patients with the appliance had eruption of the maxillary molars restrained by 0.41-mm.

Treatment in Nongrowing Patients

Management of adult patients with vertical maxillary excess and excessive vertical dimension has been addressed primarily through orthognathic surgery.[98] Surgical procedures to address long face patients have been associated with acceptable treatment outcomes and long-term stability.[99,100] However, the introduction of skeletal anchorage devices has been a major shift in orthodontics, enabling predictable, effective, and efficient tooth movements with direct occlusal and skeletal benefit to long face patients.[101,102] The molars can be intruded directly from TADs to correct the vertical dimension without the need for compliance by the patient.[103–105]

A major advantage of molar intrusion with TADs is the favorable skeletal changes that enhance a patient's dentofacial esthetics (Fig. 9-20). With conventional orthodontics in patients with anterior open bite, closure of the overbite is achieved mainly through dentoalveolar changes; however, the skeletofacial complex may worsen because of extrusive mechanics. On the other hand, TADs target the intrusion of the posterior segment, which is often the cause of the increased vertical dimension.

The suggested magnitude of force for molar intrusion is about 50 to 200 g per tooth. For en masse intrusion of premolars and molars, a force of approximately 200 to 400 g has been suggested. The rate of intrusion of a single maxillary molar is 0.75-mm per month, whereas the rate for en masse intrusion of a posterior segment is 0.5-mm per month. Usual time for intrusion of maxillary molars is 5 to 7 months for a mean intrusion of 2- to 4-mm.[106] Sugawara et al.[107] reported mean intrusions of 1.7-mm and 2.8-mm for mandibular first molars and second molars, respectively, when mini-plates were used.

Molar intrusion can be accomplished with different types of TADs. However, before anchorage devices are placed, defining the desired tooth movement in three dimensions of

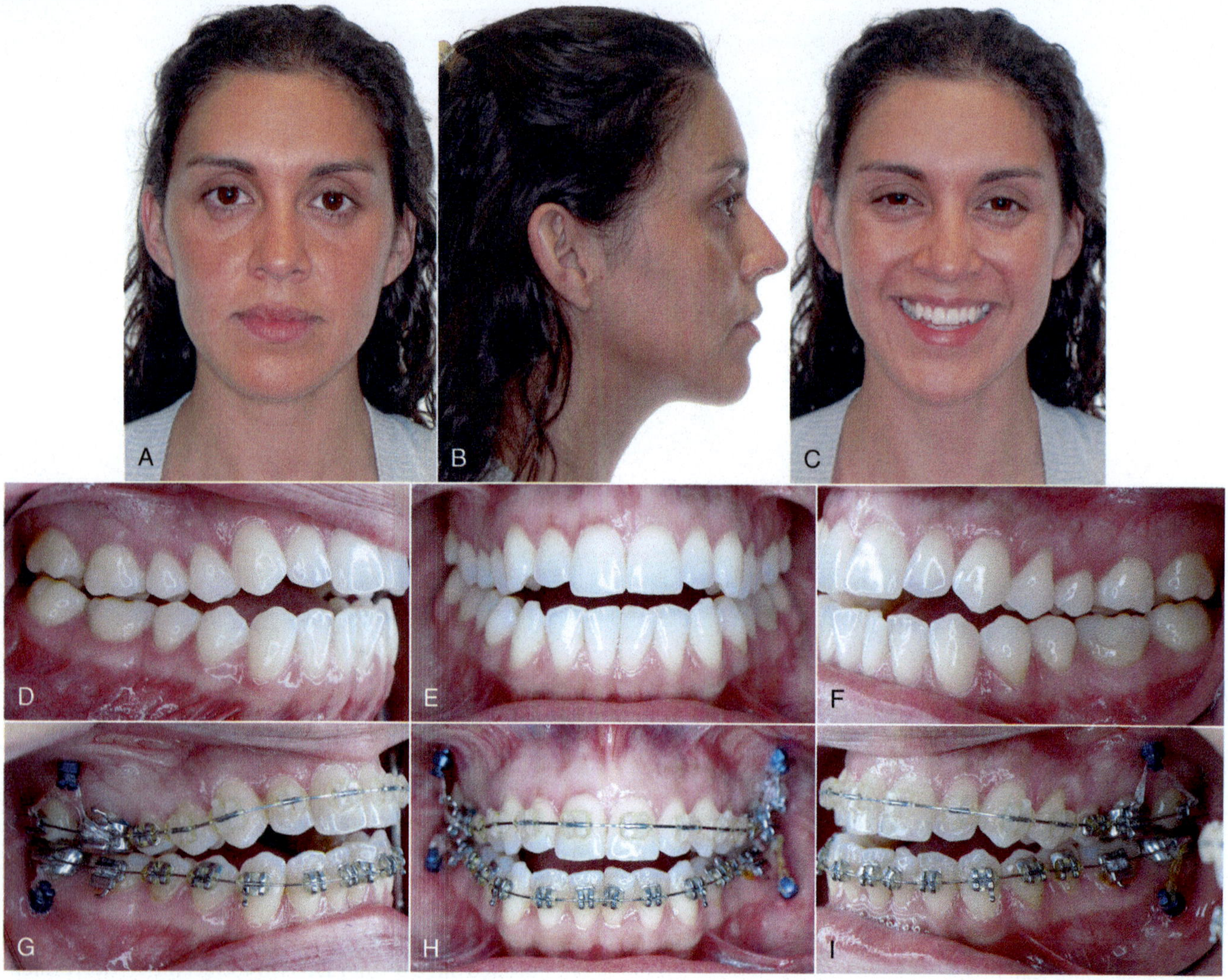

Figure 9-20 Adult patient with a moderate skeletal anterior open bite treated with temporary anchorage devices (TADs). **A–C,** Extraoral views show increased lower facial height and adequate incisor display at smile. **D–F,** Anterior open bite with occlusal planes that diverge anteriorly from the second molars. **G–I,** Four TADs (two in the infrazygomatic crest and two in the external oblique ridge) were placed to assist in the intrusion of the first and second molars.

space is important. The line of force for molar intrusion determines the number of mini-implants, buccal or palatal placement, direct anchorage or indirect anchorage, and anatomic location of TAD placement. Locating the center of resistance (C_{RES}) of the active unit is important to produce a force system designed for intended tooth movement. According to holographic studies,[108] the C_{RES} of upper dentition is located near the key ridge. However, according to a finite element study,[109] the C_{RES} of maxillary dentition is 11-mm from the tip of the cusp of the second premolar.

In another finite element study, Çifter and Saraç[110] evaluated three methods of using mini-implants for intrusion of segmental maxillary posterior teeth. Balanced intrusion with minimal buccal tipping occurred when buccal and palatal forces were applied simultaneously via mini-screws. In other models with one or two transpalatal arches and a buccal line of force application via mini-screws, vestibular tipping was greater. Mesiodistal cant also occurred in a model in which one palatal arch was modeled along with application of one-point buccal intrusive force. To minimize the bowing effect vertically, Çifter and Saraç[110] recommend establishing uniform stress distribution along the posterior segments by using separate force applications and differential force levels for the molar and premolar sites. Furthermore, because of the dynamic nature of biomechanical force systems after the initial tooth movement, appropriate changes in the magnitude and direction of force are necessary during treatment to prevent side effects in second and third order.

Buschang et al.[103] intruded the maxillary and/or maintained the mandibular posterior teeth in a controlled manner by using two mini-screws palatally in the parasagittal region mesial to the first molar in the upper arch and two mini-screws in the lower arch between the second premolar and the first molar. Maxillary molars and premolars were rigidly held by a rapid palatal expander. A lower lingual arch was used along with a 0.016-inch × 0.022-inch stainless steel archwire. The primary advantage of this approach was that during the intrusion of maxillary posterior teeth, mandibular molars were either intruded or maintained, thereby preventing them from compensatory eruption in response to

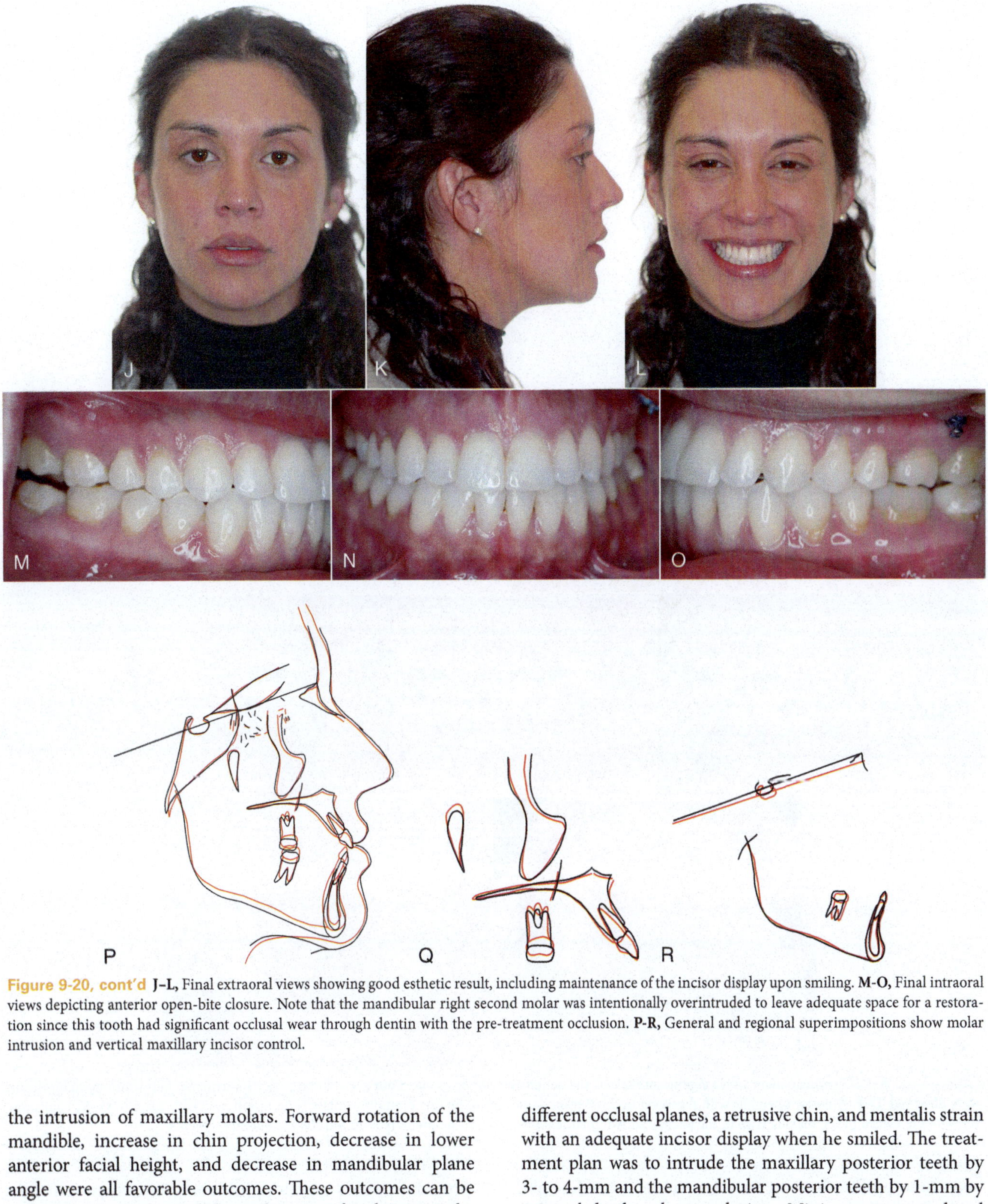

Figure 9-20, cont'd **J–L,** Final extraoral views showing good esthetic result, including maintenance of the incisor display upon smiling. **M-O,** Final intraoral views depicting anterior open-bite closure. Note that the mandibular right second molar was intentionally overintruded to leave adequate space for a restoration since this tooth had significant occlusal wear through dentin with the pre-treatment occlusion. **P-R,** General and regional superimpositions show molar intrusion and vertical maxillary incisor control.

the intrusion of maxillary molars. Forward rotation of the mandible, increase in chin projection, decrease in lower anterior facial height, and decrease in mandibular plane angle were all favorable outcomes. These outcomes can be achieved in patients with hyperdivergent facial patterns by clockwise rotation of the maxillary occlusal plane and counterclockwise rotation of the mandibular occlusal plane.

Figure 9-21 shows the management of an adolescent with Class II skeletal open-bite malocclusion with intrusion of maxillary and mandibular posterior teeth. He had an anterior open bite of 8-mm, a large interlabial gap of 9-mm, two different occlusal planes, a retrusive chin, and mentalis strain with an adequate incisor display when he smiled. The treatment plan was to intrude the maxillary posterior teeth by 3- to 4-mm and the mandibular posterior teeth by 1-mm by using skeletal anchorage devices. Mini-screws were placed palatally, mesial to the upper second molar, and between the premolars buccally. Additionally, two mini-implants were placed mesial to the mandibular second molars. To increase the rigidity of the segments, transpalatal and lingual arches were fabricated. Positive overbite with a leveled maxillary occlusal plane, increased chin projection, improvement in

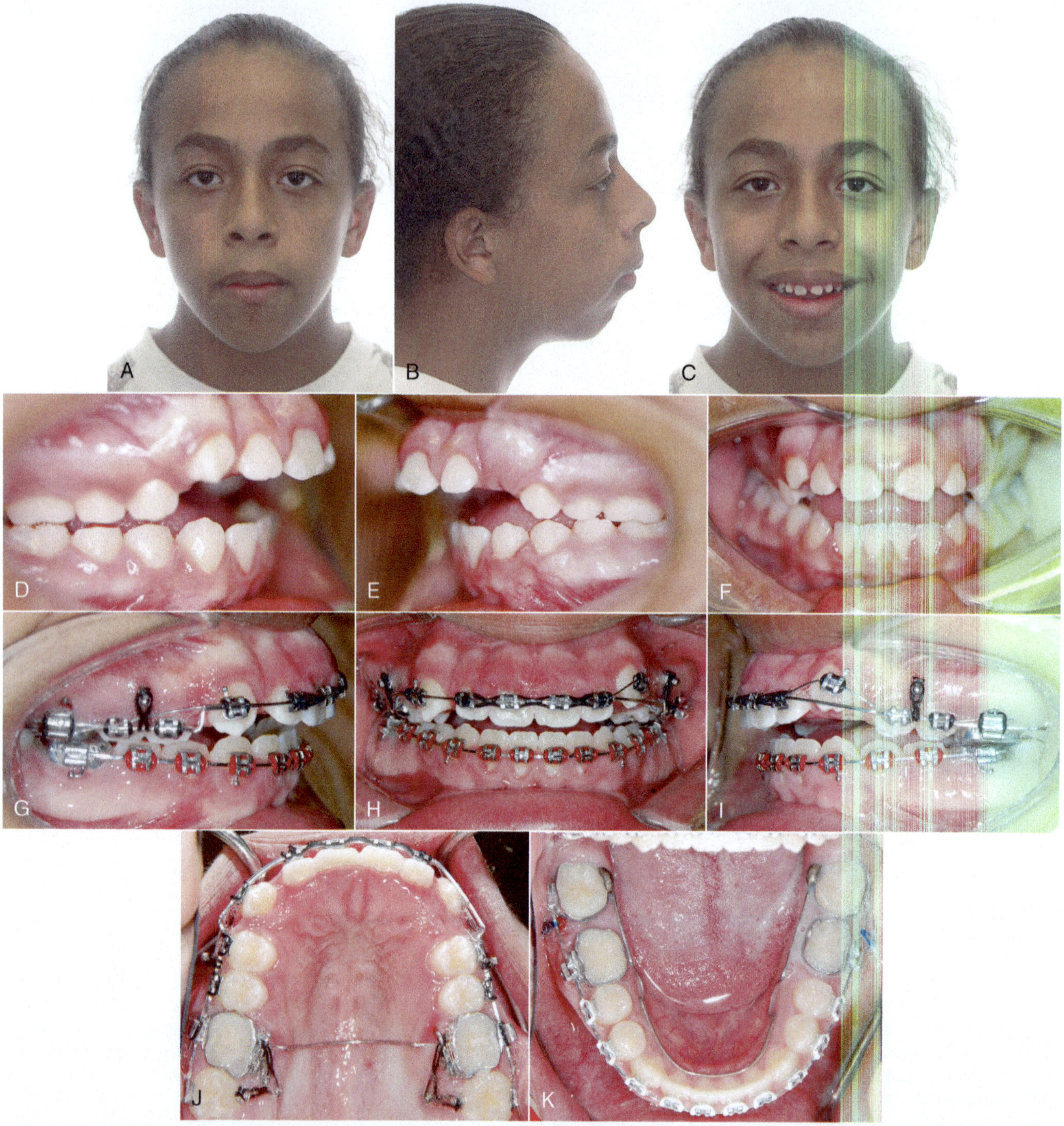

Figure 9-21 **A–C,** Growing patient with a significant skeletal and dental anterior open bite. Poor mandibular projection and mentalis strain upon lip closure were observed. **D–F,** Anterior open bite with divergent occlusal planes anterior to the first premolars. Class II occlusion noticed bilaterally. **G–K,** Four mini-screws were placed in the maxilla (two in the palate and two interdentally between the premolars) to intrude the buccal segments.

soft tissue profile, decrease in lower anterior facial height, and interlabial gap with improvement in mentalis strain were achieved.

Orthognathic Surgery

A segmental Le Fort I osteotomy is routinely performed to reduce the vertical maxillary excess in patients with two maxillary occlusal planes and a transverse deficiency. This procedure allows superior positioning and expansion of the maxilla (Fig. 9-22). At the same time, the occlusal plane is leveled. In one study, three degrees of forward autorotation of the mandible was achieved when the maxilla was impacted 1.3-mm posteriorly and 3-mm anteriorly.[111] The autorotation increased the sella-nasion B point (SNB) angle, decreased the anterior facial height, and decreased the angle of facial divergence (mandible plane angle) with minor forward

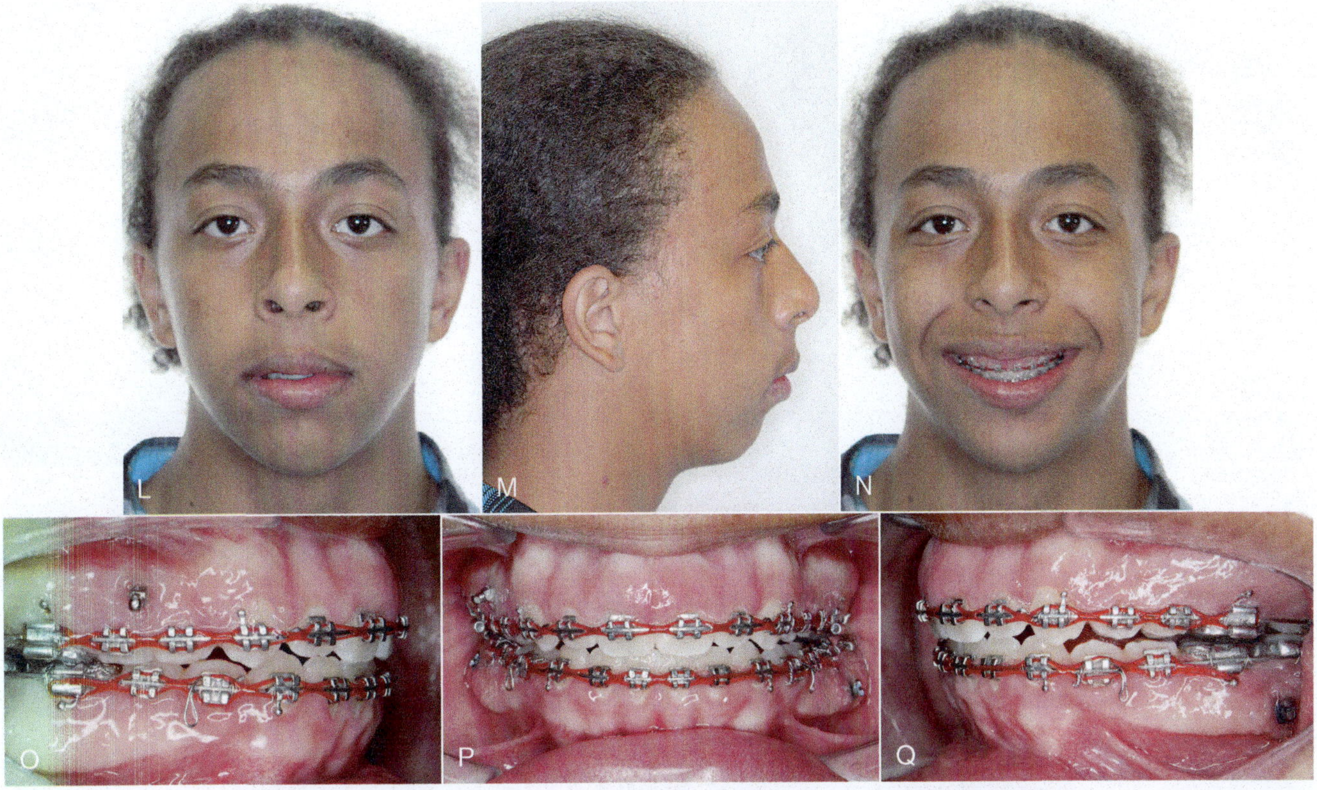

Figure 9-21, cont'd **L–N,** Progress showing improved lip seal and intrusion of the buccal segments with maintenance of the incisor display at smile. **O–Q,** Two mini-screws were added to the mandible between the first and second molars bilaterally to prevent supraeruption of the lower molars. Good overbite observed with a Class I occlusion after posterior intrusion in this growing patient.

movement of the pogonion. In addition to a Le Fort I osteotomy, mandibular surgery may be performed to correct any associated mandibular deformity.

The timing of surgical intervention is critical in a young adolescent because the subsequent effects of orthognathic surgery on the dentofacial complex are poorly understood and controversial. Washburn et al.[112] evaluated surgical superior repositioning of the maxilla in 16 growing individuals. Stable dental, skeletal, and esthetic results were still apparent after 3 years of follow-up. The authors suggest that early surgical intervention may have a favorable effect on excessive growth in patients with vertical maxillary excess. Nanda et al.[113] had similar results in studies in animals. Mojdehi et al.[111] and Mogavero et al.[114] retrospectively assessed growth changes in the maxilla and mandible after Le Fort I osteotomy. Early surgery did not normalize or inhibit the vertical pattern of growth and the growth after surgery was comparable to growth in an untreated control sample. In a consensus conference[115] on the timing of facial osteotomies, the participants recommended that most of the surgical procedures be done after completion of growth. Early surgical intervention can be an exception to the rule for psychosocial reasons,[115] especially for patients with problems in the vertical dimension, but the patients and their parents must be informed that additional surgery may be necessary later.[114]

Extractions for Open-Bite Closure

Different types of extraction patterns have been suggested to correct anterior open bites, including extracting the second molars, extracting the first molars, extracting the second premolars, and extracting the first premolars.[116] The extraction pattern is individually tailored to the patient to extrude the anterior segment, move the posterior teeth anteriorly (wedge effect),[15,117] or achieve a combination of the two.

Second Molar Extractions

The extraction of second molars has been suggested as a practical option in patients who have an anterior open bite with contact solely on these teeth and divergent occlusal planes (wedge effect; Fig. 9-23).[15] Although this option is feasible, the magnitude of divergence of the occlusal plane is the limiting factor to full overbite correction. A potential problem, depending on the age of the patient, is the necessary continual monitoring of the third molars until full eruption and correct positioning in the arch are achieved.[118] However, this method provides an advantage over the other extraction patterns because no space closure is needed and vertical forces are not likely to be generated (see Premolar Extractions later in this chapter). Interestingly, patients with this anterior open-bite pattern (divergent occlusal planes with only the second molars contacting) are generally considered surgical patients.

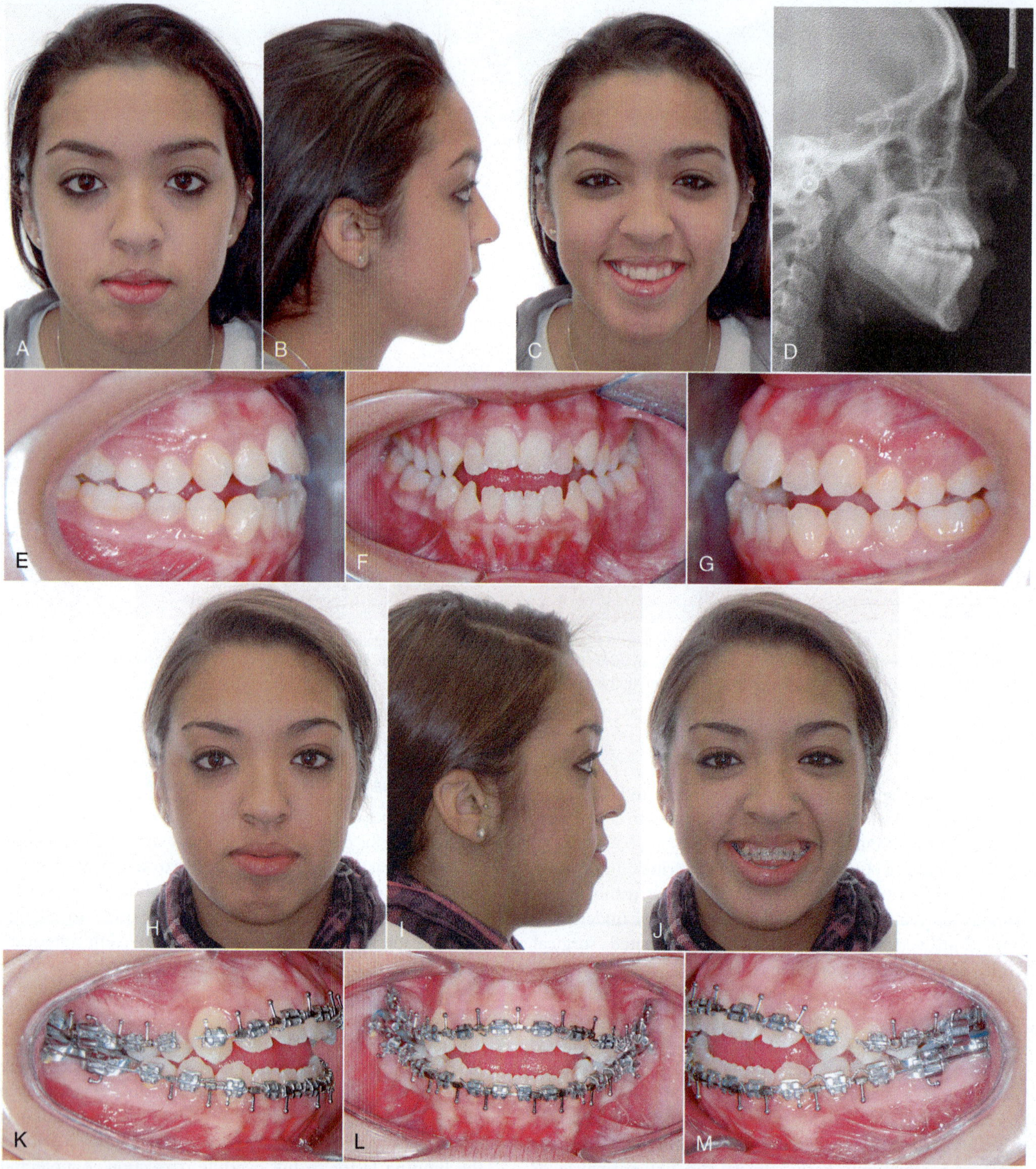

Figure 9-22 **A–D,** Patient with skeletal open-bite characteristics. **E–G,** Anterior open bite with diverging occlusal planes from the first premolar and bilateral posterior crossbite. **H–M,** Presurgical extraoral and intraoral views after segmental leveling for a three-piece maxilla Le Fort I osteotomy.

First Molar Extractions

Typically, first molars are extracted only if they are compromised by extensive decay. In theory, this treatment alternative should contribute to closure of an anterior open bite, and in one study[119] this extraction pattern maintained or slightly reduced the vertical skeletal relationships. However, in most patients the second molar replaces the first molar and the anterior open bite is not resolved. As the molar is protracted into the extraction space, extrusion of the distal aspect usually occurs because of poor mechanics, thereby increasing or maintaining the anterior open bite. Overall, if this extraction option is considered, space closure mechanics are the deciding factor in the success of the overbite correction.[117,120]

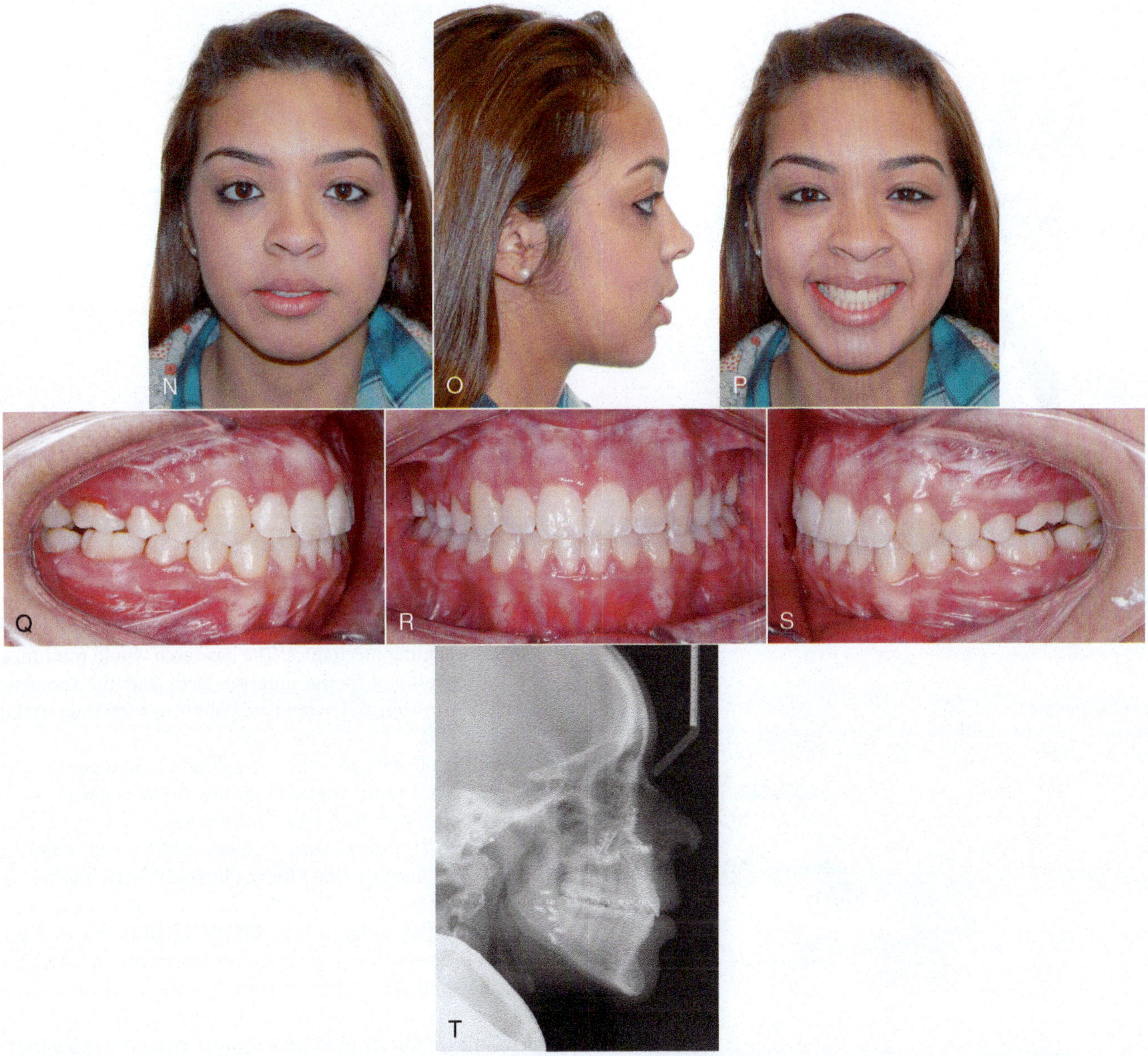

Figure 9-22, cont'd **N–T,** Final records after maxillary impaction with expansion and mandibular setback. Improved facial and smile esthetics and correction of the anterior open bite.

This treatment alternative is most effective if proper timing is considered. If the second molars have not erupted and if the only contact is between the first molars, extraction of the first molars would eliminate the increased vertical height and the second molars could not erupt beyond the newly established vertical height.

Premolar Extractions

Extractions of the first or second premolars are the most commonly considered alternatives for the treatment of anterior open bites associated with crowding and/or overjet. Deciding which premolars to extract depends on the amount of incisor retraction. In patients who have premolars extracted, extrusion of the anterior segment rather than the wedge effect aids in closing the open bite. This treatment alternative works well in patients with occlusal planes that diverge anteriorly from the first or second premolars. The mechanics are easier when the anterior teeth are flared (the usual situation in this type of divergence of the occlusal plane).[121] A single distal force (ideally controlled tipping) will produce lingual tipping of the incisor crowns. Because the center of rotation (C_{rot}) is close to the apex, the net effect is extrusion and retraction of the incisors to close the bite (Fig. 9-24).

Biomechanics of Space Closure in Open Bites

Although the biomechanics of space closure is discussed more fully in Chapter 6, specific aspects that pertain to anterior open bite are reviewed here.

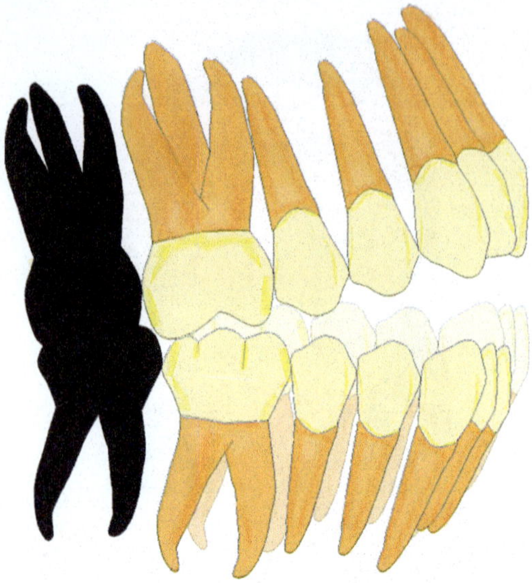

Figure 9-23 Anterior open bite with occlusal planes diverging from the second molars anteriorly. All second molars are extracted for correction of the open bite. The magnitude of the open-bite correction is dependent on the angle of divergence of the upper and lower occlusal planes. Full correction of the anterior open bite may not be obtained in extremely divergent occlusal planes.

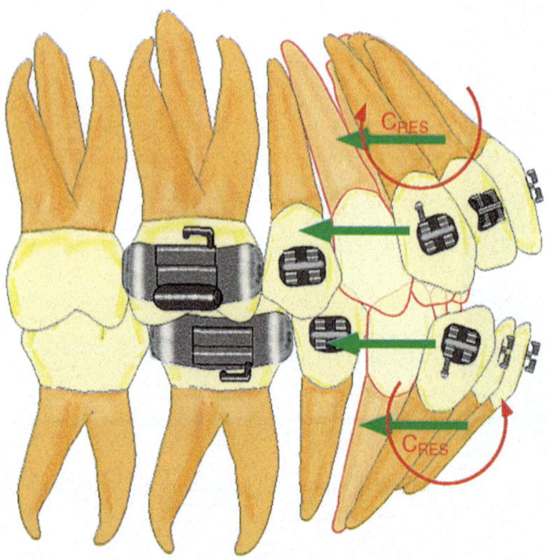

Figure 9-24 Controlled tipping of the upper incisors produced by a distal force results in extrusion of the incisal edge and reduction of the amount of labial incisor inclination.

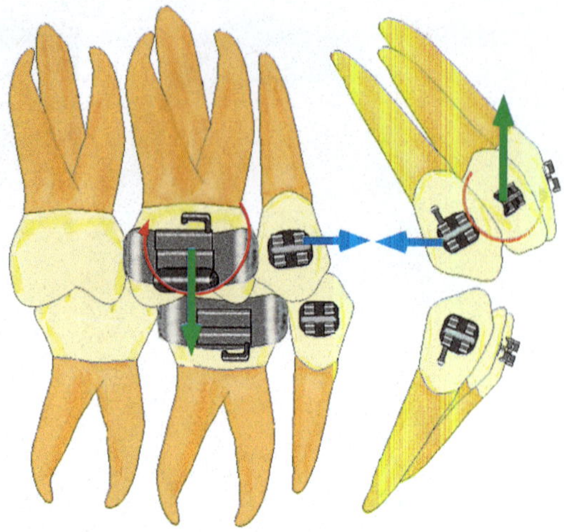

Figure 9-25 Differential moment force system in group A space closure is unfavorable for anterior open-bite correction. Vertical forces tend to accentuate the open bite.

Group A Space Closure Mechanics

Group A space closure is the most difficult to perform in patients with an anterior open bite if non-TAD-supported intraoral anchorage is desired. The use of differential moments to maintain anchorage in the force system results in a large moment and an extrusive force posteriorly. Anteriorly, a smaller moment and an intrusive force are generated. This force system is highly undesirable in patients with an open bite.[122] Figure 9-25 shows how the vertical forces are antagonistic with group A space closure. An alternative would be to use a one-couple system (intrusion arch) in which a couple is created at the level of the molar and an additional base archwire (0.018-inch stainless steel) is placed for canine sliding mechanics. The base arch would minimize the intrusive force in the anterior teeth and the moment from the intrusion arch would contribute to anchorage in the posterior end.

Another alternative is the extension of a rigid power arm from the band of the molar gingivally to its center of resistance (C_{RES}). From this arm a force is extended incisally to the canine. The same base archwire (0.018-inch stainless steel) as that just described for the intrusion arch mechanics can be used (Fig. 9-26). The effect would be differential tooth movement; the molar will bodily translate (more difficult tooth movement to achieve therefore it enhances anchorage) with the application of the force at the C_{RES} and the canine will tip (easier type of tooth movement). Although the mechanics of this method have positive effects on anchorage, the vector of the force has a slight negative extrusive component on the molar and a slight intrusive component on the canine.

Perhaps the best approach in space closure when group A anchorage is needed is the use of skeletal anchorage. The mini-screw or mini-plate can be used not only to prevent loss of molar anchorage but also to achieve intrusion of the posterior teeth if required.

Group B Space Closure Mechanics

Mechanically, Group B space closure is the simplest.[123] No vertical forces are generated and only two equal and opposite moments are needed (Fig. 9-27). Careful monitoring is essential to ensure that equal moment to force ratios are delivered to the anterior and posterior segments. If a high magnitude of force in relation to the moment is delivered in the posterior end, excessive crown tipping will result, extruding the distal cusps of the molar and possibly increasing the open bite.

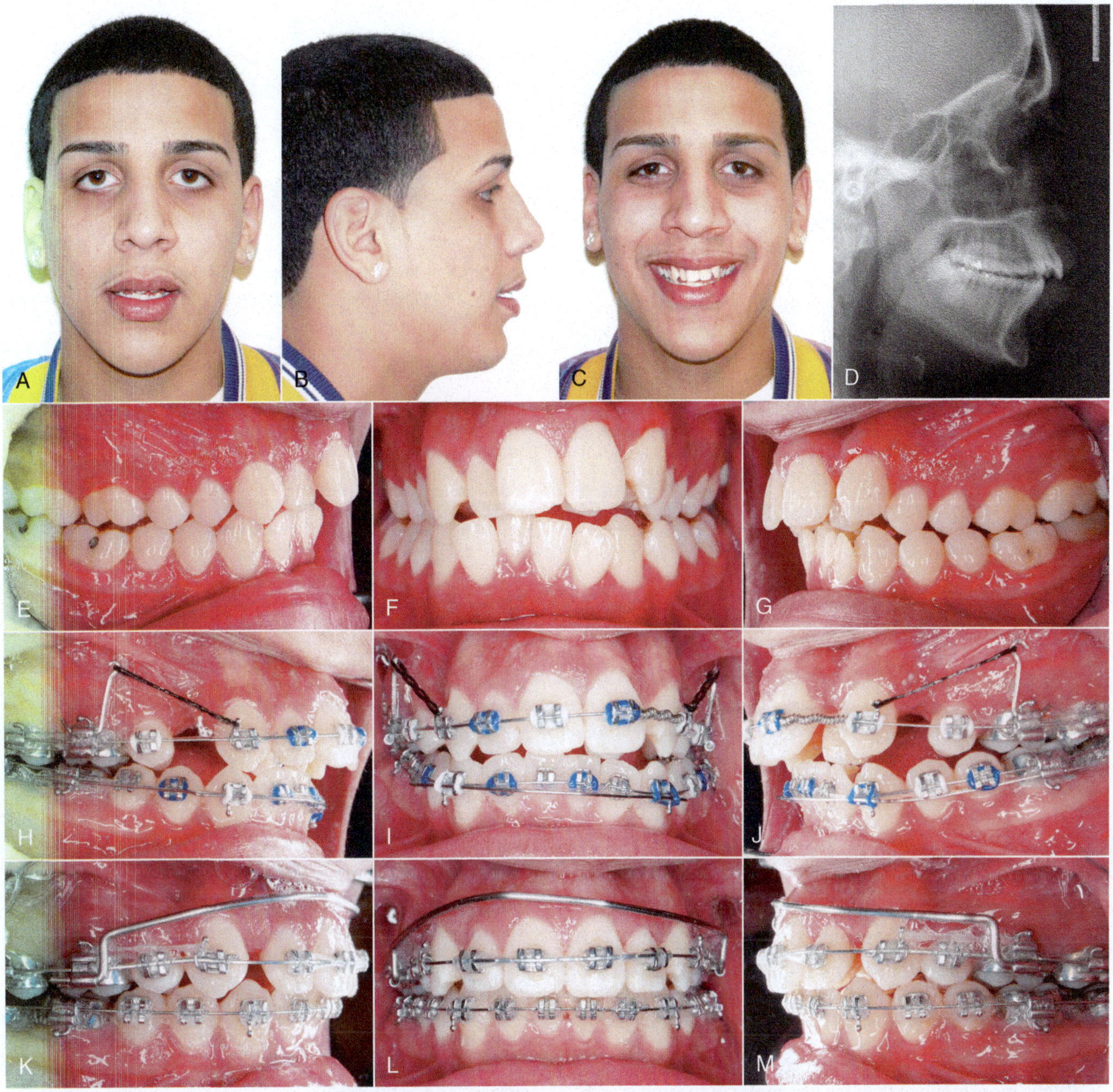

Figure 9-26 Alternative mechanics for Group A space closure. **A–G,** Initial records of a patient with a mild anterior open bite and a full cusp molar Class II occlusion. **H–J,** Retraction force extended from power arms in the maxillary first molars (promotes translation) to the crown of the canines (promotes tipping), resulting in differential anchorage. **K–M,** Progress showing canine retraction to Class I with minimal anchorage loss. Large-dimension labial bar from molar to molar was placed temporarily after the patient lost the transpalatal arch.

Group C Space Closure Mechanics

Group C space closure mechanics are the most favorable for correction of an anterior open bite. Intraoral anchorage by means of differential moments yields a consistent force system. Figure 9-28 shows a larger moment in the anterior segment and an extrusive force that will maintain the anteroposterior position of the incisor. A smaller moment in the posterior area and an intrusive force will allow this segment to tip as a mesial force is applied. The vertical forces will aid in closure of the anterior open bite.

Temporary anchorage devices such as mini-screws are also greatly indicated in this anchorage situation. Because the posterior teeth are protracted (if direct anchorage is used), the force vector has an intrusive component on these teeth that is beneficial to correction of the open bite.

Bonding Second Molars

Traditionally, orthodontists have thought that bonding the second molars in a patient with an open bite most likely would result in an increased open bite.[124] The reason for this

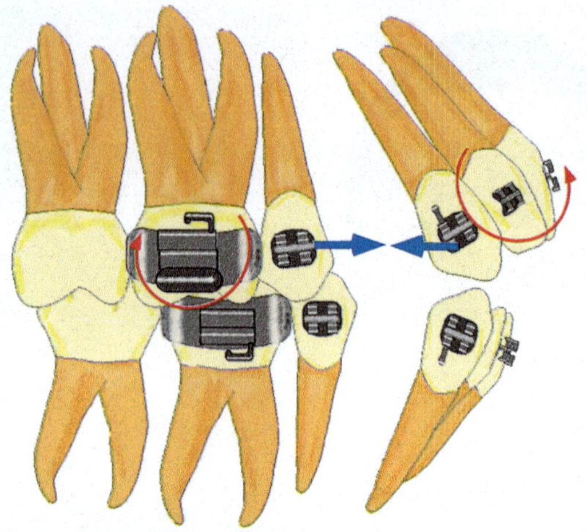

Figure 9-27 Mechanics for Group B space closure. Equal and opposite moments are favorable in anterior open-bite patients since no vertical forces are generated. Adequate moment to force ratios of approximately 10 to 1 are desired to prevent tipping of the posterior segments.

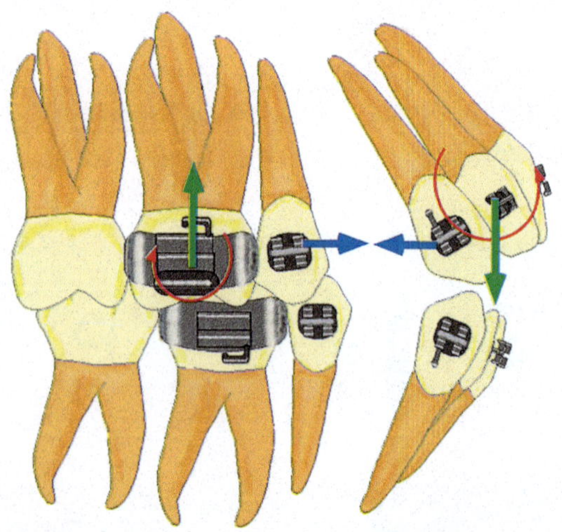

Figure 9-28 Mechanics for Group C space closure are the most favorable for open-bite correction. Vertical forces are consistent with the open-bite correction in the anterior (extrusive) and posterior (intrusive) segments.

is that as the second molar is incorporated into the arch, it is usually more gingival than the first molar in the upper arch and more occlusal in the lower arch (curve of Spee). When a straight wire is placed, a step geometry is generated, causing the lower first molar to supraerupt. Although the second molar experiences an intrusive force, intrusion seldom occurs, probably because of the magnitude of the force, which is lower than the threshold needed for intrusion. Additionally, a tip-forward moment is generated in the anterior segment that can open the bite (Fig. 9-29). In the upper arch the effect is extrusion of the second molar. If this extrusive force is not negated by the muscle forces, the mandible will rotate downward and backward (aggravating the open bite). The anterior moment generated is favorable for closure of the open bite but may be unfavorable for the esthetic objective, because the visibility of the incisor (incisor display) when the patient smiles will increase (Fig. 9-30). In summary, if alignment of the second molar is needed, care must be taken to engage the second molar passively in the second order.[124]

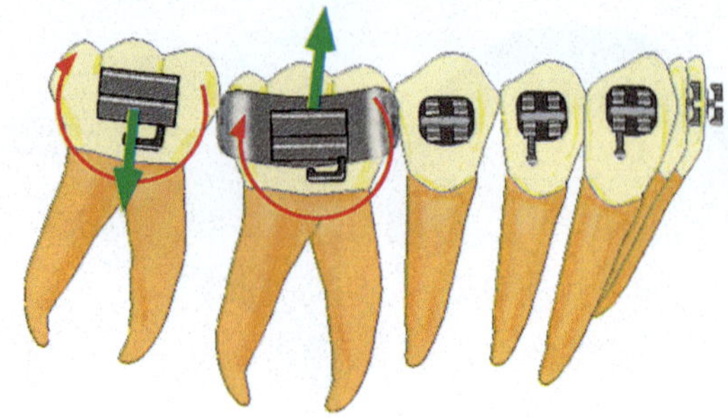

Figure 9-29 Force system resulting from bonding the lower second molars. The vertical forces and moments are antagonistic to the open-bite correction.

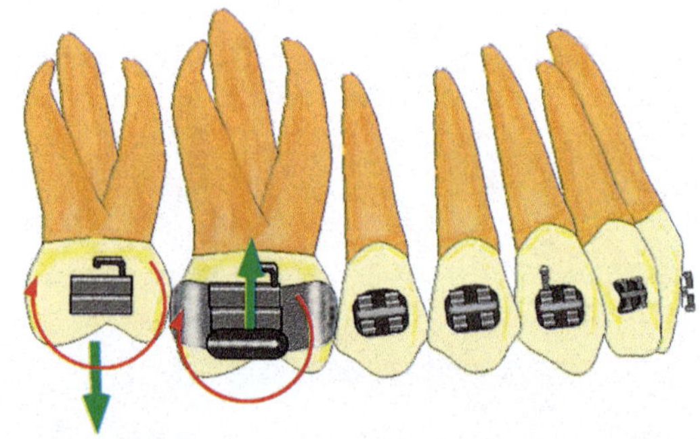

Figure 9-30 Force system resulting from bonding the upper second molars. Extrusive force generated in the upper second molars will accentuate the open bite. The anterior moment can cause overeruption of the incisors in detriment of the smile esthetics.

ESTHETICS AND OPEN BITE

The three major esthetic factors to consider when planning the correction of an open bite are the incisor display, the occlusal plane, and the interlabial gap. In patients with anteriorly divergent occlusal planes, deciding which occlusal plane to treat is important.[125] Depending on the decision, the treatment will be either orthodontics or a combination of surgery and orthodontics.

The functional occlusal plane in a patient with an open bite with two divergent occlusal planes anterior to the premolars is the limiting factor to the amount of correction that can be obtained with orthodontics. This functional occlusal plane dictates the position of the upper incisors within a 1- to 2-mm range vertically. The incisors must be erupted to this level to achieve a positive overbite. If the amount of incisor display at rest and during smiling is reduced, extrusion of the upper incisors is maintained until an acceptable level of display is achieved. Correction of the remaining amount of overbite can be achieved by extruding the lower incisors. In some instances this extrusion will accentuate the lower curve of Spee in an effort to obtain a positive overbite yet avoid excessive extrusion of the upper incisors.

To achieve additional vertical correction of the anterior segments, the functional occlusal plane must be modified by

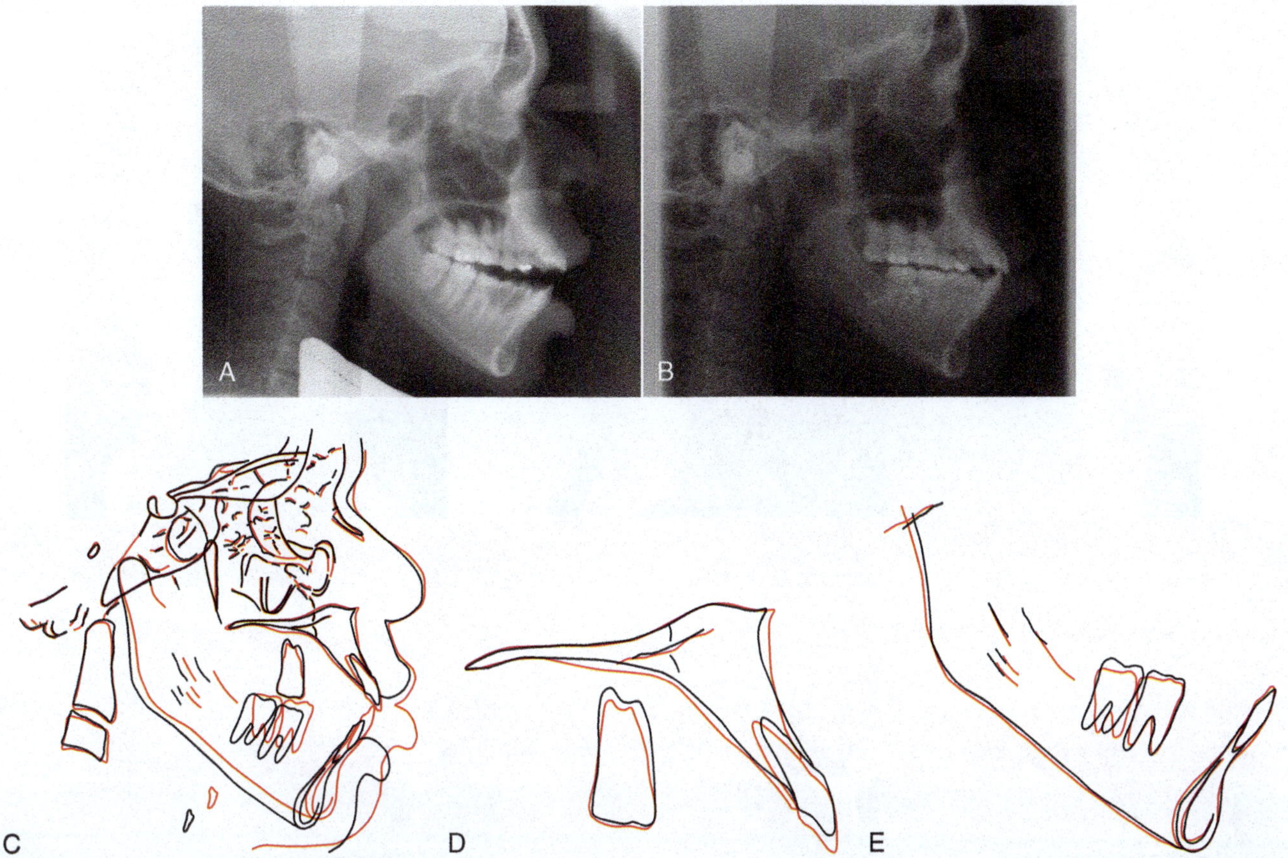

Figure 9-31 **A,** Pretreatment lateral cephalogram. **B,** Posttreatment lateral cephalogram. **C-E,** Superimposition showing counterclockwise rotation of the lower occlusal plane by intruding the lower molars via use of skeletal anchorage only in the lower arch. The net result is anterior open-bite reduction with mandibular autorotation.

using either a clockwise (steepening) or a counterclockwise movement. Steepening the occlusal plane can be somewhat easily achieved, although it is rarely desired. The reverse movement (counterclockwise rotation) is often indicated in skeletal open bites (Fig. 9-31) but unfortunately it can rarely be achieved by orthodontic means only. The long face patient with adequate or excessive gingival display and an anterior open bite is a good example of a patient for whom a counterclockwise rotation of the mandibular occlusal plane is recommended (Fig. 9-32). In this type of patient the upper incisors should be maintained or intruded and the upper occlusal plane should be either intruded or rotated in a clockwise direction.

Treatment planning for a patient with divergent occlusal planes from molar to molar requires careful consideration of the esthetics and the occlusion. A treatment occlusal plane must be selected between the upper plane, the lower plane, or an intermediate plane of occlusion. Generally, the upper plane, or a constructed plane bisecting the upper and lower occlusal planes, is considered. The lower occlusal plane is seldom used because doing so usually results in excessive incisor display and considerable extrusion of the upper buccal segments.

The upper occlusal plane is selected if the vertical relationship at the incisor (incisor display) and molar level is good. A surgical procedure is needed to rotate the mandible in a counterclockwise direction to match the upper plane. Because of the long-term instability of this surgical movement, a two-jaw surgery is usually done. The maxilla is impacted posteriorly with a center of rotation around the upper incisal edge. Some autorotation of the mandible follows and a minimal additional surgical counterclockwise rotation is performed to correct the anterior open bite. These movements can also be achieved to a lesser degree by using skeletal anchorage and orthodontics for molar intrusion.

The final major aspect related to esthetics in patients with an open bite is the interlabial gap. Excessive interlabial gap is one of the most notorious soft tissue characteristics of patients with skeletal open bites. This problem can be addressed in two ways. First, the interlabial gap can be reduced by retracting the upper and lower incisors, although the magnitude of the vertical lip change in response to the incisor retraction can be unpredictable. The other alternative is to reduce the posterior facial height.

During growth, the posterior facial height can be decreased by the methods described earlier that control the dentoalveolar molar eruption. Once growth ceases, the interlabial gap can be reduced by using molar intrusion (via maxillary impaction with mandibular autorotation or implants) or sliding genioplasty. Sliding genioplasty provides an additional advantage in patients with vertical dysplasia. The procedure not only reduces the anterior vertical height but also

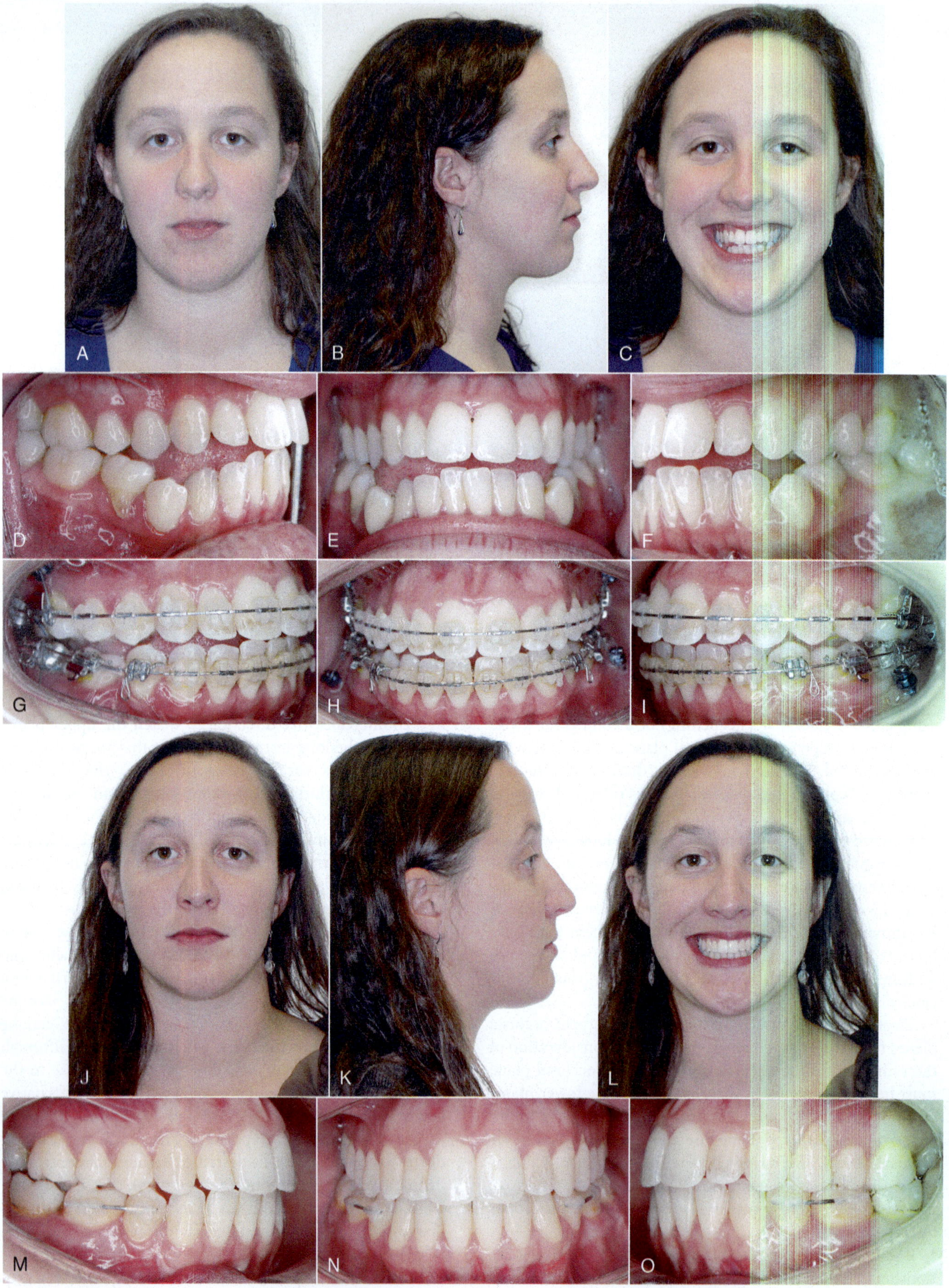

Figure 9-32 **A–F,** Lateral and anterior open bite in an adult patient with congenitally missing second premolars. **G–I,** Treatment plan included closure of the remnant space after extraction of the deciduous second molars and four mini-screws to intrude the posterior segments. **J–O,** Final records show improved smile esthetics without increasing the incisor display at smile. Gingival display of the maxillary buccal segments was reduced and a good smile arc was obtained. Adequate overbite and buccal occlusion were achieved.

allows a more anterior positioning of the chin (limited invasive surgical procedure with good esthetic result) (see Chapter 21).

Finally, of note, the interlabial gap per se is not an indication of vertical skeletal dysplasia. Evaluating the length and characteristics of the lips is important because lip lengthening procedures can be used to reduce the interlabial gap in patients who do not have vertical skeletal excess.[126]

STABILITY AND RETENTION

The management and retention of the obtained results brought about by treatment of the malocclusion in the vertical dimension are challenging because the etiology is multifactorial, involving hereditary, skeletal, dental, respiratory, and habitual factors.[127] The stability of treatment in growing and nongrowing patients with hyperdivergent facial patterns depends on the clinician's ability to address the cause of the malocclusion. Elimination of habits, weak musculature, and respiratory obstructions might decrease the rate and severity of relapse. Various protocols have been used, with a 67% to 100% success rate, in the early management of patients with hyperdivergent facial patterns.[128] Although these appliances have been effective in correcting the skeletal open bite in growing patients, long-term follow-up studies are lacking. Because the hyperdivergent growth pattern is established early and subsequently maintained until adulthood, only long-term clinical studies will help in precisely understanding the consequences of early treatment in the growth of these patients.[129]

In a 10-year follow-up[130] of patients with anterior open bite who were treated orthodontically, 35% of treated patients had a relapse of 3-mm or more. The relapse group had deficient mandibular anterior dental height, deficient upper anterior facial height, increased lower anterior facial height, and deficient posterior facial height. However, the amount of open bite, the angle of facial divergence (mandibular plane angle), and other parameters before treatment were not found to be valid predictors for post-treatment relapse. In one study[131] the long-term stability of the corrected open bite was greater in patients treated with extraction than in patients who did not have extraction. However, the open bite was not the reason for extraction in these patients. Among the extraction group, 74% of the patients had a stable open-bite correction 8 years after treatment.[132]

Analysis of various long-term studies indicates that orthognathic surgery is an effective method for the management of anterior open bite. Superior repositioning of maxilla by one-piece Le Fort I osteotomy is considered one of the most stable procedures in the hierarchy of stability. Whenever indicated, even the three-piece Le Fort I osteotomy is a stable procedure.[133] According to a meta-analysis,[127] correction of an open bite via surgery is prone to some amount of relapse, although the long-term stability was greater than 75%. Possible reasons for postoperative relapse are preoperative orthodontic treatment, type of surgery, type of surgical fixation, condylar positioning during bimaxillary surgery, growth after surgery, and finally the soft tissue adaptation.[134] Moderate skeletal changes after surgery are common in the long-term; however, minimal effects in the overbite are due to compensatory eruption of the incisors.[134]

The introduction of TADs has enabled orthodontists to intrude the maxillary and mandibular molars, correcting the anterior open bite nonsurgically and obtaining adequate long-term stability (Fig. 9-33). Lee and Park,[135] who used mini-screws to intrude maxillary molars, reported a 10.36% relapse rate for the intruded molars and an 18% relapse of overbite after 18 months in retention. Sugawara et al.[107] reported a 30% relapse rate after intrusion of mandibular molars 12 months after treatment. In a 3-year long-term stability study by Baek et al.[136] in patients who had intrusion of maxillary molars, the relapse rates were 23% for intruded molars and 17% for overbite. A total of 80% of the relapse of maxillary molars occurred in the first year of retention. Relapse of maxillary molars after treatment leads to clockwise rotation of the mandible, an increase in anterior facial height, and a change in the pogonion in a downward and backward direction. However, compensatory eruption of maxillary anterior teeth occurred during the first and third years, events that subsequently maintained the overbite. The major relapse of maxillary molars occurs in the first year after intrusion with mini-screws.

An effective method of retention is recommended to improve the long-term stability of molar intrusion with skeletal anchorage. However, an appropriate protocol for retention of an intruded tooth is lacking. Baek et al.[136] advocate using an active retainer, which consists of a clear vacuum-formed retainer with buttons attached to either the buccal or the palatal side of the maxillary molar. Elastics can be engaged from the mini-screws or mini-plates to the buttons.

Positioners are routinely suggested during the retention phase. The elasticity of positioners between the molars applies an intrusive force through daily chewing exercises.[137] Deguchi et al.[138] recommend the use of myofunctional appliances because muscular imbalance has also been attributed to relapse of a treated anterior open bite. Masticatory muscle exercise involving a chewing gum or soft bite wafer during retention might aid in retaining the obtained result.[139]

SUMMARY

The etiology of the long face and anterior open-bite malocclusions is multifactorial. Distinguishing between a dentoalveolar and a skeletal open bite is important. Treatments to correct this malocclusion rely mainly on the molar vertical control and/or extrusion of the anterior segments in growing patients. With the advent of implant anchorage, skeletofacial changes can also be obtained with molar intrusion in nongrowing patients. If esthetic results are desired in patients with severe long face morphology, surgical options should be explored. Although all of these treatments provide the possibility of attaining satisfactory outcomes, long-term stability remains the major challenge regardless of the therapy chosen.

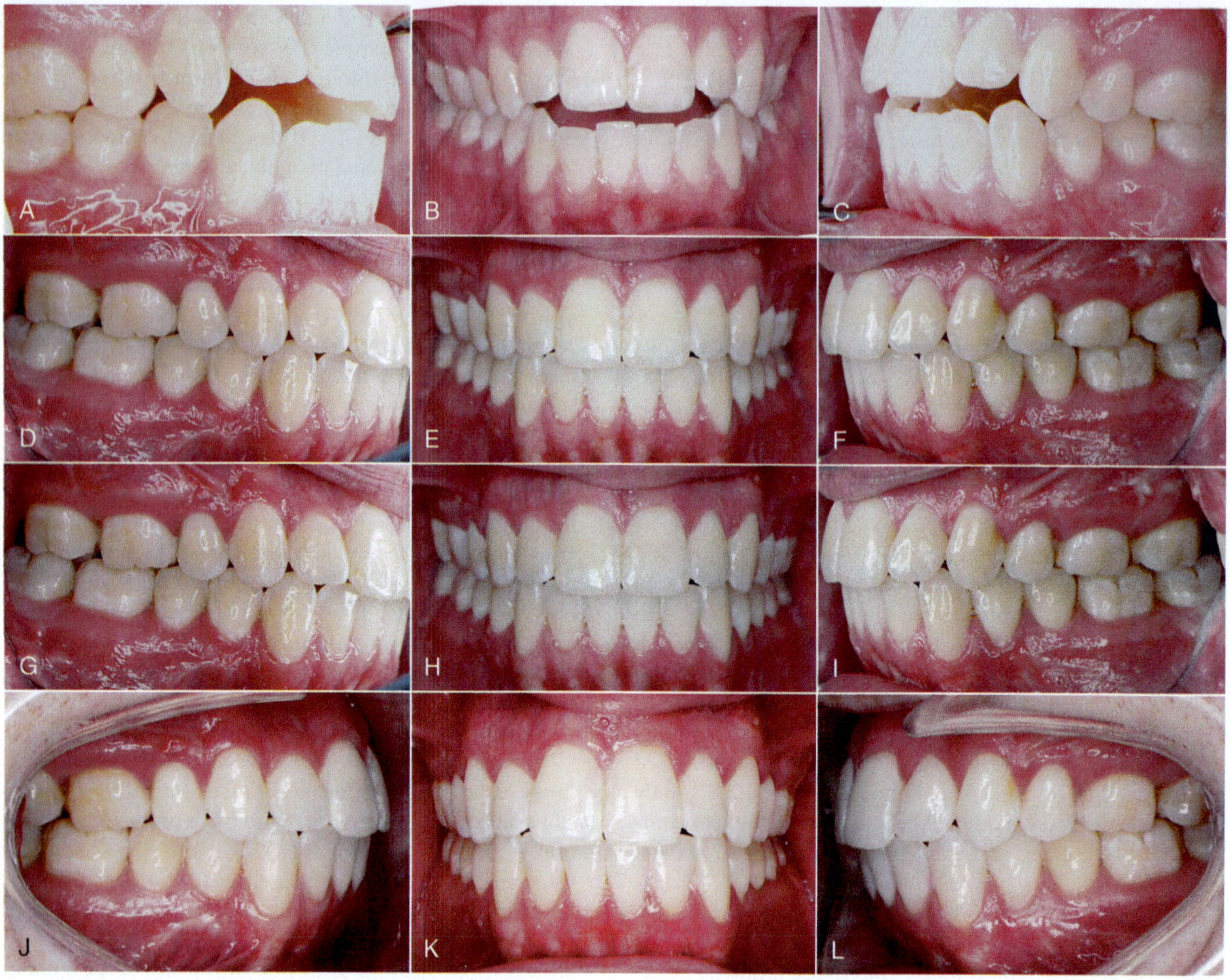

Figure 9-33 **A–C,** Pre-treatment intraoral views of a patient with an anterior open bite that relapsed after orthodontic treatment. **D–F,** Final intraoral views of the patient treated by intrusion of upper and lower buccal segments by means of skeletal anchorage without extrusion of the incisors. **G–I,** Intraoral views 1 year after debonding show very good stability of the anterior open-bite correction. **J-L,** Intraoral views 3 years after debonding show very good stability of treatment.

REFERENCES

1. Ellis E 3rd, McNamara JA Jr. Components of adult Class III open-bite malocclusion. *Am J Orthod.* 1984;86(4):277–290.
2. Sassouni V, Nanda S. Analysis of dentofacial vertical proportions. *Am J Orthod.* 1964;50(11):801–823.
3. Schudy FF. Cant of the occlusal plane and axial inclinations of teeth. *Angle Orthod.* 1963;33(2):69–82.
4. Sassouni V. A classification of skeletal facial types. *Am J Orthod.* 1969;55(2):109–123.
5. Schudy FF. Vertical growth versus anteroposterior growth as related to function and treatment. *Angle Orthod.* 1964;34(2):75–93.
6. Nanda SK. Patterns of vertical growth in the face. *Am J Orthod Dentofacial Orthop.* 1988;93(2):103–116.
7. Parker JH. The interception of the open bite in the early growth period. *Angle Orthod.* 1971;41(1):24–44.
8. Björk A. Prediction of mandibular growth rotation. *Am J Orthod.* 1969;55(6):585–599.
9. Mizrahi E. A review of anterior open bite. *Br J Orthod.* 1978;5(1): 21–27.
10. Ngan P, Fields HW. Open bite: a review of etiology and management. *Pediatr Dent.* 1997;19(2):91–98.
11. Schendel SA, Eisenfeld J, Bell WH, Epker BN, Mishelevich DJ. The long face syndrome: vertical maxillary excess. *Am J Orthod.* 1976; 70(4):398–408.
12. Dung DJ, Smith RJ. Cephalometric and clinical diagnoses of open bite tendency. *Am J Orthod Dentofacial Orthop.* 1988;94(6):484–490.
13. Isaacson JR, Isaacson RJ, Speidel TM, Worms FW. Extreme variation in vertical facial growth and associated variation in skeletal and dental relations. *Angle Orthod.* 1971;41(3):219–229.
14. Cangialosi TJ. Skeletal morphologic features of anterior open bite. *Am J Orthod.* 1984;85(1):28–36.
15. Kim YH. Anterior openbite and its treatment with multiloop edgewise archwire. *Angle Orthod.* 1987;57(4):290–321.
16. Vargervik K, Miller AJ, Chierici G, Harvold E, Tomer BS. Morphologic response to changes in neuromuscular patterns experimentally induced by altered modes of respiration. *Am J Orthod.* 1984;85(2): 115–124.
17. Harvold EP, Tomer BS, Vargervik K, Chierici G. Primate experiments on oral respiration. *Am J Orthod.* 1981;79(4):359–372.
18. Vig KWL. Nasal obstruction and facial growth: the strength of evidence for clinical assumptions. *Am J Orthod Dentofacial Orthop.* 1998;113(6):603–611.

19. Fields HW, Warren DW, Black K, Phillips CL. Relationship between vertical dentofacial morphology and respiration in adolescents. *Am J Orthod Dentofacial Orthop.* 1991;99(2):147–154.
20. Shanker S, Fields HW, Beck F, Vig P, Vig K. A longitudinal assessment of upper respiratory function and dentofacial morphology in 8- to 12-year-old children. *Semin Orthod.* 2004;10:45–53.
21. Souki BQ, Pimenta GB, Franco LP, Becker HMG, Pinto JA. Changes in vertical dentofacial morphology after adeno-/tonsillectomy during deciduous and mixed dentitions mouth breathing children—1 year follow-up study. *Int J Pediatr Otorhinolaryngol.* 2010;74(6):626.
22. Alves M Jr, Franzotti ES, Baratieri C, et al. Evaluation of pharyngeal airway space amongst different skeletal patterns. *Int J Oral Maxillofac Surg.* 2012;41(7):814–819.
23. Grauer D, Cevidanes LSH, Styner MA, Ackerman JL, Proffit WR. Pharyngeal airway volume and shape from cone-beam computed tomography: relationship to facial morphology. *Am J Orthod Dentofacial Orthop.* 2009;136(6):805–814.
24. Joseph AA, Elbaum J, Cisneros GJ, Eisig SB. A cephalometric comparative study of the soft tissue airway dimensions in persons with hyperdivergent and normodivergent facial patterns. *J Oral Maxillofac Surg.* 1998;56(2):135–139; discussion 139–140.
25. Muto T, Yamazaki A, Takeda S. A cephalometric evaluation of the pharyngeal airway space in patients with mandibular retrognathia and prognathia, and normal subjects. *Int J Oral Maxillofac Surg.* 2008; 37(3):228–231.
26. Muto T, Yamazaki A, Takeda S, et al. Relationship between the pharyngeal airway space and craniofacial morphology, taking into account head posture. *Int J Oral Maxillofac Surg.* 2006;35(2):132–136.
27. Guijarro-Martinez R, Swennen G. Cone-beam computerized tomography imaging and analysis of the upper airway: a systematic review of the literature. *Int J Oral Maxillofac Surg.* 2011;40(11):1227–1237.
28. Alves M, Baratieri C, Nojima LI, Nojima MCG, Ruellas ACO. Three-dimensional assessment of pharyngeal airway in nasal-and mouth-breathing children. *Int J Pediatr Otorhinolaryngol.* 2011;75(9): 1195–1199.
29. Alsufyani N, Flores-Mir C, Major P. Three-dimensional segmentation of the upper airway using cone beam CT: a systematic review. *Dentomaxillofac Radiol.* 2012;41(4):276–284.
30. Pepicelli A, Woods M, Briggs C. The mandibular muscles and their importance in orthodontics: a contemporary review. *Am J Orthod Dentofacial Orthop.* 2005;128(6):774–780.
31. Van Spronsen P. Long-face craniofacial morphology: cause or effect of weak masticatory musculature? *Semin Orthod.* 2010;16: 99–117.
32. Proffit W, Fields H, Nixon W. Occlusal forces in normal- and long-face adults. *J Dent Res.* 1983;62(5):566–570.
33. Ingervall B, Helkimo E. Masticatory muscle force and facial morphology in man. *Arch Oral Biol.* 1978;23(3):203–206.
34. Proffit W, Fields H. Occlusal forces in normal- and long-face children. *J Dent Res.* 1983;62(5):571–574.
35. Rowlerson A, Raoul G, Daniel Y, et al. Fiber-type differences in masseter muscle associated with different facial morphologies. *Am J Orthod Dentofacial Orthop.* 2005;127(1):37–46.
36. Miyamoto K, Yamada K, Ishizuka Y, Morimoto N, Tanne K. Masseter muscle activity during the whole day in young adults. *Am J Orthod Dentofacial Orthop.* 1996;110(4):394–398.
37. Boom H, Van Spronsen P, Van Ginkel F, et al. A comparison of human jaw muscle cross-sectional area and volume in long- and short-face subjects, using MRI. *Arch Oral Biol.* 2008;53(3):273–281.
38. Ueda HM, Ishizuka Y, Miyamoto K, Morimoto N, Tanne K. Relationship between masticatory muscle activity and vertical craniofacial morphology. *Angle Orthod.* 1998;68(3):233–238.
39. Bishara SE, Ortho D, Jakobsen JR. Longitudinal changes in three normal facial types. *Am J Orthod.* 1985;88(6):466–502.
40. Nanda SK. Growth patterns in subjects with long and short faces. *Am J Orthod Dentofacial Orthop.* 1990;98(3):247–258.
41. Winders RV. Forces exerted on the dentition by the perioral and lingual musculature during swallowing. *Angle Orthod.* 1958;28: 226–235.
42. Proffit WR. The etiology of orthodontic problems. In: Proffit WR, ed. *Contemporary Orthodontics.* 3rd ed. St. Louis, MO: Mosby; 2000: 113–144.
43. Larsson E. Dummy- and finger-sucking habits with special attention to their significance for facial growth and occlusion. 4. effect on facial growth and occlusion. *Sven Tandlak Tidskr.* 1972;65(12):605–634.
44. Welch KC, Foster GD, Ritter CT, et al. A novel volumetric magnetic resonance imaging paradigm to study upper airway anatomy. *Sleep.* 2002;25(5):532–542.
45. Wolford LM, Cottrell DA. Diagnosis of macroglossia and indications for reduction glossectomy. *Am J Orthod Dentofacial Orthop.* 1996; 110(2):170–177.
46. Proffit WR. Equilibrium theory revisited: factors influencing position of the teeth. *Angle Orthod.* 1978;48(3):175–186.
47. Akin E, Sayin MO, Karaçay S, Bulakbaşi N. Real-time balanced turbo field echo cine-magnetic resonance imaging evaluation of tongue movements during deglutition in subjects with anterior open bite. *Am J Orthod Dentofacial Orthop.* 2006;129(1):24.
48. Fukuta O, Braham RL, Yokoi K, Kurosu K. Damage to the primary dentition resulting from thumb and finger (digit) sucking. *ASDC J Dent Child.* 1996;63(6):403–407.
49. Cozza P, Baccetti T, Franchi L, Mucedero M, Polimeni A. Sucking habits and facial hyperdivergency as risk factors for anterior open bite in the mixed dentition. *Am J Orthod Dentofacial Orthop.* 2005; 128(4):517–519.
50. McElroy S. *Bjork Predictors of Mandibular Rotation and Their Relationship to Anterior Open Bite Treatment.* Farmington, CT: University of Connecticut; 1998.
51. Proffit WR, Fields HW. Orthodontic treatment planning: from problem list to specific plan. In: Proffit WR, ed. *Contemporary Orthodontics.* 3rd ed. St. Louis, MO: Mosby; 2000:196–239.
52. Wolford LM, Cardenas L. Idiopathic condylar resorption: diagnosis, treatment protocol, and outcomes. *Am J Orthod Dentofacial Orthop.* 1999;116(6):667–677.
53. Ronchezel MV, Hilario MO, Goldenberg J, et al. Temporomandibular joint and mandibular growth alterations in patients with juvenile rheumatoid arthritis. *J Rheumatol.* 1995;22(10):1956–1961.
54. Hartsfield JK. Development of the vertical dimension. *Semin Orthod.* 2002;8(3):113–119.
55. Nanda SK. Patterns of vertical growth in the face. *Am J Orthod Dentofacial Orthop.* 1988;93(2):103–116.
56. Bishara SE. Facial and dental changes in adolescents and their clinical implications. *Angle Orthod.* 2000;70(6):471–483.
57. Klocke A, Nanda RS, Kahl-Nieke B. Anterior open bite in the deciduous dentition: longitudinal follow-up and craniofacial growth considerations. *Am J Orthod Dentofacial Orthop.* 2002;122(4):353–358.
58. Ari-Viro A, Wisth PJ. An evaluation of the method of structural growth prediction. *Eur J Orthod.* 1983;5(3):199–207.
59. Lee RS, Daniel FJ, Swartz M, Baumrind S, Korn EL. Assessment of a method for the prediction of mandibular rotation. *Am J Orthod Dentofacial Orthop.* 1987;91(5):395–402.
60. Klein ET. The thumb-sucking habit: meaningful or empty? *Am J Orthod.* 1971;59(3):283–289.
61. AlEmran SE. A new method in reminder therapy technique for ceasing digit sucking habit in children. *J Clin Pediatr Dent.* 2000; 24(4):261–263.
62. Sayin MÖ, Akin E, Karaçay S, Bulakbasi N. Initial effects of the tongue crib on tongue movements during deglutition. *Angle Orthod.* 2006;76(3):400–405.
63. Taslan S, Biren S, Ceylanoglu C. Tongue pressure changes before, during and after crib appliance therapy. *Angle Orthod.* 2010;80(3): 533–539.

64. Cozza P, Baccetti T, Franchi L, McNamara JA. Treatment effects of a modified quad-helix in patients with dentoskeletal open bites. *Am J Orthod Dentofacial Orthop*. 2006;129(6):734–739.
65. Cayley AS, Tindall AP, Sampson WJ, Butcher AR. Electropalatographic and cephalometric assessment of myofunctional therapy in open-bite subjects. *Aust Orthod J*. 2000;16(1):23–33.
66. Frankel R, Frankel C. A functional approach to treatment of skeletal open bite. *Am J Orthod*. 1983;84(1):54–68.
67. Wang J, Goodger NM, Pogrel MA. The role of tongue reduction. *Oral Surg Oral Med Oral Pathol Oral Radiol Endod*. 2003;95(3):269–273.
68. Linder-Aronson S, Woodside DG, Lundstrom A. Mandibular growth direction following adenoidectomy. *Am J Orthod*. 1986;89(4):273–284.
69. Linder-Aronson S, Woodside DG, Hellsing E, Emerson W. Normalization of incisor position after adenoidectomy. *Am J Orthod Dentofacial Orthop*. 1993;103(5):412–427.
70. Nanda R, Marzban R, Kuhlberg A. The Connecticut Intrusion Arch. *J Clin Orthod*. 1998;32(12):708–715.
71. Isaacson RJ, Lindauer SJ. Closing anterior open bites: the extrusion arch. *Semin Orthod*. 2001;7:34–41.
72. Kim YH, Han UK, Lim DD, Serraon ML. Stability of anterior open-bite correction with multiloop edgewise archwire therapy: a cephalometric follow-up study. *Am J Orthod Dentofacial Orthop*. 2000;118(1):43–54.
73. Cozza P, Mucedero M, Baccetti T, Franchi L. Early orthodontic treatment of skeletal open-bite malocclusion: a systematic review. *Angle Orthod*. 2005;75(5):707–713.
74. Worms FW, Meskin LH, Isaacson RJ. Open-bite. *Am J Orthod*. 1971;59(6):589–595.
75. Baumrind S, Korn EL, Molthen R, West EE. Changes in facial dimensions associated with the use of forces to retract the maxilla. *Am J Orthod*. 1981;80(1):17–30.
76. Brown P. A cephalometric evaluation of high-pull molar headgear and face-bow neck strap therapy. *Am J Orthod*. 1978;74(6):621–632.
77. Cook AH, Sellke TA, BeGole EA. Control of the vertical dimension in Class II correction using a cervical headgear and lower utility arch in growing patients: part I. *Am J Orthod Dentofacial Orthop*. 1994;106(4):376–388.
78. Ulger G, Arun T, Sayinsu K, Isik F. The role of cervical headgear and lower utility arch in the control of the vertical dimension. *Am J Orthod Dentofacial Orthop*. 2006;130(4):492–501.
79. Haralabakis NB, Sifakakis IB. The effect of cervical headgear on patients with high or low mandibular plane angles and the "myth" of posterior mandibular rotation. *Am J Orthod Dentofacial Orthop*. 2004;126(3):310–317.
80. Burke M, Jacobson A. Vertical changes in high-angle Class II, Division 1 patients treated with cervical or occipital pull headgear. *Am J Orthod Dentofacial Orthop*. 1992;102(6):501–508.
81. Altuna G, Woodside DG. Response of the midface to treatment with increased vertical occlusal forces: treatment and posttreatment effects in monkeys. *Angle Orthod*. 1985;55(3):251–263.
82. Iscan HN, Sarisoy L. Comparison of the effects of passive posterior bite-blocks with different construction bites on the craniofacial and dentoalveolar structures. *Am J Orthod Dentofacial Orthop*. 1997;112(2):171–178.
83. Dellinger EL. A clinical assessment of the Active Vertical Corrector: a nonsurgical alternative for skeletal open bite treatment. *Am J Orthod*. 1986;89(5):428–436.
84. McNamara JA Jr. An experimental study of increased vertical dimension in the growing face. *Am J Orthod*. 1977;71(4):382–395.
85. Pearson LE. Vertical control in treatment of patients having backward-rotational growth tendencies. *Angle Orthod*. 1978;48(2):132–140.
86. Pearson LE. Case report KP: treatment of a severe openbite excessive vertical pattern with an eclectic non-surgical approach. *Angle Orthod*. 1991;61(1):71–76.
87. Pearson LE. Vertical control in fully-banded orthodontic treatment. *Angle Orthod*. 1986;56(3):205–224.
88. Iscan HN, Dincer M, Gultan A, Meral O, Taner-Sarisoy L. Effects of vertical chincap therapy on the mandibular morphology in open-bite patients. *Am J Orthod Dentofacial Orthop*. 2002;122(5):506–511.
89. Parks LR, Buschang PH, Alexander RA, Dechow P, Rossouw PE. Masticatory exercise as an adjunctive treatment for hyperdivergent patients. *Angle Orthod*. 2007;77(3):457–462.
90. English JD, Olfert KDG. Masticatory muscle exercise as an adjunctive treatment for open bite malocclusions. *Semin Orthod*. 2005;11(3):164–169.
91. Spyropoulos M. An early approach for the interception of skeletal open bite: a preliminary report. *J Pedod*. 1985;9(3):200.
92. Ingervall B, Bitsanis E. A pilot study of the effect of masticatory muscle training on facial growth in long-face children. *Eur J Orthod*. 1987;9(1):15–23.
93. Insoft MD, Hocevar RA, Gibbs CH. The nonsurgical treatment of a Class II open bite malocclusion. *Am J Orthod Dentofacial Orthop*. 1996;110(6):598–605.
94. Yamaguchi K. Etiological and therapeutic considerations with open bite. In: Nanda R, Kapila S, eds. *Current Therapy in Orthodontics*. 1st ed. St. Louis, MO: Mosby; 2010:159–170.
95. Bakke M, Siersbaek-Nielsen S. Training of mandibular elevator muscles in subjects with anterior open bite. *Eur J Orthod*. 1990;2:502.
96. DeBerardinis M, Stretesky T, Sinha P, Nanda RS. Evaluation of the vertical holding appliance in treatment of high-angle patients. *Am J Orthod Dentofacial Orthop*. 2000;117(6):700–705.
97. Chiba Y, Motoyoshi M, Namura S. Tongue pressure on loop of transpalatal arch during deglutition. *Am J Orthod Dentofacial Orthop*. 2003;123(1):29–34.
98. Kuroda S, Sakai Y, Tamamura N, Deguchi T, Takano-Yamamoto T. Treatment of severe anterior open bite with skeletal anchorage in adults: comparison with orthognathic surgery outcomes. *Am J Orthod Dentofacial Orthop*. 2007;132(5):599–605.
99. Proffit WR, Bailey LJ, Phillips C, Turvey TA. Long-term stability of surgical open-bite correction by Le Fort I osteotomy. *Angle Orthod*. 2000;70(2):112–117.
100. Swinnen K, Politis C, Willems G, et al. Skeletal and dento-alveolar stability after surgical-orthodontic treatment of anterior open bite: a retrospective study. *Eur J Orthod*. 2001;23(5):547–557.
101. Leung MTC, Lee TCK, Rabie ABM, Wong RWK. Use of miniscrews and miniplates in orthodontics. *J Oral Maxillofac Surg*. 2008;66(7):1461–1466.
102. Lin JC, Yeh CL, Liou EJ, Bowman SJ. Treatment of skeletal-origin gummy smiles with miniscrew anchorage. *J Clin Orthod*. 2008;42(5):285–296.
103. Buschang PH, Carrillo R, Rossouw PE. Orthopedic correction of growing hyperdivergent, retrognathic patients with miniscrew implants. *J Oral Maxillofac Surg*. 2011;69(3):754–762.
104. Sherwood KH, Burch JG, Thompson WJ. Closing anterior open bites by intruding molars with titanium miniplate anchorage. *Am J Orthod Dentofacial Orthop*. 2002;122(6):593–600.
105. Umemori M, Sugawara J, Mitani H, Nagasaka H, Kawamura H. Skeletal anchorage system for open-bite correction. *Am J Orthod Dentofacial Orthop*. 1999;115(2):166–174.
106. Kravitz N, Kusnoto B, Tsay T, Hohlt W. The use of temporary anchorage devices for molar intrusion. *J Am Dent Assoc*. 2007;138(1):56.
107. Sugawara J, Baik UB, Umemori M, et al. Treatment and posttreatment dentoalveolar changes following intrusion of mandibular molars with application of a skeletal anchorage system (SAS) for open bite correction. *Int J Adult Orthodon Orthognath Surg*. 2002;17(4):243.
108. Billiet T, De Pauw G, Dermaut L. Location of the centre of resistance of the upper dentition and the nasomaxillary complex: an experimental study. *Eur J Orthod*. 2001;23(3):263–273.

109. Jeong GM, Sung SJ, Lee KJ, Chun YS, Mo SS. Finite-element investigation of the center of resistance of the maxillary dentition. *Korean J Orthod.* 2009;39(2):83–94.

110. Çifter M, Saraç M. Maxillary posterior intrusion mechanics with mini-implant anchorage evaluated with the finite element method. *Am J Orthod Dentofacial Orthop.* 2011;140(5):e233–e241.

111. Mojdehi M, Buschang PH, English JD, Wolford LM. Postsurgical growth changes in the mandible of adolescents with vertical maxillary excess growth pattern. *Am J Orthod Dentofacial Orthop.* 2001;119(2):106–116.

112. Washburn MC, Schendel SA, Epker BN. Superior repositioning of the maxilla during growth. *J Oral Maxillofac Surg.* 1982;40(3):142–149.

113. Nanda R, Bouayad O, Topazian RG. Facial growth subsequent to Le Fort I osteotomies in adolescent monkeys. *J Oral Maxillofac Surg.* 1987;45(2):123–136.

114. Mogavero FJ, Buschang PH, Wolford LM. Orthognathic surgery effects on maxillary growth in patients with vertical maxillary excess. *Am J Orthod Dentofacial Orthop.* 1997;111(3):288–296.

115. Freihofer HPM, Björk G, Jönsson E, Kuijpers-Jagtman AM. Timing of facial osteotomies: a consensus conference. *Oral Surg Oral Med Oral Pathol.* 1994;78(4):432–436.

116. Cusimano C, McLaughlin RP, Zernik JH. Effects of first bicuspid extractions on facial height in high-angle cases. *J Clin Orthod.* 1993;27(11):594–598.

117. Kusnoto B, Schneider BJ. Control of vertical dimension. *Semin Orthod.* 2000;6(1):33–42.

118. Bishara SE, Ortho D, Burkey PS. Second molar extractions: a review. *Am J Orthod.* 1986;89(5):415–424.

119. Aras A. Vertical changes following orthodontic extraction treatment in skeletal open bite subjects. *Eur J Orthod.* 2002;24(4):407–416.

120. Vaden JL. Nonsurgical treatment of the patient with vertical discrepancy. *Am J Orthod Dentofacial Orthop.* 1998;113(5):567–582.

121. Sarver DM, Weissman SM. Nonsurgical treatment of open bite in nongrowing patients. *Am J Orthod Dentofacial Orthop.* 1995;108(6):651–659.

122. Braun S. Biomechanical considerations in the management of the vertical dimension. *Semin Orthod.* 2002;8(3):149–154.

123. Nanda R, Kuhlberg A. Biomechanical basis of extraction space closure. In: Nanda R, ed. *Biomechanics in Clinical Orthodontics*. Philadelphia, PA: WB Saunders; 1996:156–187.

124. Beane RA Jr. Nonsurgical management of the anterior open bite: a review of the options. *Semin Orthod.* 1999;5(4):275–283.

125. Burstone CJ, Marcotte MR. *The Treatment Occlusal Plane: Problem Solving in Orthodontics*. Chicago, IL: Quintessence Publishing Co, Inc; 2000:31–50.

126. Sarver D, Rousso D, White R. Adjunctive esthetic surgery. In: Proffit WR, ed. *Contemporary Treatment of Dentofacial Deformity*. St. Louis, MO: Mosby; 2003:394–415.

127. Greenlee GM, Huang GJ, Chen SSH, et al. Stability of treatment for anterior open-bite malocclusion: a meta-analysis. *Am J Orthod Dentofacial Orthop.* 2011;139(2):154–169.

128. Cozza P, Mucedero M, Baccetti T, Franchi L. Early orthodontic treatment of skeletal open-bite malocclusion. *Angle Orthod.* 2005;75(5):707–713.

129. Buschang PH, Sankey W, English JP. Early treatment of hyperdivergent open-bite malocclusions. *Semin Orthod.* 2002;8(3):130–140.

130. Lopez-Gavito G, Wallen TR, Little RM, Joondeph DR. Anterior open-bite malocclusion: a longitudinal 10-year postretention evaluation of orthodontically treated patients. *Am J Orthod.* 1985;87(3):175–186.

131. Janson G, Valarelli FP, Beltrão RTS, de Freitas MR, Henriques JFC. Stability of anterior open-bite extraction and nonextraction treatment in the permanent dentition. *Am J Orthod Dentofacial Orthop.* 2006;129(6):768–774.

132. de Freitas MR, Beltrão RTS, Janson G, Henriques JFC, Cançado RH. Long-term stability of anterior open bite extraction treatment in the permanent dentition. *Am J Orthod Dentofacial Orthop.* 2004;125(1):78–87.

133. Kretschmer WB, Baciut G, Baciut M, Zoder W, Wangerin K. Stability of Le Fort I osteotomy in bimaxillary osteotomies: single-piece versus 3-piece maxilla. *J Oral Maxillofac Surg.* 2010;68(2):372–380.

134. Ding Y, Xu TM, Lohrmann B, Gellrich NC, Schwestka-Polly R. Stability following combined orthodontic-surgical treatment for skeletal anterior open bite: a cephalometric 15-year follow-up study. *J Orofac Orthop.* 2007;68(3):245–256.

135. Lee H, Park Y. Treatment and posttreatment changes following intrusion of maxillary posterior teeth with miniscrew implants for open bite correction. *Korean J Orthod.* 2008;38(1):31–40.

136. Baek MS, Choi YJ, Yu HS, et al. Long-term stability of anterior open-bite treatment by intrusion of maxillary posterior teeth. *Am J Orthod Dentofacial Orthop.* 2010;138(4):396.e1–396.e9.

137. Kesling HD. The philosophy of the tooth positioning appliance. *Am J Orthod Oral Sur.* 1945;31(6):297–304.

138. Deguchi T, Kurosaka H, Oikawa H, et al. Comparison of orthodontic treatment outcomes in adults with skeletal open bite between conventional edgewise treatment and implant-anchored orthodontics. *Am J Orthod Dentofacial Orthop.* 2011;139(4):S60–S68.

139. Masumoto N, Yamaguchi K, Fujimoto S. Daily chewing gum exercise for stabilizing the vertical occlusion. *J Oral Rehabil.* 2009;36(12):857–863.

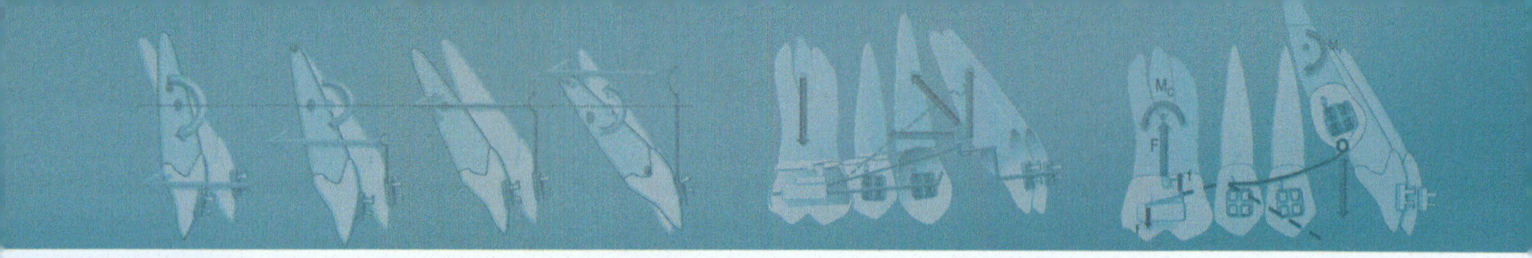

CHAPTER 10

Molar and Incisor Positioning to Achieve Occlusal and Esthetic Objectives

Bin Cai and Xiao-Guang Zhao

The goal of orthodontic treatment is a balanced oral system with functional occlusion, a healthy oral-dental structure, and improved facial appearance. To achieve this goal the stable elements in the original oral structures must be maintained while new elements are established gradually through a multistep process.

A prerequisite to orthodontic treatment is a clear understanding of the critical components in a stable occlusal system. In the 1900s Angle emphasized the importance of maxillary first molars as the center of occlusion.[1] In the 1950s Tweed identified the Tweed triangle and proposed that the mandibular incisors should be upright in relation to the mandibular plane.[2] Later, in the 1970s, Andrews, developer of the straight-wire appliance, put forward his six keys to occlusion and declared that all teeth should be positioned within the center of bone with reference to the WALA ridge (discussed later in the chapter).[3]

The belief systems introduced by these three thinkers can be regarded as the "philosophies of orthodontics" and they form the foundation for all modern-day orthodontics.

The pyramid depicted in Figure 10-1 shows the relationship between philosophy, technique, appliance, and objective in orthodontic practice. The upper layers of the pyramid are based on the lower layers whereas the realization of the lower layers depends on the upper ones. Reviewing the historical development of orthodontics contributes to an understanding of these relationships. In the holistic approach to orthodontic treatment, these comprehensive philosophies are always considered when choosing appropriate techniques and appliances for individual patients.

THE IMPORTANCE OF MAXILLARY FIRST MOLARS

The permanent first molars are the largest and strongest teeth in the human mouth and are located near the anteroposterior center of each arch (Fig. 10-2). The loss of a permanent molar allows movement and tipping of the teeth on either side of the mouth and disrupts the continuity of the arch.[4] Angle[1] was convinced that the key to occlusion is the relative position of the first molars. He claimed that in normal occlusion the mesiobuccal cusp of the maxillary first molar occludes with the buccal groove of the mandibular first molar.[1] When he developed his classification of malocclusion, he noticed that the position of the first molars relative to the jaws is more reliable than that of other teeth because the molars are less restrained in taking their positions.[1]

In addition, a strong ridge extends upward from the socket of the maxillary first molars to the zygomatic process of the maxilla[5,6] (Fig. 10-3). The occlusal force on the teeth could be distributed along this bony ridge. Therefore the maxillary first molar should stay in its original position (where it erupted) during and after orthodontic treatment in order to maintain its relationship with the strong bony ridge. The mesial and distal (sagittal) movements of the molar should be limited to 2-mm in each direction. Limiting mesial movement of the maxillary first molar preserves the extraction space for relieving anterior crowding or retracting protruded anterior teeth. The tip-back bend in the Begg technique is a solution for achieving good sagittal control of maxillary first molars and can be applied with modern appliances (Fig. 10-4). Current techniques with microimplants provide more reliable anchorage control because of their absolute immobility and direct application of force (Fig. 10-5).

The transverse position of the maxillary first molars is of the same importance. In his six keys to occlusion, Andrews emphasizes that the mesiolingual cusp of the maxillary first molar, the largest functional cuspid in the mouth, should occlude in the central fossa of the mandibular first molar.[7] More than 80-mm^2 of efficient chewing surface is gone when a first molar is lost.[4] Any excessive transverse change of a maxillary first molar, including lingual or buccal displacement, lingual or buccal tipping, and mesial or distal rotation, will result in not only the reduction of chewing surface but

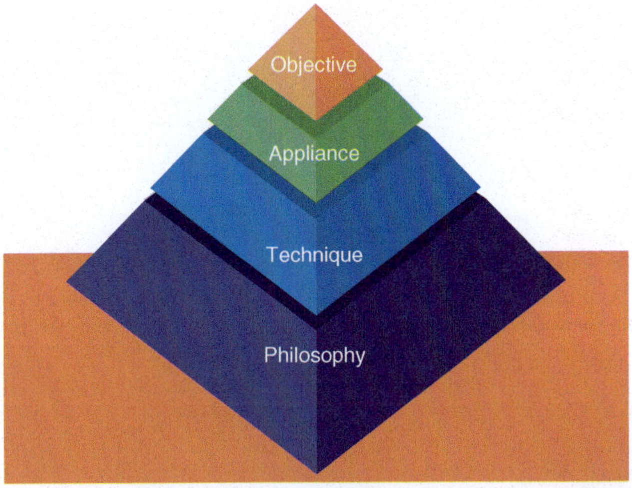

Figure 10-1 The pyramid relationship between philosophy, technique, appliance, and objective in orthodontic treatment.

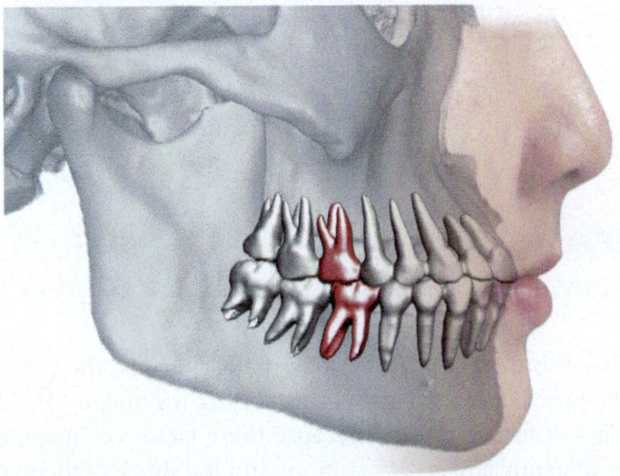

Figure 10-2 The position and the importance of the permanent first molars.

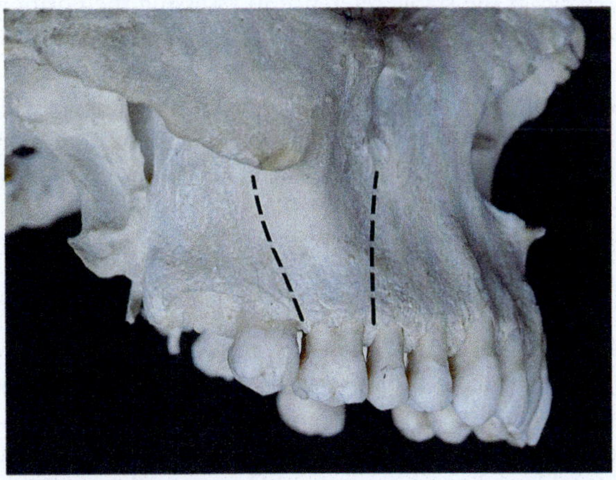

Figure 10-3 The maxillary first molars stand on the strong ridge extending the zygomatic process of the maxilla.

also mandibular backward compensatory displacement or clockwise rotation, which will destroy the balanced occlusion. Therefore the adequate inter-molar width should be kept during the treatment. Especially in extraction cases, the mesial rotation and buccal tipping of maxillary first molars during space closing should be prevented.

Any fixed appliance or orthodontic technique in use today is likely to cause the posterior teeth to extrude. The vertical control of the maxillary first molar is essential to maintaining the inclination of the functional occlusal plane and preventing the downward-backward rotation of the mandible in Class II cases, especially those with high mandibular plane angle. This clockwise rotation does harm to the patient's facial profile as well as the temporomandibular joint (TMJ) function. Methods of vertical control include micro-implants, transpalatal arch, and high-pull headgear.

No matter what kind of additional appliance is used to enforce the anchorage of the maxillary first molar and to keep the molar's position in three dimensions, all techniques have certain things in common to ensure that the treatment is carried out smoothly. These include selection of a suitable archwire, the form of the archwire, light activation force during space closure, and appropriate mechanism of space closure (see Case Report).

THE UPRIGHTING OF MANDIBULAR INCISORS

Before orthodontic treatment starts, an attempt should be made to identify an ideal incisor position that will benefit the periodontal tissues and TMJs and retain tooth alignment. The position of the mandibular incisors is of paramount importance. However, crowding and periodontal recession always occur in the field of the mandibular incisors, because these teeth are vulnerable to the tendency of posterior teeth to move forward and the biting force from the maxillary incisors.

In the 1950s Tweed[7] reported that the inclination of mandibular incisors was critical to facial esthetics and the stability of treatment results. He claimed that the incisor mandibular plan angle (IMPA) should be 85 to 95 degrees; approximately 90 degrees was designated the norm. In addition, we found the mandibular incisors always stand in an upright position with their roots in the center of the bone in the patients with congenital anodontia or general space in the anterior segment of their mandibular arch (Fig. 10-6).

Some studies have shown periodontal recession after excessive orthodontic proclination of the mandibular incisors, especially in patients with severe skeletal discrepancy.[8–10] However, other studies showed no association between the degree of proclination of the mandibular incisors during therapy with fixed appliances and gingival recession or attachment loss.[11–13] Possible reasons for the conflicting conclusions may be the methodological differences, including differences in sample age groups, pre-treatment periodontal condition, treatment methods, postoperative observation periods, and the means of evaluating periodontal parameters. Even though it is not clear whether proclination of the mandibular incisors results in periodontal sequelae, most orthodontists are convinced that uprighting the mandibular incisors benefits the patient's periodontal health, helps to

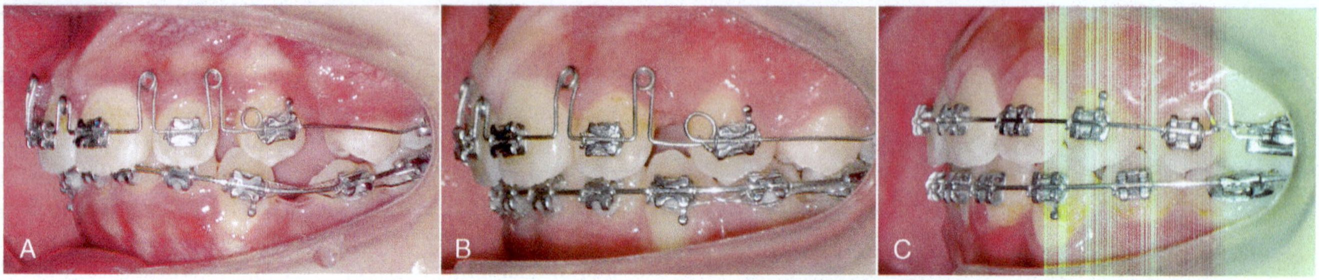

Figure 10-4 Straight-wire appliance (Mini Uni-Twin, 3M/Unitek, Monrovia, CA) is used with the Begg technique to realize effective and efficient tooth movement. **A,** Before the distalization of maxillary canines. **B,** After the distalization of maxillary canines after 3 months. **C,** After space closure in maxillary and mandibular arches.

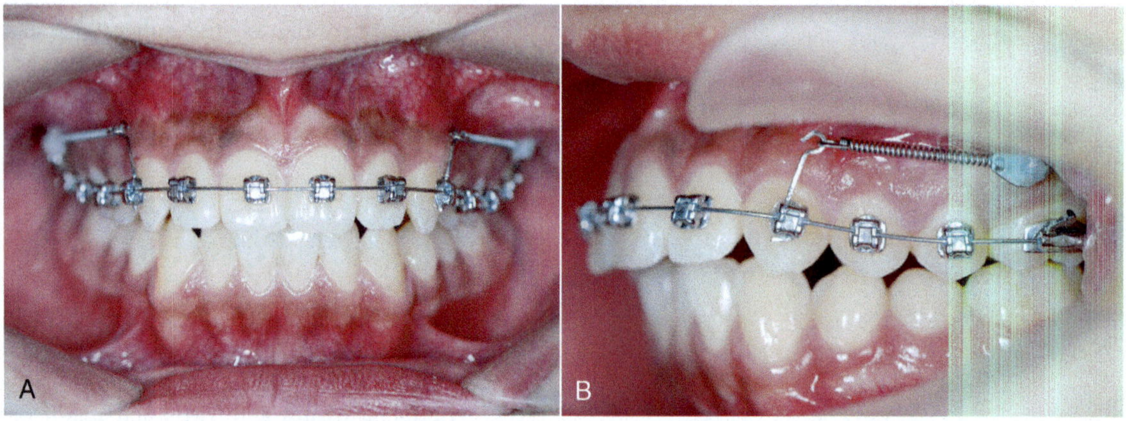

Figure 10-5 Micro-screw is used to distalize the maxillary arch via directional force application of the canine. **A,** Frontal view. **B,** Lateral view.

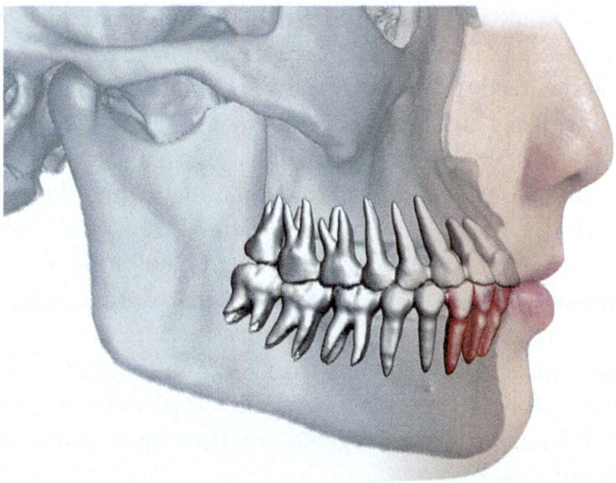

Figure 10-6 The mandibular incisors stand upright in the mandibular plane.

ensure the stability of the reconstructed structure, and improves the facial appearance.

Uprighting the mandibular incisors does not mean making them stand perpendicular to the mandibular plane. Orthodontic treatment should not be limited to the mechanical phases. The target position of mandibular incisors should be the buccolingual center of bone. The IMPA varies according to differences in the angle of the mandibular plane. In patients with a high angle the IMPA should be smaller, less than 90 degrees. In patients with a low angle the IMPA should be larger, greater than 90 degrees.

In the treatment of various malocclusions, the position and proclination of maxillary incisors are major issues in terms of facial esthetics because these factors contribute to the dynamic and static positions and the shape of the maxillary lip (Fig. 10-7). The essential role of the maxillary incisors was also noticed by Andrews and Andrews.[3] They used the forehead as the stable reference in assessing the position of the maxillary incisors. However, when we make a treatment plan for a patient with moderate skeletal discrepancy between the maxillary and mandibular jaws, the prime maxillary incisor position always conflicts with the upright position of mandibular incisors. In this instance a compromise may be necessary in order to avoid orthognathic surgery.

MASTER AND SLAVE ARCHES

As mentioned, the goal of orthodontic treatment is to establish a new balanced oral system with functional occlusion. The procedure is like doing a model setup when a treatment plan is made. Orthodontists should decide which teeth must stay stable and which teeth should be primarily repositioned. Then the rest of the teeth can be set sequentially until the final occlusion is established. In orthodontic treatment the maxillary first molars are usually kept stable in three dimensions. The upright position of the mandibular incisors should be set as early as possible, especially in patients with Class I or Class II malocclusion.

The concept of master and slave arches is useful in planning treatment. The "master arch" is the arch that is more

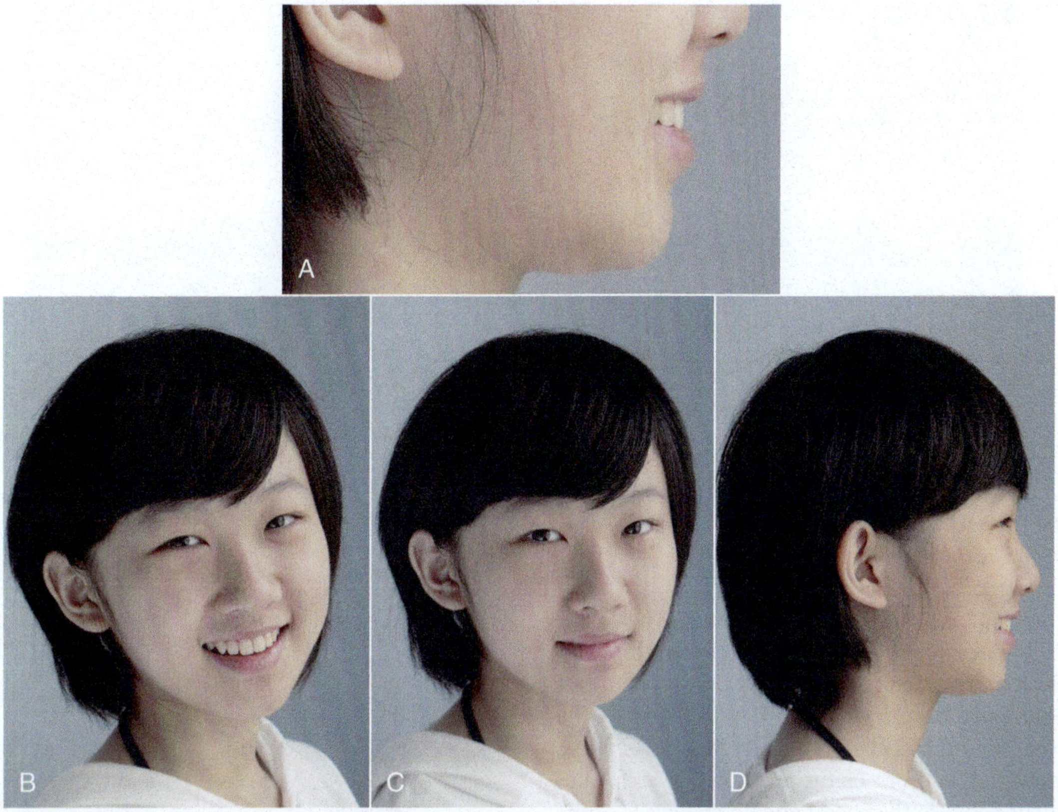

Figure 10-7 The position and proclination of the maxillary incisors are critical factors in terms of facial esthetics. **A,** Magnification of the lower one-third in facial profile with smile. **B,** Frontal facial photograph with smile. **C,** Frontal facial photograph without smile. **D,** Lateral facial photograph with smile.

stable during the relative movement of inter-arches. It is always established first and then it is fixed with a rigid archwire. The movement of teeth in the "slave arch" is always achieved gradually. Usually the extraction space in the master arch is closed earlier than in the slave arch.

In the treatment of patients with Class I or Class II malocclusion, the mandibular arch is considered the master arch. The mandibular incisors are always stabilized in an upright position as early as possible. The remaining treatment focuses on positioning the mandibular incisors, including establishing Class I canine relationships; closing the extraction space; and achieving normal overbite and overjet. The mandibular arch is chosen as the master arch for another reason as well. Angle[1] proposed that the mandibular arch is a more important factor in the oral system during the physical development of occlusion. Harmony between the maxillary and mandibular arches and the teeth in the arches is also powerfully promoted by the normal action and reaction of the arches with each other. Because the teeth of the mandibular arch erupt before those of the maxillary arch and are consequently somewhat fixed in their positions before their antagonists appear, it follows that the mandibular arch is the form over which the maxillary arch is molded; otherwise the harmony between the arches will be broken. In other words, the mandibular arch exerts a controlling influence over the form of the maxillary arch and the positions of the teeth in the arches. Of course, the maxillary arch has an effect on the mandibular arch but unquestionably the mandibular arch, not the maxillary arch, is the more important factor.

In the treatment of Class III malocclusion, because of the dental compensation for the skeletal discrepancy the anterior segment of the mandibular arch always must be moved distally. Therefore the mandibular arch becomes the slave arch and the maxillary arch acts as the master arch. During treatment the maxillary arch could be aligned before the mandibular arch is aligned and it should be stabilized with a rigid wire. Then Class III elastics with light force could be used to establish a Class I relationship between the canines and to correct an anterior crossbite. In patients who need maxillary expansion, the expander could be used as a stable structure with soldered hooks and intermaxillary elastics.

KEEPING THE TEETH IN THE CENTER OF THE BONE

Effective and efficient movement of the teeth can be achieved when the teeth are kept in the buccolingual center of the bone along the way (Fig. 10-8). After treatment the teeth should be repositioned in the center of the bone so that the occlusal force is distributed physiologically into the bone and stability is better.

Orthodontic treatments are carried out by the interaction between the brackets and the archwires, so the positions of the teeth are determined by the forms of the archwires. The size and form of the dental arches are considered an essential element in orthodontic treatment because the arches influence smile esthetics, space available, function of the occlusion, and the long-term stability of the dentition.[14-16] A

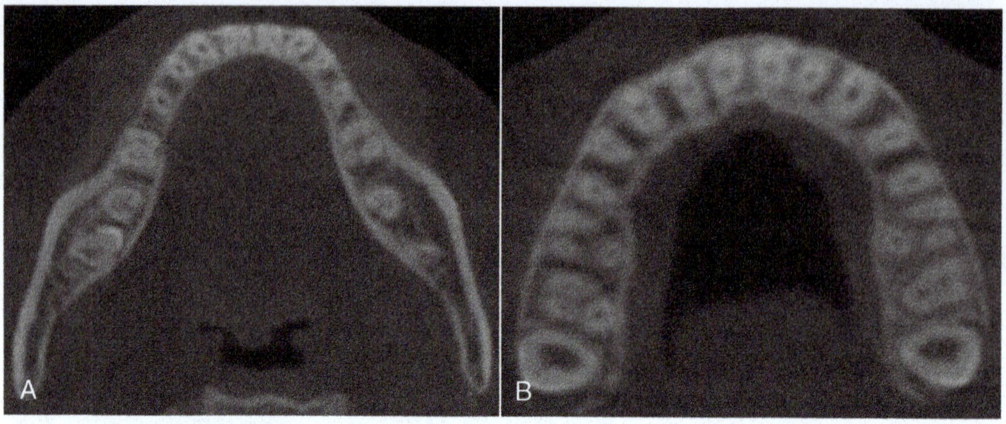

Figure 10-8 The roots of the mandibular and maxillary teeth are kept in the buccolingual center of the bone. **A,** The roots in the mandible. **B,** The roots in the maxilla.

nature dental arch form is initially established by the configuration of the bony ridge and by tooth eruption, perioral muscles, and intraoral functional forces.[16]

In the studies of the forms of dental arches, Angle proposed the line of occlusion (LO).[1] When the teeth are in normal occlusion, their greatest number of points of contact will lie along an imaginary line passing over the points of the buccal cusps of the molars and premolars, the incisal edges of the canines and incisors of the mandibular arch, and along the sulcus between the buccal and lingual cusps of the maxillary molars and premolars, then forward, crossing the lingual ridge of the canines and the marginal ridges of the incisors at a point about one-third the length of their crowns from their incisal edges. This is LO, which is the line of the greatest normal occlusal contact. In the mandibular arch, the buccal cusps are the functional cusps in the posterior teeth; the lingual cusps are the functional cusps in the maxillary arch. Similar to the LO, another line, the lingual line of occlusion (LLO) named by us, can be visualized as running through the lingual cusps of molars and premolars in the maxillary arch and through the sulcus between the buccal and lingual cusps of the mandibular molars and premolars. In the evaluation of a treatment's outcome, a single line of occlusion is not adequate because the teeth could vary in the buccolingual inclination. When the LO is used along with the LLO, both functional occlusal lines form a plane, which will fix the teeth in three dimensions. Any functional cusp deviating from the lines could be observed easily (Fig. 10-9).

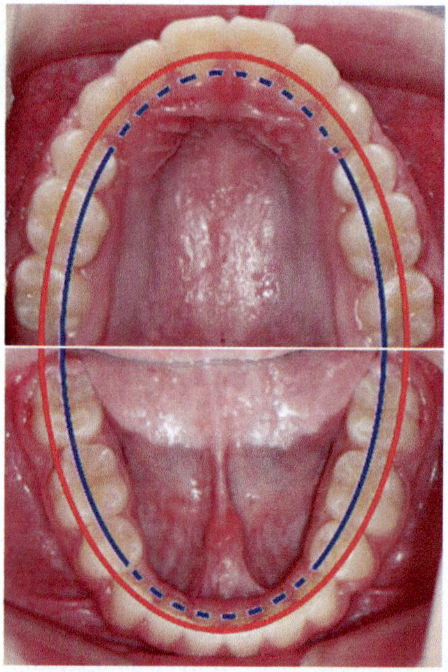

Figure 10-9 A treated case with four first premolars extracted. The red line is the line of occlusion (LO) proposed by Angle that can be used in the evaluation of treatment results. The blue line is the lingual line of occlusion (LLO), which can be used in conjunction with the LO in the assessment of treatment outcomes.

The alveolar ridge in the dental casts has been advocated as the reference for the fabrication of archwires to avoid changes in the dimensions of the transverse dental arch.[3,17] Andrews and Andrews[3] discovered the WALA ridge (Fig. 10-10), an anatomic ridge on the mandibular alveolar process that delimits the soft tissue band immediately superior to the mucogingival junction. The WALA ridge, named after Will Andrews and Larry Andrews, can be used as a referent for determining the shape of the arch and the archwire. The WALA ridge approximates the superior-inferior position of the horizontal centers of rotation of teeth in an arch; therefore this landmark is an adequate guideline for positioning the crowns and roots of teeth over the buccolingual borders of the basal bone.[3] Previous studies claimed that the standard distances between the dental crowns (facial axis [FA] points) and the WALA ridge would reflect the buccolingual inclination of the teeth and directly influence the treatment plan. The WALA ridge is a reliable landmark for determining an optimal shape of the dental arch.[3,18] However, the distance between the FA points of the teeth and the WALA ridge is not adequate for positioning the crowns. The reason is similar to that for the LO: the buccolingual inclination of the teeth could vary with a fixed FA-WALA distance. Therefore using the two functional occlusal lines (LO and LLO) in the evaluation of the transverse position of teeth in orthodontic treatment is recommended.

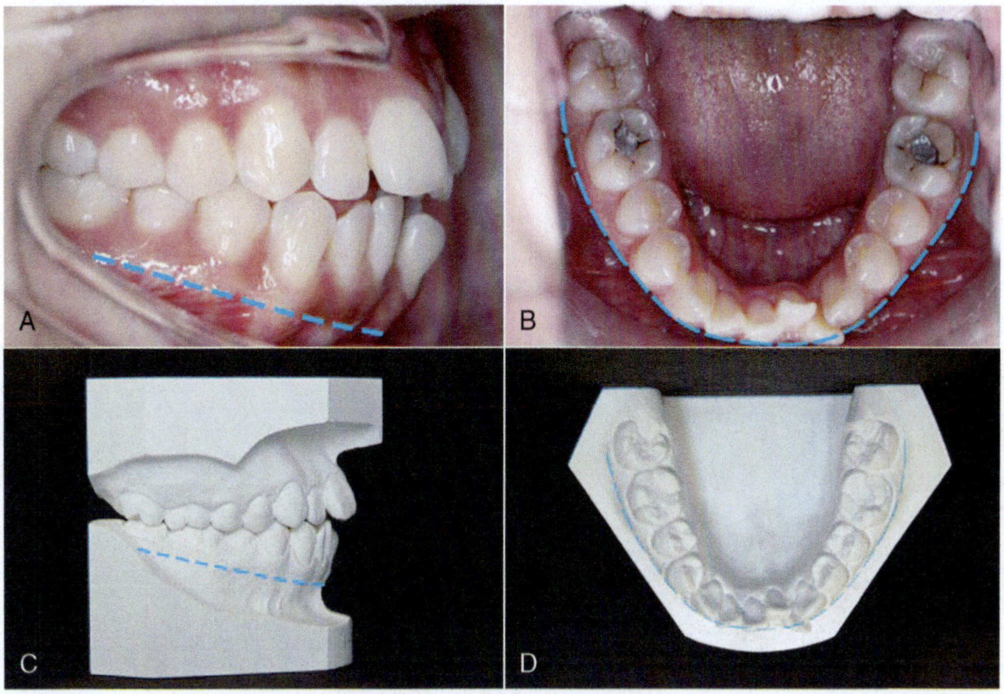

Figure 10-10 WALA ridge observed in (**A and B**) intraoral photographs and (**C and D**) dental casts.

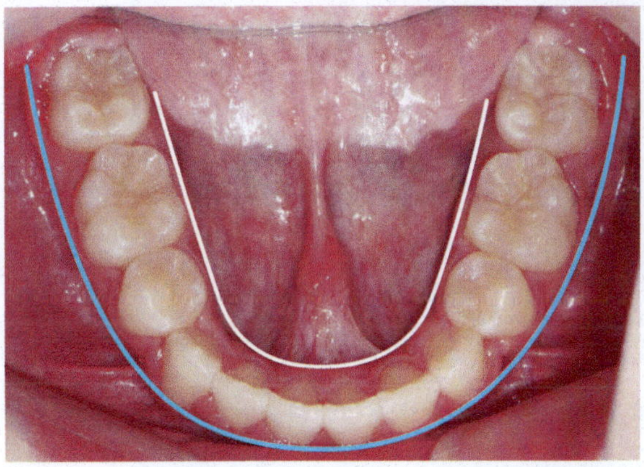

Figure 10-11 The buccolingual borders of the mandible in clinical observation.

Furthermore, in clinical observation the buccolingual borders of the mandible can be visualized in the mandibular occlusal view (Fig. 10-11). The labial border overlaps at the WALA ridge. Even though various malocclusions exist, most mandibular teeth, especially the posterior ones, stand between the two borders. These borders are supposed to be the functional range of the mandible. The mandibular teeth should be positioned within this range. In conclusion, the teeth should be moved and positioned within the buccolingual bony borders and the two functional occlusal lines should be formed and maintained once the teeth are aligned.

Some investigators have attempted to establish templates of the dental arches that represent the majority of dental arch forms, suggesting the use of prototypes or references to help provide the parameters for fabricating archwires or selecting preformed ones.[14,17,19,20] However, Trivino et al.[16] analyzed 63 mandibular models of Brazilian patients by organizing the models into eight groups and did not find one ideal arch form that could represent the normal dental arches.

The arch form, which is customized for each patient, should be determined before the orthodontic treatment begins and should be kept throughout the treatment (Fig. 10-12). This arch form should be built on the basis of a visualized final dental arch according to the pre-treatment dental structures, such as intercanine width and the WALA ridge. The mandibular intercanine width increases significantly with the changes in dentition that occur during treatment but does not increase in the permanent dentition after 12 years of age.[15] The expansion of the mandibular arch seems applicable in a growing child. However, distinguishing between the results of expansion and natural growth in a patient is difficult. No evidence indicates that appliances can stimulate "growth" beyond that which would occur normally. Stable expansion of the mandibular intercanine width is unlikely unless the canines are displaced lingually by the occlusion.[15] The original intercanine width should be preserved. However, the steadiness of the dental arch form does not mean that the form of the archwire should be fixed throughout treatment. Appropriate modification should be made according to the expected tooth movement. For example, during space closure with sliding mechanics in extraction cases, the excessive curve of Spee in the maxillary arch and the reverse curve of Spee in the mandibular arch along with mild expansion in the region of extraction should be made in the archwires to compensate for the tendency for tipping and the rotation of the adjacent teeth to the extraction space (Fig. 10-13).

In orthodontic treatment, archwires are used as a track to guide the movement of the teeth. The shape of the track must

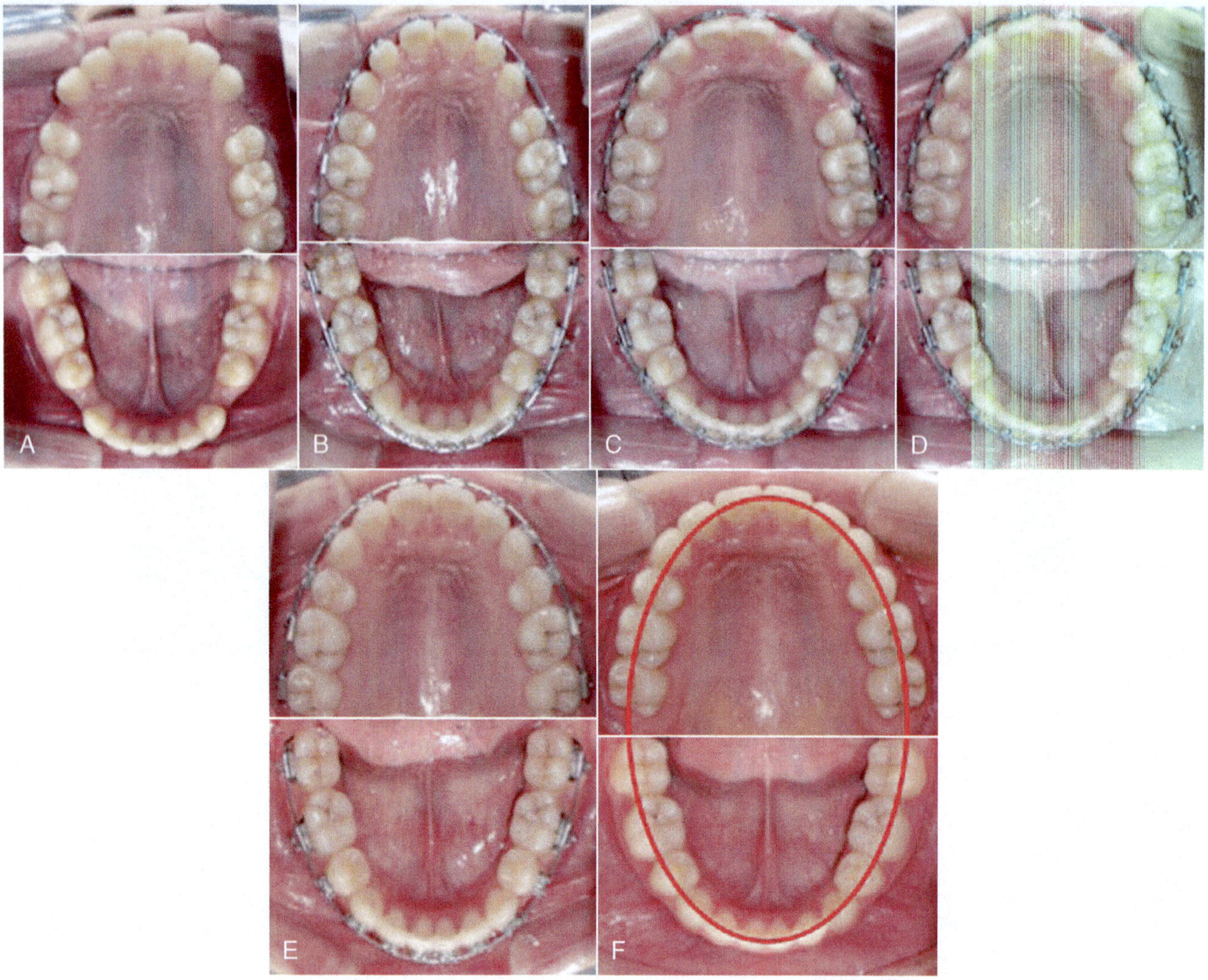

Figure 10-12 **A–F,** The customized arch forms were kept throughout all treatment procedures.

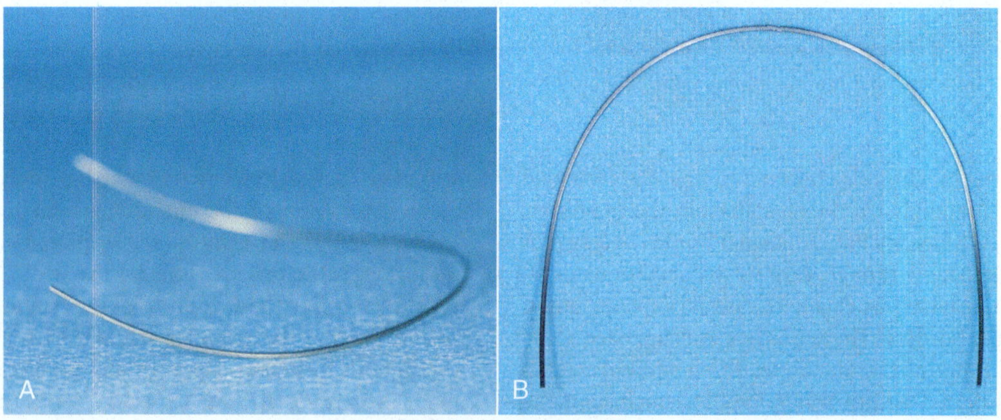

Figure 10-13 **A and B,** An archwire form used for space closure in extraction cases.

be set properly so that the teeth can be moved effectively in the buccolingual center of alveolar bone. In addition, coordination of the maxillary and mandibular arch forms is critical throughout treatment. Only with good coordination can the mandible be located correctly in the sagittal dimension.

A holistic consideration of orthodontic treatment consists of, but is not limited to, the ideas discussed in this chapter. The ideas are interrelated and should be recognized so that orthodontic treatment can be carried out smoothly and in a simple and efficient way.

Text continued on p. 195

CASE REPORT

An 11-year-old girl had crooked and proclined front teeth. She had a convex profile and a deep mentolabial fold. Her mandible was retrognathic. Severe proclined maxillary incisors were obvious in photographs that showed her smiling (Fig. 10-14). Intraoral photographs indicated a half-cusp Class II canine relationship on the left and a one-cusp Class II canine relationship on the right, with a deep overbite and a 10-mm overjet. Extraction was indicated because of the proclined maxillary anterior teeth and 3-mm crowding in the maxillary arch and the excessive curve of Spee and 2-mm crowding in the mandibular arch (Fig. 10-15).

Treatment Procedure

Treatment started with extraction of the four first premolars. The following treatment strategies were considered simultaneously:

1. The first goal was to stabilize the maxillary first molars in three dimensions, so that the inclination of the functional occlusal plane could be stabilized. We used an Australian 0.016-inch wire with 30-degree tip-back bends mesial to the first molars to reinforce the anchorage and stabilize their position in three dimensions (Fig. 10-16).
2. In patients with Class II occlusion, the mandibular arch is used as the master template and therefore rigid wires should be placed in the arch as soon as possible. The mandibular canines were laced back from the beginning to create space to resolve anterior crowding and level the curve of Spee, so that proclination of mandibular incisors was prevented (see Fig. 10-16; Fig. 10-17).
3. The maxillary canines were distalized as early as possible to establish the Class I canine

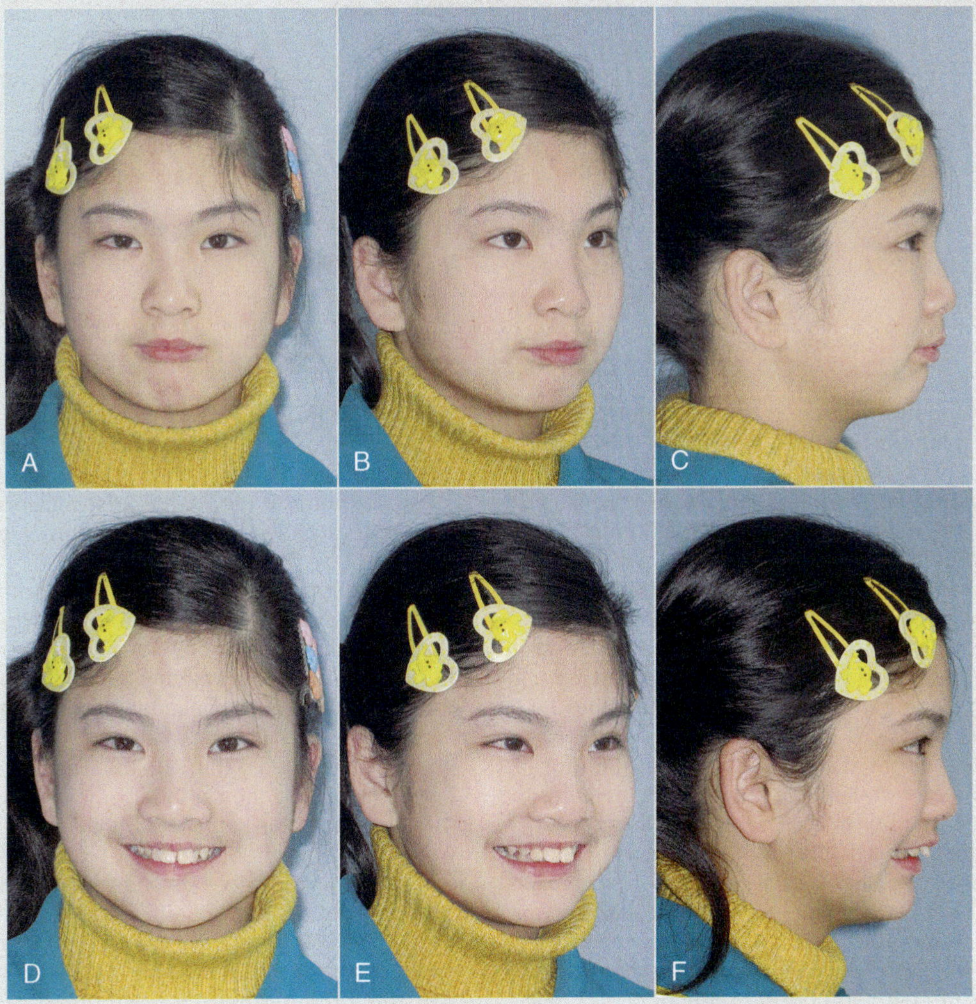

Figure 10-14 A–F, Pre-treatment facial views.

Continued

CASE REPORT—cont'd

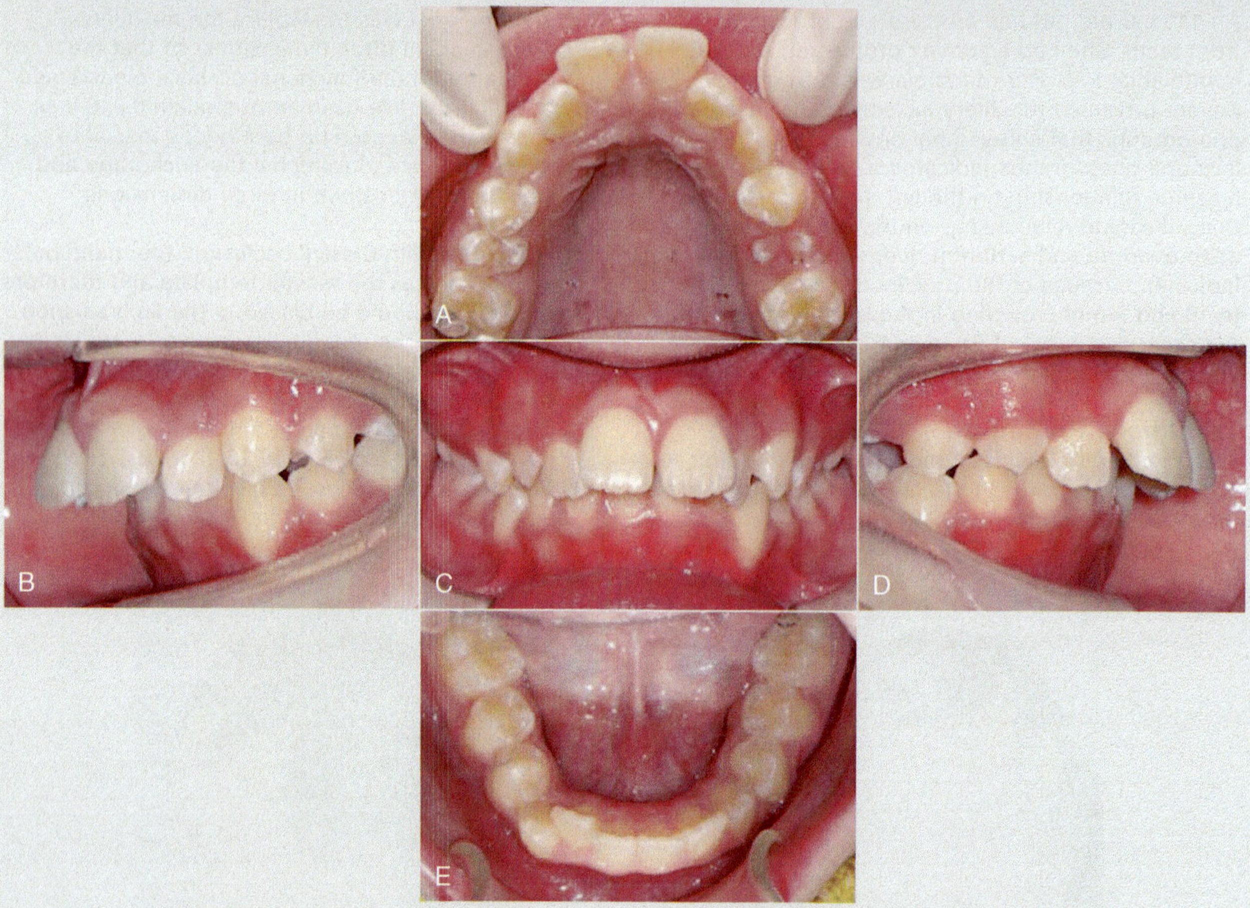

Figure 10-15 **A–E,** Pre-treatment intraoral views.

relationship and to stabilize the inter-arch structures. Initially we used Australian 0.016-inch wire with multiple helical vertical loops among maxillary anterior teeth and circle loops flush mesial to the canines, so that the resolution of anterior crowding and distalization of the canines could be realized simultaneously. During this stage Class II elastics, between mandibular first molars and the vertical loops distal to the lateral incisors, were used with light force, around 2 oz. The flush circle bend then pushed the canine distally (see Figs. 10-16 and 10-17).

4. Stable arch widths were maintained throughout the treatment with suitable customized archwire forms. The functional occlusal lines and the relationship between the teeth and the bony borders were checked at every visit.
5. High-torque brackets were used in the maxillary arch (22-degree torque for the maxillary central incisors) because the maxillary incisors were prone to retroclination during retraction. Low-torque brackets were chosen for the mandibular arch (–6-degree torque for the mandibular incisors) because the negative torque prescription in the mandibular incisors could counteract the side effect of anterior proclination caused by Class II elastics.

The treatment was carried out smoothly, with stable key structures in both arches. When the Class I canine relationship was established with the successful distalization of maxillary canines, the mandibular arch was stabilized without space (see Fig. 10-17). The facial appearance and profile improved markedly (Fig. 10-18). The rest of the work involved closing the remaining general space in the maxillary anterior segment. Maxillary premolars were then bracketed. Later, a rigid rectangular wire with a moderate curve of Spee was used with the activation of a power chain. Meanwhile the form of the maxillary archwire was modified a little (a slight increase in the intercanine width) to prevent constriction during space closure (Fig. 10-19).

CASE REPORT—cont'd

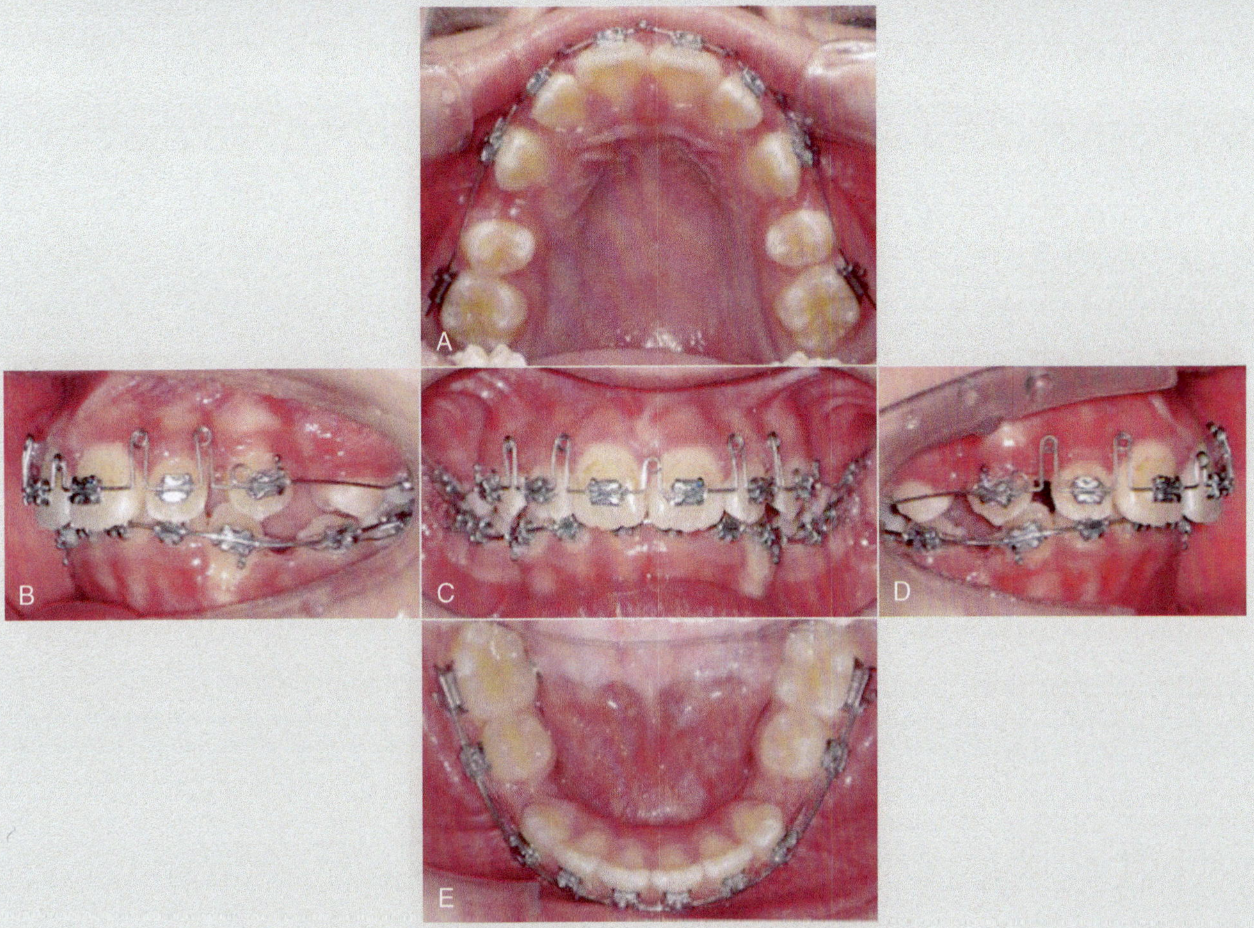

Figure 10-16 **A–E,** Intraoral views at the beginning of the treatment.

Treatment Results

At the end of treatment the space was closed successfully and normal overbite and overjet were established. After the eruption of maxillary second molars, the patient was ready to have the dental appliances removed (Fig. 10-20). Finally, a new balanced dentofacial structure was realized. The occlusion fulfilled the six keys proposed by Andrews[7] (Fig. 10-21). The maxillary anterior teeth had ideal inclination and proclination, factors critical to facial esthetics (Fig. 10-22). The maxillary and mandibular arch forms were maintained properly during and after treatment (Fig. 10-23). In the post-treatment cephalogram, the mandibular incisors were seen standing in the center of the symphysis (Fig. 10-24). A balanced facial appearance and straight facial profile were achieved and the patient was quite satisfied (Fig. 10-25). The total treatment lasted 24 months.

Continued

CASE REPORT—cont'd

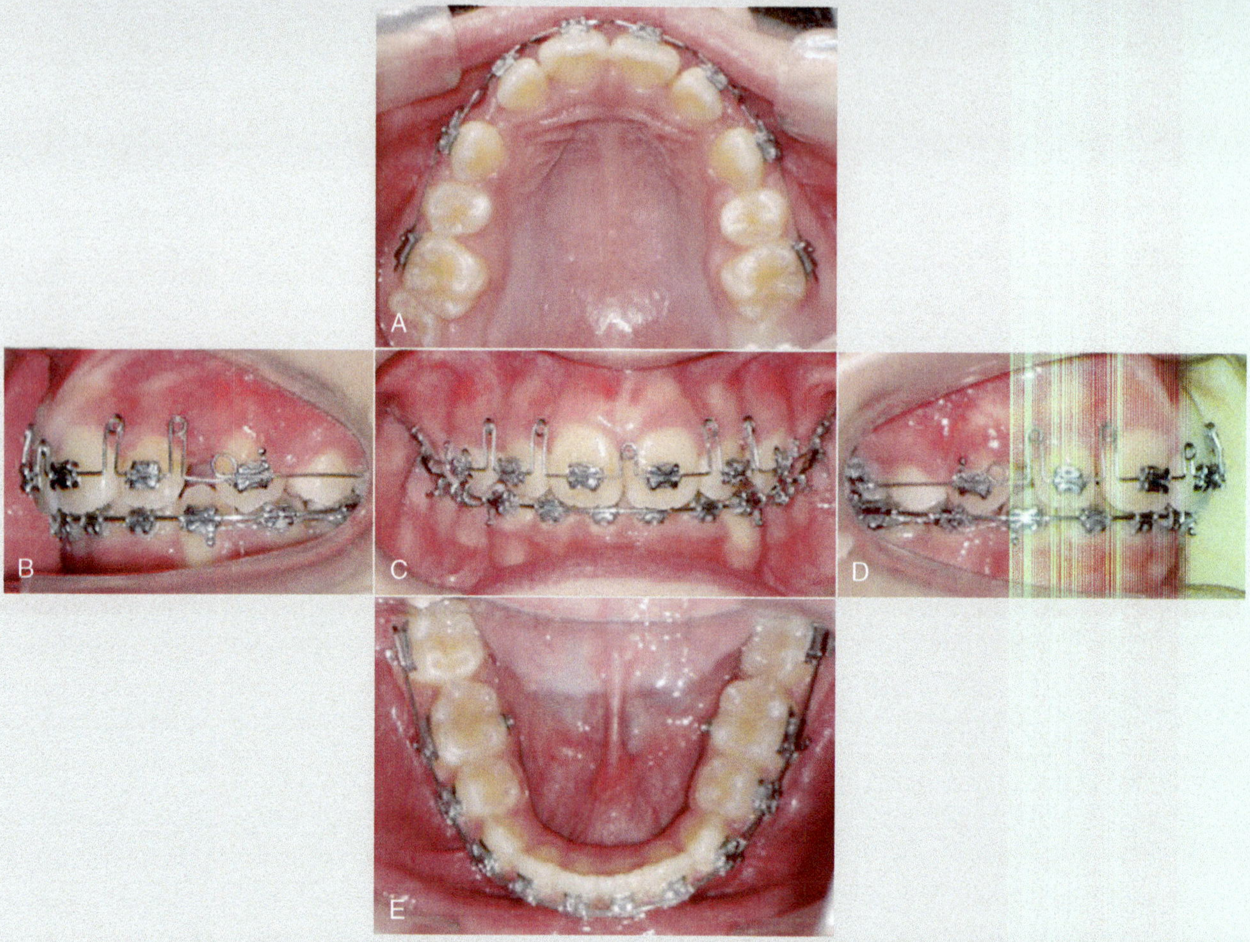

Figure 10-17 **A–E,** Intraoral views after the distalization of the maxillary canines. The mandibular arch was stabilized as the master arch.

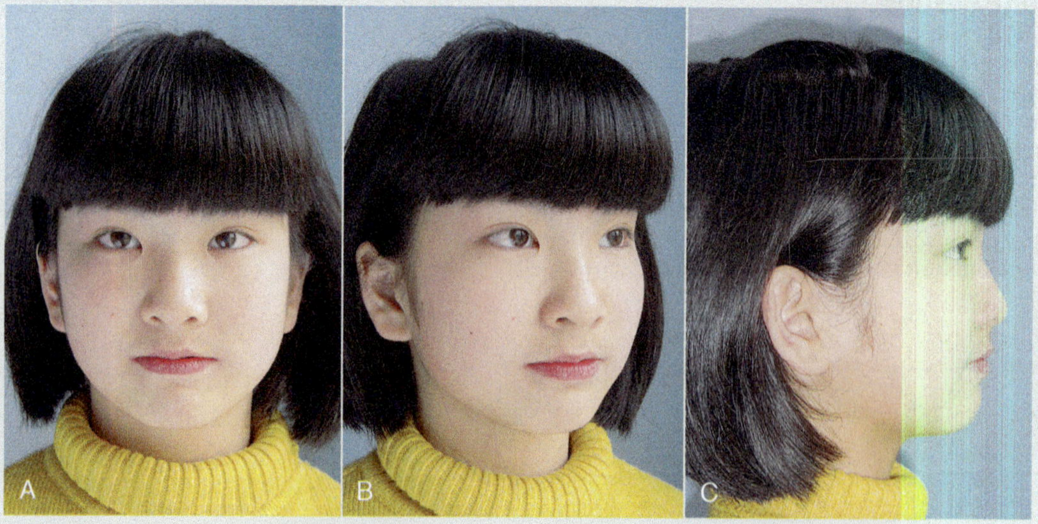

Figure 10-18 **A–C,** Facial views during the treatment after the canines were distalized.

CASE REPORT—cont'd

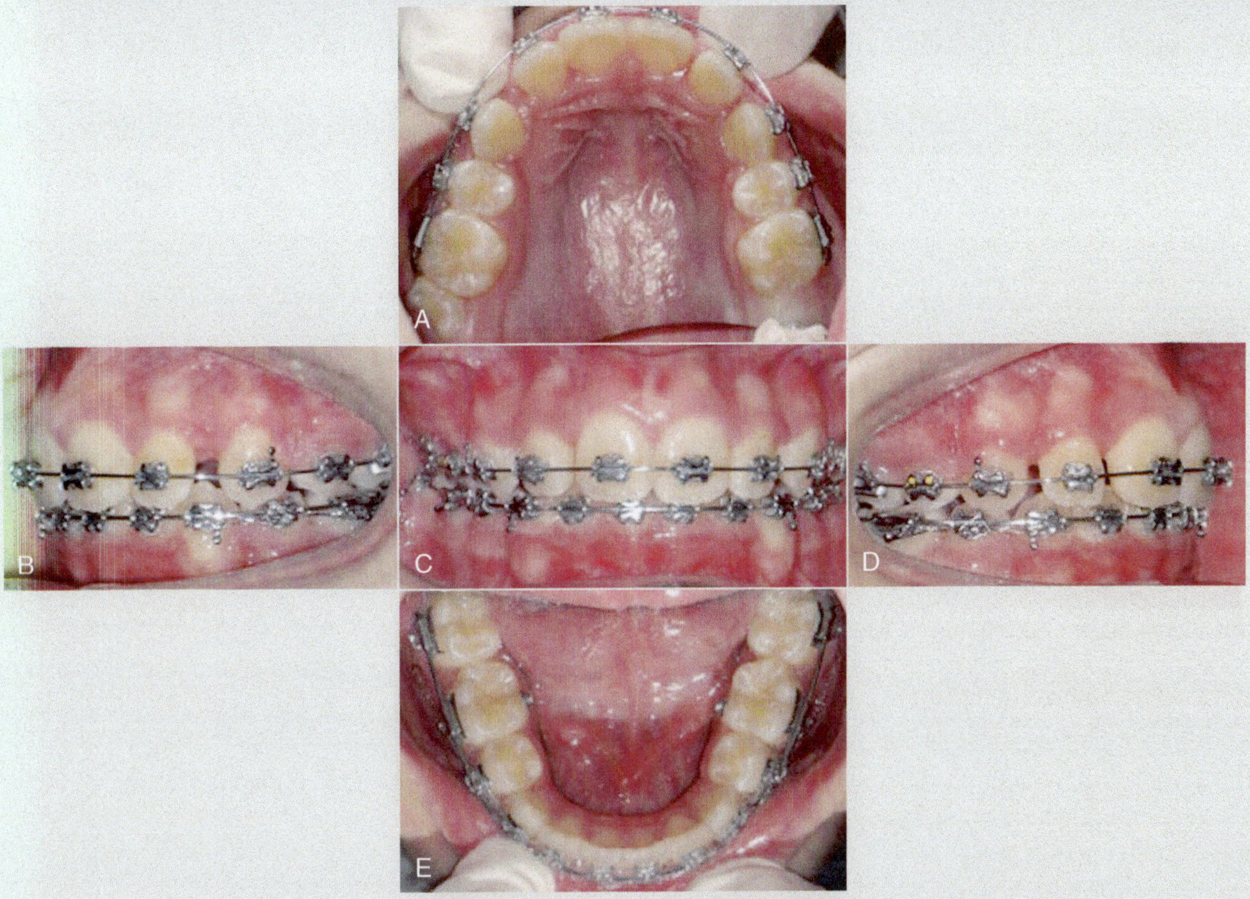

Figure 10-19 **A–E,** Intraoral views during the treatment when maxillary premolars were incorporated and aligned.

Continued

CASE REPORT—cont'd

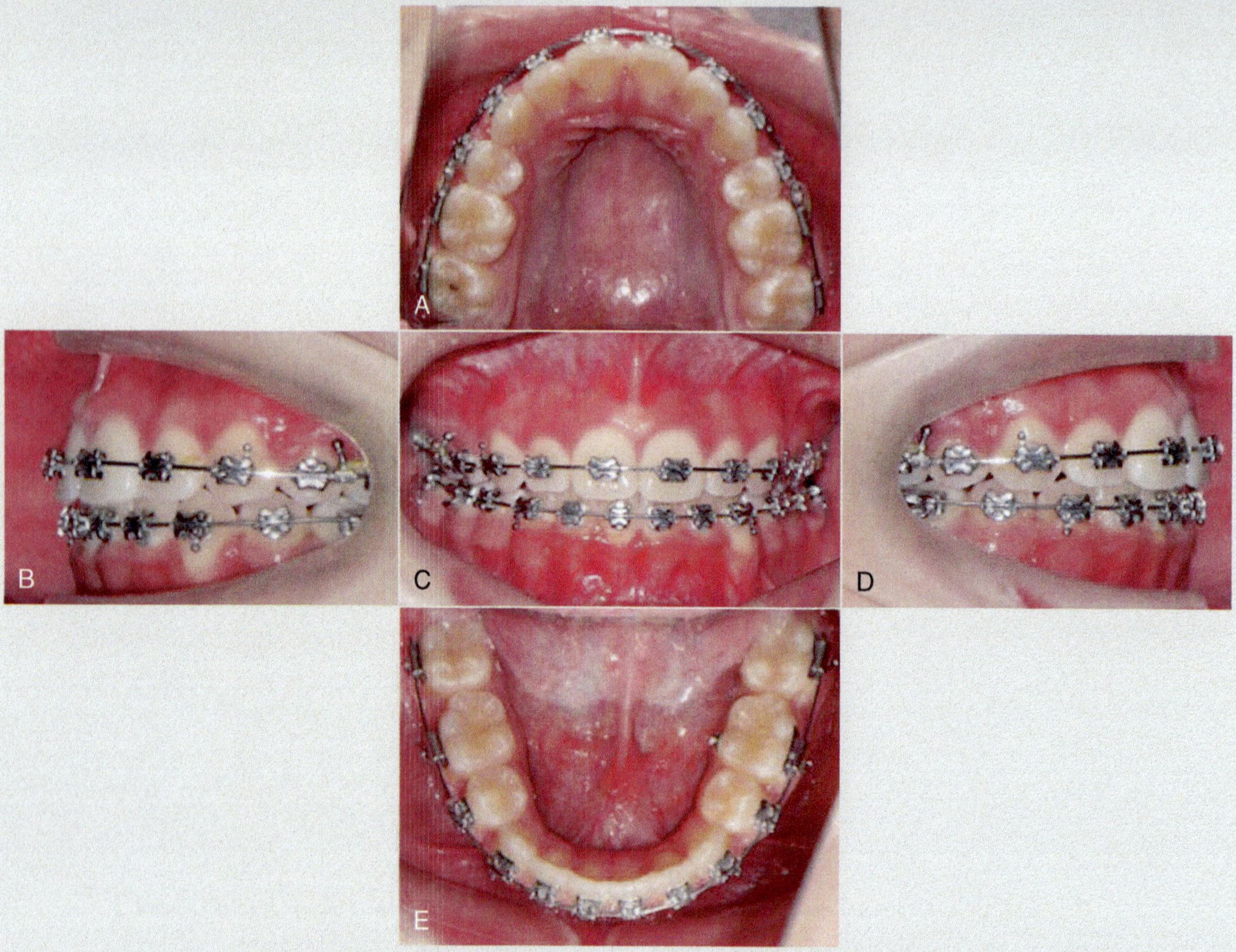

Figure 10-20 A–E, Intraoral photographs during treatment when the extraction space was closed and the maxillary second molars were included.

CASE REPORT—cont'd

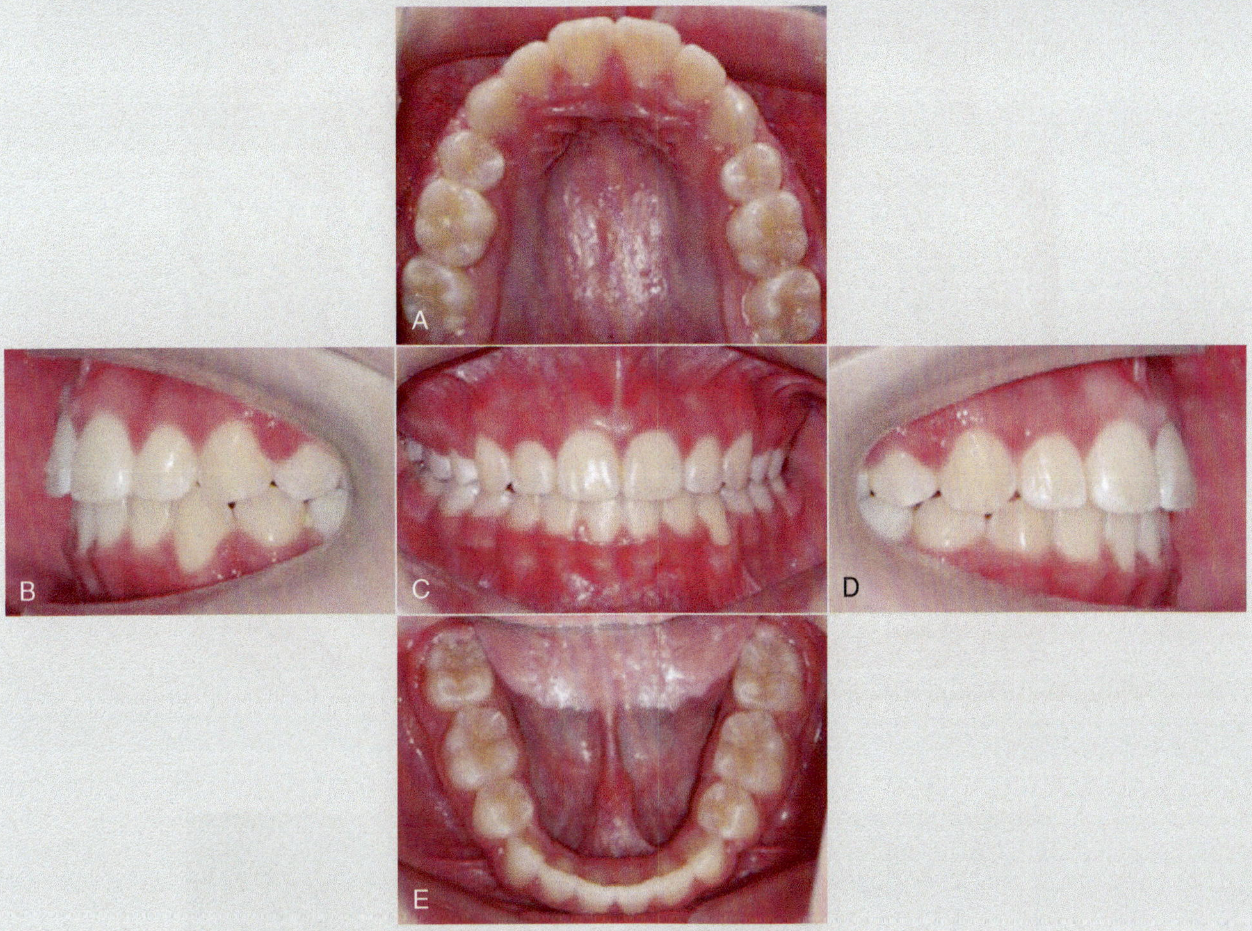

Figure 10-21 **A–E,** Post-treatment intraoral views.

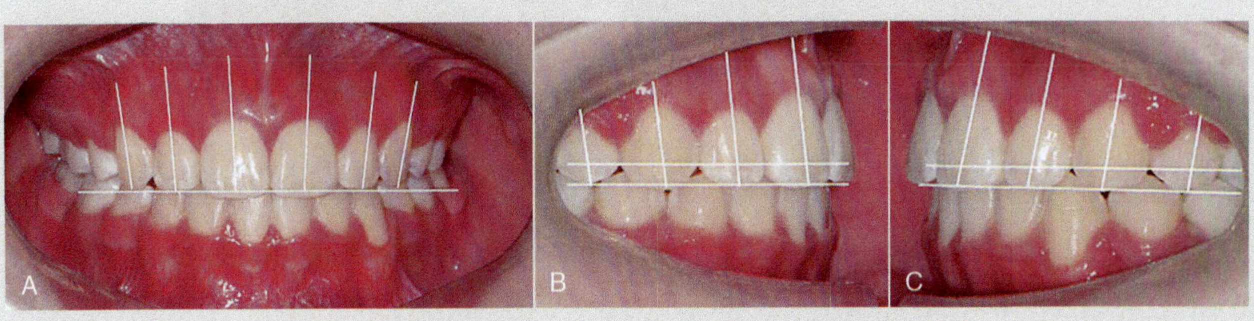

Figure 10-22 **A–C,** Proper inclination of maxillary teeth after treatment.

Continued

CASE REPORT—cont'd

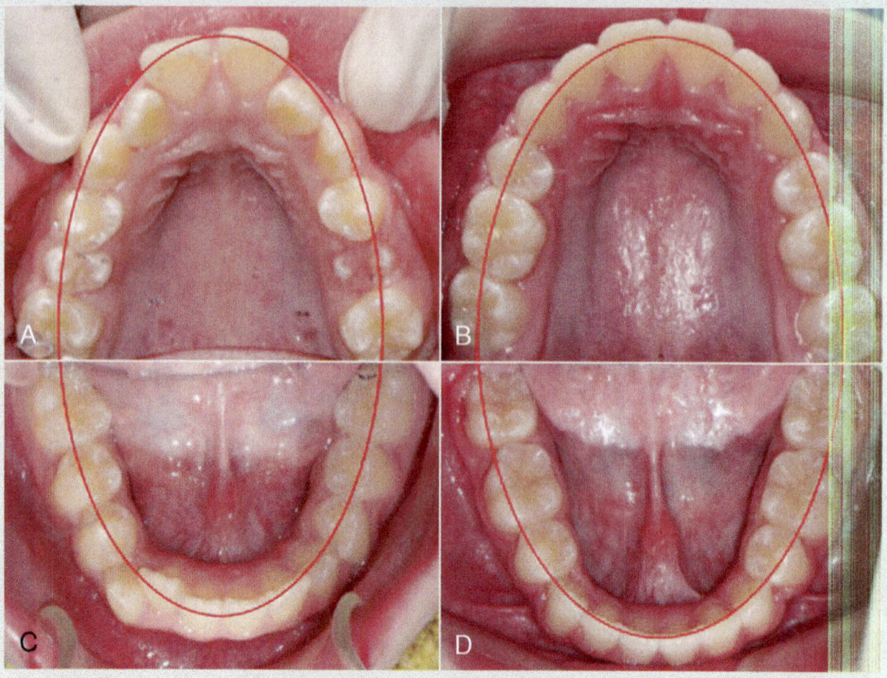

Figure 10-23 Comparison of arch forms before and after treatment. **A and C,** Before treatment. **B and D,** After treatment.

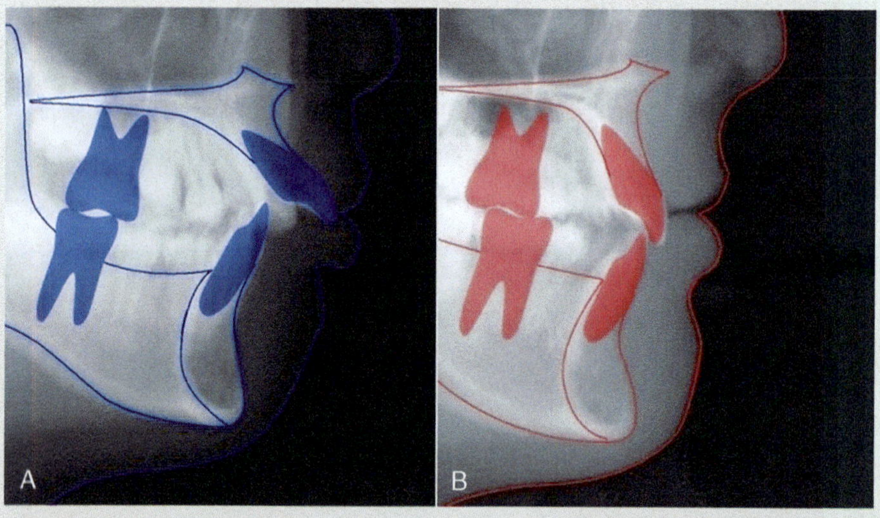

Figure 10-24 Incisor inclination before and after treatment. **A,** Before treatment. **B,** After treatment.

CASE REPORT—cont'd

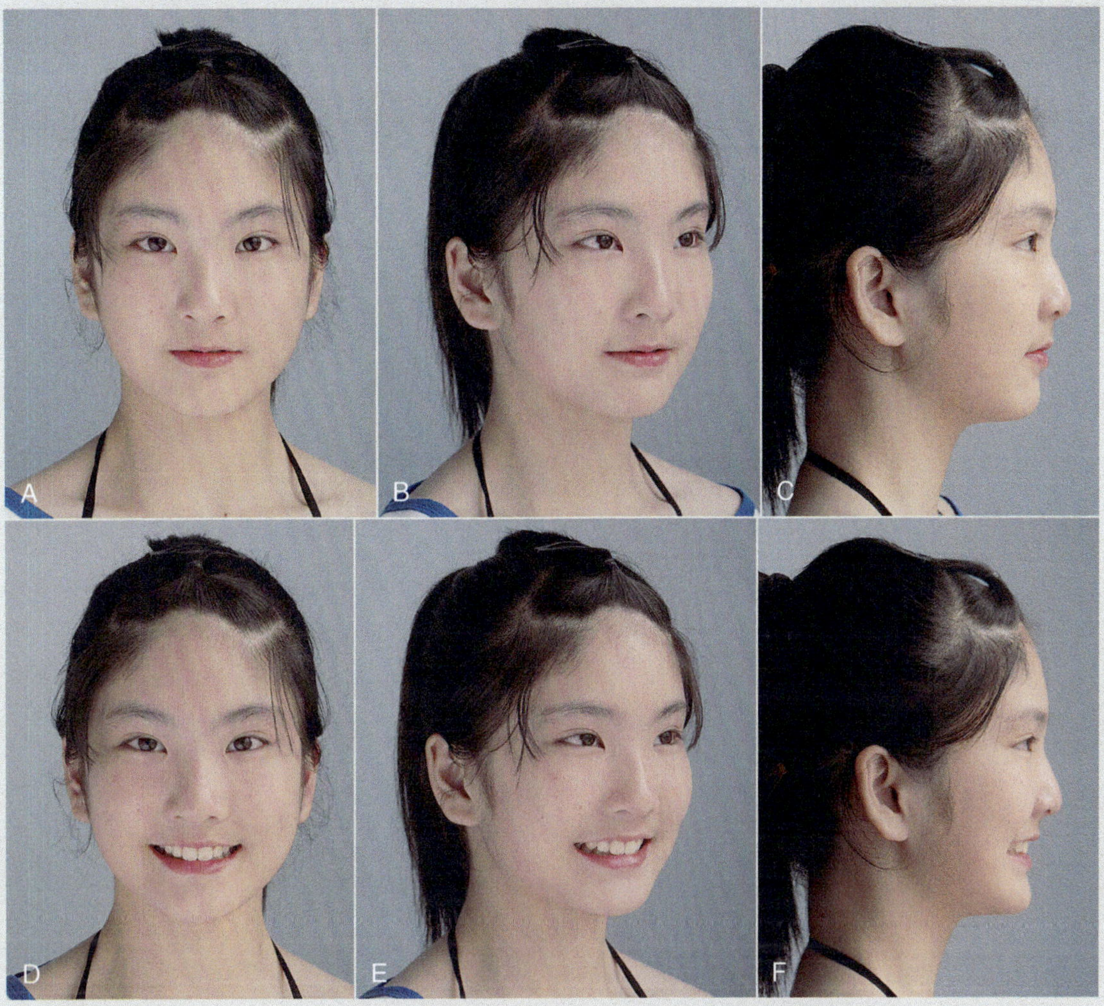

Figure 10-25 **A–F,** Facial views after treatment.

SUMMARY

This chapter introduced a holistic philosophy that combines the critical components of molar and incisor positioning, master and slave arches, and keeping the teeth in the center of bone. All these should be considered simultaneously throughout the active orthodontic treatment. With a case presentation of a Class II patient, we explained how the objectives were realized under the guidance of the holistic philosophy.

REFERENCES

1. Angle EH. *Treatment of Malocclusion of the Teeth and Fractures of the Maxillae, Angle's System*. 6th ed. Philadelphia, PA: S.S. White Dental Manufacturing; 1900.
2. Tweed CH. The Frankfort-mandibular incisor angle (FMIA) in orthodontic diagnosis, treatment planning and prognosis. *Angle Orthod*. 1954;24:121–169.
3. Andrews LF, Andrews WA. *The Syllabus of the Andrews Orthodontic Philosophy*. 9th ed. San Diego, CA: L.F. Andrews Foundation; 2001.
4. Scheid RC, Woelfel JB. *Woelfel's Dental Anatomy: Its Relevance to Dentistry*. 7th ed. Philadelphia, PA: Lippincott Williams & Wilkins; 2007.
5. Gray H, Lewis WH. *Anatomy of the Human Body*. 20th ed. Philadelphia, PA: Lea & Febiger; 1918.
6. Gray H. *Anatomy of the Human Body* (Bartleby.com edition), 2000. Accessed at www.bartleby.com/107.
7. Andrews LF. The six keys to normal occlusion. *Am J Orthod*. 1972; 62:296–309.
8. Dorfman HS. Mucogingival changes resulting from mandibular incisor tooth movement. *Am J Orthod*. 1978;74:286–297.
9. Artun J, Krogstad O. Periodontal status of mandibular incisors following excessive proclination: a study in adults with surgically treated mandibular prognathism. *Am J Orthod Dentofacial Orthop*. 1987;91:225–232.
10. Yared KF, Zenobio EG, Pacheco W. Periodontal status of mandibular central incisors after orthodontic proclination in adults. *Am J Orthod Dentofacial Orthop*. 2006;130:6.e1–8.
11. Ruf S, Hansen K, Pancherz H. Does orthodontic proclination of lower incisors in children and adolescents cause gingival recession? *Am J Orthod Dentofacial Orthop*. 1998;114:100–106.

12. Djeu G, Hayes C, Zawaideh S. Correlation between mandibular central incisor proclination and gingival recession during fixed appliance therapy. *Angle Orthod.* 2002;72:238–245.
13. Melsen B, Allais D. Factors of importance for the development of dehiscences during labial movement of mandibular incisors: a retrospective study of adult orthodontic patients. *Am J Orthod Dentofacial Orthop.* 2005;127:552–561.
14. Ricketts RM. A detailed consideration of the line of occlusion. *Angle Orthod.* 1978;48:274–282.
15. Lee RT. Arch width and form: a review. *Am J Orthod Dentofacial Orthop.* 1999;115:305–313.
16. Trivino T, Siqueira DF, Scanavini MA. A new concept of mandibular dental arch forms with normal occlusion. *Am J Orthod Dentofacial Orthop.* 2008;133:10.e5–22.
17. Strang RHW. Factors associated with successful orthodontic treatment. *Am J Orthod.* 1952;38:790–800.
18. Trivino T, Siqueira DF, Andrews WA. Evaluation of distances between the mandibular teeth and the alveolar process in Brazilians with normal occlusion. *Am J Orthod Dentofacial Orthop.* 2010;137:308.e1–4.
19. Interlandi S. New method for establishing arch form. *J Clin Orthod.* 1978;12:843–845.
20. Lee SJ, Lee S, Lim J, Park HJ, Wheeler TT. Method to classify dental arch forms. *Am J Orthod Dentofacial Orthop.* 2011;140:87–96.

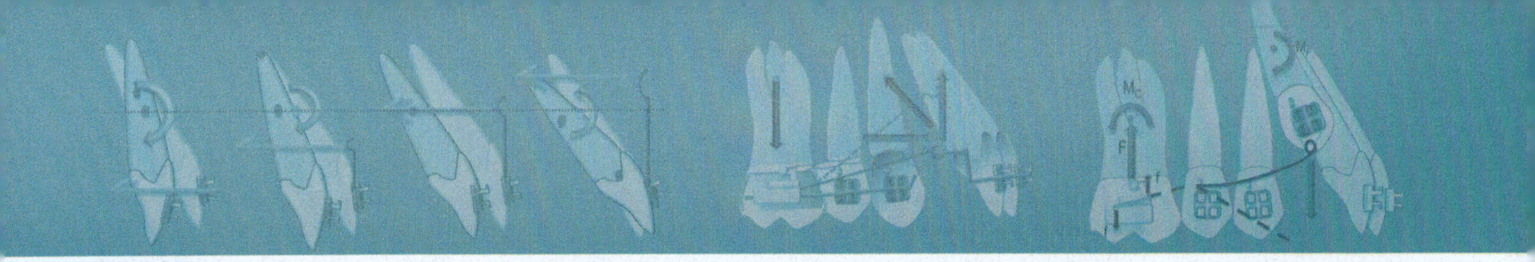

CHAPTER 11

Strategies for Treatment of Adolescent Patients with Class II Malocclusions

Urban Hägg and Ricky Wing Kit Wong

A German anatomist named Wilhem Roux (1850–1924) was the first to investigate the influence of natural forces and functional stimulation on form, and his work became the foundation for the principles of functional orthodontic appliances.[1] In 1889 Roux asked, "How many thousands of children afflicted with jaw-borne deformities have had to tolerate useless appliances ... before the infinite number of failures tend to deepening knowledge?"[2]

This question is still relevant today. We ask: Are there orthodontic devices currently in use that can deliver predictable and positive outcomes in the treatment of jaw-borne deformities such as skeletal Class II malocclusion? To answer this question, several randomized clinical trials (RCTs) have been conducted in recent years to study mixed dentition patients with Class II characteristics. In these studies subjects were divided into two groups: one group underwent early-stage (Phase 1) treatment using growth modification devices and the other group was the control group. Later, the patients in both groups underwent a phase of fixed appliance treatment, with and without extractions (this was Phase 2 for those who had had the Phase 1 treatment). By comparing the changes observed in patients during the Phase 1 treatment with the growth changes observed in the control group, one could estimate the effects of the treatment and also make comparisons between the groups treated with various "growth modificators." No matched controls were available to estimate the treatment effects of the group undergoing fixed appliance therapy because it was considered unethical to delay treatment any further. Consequently it was at best possible to estimate and compare the treatment effects during the early phase; that is, to compare the treatment changes in the groups that had observation followed by a fixed appliance phase with the group that had a combination of growth modification and a fixed appliance. It was reported that in the groups that had undergone the Phase 1 treatment with growth modification devices, there was some effect on the sagittal jaw–base relationship with restraint, forward growth of the maxilla, and/or enhanced growth of the mandible.[3,4] However, the possible advantage of these effects did not remain after the treatment with a fixed appliance when compared to the group that had fixed appliance only.

One study concluded that there were "remarkably similar outcomes with and without early phase 1 treatment,"[5] while another study reported "an inferior final occlusal result" with the two-stage approach.[6] A recent meta-analysis[7] concluded that the "effectiveness of functional appliances on mandibular growth in the short term ... provided in early adolescence ... probably was not very clinically significant." In conclusion, based on the reports from recent RCTs it seems that a number of orthodontic devices and concepts aimed at treating jaw discrepancies in the last century have had minimal to no benefit when used early.

DENTOFACIAL CHARACTERISTICS OF CLASS II MALOCCLUSION

Definition of Class II Malocclusion

The original definition of Class II malocclusion by Angle[8] was based on the sagittal dental arch relationship of the permanent dentition based primarily on the original position of the first permanent molars. Class II malocclusion as defined by Angle had a bilateral distal molar relationship and, based on the position of the maxillary incisors, was divided into two divisions: Division 1 and Division 2, with proclined and retroclined maxillary incisors, respectively. Cases with a unilateral distal molar relationship were classified as Class II (Division 1 or 2) subdivision. This definition, still widely used, is limited to the sagittal dental arch relationship only, not taking into account the vertical and transversal dental arch relationships or the jaw-base relationship.

Consequently, the original definition of Angle Class II malocclusion comprises subjects with a very wide range of dentofacial features, which have to be recognized in the orthodontic diagnosis and problem lists, treatment objectives, and treatment plans. Class II malocclusion is common in all ethnic groups and is reported as present in 10% to 25% of the general population.[9]

Differential Diagnosis of Class II Malocclusion

The distal relationship between the first permanent molars could be due to mesial rotation of the maxillary first permanent molars, maxillary dentoalveolar protrusion, a skeletal Class II jaw relationship, or a combination of all of these factors. Giuntini et al.[10] reported that 80% of subjects with a Class II molar relationship had mesially rotated first maxillary molars. Based on conventional cephalometric analysis the average dentofacial pattern in subjects with Angle Class II malocclusion is skeletal Class II (increased A point nasion B point [ANB] angle) usually with a retrognathic mandible but with normal positioning of the maxilla in Caucasians[11,12] and maxillary protrusion in Chinese.[13] However, a population study of Chinese patients demonstrated that only about one-third of the subjects with a Class II dental arch relationship were true skeletal Class II judged from the ANB angle or Wits appraisal, whereas about 1 in 10 subjects with Class I dental arch relationship had a skeletal Class II jaw relationship.[14] The lower face height[11] can be normal but is often increased (vertical maxillary excess), although it can also be decreased (vertical maxillary deficiency). Clinically, subjects with Class II malocclusion often have a convex profile, whereas others have straight profiles. Lips can be incompetent, especially in subjects with increased lower face height, or "overcompetent" in those with decreased lower face height. The maxillary incisors show at rest in subjects with Class II malocclusion and the smile may vary from excessive (gummy smile) to "not showing at all."

GROWTH PATTERN

Dentofacial growth is a very complex process. In the clinical context it is important to realize that the positioning of the mandible depends not only on condylar growth but also on the growth rotation of the mandible,[15] which is influenced by the growth direction and rotation of the maxilla and even that of the midface. Consequently the positioning of the mandible over a given amount of time depends on the growth rate and direction of the condyle and, in addition, that of the maxilla and midface. Subjects with vertical growth of the condyle will exhibit an anterior rotation pattern but the existence or lack of incisal contact affects the positioning of the mandible and the size of the lower face height. In subjects with both vertical condylar growth and incisal contacts the rotation center is located at the incisors, whereas in those with no incisal contacts the rotation center will be located more posteriorly (i.e., at the first premolars).[15] In the latter group the facial height will be relatively shorter and the chin prominence relatively marked. In subjects with sagittal growth direction of the condyle there will be posterior rotation of the mandible and the rotation center will be located at the molar region; these subjects will have a relatively larger lower anterior face height and the mandible will be positioned relatively less forward. Consequently some subjects with Class II malocclusion have a favorable, unchanged, or worsening sagittal jaw relationship. In orthodontic treatment it is important to use appliances in such a way that the facial esthetics, the positioning of the maxilla and mandible, and the jaw relationship do not deteriorate. Fortunately many Class II subjects have an inherent favorable growth pattern and the prognosis for improvement is good or fair in such cases.[3,16] In other subjects the prognosis is poor because of their inherent unfavorable growth pattern. Unfortunately many devices used to treat Class II malocclusion have negative effects on the face; that is, while they improve the occlusal relationship, they might ruin a tentatively favorable growth pattern, seriously worsening the treatment outcome in those with a poor inherent growth pattern. In such cases the growth pattern is often blamed for undesirable treatment outcomes when in fact it is more likely that the orthodontic devices are to blame.

Is it possible that a definite Class II malocclusion improves markedly with growth only? In a longitudinal study of untreated skeletal Class II subjects followed from 12 to 23 years of age, the average change in overjet was a reduction of only 1-mm but the sample comprised subjects with greatly improved occlusion, those in whom there was minimal change, and those who became considerably worse.[17] The classical study by Björk and Skieller[18] in which 21 untreated subjects were followed during adolescence included subjects with Class II malocclusion. The occlusion was greatly improved and "normalized" in Case 5, whereas it got much worse in Case 12. The records of these two cases[18] illustrated how the positioning of the mandible is related to the vertical growth of the maxilla, rather than primarily to the amount of condylar growth. In the subject with worsening Class II malocclusion (Case 12), the condylar growth was almost twice as great as in the Case 5 subject, who showed improved occlusion. However, the Case 5 subject had little vertical facial growth whereas the Case 12 subject had marked vertical growth of the face.

Figures obtained from this sample of 21 untreated subjects demonstrated that conventional cephalometric variables did not express condylar growth well. There was no significant association between the amount of condylar growth and change in mandibular prognathism expressed with the sella-nasion B point (SNB) angle ($r = 0.15$) and only a moderate association when expressed linearly[19] parallel to the upper occlusal plane ($r = 0.69$). Clinicians still attempt to predict mandibular positioning in patients based on certain features of the dentofacial morphology assessed from lateral head films, despite the fact that Baumrind et al.[20] demonstrated almost 30 years ago that such predictions were no better than chance. (For more information, see Hägg and Attström[21] and Meikle.[22])

The treatment options for Class II malocclusion are growth modification, camouflage treatment, and orthognathic surgery. Growth modification aims to influence the growth of the mandible and maxilla; that is, to reduce the skeletal Class II jaw-base relationship by enhancing mandibular and/or restraining maxillary forward positioning while at the same time controlling the lower face height. The treatment plan must be individualized and the position of the maxillary and mandibular incisors carefully evaluated. In many subjects maxillary incisors might appear protruded when they are in fact in a correct position that should be maintained to allow the lower jaw to come forward sufficiently. If maxillary incisors are to be retroclined, this might prevent forward positioning of the mandible. Changing the position of the incisors could potentially modify and compromise the growth changes.

Orthognathic surgery is a versatile and effective way to treat skeletal Class II malocclusion, with surgery of one or both jaws. Surgery of the maxilla, in one or several pieces with or without extraction of teeth, makes it possible to move the maxilla in all three planes. Any movement of the maxilla in the vertical plane affects the position of the mandible in both the vertical and the sagittal planes. Usually mandibular surgery aims to make the mandible longer and position it forward. Subapical surgery of the anterior mandibular segment allows for decompensation of the inclination of mandibular incisors and correction of the curve of Spee. This surgery in combination with extractions of two premolars provides space to place the alveolar segment with its six anterior teeth posteriorly over the mandibular base. In this way a chin prominence is created, allowing for correction of dentoalveolar compensation and an increase of the overjet, which subsequently allow for more forward positioning of the mandible and increased mandibular prognathism. However, there is the potential for relapse in any orthognathic procedure. The average sagittal relapse rate after bilateral sagittal split osteotomy (BSSO) has been reported to be about one-third, and the larger the movements the greater is the risk for substantial relapse.[23] In recent years distraction osteogenesis (DO) has been introduced to increase the length of the mandibular body gradually in an effort to produce more stable results, but the relapse rate associated with this approach appears to be very similar to that of BSSO.[24]

LIMITATIONS OF TREATMENT

Treatment objectives should be realistic and should aim to improve the patient's appearance rather than achieve "ideal" norms. Even with accurate problem lists, realistic treatment objectives, and skillful treatment, there are definite treatment limitations to both growth modification and orthognathic surgery in subjects with skeletal Class II malocclusion. The role of the individual subject's soft tissue "envelope" must be considered carefully during planning and treatment. Depending on the choice of orthodontic devices and the way in which they are used, there is a risk that treatment could make the patient's appearance worse. This is the case when there is a lack of vertical control, especially in the molars. Subsequently, the mandible rotates posteriorly and the lower face height increases, which prevents maximum forward positioning of the mandible.

GROWTH MODIFICATION

Recent RCTs on Class II treatment have not demonstrated any positive effect on the mandible following treatment with "growth modification devices." Tulloch et al.,[5] who compared one-phase treatment (i.e., fixed appliance only) and two-phase treatment (i.e., a first phase with bionator or headgear followed by a second phase with fixed appliance), stated that there were "remarkably similar outcomes of treatment with and without early phase 1 treatment." Later, O'Brien et al.[6] concluded that "there are definite disadvantages to the 2-stage approach (Twin-block and fixed appliance) … increased burden, appointments, costs, length of treatment and an inferior final occlusal result." The American Association of Orthodontists' Council on Scientific Affairs[25] concluded that "functional appliances do not increase horizontal mandibular growth in the long term" and in a recent meta-analysis[7] it was stated that "effectiveness of functional appliances on mandibular growth in the short term … provided in early adolescence … [were] probably not very clinically significant." So it seems that the outcomes of the RCTs have finally answered the question raised by Roux in 1889: "How many thousands of children afflicted with jaw-bone deformities have had to tolerate useless appliances … before the infinite number of failures tend to deepening knowledge?"[2] However, others are skeptical of the reports from the RCTs. For example, Darendeliler[26] wrote, "it is irresponsible to say there is no difference between treatment modalities" and others, such as Johnston[27] and Meikle,[22] have questioned the suitability of RCTs in the orthodontic context.

Can treatment modify any part of the body? It is well-documented that it is possible to modify the shape of the foot, head, and neck. Why should it not be possible to modify the growth of the face, including the mandible? In the clinical context, in treatment of mandibular retrognathism one should distinguish between enhancement of condylar growth and positioning of the mandible. Enhancement of condylar growth increases the length of the mandible but does not necessarily result in forward positioning of the mandible (i.e., increase in mandibular prognathism). The positioning of the mandible depends not only on condylar growth and the growth rotation of the mandible,[15] but also on the growth and rotation of the maxilla and even that of the midface. A common effect from orthodontic treatment is extrusion of molars, which causes backward rotation of the mandible and lengthening of the lower face height,[28] and most functional appliances and cervical headgear cause downward rotation of the maxilla, which also affects the position of the mandible, suggesting that vertical control of the maxilla and the molars could be critical for the positioning of the mandible.

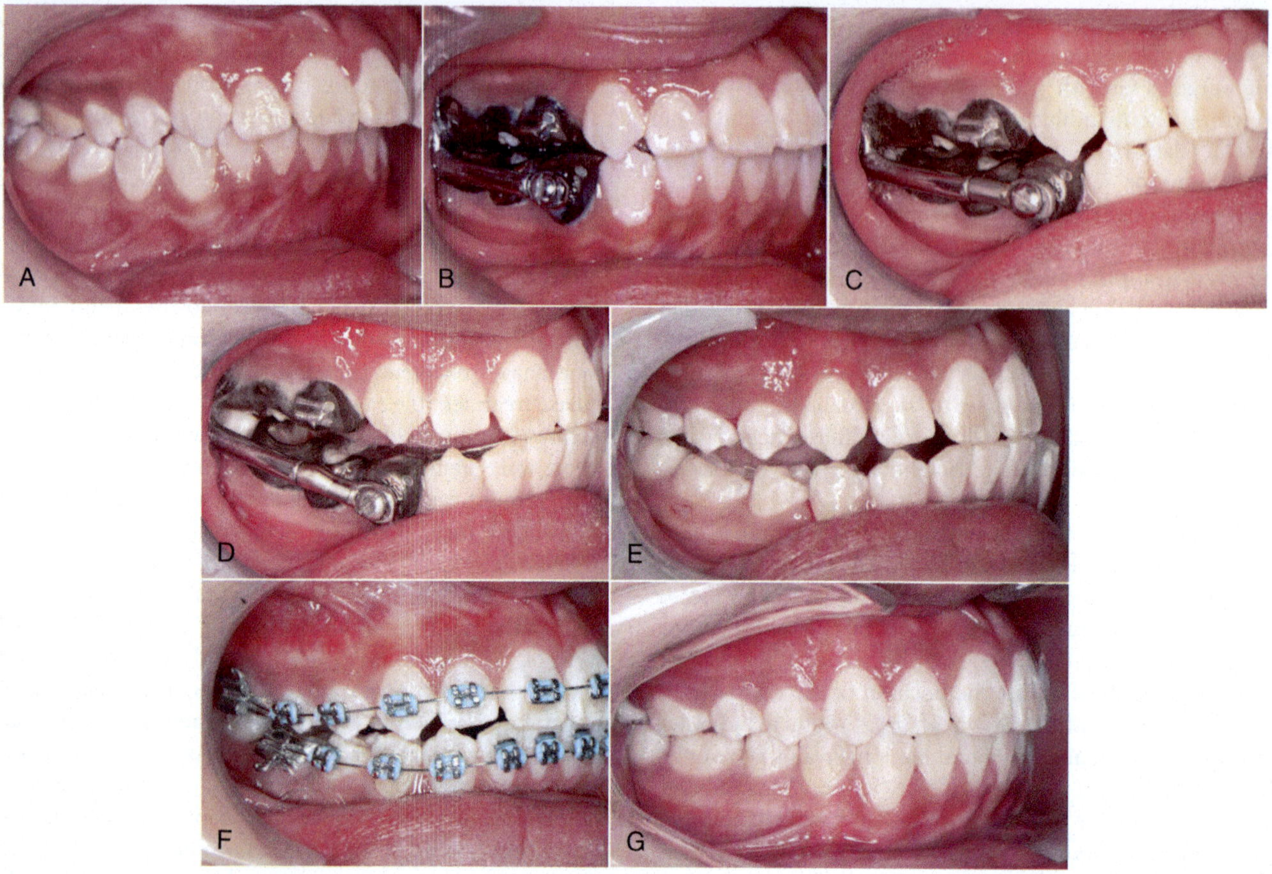

Figure 11-1 Growth modification fixed treatment of Class II malocclusion. **A,** Before treatment. **B,** Herbst appliance, first advancement. **C,** Herbst appliance, second advancement. **D,** Herbst appliance, third advancement. **E,** After 18 months, Herbst appliance. **F,** Fixed appliance use. **G,** After treatment.

BIOMECHANICS OF FUNCTIONAL APPLIANCES

At the beginning of the chapter, we described the functional orthodontic appliance. One example shown in Figure 11-1 is a Herbst appliance, which holds the mandible in a more anterior position when the jaw closes. The result is shown from A-G. In this section, the biomechanics of these functional appliances will be discussed.

Mandibular and Glenoid Fossa Growth Enhancement

The mandibular condyle is held away from its normal articular position, causing stimulation of growth at the mandibular condyle and remodeling of the glenoid fossa.[29] This contributes to the skeletal component for Class II correction. The direction of condylar growth can be favorable (backward) or unfavorable (upward).

Maxillary Growth Inhibition

Intermaxillary force delivered by the labial bow and sometimes by the acrylic cap to the maxillary dental arch delivers an orthopedic force to the maxilla that serves to inhibit downward and forward growth of the maxilla. This, together with the growth enhancement discussed above, contributes to the skeletal correction of the increased overjet and the Class II buccal occlusal relationship.[30]

Posterior Biteplate Effect

When a large bite opening is used, stretching forces are developed within the connective tissue and transmitted to the appliance, and thereby to the teeth and bones. This inhibits the vertical growth of maxilla and eruption of teeth so that downward rotation of the mandible is minimized. The amount of posturing or opening depends on whether a "myodynamic" or "myotonic" effect is desired.[30] In the myodynamic approach a small amount of forward posturing (mandible postured forward 5- to 6-mm and opened 2- to 3-mm beyond the rest position) stretches the muscle fibers and stimulates their continued contraction, which in turn brings the mandible back into the rest position.[30] In the myotonic approach the mandible is postured forward or opened vertically by a much greater amount. The muscles and soft tissues are stretched to a greater degree than with myodynamic appliances (mouth opening 8- to 10-mm or more beyond the rest position) so that the inherent elasticity of the tissues will create traction on the mandible.[30] The horizontal and vertical growth of the maxilla may also be retarded when using functional appliances in combination with high-pull headgear.[31] This is particularly suitable if there is midfacial prognathism.

Guidance of Eruption

By selectively using anterior or posterior occlusal stops or facets, eruption of teeth can be guided or stopped so that the arches can be leveled, molar relationships can be corrected, and buccal expansion can be encouraged.[30] Using the Andresen appliance,[32] tooth eruption is guided by facets cut into the lingual acrylic. In the upper arch the acrylic contacts the posterior teeth on their mesiopalatal aspects, with flutes sloping distally so that the teeth erupt distally. The lower posterior teeth contact acrylic on their distolingual aspect, with flutes sloping mesially to encourage their mesial eruption. The lingual acrylic can also be trimmed to encourage buccal expansion. In deep bite cases, capping the lower anteriors prevents their further eruption but leaving the lower posterior teeth free allows their continued eruption and thus levels the occlusal plane.[30] Conversely, using posterior bite blocks would prevent continued eruption of the posterior teeth while allowing the incisors to erupt. These can be used to treat anterior open-bite cases.[30] In hemifacial micrognathia, asymmetrical functional appliances with posterior bite blocks on the unaffected side encourage catch-up growth on the affected side.[30] Alternation of the buccal occlusion can be achieved by the selective inhibition of tooth eruption. In general the upper teeth erupt downward and forward and the lower teeth erupt vertically. Therefore to guide eruption and correct a sagittal discrepancy, occlusal stops can be placed on the upper molars and not on the lower molars. The downward and forward eruption of the upper molars is prevented while the lower molars are free to erupt upward and forward. This encourages correction of a Class II molar relationship.[33]

Stimulation of Bone Deposition in Areas Where the Periosteum is Stretched

When using the Frankel appliance, the buccal shields are extended well into the buccal sulci around point A. This, as postulated by Frankel, stretches the periosteum and promotes bone deposition with simultaneous relocation of muscle attachment in that area, thereby aiding in the correction of Class III malocclusion.[34]

Class II Elastic Effect

When the functional appliance is in place, it causes the mandible to be postured forward and held open in relation to the rest position. In this way the masticatory muscles are stimulated to retract the mandible to its original rest position and then intermaxillary forces are transmitted to the teeth of both dental arches through the appliance. This produces distal movement of the maxillary teeth and mesial movement of the mandibular teeth. If a labial bow is incorporated, class II traction will apply a distally directed force on the upper incisors via the labial bow and tend to tip the teeth palatally.[30]

Altering Soft Tissue Forces

The teeth are in a position of soft tissue balance between the lips and tongue anteriorly and the cheeks and tongue posteriorly. By using shields buccally or lingually the influence of the soft tissues can be eliminated on one side, thus altering the equilibrium and encouraging the teeth to take up a new position. One example is expansion of the dental arches by eliminating the forces of the lip and cheek muscles through use of buccal shields and leaving the tongue musculature unopposed. Another example is the lingual acrylic shield in the Andresen appliance, which prevents the resting tongue from lying between the teeth so that eruption is enhanced. A third example is anterior lingual shields used to prevent the tongue coming forward between the incisor teeth in open-bite cases. Functional appliances may also be used to modify lip form and activity and elimination of abnormal functions like breathing, swallowing and habit.[30] Further research is needed to investigate these actions.

WHAT CONCLUSIONS CAN BE DRAWN FROM RCTs ABOUT THE TREATMENT OF CLASS II MALOCCLUSION?

The best evidence of the effects of treatment on Class II malocclusion comes from systematic reviews based on actual RCTs. Meikle[22] has suggested that it is impossible to conduct a valid RCT in the setting of clinical orthodontics, concluding that there are simply too many variables that must be taken into account. None of the published RCTs have addressed the complexity of the problem of Class II malocclusion but rather have adopted the view that RCTs can be conducted by considering only a few simple, usually cephalometric, variables.

Limitations of the Sampling Criteria

The sampling criteria used in the RCTs are indeed very simple. Typically they include the size of the overjet, whether subjects are in the mixed dentition group, whether they have no severe vertical discrepancies,[5,6] whether they are Class II molar cases (including those with subdivision),[35] and whether they are Class II molar cases with an ANB angle >4.5 degrees.[36] Controls were not included in one study[36] and were included only for the first phase of treatment in the other studies.[5,6,35] The observation period was not standardized in one study,[35] since theF planned observation period was 24 months, but in patients in whom the treatment objectives were met records were kept at an earlier stage. In another study[5] follow-up records were taken after 15 months but all data were annualized (for 12 months), assuming that treatment changes were linear, which they are not.[37,38]

Drawbacks of Using Simple Sampling Criteria

The adoption of simple sampling criteria of dentofacial morphology is likely to result in very inhomogeneous samples. For example, in the sample obtained by Tulloch et al.[5] the youngest subject was 7.7 years old whereas the oldest subject was nearly 5 years older (12.4 years); in addition, the size of the overjet varied from 7-mm to more than twice that size, 1 in 10 subjects had a Class I molar relationship at the start of treatment (i.e., the dental arch relationship was Class I rather than Class II), and the jaw-base relationship assessed from the ANB angle varied from mild skeletal Class III (0.4 degrees, −1.4 standard deviations [SD]) to extremely severe Class II (12.2 degrees, +3.7 SD).

In general, not many details of either the dentofacial morphology or treatment changes were reported in those RCTs. To identify subjects in need of growth modification one should instead assess the subject's profile, specifically looking for a convex profile when the subject is assessed with the head in natural head posture, rather than the size of the overjet, the molar relationship, or the ANB angle, all of which have obvious and definite shortcomings in identifying subjects with sagittal jaw–base relationship. As clearly demonstrated by Björk and Palling,[39] the size of the overjet could be due to one or more of the following factors: angulation of the incisors and/or alveolar processes in both jaws and the sagittal position of the maxilla and/or mandible. Class II molar relationship more often seems to be associated with normal jaw-base relationship than skeletal Class II[14] and could be due to mesially rotated maxillary molars in many subjects.[10] The ANB angle does not necessarily reflect on the true sagittal jaw relationship.[40,41] The data for boys and girls were pooled in all studies, even though it is well-known that the timing of the pubertal growth spurt and the growth rates within it differ markedly between the sexes.[42,43]

Evaluation of Growth, Treatment Changes, and Treatment Effects

The evaluation of growth, treatment changes, and treatment effects is made from study casts using indices that attempt to reflect occlusal conditions and conventional cephalometric methods based on measurements of angles and distances. The effect on or change in mandibular prognathism[5,35,36] was described in terms of observed changes in the SNB angle,[44,45] ignoring the fact that the SNB angle is a very poor indicator of the sagittal position of the mandible because the nasion (N) moves forward and masks much of the actual forward positioning of the mandible.[45,46] Other factors that influence the SNB angle are the length and angulation of sella-nasion (SN) and the angulation of the occlusal plane.[40,41] It is obvious that a change expressed by an angular measurement on the maxillary level is about half of that on the mandibular level with the very same angular change, if one uses linear measurements. O'Brien et al.[6] used linear measurements (i.e., Sagittal-Occlusal [SO] analysis[19]) to describe sagittal effect and change of the mandible. This approach gives more valid information about the change in position of the mandible compared to that of the SNB angle but it still exaggerates the actual change in position of the mandible since the reference plane used, the upper occlusal plane, is inclined, on average, about 14 degrees to the true horizontal plane with a marked individual variation (0 to 30 degrees; see Wu et al.[47]). None of the RCTs took the head posture into account when describing the treatment effect and changes; therefore all of the results are potentially biased since they do not report the changes in the jaws in relation to the true horizontal and vertical planes.

Other Issues Affecting the Success of RCTs

Patient compliance and dropout rates are taken into account in some RCTs[6,35,36] but not in the one by Tulloch et al.[5] The noncompliance rates were reported to be 25% to 40% for removable functional appliances, 15% to 30% for headgear, and 15% for fixed functional appliances. As well, noncompliance rates were reported to be higher in older children and to differ between boys and girls. The reported noncompliance rate for both Twin Block and Herbst appliances was very much higher in one RCT[4] than in other studies conducted by clinicians very experienced with these devices.[43,48] In fact, the clinicians' prior experience with the devices used in the RCTs varied from no previous experience to many years of experience with the devices (e.g., in the Manchester RCT[4] the clinicians had practically no prior experience with the Herbst appliance but were all very familiar with the Twin Block). Herbst[49] admitted that the handling of his appliance required some experience. The high failure rate and comparatively short treatment with the Herbst appliance in that study[4] might reflect on the lack of experience among the clinicians. The difference in design of the Twin Block and the management and selection of patients in an efficiently run practice compared to a series of public authority clinics might explain why the failure rate was about four times higher in the latter setting.[48]

According to a recent systematic review[7] based on a series of RCTs, there was not much clinical effect from functional appliances. The authors concluded that "functional appliance treatment provided in early adolescence … small beneficial changes in the skeletal pattern probably not very clinical significant." In a prospective study it has been demonstrated that the timing of treatment is critical, since at least one fixed functional appliance, the Herbst appliance, seemed to have the potential to enhance and redirect growth of the mandible[38,50,51] so the more basic growth, the more growth to redirect.[52,53] The timing and length of treatment seem to be of particular importance. It has been reported that the mandibular growth rate at or just after the pubertal maximum of standing height is twice that of 1 to 2 years prior to that growth event and three times that of 3 years prior to that growth event. However, the period during which functional appliances were used in the RCTs in all boys and in most girls is the juvenile period, when the condylar growth rate can be as low as 0.5-mm per year, rather than adolescence.[52] In the RCTs early treatment with growth modification of Class II was conducted when most patients' growth rate was comparatively low and followed by fixed appliance treatment during a period with a higher growth rate and potentially unfavorable growth pattern that cannot be managed easily with a fixed appliance. It seems wiser to delay the phase of growth modification until the patient experiences maximum growth, when there is more growth to affect. During the first phase of treatment clinicians should use devices that are effective in redirecting mandibular growth for a sufficiently long time and thereafter use "effective-active" retention devices until the growth rate slows, at which time the second phase of treatment with fixed appliances begins (see Fig. 11-1). A fixed "growth modificator" such as the Herbst appliance adds, on average, only a modest amount to the basic condylar growth. Consequently, any enhancement of forward position of the mandible will depend on the total amount and direction of condylar growth, in which vertical control of the jaws and teeth is critical.

SUMMARY

A large proportion of young patients undergoing orthodontic treatment have Class II malocclusion. However, individuals with Class II malocclusion can differ greatly in their dentoskeletal-facial morphology and growth pattern. Consequently there is no simple formula of one treatment that fits all. Studying the growth pattern of a young patient might make it possible to identify whether the patient is a poor, average, or good grower, information that should be an important component of the individual patient's treatment plan. Based on the information obtained, the clinician can then decide whether the patient should be treated with growth modification, camouflage treatment, or orthognathic surgery.

REFERENCES

1. Wahl N. Orthodontics in 3 millennia: chapter 9: functional appliances to midcentury. *Am J Orthod Dentofacial Orthop*. 2006;129:829–833.
2. Levrini A, Favero L. *The Masters of Functional Orthodontics*. Carol Stream, IL: Quintessence Publishing Co; 2004:416.
3. Tulloch JF, Phillips C, Proffit WR. Benefit of early Class II treatment: progress report of a two-phase randomized clinical trial. *Am J Orthod Dentofacial Orthop*. 1998;113:62–72.
4. O'Brien K, Wright J, Conboy F, et al. Effectiveness of early orthodontic treatment with the Twin-block appliance: a multicenter randomized, controlled trial, part 1: dental and skeletal effects. *Am J Orthod Dentofacial Orthop*. 2003;124:234–243.
5. Tulloch JF, Proffit WR, Phillips C. Outcomes in 2-phase randomized clinical trial of early Class II treatment. *Am J Orthod Dentofacial Orthop*. 2004;125:657–667.
6. O'Brien K, Wright J, Conboy F, et al. Early treatment for Class II division 1 malocclusion with the Twin-block appliance: a multi-center, randomized, controlled trial. *Am J Orthod Dentofacial Orthop*. 2009; 135:573–579.
7. Marsico E, Gatto E, Burrascano M, Matrese G, Cordasco G. Effectiveness of orthodontic treatment with functional appliances on mandibular growth in the short term. *Am J Orthod Dentofacial Orthop*. 2011; 139:24–36.
8. Angle EH. Classification of malocclusion. *Dental Cosmos*. 1899;248–264, 350–357.
9. Proffit WR. Malocclusion and dentofacial deformity in contemporary society. In: Proffit WR, Fields HW, Sarver DM, eds. *Contemporary Orthodontics*. 5th ed. St. Louis, MO: Mosby; 2012:8.
10. Giuntini V, Baccetti T, Defraia E, et al. Mesial rotation of upper first molars in Class II division 1 malocclusion in the mixed dentition: a controlled blind study. *Prog Orthod*. 2011;12:107–113.
11. McNamara JA. Components of class II malocclusion in children 8–10 years of age. *Angle Orthod*. 1981;51:177–202.
12. Pancherz H, Zieber K, Hoyer B. Cephalometric characteristics of Class II division 1 and Class II division 2 malocclusions: a comparative study in children. *Angle Orthod*. 1997;67:111–120.
13. Lau JW, Hagg U. Cephalometric morphology of Chinese with Class II division 1 malocclusion. *British Dent J*. 1999;186:188–190.
14. Zhou L, Mok CW, Hagg U, et al. Anteroposterior dental arch and jaw-base relationships in a population sample. *Angle Orthod*. 2008;78; 1023–1029.
15. Björk A. Variations in the growth pattern of the human mandible: longitudinal radiographic study by the implant method. *J Dent Res*. 1963;42:400–411.
16. Klocke A, Nanda RS, Kahl-Nieke B. Skeletal Class II patterns in the primary dentition. *Am J Orthod Dentofacial Orthop*. 2002;212: 596–601.
17. Feldmann I, Lundstrom F, Peck S. Occlusal changes from adolescence to adulthood in untreated patients with Class I Division 1 deepbite malocclusion. *Angle Orthod*. 1999;69:33–38.
18. Björk A, Skieller V. Facial development and tooth eruption: an implant study at the age of puberty. *Am J Orthod*. 1972;62:49–58.
19. Pancherz H. The mechanism of Class II correction in Herbst appliance treatment: a cephalometric investigation. *Am J Orthod*. 1982;82: 104–113.
20. Baumrind S, Kom EL, West EE. Prediction of mandibular rotation: an empirical test of clinician performance. *Am J Orthod*. 1984;86: 371–385.
21. Hägg U, Attström K. Mandibular growth estimated by four cephalometric measurements. *Am J Orthod*. 1992;102:146–152.
22. Meikle M. Guest editorial: what do prospective randomized clinical trials tell us about the treatment of Class II malocclusions? A personal viewpoint. *Eur J Orthod*. 2005;27:105–114.
23. Mobarak KA, Espeland L, Korgstad O, Lyberg T. Mandibular advancement surgery in high-angle and low-angle Class II patients: different long-term responses. *Am J Orthod Dentofacial Orthop*. 2001;119: 368–381.
24. Ow A, Cheung LK. Skeletal stability and complications of bilateral sagittal split osteotomies and mandibular distraction osteogenesis: an evidenced-based review. *J Oral Maxillofac Surg*. 2009;67:2344–2353.
25. Council on Scientific Affairs (COSA). Functional appliances and long-term effects on mandibular growth. *Am J Orthod Dentofacial Orthop*. 2005;128:271–272.
26. Darendeliler MA. Validity of randomized clinical trials in evaluating the outcome of Class II treatment. *Semin Orthod*. 2006;12:67–79.
27. Johnston LE. Let them eat the cake: the struggle between form and substance in orthodontic clinical investigation. *Clin Orthod Res*. 1998;1:88–93.
28. Nelson B, Hansen K, Hägg U. Overjet reduction and molar correction in fixed appliance treatment of class II division I malocclusion: sagittal and vertical components. *Am J Orthod Dentofacial Orthop*. 1999;115: 13–23.
29. McNamara JA. Neuromuscular and skeletal adaptations to altered function in the orofacial region. *Am J Orthod*. 1973;64:578–606.
30. Turner PJ. Functional appliances: a systemic approach. *Dent Update*. 1991;3:72–76.
31. Graber TM, Rakosi T, Petrovic AG. *Dentofacial Orthopaedics with Functional Appliances*. St. Louis, MO: CV Mosby; 1985.
32. Graber TM, Neumann B. *Removable Orthodontic Appliances*. Philadelphia, PA: WB Saunders; 1977.
33. Harvold EP, Vargervik K. Morphogenetic response to activator treatment. *Am J Orthod*. 1971;60:478–490.
34. Frankel R. A functional approach to orofacial orthopaedics. *Br J Orthod*. 1980;7:41–51.
35. Keeling SD, Wheeler TT, King GJ, et al. Anterioposterior skeletal and dental changes after early Class II treatment with bionators and headgear. *Am J Orthod Dentofacial Orthop*. 1998;113:40–50.
36. Ghafari J, Shofer FS, Jacobsson-Hunt U, Markowitz DL, Laster LL. Headgear versus function regulator in the early treatment of Class II, division 1 malocclusion: a randomized clinical trial. *Am J Orthod Dentofacial Orthop*. 1998;113:51–61.
37. Hägg U, Du X, Rabie ABM. Initial and late treatment effect of headgear-Herbst appliance with mandibular step-by-step advancement. *Am J Orthod Dentofacial Orthop*. 2002;122:477–485.

38. Hägg U, Rabie ABM, Bendeus M, et al. Condylar growth and mandibular positioning with stepwise versus maximum jumping. *Am J Orthod Dentofacial Orthop*. 2008;134:525–536.
39. Björk A, Palling M. Adolescent age changes in sagittal jaw relation, alveolar prognathy, and incisal inclination. *Acta Odontol Scand*. 1955; 12:201–232.
40. Jacobsson A. The "Wits" appraisal of jaw disharmony. *Am J Orthod*. 1975;67:125–138.
41. Jacobsson A. Application of the "Wits" appraisal. *Am J Orthod*. 1976; 70:179–185.
42. Hägg U, Taranger J. Maturation indicators and the pubertal growth spurt. *Am J Orthod*. 1982;82:299–309.
43. Pancherz H, Hägg U. Dentofacial orthopaedics in relation to somatic maturation: an analysis of 70 consecutive cases treated with the Herbst appliance. *Am J Orthod*. 1985;88:273–287.
44. Björk A. The face in profile: an anthropological x-ray investigation on Swedish children and conscripts. *Sv Tandl Tidskr*. 1947;40:5B.
45. Downs WB. Analysis of the dentofacial profile. *Am J Orthod*. 1956; 26:191–212.
46. Taylor CM. Changes of the relationship of nasion, point A, point B and the effect upon ANB. *Am J Orthod*. 1969;56:143–163.
47. Wu JYC, Hagg U, Wong RWK, McGrath C. The natural head posture horizontal vs conventional cephalometric. *Angle Orthod*. 2013; submitted.
48. Clark WJ. *New horizons in orthodontics and dentofacial orthodopedics: aspects of Twin Block functional therapy [PhD thesis]*. Dundee, Scotland: University of Dundee; 2009.
49. Herbst E. *Dreissiger Erfahrungen mit dem Retentions-Schanier Zhanarztl Rundschau*. [Thirty years experience with the retention-joint (Herbst appliance)]. 1934;43:1515–1524, 1563–1568, 1611–1616. Translation into English by Bachmeyer D, University of Toronto.
50. Hägg U. Change in mandibular growth direction by means of a Herbst appliance? A case report. *Am J Orthod*. 1992;102:456–463.
51. Pancherz H, Fackel U. The skeletofacial growth pattern pre- and post-dentofacial orthopedics: a long-term study of Class II malocclusions treated with the Herbst appliance. *Eur J Orthod*. 1990;12:209–218.
52. Björk A. Timing of interceptive orthodontic measures based on stages of maturation. *Trans Eur Orthod Soc*. 1972;61–74.
53. Hägg U, Pancherz H, Taranger J. Pubertal growth and orthodontic treatment. In: Carlson DS, Ribbens KA, eds. *Craniofacial Growth during Adolescence*. Monograph 20, Craniofacial Growth Series. Ann Arbor, MI: Center for Human Growth and Development, The University of Michigan; 1987:87–115.

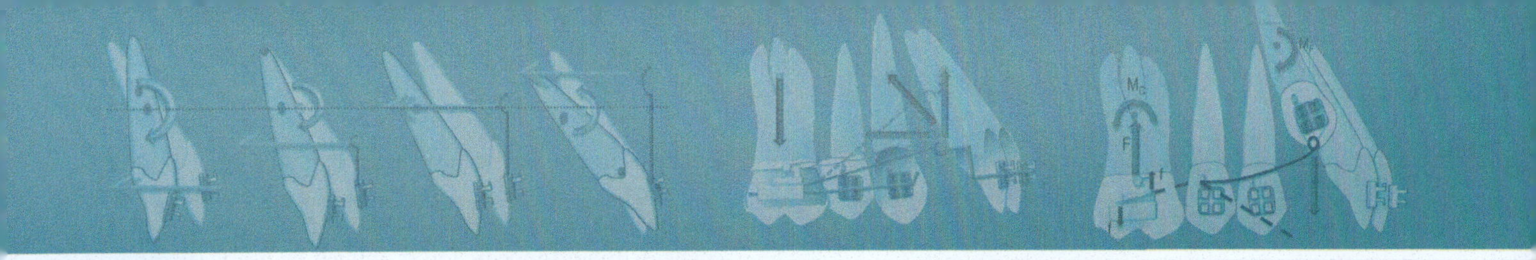

CHAPTER 12

Nonextraction Class II Correction

Ram S. Nanda, Tarisai C. Dandajena, and Ravindra Nanda

Nonextraction treatment has gained in popularity in the orthodontic community since the second half of the twentieth century. This is due to the paradigm shift from focusing on the dentition to appraising the whole face. The careful selection of patients and timing of treatment are essential to the success of nonextraction treatment. When planning nonextraction treatment, we opt to use early treatment, redirection of growth, saving leeway space, guidance of eruption, and mechanics that aim to achieve distal movement of the maxillary molars. For a successful outcome, it is necessary before the initiation of treatment to take into consideration the type of malocclusion, facial type, required arch perimeter, individual growth, and motivation of the patient.

Class II, Division 1 malocclusion has been described as the most frequent treatment problem in orthodontic practice. It is estimated that about 35% of American children have Class II malocclusions. Distal movement of the maxillary first molars is a common goal in the treatment of the Class II molar relationship and in the resolution of tooth size–arch length discrepancy in the maxillary arch.

Early treatment is the key to successful treatment of Class II malocclusions. During the 1940s and 1950s Kloehn[1] suggested the use of headgear during the transitional dentition to correct molar relations. In the 1960s Ricketts et al.[2] promoted the bioprogressive philosophy, which used utility arches, quad helix, and cervical facebow headgear among several other innovative appliance systems. However, the real impetus behind nonextraction treatment was the realization that for far too long orthodontists had focused on the placement of the denture on the basal bone without sufficient regard to the facial integument. Research findings on long-term retention of treated dentitions revealed that relapse was common in both extraction and nonextraction treatment modalities. Cetlin and Ten Hoeve[3] showed stable results for nonextraction treatment of patients with severe malocclusions. The thickness of facial soft tissue integument varies among individuals and its growth pattern is specific to individuals throughout their lifespan and not just during the period of active growth.[4] In view of these findings, the nonextraction treatment modality has become a treatment of choice for select groups of patients.

PATIENT SELECTION

Patients need to be carefully selected for nonextraction treatment. Prospective patients to be treated using maxillary molar distalization techniques should exhibit a Class II dental relation or a minor skeletal Class II relation. A Class II relationship with mesial migration of maxillary molars due to premature loss of the primary molar is preferred. The patient should have minimal or no mandibular arch length discrepancy, preferably with mesofacial or brachyfacial types, and potential remaining growth. A low mandibular plane angle is most suitable because in high angle the distal movement of molars will tend to open the bite due to the extrusive force component. Even a full Class II relationship can be corrected if treated earlier. Recently, Kim et al.[5] have shown that an occlusion established at an early age is more likely to be maintained despite the differential growth of the jaws.

A variety of appliances has been used, including ones that require patient cooperation and ones that do not.

BIOMECHANICAL PRINCIPLES

The adequate force for distal movement of the molars is in the range of 150 to 250 g. The type of movement can be either translation or controlled tipping followed by uprighting. Translation movement requires the force to pass through the center of resistance (see Chapter 4). Therefore, when using any type of appliance, it is necessary to evaluate the force system of that appliance and to be informed about the side effects. Anchorage considerations include extrusion of molars and mesial movement of the anterior segment. To obtain the maximum benefit the distal resistance (the presence of second or third molars), growth in the tuberosity region, and functional interferences should be checked.

TREATMENT MODALITIES FOR MAXILLARY MOLAR DISTALIZATION

Several treatment modalities exist for the distal movement of the maxillary molars. These can be with either fixed or removable appliances, and intraoral or extraoral. The extraoral approach can use cervical, occipital, or high-pull headgear. The intraoral mechanics can be inter-arch or intra-arch. Of the inter-arch appliances, the Herbst, Twin Force bite corrector, Jasper jumper, and SAIF spring constitute fixed functional appliances that do not require patient compliance. Class II elastics with the jig and bimetric arch (Wilson appliance) require patient compliance. The transpalatal arch, coil springs, repelling magnets, K-loop,[7] pendulum, Jones jig, and distal jet are intra-arch appliances. These appliances can be used as single entities or combined with another appliance. Some of these appliances are discussed below.

Headgear

Kingsley[8] first introduced the extraoral method of applying traction to the maxillary arch to retract maxillary incisors. Later, Angle[9] described and illustrated the headgear he used in the treatment of patients with Class II, Division 1 malocclusion. Both Kingsley and Angle used astonishingly modern-looking appliances, apparently with reasonable success. At the beginning of the twentieth century, the introduction of intermaxillary elastics resulted in the discontinuation of extraoral anchorage. This was not due to its ineffectiveness, but rather because it was considered an unnecessary complication.

By 1920 Angle and his followers were convinced that Class II and III elastics not only moved teeth but also caused significant skeletal changes, stimulating the growth of one jaw while restraining the other. If intraoral elastics could produce a true stimulation of mandibular growth while simultaneously restraining the maxilla, there would be no reason either to ask a patient to wear an extraoral appliance or to initiate treatment while waiting for the permanent teeth to erupt.

When cephalometric evaluations became available in the 1940s, they did not support the idea that significant skeletal changes occurred in response to intraoral forces. In 1936 Oppenheim[10] strongly advocated extraoral anchorage therapy. Later, Kloehn[1] demonstrated impressive results with headgear in the early treatment of Class II malocclusion. He stated that, during the transitional dentition, cervical traction can retard or even halt the forward growth of the maxilla and assist in moving maxillary teeth distally to correct developing Class II relationships.

While the distal movement of the molars by headgear may not be questionable, the changes that take place within the temporomandibular joint (TMJ) complex have not been well explained. Animal studies have shown remodeling of the condyle-glenoid fossa complex: apposition in the posterior compartment and resorption in the anterior compartment.[11–13] Cephalometric studies have shown little or no change in the size of the mandible with the use of functional appliances such as headgear. It is possible that the lateral cephalogram is not sensitive enough to isolate these changes. The orthopedic forces applied by headgear cannot be ignored, however.

Extraoral traction has some demonstrable important advantages. These include maximum anchorage, ability to adjust the force levels, and control of bodily or tipping movement. It can assist in correcting transverse deficiencies by expanding the inner bow. The extrusive component of the cervical headgear will allow for bite opening in deep bite patients. If vertical control is a concern in a high-angle patient, a high-pull facebow headgear will control the extrusive force component.

There are limitations in the use of extraoral traction, of which the need for patient compliance is perhaps the most important. Besides compliance, the type of force delivered by the appliance is intermittent, with tooth movement usually being slower. We have found that prolonged use of headgear can delay the eruption of maxillary second molars or even lead to their impaction. This may not be a problem if treatment is initiated at the appropriate age of 9 years and for a limited time. In such cases the second molars need to be monitored if treatment is completed prior to their eruption. Extraction of the second molars may be considered if the presence of the third molars is radiographically documented. Despite these limitations, extraoral traction is perhaps one of the most effective ways to obtain distal movement of maxillary molars and a successful nonextraction treatment plan.

A decision to extract the second molars may be made in severe Class II cases where maximum retraction of the first molars is required. As mentioned, radiographic documentation for the presence of the third molars is important. Figure 12-1 documents a case in which extraction of the maxillary second molars was performed prior to their eruption. A mandibular lip bumper engaged to the mandibular first molar bands was used to align and unravel the minor mandibular crowding. The maxillary premolars were allowed to passively drift back. Retraction of the anterior segment, however, required active mechanics and this was accomplished using a T-loop. Class II elastics were used for 1 month. During this process the headgear was used as anchorage and the patient wore it only at bedtime.

The headgear may be used effectively in cases of asymmetrical Class II correction. In such cases there is asymmetrical adjustment of the outer bow, one side being longer than the other.[14,15] The longer arm of the outer bow will be placed on the side where correction of the Class II molar relationship is desired. Asymmetrically positioning the center of the outer bows while the arms are kept the same length may not achieve the same results as altering the lengths of the outer bows. This is because in the first instance the force applied will pass through the center, while in the latter instance there is an asymmetrical distribution of the moments. The greater moment is applied to the longer side.[14,15] Of importance, however, is the need for patient compliance.

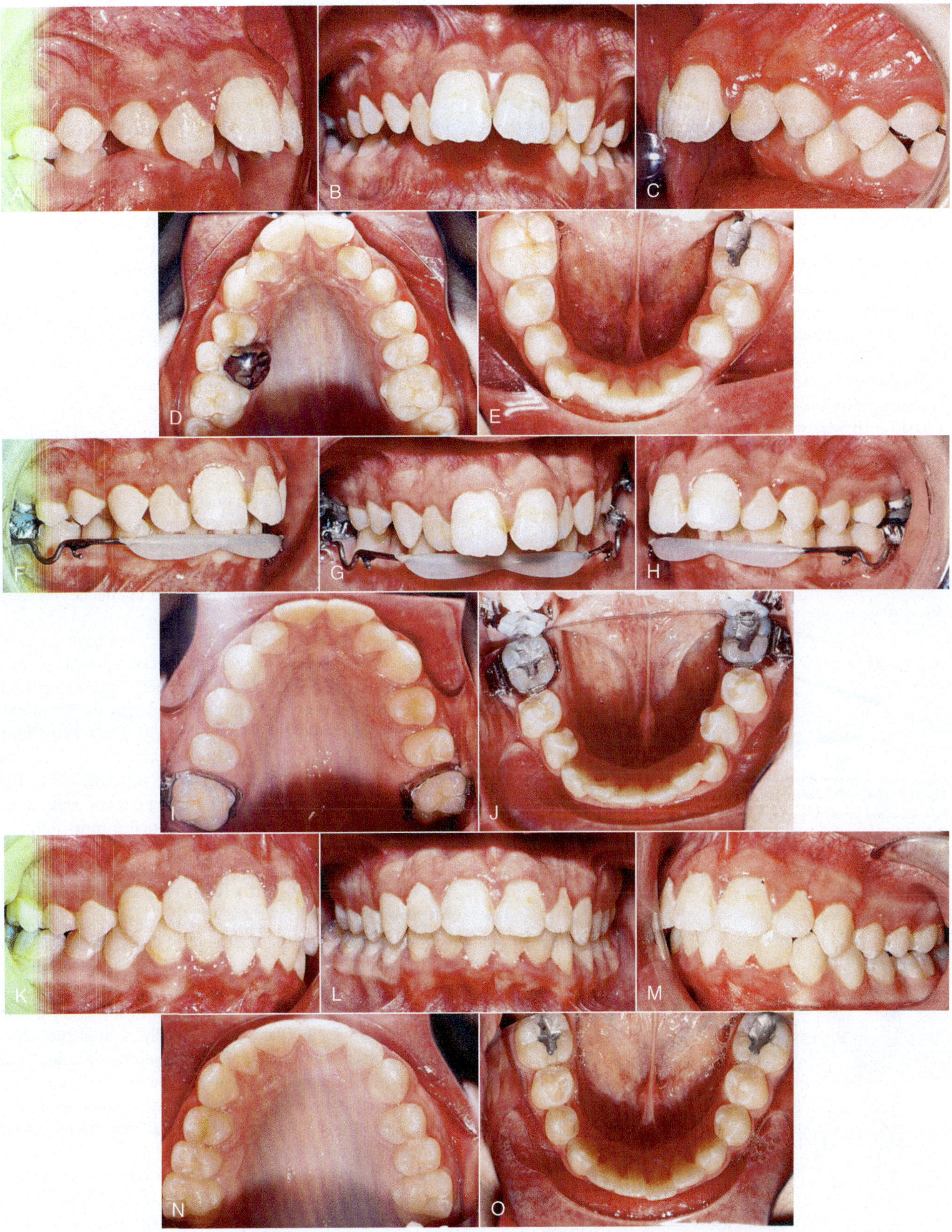

Figure 12-1 Headgear treatment. **A–E,** Pre-treatment intraoral photographs. A stainless steel crown is present on the exfoliating maxillary left second primary molar. **F–J,** Progress photographs show the lip bumper in place. **K–O,** Intraoral photographs 1 month post-treatment. Total treatment time was 23 months.

Care should be taken to adjust the facebow so as to achieve the desired result. In open bite, for example, care should be taken to avoid extrusion of the molars, while in cases of low mandibular plane angle extrusion of the molars may be a desired consequence. In such patients, then, application of the force above the center of resistance with the strap pulling down and backward will produce extrusion with distal movement.[16] Figure 12-2 shows the various movements that can be obtained using the facebow headgear depending on the point of force application.[16]

Vertical Holding Appliance

Some clinicians and investigators have sought ways to augment the extraoral traction. One method is the combined use of a vertical holding appliance (VHA)[17,18] and high-pull headgear. The VHA (Fig. 12-3) has been recommended for treatment of high-angle patients where there is an important need to control the vertical dimension. It is fabricated from a 0.040-inch wire with a helix just distal to each maxillary first molar. Two more helices are placed at the center of the appliance, and these are separated by a V-bend to which is molded an acrylic button the size of a dime. The most mesial portion of this appliance (i.e., the acrylic button) should lie on a line that connects the mesial margins of the maxillary first molars. The button should also be 2- to 5-mm away from the palate. The VHA achieves the treatment objectives by way of an intrusive and distally directed force. The result is intrusion and distal movement of the molars. This is a fixed functional appliance since the forces are achieved from the functional activity of the tongue. In a study conducted at the University of Oklahoma,[19] excellent results were achieved using the VHA compared to other methods.

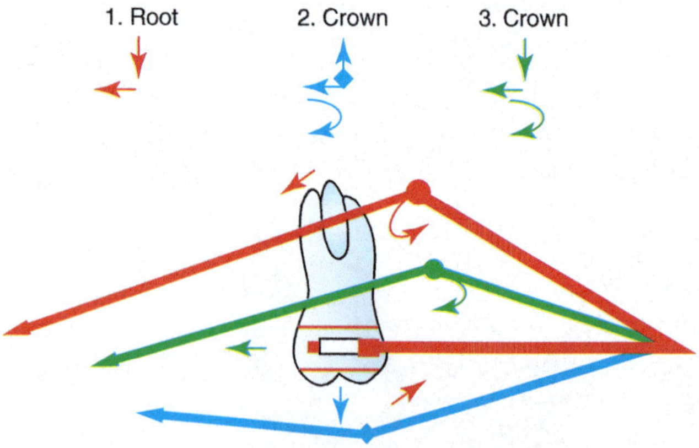

Figure 12-2 Forces and moments generated by the facebow headgear. **1,** Force is above the center of resistance—the result is extrusion, mesial moment, and distal movement of the root. **2,** Force is below the center of resistance in an upward direction—the effect is distal crown movement, clockwise moment, and an intrusive effect. **3,** Force is below the center of resistance in a downward direction—the effect is extrusion, distal crown movement, and clockwise moment.

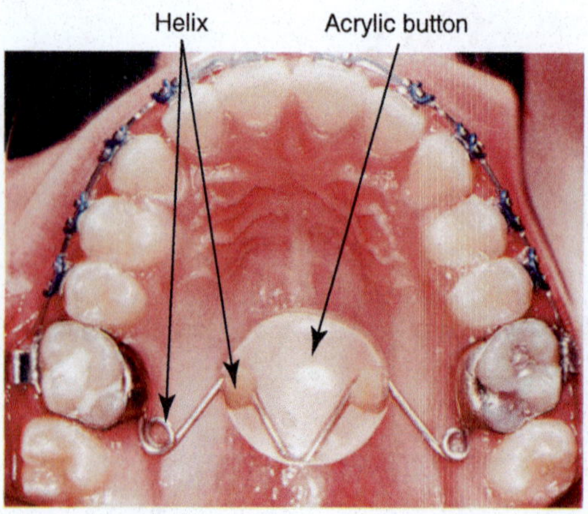

Figure 12-3 Vertical holding appliance (VHA). The first set of helices is positioned distal to the maxillary first molar and the second set is under the acrylic but not inside it. Only the V-bend attaches the 0.040-inch wire to the acrylic.

Though initially recommended for use in combination with headgear, we have noted that the VHA on its own is useful for correction of Class II malocclusion. Figure 12-4 documents a patient whose initial treatment plan was for treatment with a straight-pull facebow headgear, but she declined to use it. The patient was put under observation for 6 months while the VHA was cemented to the maxillary first molars. A fixed lingual arch (FLA) was also cemented to the mandibular arch for maintenance of the leeway space. Even though the leeway space may not always be available,[19] the FLA can be used to control the vertical dimension during the growth period.[20] After 6 months, correction of the Class II malocclusion was observed. No other appliance was used during this period.

Although the forces generated by the VHA have not been measured, measurement of the forces applied to the transpalatal arch (TPA) from the tongue[20] suggest that these forces may reach very high levels considering the size of the Nance button to which the 0.040-inch wire is attached. Chiba et al.[21] noted that maximum pressure was applied to the TPA during deglutition when the appliance was engaged to the maxillary second molars. Also, this pressure was at its maximum when the TPA was positioned 6-mm from the palate.

Cervical Facebow with Removable Maxillary Plate

Cetlin has proposed the treatment of Class II relationships using a combination of TPAs (Fig. 12-5), cervical headgear, and a removable maxillary plate with auxiliary springs. This treatment modality requires correction of maxillary molar rotations (which in Class II are usually rotated mesiolingually) prior to distal movement and then distalization. The derotation of the molars in a distobuccal direction may produce a space gain of as much as 2- to 3-mm on each side. Once the rotations are corrected, distal movement can be initiated. The distal movement of the maxillary molars is achieved by means of a removable maxillary plate to which is attached some auxiliary springs. The springs deliver a distally directed force of approximately 30 g that is augmented by a cervical-pull facebow headgear with approximately 150 g of force. Once again, the outer bows of the facebow must be positioned such that the side effects from the headgear are minimized. No extrusive forces should be applied

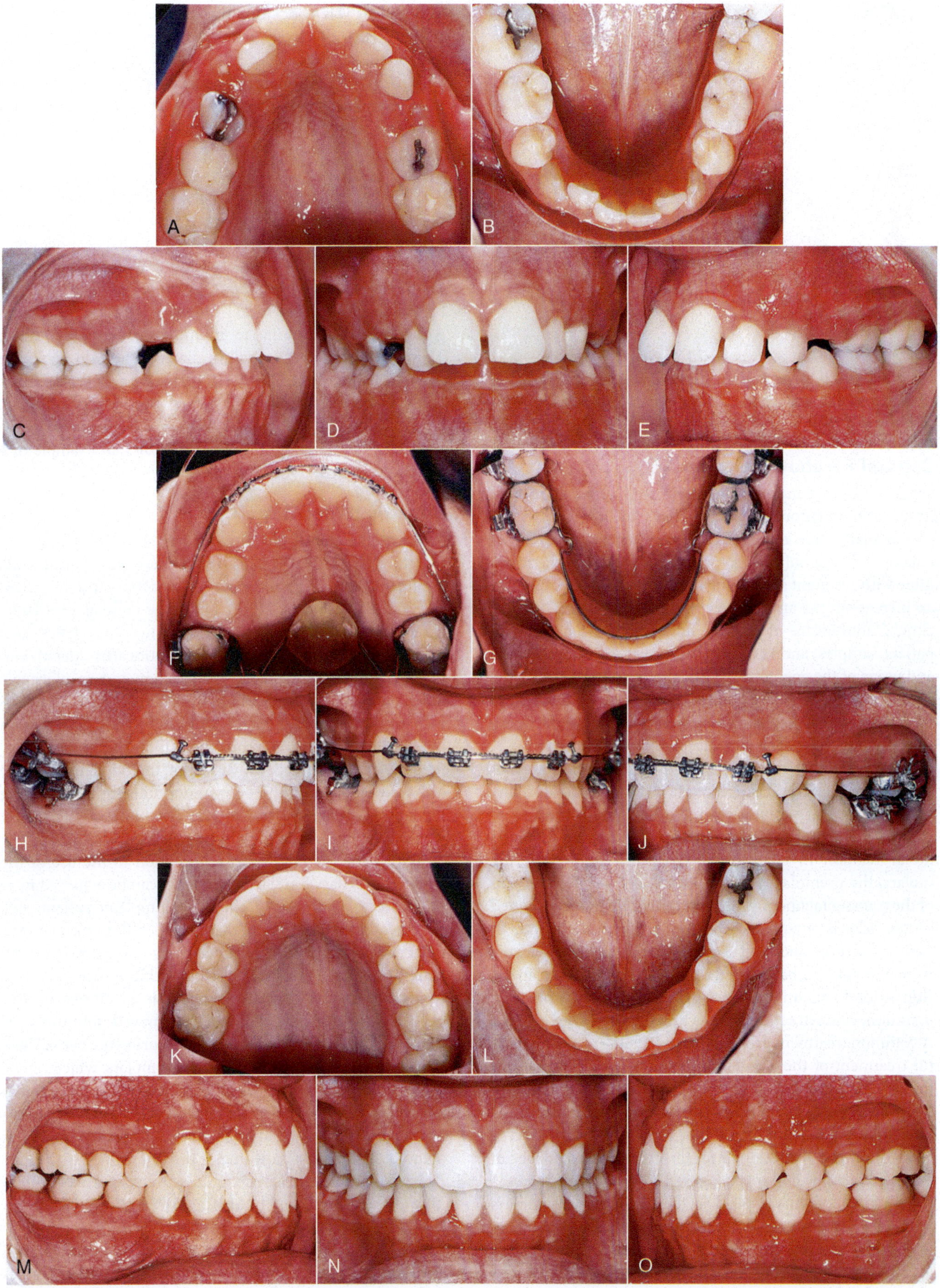

Figure 12-4 Class II, Division 1 malocclusion treated with a vertical holding appliance (VHA). **A–E,** Pre-treatment intraoral photographs of a Class II, Division 1 subdivision left malocclusion. **F–J,** Progress photographs showing a VHA cemented to the maxillary first molars and a fixed lingual arch (FLA) cemented to the mandibular first molars. These photographs were taken 6 months after delivery of the VHA and FLA. **K–O,** Final records at completion of treatment.

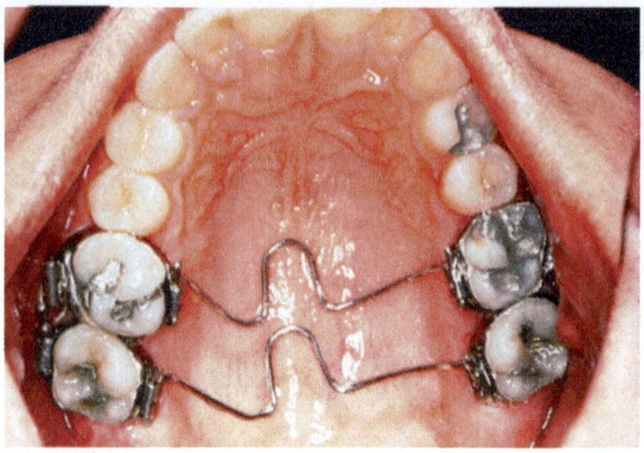

Figure 12-5 Transpalatal arches for molar derotation prior to distalization. (Courtesy of Dr. Norman Cetlin, Boston, MA.)

when extrusion is not desired, as these will result in opening of the bite from extrusion of the molars and clockwise rotation of the mandible.

Cervical Facebow Headgear

Some studies on molar distalization with cervical facebow headgear have reported negative effects, including extrusion of maxillary first molars, downward anterior tipping of palatal and occlusal planes, posterior rotation of the mandible with resultant steepening of the mandibular plane, and an increase in the anterior lower face height. Many of these clinical studies are of variable duration, some have small patient samples, and some lack information on compliance and usage of the appliance. The credibility of these studies is further compromised by poor documentation of force magnitude, direction of force, duration of force application, physiological age of the patients, and biological response.

Kloehn popularized and reported the successful usage of the cervical facebow headgear.[1] He demonstrated in many patients that this was an important and useful method of maxillary molar distalization and correction of Class II molar relation in developing dentitions. Along with the molars, the premolars also drifted distally through the pull of the transseptal fibers. A retrospective study was conducted on the records of patients treated by Dr. John S. Kloehn.[22,23] Eighty-five pre- and post-treatment records were selected from 125 patients based on the Class II first molar relationship prior to treatment on the transitional or permanent dentition, nonextraction treatment, and good cooperation. A common treatment protocol that was followed for successful treatment of these patients was alternate adjustment of the outer facebow below or above the line of occlusion every 6 to 12 weeks. The outer bow is bent downward during the first 6 to 12 weeks and then it is bent upward for a period of equal duration. The rationale for this treatment protocol can be appreciated by looking at Figure 12-2, which analyzes the forces and moments applied to the maxillary first molars with each adjustment. With this treatment regimen, there was no change in the anterior face height. However, an average tipping of the palatal plane of 1.5 degrees was observed, an indication of the orthopedic effect of the headgear. It was concluded that the cervical-pull headgear can be used effectively for maxillary molar distalization without detrimental effects. However, patient compliance with the treatment regimen is a serious issue, as social and peer pressures on children make it almost impossible for them to accept the facebow headgear regimen.

Jig

Another appliance that can be used with either patient compliance or patient noncompliance is the jig. The jig can be easily fabricated at chairside and used to correct either bilateral or unilateral Class II, Division 1 malocclusions (Fig. 12-6). In patients with poor compliance, the appliance can be tied in using long nickel-titanium (Ni-Ti) coil springs with an external tubing to minimize patient discomfort. These springs are very small in diameter and do not cause more discomfort than the SAIF springs. The SAIF spring is bulky, compared to the Ni-Ti spring (Fig. 12-7), and it can be tied from the mandibular first or second molar to the maxillary canine hook. Figure 12-6 shows an example of a patient treated with a unilateral jig.

Bimetric (Wilson) Arch

Wilson[24] introduced the bimetric arch into the orthodontic literature in 1955 at a time when there was considerable argument between proponents of extraction and of nonextraction with expansion. The appliance consists of a labial arch made of a 0.040-inch posterior section and a 0.020-inch anterior section. Hooks for Class II elastics are soldered onto the anterior end of the 0.040-inch section and an adjustable omega loop is placed in the premolar region of the 0.040-inch section. The appliance is activated by placement of an open coil spring between the omega loop and the maxillary first molar. Continued activation of the appliance can be achieved by opening the omega loop, thereby compressing the open coil against the molar. The bimetric arch, as it would look in the mouth, is shown in Figure 12-8.

With patient compliance, a limitation to the use of the appliance, a Class I molar relationship can be achieved in as little as 6 to 12 weeks.[25-27] In a noncompliant patient, side effects can lead to flaring of the incisors.[27] Both distal movement and distal tipping of the maxillary molars are observed with the Wilson appliance.[25,27] Upon achievement of a Class I relationship, the second premolar can be allowed to drift back and the appliance may not be removed until this relationship is achieved.[27] Of importance during the use of Class II elastics is stability of the mandibular molars, which can be achieved in one of three ways: FLA, removable lingual arch (RLA), or lip bumper. The lip bumper has the added advantage of uprighting the mandibular molars and unraveling mandibular anterior crowding, if present.

FIXED NONCOMPLIANCE APPLIANCES

To overcome the problem of patient compliance, several fixed noncompliance appliances have been introduced, especially during the last two decades. These include the Herbst,

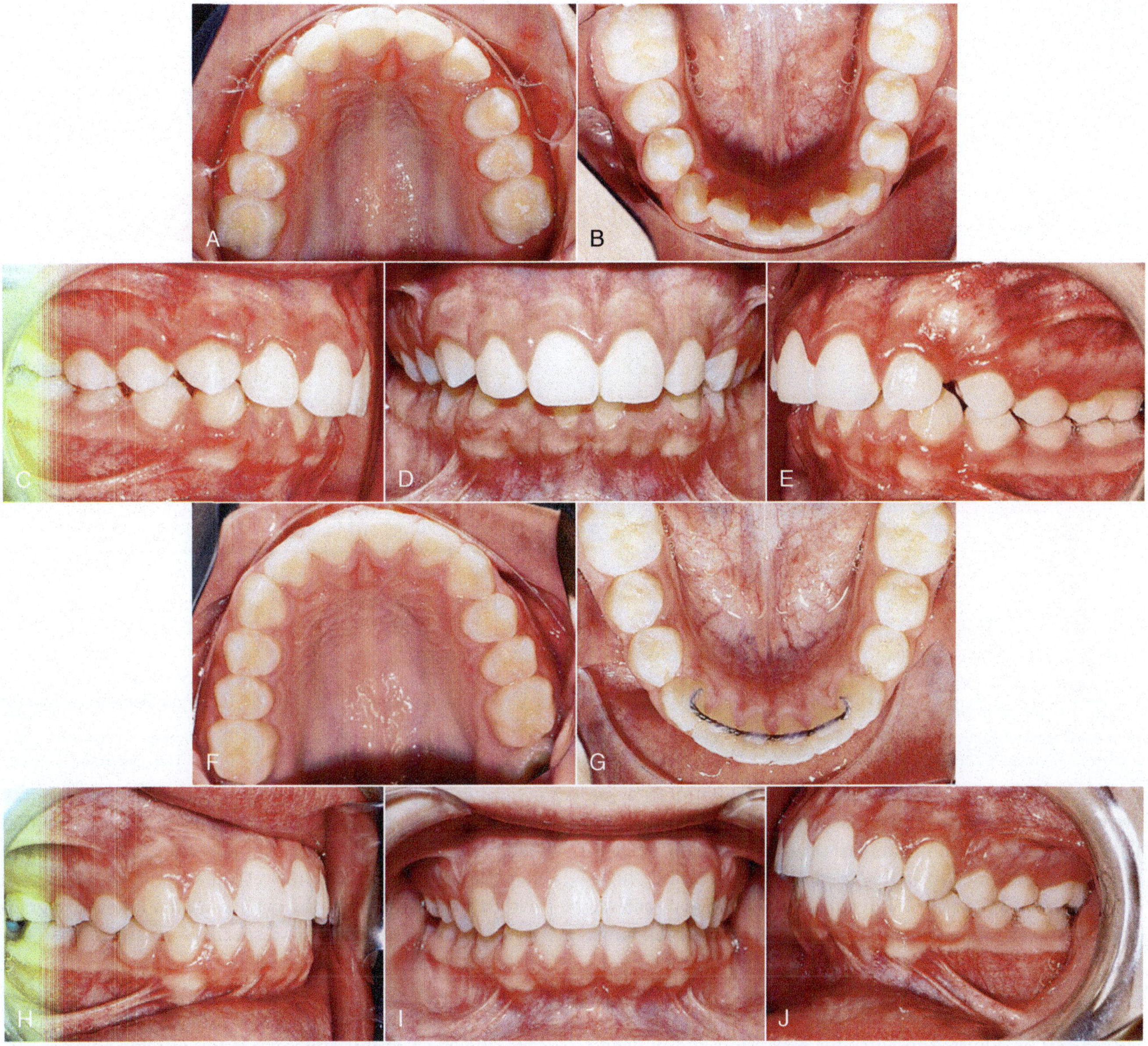

Figure 12-6 Patient with a unilateral Class II, Division 1 malocclusion treated with a jig. The maxillary left canine was blocked out and could not erupt. **A–E,** Pre-treatment records showing Class II, Division 1 subdivision left. **F–J,** Final records after 12 months of treatment. No exposure of the unerupted canine was performed and the canine erupted as soon as space was created.

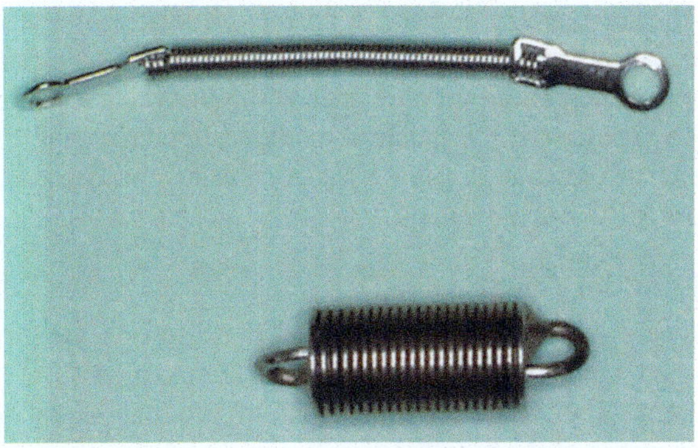

Figure 12-7 Size difference between the SAIF (*bottom*) and nickel-titanium (Ni-Ti) springs (*top*). In cases involving noncompliant patients, these springs can be tied in to correct a Class II malocclusion. The SAIF spring is bulky compared to the Ni-Ti spring.

Twin Force bite corrector, repelling magnets, pendulum appliance, compressed stainless steel or Ni-Ti springs, Jones jig, and distal jet. The majority of these appliances have been reported to achieve the same amount of molar distalization as the headgear. They also have side effects that need to be considered.

Pendulum Appliance

Hilgers[28] introduced an appliance for Class II correction in the noncompliant patient to expand the maxilla and simultaneously rotate and distalize the maxillary first molars. The pendulum appliance provides the clinician with the ability to distalize molars unilaterally and bilaterally. The type of force delivered is continuous and it requires minimal patient cooperation.

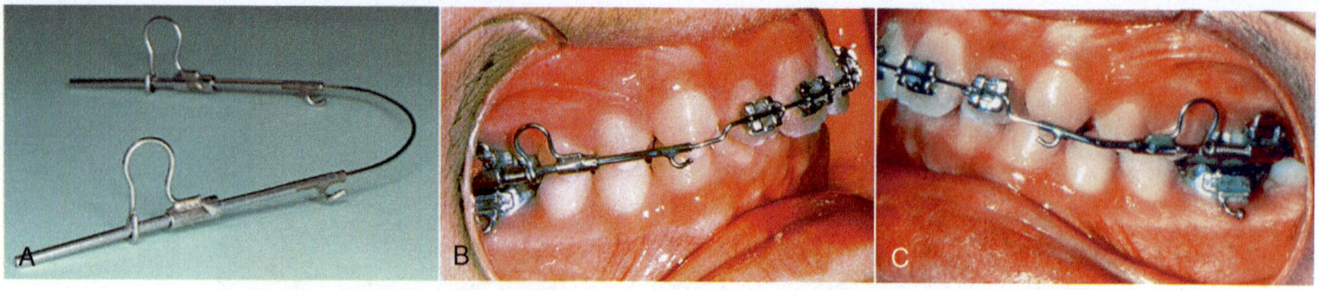

Figure 12-8 **A,** Bimetric arch (Wilson appliance). **B and C,** Bimetric arch engaged and activated.

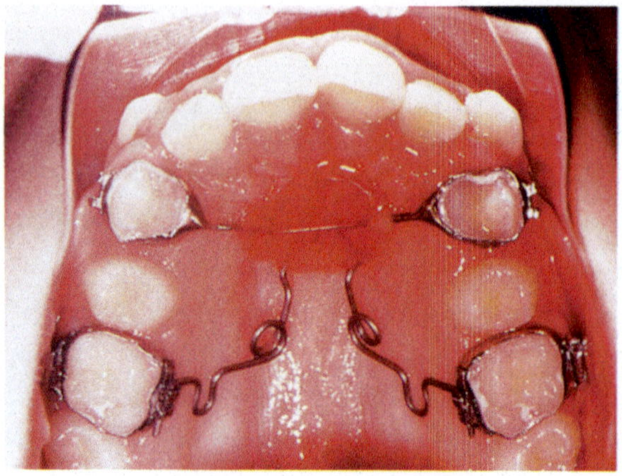

Figure 12-9 Pendulum appliance.

TABLE 12-1 Effects of the Pendulum Appliance

	Sagittal Change		
Tooth		Medial mvt (mm) Tipping (degrees)	Vertical Change Extrusion (mm)
First premolar	2.55 ± 1.9	1.29 ± 7.52	1.7 ± 1.36
	Distal mvt (mm)		
First molar	3.37	8.36 ± 8.37	0.1 ± 1.29
Second molar	2.27 ± 1.44	11.99 ± 1.9	0.47 ± 1.36

mvt, Movement.
Adapted from Ghosh J, Nanda RS. Evaluation of an intraoral maxillary molar distalization technique. *Am J Orthod Dentofacial Orthop.* 1996;110:639–646.

The appliance consists of a palatal acrylic button that is about 25-mm in diameter with distalization springs made of 0.032-inch beta-titanium wire that originate from the palatal acrylic and are engaged in lingual sheaths on maxillary first molar bands (Fig. 12-9). It is bonded to the first and second premolars with wires embedded in the acrylic. It needs only a one-time activation of 60 to 70 degrees, producing a force of 230 g per side. It produces a swinging arch, or pendulum of force, from the palate to the molars. A loop within each spring can be adjusted to allow for expansion and prevent any tendency for the maxillary molar to move lingually into a crossbite. Once the molars are distalized, they may be stabilized with a Nance button attached to the maxillary first molars, a headgear, or a fixed appliance, along with a maxillary utility archwire or a stopped continuous archwire. Usually after molar distalization, the second premolar is released from the anchor unit and allowed to drift distally. According to Hilgers,[28] it is not unusual to see as much as 5-mm of distal molar movement in 3 to 4 months of treatment with this appliance.

Evaluation of the treatment effects has shown that there is a difference in response between patients with erupting second molars and those with second molars in occlusion. Patients with erupted second molars will experience an extrusion of these teeth with subsequent opening of the bite, which is observed by an increase in the mandibular plane angle, increased lower anterior face height, and a reduced overbite.[29,30] Table 12-1 shows some of the results observed from a cephalometric analysis of patients treated with the pendulum appliance. The response differs between individuals with a low and a high mandibular plane angle. In another study, patients in the angle >25 degrees group showed an increase in the lower anterior vertical height (4.13-mm) that was greater than that in the patients in the low and average groups (1.97- and 2.84-mm, respectively).[29]

A common finding in studies that have evaluated the pendulum appliance is distal tipping of the maxillary first molars and anterior tipping of the premolars.[29,30] An important side effect of this appliance is undesirable anterior displacement of anterior teeth. However, this appliance presents an effective method for molar distalization with minimal dependence on patient compliance.[31] Other advantages include ease of fabrication, one-time activation, adjustment of the springs if necessary to correct minor transverse and vertical molar positions, and patient acceptance. Modifications of the pendulum appliance with removable arms have been introduced.[32–34] Such a modified appliance makes it easier to adjust and stabilize the appliance upon completion of molar distal movement.

Distal Jet

Carano and Testa[35] first described the distal jet as a fixed lingual appliance that required no compliance from the patient. They claimed that it could produce translatory movement of the maxillary molars in 4 to 6 months.

The original appliance[35] has had some modification[36,37] and now consists of a bilateral piston and tube arrangement (Fig. 12-10). The tube is embedded in an acrylic palatal

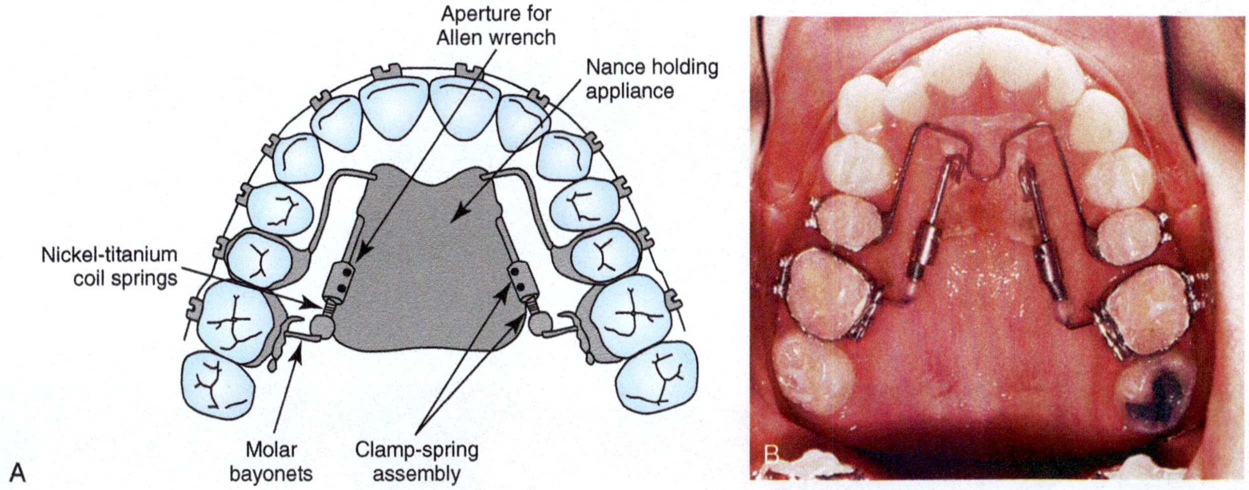

Figure 12-10 **A,** Schematic and **(B)** photograph of the distal jet appliance in a patient's mouth.

button supported by attachments to the first or second premolars. This tube extends distally, adjacent to the palatal tissues and parallel to the occlusal plane, to the first molars. A bayonet wire inserted into the lingual sheath on the first molar bands extends into the tube, much like a piston. A superelastic Ni-Ti open coil spring is placed around this piston and tube arrangement, along with an activation collar used to compress the spring distally. This collar is pushed distally to compress the coil spring once every 4 to 6 weeks during distalization. The mesial set screw in the collar is locked onto the tube with a small Allen wrench in an aluminum handle.

Upon completion of distalization of the molars, the appliance is converted to a palatal holding arch by removing the coil spring (peeling it off the tube with utility pliers) and locking the activation collar over the junction of the tube and piston; the mesial set screw is locked onto the tube and the distal set screw is locked onto the piston, thereby creating a solid support from the first molars to the Nance button. The supporting wire is then sectioned from the premolars and the Nance button with a dental handpiece and a burr.

Other than clinical reports from users of the appliance,[36–38] no research has clearly documented the effects of the distal jet. Studies conducted at the University of Oklahoma[39,40] revealed that the distal jet was indeed a good tool for distalizing maxillary molars but there could also be anchorage loss during its use, although less than reported for other appliances such as the pendulum. Minimal tipping of the maxillary molars was observed during the treatment period due to the force application near the center of resistance of the maxillary molars. The patients evaluated were in their growth period and some of the distalization achieved was lost during retraction of the anterior teeth. However, this was compensated for by anterior movement of the mandibular molars. Upon completion of distalization of the molars and during the rest of the treatment phase, it is necessary to use some other appliance to hold the molars back.[37,38] A Jasper jumper[41,42] or a short Twin Force bite corrector[6] may serve this purpose well since neither requires compliance by the patient.

Jones Jig Appliance

The Jones jig appliance[43] is an intraoral noncompliance distalization appliance (Fig. 12-11). It has a modified Nance appliance banded to the second bicuspids, with the Jones jig assemblies tied in place. It consists of a palatal acrylic button of 0.50-inch diameter anchored to the second premolar with a bonded 0.036-inch wire. One arm of the jig fits into a 0.045-inch headgear tube and the second arm fits into a 0.018-inch tube on the first molar. The activation is delivered from the Ni-Ti coil spring tied to the second premolar bracket. The force applied is between 70 and 75 g and average treatment time is 6.35 ± 2.75 months.

Despite reports of successful correction of Class II malocclusions with the Jones jig, there has been no comprehensive study of molar movement and loss of anchorage during the use of this appliance. To validate its effectiveness, a study was conducted on the patients treated in the office of Dr. Richard Jones, the clinician credited with the design and use of this appliance.[44] The sample of 72 patients (26 male and 46 female) was unique. The average age before treatment was 13.8 ± 4.38 years. The results showed molar correction for Class II to Class I malocclusions due primarily to distal movement of the molars. The mean maxillary first molar distal movement was 2.51-mm, with distal tipping of 7.53 degrees. The mean reciprocal mesial movement of the maxillary premolar was 2.0-mm, with mesial tipping of 4.76 degrees. The maxillary first molar extruded 0.14-mm while the maxillary premolar extruded 1.88-mm. The maxillary second molars also moved 2.02-mm and tipped distally 7.89 degrees. Table 12-2 shows the sagittal and vertical movements that accompany the molar distalization procedure with the Jones jig. The changes are highly variable, a factor that should be noted when considering treatment options.

Although the Jones jig appliance can distalize maxillary first molars effectively, it has negative effects on the anchor

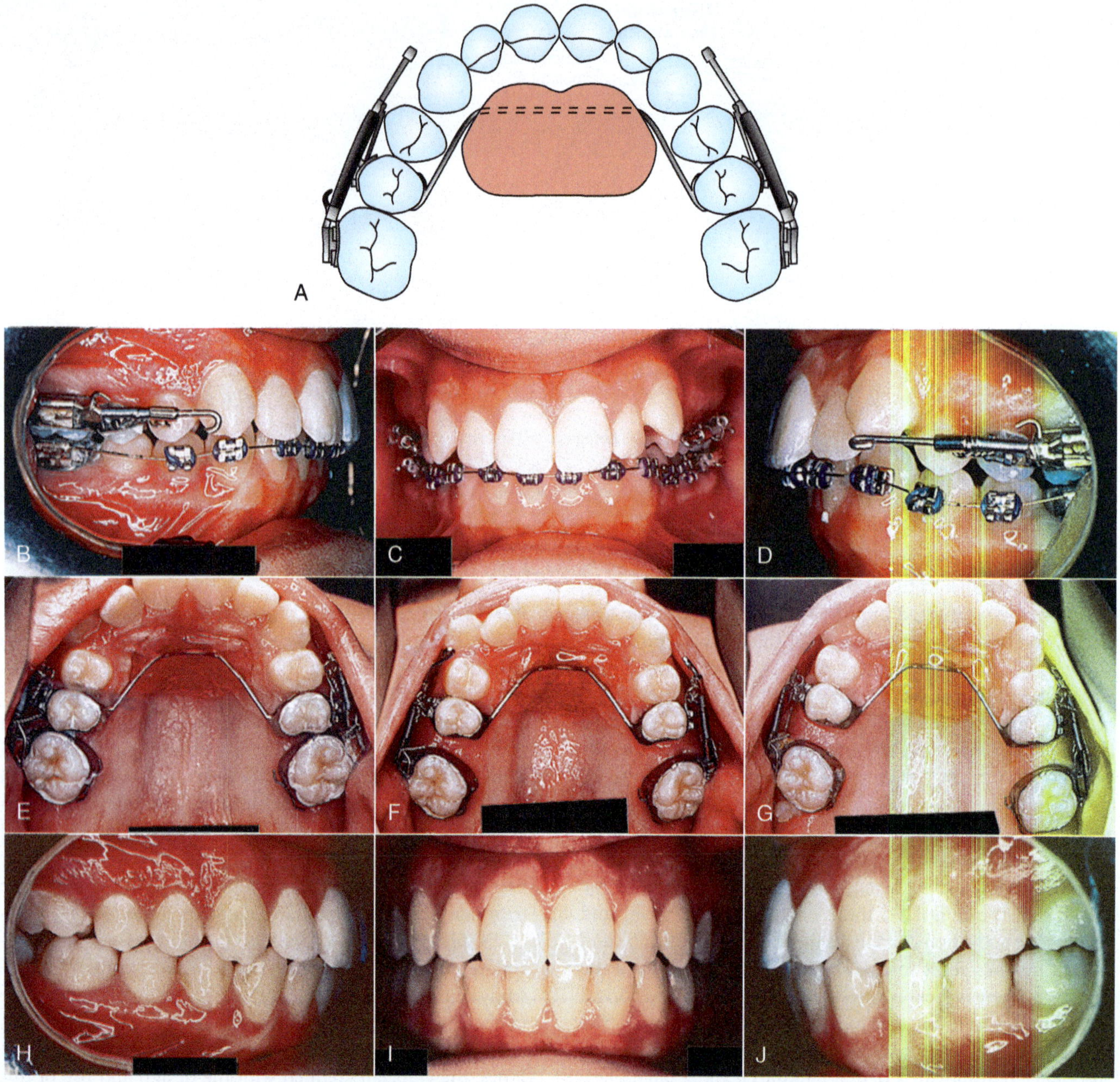

Figure 12-11 Jones jig appliance. **A,** Schematic of the modified Nance appliance banded to the second bicuspids with the Jones jig assemblies tied into place. **B–D,** Pre-treatment photographs of a patient with a Class II, Division 1 malocclusion, showing the activated appliance. **E-G,** Intraoral palatal photographs at (*from left to right*) initial delivery (0 months), 2 months, and 4 months of appliance activation. **H–J,** Treatment completion. Total treatment time was 24 months. The majority of the time was spent distalizing the premolars, canines, and incisors.

TABLE 12-2 Sagittal and Vertical Changes with Jones Jig Treatment

	Sagittal Change		
Tooth		**Distal mvt (mm) Tipping (degrees)**	**Vertical Change Extrusion (mm)**
First molar	2.16 ± 1.35	7.53 ± 4.57	0.1 ± 1.3
Second molar	1.79 ± 1.55	8.03 ± 6.65	0.71 ± 1.96
	Mesial mvt (mm)		
Second premolar	2.36 ± 1.99	5.89 ± 5.19	1.82 ± 1.44 1.46 ± 1.61 Increase anterior face height

mvt, Movement.

unit.[44,45] Compared to the headgear, however, it has the advantage of accelerated distal molar movement within a short time span.[45] Upon completion of distalization, proper anchorage must be used to maintain the molar relationship. Suitable anterior retraction mechanics must be used to achieve this goal. The use of full palatal coverage combined with short Class II elastics to reinforce posterior anchorage could possibly minimize the reciprocal anchorage loss of the molar anchor units during anterior segment retraction. An option that should be considered is nighttime headgear wear, which can be tolerated, especially by the young patient.

INTERMAXILLARY CLASS II MALOCCLUSION CORRECTION APPLIANCES

Several intermaxillary fixed noncompliant appliances have been proposed and used over the last two decades.[6,12,13,41,42,46–48] The advantage of these appliances is that they allow forward displacement of the mandible and a distal force on the maxillary teeth as well as an anterior force on the mandibular dentition. The net result of these three force vectors is correction of a Class II malocclusion. The common disadvantages of intermaxillary appliances are undesirable steepening of the occlusal plane with concomitant flaring of the lower incisors and distal tipping along with extrusion of the maxillary incisors.

Herbst Appliance

The Herbst appliance was developed in the early 1900s and reintroduced by Pancherz[46,47] in the mid-1970s. Pancherz showed that a 6-month Herbst treatment in prepeak pubertal patients with a Class II, Division 1 malocclusion resulted in a Class I occlusion relationship. However, he reported that improvement in occlusion was equally due to skeletal and dentoalveolar changes: a Class II molar correction averaging 6.7-mm resulted from a 2.2-mm increase in mandibular length, a 1.8-mm mesial movement of mandibular incisors, and a 2.8-mm distal movement of maxillary molars.

Pancherz and Hägg[48] found that sagittal growth at the condyle in patients treated with the Herbst appliance at the peak in pubertal growth was twice that observed in patients treated 3 years before or 3 years after the peak. Other studies[49,50] have shown that greater percentages of molar and overjet correction were dentoalveolar in nature in postpubertal patients with greater lower incisor flaring.

Jasper Jumper

Fixed intermaxillary appliances such as the Jasper jumper incorporate active pushing force on the maxillary molars and mandibular dentition. In a clinical study Rankin[51] reported greater dentoalveolar effects than skeletal effects. The Class II correction was obtained from mesial movement of lower molars and a significant flaring of the lower incisors. Jasper and McNamara[42] concluded that the skeletal and dental components of Class II correction were approximately equal, whereas Weiland and Bantleon[41] attributed only 38% of molar correction to skeletal changes. The majority of the studies on this appliance have shown that Class II correction is attributed to a slight increase in mandibular length, a significant posterior movement of the maxillary posterior segments, and proclination of the lower incisors.[52,53]

SUMMARY

Headgear is perhaps the most useful appliance for maxillary molar distalization if used in the early treatment of Class II malocclusions. Kim et al.[5] have shown that the occlusion established early during the growth phase is most likely to be maintained throughout life. Based on this and the premise that children are more compliant before adolescence, the headgear becomes a versatile appliance for treatment of Class II malocclusions. Its effect is twofold: (1) distal movement of the maxillary molars and (2) an orthopedic effect on the maxilla that restrains growth.

Both extraoral and intraoral inter-arch appliances require patient compliance, which may sometimes pose difficulty. Intermaxillary appliances that use the mandibular arch as anchorage may have protrusive effects on the mandibular teeth. All investigations that have evaluated intraoral arch noncompliance appliances for molar distalization have come to surprisingly similar conclusions on the behavior of both the distal segment and the anterior anchor unit. The intramaxillary arch appliances, which have gained in popularity because they do not require patient compliance to distalize molars, show loss of anchorage whereby the premolars move mesially with concomitant protrusion of the maxillary incisors. This suggests that no matter which intraoral appliance is used, it behooves the clinician to avoid round tripping in retraction of maxillary anterior teeth.

It is necessary that the molars are held back with some other form of appliance upon completion of distalization. The use of a Nance palatal arch or TPAs has proven not to resist the anchorage loss during the subsequent retraction of the anterior segment.

REFERENCES

1. Kloehn SJ. Orthodontics: force or persuasion. *Angle Orthod.* 1953;23:56–66.
2. Ricketts RM, Bench RW, Gugino CF, Hilgers JJ, Schulhof RJ. *Bioprogressive Therapy.* Denver, CO: Rocky Mountain Orthodontics; 1979.
3. Cetlin NM, Ten Hoeve A. Nonextraction treatment. *J Clin Orthod.* 1983;17:396–413.
4. Macho GA. Cephalometric and craniometric age changes in adult humans. *Ann Hum Biol.* 1986;14:49–61.
5. Kim YE, Nanda RS, Sinha PK. Transition of molar relationships in different skeletal growth patterns. *Am J Orthod Dentofacial Orthop.* 2002;121:280–290.
6. Campbell E. A *prospective clinical trial and mechanical analysis of a push type fixed intermaxillary Class II correction appliance* [master's thesis]. Storrs, CT: University of Connecticut, 2003.
7. Kalra V. The K-loop distalizing appliance. *J Clin Orthod.* 1995;29:298–301.
8. Kingsley NW. *Treatise on Oral Deformities.* New York, NY: Appleton & Co; 1880.
9. Angle EH. *Treatment of Malocclusion of the Teeth.* Philadelphia, PA: SS White Dental Manufacturing Co; 1907.

10. Oppenheim A. Biologic orthodontic therapy and reality. *Angle Orthod.* 1936;6:69–79.
11. Rabbie ABM, Leung FYC, Chayanupatkul A, Hägg U. The correlation between neovascularization and bone formation in the condyle during forward mandibular positioning. *Angle Orthod.* 2002;72: 431–438.
12. Voudouris JC, Woodside DG, Altuna G, Kuftinec MM, Angelopoulos G, Bourque PJ. Condyle–fossa modifications and muscle interactions during Herbst treatment, part 1: new technological methods. *Am J Orthod Dentofacial Orthop.* 2003;123;604–613.
13. Voudouris JC, Woodside DG, Altuna G, et al. Condyle–fossa modifications and muscle interactions during Herbst treatment, part 2: results and conclusions. *Am J Orthod Dentofacial Orthop.* 2003;124:13–29.
14. Haack DC, Weinstein S. The mechanics of centric and eccentric cervical traction. *Am J Orthod.* 1958;44:346–357.
15. Hershey GH, Houghton CW, Burstone CJ. Unilateral face-bows: a theoretical analysis. *Am J Orthod.* 1981;79:229–249.
16. Contasti GI, Legan HL. Biomechanic guidelines for headgear application. *J Clin Orthod.* 1982;16:308–312.
17. Wilson MD. Vertical control of maxillary molar position with a palatal appliance [thesis]. Oklahoma City, OK: Health Sciences Center, University of Oklahoma; 1996.
18. DeBerardinis M, Stretesky T, Sinha PK, Nanda RS. Evaluation of the vertical holding appliance in treatment of high-angle patients. *Am J Orthod Dentofacial Orthop.* 2000;117:700–705.
19. Nanda RS, Chawla JM. Variability of leeway space in Lucknow children. *Ind Dental J.* 1973;45:99–108.
20. Villalobos FJ, Sinha PK, Nanda RS. Longitudinal assessment of vertical and sagittal control in the mandibular arch by the mandibular fixed lingual arch. *Am J Orthod Dentofacial Orthop.* 2000;118:366–370.
21. Chiba Y, Motoyoshi M, Namura S. Tongue pressure on loop of transpalatal arch during deglutition. *Am J Orthod Dentofacial Orthop.* 2003;123: 29–34.
22. Hubbard GW. A cephalometric evaluation of non-extraction cervical headgear treatment in Class II malocclusion [thesis]. Oklahoma City, OK: Health Sciences Center, University of Oklahoma; 1992.
23. Hubbard GW, Nanda RS, Currier GF. A cephalometric evaluation of non-extraction cervical headgear treatment in Class II malocclusion. *Angle Orthod.* 1994;60:359–370.
24. Wilson WL. Variations of labiolingual therapy in Class II cases. *Am J Orthod.* 1955;41:852–871.
25. Muse DS, Fillman MJ, Emmerson WJ, Mitchell RD. Molar and incisor changes with Wilson rapid molar distalization. *Am J Orthod Dentofacial Orthop.* 1993;104:556–565.
26. Harnick DJ. Case report: Class II correction using a modified Wilson bimetric distalizing arch and maxillary second molar extraction. *Angle Orthod.* 1998;68:275–280.
27. Ücem TT, Yüksel S, Okay C, Gülsen A. Effects of a three-dimensional bimetric maxillary distalizing arch. *Eur J Orthod.* 2000;22:293–298.
28. Hilgers JJ. The pendulum appliance for Class II non-compliance. *J Clin Orthod.* 1992;26:706–714.
29. Ghosh J, Nanda RS. Evaluation of an intraoral maxillary molar distalization technique. *Am J Orthod Dentofacial Orthop.* 1996;110: 639–646.
30. Bussick TJ, McNamara JA Jr. Dentoalveolar and skeletal changes associated with the pendulum appliance. *Am J Orthod Dentofacial Orthop.* 2000;117:333–343.
31. Wong AMK, Rabie ABM, Hägg U. The use of pendulum appliance in the treatment of Class II malocclusion. *Br Dent J.* 1999;187:367–370.
32. Scuzzo G, Pisani F, Takemoto K. Modified molar distalization with a modified pendulum appliance. *J Clin Orthod.* 1999;33:645–650.
33. Scuzzo G, Takemoto K, Pisani F, Della VS. The modified pendulum appliance with removable arms. *J Clin Orthod.* 2000;34:244–246.
34. Byloff FK, Kärcher H, Clar E, Stoff F. An implant to eliminate anchorage loss during molar distalization: a case report involving the Graz implant-supported pendulum. *Int J Adult Orthodon Orthognath Surg.* 2000;15:129–137.
35. Carano A, Testa M. The distal jet for upper molar distalization. *J Clin Orthod.* 1996;30:374–380.
36. Bowman SJ. Modifications of the distal jet. *J Clin Orthod.* 1998;32: 549–556.
37. Quick AN, Harris AMP. Molar distalization with a modified distal jet appliance. *J Clin Orthod.* 2000;34:419–423.
38. Bowman SJ. Class II combination therapy (distal jet and jasper jumpers): a case report. *J Orthod.* 2000;27:213–218.
39. Patel A. Analysis of the distal jet appliance for maxillary molar distalization [thesis]. Oklahoma City, OK: Health Sciences Center, University of Oklahoma; 1999.
40. Ngantung V, Nanda RS. Posttreatment evaluation of the distal jet appliance. *Am J Orthod Dentofacial Orthop.* 2001;120:178–185.
41. Weiland FJ, Bantleon H. Treatment of Class II malocclusions with the Jasper Jumper appliance—a preliminary report. *Am J Orthod Dentofacial Orthop.* 1995;108:341–350.
42. Jasper JJ, McNamara JA. The correction of interarch malocclusions using a fixed force module. *Am J Orthod Dentofacial Orthop.* 1995;108: 641–650.
43. Jones RD, White MJ. Rapid Class II molar correction with an open-coil jig. *J Clin Orthod.* 1992;26:661–664.
44. Brickman CD, Sinha PK, Nanda RS. Evaluation of the Jones jig appliance for distal molar movement. *Am J Orthod Dentofacial Orthop.* 2000;118:526–534.
45. Haydar S, Üner O. Comparison of Jones jig molar distalization with extraoral traction. *Am J Orthod Dentofacial Orthop.* 2000;117:49–53.
46. Pancherz H. Treatment of Class II malocclusions by jumping the bite with the Herbst appliance. *Acta Odotol Scand.* 1980;38:187–200.
47. Pancherz H. The mechanism of Class II correction in Herbst appliance treatment: a cephalometric investigation. *Am J Orthod.* 1982;82: 104–113.
48. Pancherz H, Hägg U. Dentofacial orthopedics in relation to chronologic age, growth period and skeletal development: an analysis of 72 male patients with Class II division 1 malocclusion treated with Herbst appliance. *Eur J Orthod.* 1988;10:169–176.
49. Croft RS, Buschang PH, English JD, Meyer R. A cephalometric and tomographic evaluation of Herbst treatment in the mixed dentition. *Am J Orthod Dentofacial Orthop.* 1999;116:435–443.
50. Konik M, Pancherz H, Hansen K. The mechanism of Class II correction in late Herbst treatment. *Am J Orthod Dentofacial Orthop.* 1997;112: 87–91.
51. Rankin T. Correction of Class II malocclusions with a fixed functional appliance [thesis]. Storrs, CT: University of Connecticut; 1990.
52. Cash RG. Adult non-extraction treatment with Jasper Jumper. *J Clin Orthod.* 1991;25:443.
53. Cope JB. Quantitative evaluation of craniofacial changes with Jasper Jumper therapy. *Angle Orthod.* 1994;64:113.

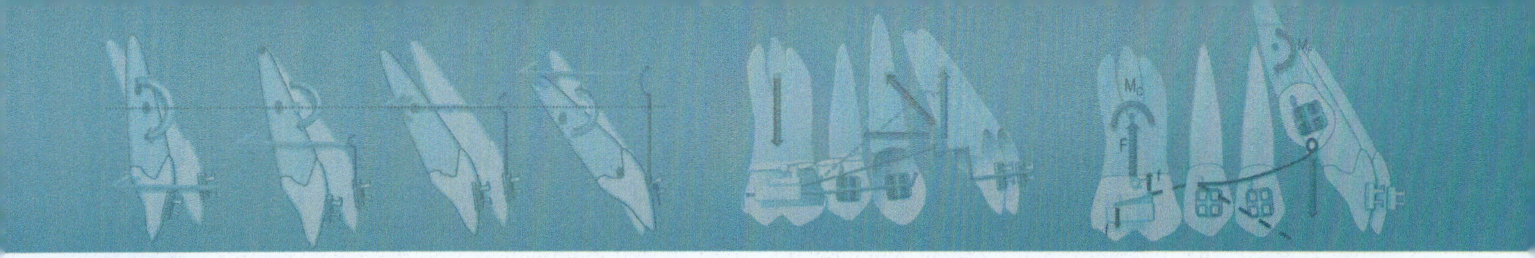

CHAPTER 13

Class II Correction with an Intermaxillary Fixed Noncompliance Device: Twin Force Bite Corrector

Aditya Chhibber, Madhur Upadhyay, and Ravindra Nanda

Morphogenesis and the development of the face is one of the most complex processes in human development. The role of nature versus nurture has long been debated. Proponents of genetic theory claim that growth patterns may arise from the activation and repression of genes that regulate the metabolic activity of differentiated cells, while proponents of epigenetic theories believe that growth control factors may lie in sutures,[1] cartilage,[2] or functional matrices[3] surrounding the craniofacial structures. Others believe that it is the confluence of genetics and external environmental factors that ultimately determines the size, shape, and location of craniofacial structures.[4]

The role of heredity in the development of one's phenotypical appearance has been examined through observational studies of monozygotic or dizygotic twins, who have greater similarity in appearance than unrelated individuals.[5] The question always has been whether and to what degree the external environment can influence the genetically predisposed size, shape, and direction of growth of craniofacial structures. While some studies[6] suggest that the presence of malocclusion can be greatly influenced by environmental factors, others believe its cause is multifactorial.[5] Even though it is reported that both Class II and Class III malocclusions may have strong familial tendency,[7,8] it may be difficult to estimate the influence of environmental factors in modifying craniofacial growth because the heritability studies of occlusion are typically based on twins and siblings who did not receive orthodontic treatment.

Class II malocclusion is one of the most common problems presenting to orthodontists. Skeletally, a prognathic maxilla, a retrognathic mandible, or a combination of the two is a possible etiology for this malocclusion. Studies in the literature[9–12] report that Class II malocclusion is more commonly associated with mandibular retrognathism than with maxillary prognathism. Stahl et al.[13] reported that features of a skeletal Class II occlusion develop early in the deciduous dentition and do not tend to self-correct with age, implying that some sort of intervention is necessary to achieve correction. Depending on the patient's growth status, treatment options commonly include use of functional appliances or fixed functional appliances (FFAs) to enhance mandibular growth, headgear to restrict maxillary growth, camouflage by extraction of upper and/or lower premolars, or surgical correction of the underlying skeletal discrepancy in patients in whom facial growth has been completed.[14] The goal of either orthodontic intervention or orthognathic surgery is generally to improve the patient's dental and facial esthetics, dental function, self-image, and quality of life.

The term *functional appliance* refers to a group of appliances that posture the mandible forward in an attempt to stimulate mandibular growth. Historically, the use of functional appliances began with Kingsley's vulcanite biteplate but probably was first propagated by Anderson with the use of the Activator appliance.[15] Since then, numerous functional appliances have been reported in the literature, with the most popular being the Activator, Bionator, and the Twin Block appliance. However, despite the use of functional appliances for more than a century, there is still considerable debate over the effectiveness of such mandibular anterior repositioning appliances in stimulating skeletal mandibular growth.[16] Studies[17–19] on experimental animals such as rats, mice, and primates depict a clear increased mandibular growth potential with the use of such appliances. However, similar experiments with these bite-jumping appliances to enhance mandibular skeletal growth in human subjects did not yield comparable results. The results of randomized clinical trials[20–22] have shown that with the use of functional appliances there is an initial increase in the mandibular growth response that is greater than that seen in the control sample; however, in the long-term, when patients treated with functional appliances were compared to untreated control subjects, the difference in the overall mandibular length was statistically insignificant.

Typically a functional appliance is advocated for a minimum of 12 hours per day for 6 to 9 months to observe dentoskeletal changes. Thus patient compliance is critical to the success of removable functional appliances.[23,24] In general, the factors associated with patient compliance are age, nature of the treatment delivered, and psychosocial characteristics of the individual patient. It has been reported that compliance with treatment is better in adults than in children and that younger children are more compliant with treatment than are adolescents.[25] Since most growth modulation procedures are undertaken in the adolescent phase, proficient patient compliance may be difficult to obtain in certain patients. Removable appliances such as headgear and functional appliances are usually rejected by patients due to discomfort, pain, restriction, and constraints on physical activity and movement.[26] In a study on patient compliance with functional appliances monitored microelectronically, Sahm et al.[27] reported that the patients wore the functional appliances far less than recommended to obtain dentoskeletal changes.

To eliminate patient compliance for Class II correction, the use of non–patient-compliance-based FFAs was first propagated by Emil Herbst in 1905 with the Herbst appliance. The appliance never really gained popularity until Pancherz revived it in the 1970s. Since then there have been numerous modifications of the rigid Herbst appliance[28] and various other FFAs[29–32] have also been reported in the literature. These FFAs may be broadly classified as rigid, flexible, and semirigid fixed functional appliances. The major difference between functional appliances and FFAs is that the mandible is forcefully postured in an anterior position with FFAs with the help of inter-arch anchorage using the maxillary denture base as the anchor unit.

Using the concept of equilibrium,[33] it can be understood that when a rigid FFA is placed in the mouth, the appliance is in static equilibrium. This essentially means that when there is a mesial or forward directed force on the lower arch, there exists an equal and opposite distal or backward directed force on the upper arch. This effect has been proved by cephalometric studies as the "headgear effect"[34,35] of FFAs. Apart from the "skeletal" effects on the denture bases, effects on the dentition such as retroclination of maxillary incisors,[36] proclination of mandibular incisors,[36–38] distalization of upper molars and mesialization of lower molars,[37,38] and clockwise rotation of the occlusal plane[38] have also been observed with FFAs. Thus Class II correction with FFAs is reported to be due to a combination of skeletal and dental effects.

DIAGNOSIS AND TREATMENT PLANNING

To accurately diagnose a patient, detailed information is gathered through a chief complaint, medical and dental history, clinical examination, and records that include extraoral and intraoral photographs, models, and radiographic images. An accurate interpretation of the data obtained from all clinical examinations and diagnostic records is made to develop a problem list, on the basis of which treatment objectives are identified and an individualized treatment plan is formulated for each patient.

Cephalometric Analysis

Orthodontists usually judge skeletal and dental relationships through cephalometric analysis, in which the patient's characteristics are compared to norms that differ among patient populations based on age, sex, and race. Cephalometric analysis can be performed to evaluate the cranial base, the relationship of the maxilla to the cranial base, the mandible's size and position relative to the cranial base, the relationship between the maxilla and the mandible, the vertical dimension, maxillary and mandibular dentition, and soft tissue. Table 13-1 provides an example of such analysis. Although the absolute numbers obtained in a cephalometric analysis provide basic information regarding an individual patient, there may be limitations to restricting diagnosis of a patient to numbers only.

A relatively easy, quick, and reliable way to assess the outcome with a functional appliance or FFA is a visualized treatment objective (VTO). The patient is asked to posture the mandible forward, obtaining anterior incisal contact with the posterior teeth in a Class I or super Class I relationship. If the profile of the patient improves, it indicates that the patient may be a good candidate for functional jaw orthopedics (Fig. 13-1). If on posturing the mandible forward the profile does not show improvement, the patient may not be an ideal candidate for a functional appliance and other methods for Class II could be considered or a prefunctional orthodontic phase may be required (Fig. 13-2). As a general rule, a functional appliance (FFA) is most ideally indicated in growing Class II patients who are essentially mandibular deficient, with an average to flat mandibular plane angle and upright lower anterior teeth over the mandibular basal bone with minimal to moderate crowding.

TWIN FORCE BITE CORRECTOR APPLIANCE

The Twin Force bite corrector (TFBC) appliance[39–42] is a hybrid fixed push-type, semirigid FFA clamped to archwires in both the upper and the lower arches bilaterally. Each unit is made up of two 15-mm telescopic parallel cylinders (Fig. 13-3). Within the cylinder is a nickel-titanium (Ni-Ti) coil spring that is activated when the patient occludes. A plunger is incorporated at the end of each cylinder on both ends. At the end of each plunger, hex nuts are present to attach the appliance to the archwires mesial to the upper molars and distal to the lower canine. At full compression a force of approximately 210 g is delivered on each side by compression of the coil spring. This force is synergistic to the indirectly applied force by the muscles of mastication due to the forced anterior repositioning of the mandible.

TABLE 13-1 Cephalometric Facial Analysis of Patient EE

	Value	Norm	SD
Cranial Base			
Anterior cranial base (SN) (mm)	61.8	73.5	3
Posterior cranial base (S-Ar) (mm)	34.4	33.2	4
Maxilla to Cranial Base			
SNA (degree)	80.9	82	3.5
Midface length (Co-A) (mm)	82.4	90.5	4
Maxillary length (ANS-PNS) (mm)	48.8	51.6	4.3
Mandible to Cranial Base			
SNB (degree)	72.5	80.9	3.4
Facial angle (FH-NPo) (degree)	85.7	87.7	3
Mandibular length (Co-Gn) (mm)	101.5	116.9	4
Mandibular length (Go-Gn) (mm)	72.9	65.9	5.5
Ramus height (Ar-Go) (mm)	32.8	44.5	4.5
Maxilla to Mandible			
ANB (degree)	8.4	1.6	1.5
Wits appraisal (mm)	5.9	−1	1
Mx/Md diff (Co-Gn–Co-A) (mm)	14.5	22.3	4
Vertical			
Angle of facial convexity (degree)	158.6	171.5	3.5
FMA (MP-FH) (degree)	27.8	24.8	4.5
MP-SN (degree)	40.4	33	6
Y axis–Downs (SGn-FH) (degree)	61.7	60.6	3.4
Occlusal plane to SN (degree)	20.8	14.4	2.5
LAFH (ANS-Me) (mm)	60.5	63	5
UAFH/LAFH ratio (N-ANS/ANS-Me) (%)	84.3	80	7
PFH/AFH (%)	59.3	62.2	N/A
Saddle/sella angle (SN-Ar) (degree)	129.4	124	5
Articular angle (degree)	147.7	143	6
Vertical—cont'd			
Gonial/jaw angle (Ar-Go-Me) (degree)	124.9	124.8	6.7
Sum of angles (Jarabak) (degree)	400.4	392.5	6
Other			
FH-SN (degree)	12.6	6	4
Maxillary Dentition			
U1-FH (degree)	113.1	111	6
U1-SN (degree)	100.5	102.5	5.5
U1-PP (mm)	26.5	26	3
U6-PP (mm)	18.3	19	2
Mandibular Dentition			
L1-APo (mm)	2	2.7	1.7
IMPA (L1-MP) (degree)	96.7	95	7
L1-MP (mm)	36.7	40.8	1.8
L6-MP (mm)	25.2	32.1	1.9
Maxillomandibular Dental			
Inter-incisal angle (U1-L1) (degree)	122.4	130	6
Soft Tissue			
Upper facial height (G-SN) (mm)	64.6	62.5	2.5
Lower facial height (SN-Me) (mm)	60.7	62.5	2.5
Nasolabial angle (Col-Sn-UL) (degree)	112.5	102	8
Upper lip to E-plane (mm)	2.2	−4.3	2
UL protrusion (UL-SnPg′) (mm)	6.5	4.4	2
Lower lip to E-plane (mm)	1.9	−2	2
LL protrusion (LL-SnPg′) (mm)	4.2	3.8	2
Soft tissue convexity (degree)	125.9	134.5	4

A, A point; *AFH,* anterior facial height; *ANB,* A point nasion B point; *ANS,* anterior nasal spine; *APo,* A point to pogonion; *Ar,* articulare; *Co,* condylion; *Col,* columella; *FH,* Frankfurt plane; *G,* glabella; *Gn,* gnathion; *Go,* gonion; *IMPA,* incisor mandibular plane angle; *L1,* lower incisor; *L6,* lower molar; *LAFH,* lower anterior facial height; *LL,* lower lip; *Me,* menton; *MP,* mandibular plane; *N,* nasion; *PFH,* posterior facial height; *Pg′,* soft tissue pogonion; *PNS,* posterior nasal spine; *PP,* palatal plane; *SD,* standard deviation; *Sn,* subnasale; *SN,* sella-nasion; *SNA,* sella-nasion A point; *SNB,* sella-nasion B point; *U1,* upper incisor; *U6,* upper molar; *UAFH,* upper anterior facial height; *UL,* upper lip.
Cephalometric facial analysis analyzing cranial base, maxilla to cranial base, mandible to cranial base, maxilla-mandibular relation, vertical relation, maxillary and mandibular dentition, and soft-tissue analysis.

Looking at the individual force components exerted by the appliance, there is an intrusive and distal component of force on the maxillary posterior segment and a mesial and intrusive force component on the lower anterior segment. Since the point of force application is away from the estimated center of resistance (C_{RES}) of the maxillary and mandibular denture bases,[43] a clockwise moment is generated (Fig. 13-4, A). A unique feature of the TFBC appliance is that since the point of force application is closer to the C_{RES} of the maxillary dentition, compared to other traditional FFAs where the point of force application in the maxillary arch is distal to the upper molar (Fig. 13-4, B), a lesser clockwise moment is generated with the appliance on the maxillary arch. Also, since the appliance is clamped to the archwire, the intrusive component of the spring force is probably redistributed along the entire denture base. In addition, since the force is applied buccal to the C_{RES} of the maxillary molar, estimated to be at the center of the trifurcation of the maxillary molar, a buccal expansive force is experienced (Fig. 13-5).

Treatment Protocol

Pre-treatment records for a patient are obtained (Fig. 13-6) and after the initial leveling and alignment phase, the archwires are progressively increased to 0.019 × 0.025-inch stainless steel in the upper arch and 0.021 × 0.025-inch stainless steel in the lower arch (Fig. 13-7, A–C). Both archwires are cinched to consolidate the arches into a single unit to avoid

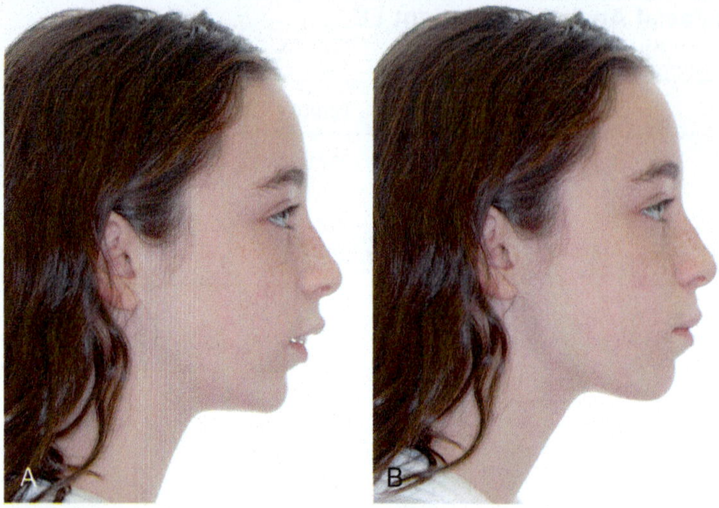

Figure 13-1 **A,** Profile view of Class II patient before treatment. **B,** Visualized treatment objective (VTO). Patient is asked to posture the mandible forward to estimate improvement in the soft tissue profile. Note the improvement in the soft tissue profile of the patient.

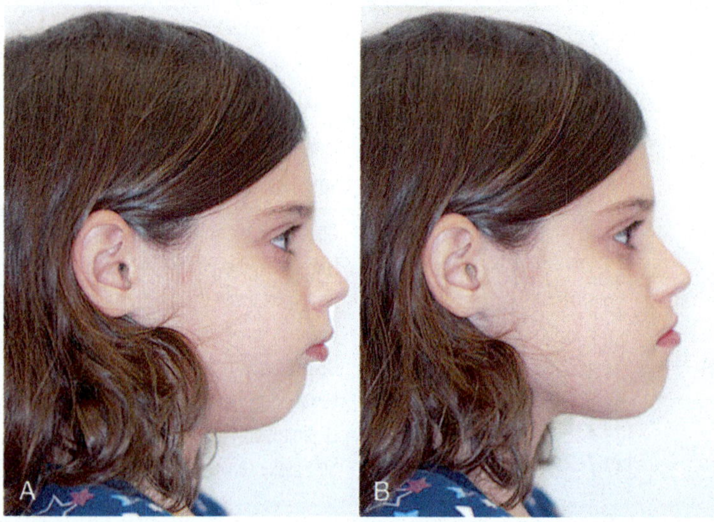

Figure 13-2 **A,** Profile view of Class II patient before treatment. **B,** Visualized treatment objective (VTO) of the patient. Note that the soft tissue profile of the patient is not improved, indicating that the patient may not be an ideal case for functional appliances.

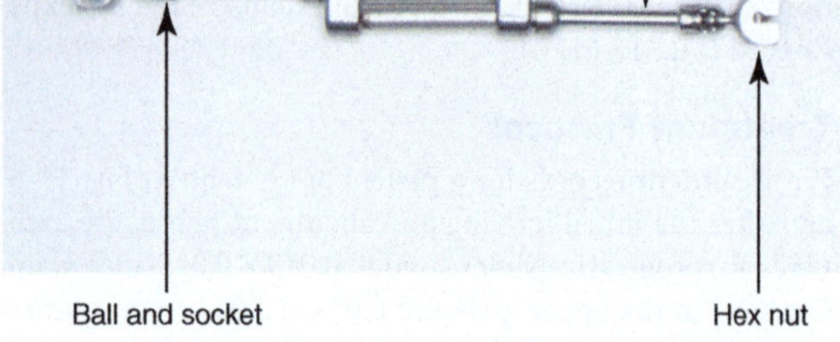

Figure 13-3 Components of the Twin Force bite corrector (TFBC) appliance.

any spaces developing or flaring of the incisors. Additionally, to minimize lower incisor flaring, MBT bracket prescription with −6-degree torque lower anterior brackets is advised. A 0.032-inch × 0.032-inch transpalatal arch is placed to counteract the buccal forces exerted by the TFBC appliance. The standard TFBC version is attached by the hex nuts to the archwires mesial to the maxillary molars and distal to the lower canines, posturing the mandible forward in an anterior edge-to-edge relationship (Fig. 13-7, D–F).

After 3 to 4 months of appliance placement, the patient usually has an overcorrected Class I molar and canine relationship. This helps to overcompensate for any relapse that may occur after appliance removal (Fig. 13-7, G–I). Appropriate finishing and detailing is performed and the patient is subsequently debonded (Fig. 13-8). The retention protocol involves a fixed lingual retainer for the lower arch and a removable wrap-around retainer for the upper arch.

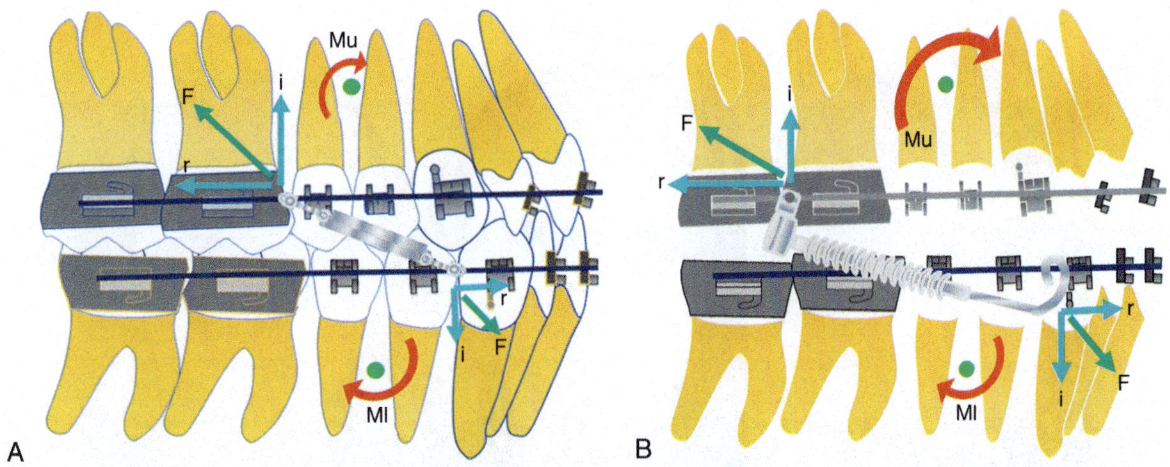

Figure 13-4 Force system with **(A)** Twin Force bite corrector (TFBC) appliance and **(B)** conventional fixed functional appliance (FFA). *F,* Total force; *i,* vertical (intrusive) component; *Ml,* moment created on the lower arch; *Mu,* moment created on the upper arch; *r,* horizontal component.

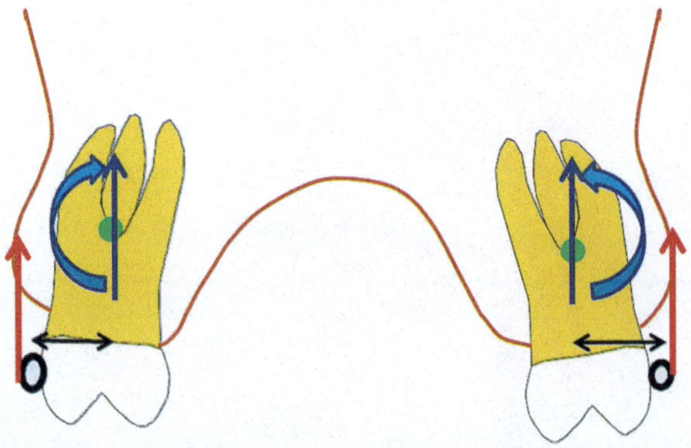

Figure 13-5 Force system with Twin Force bite corrector (TFBC) appliance in transverse dimension. Force applied by the TFBC appliance is depicted in red. Equivalent force system at the center of resistance of the molar is depicted in blue.

Effects of the TFBC Appliance

In an unpublished study[44] conducted at the University of Connecticut Health Center to analyze the effects of the TFBC appliance, a comparison was done between 20 subjects who received the TFBC appliance and an untreated Class II sample derived from the Denver growth study. The patients were matched for age, sex, and maturation status. The skeletal and dental results (Figs. 13-9 and 13-10, respectively) showed that during the 3-month period of using the TFBC appliance, A point in the maxilla moved 0.5-mm posteriorly under the distal force of the appliance and 1.7-mm inferiorly by the clockwise moment acting on the upper arch (compared to 0.1-mm anterior and 0.4-mm inferior movement in the control sample). The absolute length of the maxilla (anterior nasal spine [ANS]–posterior nasal spine [PNS]) was similar in both groups. The palatal plane rotated clockwise 0.5 degree in the TFBC sample compared to 0.1 degree in the control sample. The mandibular length (Ar-Pog) increased significantly—2.1-mm in the TFBC sample compared to 0.7-mm in the control sample—which could be attributed to a combination of growth and forward posturing of the mandible under the influence of the TFBC appliance. Dentally, the upper incisors showed distal crown tipping of −7.0 degrees in the TFBC sample compared to 0.1 degree mesial tipping in the control sample. The upper molar distalized −0.7-mm and intruded −1.1-mm in the TFBC group; in the control group the upper molar mesialized 0.3-mm and extruded 0.2-mm. The lower incisors flared 7.3 degrees and mesialized 2.6-mm in the TFBC group compared to no movement in the control group. The lower molar mesialized 1.8-mm in the TFBC group whereas in the control group the molar mesialized only 0.2-mm. Therefore the Class II correction was due to a combination of skeletal and dental effects.

Treatment Timing with the TFBC Appliance

The question of optimal timing for Class II correction has always been of significant interest as well as controversial. Traditionally, removable functional appliances are advocated "early" for mandibular-deficient growing Class II patients while rigid FFAs are considered more appropriate toward the end of the growth phase to use residual mandibular growth. While earlier studies with functional appliances[45] treated patients early for Class II correction, more recent evidence[46,47] suggests that the optimum treatment timing for removable functional appliances appears to be during or slightly after the onset of the pubertal peak in growth velocity. With the rigid FFAs, such as the Herbst appliance, Ruf and Pancherz[48] and Pancherz and Hägg[49] found them to be most effective in the treatment of young adults during their peak height velocity stage of growth.

In contrast to functional appliances or rigid FFAs, treatment outcomes produced by semirigid FFAs, such as the TFBC appliance, might be different. A study[50] was designed to determine the best possible time to use semirigid FFAs such as the TFBC appliance. Patients were divided into two groups: prepubertal and postpubertal, based on skeletal maturity at the beginning of treatment (Fig. 13-11). All subjects in the group treated early experienced their pubertal

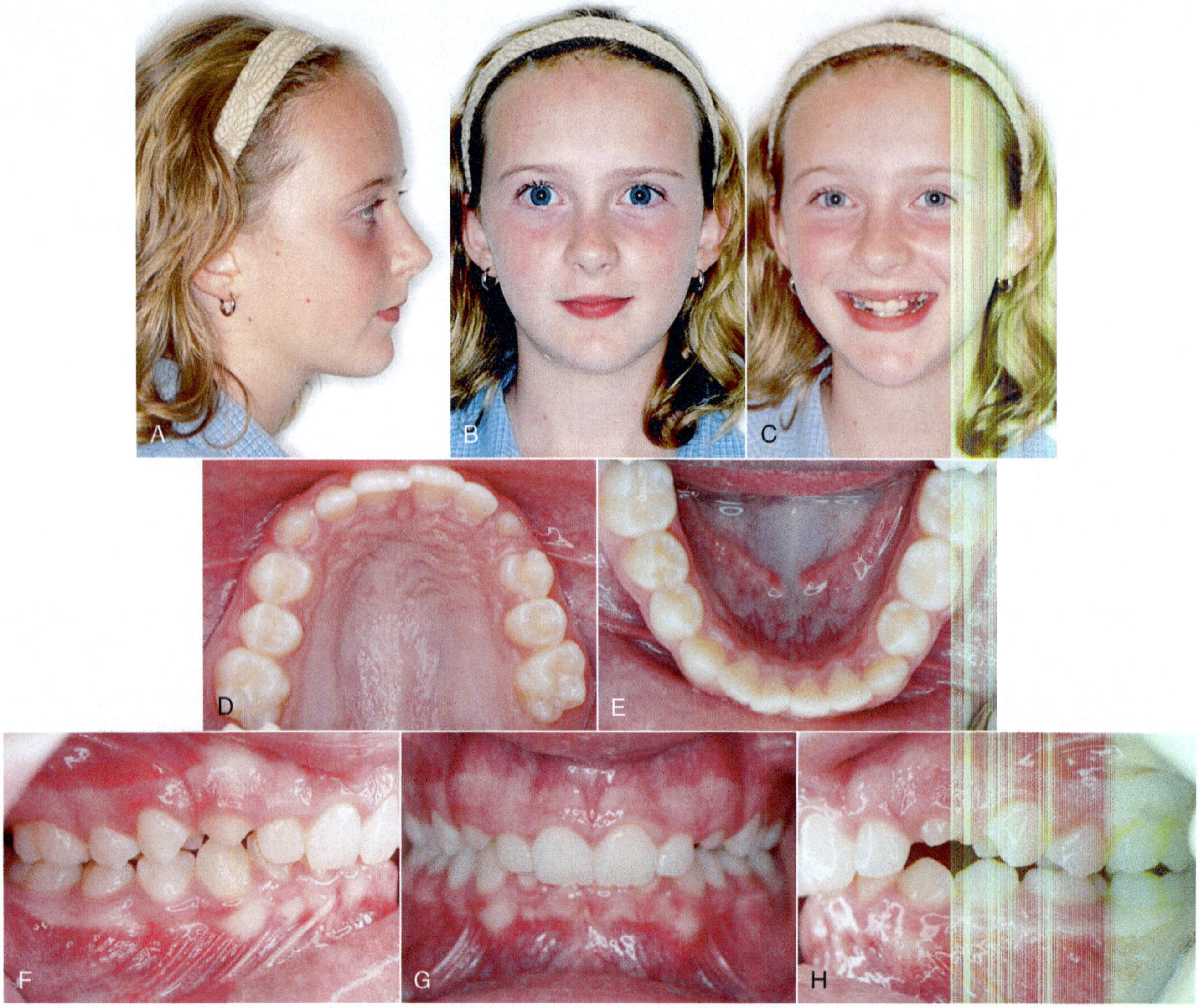

Figure 13-6 Pre-treatment records of Class II patient treated with the Twin Force bite corrector (TFBC) appliance. **A–C,** Facial views. **D–H,** Intraoral views.

growth spurt during treatment, while treatment was initiated after the pubertal growth spurt in subjects in the group treated late. The demographics of the patient population in both groups are depicted in Figure 13-12.

At the beginning of treatment there were significant differences in linear maxillary and mandibular skeletal parameters between the early and late treatment groups (Table 13-2), which could be explained by the fact that patients were developmentally less mature in the prepubertal group than in the postpubertal group. During treatment (Fig. 13-13) there was an increase in the differential jaw growth, which was significantly greater in prepubertal patients than postpubertal patients, most likely because patients in the prepubertal group were developmentally less mature than those in the postpubertal group, predisposing them to greater growth during treatment and a longer treatment time. However, when the prepubertal and postpubertal groups were compared at the end of treatment, when growth was complete (Table 13-3), no significant differences were observed. The final skeletal outcomes were similar in both groups whether treatment was initiated before or after the growth spurt.

For dental measurements, regional superimpositions of the maxilla were performed along the palatal cortex by registering on the bony internal details and the superior and inferior surfaces of the hard palate. The mandible was superimposed posteriorly on the outline of the mandibular canal and anteriorly on the anterior contour of the chin and internal bony structures of the symphysis. There was similar dentoalveolar correction in both groups. The contribution of skeletal and dental effects for overjet correction, whether the treatment was initiated early or late, was similar (Fig. 13-14). A possible reason for this is that semirigid FFAs rely on all teeth being present to attach the appliance and therefore significant time is spent waiting for teeth to erupt. If treatment efficiency is assumed to be a function of treatment duration, then the postpubertal group fared significantly

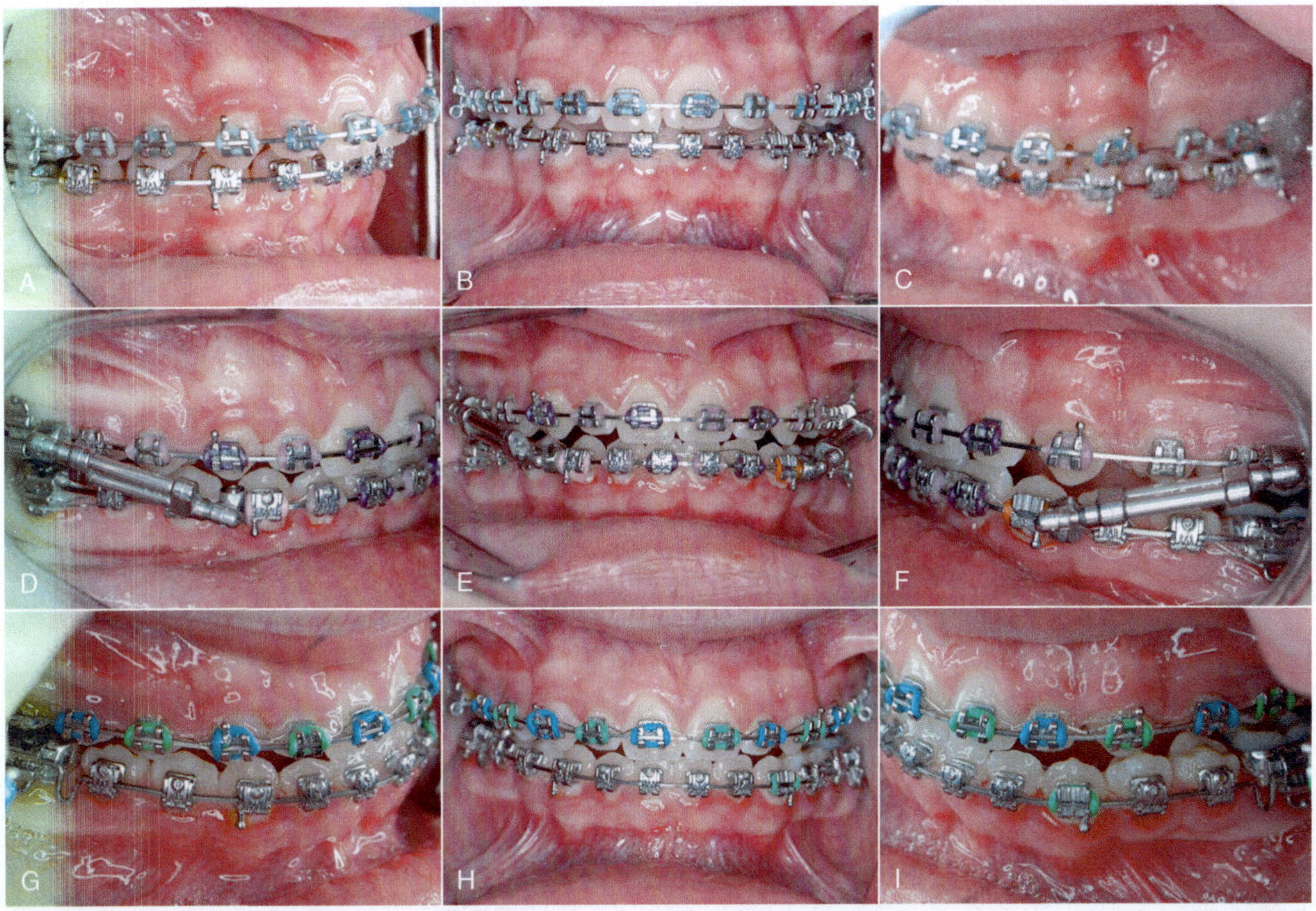

Figure 13-7 **A–C,** Clinical setup before placement of an appliance. **D–F,** Placement of the Twin Force bite corrector (TFBC) appliance. **G-I,** Removal of the appliance with overcorrection achieved.

better because treatment time for that group (2.75 ± 1.07 years) was significantly less than for the prepubertal group (3.67 ± 1.45 years) (Fig. 13-15). The longer treatment duration in prepubertal patients may be attributed to the time spent waiting for the eruption of permanent teeth, which prolongs the overall treatment time. The outcomes of the study demonstrated that although there might be differences in the dentoskeletal changes produced during treatment (see Fig. 13-13) between the two groups, the final results at the end of treatment were remarkably similar (see Table 13-3). This makes the postpubertal phase the preferred phase for Class II intervention with the TFBC appliance.

Contribution of the TFBC Appliance to Overall Class II Correction

From the previous study,[50] we observed that there was mesialization and extrusion of the upper molar in both prepubertal and postpubertal groups with use of the TFBC appliance, while from the mechanics section we know that a distal and intrusive force is exerted on the upper molar from the TFBC appliance. This leads us to question which effects of the TFBC appliance are stable and contribute to overall Class II correction and which effects are unstable and transient effects that relapse after removal of the FFA and do not contribute to overall Class II correction.

We conducted a study in which lateral cephalograms taken at four different time points—pre-treatment (T1), pre-TFBC appliance placement (T2), after removal of TFBC appliance (T3), and post-treatment (T4)—in 27 successfully treated Class II cases were analyzed. A mean difference of T3-T2 gave us the specific effects of the TFBC appliance and a difference of T4-T3 gave us the changes that occur after removal of the TFBC appliance until the end of treatment (Fig. 13-16).

A comparison of the observations showed that skeletally there was no difference in the rate of differential jaw growth during the TFBC appliance phase or after the appliance was removed (Fig. 13-17). Clockwise canting of the occlusal plane appears to be a transient effect of the TFBC appliance, as during the appliance phase clockwise canting was observed but after removal of the appliance, during the finishing stage of treatment, the occlusal plane reverted completely and did not contribute to overall Class II correction. During the appliance phase there was an overjet correction of 5.69-mm but after removal of the appliance about 2.2-mm (38%) of overjet correction relapsed.

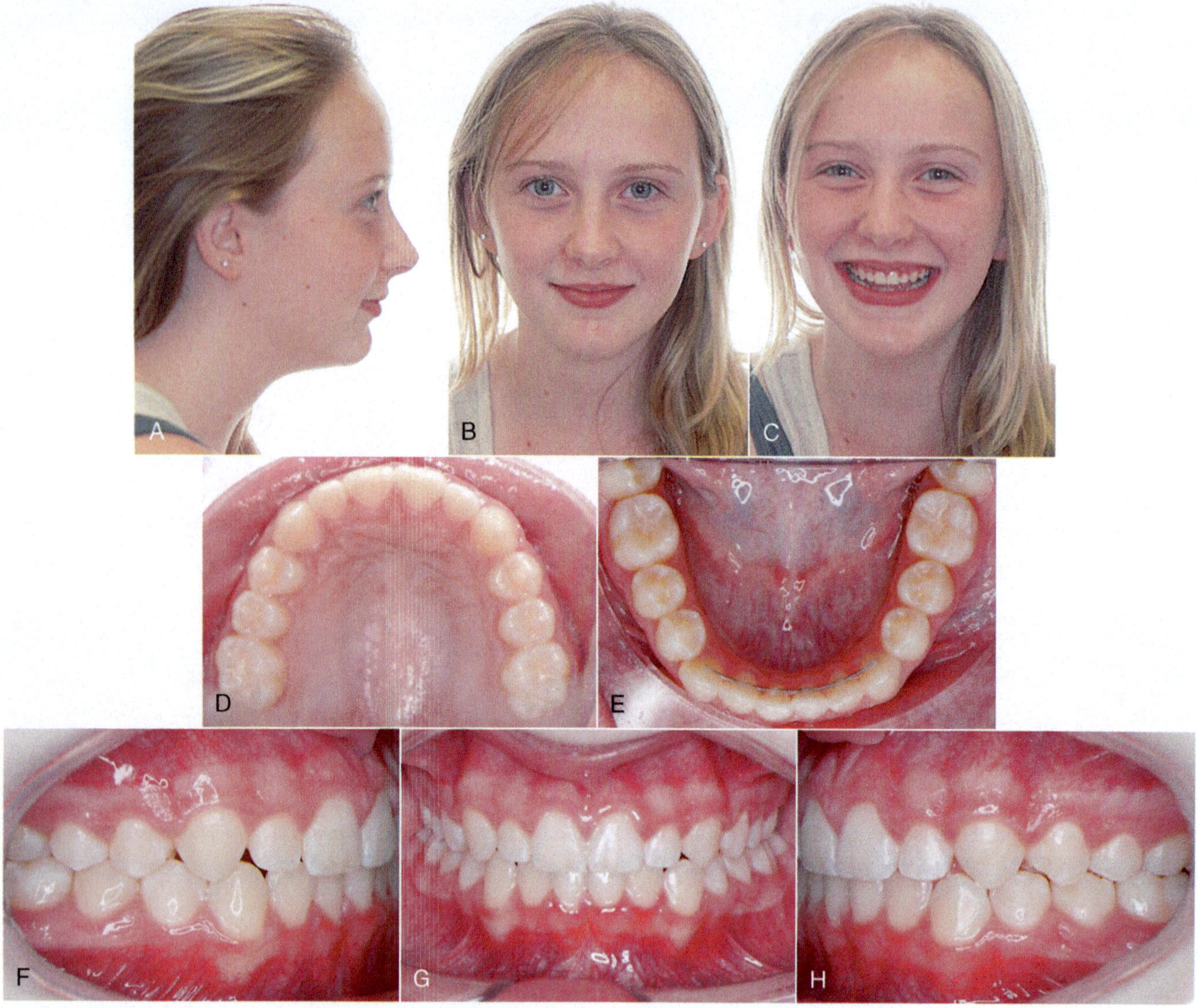

Figure 13-8 Post-treatment **(A–C)** extraoral and **(D–H)** intraoral photographs.

Dental measurements were made by regional superimpositions (Figs. 13-18 and 13-19). In the anteroposterior and vertical dimensions, the distalization and intrusion of the upper molar under the influence of the TFBC appliance relapsed after removal of the appliance during the finishing stages. Significant relapse of the distalization of the upper incisors was observed. This possibly may be attributed to the natural tendency of teeth to drift mesially and occlusally with growth.[51] Similar observation of the upper molars moving mesially and extruding in the entire treatment duration after use of a FFA has been reported with other FFAs.[34,52,53] It could also be hypothesized that since the point of force application was away from the C_{RES} of the maxillary molar, there was tipping of the molar under the influence of the force of the TFBC appliance with distal movement of the crown and the root staying in its initial position. After removal of the distal force on the crown under the influence of the TFBC appliance, the crown reverted to its original position since the root may not have distalized.

The dental changes of mesialization and extrusion of the lower molar, however, were very stable effects. The mesial movement of the lower molar during the TFBC appliance phase did not show any changes in the finishing stages. Similarly, extrusion of the lower molar during the TFBC appliance phase due to the clockwise moment exerted by the appliance was a stable effect and did not revert in the finishing stages. This could perhaps be due to the fact that the natural direction of eruption of teeth is mesial and upward in the lower dentition and the patients were growing Class II patients in whom the teeth may have erupted into the intermaxillary growth space.

Thus dental effects on the maxillary arch of distalization and intrusion of the upper molars and canting of the occlusal plane were unstable effects of the TFBC appliance and did not contribute to overall overjet correction whereas mesial movement and extrusion of the lower molars under the influence of the TFBC appliance were stable effects and contributed to overall Class II correction.

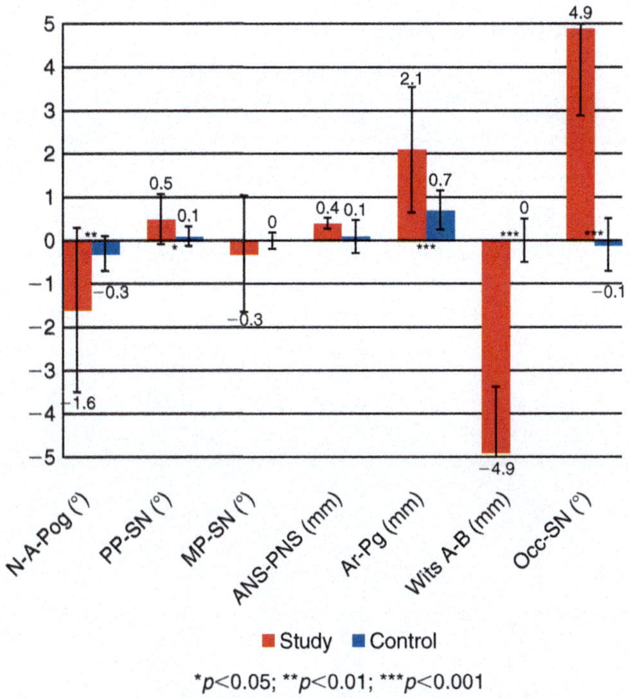

Figure 13-9 Skeletal observations of a study sample treated with the Twin Force bite corrector (TFBC) appliance compared to an untreated Class II control sample matched for age, sex, and cervical vertebral maturation stage (CVMS). *ANS-PNS (mm),* Anterior nasal spine to posterior nasal spine; *Ar-Pg (mm),* articulare to pogonion; *MP-SN (°),* mandibular plane (gonion-gnathion) to sella-nasion; *N-A-Pog (°),* nasion – A point – pogonion; *Occ-SN (°),* occlusal plane to sella-nasion; *PP-SN (°),* palatal plane to mandibular plane (gonion-gnathion); *Wits A-B (mm),* Wits occlusal plane changes.

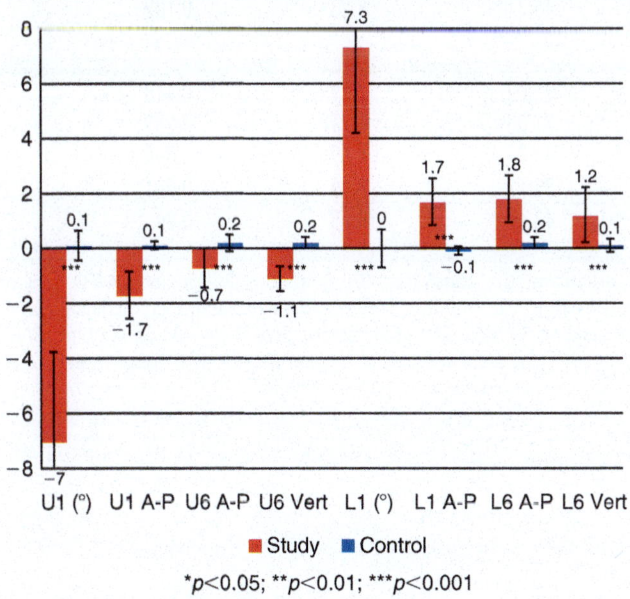

Figure 13-10 Regional superimposition observations of the dental effects of the Twin Force bite corrector (TFBC) appliance compared to the untreated Class II control sample. *L1 (°),* Angular change in lower incisor inclination; *L1 A-P,* linear changes in lower incisor position; *L6 A-P,* linear changes in lower molar position; *L6 Vert,* vertical changes in lower molar position; *U1 (°),* angular change in upper incisor inclination; *U1 A-P,* linear changes in upper incisor position; *U6 A-P,* linear changes in upper molar position; *U6 Vert,* vertical changes in upper molar position.

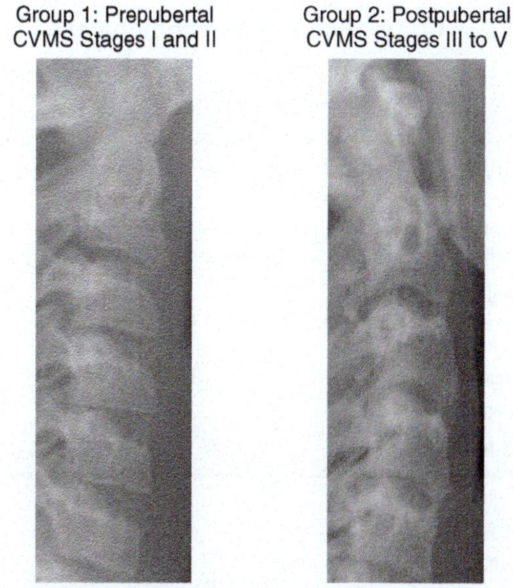

Figure 13-11 Sample distribution. Patients in cervical vertebral maturation stages (CVMS) I and II, at which the growth spurt had not yet occurred, were grouped into the prepubertal group. Patients in CVMS stages III to V were grouped into the postpubertal group. Based on modified CVMS staging.

	Prepubertal		Postpubertal		
Variable	n=23		n=18		
CVMS	I	II	III	IV	V
Pre-treatment age (y)	12.44 ± 1.59		13.76 ± 1.44		
Sex (n) Male	9	8	3	3	
Female	4	2	4	7	1
Total	13	10	7	10	1
Treatment time (y)	3.67 ± 1.45		2.75 ± 1.07		

Figure 13-12 Demographics of the study sample. *CVMS,* Cervical vertebral maturation stage; *y,* years.

Long-Term Effects of Treatment with the TFBC Appliance

Retention of orthodontic correction of any type of malocclusion is a challenge. Relapse of orthodontic treatment is a common problem reported in the literature.[54] Therefore assessment of the outcomes of any FFA in the long-term helps to establish the efficacy and efficiency of such appliances for Class II correction. Pancherz[55] studied the long-term retention related to the rigid Herbst appliance and concluded that most of the relapse could be attributed to dental changes or unstable occlusal relationships that exist at the end of treatment with such appliances.

In a study of the long-term effects of the TFBC appliance, 23 nonextraction Class II, Division 1 patients with a mean age of 12.01 ± 1.24 years at the beginning of treatment were treated with the TFBC appliance and evaluated a minimum

Text continued on p. 231

TABLE 13-2 Comparison of Morphological Characteristics of Patients at Beginning of Treatment

	Prepubertal (n = 23)		Postpubertal (n = 18)		
	Mean	SD	Mean	SD	P value
Maxillary Skeletal					
SNA (degree)	81.54	4.7	82.33	2.82	0.527
Co-A (mm)	96.1	4.77	99.78	6.81	0.043*
Mandibular Skeletal					
SNB (degree)	75.48	3.68	77.03	2.7	0.138
Co-Gn (mm)	114.54	7.17	122	7.65	0.002*
Go-Gn (mm)	74.72	4.57	80.64	6.33	0.001*
Maxilla-Mandible					
ANB (degree)	6.08	2.27	5.36	2.15	0.301
Co-Gn–Co-A (mm)	5.26	2.3	3.22	2.35	0.007*
Overjet (mm)	6.66	2.66	5.86	2.69	0.339
Vertical Skeletal					
SN-GoGn (degree)	31.88	5.06	31.67	4.5	0.887
UFH/LFH (%)	82.35	5.72	77.89	8.24	0.042*
PFH/AFH (%)	64.19	4.41	64.93	3.52	0.561
PP-SN (degree)	8.02	2.7	6.86	2.56	0.164
Occ-Sh (degree)	12.76	3.61	12.06	3.98	0.549
Ar-Go-Me (degree)	128.86	5.86	126.44	4.45	0.15
Maxillary Dentoalveolar					
U1-SN (degree)	103.8	8.22	101.47	8.76	0.378
U1-Sv (mm)	77.5	5.58	79.28	7.2	0.367
U1-PP (mm)	21.16	2.81	23.69	3.18	0.009*
U6-PP (mm)	18.72	2.03	20.69	2.78	0.01*
U6-Sv (mm)	44.18	4.94	46.31	5.23	0.182
Mandibular Dentoalveolar					
IMPA (degree)	97.7	6.97	96.03	7.19	0.448
L1-Sv (mm)	68.78	6.08	71.03	6.71	0.259
L1-MP (mm)	38.24	3.14	41.72	4.69	0.006*
L6-MP (mm)	29.72	2.26	32.72	3.49	0.001*
L6-Sv (mm)	41.9	4.83	43.67	4.75	0.24

A, A point; *AFH,* anterior facial height; *ANB,* A point nasion B point; *Ar,* articulare; *Co,* condylion; *Gn,* gnathion; *Go,* gonion; *IMPA,* incisor mandibular plane angle; *L1,* lower incisor; *L6,* lower molar; *LFH,* lower facial height; *Me,* menton; *MP,* mandibular plane; *Occ,* occlusal plane; *PFH,* posterior facial height; *PP,* palatal plane; *SD,* standard deviation; *Sh,* sella horizontal; *SN,* sella-nasion; *SNA,* sella-nasion A point; *SNB,* sella-nasion B point; *SN-GoGn,* sella-nasion to mandibular plane (gonion-gnathion); *Sv,* sella vertical; *U1,* upper incisor; *U6,* upper molar; *UFH,* upper facial height.

*$p < 0.05$.

TABLE 13-3 Comparison of Prepubertal and Postpubertal Patients at End of Treatment

	Prepubertal (n = 23)		Postpubertal (n = 18)		
	Mean	SD	Mean	SD	P value
Maxillary Skeletal					
SNA (degree)	80.32	4.76	81.11	2.97	0.538
Co-A (mm)	99.9	5.12	101.44	7.34	0.420
Mandibular Skeletal					
SNB (degree)	77.02	4.51	77.31	2.61	0.811
Co-Gn (mm)	123.68	7.91	126.94	9.05	0.216
Go-Gn (mm)	80.79	5.95	85.81	7.92	0.022*
Maxilla-Mandible					
ANB (degree)	3.34	2.17	3.72	2.14	0.569
Co-Gn—Co-A (mm)	23.78	4.80	25.44	4.84	0.270
Overjet (mm)	2.52	0.94	1.86	0.78	0.019*
Vertical Skeletal					
SN-GoGn (degree)	31.02	6.03	31.72	5.02	0.689
UFH/LFH (%)	80.76	8.99	76.51	8.25	0.121
PFH/AFH (%)	66.26	7.76	65.55	4.18	0.728
PP-SN (degree)	8.7	2.78	8.25	2.82	0.605
Occ-Sh (degree)	10.28	4.23	10.69	4.38	0.756
Ar-Go-Me (degree)	127.74	6.71	125.03	4.59	0.146
Maxillary Dentoalveolar					
U1-SN (degree)	104.5	7.11	103.28	6.15	0.560
U1-Sv (mm)	78.76	7.00	79.58	6.50	0.697
U1-PP (mm)	23.1	2.70	25.36	2.41	0.007*
U6-PP (mm)	21.14	2.20	22.86	3.12	0.039*
U6-Sv (mm)	47.02	5.33	47.69	5.35	0.685
Mandibular Dentoalveolar					
IMPA (degree)	99.2	6.93	102.33	7.28	0.159
L1-Sv (mm)	73.44	7.35	74.53	6.73	0.623
L1-MP (mm)	41.38	3.87	43.39	5.68	0.175
L6-MP (mm)	34.64	3.20	36.81	4.30	0.065
L6-Sv (mm)	47.5	5.71	47.56	5.28	0.974

A, A point; *AFH,* anterior facial height; *ANB,* A point nasion B point; *Ar,* articulare; *Co,* condylion; *Gn,* gnathion; *Go,* gonion; *IMPA,* incisor mandibular plane angle; *L1,* lower incisor; *L6,* lower molar; *LFH,* lower facial height; *Me,* menton; *MP,* mandibular plane; *Occ,* occlusal plane; *PFH,* posterior facial height; *PP,* palatal plane; *SD,* standard deviation; *Sh,* sella horizontal; *SN,* sella-nasion; *SNA,* sella-nasion A point; *SNB,* sella-nasion B point; *SN-GoGn,* sella-nasion to mandibular plane (gonion-gnathion); *Sv,* sella vertical; *U1,* upper incisor; *U6,* upper molar; *UFH,* upper facial height.

*$p < 0.05$.

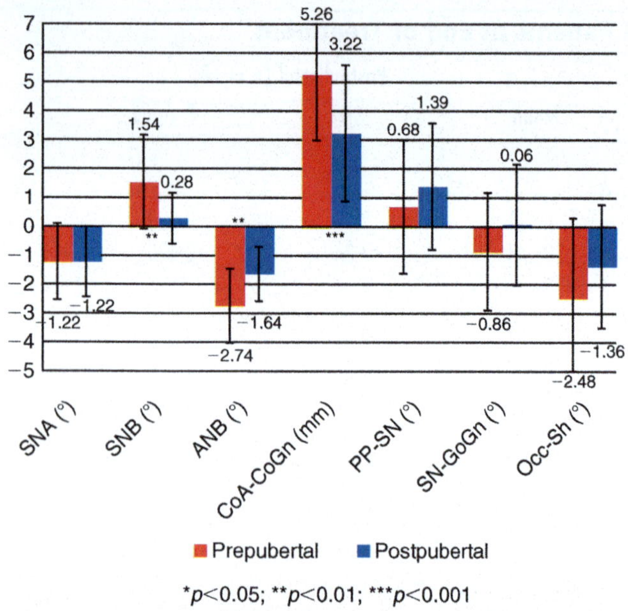

Figure 13-13 Skeletal observations in prepubertal patients compared to postpubertal patients. *ANB (°)*, A point–nasion–B point; *CoA-CoGn (mm)*, differential jaw growth, condylion to A point–condylion to gnathion; *Occ-Sh (°)*, occlusal plane to sella horizontal (constructed 7 degrees upward from sella-nasion at nasion point); *PP-SN (°)*, palatal plane to sella-nasion; *SNA (°)*, sella-nasion A point; *SNB (°)*, sella-nasion B point; *SN-GoGn (°)*, sella-nasion to mandibular plane (gonion-gnathion).

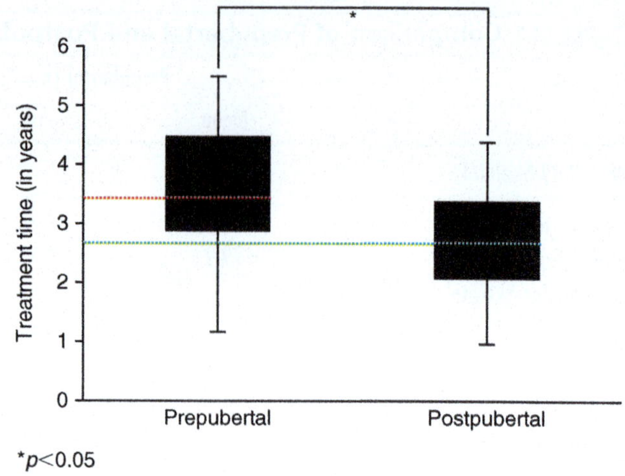

Figure 13-15 Comparison of treatment efficiency based on treatment time in prepubertal and postpubertal groups.

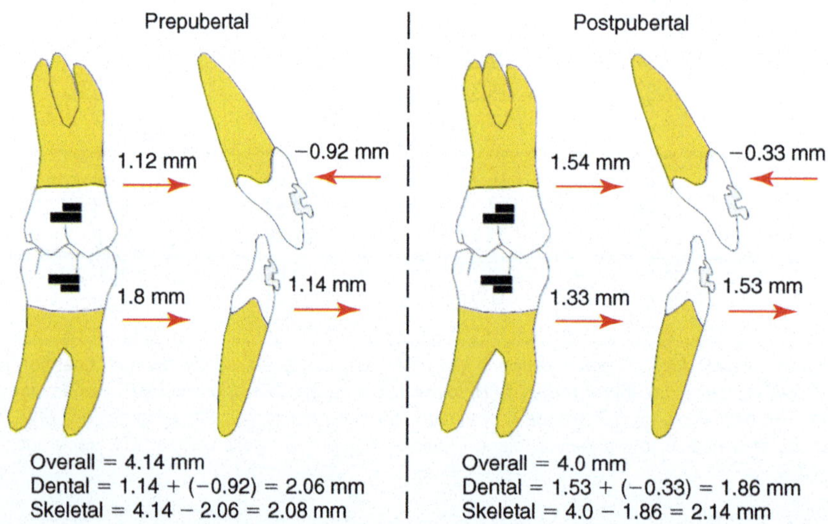

Figure 13-14 Comparison of overjet correction between prepubertal and postpubertal Class II patients treated with the Twin Force bite corrector (TFBC) appliance.

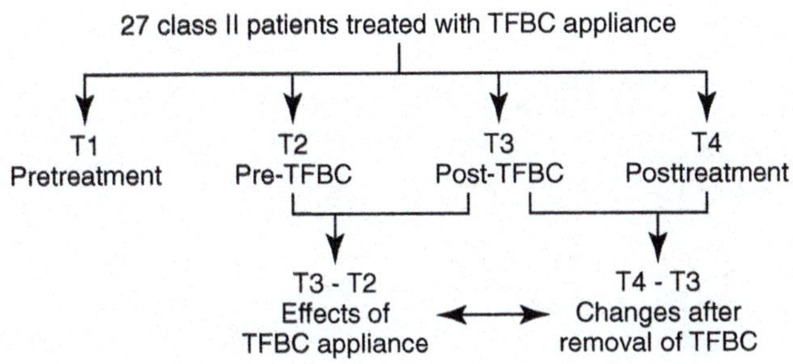

Figure 13-16 Demographics of study examining the contribution of the Twin Force bite corrector (TFBC) appliance to overall Class II correction.

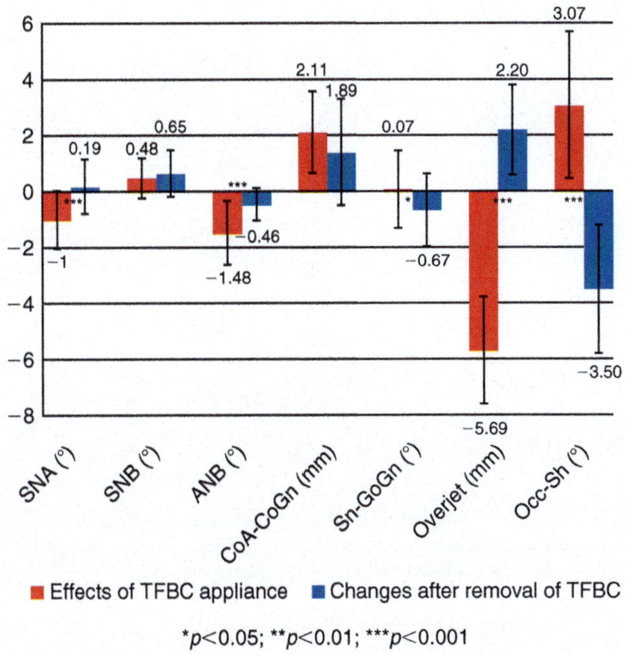

Figure 13-17 Skeletal observations during the Twin Force bite corrector (TFBC) appliance phase compared to skeletal changes that occurred after removal of the TFBC appliance. *ANB (°)*, A point-nasion-B point; *CoA-CoGn (mm)*, differential jaw growth, condylion to A point–condylion to gnathion; *Occ-Sh (°)*, occlusal plane to sella horizontal (constructed 7 degrees upward from sella-nasion at nasion point); *Overjet (mm)*, overjet changes measured from incisal edge of the maxillary incisor to most labial surface of the mandibular incisor; *SNA (°)*, sella-nasion A point; *SNB (°)*, sella-nasion B point; *SN-GoGn (°)*, sella-nasion to mandibular plane (gonion-gnathion).

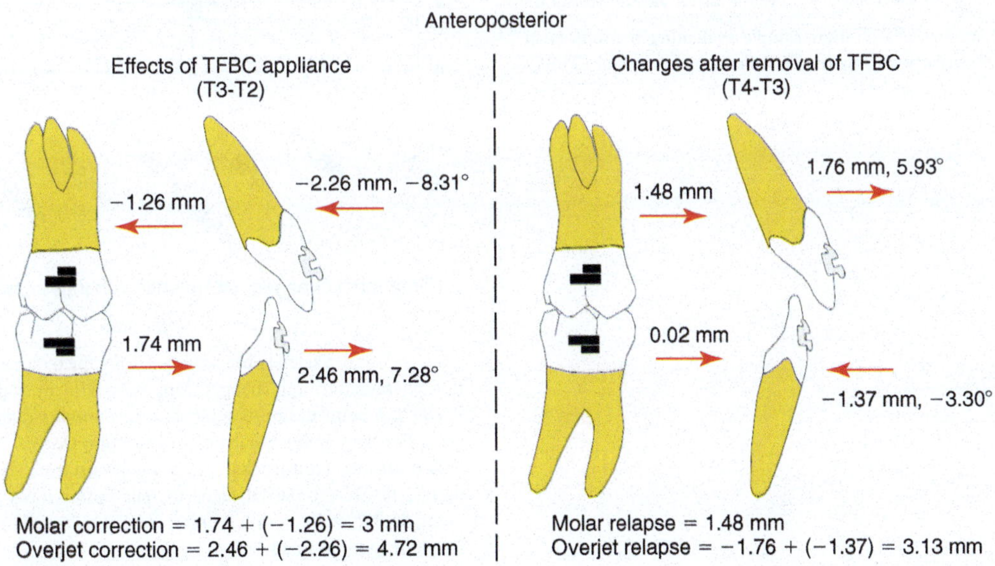

Figure 13-18 Dental changes in the anteroposterior dimension during the Twin Force bite corrector (TFBC) appliance phase and after removal of the appliance. Linear measurements showing a negative (−) sign are synonymous with distal, backward, or intrusive movement to a relevant reference line, while a positive (+) value indicates forward, mesial, or extrusive movement.

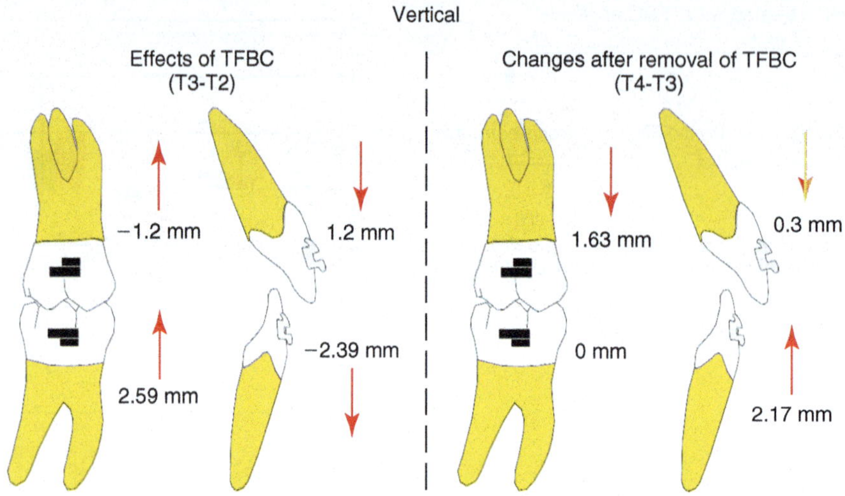

Figure 13-19 Dental changes in the vertical dimension during the Twin Force bite corrector (TFBC) appliance phase and after removal of the appliance. Linear measurements showing a negative (−) sign are synonymous with distal, backward, or intrusive movement to a relevant reference line, while a positive (+) value indicates forward, mesial, or extrusive movement.

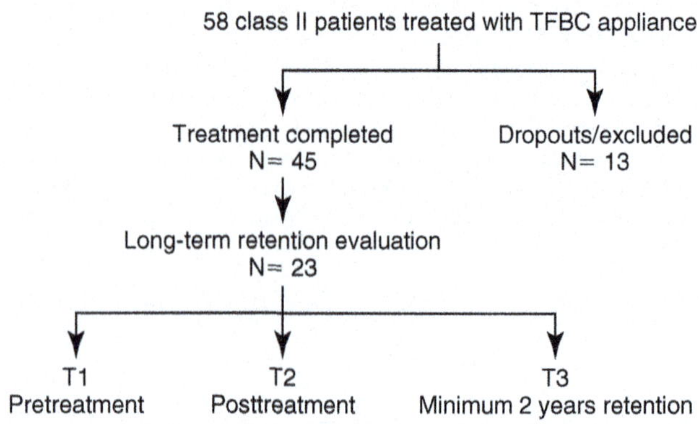

Figure 13-20 Demographics of study sample evaluating the long-term retention of Class II correction using the Twin Force bite corrector (TFBC) appliance.

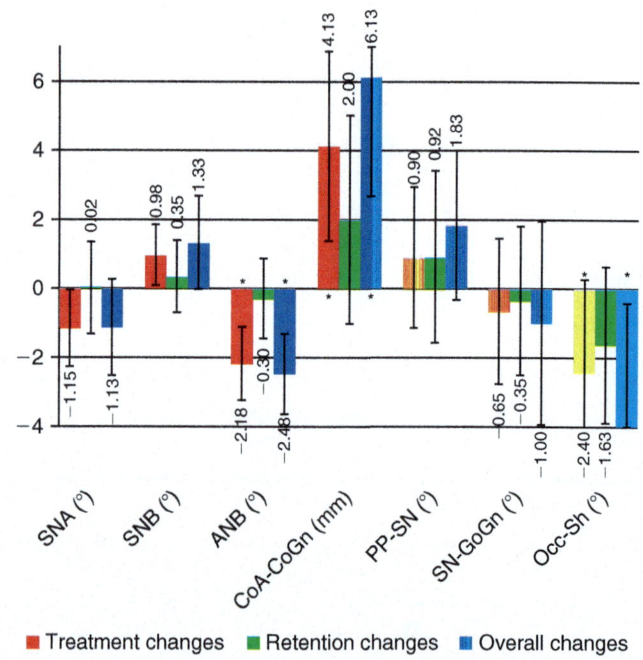

Figure 13-21 Skeletal observations during the treatment phase and retention phase and overall changes from pre-treatment to the retention phase. *ANB (°)*, A point-nasion-B point; *CoA-CoGn (mm)*, differential jaw growth, condylion to A point–condylion to gnathion; *Occ-Sh (°)*, occlusal plane to sella horizontal (constructed 7 degrees upward from sella-nasion at nasion point); *PP-SN (°)*, palatal plane to sella-nasion; *SNA (°)*, sella-nasion A point; *SNB (°)*, sella-nasion B point; *SN-GoGn (°)*, sella-nasion to mandibular plane (gonion-gnathion).

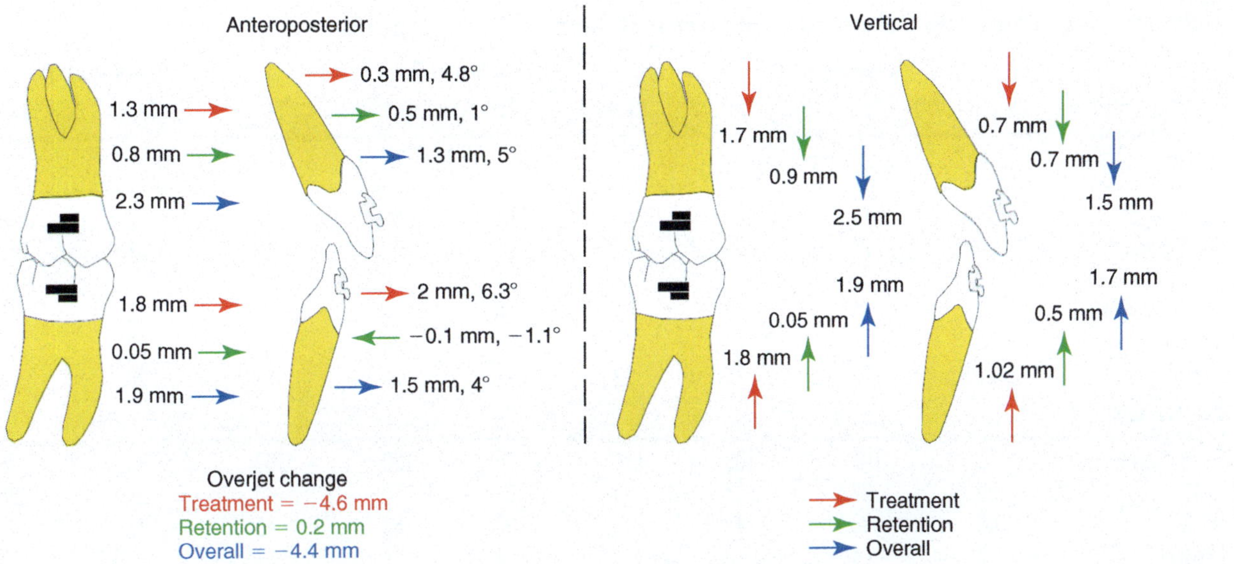

Figure 13-22 Dental observations in the anteroposterior and vertical dimensions during treatment and the retention phase and overall changes from pretreatment to the retention phase.

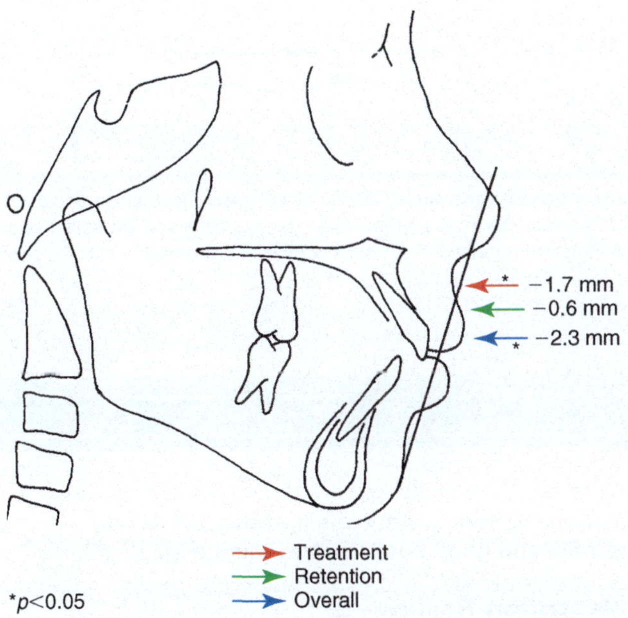

Figure 13-23 Significant soft tissue changes observed at three time points (treatment, retention, and overall). The only significant change observed was the retraction of the upper lip in the treatment phase and overall observation.

of 2 years after appliance removal using lateral cephalograms obtained at three time points: before orthodontic treatment (T1), at completion of treatment (T2), and at least 2 years after the removal of all fixed appliances (T3) (Fig. 13-20).

Skeletally, there was a nonsignificant headgear effect on the maxilla with reduction of the sella-nasion A point (SNA) angle during overall treatment (Fig. 13-21). In the retention evaluation there was no angular change in the SNA angle. In the mandible there was also a nonsignificant increase in the sella-nasion B point (SNB) angle, with nonsignificant change in the retention evaluation. However, the differential A point nasion B point (ANB) angle change was significant in the overall treatment and did not decrease significantly in the retention phase. The differential jaw growth, condylion to gnathion -condylion to A point- CoGn- (CoA-CoGn) was significant in the overall treatment and there was a nonsignificant increase in the retention phase. The occlusal plane decreased by −2.4 degrees in the overall treatment evaluation and further decreased by −1.62 degrees during the retention phase.

Dentally, based on regional superimpositions for the maxilla and mandible (Fig. 13-22), the overjet decreased by -4.65-mm in the overall treatment and in the retention phase was stable with a marginal increase of 0.22-mm. The upper incisor mesialized 0.3-mm after the end of orthodontic treatment and further mesialized 0.5-mm in the retention evaluation. Both the upper and the lower molars mesialized and extruded during the overall treatment changes. In the retention evaluation the upper molar further mesialized and extruded. The forward movement and extrusion of the lower molar showed negligible changes in the retention phase. The lower incisor flared 2.8-mm and 6.98 degrees in the overall treatment and relapsed 0.1-mm and 1.13 degrees in the retention phase, showing minor relapse tendencies. In the soft tissue profile outcome (Fig. 13-23) the only significant difference observed was retrusion of the upper lip during the overall treatment; the lip further retracted during the retention phase. This could be attributed to the headgear effect on the maxilla or to the fact that with growth the reference line of the soft tissue nose and chin may move forward, causing the upper lip to appear retrusive compared to it.

CASE REPORTS

The following three case reports illustrate the effectiveness of long-term Class II correction with the TFBC appliance (see Figs. 13-24 to 13-35 and Table 13-4).

Text continued on p. 244

TABLE 13-4 Cephalometric Values for Long-Term Retention Case Reports

	Case Report 1			Case Report 2			Case Report 3		
	T1	T2	T3	T1	T2	T3	T1	T2	T3
Skeletal									
SNA (degree)	80.5	79	79	85	85	84	88	87	86
SNB (degree)	75	76	77	81	81	82	76	77	77
ANB (degree)	5.5	3	2	4	4	2	12	10	9
Occ-FH (degree)	13	9	8	12	8	6	18	15	13
SN-GoGn (degree)	26	24	23	25	24	24.5	31	32	32
FMA (degree)	21.5	20	18	22	21	20	27	28	26
Dentoalveolar									
U1-SN (degree)	102	105	105	115		120	102	96	98
U6-PP	20.5	22.5	22	18	21	20	20	21	23
U6-Sv	48	48.5	49	48	52	53	45	46	46
L1-Apog	2	4	3	3.5	4	6	1	5.5	5
IMPA (degree)	106	111	113	104		114	104	110	108
L6-MP	31.5	36	38	31	37	39	32	37	38
L6-Sv	41.5	50	49	46	51	55	44	47	47
Soft Tissue									
G-Sn-Pg (degree)	159	162	166	159		165	155	157	154
S line-Ls	4	4	3	5	0	0	6	4	5
S line-Li	3.5	3	2	3	0	1	3.5	3.5	4

ANB, A point nasion B point; *G*, glabella; *FH*, facial height; *FMA*, Frankfurt mandibular plane angle; *IMPA*, incisor mandibular plane angle; *L1*, lower incisor; *L6*, lower molar; *MP*, mandibular plane; *Occ*, occlusal plane; *PP*, palatal plane; *SN*, sella-nasion; *Sn*, subnasale; *SNA*, sella-nasion A point; *SNB*, sella-nasion B point; *SN-GoGn*, sella-nasion to mandibular plane (gonion-gnathion); *Sv*, sella vertical; *T1*, pre-treatment; *T2*, post-treatment; *T3*, retention; *U1*, upper incisor; *U6*, upper molar.

CASE REPORT 1

Patient Profile

The patient was a 12-year-old prepubertal male who presented with a chief complaint of deep bite. He was diagnosed with a Class II malocclusion due to a retrognathic mandible with full cusp Class II molars bilaterally, 100% deep bite, and 6-mm of overjet (Fig. 13-24).

Treatment Progress

After initial leveling and alignment, stiff upper (0.019-inch × 0.025-inch and lower 0.021-inch × 0.025-inch) stainless steel archwires were placed with the TFBC appliance inserted with 5-mm of activation. Three months later the patient was in a super Class I relationship and the appliance was removed. Class II elastics were used to maintain the corrections and finishing and detailing were done. The patient was debonded with improvement of the soft tissue profile and good posterior occlusion (Fig. 13-25).

Retention Review

The patient was evaluated 6 years in retention and showed stable Class I molar and canine relationship bilaterally (Fig. 13-26). Overall and regional superimpositions (Fig. 13-27) showed that, in the treatment phase, the upper molar was held in place with mesialization of the lower molar. In the retention phase, both the upper and the lower molars were very stable with negligible changes. The flaring of the lower anterior teeth caused by the TFBC appliance was found to be stable in the retention evaluation.

CASE REPORT 1—cont'd

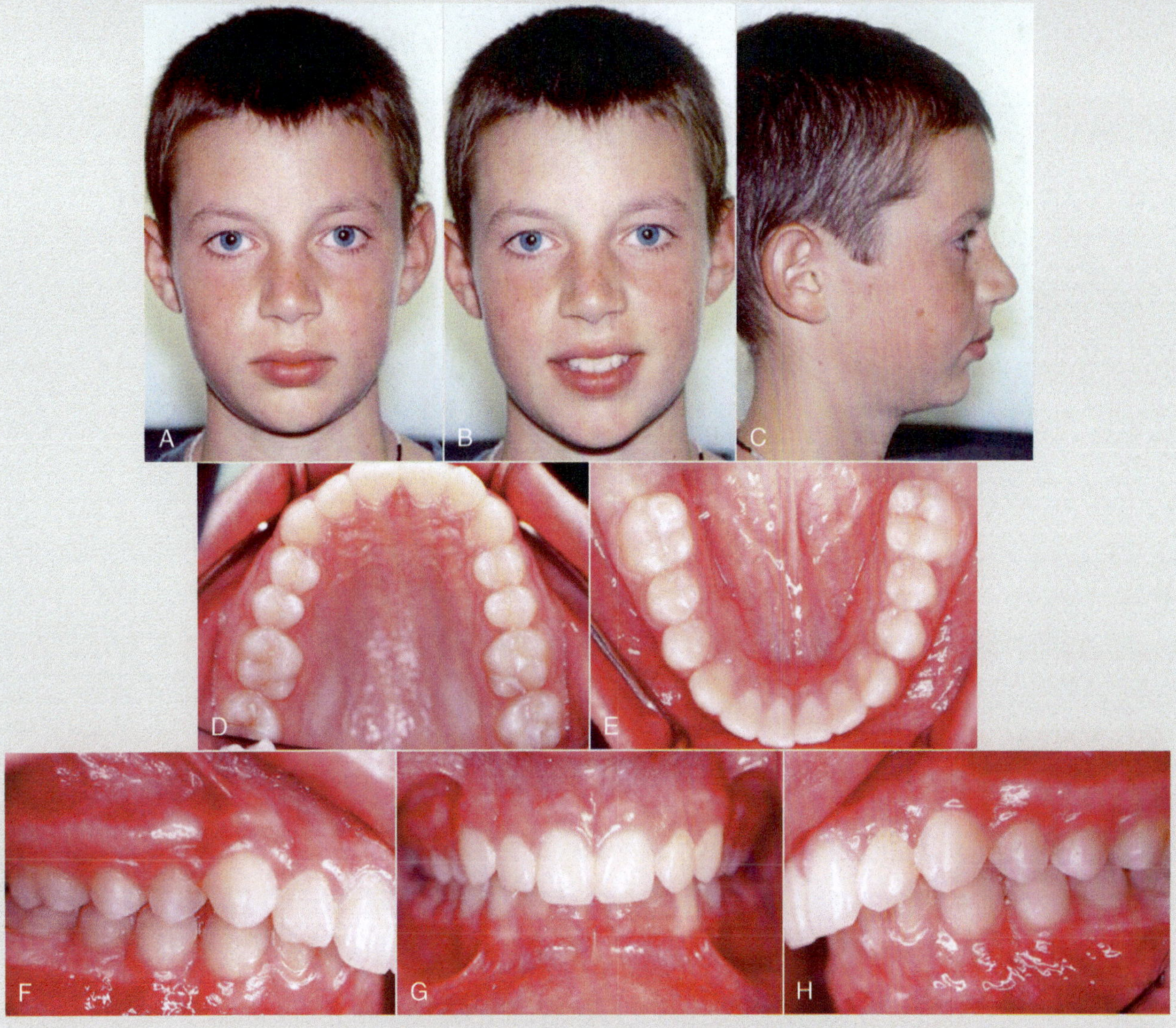

Figure 13-24 Pre-treatment records for Case Report 1. **A-C,** Facial views. **D-H,** Intraoral views.

Continued

CASE REPORT 1—cont'd

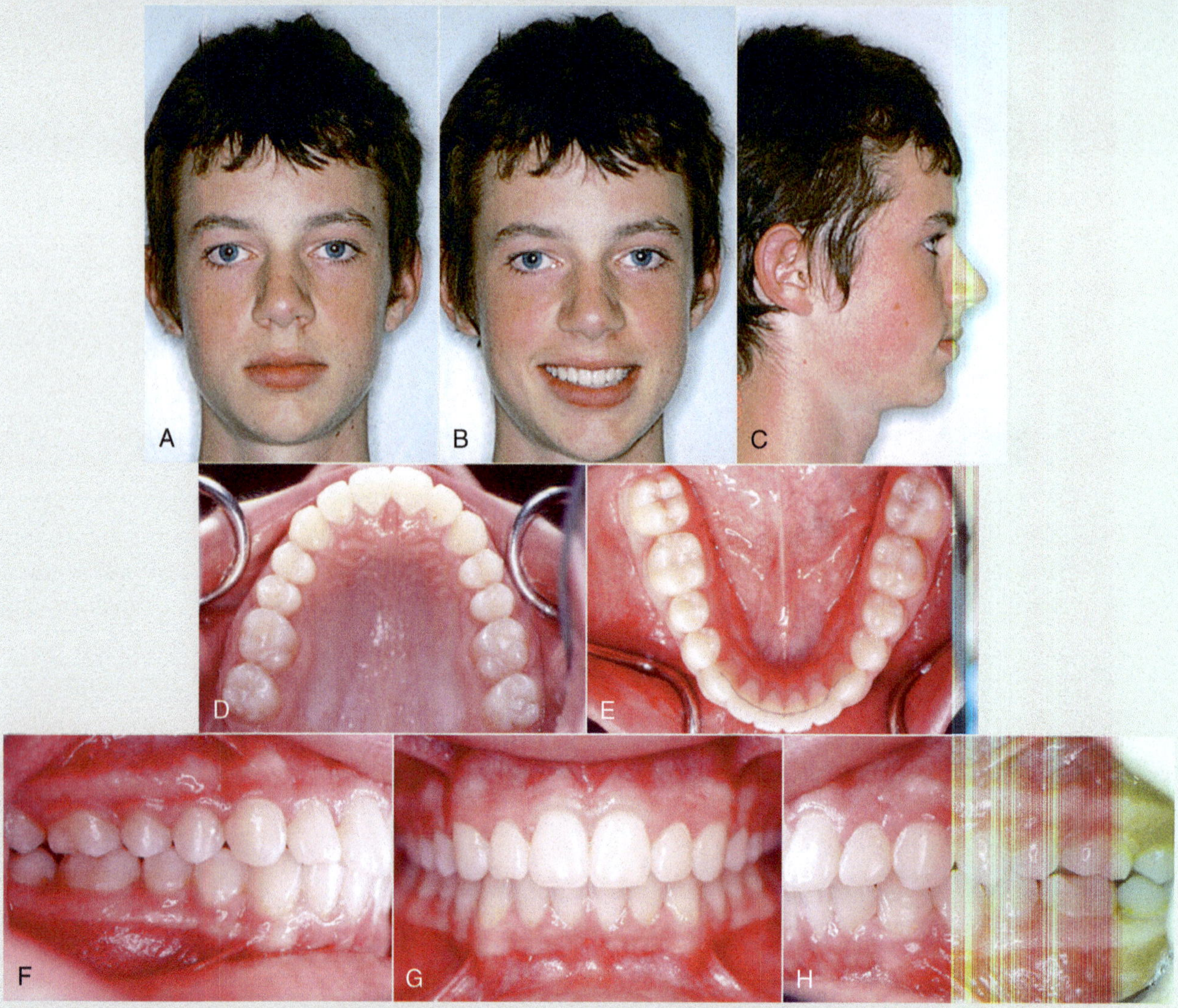

Figure 13-25 Post-treatment records for Case Report 1. **A–C,** Facial views. **D–H,** Intraoral views.

CASE REPORT 1—cont'd

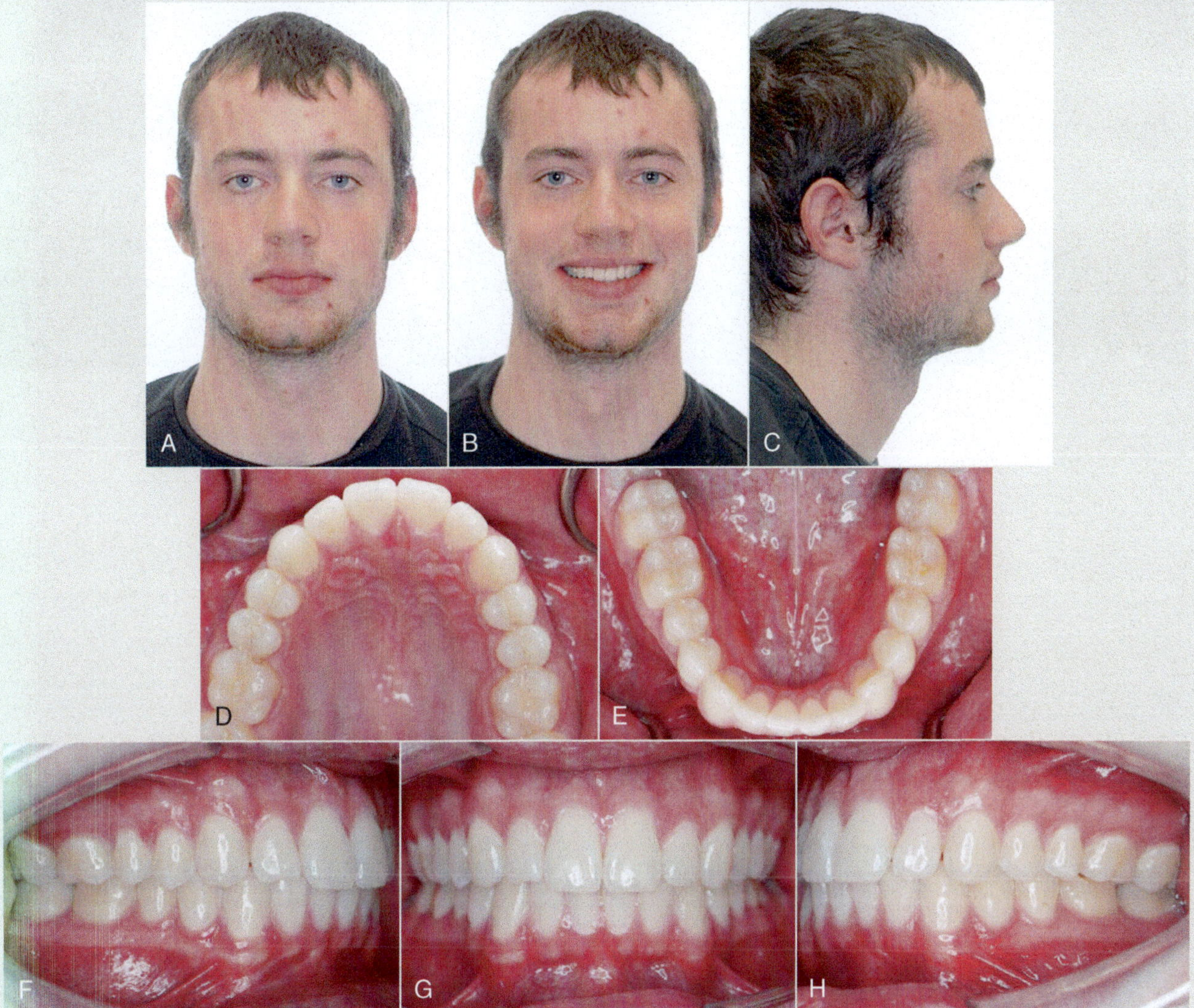

Figure 13-26 Case Report 1 retention evaluation 6 years after debonding. **A–C,** Facial views. **D–H,** Intraoral views.

Continued

CASE REPORT 1—cont'd

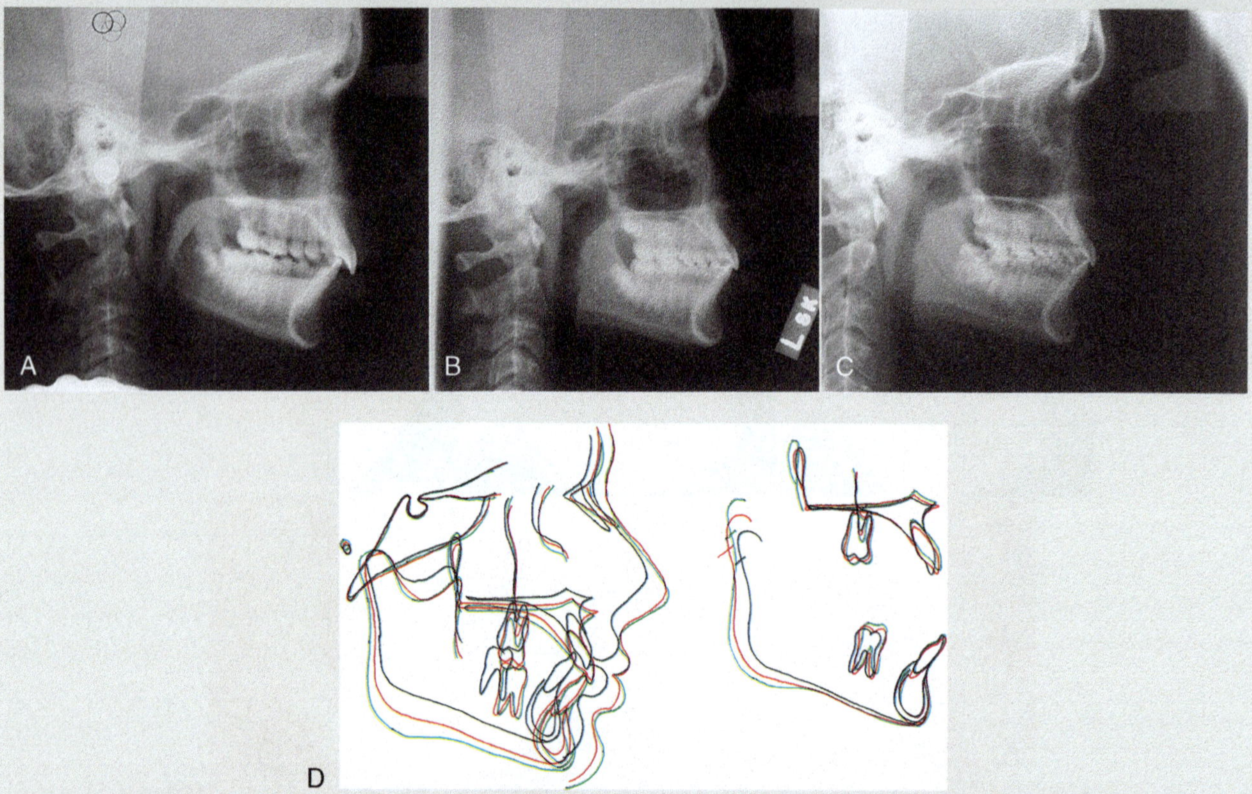

Figure 13-27 **A,** Pre-treatment lateral cephalogram. **B,** Post-treatment lateral cephalogram. **C,** Lateral cephalogram in retention. **D,** Overall and regional cephalometric superimpositions. Black is pre-treatment, red is post-treatment, and green is retention.

CASE REPORT 2

Patient Profile

The patient was an 11-year-old prepubertal male in late mixed dentition who presented with a chief complaint of crooked teeth. The patient was diagnosed with a Class II malocclusion due to a retrognathic mandible with end on molars bilaterally and minimal crowding in both the upper and the lower arches. The patient had 5-mm of overjet and 50% deep bite (Fig. 13-28).

Treatment Progress

After initial leveling and alignment, the deciduous upper left second molar was extracted and the second premolar was exposed and evaluated to be small and rotated. Subsequently, stiff upper and lower archwires were placed with the TFBC appliance for 3 months to achieve the overcorrected super Class I molar and canine relationship. The patient was debonded in good Class I molar and canine relationship (Fig. 13-29).

Retention Review

The patient was evaluated after 6 years and stable class I molar and canine relationship was observed (Fig. 13-30). However, mild relapse of the midline diastema was noted. Overall and regional superimpositions (Fig. 13-31) showed that, in the treatment phase, both the upper and the lower molars mesialized. In the retention phase, there was no change in the position of the upper and lower molars. There was significant flaring of the lower anteriors, which was stable in the retention phase.

CASE REPORT 2—cont'd

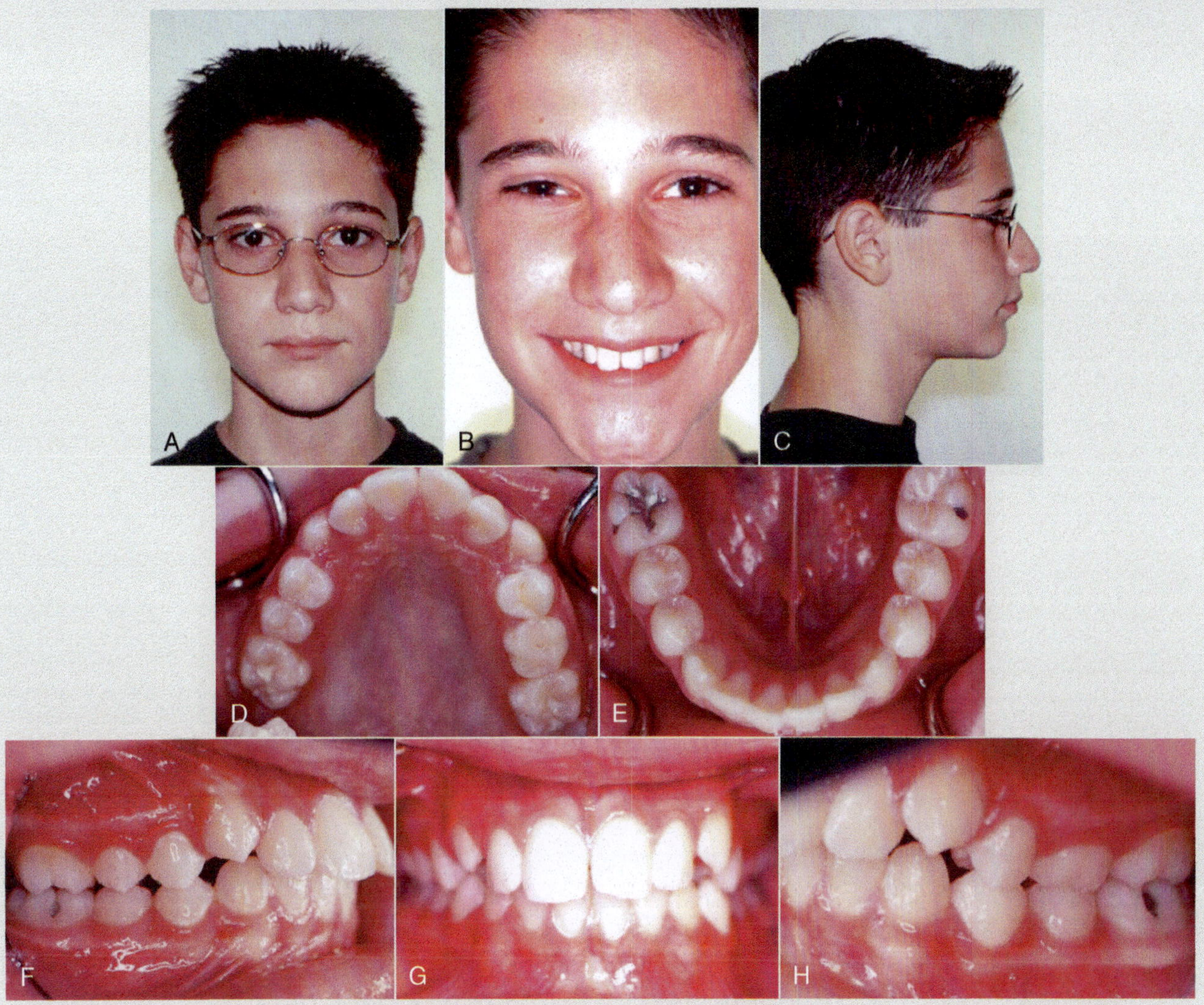

Figure 13-28 Pre-treatment records for Case Report 2. **A–C,** Facial views. **D–H,** Intraoral views.

Continued

CASE REPORT 2—cont'd

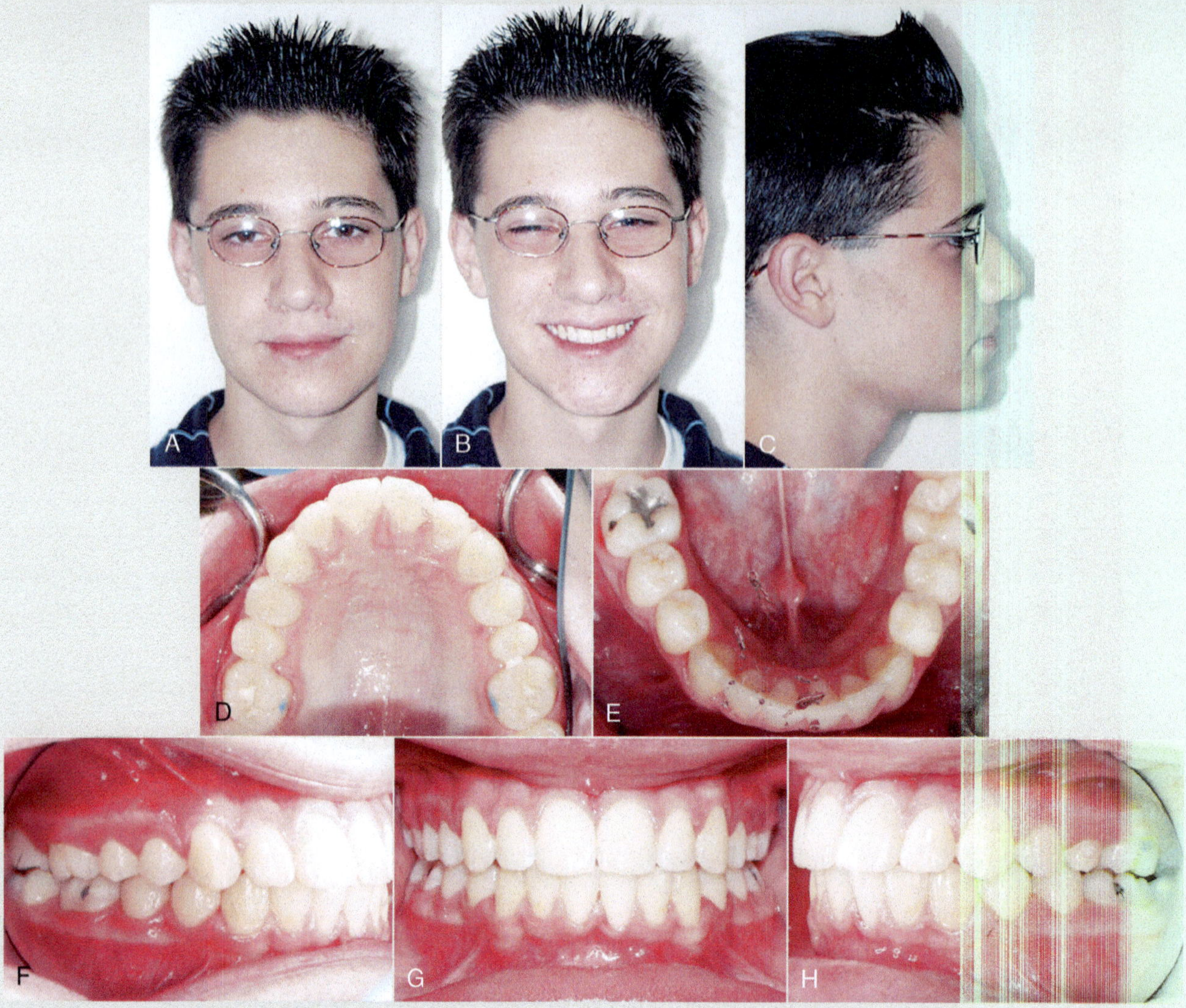

Figure 13-29 Post-treatment records for Case Report 2. **A–C,** Facial views. **D–H,** Intraoral views.

CASE REPORT 2—cont'd

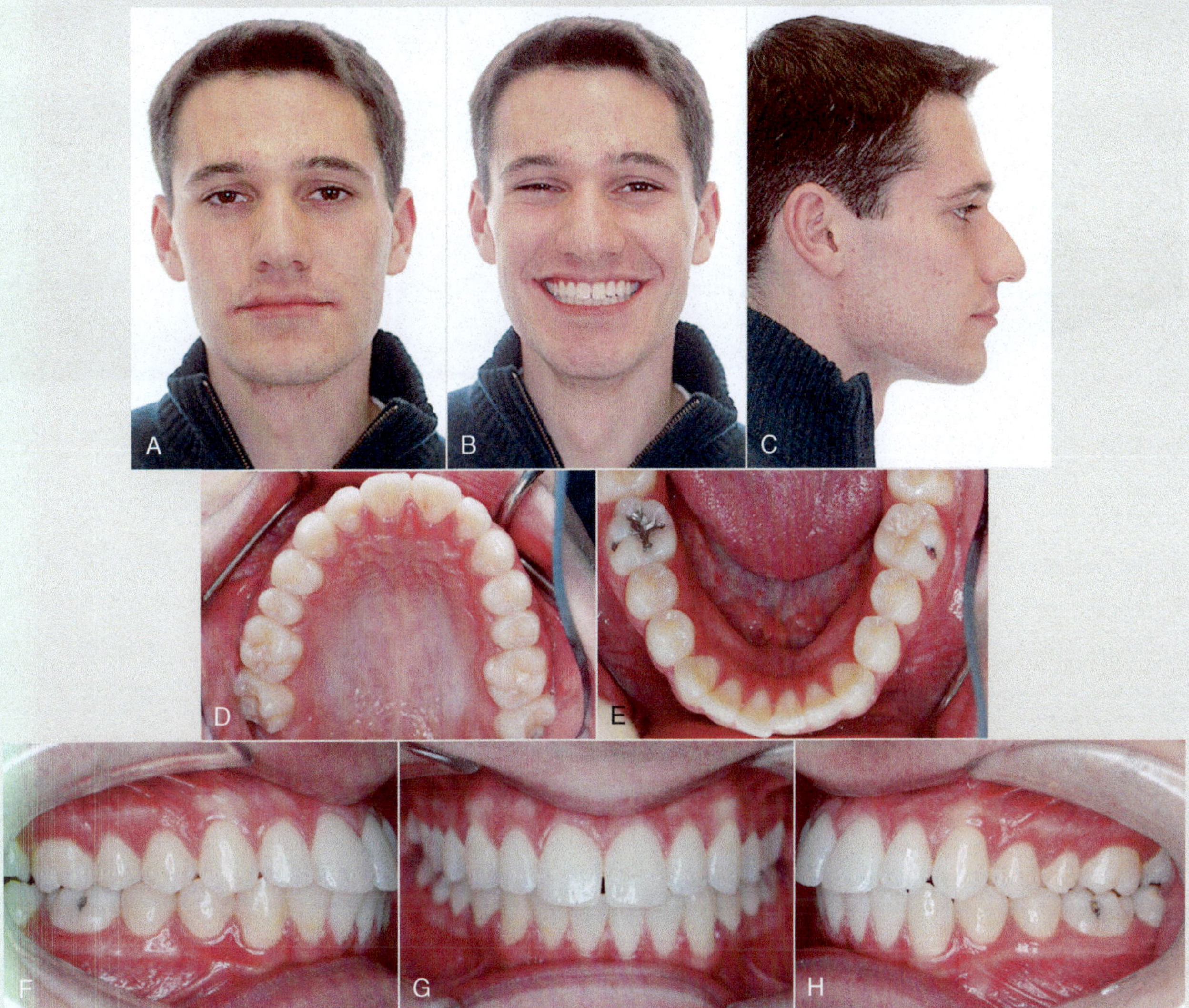

Figure 13-30 Case Report 2 retention evaluation 6 years after appliance removal. **A–C,** Facial views. **D–H,** Intraoral views.

Continued

CASE REPORT 2—cont'd

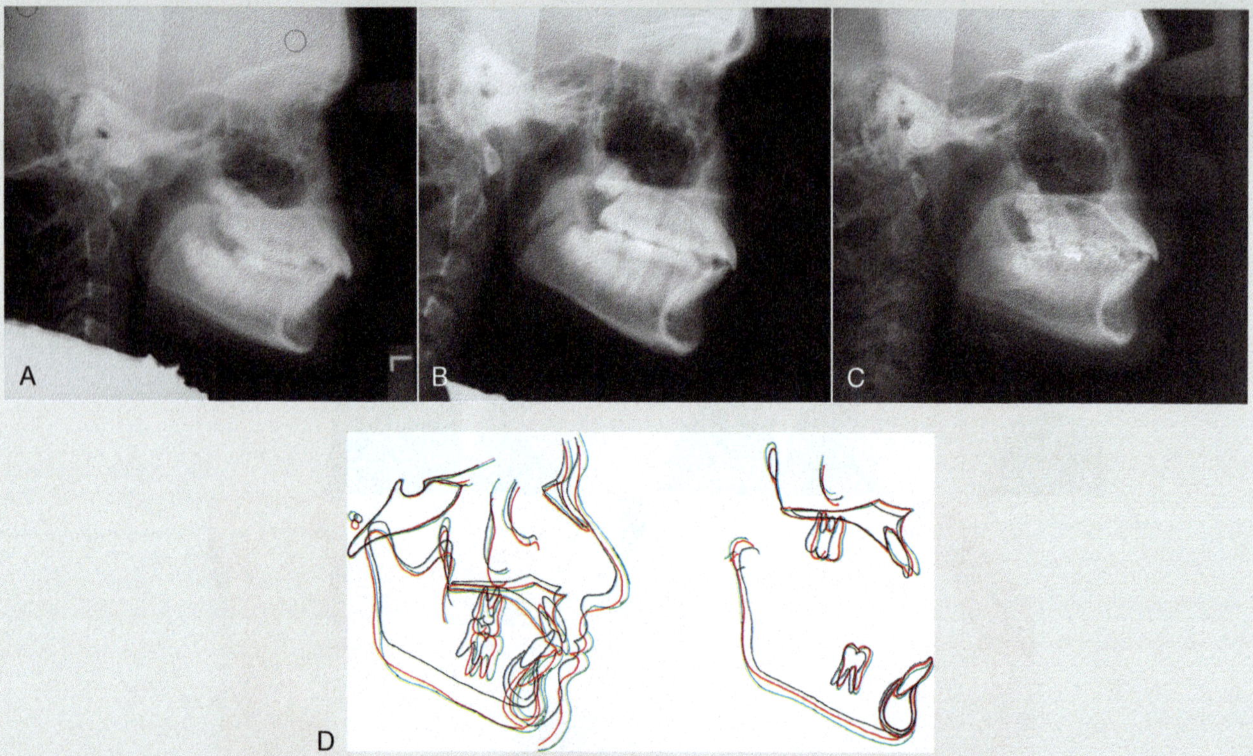

Figure 13-31 **A,** Pre-treatment lateral cephalogram. **B,** Post-treatment lateral cephalogram. **C,** Lateral cephalogram in retention. **D,** Overall and regional cephalometric superimpositions. Black is pre-treatment, red is post-treatment, and green is retention.

CASE REPORT 3

Patient Profile

The patient was an 11-year-old female who presented with a chief complaint of crowding (see Fig. 13-6A). She was diagnosed with a Class II, Division I malocclusion due to a prognathic maxilla and a retrognathic mandible with Class II molars and canines on both sides and an overjet of 7-mm, overbite of 70% with crossbite of the molars bilaterally, and a convex soft tissue profile (Fig. 13-32).

Treatment Progress

The patient presented with a severe Class II skeletal relationship with an ANB angle of 12 degrees (see Table 13-4). However, since the patient was still growing, growth modulation was attempted. There was moderate crowding in the upper arch and minimal crowding in the lower arch. Treatment began with banding of the maxillary molars and rapid maxillary expansion (RME) in the upper arch to create space for the crowding. Subsequently, the patient's upper and lower arches were set up for TFBC appliance placement. The patient was debonded after 24 months of active treatment with a Class I molar and canine relationship bilaterally (Fig. 13-33).

Retention Review

The patient was evaluated after 7 years and showed a harmonic soft tissue profile with maintenance of stable buccal occlusion bilaterally (Fig. 13-34). Overall and regional superimpositions (Fig. 13-35) showed mesial movement of both the upper and the lower molars in the treatment phase and no changes in the retention phase. Flaring of the lower anteriors was observed to be stable in the retention phase.

CASE REPORT 3—cont'd

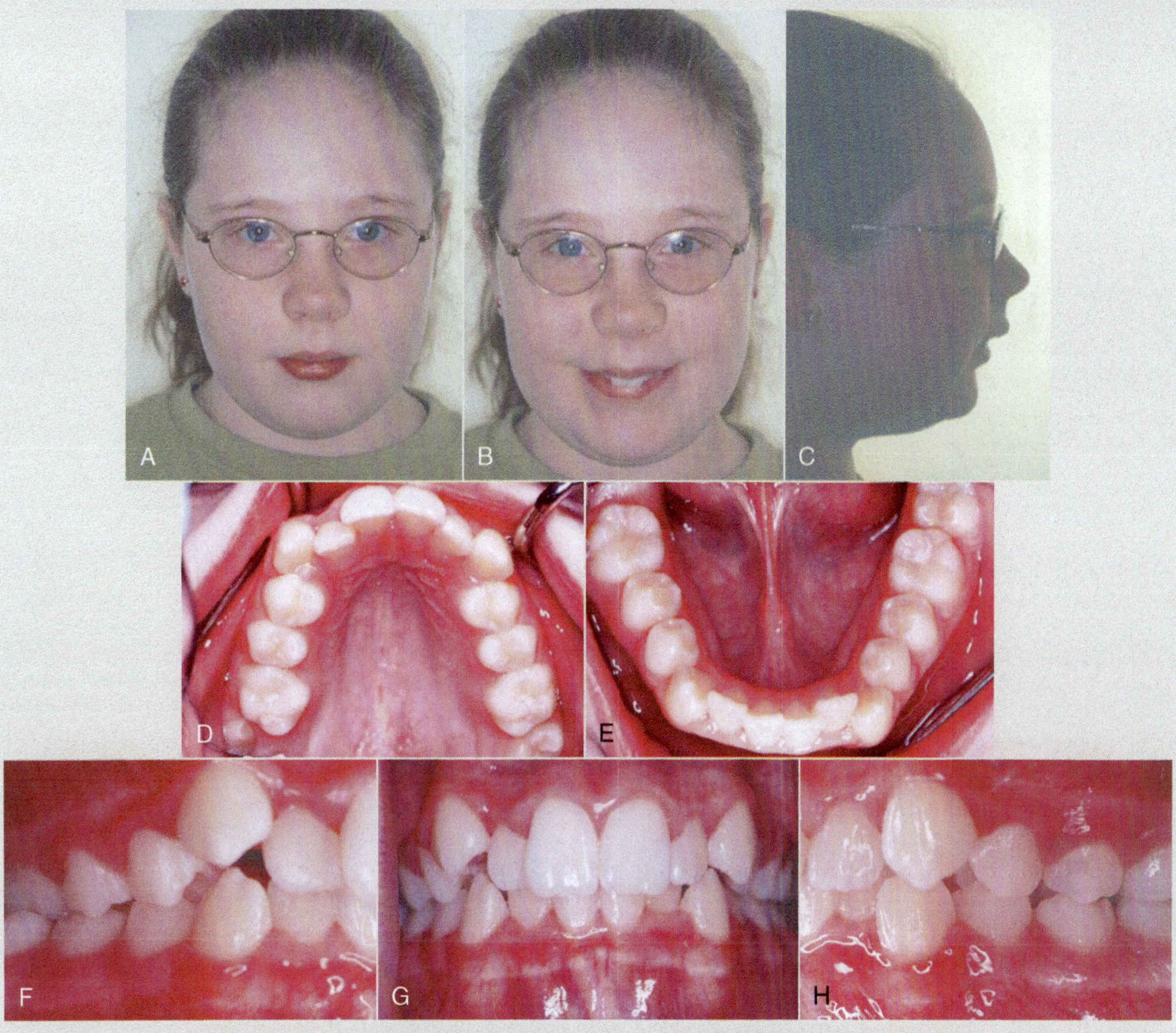

Figure 13-32 Pre-treatment records of Case Report 3. **A–C,** Facial views. **D–H,** Intraoral views.

Continued

CASE REPORT 3—cont'd

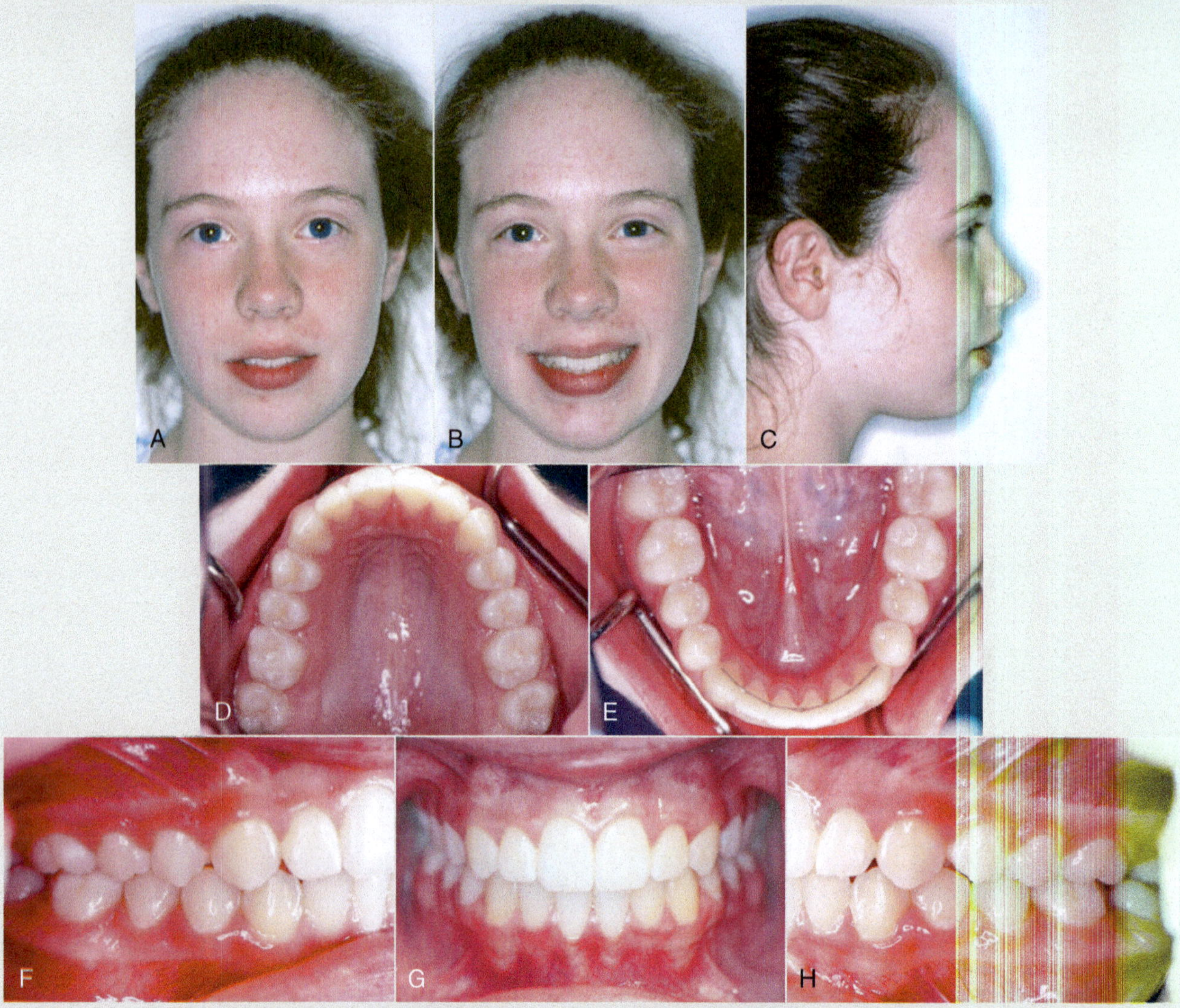

Figure 13-33 Post-treatment records for Case Report 3. **A–C,** Facial views. **D–H,** Intraoral views.

CASE REPORT 3—cont'd

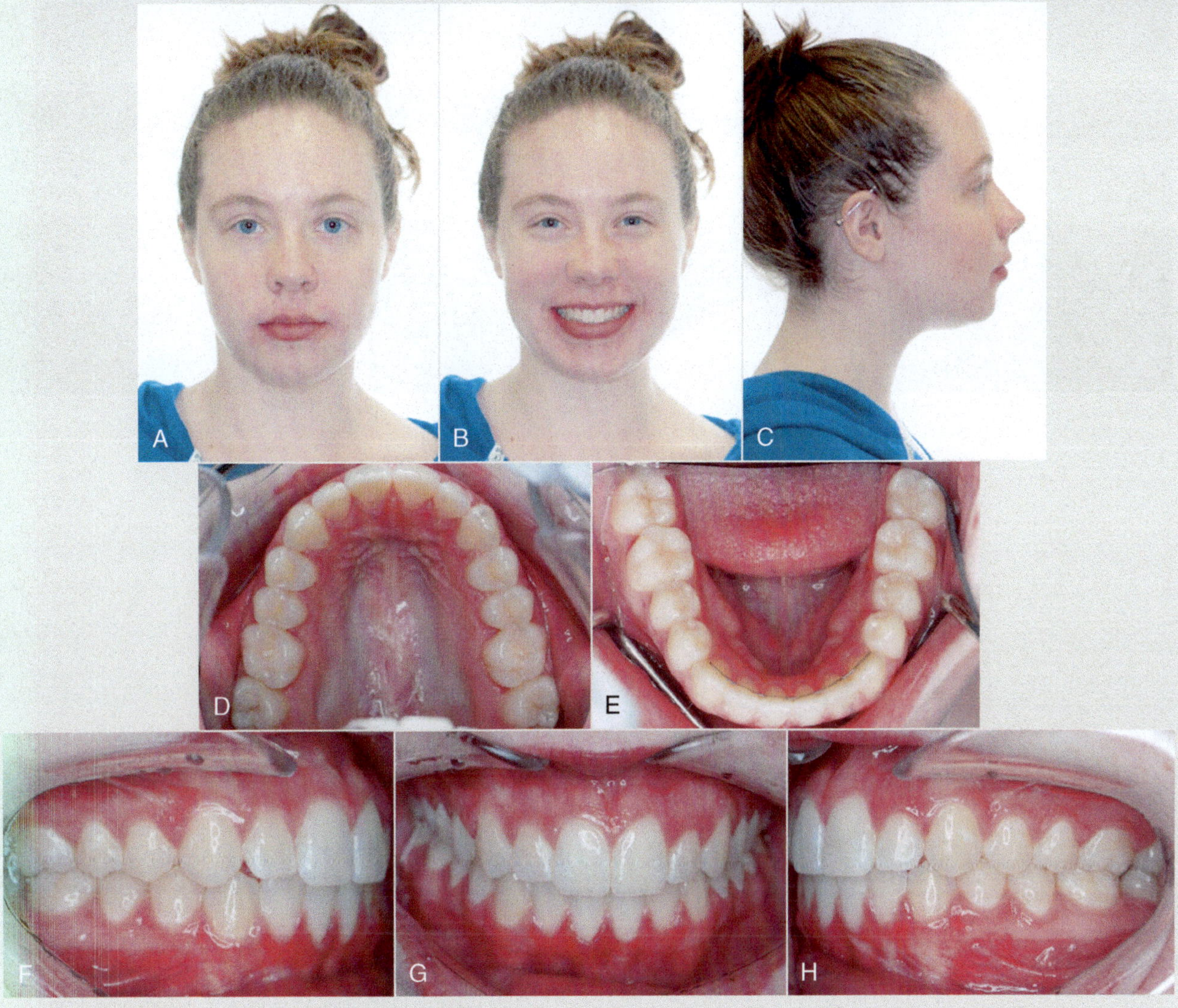

Figure 13-34 Case Report 3 retention evaluation 7 years after appliance removal. **A–C,** Facial views. **D–H,** Intraoral views.

Continued

CASE REPORT 3—cont'd

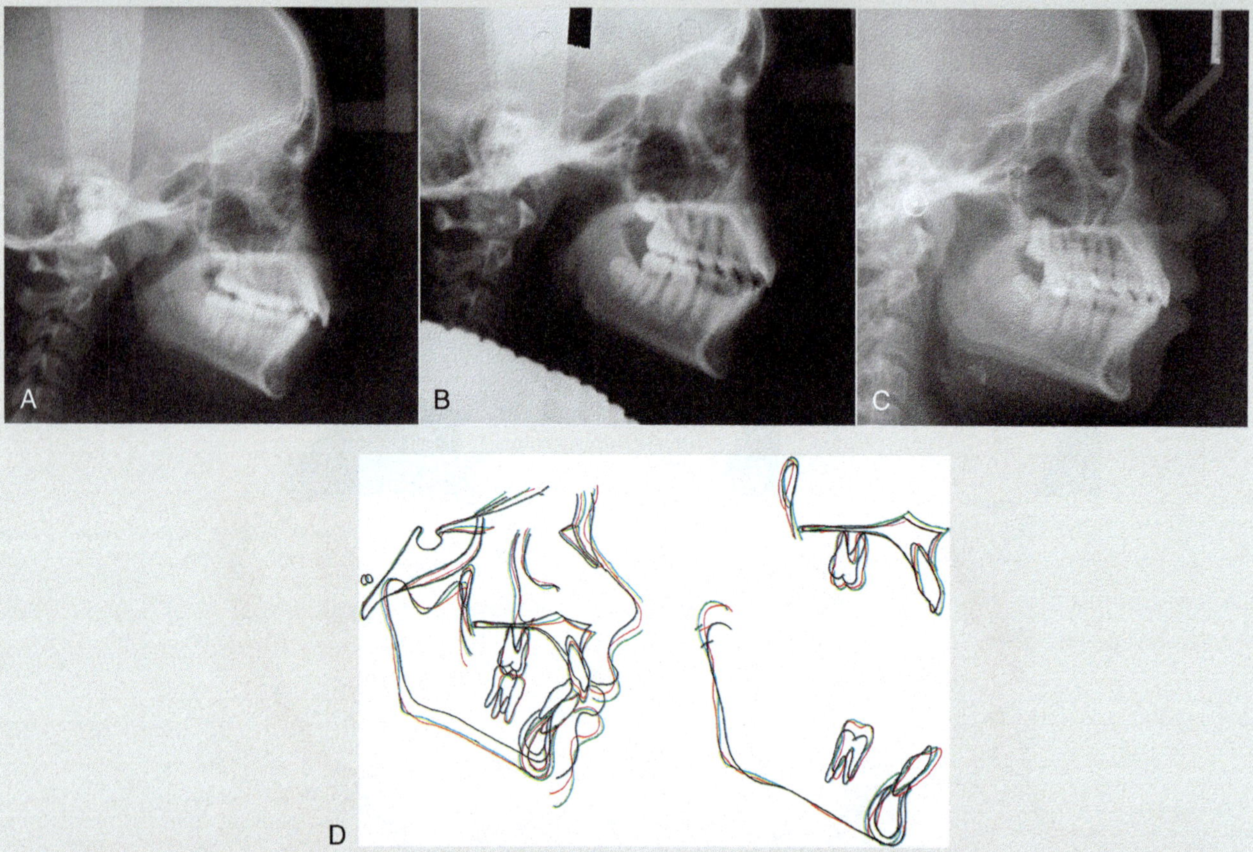

Figure 13-35 **A,** Pre-treatment lateral cephalogram. **B,** Post-treatment lateral cephalogram. **C,** Lateral cephalogram in retention. **D,** Overall and regional cephalometric superimpositions. Black is pre-treatment, red is post-treatment, and green is retention.

SUMMARY

Class II correction with the semirigid TFBC appliance appears to be predominantly a combination of dentoalveolar and mild skeletal changes. Long-term retention evaluation of Class II correction achieved with the TFBC appliance showed the correction to be stable. Dental effects of the appliance, such as occlusal plane rotation, distalization, and intrusion of the maxillary molars, appear to be transient effects that do not contribute to overall Class II correction; however, mesial movement and extrusion of the lower molar with use of the appliance appear to be stable effects in the long-term. Treatment efficiency based on overall treatment time suggests that the postpubertal phase is the preferred phase for Class II correction with the TFBC appliance.

REFERENCES

1. Weinmann JP, Sicher H. *Bone and Bones: Fundamentals of Bone Biology*. St. Louis, MO: CV Mosby; 1947.
2. Scott JH. The growth of the human face. *Proc R Soc Med*. 1954;47:91–100.
3. Moss ML, Salentijn L. The primary role of functional matrices in facial growth. *Am J Orthod*. 1969;55:566–577.
4. Van Limborgh J. A new view on the control of the morphogenesis of the skull. *Acta Morph Neerl Scand*. 1970;8:143–170.
5. King L, Harris EF, Tolley EA. Heritability of cephalometric and occlusal variables as assessed from siblings with overt malocclusions. *Am J Orthod Dentofacial Orthop*. 1993;104:121–131.
6. Kawala B, Antoszewska J, Necka A. Genetics or environment? A twin-method study of malocclusions. *World J Orthod*. 2007;8:405–410.
7. Nakasima A, Ichinose M, Nakata S, Takahama Y. Hereditary factors in the craniofacial morphology of Angle's Class II and Class III malocclusions. *Am J Orthod*. 1982;82:150–156.
8. Harris JE, Kowalski CJ. All in the family: use of familial information in orthodontic diagnosis, case assessment and treatment planning. *Am J Orthod*. 1976;69:493–509.
9. McNamara JA Jr. Components of Class II malocclusion in children 8–10 years of age. *Angle Orthod*. 1981;51:177–202.
10. Baccetti T, Franchi L, McNamara JA Jr, Tollaro I. Early dentofacial features of Class II malocclusion: a longitudinal study from the deciduous through the mixed dentition. *Am J Orthod Dentofacial Orthop*. 1997;111:502–509.
11. Ngan PW, Byczek E, Scheick J. Longitudinal evaluation of growth changes in Class II Division 1 subjects. *Semin Orthod*. 1997;3:222–231.
12. Bishara SE. Mandibular changes in persons with untreated and treated Class II Division 1 malocclusion. *Am J Orthod Dentofacial Orthop*. 1998;113:661–673.

13. Stahl F, Baccetti T, Franchi L, McNamara JA Jr. Longitudinal growth changes in untreated subjects with Class II Division 1 malocclusion. *Am J Orthod Dentofacial Orthop*. 2008;134:125–137.
14. Spalding PM. Treatment of Class II malocclusions. In: Bishara SE, ed. *Textbook of Orthodontics*. 1st ed. Philadelphia, PA: WB Saunders; 2001: 324–374.
15. Rakosi T. The activator. In: Graber TM, Rakosi T, Petrovic AG, eds. *Dentofacial Orthopedics with Functional Appliances*. 1st ed. St. Louis, MO: Mosby; 1985:150–180.
16. Bishara SE, Ziaja RR. Functional appliances: a review. *Am J Orthod Dentofacial Orthop*. 1989;95:250–258.
17. Charlier JP, Petrovic A, Stutzmann JH. Effects of mandibular hyperpropulsion on the prechondroblastic zone of young rat condyle. *Am J Orthod*. 1969;55:71–74.
18. Rabie ABM, She TT, Hägg U. Functional appliance therapy accelerates and enhances condylar growth. *Am J Orthod Dentofacial Orthop*. 2003; 123:40–48.
19. McNamara JA Jr, Bryan FA. Long-term mandibular adaptations to protrusive function: an experimental study in *Macaca mulatta*. *Am J Orthod Dentofacial Orthop*. 1987:92:98–108.
20. Tulloch JF, Phillips C, Proffit WR. Benefit of early Class II treatment: progress report of a two-phase randomized clinical trial. *Am J Orthod Dentofacial Orthop*. 1998;113:62–72.
21. Ghafari J, Shofer FS, Jacobsson-Hunt U, Markowitz DL, Laster LL. Headgear versus function regulator in the early treatment of Class II, Division 1 malocclusion: a randomized clinical trial. *Am J Orthod Dentofacial Orthop*. 1998;113:51–61.
22. Dolce C, McGorray SP, Brazeau L, King GJ, Wheeler TT. Timing of Class II treatment: skeletal changes comparing 1-phase and 2-phase treatment. *Am J Orthod Dentofacial Orthop*. 2007;132:481–489.
23. Johnson PD, Cohen DA, Aisoa L, McGorray S, Wheeler T. Attitudes and compliance of preadolescent children during early treatment of Class II malocclusion. *Clin Orthod Res*. 1998;1:20–28.
24. O'Brien K, Wright J, Conboy F, et al. Effectiveness of treatment for Class II malocclusion with the Herbst or Twin-block appliances: a randomized, controlled trial. *Am J Orthod Dentofacial Orthop*. 2003;124: 128–137.
25. Fotheringham MJ, Sawyer MG. Adherence to recommended medical regimens in childhood and adolescence. *J Paediatr Child Health*. 1995; 31(2):72–78.
26. Zentner A, Stelve V, Sergl HG. Patients' attitudes and non-compliance in orthodontic treatment. *Eur J Orthod*. 1996;18:429 (abstract).
27. Sahm G, Bartsch A, Witt E. Micro-electronic monitoring of functional appliance wear. *Eur J Orthod*. 1990;12(3):297–301.
28. Papadopoulos MA. Overview of the intermaxillary noncompliance appliances. In: Papadopoulos MA, ed. *Orthodontic Treatment of the Class II Noncompliant Patient: Current Principles and Techniques*. 1st ed. St. Louis, MO: Elsevier; 2006:21–34.
29. Pangrazio-Kulbersh V, Berger JL, Chermak DS, Kaczynski R, Simon ES, Haerian A. Treatment effects of the mandibular anterior repositioning appliance on patients with Class II malocclusion. *Am J Orthod Dentofacial Orthop*. 2003;123:286–295.
30. Heinig N, Göz G. Clinical application and effects of the Forsus spring: a study of a new Herbst hybrid. *J Orofac Orthop*. 2001;62:436–450.
31. Cope JB, Buschang PH, Cope DD, Parker J, Blackwood HO 3rd. Quantitative evaluation of craniofacial changes with Jasper Jumper therapy. *Angle Orthod*. 1994;64:113–122.
32. Stromeyer EL, Caruso JM, DeVincenzo JP. A cephalometric study of the Class II correction effects of the Eureka Spring. *Angle Orthod*. 2002;72:203–210.
33. Burstone CJ, Koenig HA. Force systems from an ideal arch. *Am J Orthod*. 1974;65:270–289.
34. Pancherz H, Anehus-Pancherz M. The headgear effect of the Herbst appliance: a cephalometric long term study. *Am J Orthod Dentofacial Orthop*. 1993;103:510–520.
35. Pancherz H. The mechanism of Class II correction in Herbst appliance treatment: a cephalometric investigation. *Am J Orthod*. 1982;82: 104–113.
36. Heinig N, Göz G. Clinical application and effects of the Forsus spring: a study of a new Herbst hybrid. *J Orofac Orthop*. 2001;62:436–450.
37. Franchi L, Alvetro L, Giuntini V, Masucci C, Defraia E, Baccetti T. Effectiveness of comprehensive fixed appliance treatment used with the Forsus Fatigue Resistant Device in Class II patients. *Angle Orthod*. 2011;81:678–683.
38. Herrera FS, Henriques JF, Janson G, Francisconi MF, de Freitas KM. Cephalometric evaluation in different phases of Jasper jumper therapy. *Am J Orthod Dentofacial Orthop*. 2011;140:e77–e84.
39. Rothenberg J, Campbell ES, Nanda R. Class II correction with the Twin Force bite corrector. *J Clin Orthod*. 2004;38:232–240.
40. Chhibber A, Upadhyay M, Uribe F, Nanda R. Long-term stability of Class II correction with the Twin Force bite corrector. *J Clin Orthod*. 2010;44:363–376.
41. Guimaraes CH Jr, Henriques JF, Janson G, et al. Prospective study of dentoskeletal changes in Class II division malocclusion treatment with twin force bite corrector. *Angle Orthod*. 2013;83:319–326.
42. Davoody AR, Feldman J, Uribe FA, Nanda R. Mandibular molar protraction with the Twin Force bite corrector in a Class II patient. *J Clin Orthod*. 2011;45(4):223–228.
43. Upadhyay M, Nanda R. Principle of biomechanics. In: Nanda R, ed. *Biomechanics in Clinical Orthodontics*. Philadelphia, PA: WB Saunders; 1997:1–22.
44. Campbell E. A prospective clinical analysis of a push-type fixed intermaxillary Class II correction appliance [Masters thesis]. Farmington, CT: University of Connecticut; 2003.
45. Jakobsson S. Cephalometric evaluation of treatment effect on Class II, Division I malocclusions. *Am J Orthod*. 1967;53:446–456.
46. Baccetti T, Franchi L, Toth LR, McNamara JA. Treatment timing for Twin-block therapy. *Am J Orthod Dentofacial Orthop*. 2000;118: 159–170.
47. Faltin K Jr, Faltin RM, Baccetti T, Franchi L, Ghiozzi B, McNamara JA Jr. Long-term effectiveness and treatment timing for Bionator therapy. *Angle Orthod*. 2003;73:221–230.
48. Ruf S, Pancherz H. Dentoskeletal effects and facial profile changes in young adults treated with the Herbst appliance. *Angle Orthod*. 1999;69: 239–246.
49. Pancherz H, Hägg U. Dentofacial orthopedics in relation to somatic maturation: an analysis of 70 consecutive cases treated with the Herbst appliance. *Am J Orthod*. 1985;88:273–287.
50. Chhibber A, Upadhyay M, Uribe F, Nanda R. Mechanism of Class II correction in prepubertal and postpubertal patients with Twin Force bite corrector. *Angle Orthod*. 2013;83(4):718–727.
51. Bishara SE, Hoppens BJ, Jakobsen JR, Kohout FJ. Changes in the molar relationship between the deciduous and permanent dentitions: a longitudinal study. *Am J Orthod Dentofacial Orthop*. 1988;93:19–28.
52. Stucki N, Ingervall B. The use of the Jasper jumper for the correction of Class II malocclusion in the young permanent dentition. *Eur J Orthod*. 1998;20:271–281.
53. Jones G, Buschang PH, Kim KB, Oliver DR. Class II non-extraction patients treated with the Forsus fatigue resistant device versus intermaxillary elastics. *Angle Orthod*. 2008;78:332–338.
54. Proffit WR. Retention. In: Profitt WR, Fields HW Jr, Sarver DM, eds. *Contemporary Orthodontics*. 4th ed. St. Louis, MO: Elsevier; 2007: 617–634.
55. Pancherz H. The nature of Class II relapse after Herbst appliance treatment: a cephalometric long-term investigation. *Am J Orthod Dentofacial Orthop*. 1991;100:220–233.

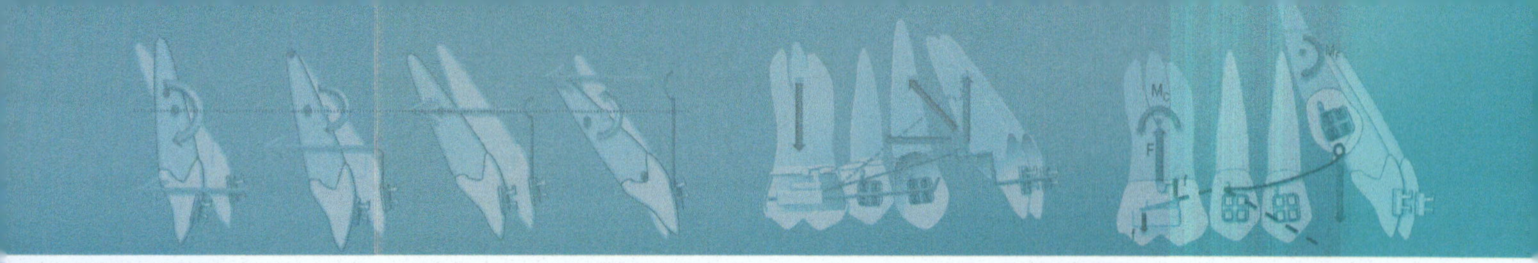

CHAPTER 14

Treatment Strategies for Developing and Nondeveloping Class III Malocclusions

Peter W. Ngan and Jae-Hyun Sung

Class III malocclusions can be broadly divided into two categories: developing and nondeveloping malocclusions. A number of authors have recommended early treatment of developing Class III malocclusions to obtain growth modification. The validity of two-phase treatment is supported by studies that show greater orthopedic effects when treatment is started in younger patients.[1,2] On the other hand, several investigators reported significant relapse for patients who resume the original growth pattern after treatment.[3] The question is whether a two-phase Class III treatment is worth the burden. If so, is early treatment suitable for all types of Class III malocclusions? In this chapter we classify developing Class III malocclusions into four categories and discuss strategies for selecting appliances to treat the various types of developing Class III malocclusions.

For Class III patients with no remaining growth, the nondeveloping malocclusions can be camouflaged by dentoalveolar tooth movement. Different approaches to camouflage a Class III malocclusion have been suggested, ranging from extraction of premolars to en masse distalization of the entire lower arch.[4] With the advent of micro-implants, it is possible to increase the range of orthodontic tooth movement without encountering the side effects associated with traditional treatment mechanics.[5,6] This chapter suggests possible treatment strategies for patients with no remaining growth who require tooth movement to camouflage skeletal discrepancies.

DIAGNOSIS AND CLASSIFICATION OF CLASS III MALOCCLUSIONS

The prevalence of Class III malocclusion varies among different ethnic groups. The prevalence in Caucasians ranges between 1% and 4% depending on the method of studying the malocclusion and the age group evaluated.[7-10] A high prevalence of Class III malocclusion has been observed in Asian populations such as Chinese (4% to 12%),[11-14] Japanese (2.3% to 13%),[15,16] and Koreans (9% to 19%).[17] A relatively high prevalence of Class III malocclusion was also reported in countries such as Saudi Arabia (9.4%)[18] and Sweden (6%).[19] This was in contrast to African Americans (0.6% to 1.2%).[20]

Individuals with Class III malocclusion and anterior crossbites may have combinations of skeletal and functional (dentoalveolar) components. Consideration of these components is essential so that the underlying cause of the discrepancy can be treated appropriately. To differentiate between skeletal and functional malocclusions, patients who present with Class III molar relationship and/or anterior crossbite should be checked for the presence of a functional shift (Fig. 14-1). First, clinicians should assess the relationship of the mandible to the maxilla to determine whether a centric relation–centric occlusion discrepancy exists. Anterior positioning of the mandible may result from abnormal tooth contact that forces the mandible forward. Patients who present with a forward shift of the mandible on closure may have a normal facial profile and Class I molar relationship in centric relation (CR) but a prognathic profile and Class III molar relationship in centric occlusion (CO), a situation referred to as "pseudo Class III malocclusion." Elimination of CO-CR shift should reveal whether it is a simple Class I malocclusion or a compensated Class III malocclusion with lingual tipping of the lower incisors. On the other hand, a patient presenting with no shift on closure, a full-step Class III molar relationship, and a mesial occlusion of the lower to upper canines most likely has a skeletal Class III malocclusion. Second, Class III patients should be evaluated in the vertical dimension for vertical hypodivergent or hyperdivergent growth pattern. This can be achieved by measuring the inclination of the occlusal plane (OP°) and the ratio of lower anterior facial height (LAFH) to total facial height (TFH). The average occlusal plane inclination is 7 degrees. Patients with OP° greater than 7 degrees are considered to have a

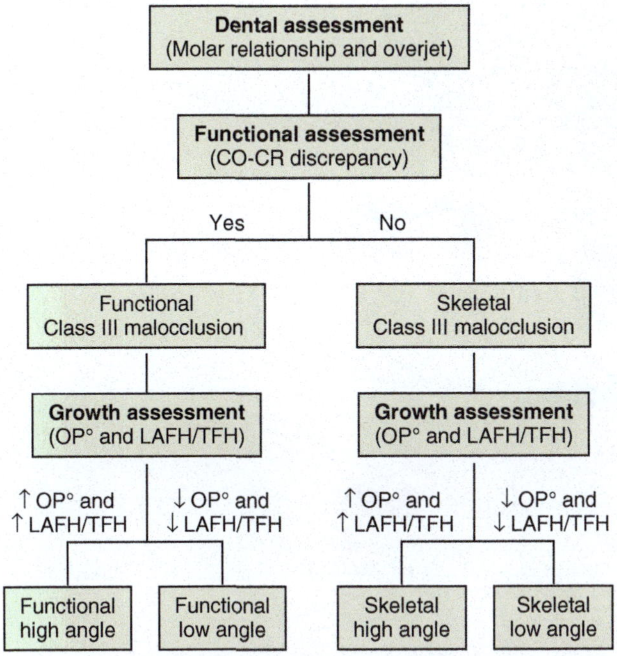

Figure 14-1 Classification of developing Class III malocclusion for early treatment. *CO*, Centric occlusion; *CR*, centric rotation; *LAFH*, lower anterior face height; *OP°*, occlusal plane inclination; *TFH*, total facial height.

hyperdivergent growth pattern or be high angle cases and those with OP° less than 7 degrees are considered to have a hypodivergent growth pattern or be low angle cases. Similarly, patients with a ratio of LAFH/TFH greater than 0.55 are high angle cases and those with a ratio less than 0.55 are low angle cases. Class III patients can then be classified into four types: functional low angle, skeletal low angle, functional high angle, and skeletal high angle. The classification of malocclusion will aid in the selection of appliances for early orthopedic treatment, as discussed in the following section (see Fig. 14-1).

TREATMENT OF DEVELOPING CLASS III MALOCCLUSION

Expansion and Partial Fixed Appliance

Correction of multiple teeth in anterior crossbite is best accomplished with a fixed appliance. An expansion appliance or maxillary lingual arch in conjunction with a partial fixed appliance can be used to correct anterior crossbite in young Class III patients.

Treatment Effects

Figure 14-2 shows an 8-year-old patient who presented with multiple teeth in anterior crossbite. A Hyrax maxillary expansion appliance was fabricated to create arch length for the alignment of the maxillary incisors. After expansion, a sequence of three archwires (0.012-inch nickel-titanium [Ni-Ti], 0.018-inch Ni-Ti, and 0.018-inch stainless steel) was used to align the maxillary incisors. A coil spring can be inserted between the maxillary lateral incisors and the first primary molars to help in the correction of crossbite. The correction is usually accomplished within 6 months and retainers are usually not necessary if overbite is adequate after crossbite correction (see Fig. 14-2).

Limitations

Several investigators reported forward movement of the maxilla with maxillary expansion. However, the effect was not consistent and was rarely more than 1.5-mm. A rapid palatal expansion (RPE) appliance in conjunction with a protraction facemask is recommended for patients diagnosed with functional hypodivergent or hyperdivergent types of Class III malocclusions.

Protraction Facemask Therapy

Treatment Effects

Meta-analysis showed that the treatment effects of using protraction facemask to correct anterior crossbite are a combination of skeletal and dental changes of the maxilla and mandible.[21] The maxilla moves downward and forward with a slight upward movement in the anterior and downward movement in the posterior palatal plane as the result of protraction force; at the same time posterior teeth extrude somewhat. As a consequence, downward and backward rotation of the mandible improves the maxillomandibular skeletal relationship in the sagittal dimension but results in an increase in lower anterior facial height. This rotation is a major contributing factor in establishing an anterior overjet improvement. A force exerted by the chin cup has been speculated to help in redirecting the mandibular downward and backward growth. Upper incisor labial inclination increased, although lower incisor inclination decreased. It is postulated that upper incisor proclination is due to mesial dental movement and lower incisor uprighting occurs as the result of pressure by the chin cup and soft tissue.

In the mixed dentition, a banded or bonded expansion appliance can be fabricated as anchorage for maxillary protraction. Patients with an increased lower face height can benefit from using a bonded expansion appliance, which provides a temporary biteplate effect. Additionally, a bonded maxillary appliance can be used in patients with a deep overbite and overclosure of the mandible to facilitate the jumping of the anterior crossbite. The expansion appliance is activated twice daily (0.25-mm per turn) by the patient or parent for 7 to 10 days. In patients with a more constricted maxilla, activation of the appliance is carried out for 2 weeks or longer.

Several facial sutures play an important role in the development of the nasomaxillary complex, including the frontomaxillary, nasomaxillary, zygomaticotemporal, zygomaticomaxillary, pterygopalatine, intermaxillary, ethmomaxillary, and lacrimomaxillary sutures.[22] Animal studies have shown that the maxillary complex can be displaced anteriorly with significant changes in the facial sutures.[23] However, maxillary protraction does not always result in forward movement of the maxilla. With the same line of force, different midfacial bones were displaced in different

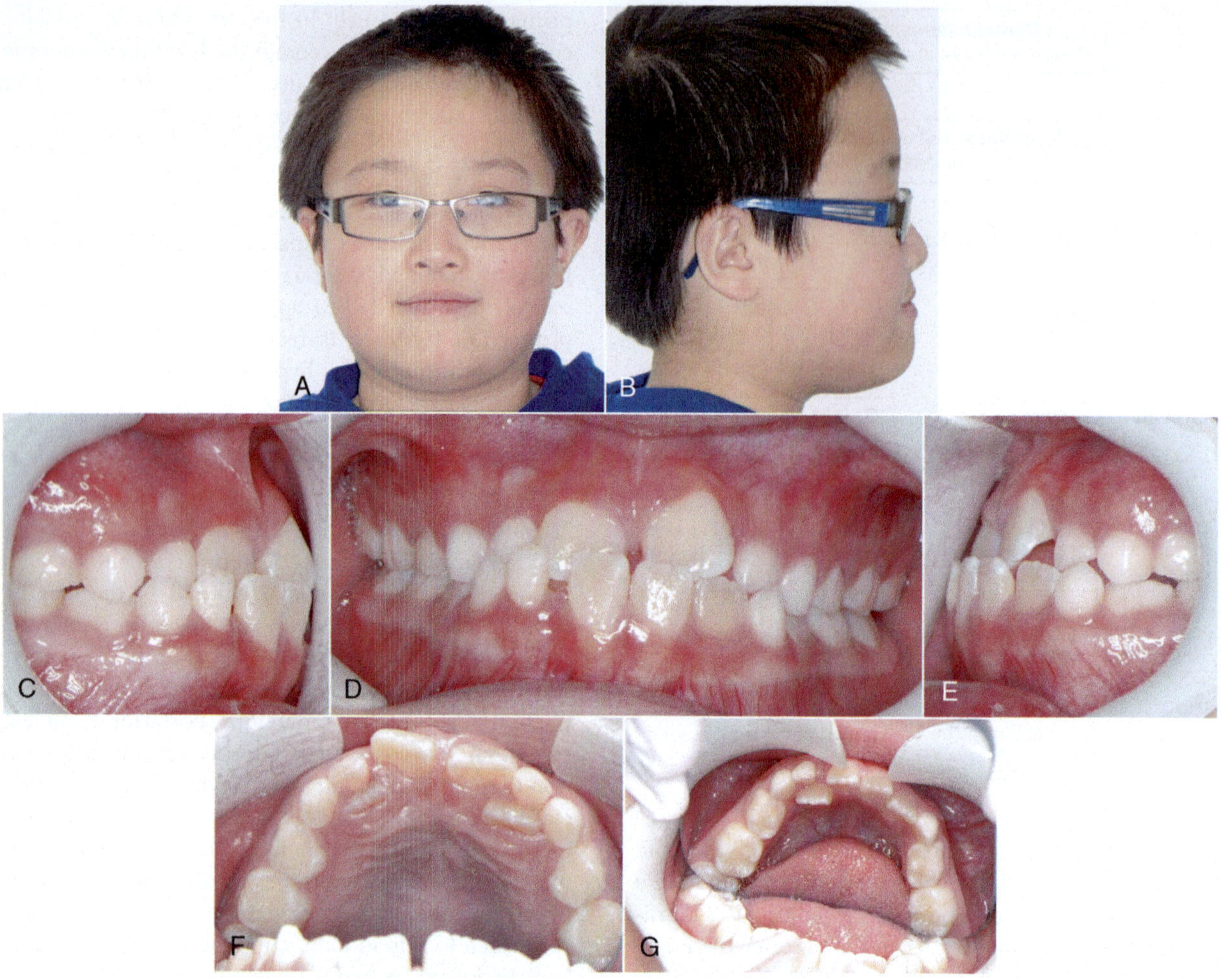

Figure 14-2 Pre-treatment **(A and B)** facial and **(C–G)** intraoral photographs of an 8-year-old patient who presented with multiple teeth in anterior crossbite.

directions depending on the moments of force generated at the sutures. The center of resistance (C_{RES}) of the maxilla was found to be located at the distal contacts of the maxillary first molars one-half the distances from the functional occlusal plane to the inferior border of the orbit. Protraction of the maxilla below the C_{RES} produces counterclockwise rotation of the maxilla, which may not be favorable for patients with open-bite tendency.[24] The facemask has an adjustable anterior wire that can accommodate a downward and forward pull on the maxilla with elastics. To minimize the tipping of the palatal plane, the protraction elastics are attached near the maxillary canines with a downward and forward pull of 30 degrees from the occlusal plane. Maxillary protraction usually requires 300 to 600 g of force per side, depending on the age of the patient. Patients are instructed to wear the appliance for 12 hours per day.

Sutural expansion and/or protraction induce new bone growth by mechanically stretching the sutures. Clinically, it has been shown that maxillary expansion can disarticulate the maxilla to allow a more favorable forward movement of the maxilla.[25–27] A well-disarticulated maxilla seems to be critical when using tooth-borne devices for orthopedic effects. A protocol of repetitive weekly alternate rapid maxillary expansion and constriction of the maxilla to disarticulate it without overexpanding has been proposed.[28] Usually it requires 7 to 9 weeks to loosen the maxilla. This protocol was modified to treat cleft lip and cleft palate patients using maxillary protraction in conjunction with Class III elastics.[29] The sutures were loosened by alternating weekly expansion and constriction for 8 weeks, a facemask was used at night to "pull" the maxilla forward, and Class III elastics were used during daytime to "hold" the result of the protraction.

Figure 14-3 shows an 8-year-old female patient who presented with a chief concern of "my bite is not right." Clinically, she presented with a concave facial profile, obtuse nasolabial angle, deficient (black) maxilla, and relatively normal mandible. Intraorally, she had an anterior crossbite and crowding in the upper arch. The upper left and right permanent canines were blocked out due to crowding. The maxillary incisors were proclined and the mandibular incisors were retroclined, compensating for the skeletal malocclusion. There was no family history of mandibular prognathism (see Fig. 14-3, A–D).

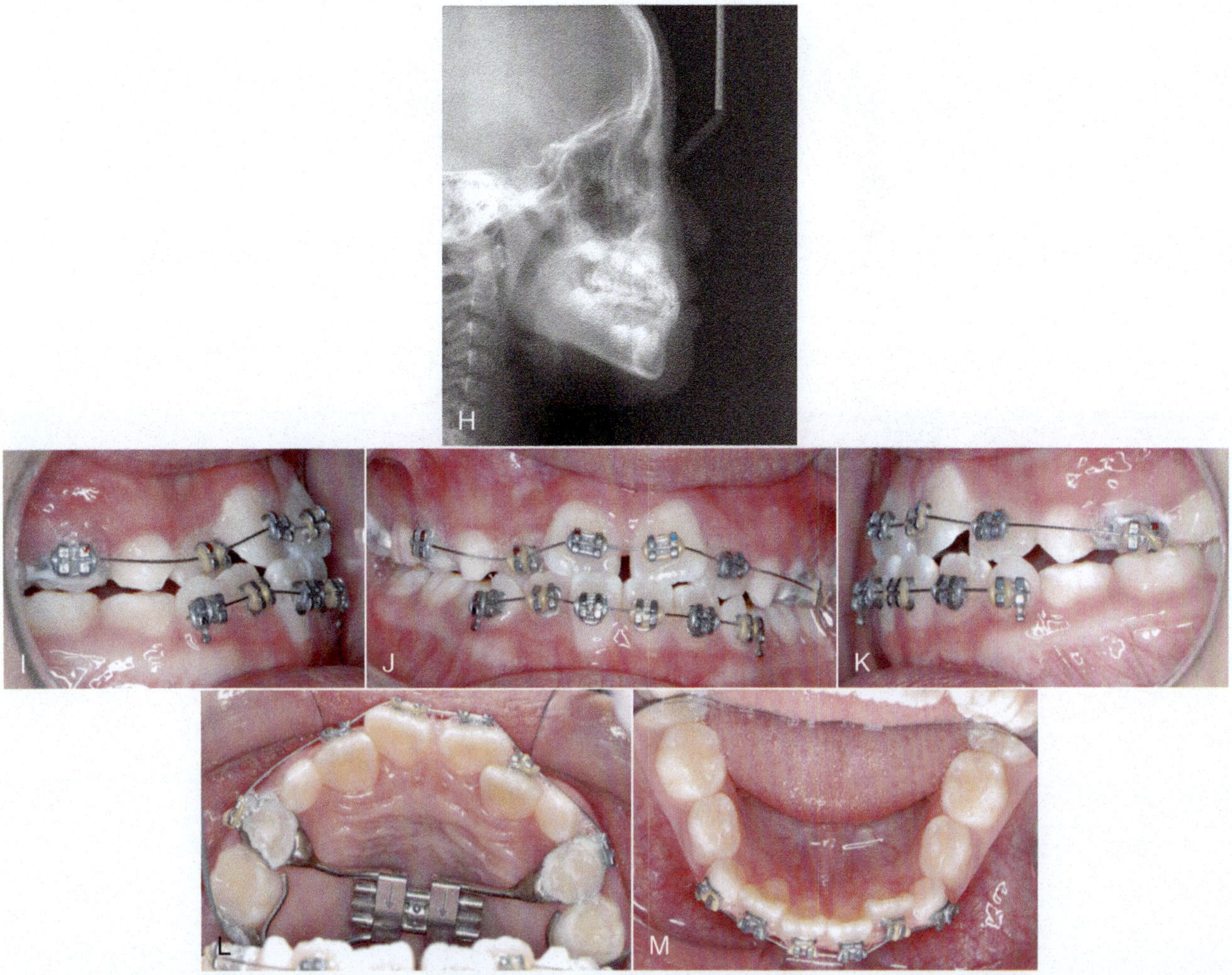

Figure 14-2, cont'd **H,** Cephalometric radiograph showing a mild skeletal growth pattern. **I–M,** A Hyrax maxillary expansion appliance was fabricated to create arch length for the alignment of the maxillary incisors. A sequence of three archwires (0.012-inch nickel-titanium [Ni-Ti], 0.018-inch Ni-Ti, and 0.018 inch stainless steel) was used to align the maxillary incisors.

Continued

Two treatment options were proposed. The first option was an early phase of orthopedic treatment to induce harmonious skeletal growth and improve facial esthetics followed by a second phase of fixed appliance to correct the remaining crowding, overjet, and overbite problems. It was thought that this option might eliminate the need for orthognathic surgery. The patient would be followed to determine the stability of the treatment. The second option was to wait until all growth was completed and determine whether the malocclusion could be camouflaged by orthodontic treatment or a combination of surgical and orthodontic treatment. The patient agreed to the first treatment option.

The Hyrax RPE appliance was constructed by using bands on the posterior teeth. Bands were fitted on the upper deciduous second molars and on the upper permanent first molars. The bands were soldered to heavy wires (0.045-inch) that were connected to a jackscrew that centered along the midline of the maxillary palate. Bilaterally, a 0.045-inch wire was soldered to the buccal aspects of the molar bands and extended anteriorly to the canine area. This buccal wire had a curve at the canine area so that elastics could be used to connect the appliance to a protraction facemask. The alternate rapid maxillary expansion and constriction protocol was used to loosen the sutures that connect the maxilla to the surrounding bones via rapid expansion and contraction on an alternating weekly basis for 7 weeks.[28] The maxilla was expanded or contracted 1-mm per day (two turns in the morning and two turns in the evening). The amount of expansion was checked after the first, second, and fifth week. The mobility of the maxilla was checked before proceeding to maxillary protraction. The maxilla could be clinically examined for mobility by holding the patient's head with one hand and rocking the anterior segment of the maxilla up and down with the other hand.

The Petit protraction facemask (Ormco Corporation, Glendora, CA.) is a one-piece construction with adjustable forehead padding, an adjustable chin cup, and an adjustable anterior bar. The adjustable components of the protraction facemask and appropriate positioning of the anterior bar (to which elastics were attached to both right and left sides) allowed for proper positioning of the chin cup for comfort on both opening and closing of the mandible. To avoid an

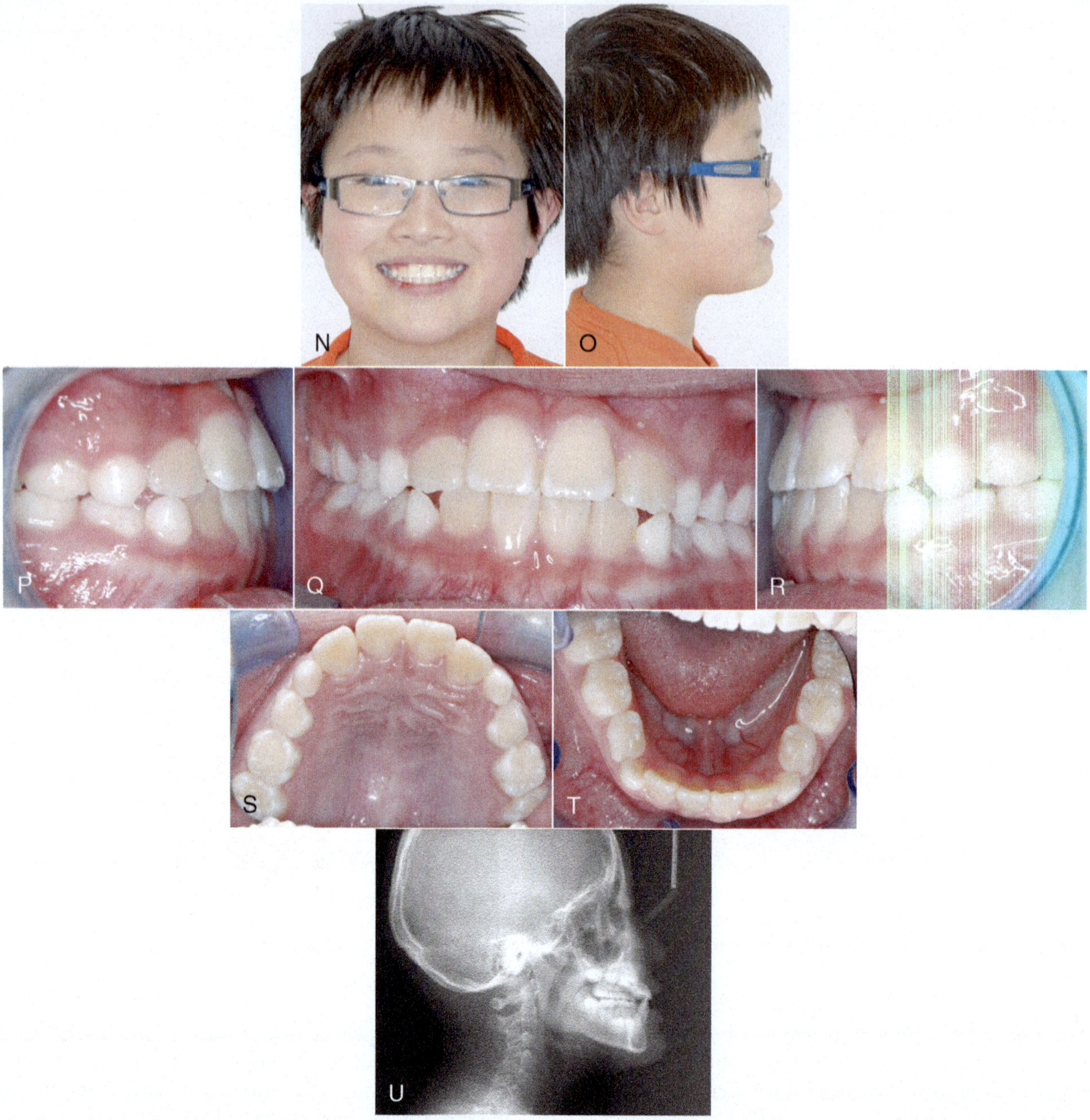

Figure 14-2, cont'd Post-treatment (**N and O**) facial and (**P–T**) intraoral photographs show the correction of anterior crossbite. **U**, Post-treatment cephalometric radiograph shows the crossbite was corrected by proclination of the maxillary incisors and retroclination of the mandibular incisors.

opening of the bite as the maxilla is protracted, the elastics were attached near the maxillary canines with a downward and forward pull of 30 degrees to the occlusal plane. A Correx gauge (Haag-Streit, Bern, Switzerland) was used to measure the elastic force between the expansion appliance and the facemask to ensure that approximately 450 g of force was generated on each side. The patient was instructed to wear the protraction facemask for 10 to 12 hours of nighttime wear. On the mandibular arch, bands were fitted on the mandibular first molars and brackets were placed on the mandibular four incisors. A 0.019-inch × 0.025-inch posted archwire with a stop loop in front of the mandibular first molar was placed so that the patient could wear Class III elastics during the day for 8 hours. Figure 14-3 shows the correction of the anterior crossbite after 4 months of maxillary protraction with the facemask at night and Class III elastics during the day. Superimposition of the pre-treatment and post-treatment radiographs shows a 4.5-mm forward movement of the A point. The patient was placed on retention with a Frankel III regulator for 1 year (see Fig. 14-3, E–M).

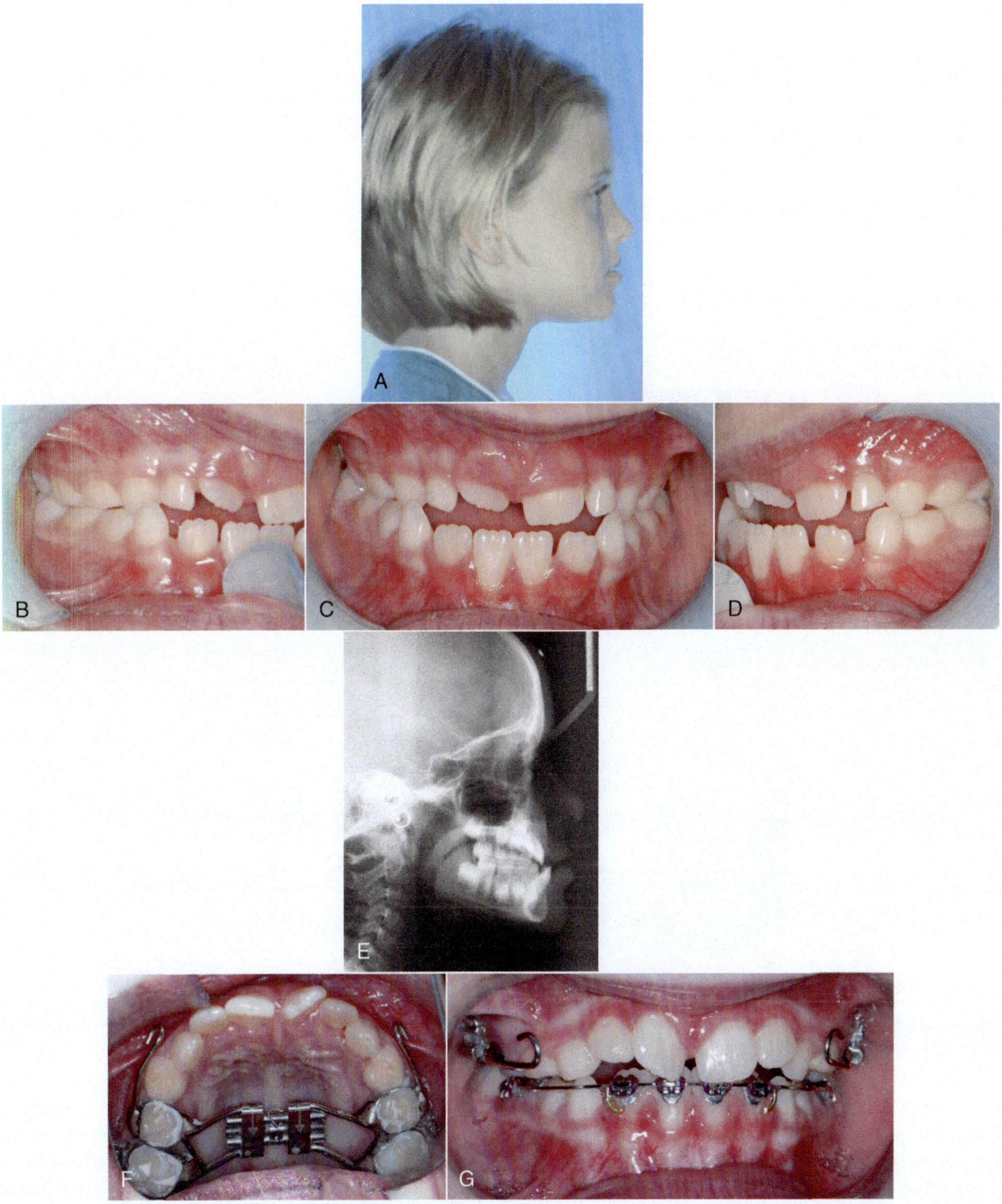

Figure 14-3 Pre-treatment **(A)** profile and **(B–D)** intraoral photographs of an 8-year-old patient who presented with a Class III malocclusion and a concave facial profile. **E,** Cephalometric radiograph shows a deficient maxilla and normal mandible. **F and G,** Patient was treated with the expansion and constriction protocol to loosen the facial sutures. This was followed by facemask treatment.

Continued

Treatment Timing

A question of clinical importance in maxillary protraction is when to start the facemask treatment. The main objective of early facemask treatment is to enhance forward displacement of the maxilla by sutural growth. Histological studies have shown that the midpalatal suture is broad and smooth during the "infantile" stage (8 to 10 years of age) and becomes more squamous and overlapping in the "juvenile" stage (10 to 13 years).[30] Biologically, the circumaxillary sutures are smooth and broad before age 8 years and become more heavily interdigitated around puberty. These findings are related to observations in clinical studies that have shown that maxillary protraction is effective in the primary mixed as well as early permanent dentitions. Several studies

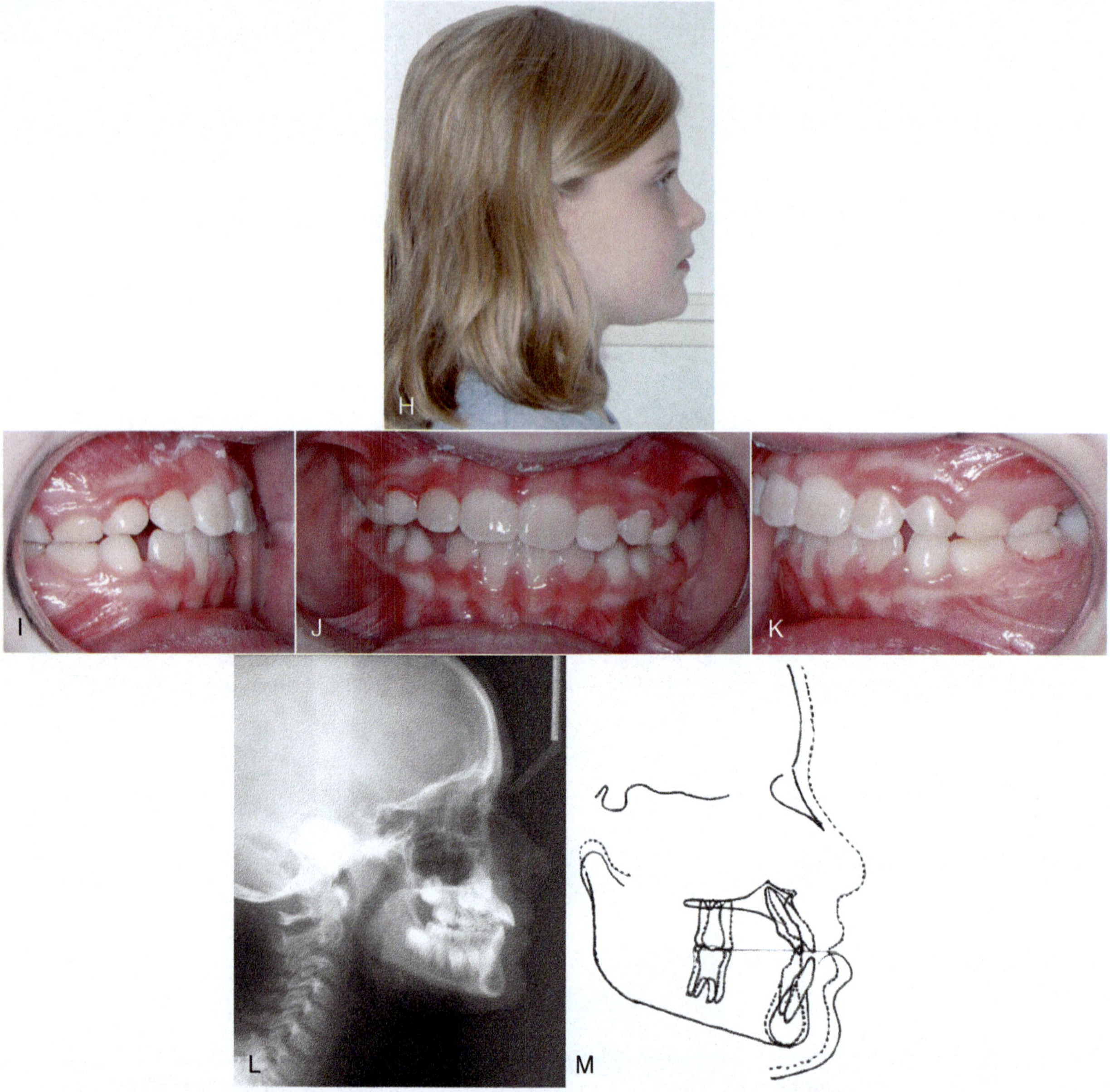

Figure 14-3, cont'd Post-treatment (**H**) profile and (**I–K**) intraoral photographs show the improvement in overbite and overjet. **L,** Post-treatment cephalometric radiograph shows the improvement in skeletal relationship. **M,** Superimposition of pre-treatment and post-treatment radiographs shows forward movement of the maxilla and downward and backward rotation of the mandible, after facemask treatment.

have suggested that a greater degree of anterior maxillary displacement can be found when treatment is initiated in the primary or early mixed dentition. The optimal time to intervene in a Class III malocclusion is at the time of the initial eruption of the maxillary incisors. A positive overjet and overbite at the end of the facemask treatment appears to maintain the anterior occlusion.

An additional question worth addressing is whether the results of early protraction treatment can be sustained when subsequent mandibular growth occurs during the pubertal growth spurt. In a prospective clinical trial, protraction facemask treatment starting in the mixed dentition was found to be stable 2 years after the removal of the appliances.[31] This probably resulted from overcorrection and the use of a functional appliance as retainer for 1 year. When these patients were followed for another 2 years, 15 of 20 patients maintained a positive overjet. In patients who relapsed to a negative overjet, the mandible outgrew the maxilla in the horizontal direction. When these patients were followed for another 4 years (8 years after treatment until about 17.5 years of age), 14 of 20 patients (67%) maintained a positive overjet. For the patients who relapsed into a reverse overjet, the mandible outgrew the maxilla by four times, compared with twice that in the stable group. These results suggest that in a random clinical trial when patients are followed until after completion of pubertal growth, two out of three patients (67%) will have a favorable outcome. About one-third of the patients might be candidates for orthognathic surgery later in life because of unfavorable growth pattern. Patients treated by protraction facemask either in the early mixed dentition or in the late mixed dentition and permanent dentition and followed up after a second phase of fixed appliance therapy demonstrated ongoing improvements in the former group but not in the latter group at the end of phase II treatment.[32] Specifically, a 1.8-mm additional forward movement of the maxilla was noted in the early treatment group as compared to the control group. In the late mixed dentition group, no significant difference in forward movement of maxilla was found after puberty as compared to the control subjects.

Utility and Limitations

Clinically, anterior crossbite can be corrected with 3 to 4 months of maxillary expansion and protraction depending on the severity of the malocclusion. Improvement in overbite and molar relationship can be expected with an additional 4 to 6 months of treatment. In a prospective clinical trial, overjet correction was found to be the result of forward maxillary movement (31%), backward movement of the mandible (21%), labial movement of the maxillary incisors (28%), and lingual movement of the mandibular incisors (20%).[31] Overcorrection of the overjet and molar relationship was highly recommended to anticipate unfavorable mandibular growth. Overbite was improved by eruption of the posterior teeth. The total facial height was increased by inferior movement of the maxilla and downward and backward rotation of the mandible. According to several clinical studies, the mean forward movement of the maxilla with 6 to 8 months of maxillary protraction is about 1- to 3-mm.[21] A meta-analysis on the effectiveness of protraction facemask treatment found that the average change in Wits appraisal was 4- to 6-mm and the average horizontal A point movement was 1- to 3-mm. The average forward movement of the A point with 8 to 12 months of maxillary protraction was 2- to 4-mm. The increase in A point nasion B point (ANB) angle ranged from 0.9 to 4.4 degrees, with a mean value of 2.8 degrees. This is well over the expected growth changes for 1 year. Variability exists among individual subjects.

Chin Cap Appliance Therapy

Treatment Effects

The objective of early treatment with the use of a chin cap is to provide growth inhibition or to redirect mandibular growth. The short-term and long-term effects of chin cap have been reported extensively in the literature.[33-37] The orthopedic effects of a chin cap on the mandible include downward and backward rotation of the mandible, closure of the gonial angle, shortening of the mandibular length, bending of the condylar neck, remodeling of the glenoid fossa, and opening of the cranial base angle. To date, there is no agreement in the literature as to whether chin cap may or may not inhibit the growth of the mandible long-term. However, Deguchi et al.[36,37] reported that the long-term use of chin cap was effective in subjects with severe skeletal Class III abnormality.

To better understand the orthopedic effects of a chin cap, the treatment results of two sisters were compared (Fig. 14-4). The older sister, SH, received orthopedic treatment with an activator and a chin cap while the younger sister, SJ,

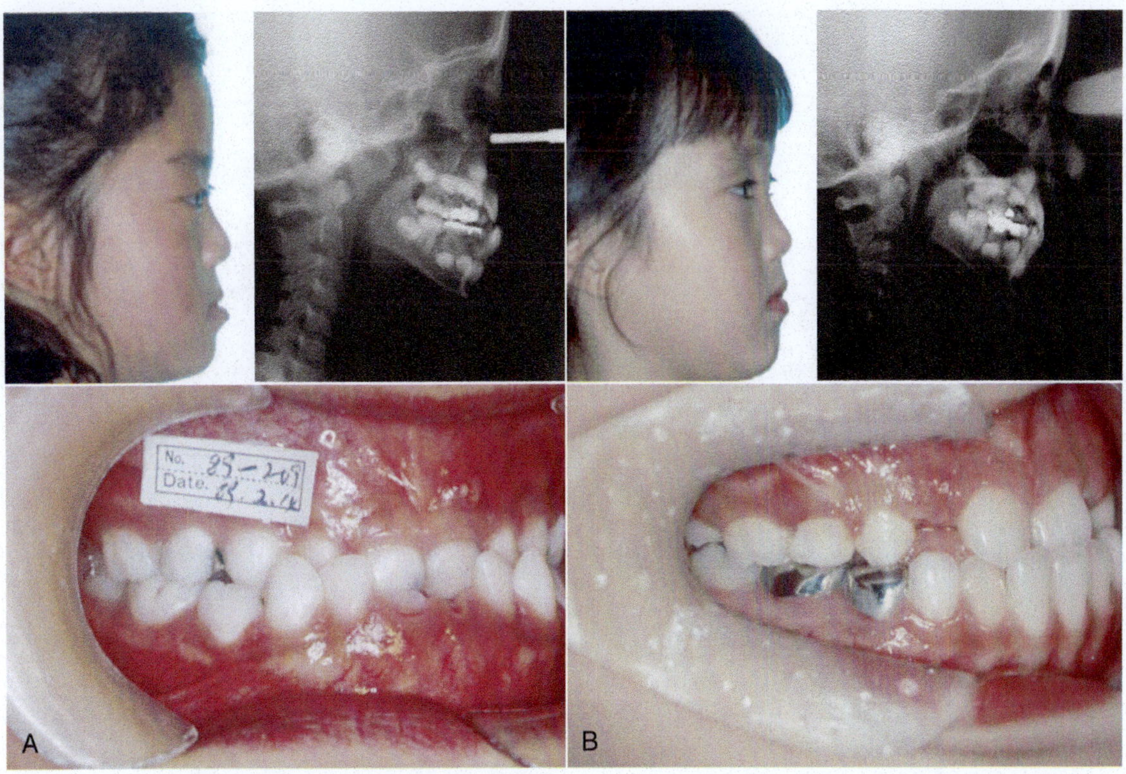

Figure 14-4 Initial facial and intraoral photographs and cephalograms of two sisters. **A,** The older sister, SH, showed a more protruded lower lip and a more severe crossbite and deep bite. She began treatment at age 6 years, 11 months. **B,** The younger sister, SJ, showed a large lower facial height, a slight crossbite, and a shallow overbite. She began treatment at age 12.

did not receive any orthopedic treatment during the growing period. SH presented at the age of 6 years, 11 months with a significant reverse overjet while SJ presented at the age of 7 years, 9 months with a mild anterior crossbite. There was no difference in the cranial base length and angle for both sisters but SH had a larger maxilla and mandible and a more prognathic chin profile than SJ (Fig. 14-5).

SH received phase I orthopedic treatment together with partial fixed appliance to align her incisors. SJ was placed on observation until permanent dentition without any orthopedic treatment due to a shallow overbite and a long lower facial height. SJ received comprehensive orthodontic treatment at 12 years of age with extraction of the lower first premolars. Figure 14-6 shows the profile and dentition of the

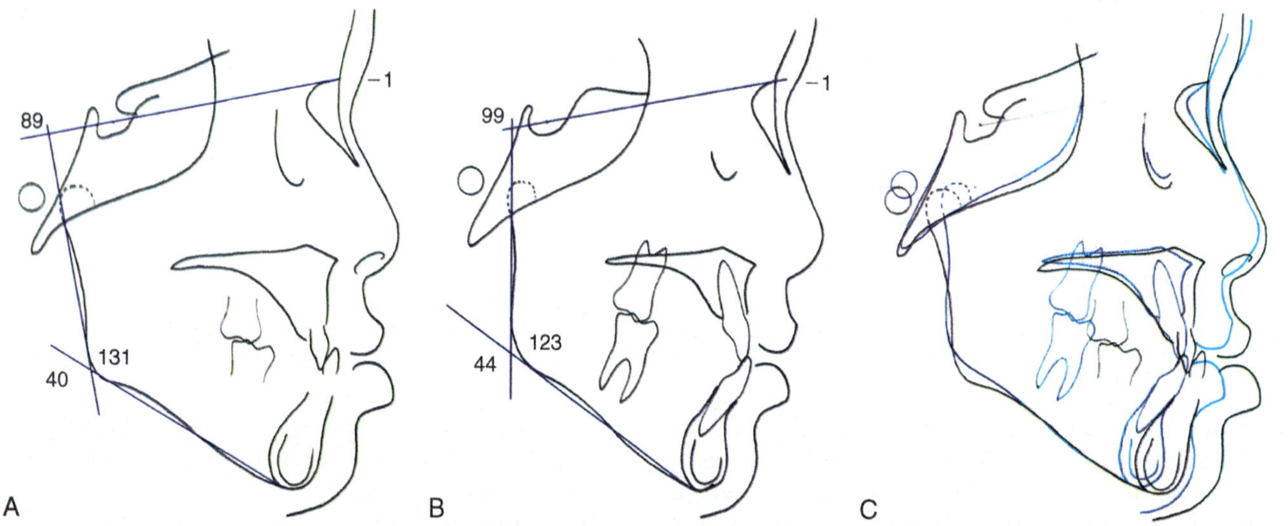

Figure 14-5 Initial cephalometric tracings and superimposition of the sisters. **A,** The older sister, SH, at the age of 6 years, 11 months: ANB angle −1, gonial angle 131, sella-nasion (SN) to mandibular plane angle 40, and SN to ramal angle 89. **B,** The younger sister, SJ, at the age of 7 years, 9 months: ANB angle −1, gonial angle 123, SN to mandibular plane angle 44, and SN to ramal angle 99. **C,** Pre-treatment cephalometric superimposition of the sisters. The black line is the older sister and the blue line is the younger sister. There is no difference in cranial base size and shape but the older sister shows a larger maxilla and mandible and a more prognathic chin than her younger sister.

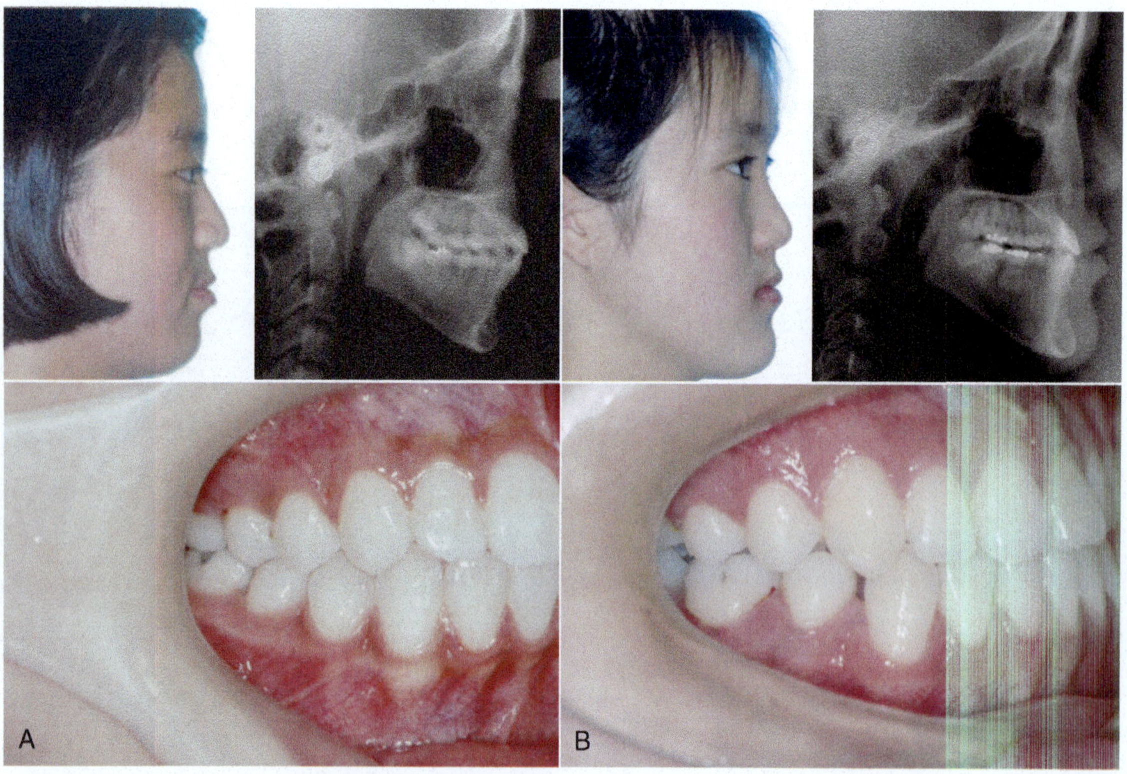

Figure 14-6 Post-treatment facial and intraoral photographs and cephalograms of two sisters. **A,** The older sister, SH, shows a slight protrusion of the lip and a Class I molar relation. **B,** The younger sister, SJ, shows a straight profile, a slightly prominent chin, and a full Class III molar relation (due to lower first premolar extraction).

two sisters after treatment. SH showed a little lower lip protrusion whereas SJ showed a straight profile after extraction therapy.

The superimpositions of the pre-treatment and post-treatment lateral cephalograms showed quite distinct differences between the growth patterns of the two sisters in terms of the cranial base angle, mandibular position, and mandibular length and shape (Fig. 14-7). SH showed a downward and backward rotation of the mandible with the chin cap treatment while SJ showed a downward and forward growth of the mandible following the normal growth pattern. In addition, the posterior cranial base bending observed in SH could be explained by the application of chin cap force.

The orthopedic effects in SH can be seen more clearly by cephalometric superimpositions of the sisters at pre-treatment and post-treatment (Fig. 14-8). There was no difference in the position of the maxilla and upper face as well as the position of the anterior cranial base at pre-treatment. However, there were distinct changes in the position of the mandible and posterior cranial base at post-treatment. The results illustrate the typical effect of chin cap therapy.

Limitations

The limitations of chin cap therapy in growing children with Class III malocclusion include long treatment time. Chin cap therapy is recommended to start early in childhood and

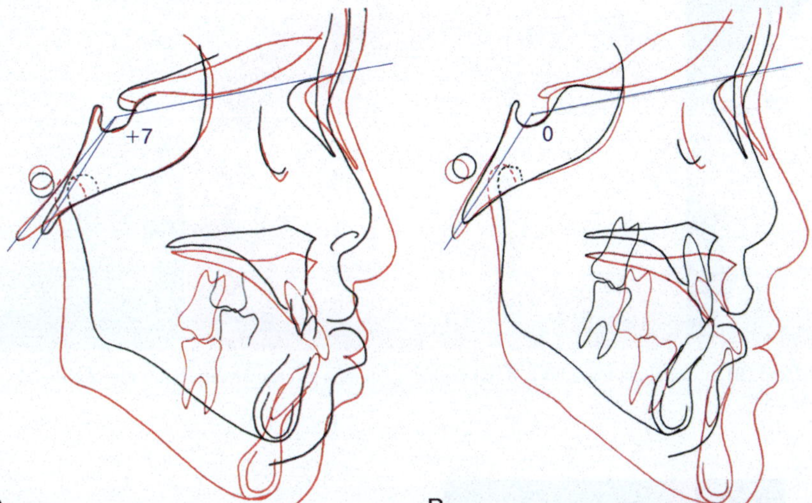

A B

Figure 14-7 Cephalometric superimpositions of two sisters at pre-treatment and post-treatment. The superimpositions show distinct differences in mandibular position after treatment. The black line is pre-treatment and the red line is post-treatment. **A,** The older sister, SH, who had chin cap treatment, shows a downward and backward rotation of the mandible. **B,** The younger sister, SJ, who had no orthopedic treatment, shows a downward forward growth, following normal mandibular growth. In addition, posterior cranial base bending was observed in SH while no change was observed in SJ.

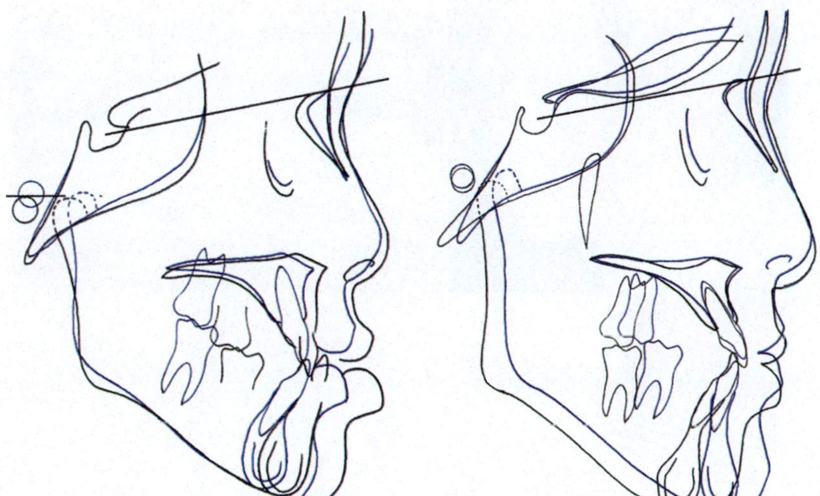

A B

Figure 14-8 Cephalometric superimpositions of two sisters at pre-treatment and post-treatment. The black line is the older sister, SH, and the blue line is the younger sister, SJ. **A,** Cephalometric superimposition at pre-treatment. **B,** Cephalometric superimposition at post-treatment. In the pre-treatment superimposition, SH *(black line)* shows a protruded mandible and chin compared to SJ *(blue line)*. However, in the post-treatment superimposition the mandible and chin of SH are behind those of SJ.

continue until growth completion. However, it is almost impossible to obtain such cooperation from patients. Another limitation is that chin cap therapy shows various responses depending on the facial pattern of patients. Therefore it is important to select cases that will show good response to the chin cap.

Figure 14-9 shows a female patient age 5 years, 5 months who presented with an anterior crossbite in the primary dentition. Cephalometric analysis showed an increase in the vertical dimension and an obtuse gonial angle. The patient was treated with a chin cap and an activator at that time. Retrospectively, early orthopedic treatment in Class III patients with hyperdivergent growth pattern is not recommended. Another unfavorable decision that was made at that time was the removal of the four first premolars to obtain proper occlusion. Therefore proper occlusal interdigitation was never achieved due to the continuous growth of the mandible. The growth discrepancy was explained to the parents and the patient accepted orthognathic surgery as the definitive treatment (Fig. 14-10).

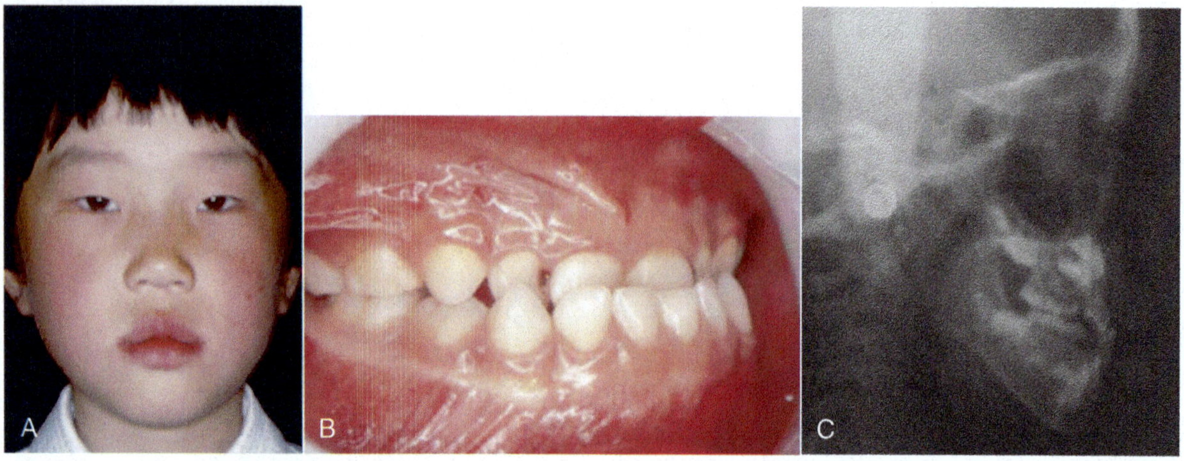

Figure 14-9 Initial **(A)** facial and **(B)** intraoral photographs and **(C)** cephalogram of a girl age 5 years, 5 months. ANB −0.5, gonial angle 142, and Frankfurt Mandibular Plane Angle (FMA) 39.

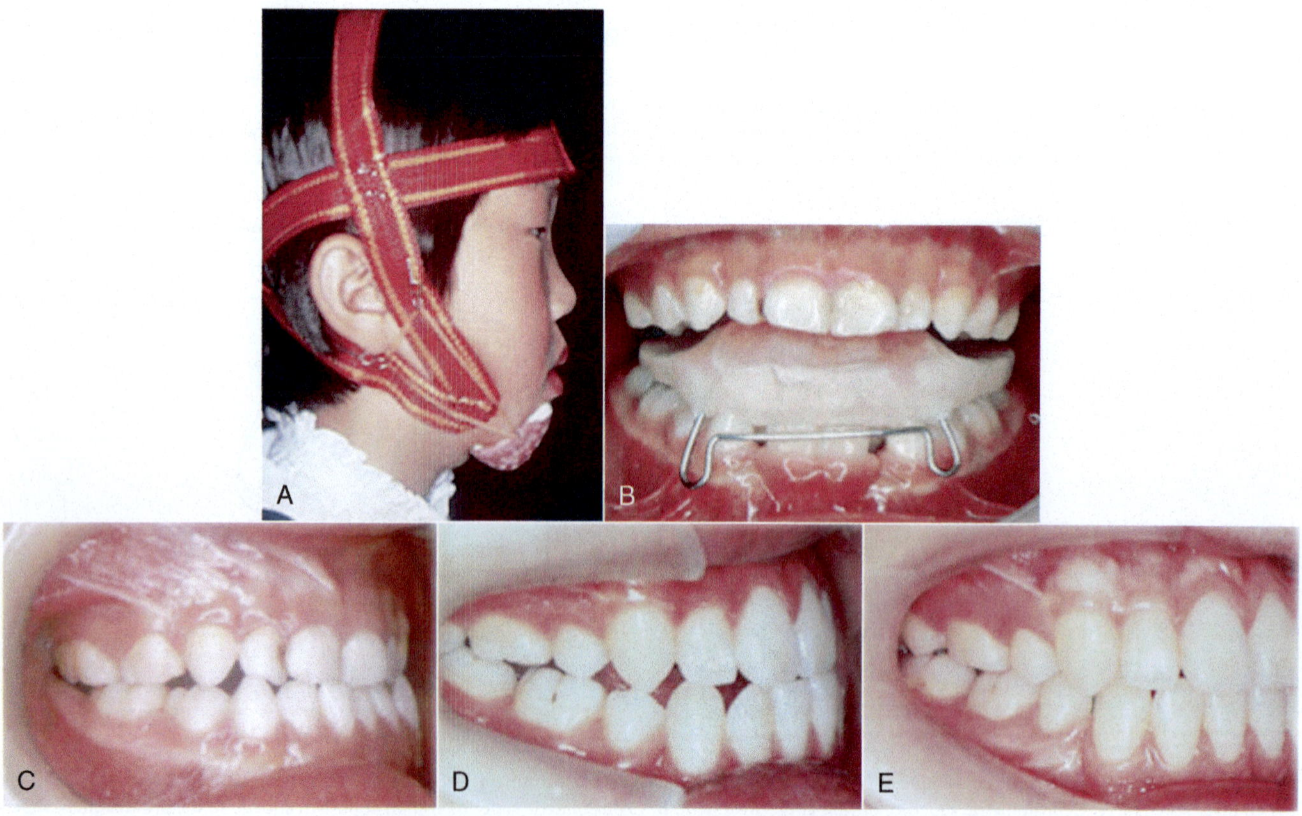

Figure 14-10 **A–C,** At age 5 years, phase I treatment was performed with activator and chin cap treatment. **D,** At age 15 years, after phase II treatment with four first premolar extractions. **E,** At age 19 years, orthognathic surgery was performed because of late mandibular growth.

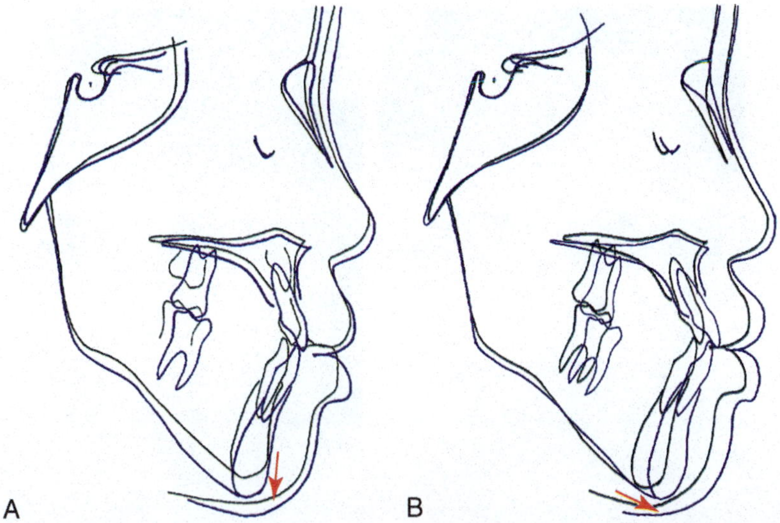

Figure 14-11 Cephalometric superimpositions of treatment progress. **A,** Mandibular changes during chin cap therapy. The black line is before chin cap therapy at age 6 years, 5 months and the blue line is after chin cap therapy at age 8 years, 1 month. **B,** Mandibular changes after stopping chin cap therapy. The black line is just after chin cap therapy at age 8 years, 1 month and the blue line is after growth without chin cap therapy at age 10 years, 1 month. Note the changes in mandibular growth direction between parts A and B.

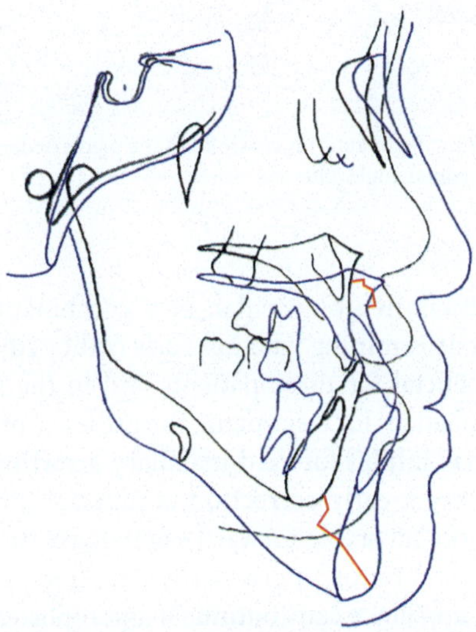

Figure 14-12 Cephalometric changes until the completion of growth. The black line is the initial stage at age 5 years and the blue line is after completion of growth at age 19 years. Note the great growth changes in the vertical dimension of the mandible. The red line indicates the changes of the A point and the gnathion during the observed period.

Two lessons can be learned from the treatment of this patient. One is that the length of treatment is too long. Despite the long orthodontic treatment, surgery is still inevitable. The other lesson is that chin cap therapy tends to increase the lower facial height. The mandible actually grew forward after the termination of chin cap therapy (Fig. 14-11). Therefore chin cap treatment is not recommended for patients with hyperdivergent growth pattern. The changes from initial to post-treatment show tremendous growth of the mandible and large vertical growth of the mandible (Fig. 14-12). These results show that individual growth of the mandible cannot be predicted.

Removable Functional Appliance Therapy

Treatment Effects of Frankel III Regulator

The Frankel III regulator (FRIII) has been used to treat young Class III patients with mild maxillary skeletal deficiency. This appliance is usually used during early mixed dentition when the maxillary incisors are erupting. The treatment effects of FRIII include a more forward movement of maxillary skeletal and dental landmarks as well as a backward rotation or repositioning of the mandible combined with an increase in lower anterior facial height.[38–41] Occlusal changes have also been noted, including proclination of maxillary incisors and lingual tipping of lower incisors. The FRIII looks quite bulky to insert in a child's mouth. However, clinical experience shows that it is a very acceptable and comfortable appliance for treatment in young patients. Most children have no resistance to wearing the FRIII for a long time. As well, the FRIII could be a good retention appliance after facemask therapy. Figures 14-13 to 14-16 illustrate a typical Class III malocclusion treated with the FRIII.

Limitations of Frankel III Regulator

The limitations of the FRIII are similar to those of chin cap therapy. The appliance requires a long treatment time as well as excellent patient cooperation.

STRATEGIES FOR APPLIANCE SELECTION

Functional low angle patients can be treated with any type of functional or orthopedic appliances depending on the patient's condition. Functional high angle patients will require appliances that can maintain the vertical dimension such as an active plate with posterior bite block, a two-piece corrector,[42,43] or a 2 × 4 torquing arch[44] (Table 14-1).

Skeletal low angle patients with mandibular prognathism can be treated using chin cap therapy and maxillary

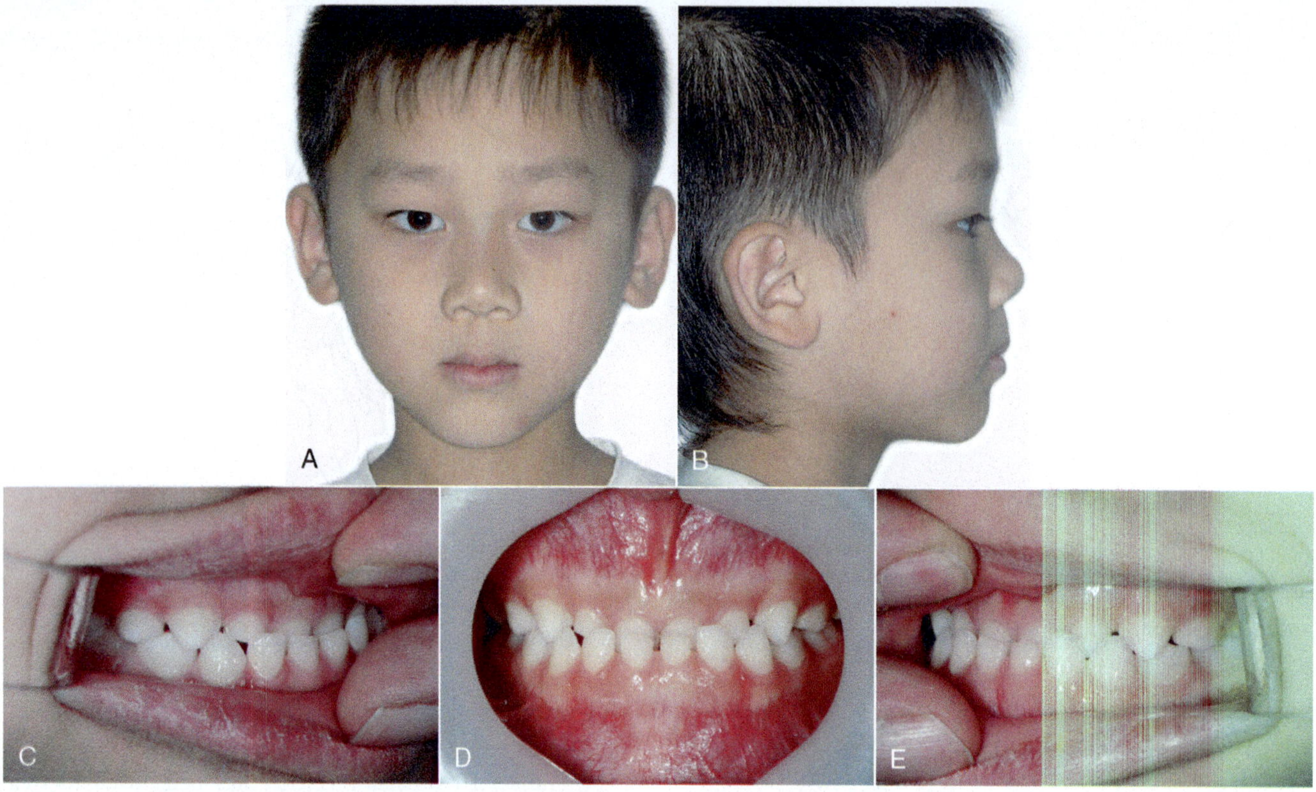

Figure 14-13 Initial (**A and B**) facial and (**C–E**) intraoral photographs of patient who presented with an anterior crossbite in the primary dentition. He was age 5 years, 4 months at first visit. ANB 0.4, Frankfurt Mandibular Plane Angle (FMA) 30, and gonial angle 130.

TABLE 14-1 Guidelines for Appliance Selection, According to Types of Growing Class III Malocclusion

Functional		Skeletal	
Low Angle Case	High Angle Case	Low Angle Case	High Angle Case
– Inclined plane – Class III activator – FRIII – Second appliance – Chin cap or facemask	– Active plate with posterior bite block – Sagittal III – Two-piece corrector – 2 × 4 torquing arch	– Chin cap – Maxillary protraction appliance (facemask)	– Observation until growth completion

protraction appliances can be used for patients with deficient maxilla. Skeletal high angle cases will not benefit from early orthopedic treatment. These patients should be kept under observation without any treatment until their growth is completed.

Figure 14-17 summarizes the treatment strategies for the developing Class III malocclusions. Developing Class III patients should be classified into categories such as functional, skeletal, or a combination of both. Understanding the causative factors such as maxillary skeletal, mandibular skeletal, dental, neuromuscular, or a combination of these will help in determining whether early orthopedic treatment will be beneficial for these patients and in the selection of suitable appliances for treatment. The presence of an anterior crossbite may inhibit forward maxillary growth and reports have shown that early correction of anterior crossbite may induce a more favorable forward sagittal growth.

After correction of anterior crossbite, treatment with an orthopedic appliance can continue if anteroposterior skeletal problems persist. However, orthopedic appliances should not be used for more than 2 to 3 years. It is better to wait until diminution of growth at around 14 years of age for girls and 17 years of age for boys than to start the treatment immediately after phase I treatment. At that time, a final decision can be made on whether to treat the patient orthodontically or by surgical treatment. Considering the difficulty of predicting late mandibular growth, it is better to delay the start of phase II treatments until cessation of growth.

TREATMENT OF NONGROWING CLASS III MALOCCLUSIONS

Nongrowing patients with mild to moderate skeletal Class III malocclusions can be camouflaged with orthodontic tooth movement. The treatment strategies include (1) conventional edgewise appliance with or without extraction, (2) multiloop edgewise archwire (MEAW) with Class III and

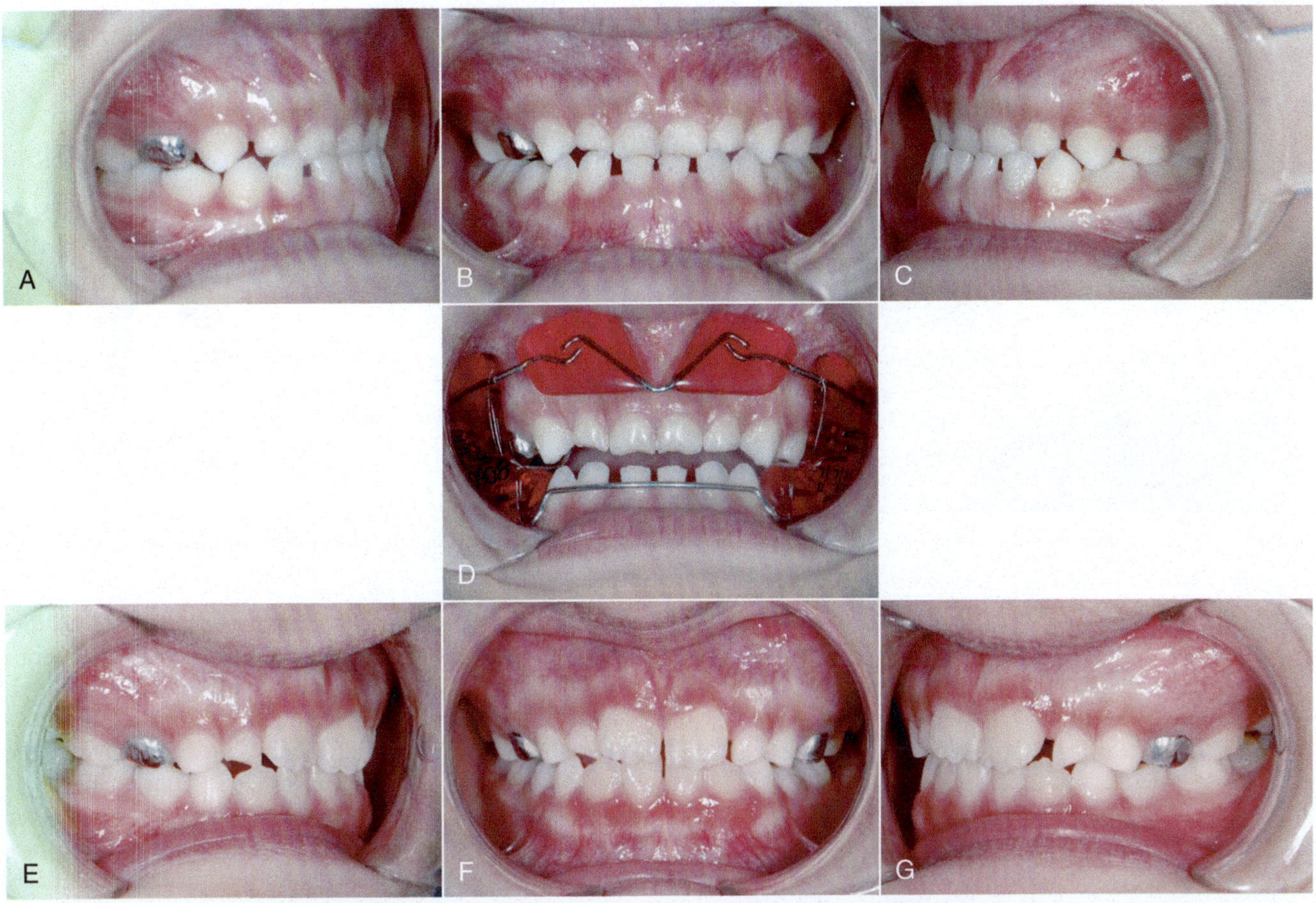

Figure 14-14 Photographs of treatment progress. **A–C,** After 6 months of using Class III activator, **(D)** the Frankel III regulator (FRIII) was delivered. **E–G,** Results after 17 months of FRIII.

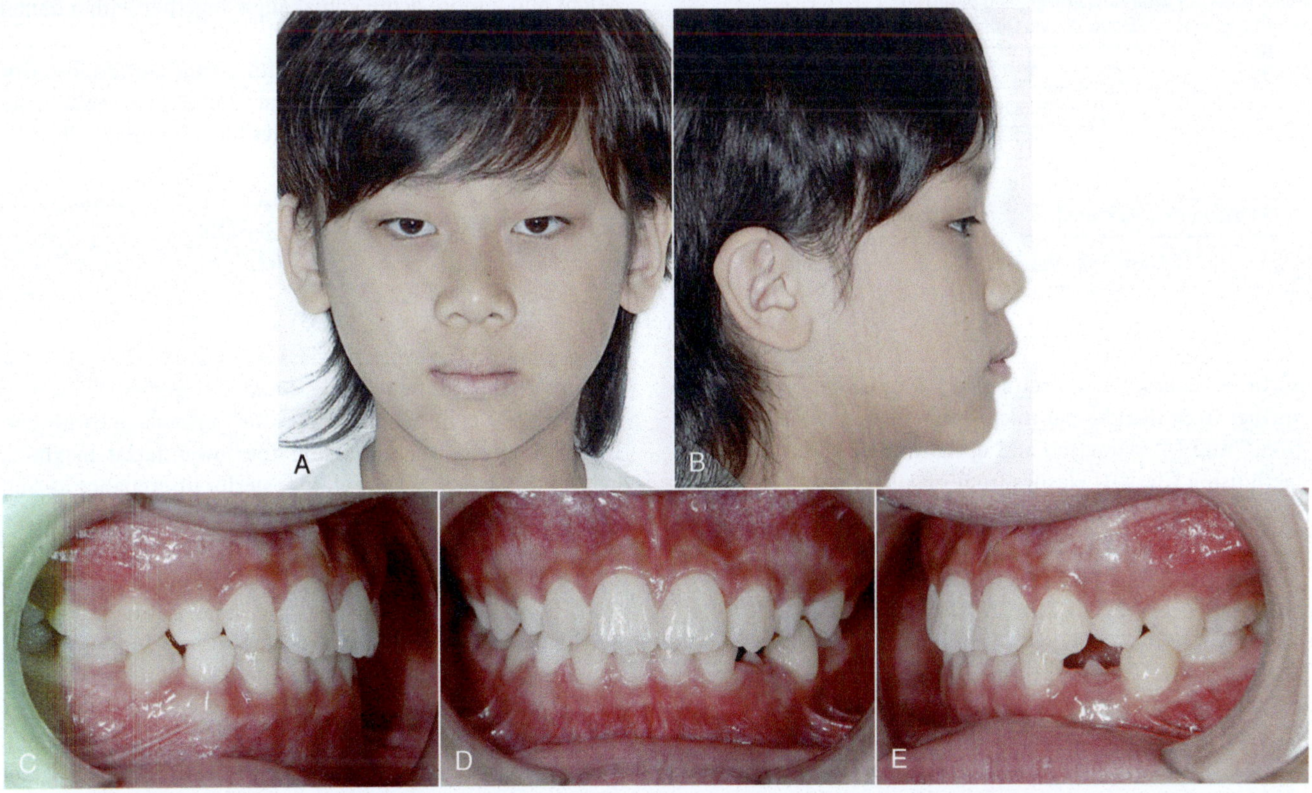

Figure 14-15 **A and B,** Facial and **(C–E)** intraoral photographs at age 9 years, 8 months. The Frankel III regulator (FRIII) was stopped and the patient was observed until growth completion.

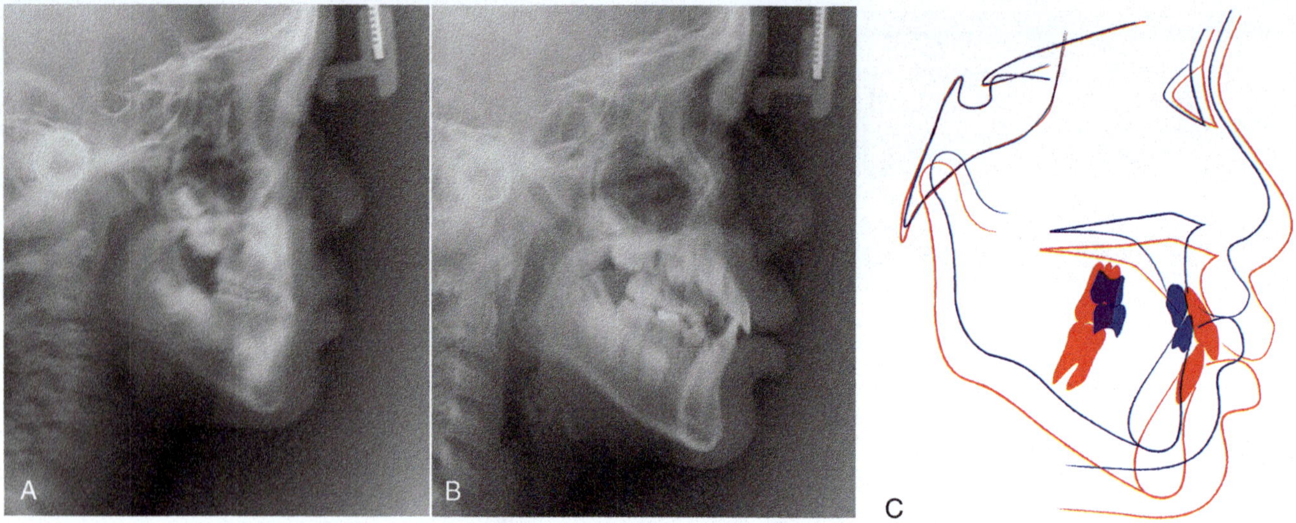

Figure 14-16 **A,** Initial cephalogram at age 5 years, 4 months and **(B)** cephalogram at age 9 years, 8 months. **C,** Superimposition of the two cephalograms.

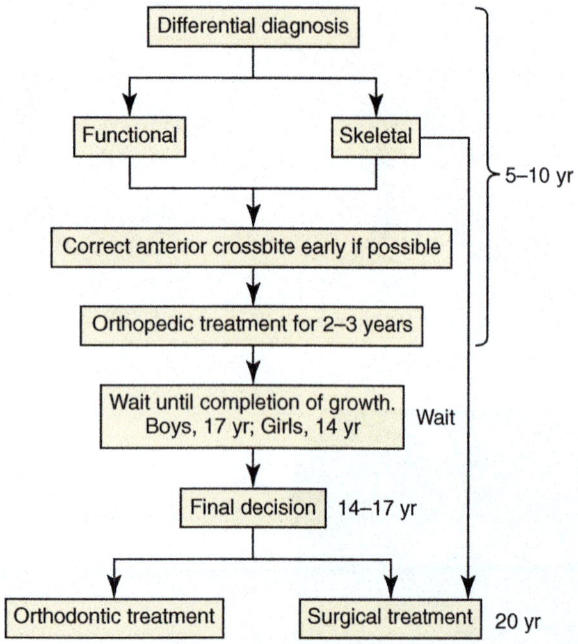

Figure 14-17 Long-term treatment protocol for a developing Class III patient.

vertical elastics,[45–47] (3) retraction of lower dentition using springs from mandibular micro-implants to the lower dentition,[48] and (4) retraction and uprighting of lower posterior teeth using Class III elastics from maxillary micro-implants to the lower dentition.[49]

DIAGNOSIS AND CLASSIFICATION OF NONGROWING CLASS III MALOCCLUSIONS

Skeletal Class III malocclusion can be classified into retruded maxilla, protruded mandible, or a combination of the two according to cephalometric analysis.[50] Generally, as growth is completed there is little or no functional shift of the mandible on closure. However, adult patients with an anterior crossbite should still check for functional shift (CO-CR discrepancy) during clinical examination. Patients with anterior crossbite can be corrected by downward and backward rotation of the mandible.

In the vertical dimension, adult Class III patients can be categorized into high angle and low angle cases.[51] High angle Class III patients are characterized skeletally by an increase in occlusal plane angle, mandibular plane angle, lower face height, and gonial angle. Dentally, they are accompanied by an open bite and an increase in clinical crown length. On the other hand, low angle cases usually show a decrease in occlusal plane angle, mandibular plane angle, and lower facial height and a more acute gonial angle together with a dental deep bite (Fig. 14-18).

In general, patients present with a mild anteroposterior skeletal discrepancy and functional CO-CR discrepancy and low angle cases are good candidates for camouflage Class III treatment with orthodontic tooth movement.

TREATMENT PRINCIPLES FOR NONGROWING SKELETAL CLASS III PATIENTS

Depending on the types of Class III malocclusion, different options and treatment goals could be applied. However, there are few common principles for camouflage treatment. In low angle cases, increasing the lower facial height is helpful in alleviating the anteroposterior discrepancy as well as reducing the deep overbite. Intermaxillary elastics or mechanics that can increase the vertical dimension can be used to achieve these goals (Figs. 14-19 to 14-22; Table 14-2). In high angle cases, mechanics that increase the lower face height should be avoided (see micro-implant anchorage cases in Class III Treatment with Micro-implant Anchorage). In the dentition, the upper incisors should not be tipped forward because the incisors are already compensated. Therefore upper incisors should be moved with root labial torque to keep or control the proper torque of the upper

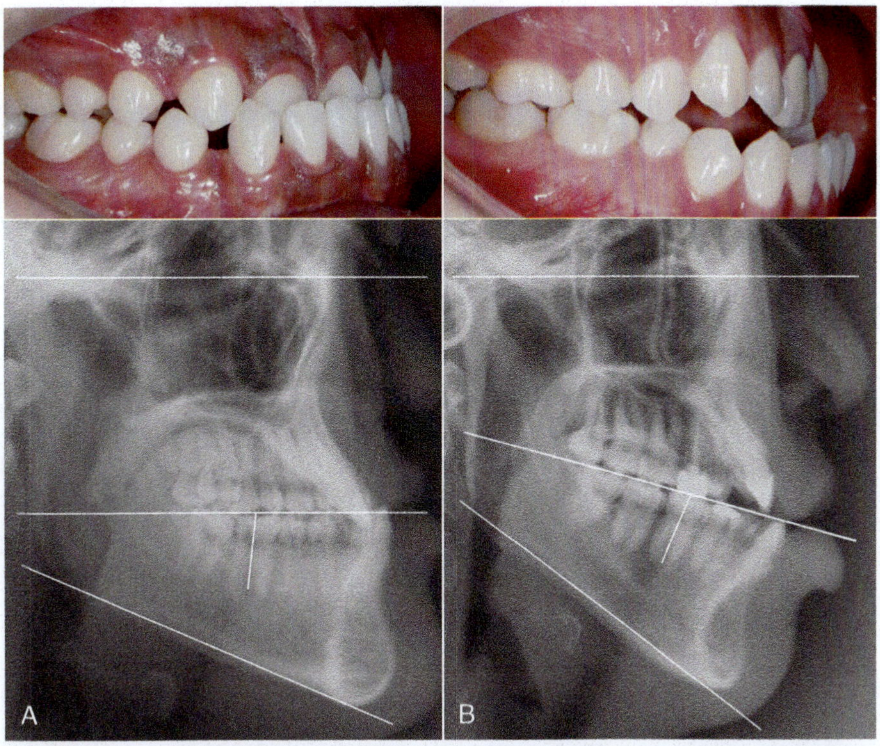

Figure 14-18 Two types of skeletal class III. **A,** Typical low angle Class III; deep overbite and flat occlusal plane. **B,** Typical high angle Class III; open bite and steep occlusal plane.

TABLE 14-2 Cephalometric Measurements of Patient CJ Compared with the Korean Norms

	Norm		Patient CJ		
	Mean	SD	Pre	CR	Post
ANB	1.5	1.8	−7.1	−4.5	−4.5
FMA	23.8	5.3	19.9	22.7	22.7
Occ. pl. a.	4.6	4.1	1.3	1.3	1.3
U1 to FH	119.0	4.6	123.4	123.4	130.0
FMIA	65.8	7.0	85.1	81.3	88.5
IMPA	86.9	7.1	75.0	76.0	68.8
Z angle	75.0	2.0	91.6	87.2	89.4

ANB, A point nasion B point; *CR,* centric relation; *FH,* Frankfurt horizontal; *FMA,* Frankfurt mandibular plane angle; *FMIA,* Frankfurt mandibular incisal angle; *IMPA,* incisor mandibular plane angle; *Occ. pl. a.,* occlusal plane angle; *Post,* post-treatment; *Pre,* pre-treatment; *SD,* standard deviation; *U1,* upper incisor.

TABLE 14-3 Cephalometric Measurements of Patient YJ Compared with the Korean Norms

	Norm	Patient YJ	Patient YJ
Measurement	Mean	Initial	Final
ANB	2.8	−2.6	−2.9
FMA	25.7	30.2	29.3
Occ. pl. a.	7.1	8.3	7.8
U1 to FH	116.6	116.5	122.1
FMIA	63.1	68.4	80.9
IMPA	85.9	81.4	69.8
Z angle	77.0	77.4	77.4

ANB, A point nasion B point; *FH,* Frankfurt horizontal; *FMA,* Frankfurt mandibular plane angle; *FMIA,* Frankfurt mandibular incisal angle; *IMPA,* incisor mandibular plane angle; *Occ. pl. a.,* occlusal plane angle; *U1,* upper incisor.

incisors. The lower incisors are usually already tipped lingually in skeletal Class III patients. However, if it is necessary to tip the lower incisors more lingually for crossbite correction, one should proceed with caution and check the width of the labial bone plate.

Conventional Edgewise Treatment with or without Extraction

The need for extraction of premolars or lower incisors depends on the severity of the malocclusion and the amount of crowding in both arches. Extraction of lower premolars is indicated only in cases where lingual tipping of the lower incisors is required without moving the upper incisors (Figs. 14-23 to 14-26; Table 14-3). Extraction of the upper second and lower first premolars is indicated in situations where space for correction of upper crowding is not necessary and extraction space is only for mesial movement of molars to correct molar relationship. Extraction of the upper and lower first premolars is indicated when there is upper and lower crowding and the first molars are almost in Angle's Class I relationship. Extraction of a lower incisor is sometimes indicated in cases with mild crowding of the lower arch or where

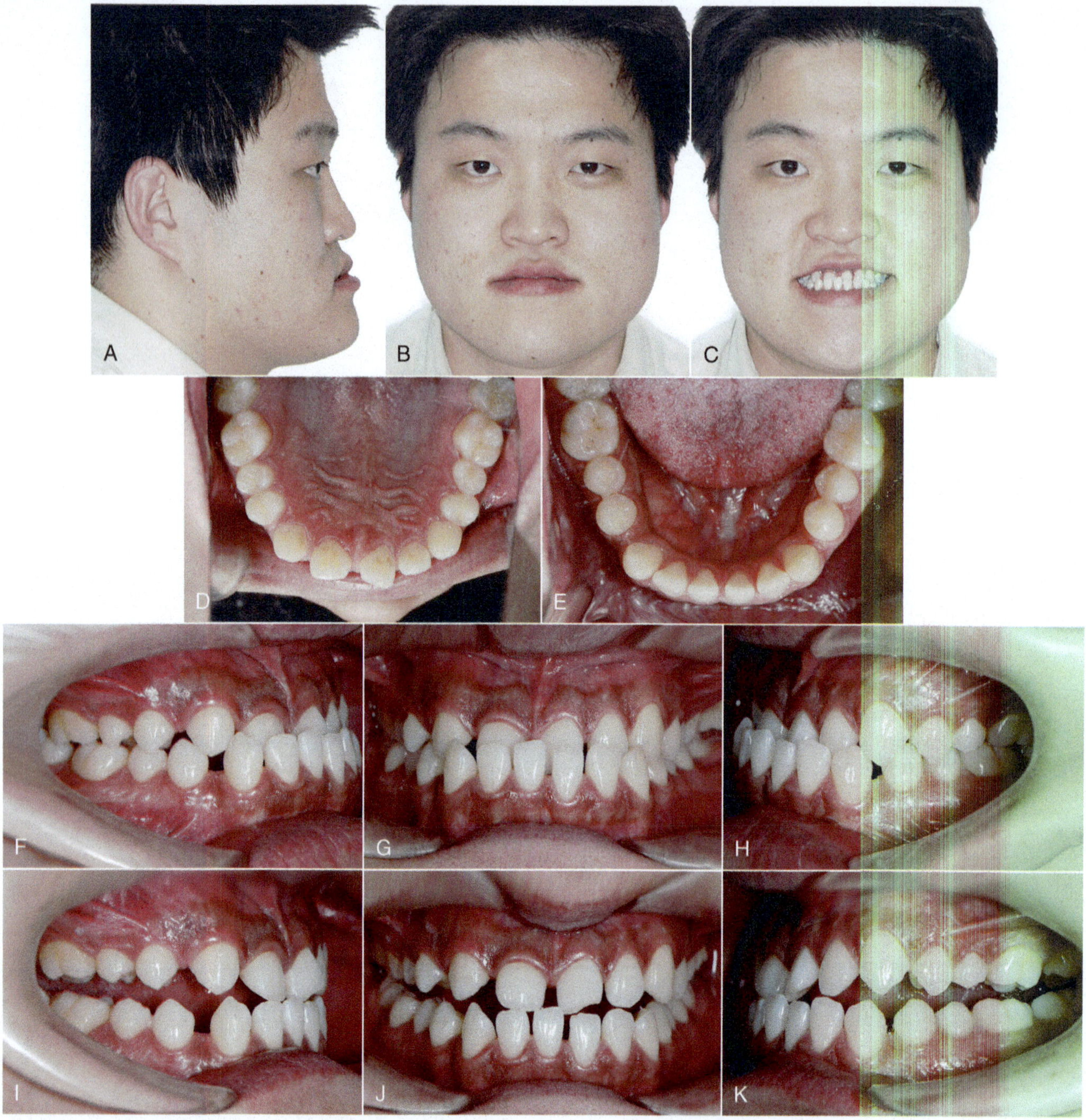

Figure 14-19 Pre-treatment facial photographs (**A–C**) and intraoral photographs taken in centric occlusion (**D–H**) and in centric relation (**I–K**) of a 22-year-old male patient, CJ. The patient shows excess space in the upper and lower arches and has a missing upper right lateral incisor. The patient wanted only orthodontic treatment. **F–H,** Centric occlusion. **I–K,** Centric relation.

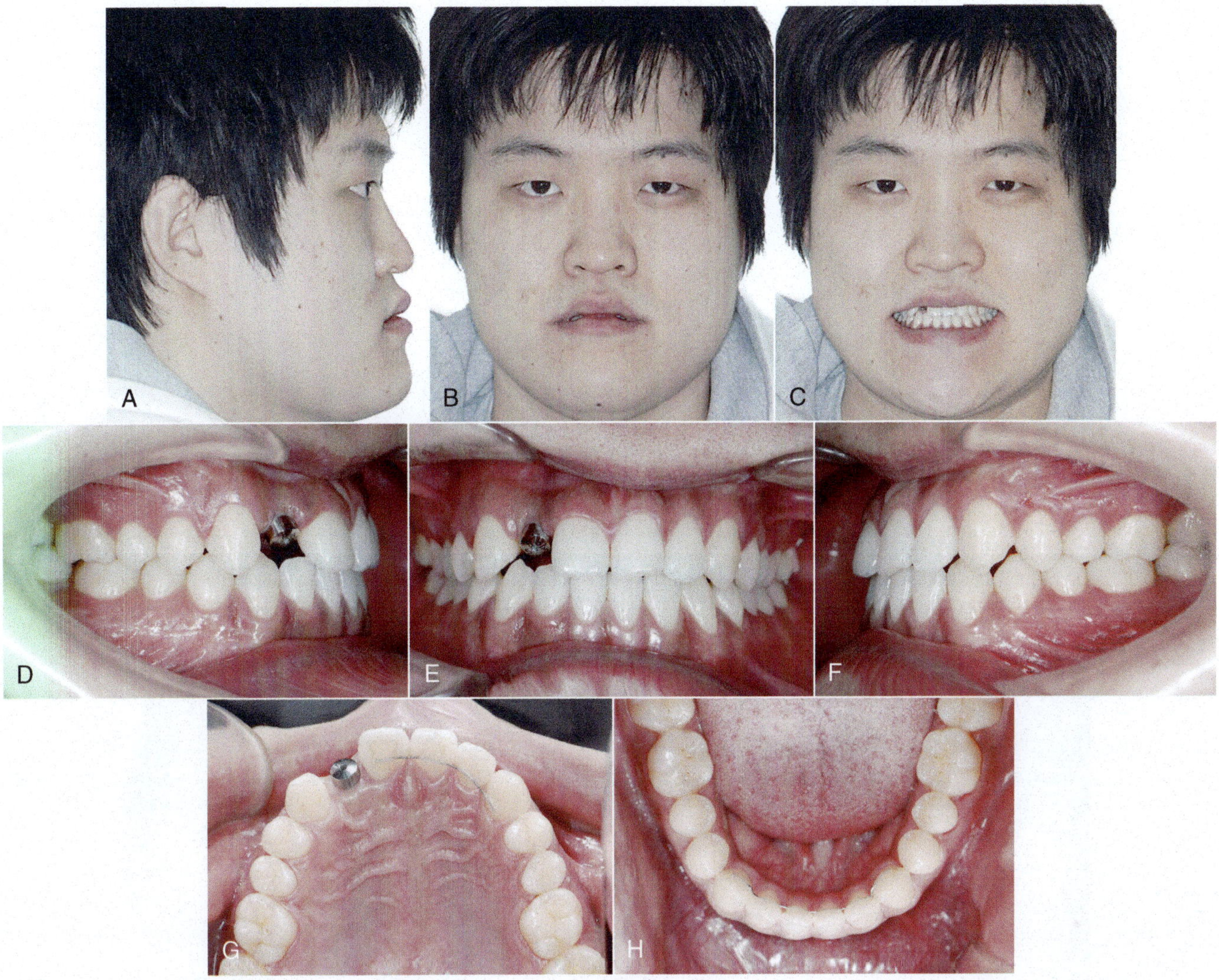

Figure 14-20 Post-treatment **(A–C)** facial and **(D–H)** intraoral photographs of CJ. Note the good Class I molar and canine relationship and occlusion. The soft tissue profile is still concave and shows a prognathic chin.

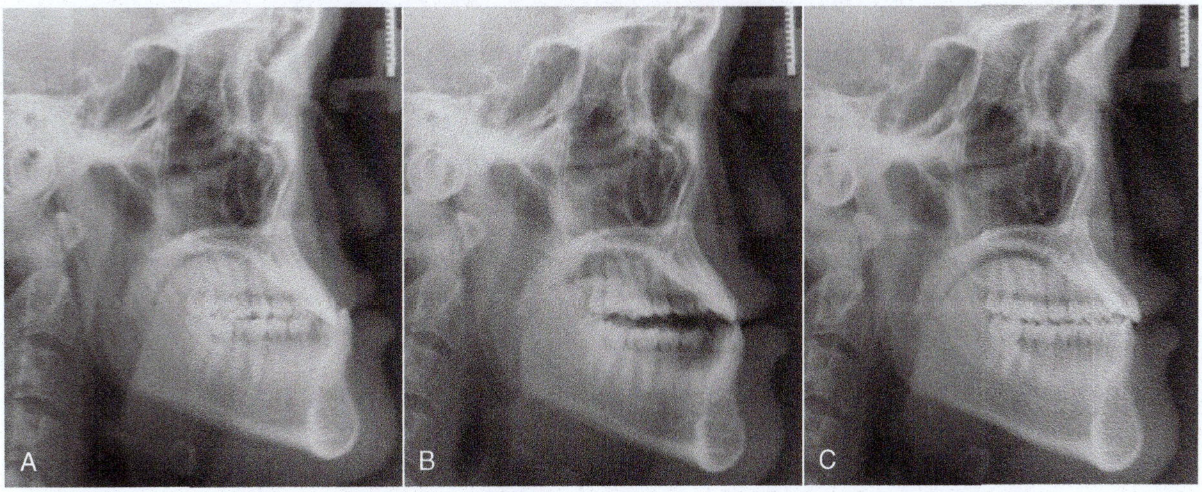

Figure 14-21 Cephalometric radiographs of CJ: **(A)** pre-treatment centric occlusion (CO), **(B)** pre-treatment centric relation (CR), and **(C)** post-treatment.

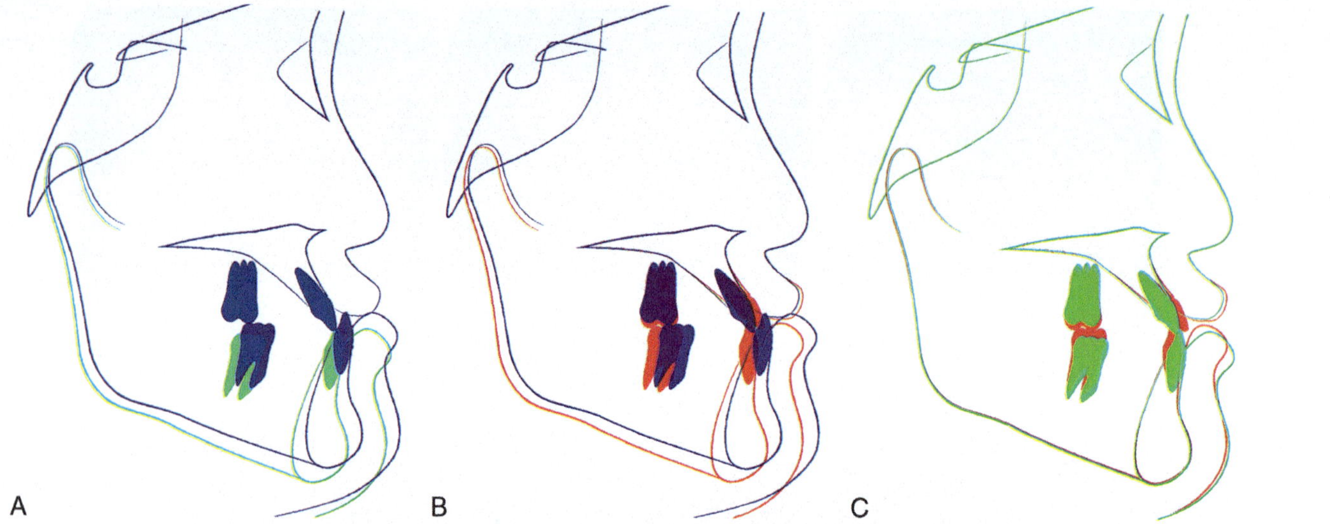

Figure 14-22 Cephalometric superimpositions of CJ. **A,** Superimposition of pre-treatment centric occlusion (CO) and centric relation (CR). **B,** Superimposition of pre-treatment and post-treatment. **C,** Pre-treatment CR and post-treatment. **A** and **B** show almost the same pattern. That means that the CR position of the mandible might be the treatment goal for this case. Note that the mandible position at post-treatment is the same as pre-treatment CR position. This post-treatment position resulted from a downward and backward rotation of the mandible, with the extrusion of the molars, lingual tipping of the lower incisors, and labial tipping of the upper incisors.

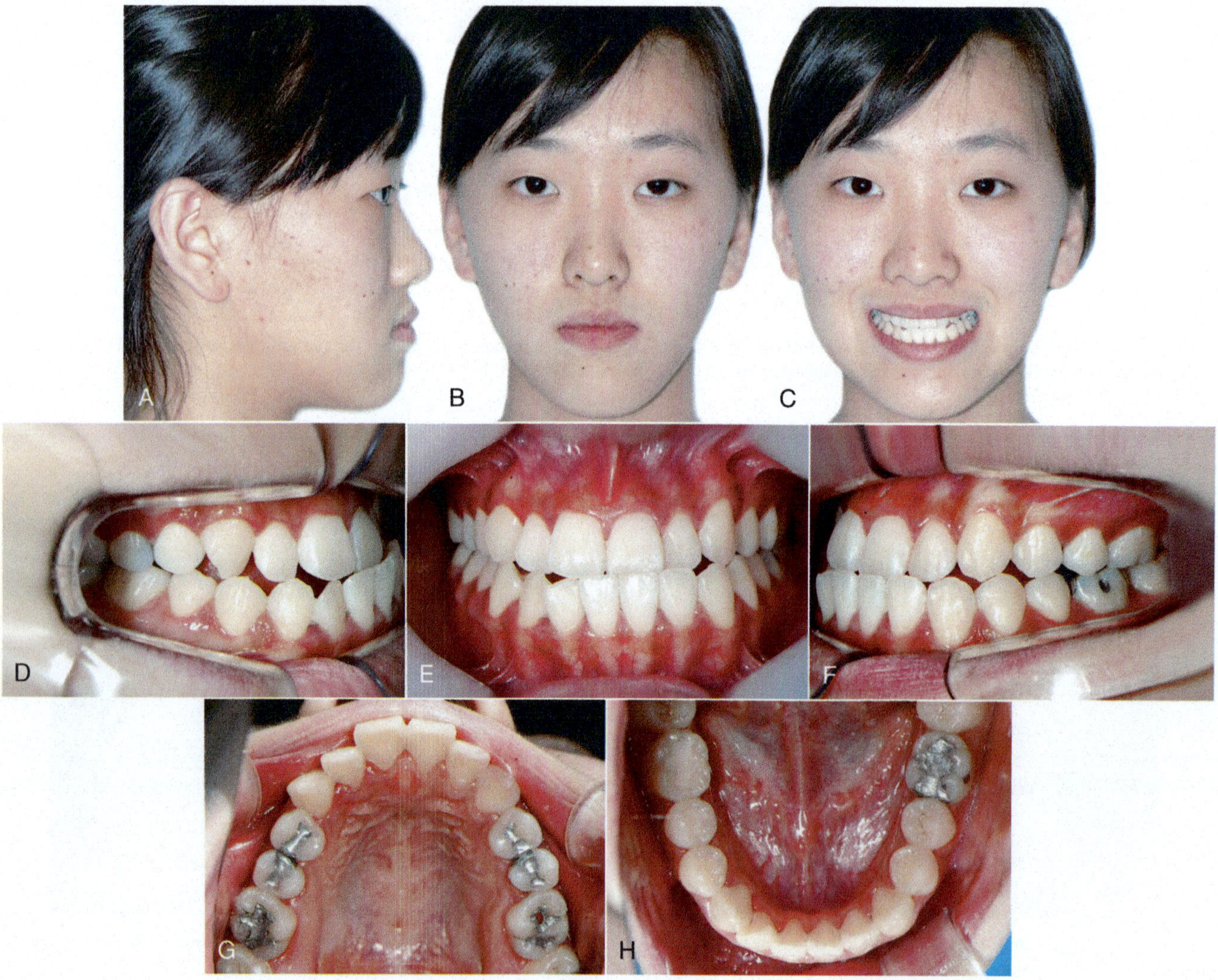

Figure 14-23 Pre-treatment **(A–C)** facial and **(D–H)** intraoral photographs of patient YJ. Facial views show lip protrusion, acute nasolabial angle, and chin deviated to left side. Intraoral views show Class III molar and canine and anterior crossbite. Lower dental midline is shifted to the left (3-mm).

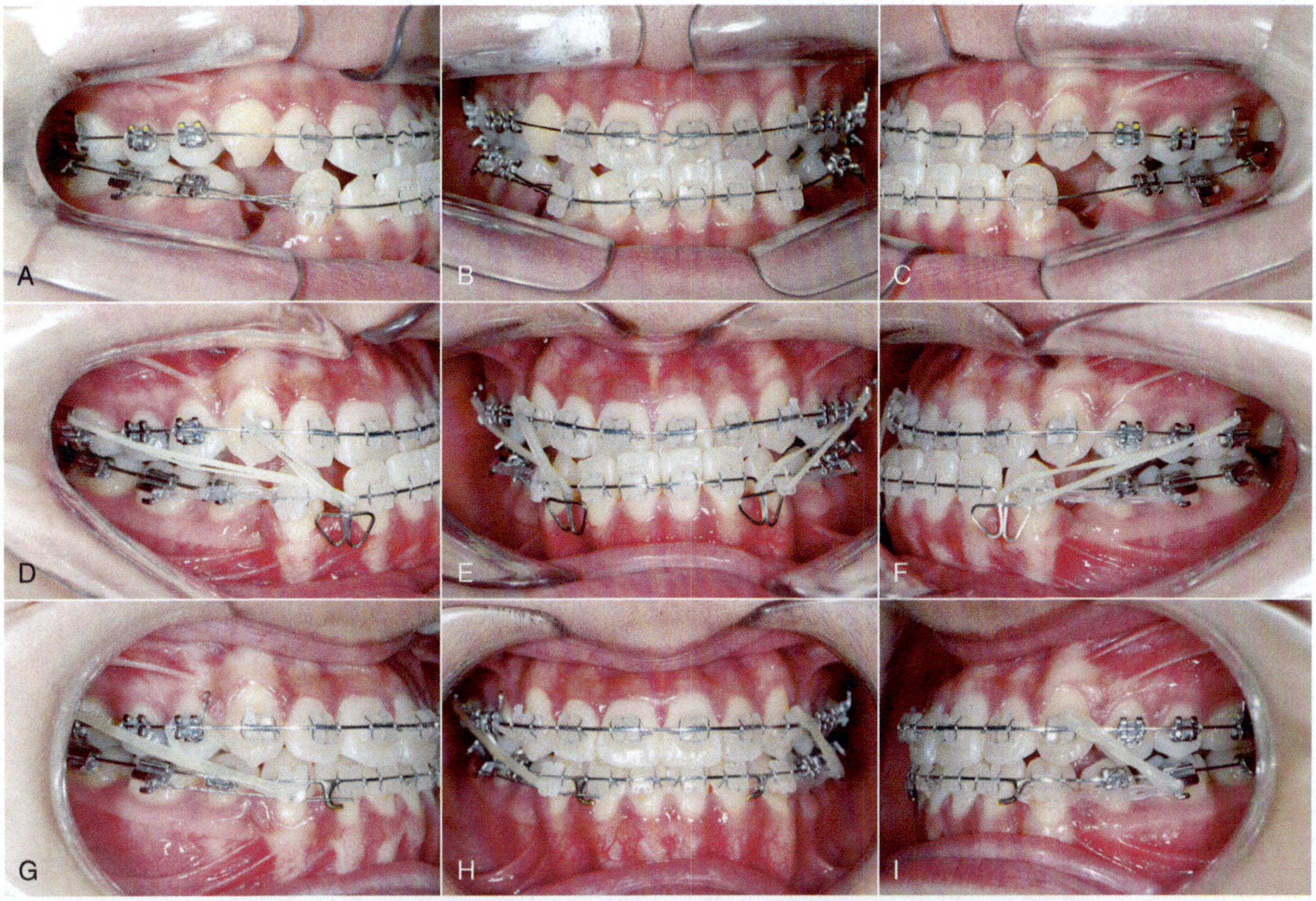

Figure 14-24 Treatment procedure for YJ. **A–C,** The lower canines were extracted, and leveling and canine retraction were done. **D–F,** The lower four incisors were retracted using a double delta arch with Class III elastics to correct the anterior crossbite. **G–I,** Final detailing with Class III and midline correction elastics.

there is presence of a Bolton tooth size discrepancy between the upper and lower incisors. Finally, nonextraction therapy can be used in low angle cases with the presence of an anterior crossbite by uprighting the lower posterior teeth or changing the occlusal plane (Figs. 14-27 to 14-30; Table 14-4). Furthermore, after the development of the microimplant anchorage (MIA) technique, high angle cases with open bite and crossbite can be treated without extraction by uprighting posterior teeth and changing the occlusal plane with the MIA technique.

Multiloop Edgewise Archwire (MEAW) Treatment Technique

The MEAW technique[45–47] was created by Dr. Young H. Kim in 1967 to treat a marked open-bite malocclusion. This technique was later found to be useful in the correction of Class III open bite in Asian countries, such as Korea and Japan. It is indicated in the treatment of mild skeletal Class III malocclusion with mesially inclined lower posterior teeth together with an open bite.

The MEAW consists of multiple L-shaped loops with a horizontal loop and vertical loop between each tooth except the four incisors (Fig. 14-31). Kim strongly recommended the use of standard edgewise twin brackets with a 0.018-inch slot and fabricating the MEAW with a 0.016-inch × 0.022-inch stainless steel archwire. The fabricated MEAW should have the configuration of an ideal arch. Then, third-order bends are incorporated into the archwire according to the required degree. Finally, the MEAW should be activated with a series of tip-back bends. The tip-back

TABLE 14-4 Cephalometric Measurements of Patient CS Compared with the Korean Norms

	Norm		Patient CS	
	Mean	SD	Pre	Post
ANB	2.8	2.3	−3.4	−2.8
FMA	25.4	6.1	18.1	19.4
Occ. pl. a.	5.9	4.6	5.9	2.8
U1 to FH	116.6	5.7	116.5	130.7
FMIA	64.8	7.2	65.5	67.5
IMPA	87.3	6.8	96.5	93.1
Z angle	77.0	2.0	79.9	85.2

ANB, A point nasion B point; *FH,* Frankfurt horizontal; *FMA,* Frankfurt mandibular plane angle; *FMIA,* Frankfurt mandibular incisal angle; *IMPA,* incisor mandibular plane angle; *Occ. pl. a.,* occlusal plane angle; *Post,* post-treatment; *Pre,* pre-treatment; *SD,* standard deviation; *U1,* upper incisor.

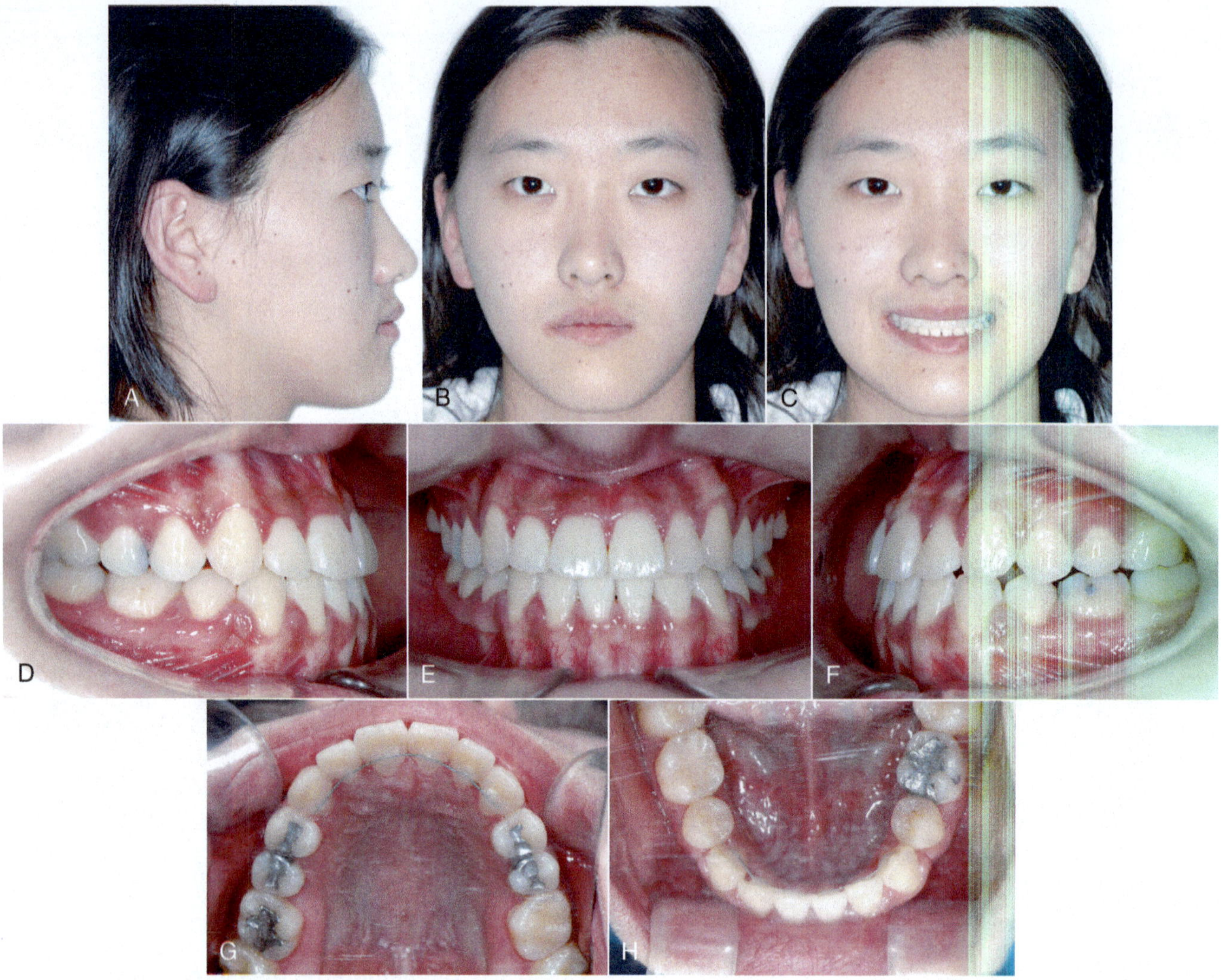

Figure 14-25 **A–C,** Post-treatment facial photographs of YJ show a retracted lip profile and deviated chin. **D–H,** Intraoral photographs show good occlusion on the right side but poor occlusion on the left side (because of skeletal asymmetry). These results demonstrate a limitation of camouflage treatment of skeletal Class III with asymmetry.

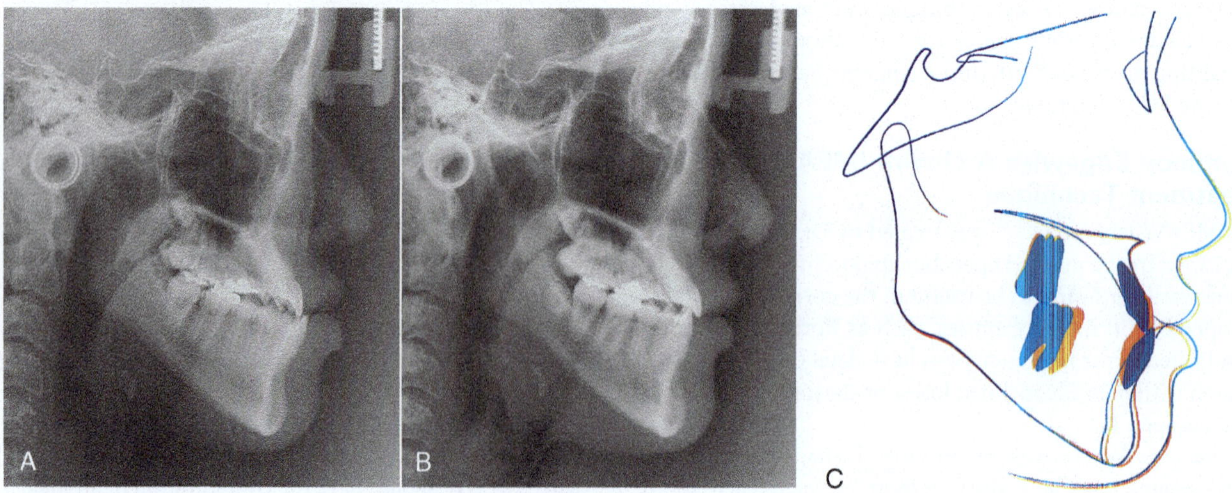

Figure 14-26 **A,** Pre-treatment and (**B**) post-treatment cephalograms of YJ. **C,** Superimposition of the pre- and post-treatment radiographs.

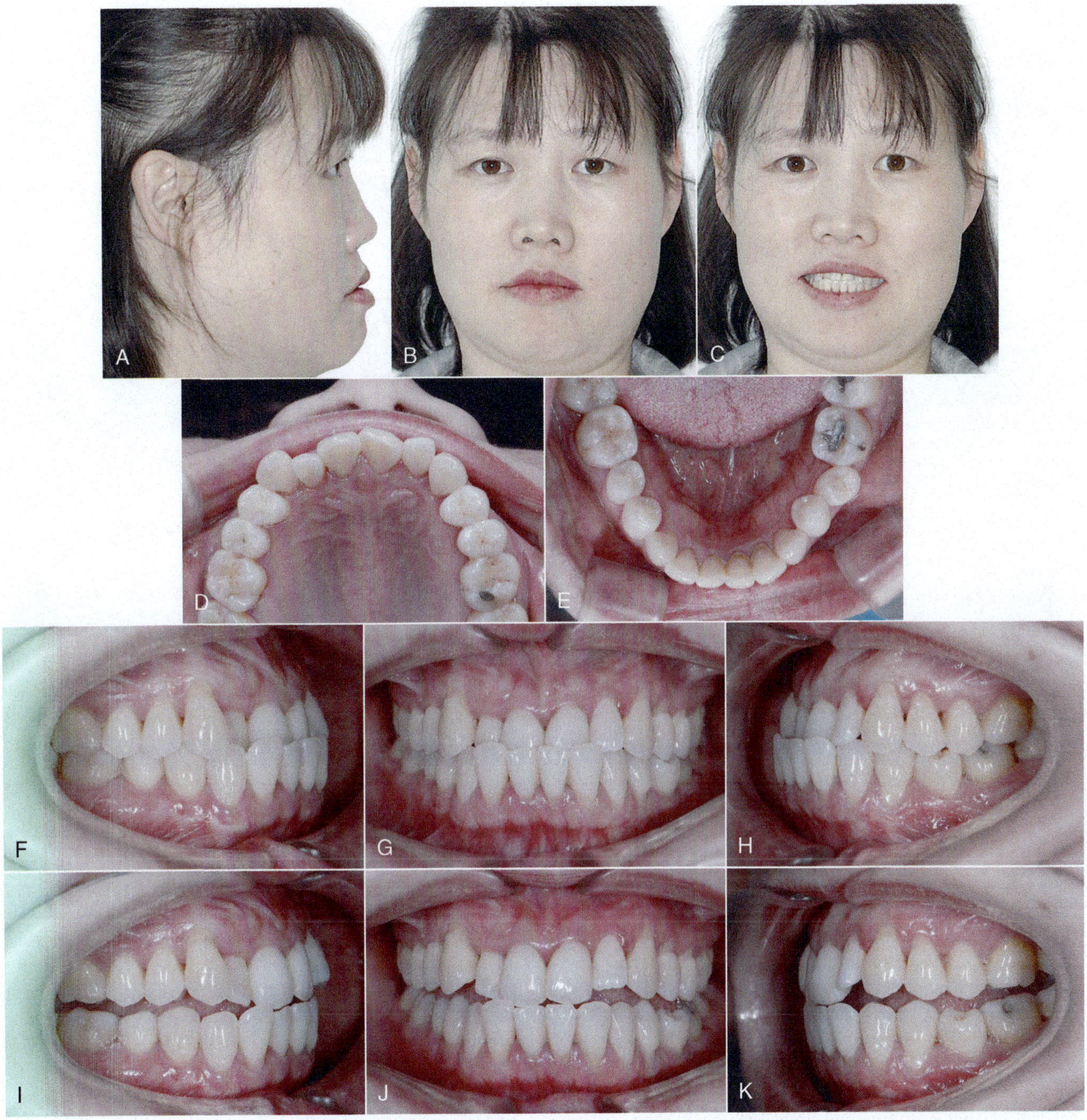

Figure 14-27 Pre-treatment facial photographs (A–C) and intraoral photographs taken in centric occlusion (F–H) and in centric relation (I–K) of a patient CS.

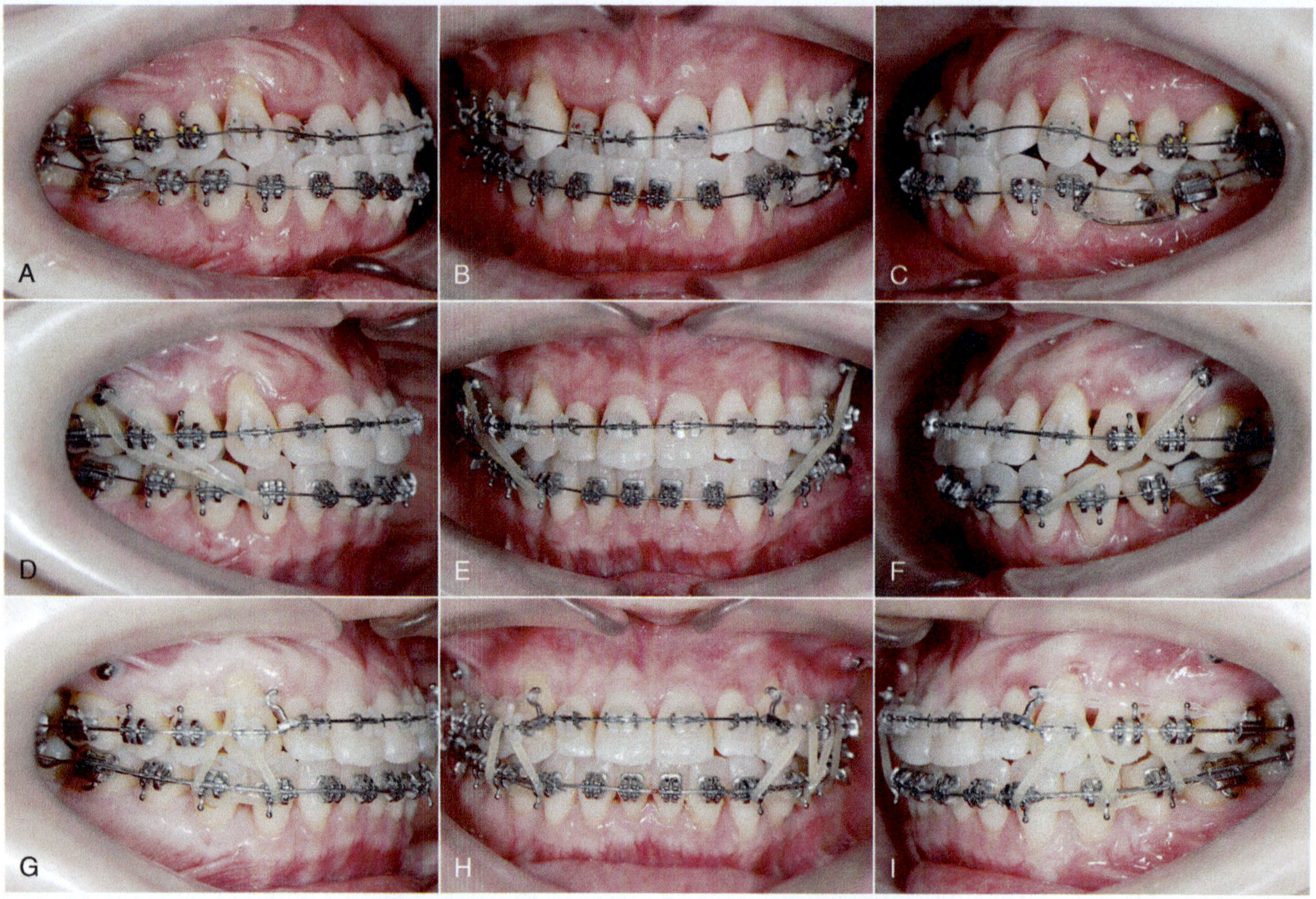

Figure 14-28 Intraoral photographs of CS showing the treatment procedures. Treatment procedures: **A-C,** Initial leveling with a 0.014-inch NiTi archwire. **D-F,** Placement of two maxillary MIA between the upper second premolars and first molars and applied Class III elastics from MIA to the lower canines. **G-I,** Vertical elastics to sock in the posterior occlusion.

bends begin at the first bicuspid and progress posteriorly to the last molars. The typical tip-back bends are 3 to 5 degrees on each tooth. The terminal wire has a 15- to 20-degree tip-back bend. The completed mandibular MEAW should show a marked reverse curve (Fig. 14-32). Heat treatment is necessary after the wires have been activated to increase the strength of the archwire. The mechanism of MEAW is a tip-back movement of the posterior teeth using Class III and vertical elastics accompanied with a tip-back bend of the archwire. Along with the tip-back activation, anterior vertical and Class III elastics produce uprighting and distal movement of the lower posterior teeth and change of the occlusal plane. This, in turn, corrects the anterior crossbite and closes the open bite.

Before applying the MEAW, all rotation, spacing, irregularities, and poorly positioned brackets should be eliminated. The stabilizing archwire made of 0.016-inch × 0.022-inch stainless steel wire is usually placed in the upper arch. However, in cases that need better interdigitation, MEAW could be placed in the upper arch.

The MEAW should have a deep reverse curve on the lower arch. Anterior vertical and Class III elastics (short or long) are necessary in order to counterbalance the intrusion force created by the archwire on the incisors and to simultaneously provide mandibular retraction (Fig. 14-33).

The long Class III elastics cause extrusion of the upper molars and produce a counterclockwise rotation of the occlusal plane and a clockwise rotation of the mandible. This can be minimized by the use of short Class III elastics. Vertical elastics (3/16 inch, 6 oz.) are placed between the upper and lower first loops or the lower first loop and upper canine hooks of the plain arch. Long Class III elastics placed from the upper last molars or first molars to the second loop of the lower arch (3/8 inch, 5 oz. or 5/16 inch, 5 oz.) would further elongate the upper molars, upright the occlusal plane, and rotate the mandible clockwise. They are used in low angle cases. However, short Class III elastics (1/4 or 3/16 inch, 5 oz.) from the upper loop or hook lying mesial to the second premolar to the lower second loop can be used in high angle cases. These elastics must be in place full-time, except when eating and brushing.

There are two common problems associated with the MEAW technique: complicated wire bending and 24-hour elastics wearing. These are illustrated in the following two cases.

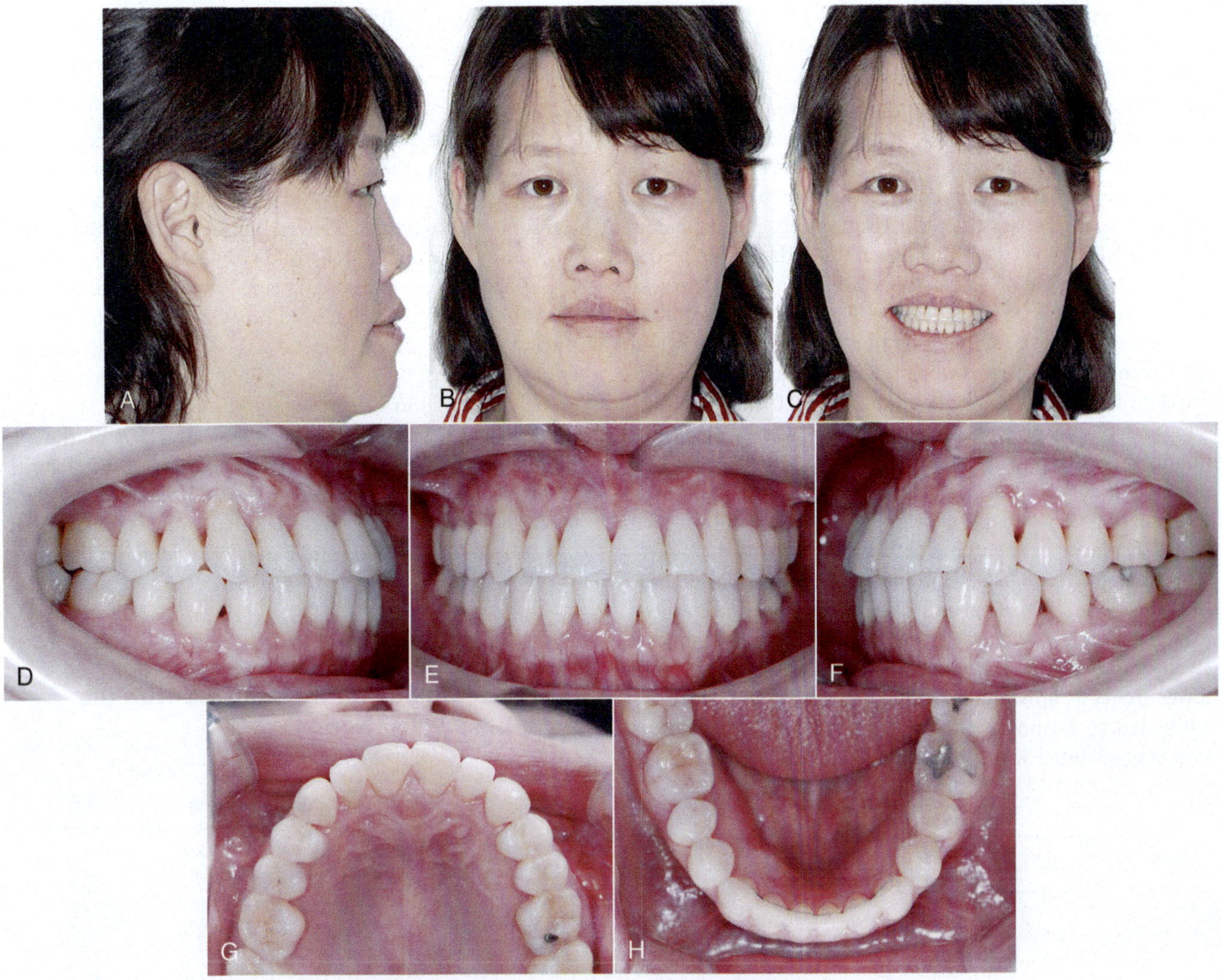

Figure 14-29 Post-treatment **(A–C)** facial and **(D–H)** intraoral photographs of CS.

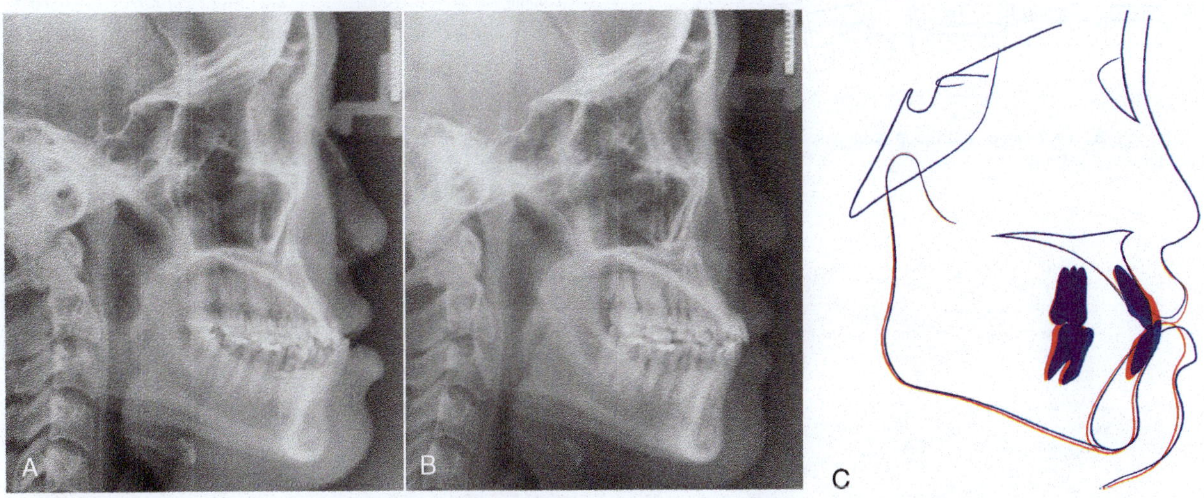

Figure 14-30 **A,** Pre-treatment and **(B)** post-treatment cephalograms of CS. **C,** Superimposition of the pre- and post-treatment radiographs.

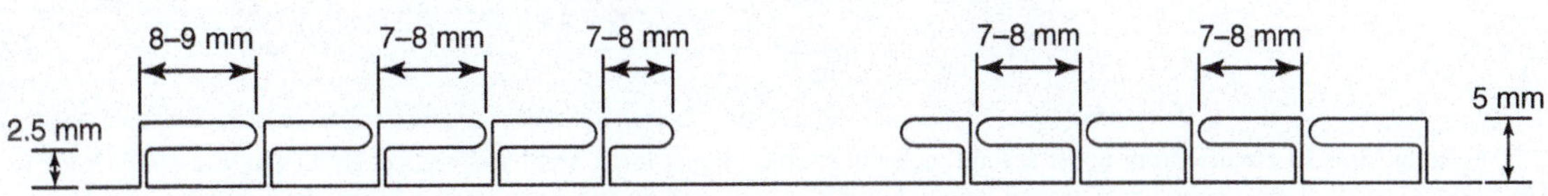

Figure 14-31 Multiloop edgewise archwire (MEAW). Components of MEAW are multiple L-loops with horizontal and vertical loops. First loop is placed just mesial to the canines. Average loop length and height are presented in diagram.

Case 1: The MEAW Technique

A 20-year-old female presented with a chief concern of an open bite and difficulty in mastication. The extraoral photographs showed a convex facial profile and a slight prominent chin. The intraoral photographs showed an open-bite malocclusion except in the molar regions. There was mild crowding in the upper and lower arches, a slight narrow maxillary arch, and a mild Class III molar relationship. The cephalometric tracing showed a mild skeletal Class III malocclusion with an ANB angle of −1.8 degrees, a FMA of 22.7 degrees, and a gonial angle of 120.1 degrees (Fig. 14-34; Table 14-5).

Standard edgewise 0.018-inch slot brackets were bonded from second premolars to second premolars and bands were fitted on the upper first molars. An initial 0.016-inch Ni-Ti wire was placed on both arches together with a precision lingual arch (0.022-inch × 0.028-inch TMA) to expand the upper arch (Fig. 14-35, A–C). After leveling and alignment, a stabilizing wire with 0.016-inch × 0.022-inch stainless steel wire was placed in the upper arch and an activated MEAW with 0.016-inch × 0.022-inch stainless steel wire was placed in the lower arch. Vertical and Class III elastics were applied (Fig. 14-35, D–F). Later, 0.016-inch × 0.022-inch stainless steel ideal arches with hooks were placed in the upper and lower arches as finishing archwire (Fig. 14-35, G–I). Figures 14-36 and 14-37 show the treatment results. Excellent occlusion was obtained with the MEAW technique. The occlusal plane was decreased with uprighting of the lower posterior teeth and a slight increase in chin prominence.

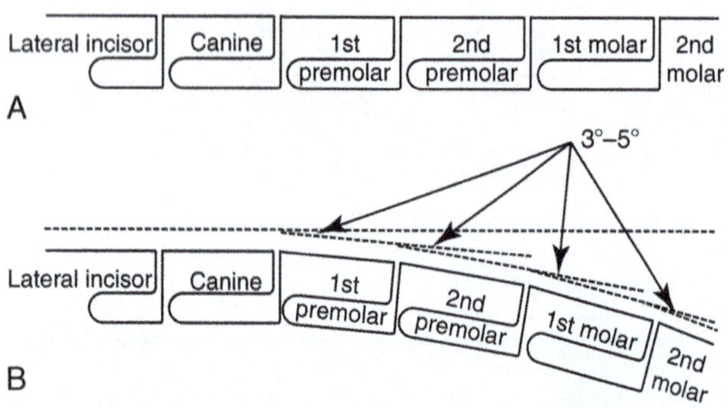

Figure 14-32 **A,** Fabricated multiloop edgewise archwire (MEAW). **B,** Lower activated MEAW.

Case 2: The MEAW Technique

An 18-year-old female presented with a chief concern of open bite and crowding. The extraoral photographs showed slight lower lip protrusion and large lower facial height. The intraoral photographs showed an open bite with severe crowding in the upper arch, mild crowding in the lower arch, a V-shaped upper arch, a U-shaped lower arch, and a mild Class III molar relationship (Fig. 14-38). The cephalometric tracing showed a mild skeletal Class III malocclusion with an ANB angle of 0.5 degrees, an FMA of 36.1 degrees, and a gonial angle of 136.4 degrees (Table 14-6).

The treatment plan consisted of extraction of the #15 tooth and 24, 34, 44 (upper left first premolar, lower left first premolar, and lower right first premolar). Standard edgewise 0.022-inch slot brackets were bonded from second premolars to second premolars and bands were fitted on the upper

TABLE 14-5 Cephalometric Measurements of Patient PS Compared with the Korean Norms

	Norm		Patient PS	
	Mean	SD	Pre	Post
ANB	2.8	2.3	−1.8	−1.5
FMA	25.4	6.1	22.7	22.8
Occ. pl. a.	5.9	4.6	9.1	4.8
U1 to FH	116.6	5.7	112.7	118.9
FMIA	64.8	7.2	77.2	76.7
IMPA	87.3	6.8	80.1	80.5
Z angle	77.0	2.0	79.1	78.9

ANB, A point nasion B point; *FH,* Frankfurt horizontal; *FMA,* Frankfurt mandibular plane angle; *FMIA,* Frankfurt mandibular incisal angle; *IMPA,* incisor mandibular plane angle; *Occ. pl. a.,* occlusal plane angle; *Post,* post-treatment; *Pre,* pre-treatment; *SD,* standard deviation; *U1,* upper incisor.

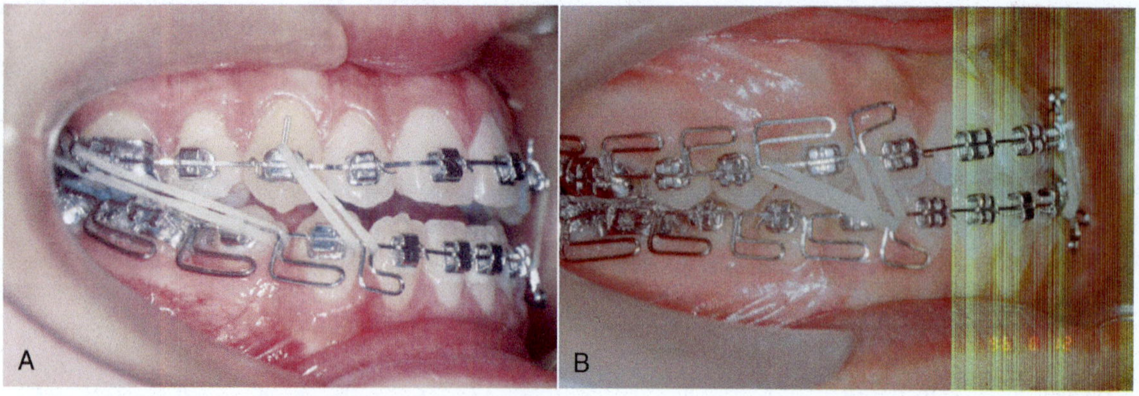

Figure 14-33 **A,** Long Class III elastics (from upper second molar to second loop of lower arch) and vertical elastics (upper canine hook to first loop in lower arch). **B,** Short Class III elastics (from upper second loop to lower first loop) and up and down elastics (from upper first loop to lower first loop).

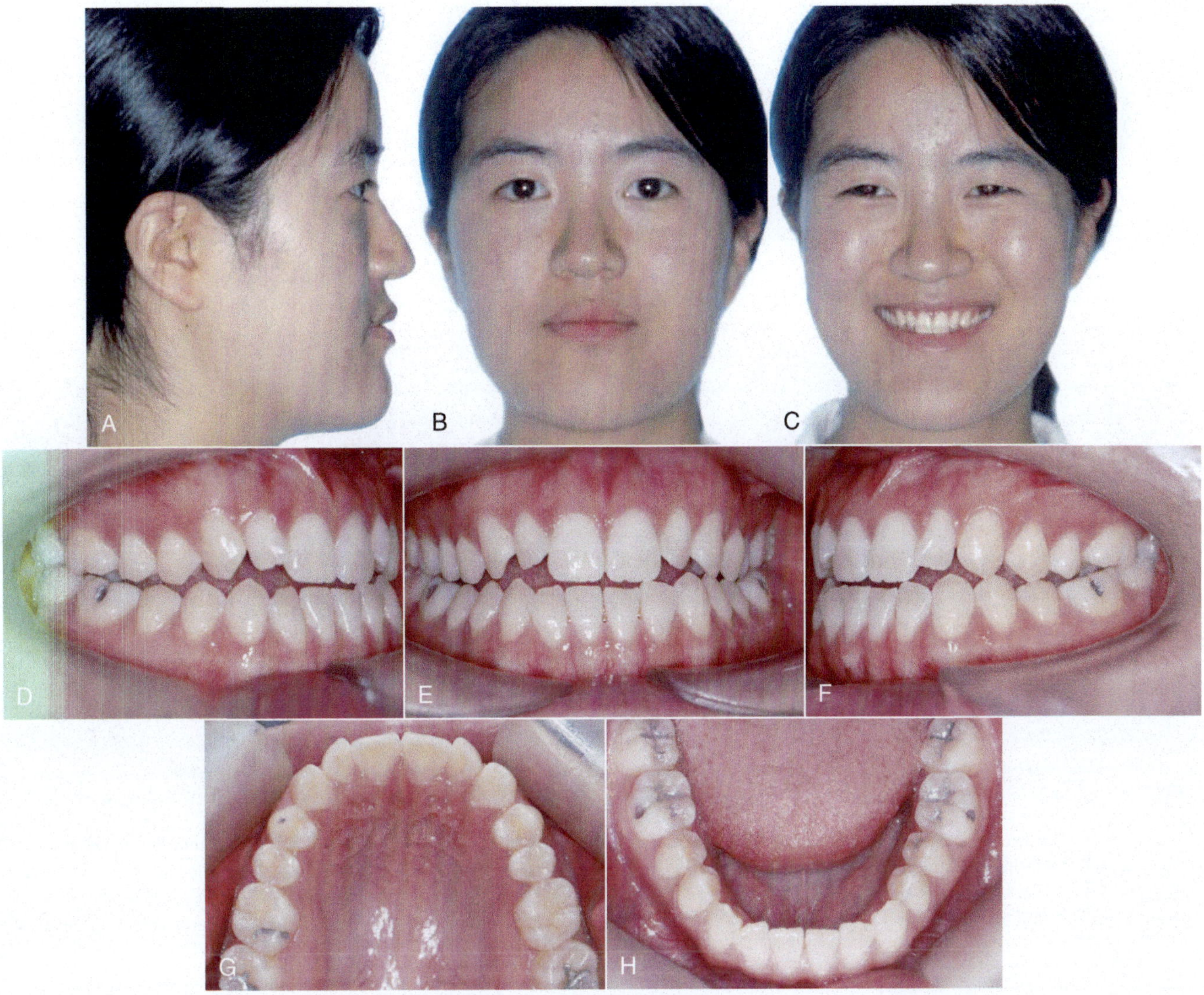

Figure 14-34 Pre-treatment **(A–C)** facial and **(D–H)** intraoral photographs of patient PS.

TABLE 14-6 Cephalometric Measurements of Patient KG Compared to the Korean Norms

	Norm		Patient KG	
	Mean	SD	Pre	Post
ANB	2.8	2.3	0.5	1.9
FMA	25.4	6.1	36.1	39.3
Occ. pl. a.	5.9	4.6	13.1	10.0
U1 to FH	116.6	5.7	126.9	112.0
FMIA	64.8	7.2	53.2	70.5
IMPA	87.3	6.8	90.6	70.3
Z angle	77.0	2.0	73.6	70.7

ANB, A point nasion B point; *FH,* Frankfurt horizontal; *FMA,* Frankfurt mandibular plane angle; *FMIA,* Frankfurt mandibular incisal angle; *IMPA,* incisor mandibular plane angle; *Occ. pl. a.,* occlusal plane angle; *Post,* post-treatment; *Pre,* pre-treatment; *SD,* standard deviation; *U1,* upper incisor.

first molars. An initial 0.016-inch Ni-Ti wire was placed on both arches (Fig. 14-39, A–C). After leveling and alignment, a stabilizing wire with 0.019-inch × 0.025-inch stainless steel wire was placed in the upper arch and an activated MEAW with 0.018-inch × 0.025-inch stainless steel wire was placed in the lower arch. Vertical (3/16 inch, 6 oz.) and Class III elastics (5/16 inch, 5 oz.) were applied (Fig. 14-39, D–F). After correction of crossbite and open bite, a MEAW with 0.018-inch × 0.025-inch stainless steel wire was placed in the upper arch to produce more detailed interdigitation in the posterior teeth (Fig. 14-39, G–I). Later, 0.019-inch × 0.025-inch stainless steel ideal arches with hooks were placed in the upper and lower arches as finishing archwire (Fig. 14-39, J–L).

The treatment results were (1) uprighting and extrusion of the lower molars, (2) decreased occlusal plane angle, (3) lingual tipping of the lower incisors, (4) extrusion of the upper and lower incisors, and (5) downward and backward

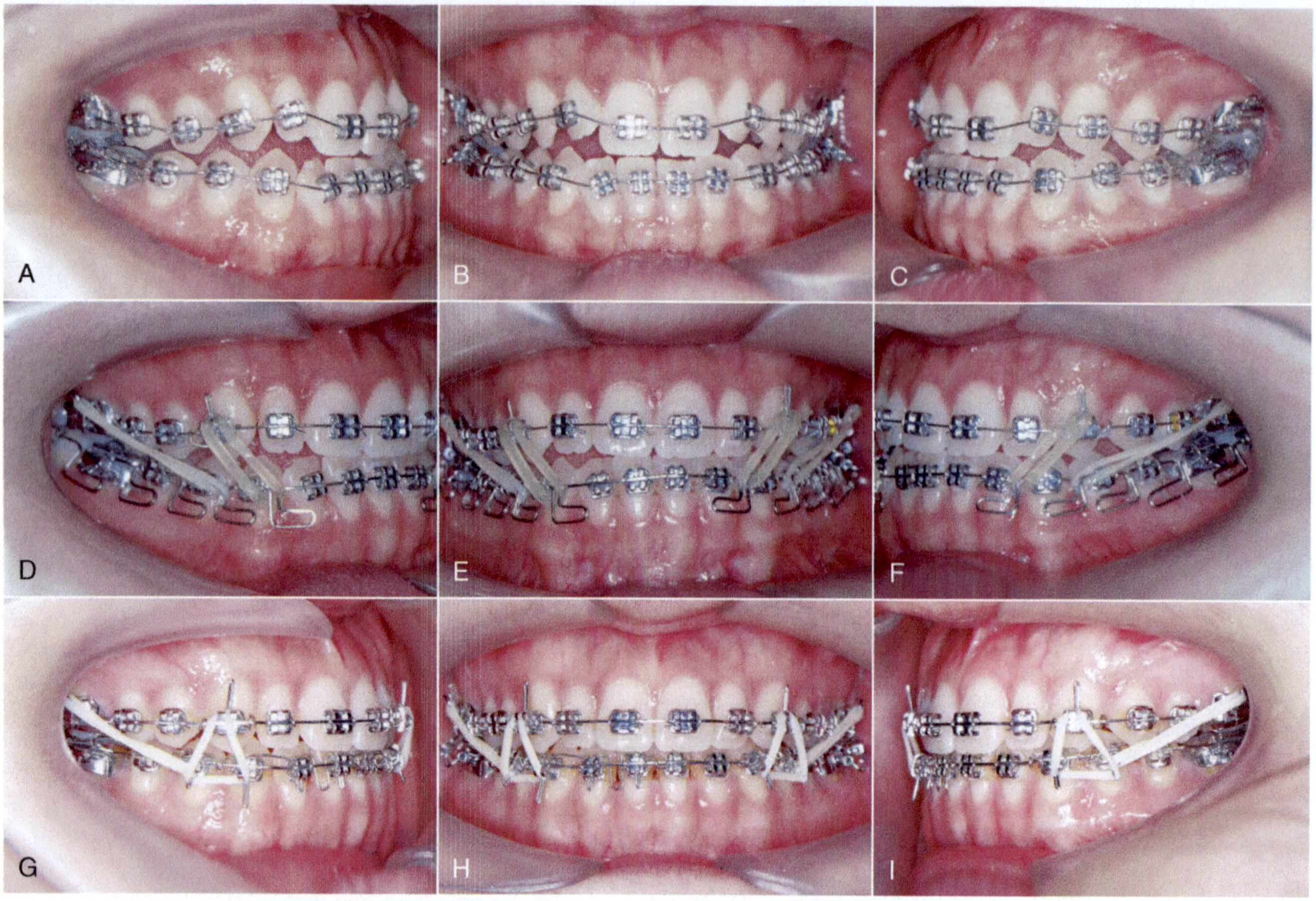

Figure 14-35 Treatment progress photographs of PS. **A–C,** Initial archwire was placed after fixed appliance was bonded and banded on upper and lower dentition. **D–F,** Stabilizing archwire was placed in upper arch and MEAW was placed in lower arch. **G–I,** Finishing stage.

rotation of the mandible with an increase in the lower facial height (Figs. 14-40 and 14-41).

CLASS III TREATMENT WITH MICRO-IMPLANT ANCHORAGE

Since the development of micro-implants,[52–54] MIA has been used to treat all types of malocclusion including Class III. MIA has been used to retract lower dentition for Class III treatment in two ways: micro-implants placed in the mandible[48] and micro-implants placed in the maxilla.[49]

Lower Micro-Implant Anchorage

The lower MIA can be used to treat mild and moderate skeletal Class III malocclusion and relapse after Class III surgery in high or low angle cases.

For retraction of the lower dentition, micro-implants can be placed in the retromolar area or in the interradicular space between the first molars and second premolars or between the second and first molars (Fig. 14-42). The retromolar area is the best site to place the micro-implants to retract lower dentition without interference of posterior teeth during retraction. However, it is difficult to place micro-implants in the retromolar area, primarily due to abundant movable soft tissue and limited space.

There are two methods of lower dentition retraction: whole dentition retraction and sequential retraction.

Whole Dentition Retraction

After leveling, a proper sized rectangular stainless steel wire attached hook between the canine and lateral incisor is placed in the lower arch, and retraction force is applied from the micro-implants to the hook using a Ni-Ti coil spring or power chain.

Problems. The clinician should pay attention to the relationship between force direction (line of action) and the C_{RES}. The line of action should pass over or on the CR of the lower dentition to retract lower dentition. Therefore the head of the micro-implants should be placed close to the cervical area. Clinically, it is very difficult to achieve this placement, especially in a case in which the clinician wants to place micro-implants in the interradicular space between 5 and 6 (between the second premolars and the first molars) or between 6 and 7 (between the first molar and second molar). Therefore the retromolar area is the best place to install

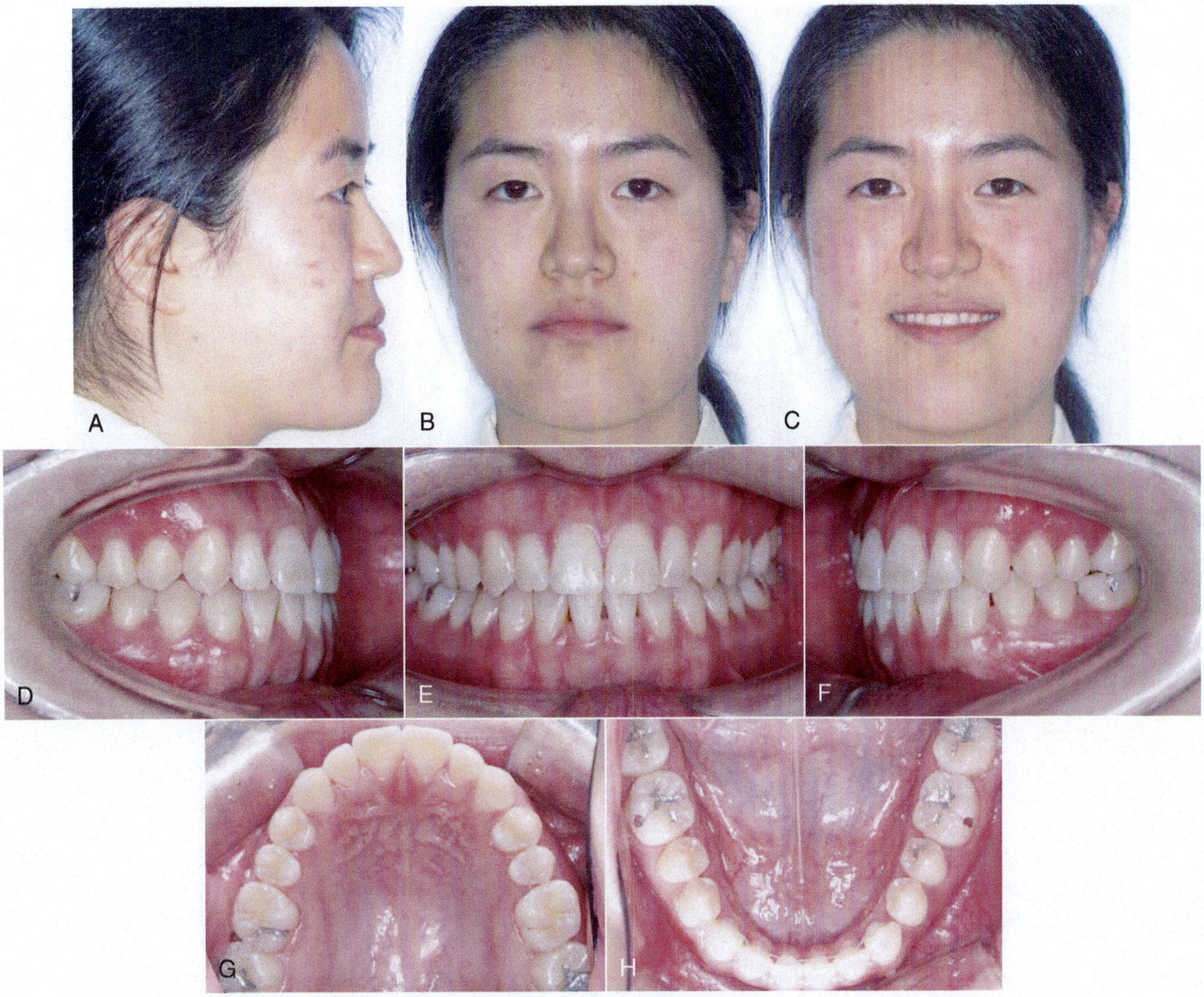

Figure 14-36 Post-treatment (**A–C**) facial and (**D–H**) intraoral photographs of PS.

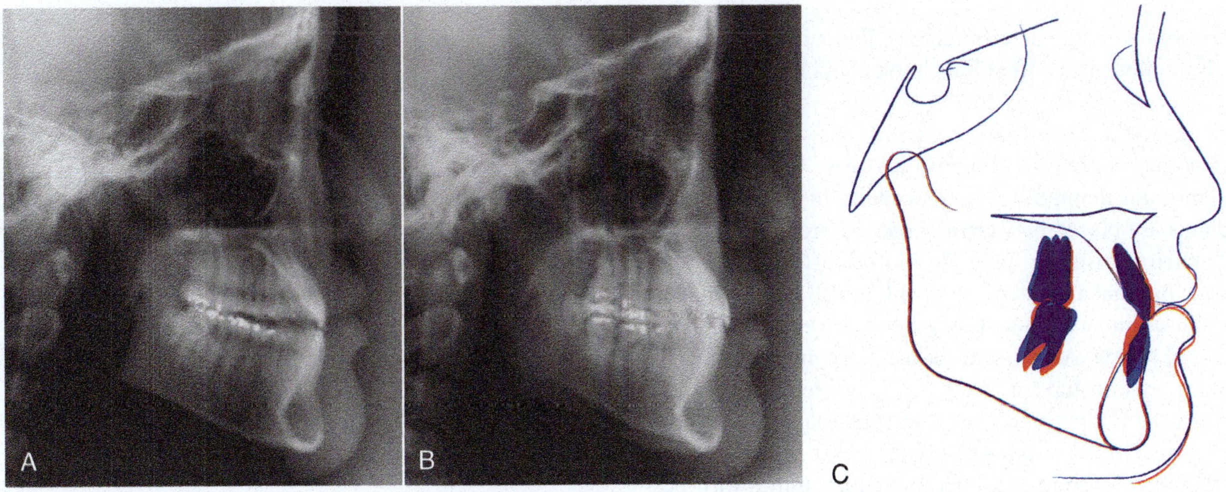

Figure 14-37 **A,** Pre-treatment and (**B**) post-treatment cephalograms of PS. **C,** Superimposition of pre-treatment and post-treatment tracings. Note the changes in the occlusal plane, with uprighting of lower molars after treatment.

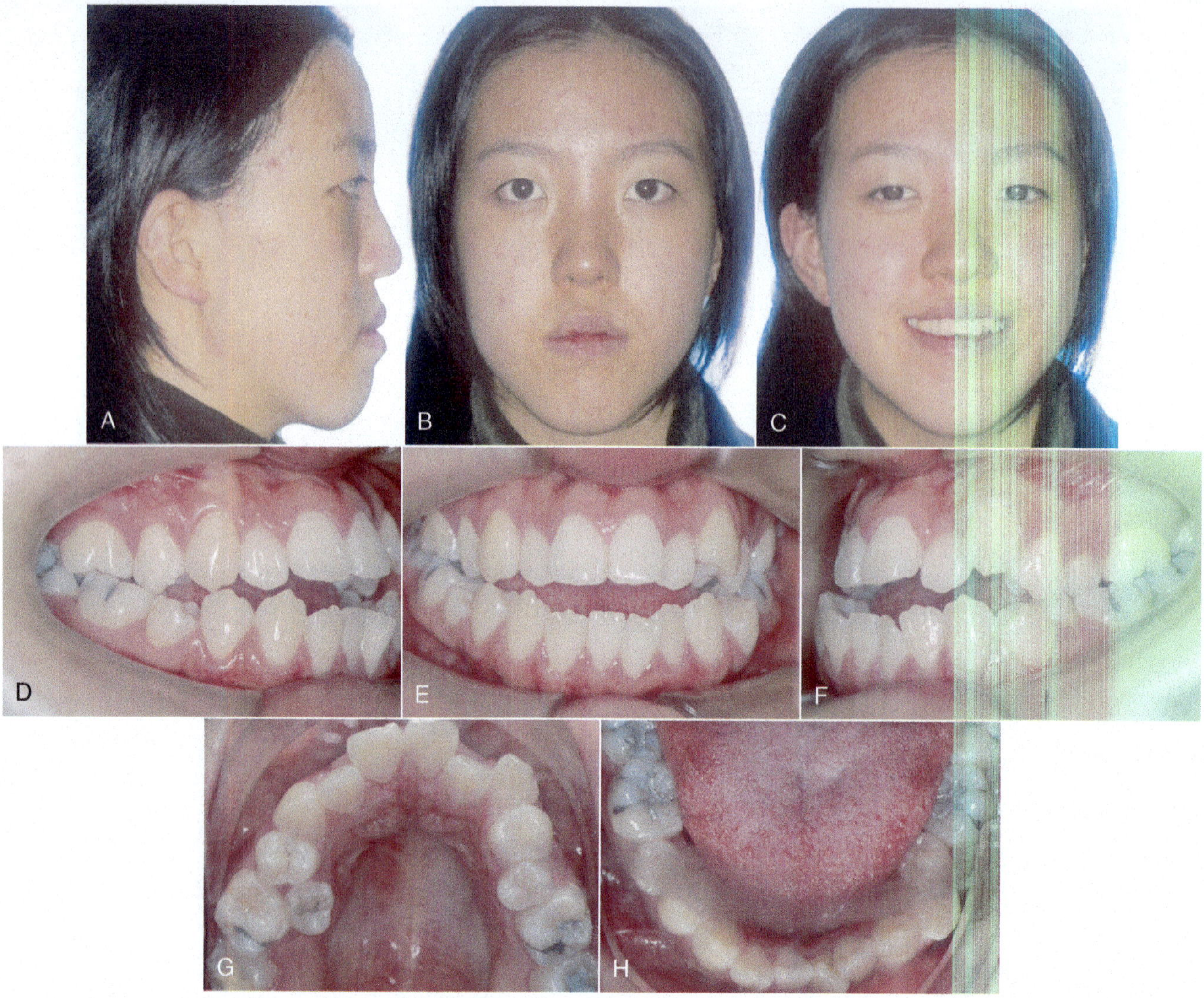

Figure 14-38 Pre-treatment (**A–C**) facial and (**D–H**) intraoral photographs of patient KG. Note that the #15 tooth is positioned palatally.

micro-implants for the retraction of lower dentition. Alternately, a mini-plate with a long hook could be used.[55]

Sequential Retraction

This option is preferred because it is easy to place micro-implants and manipulate the procedure. In general, micro-implants are placed between the second premolars and the first molars. Posterior teeth are moved distally using open coil springs that are compressed with ligature wire tied from the micro-implants to a sliding hook placed at the end of each coil spring. After posterior teeth are moved to a Class I molar relationship, micro-implants are removed and the same micro-implants are placed in the distal area and anterior teeth are retracted distally (Fig. 14-43).

The other method is to first move the canines with posterior teeth distally using coil springs or power chains from the micro-implants to the canines. Through that movement, the posterior teeth can be uprighted to gain space to align or retract the lower incisors (Figs. 14-44 to 14-47; Table 14-7).

TABLE 14-7 Cephalometric Measurements of Patient PJ Compared with the Korean Norms

	Norm		Patient PJ	
	Mean	SD	Pre	Post
ANB	1.5	1.8	−1.6	−1.6
FMA	23.8	5.3	24.4	24.3
Occ. pl. a.	4.6	4.1	5.9	4.2
U1 to FH	119.0	4.6	122.6	126.4
FMIA	65.8	7.0	71.5	77.5
IMPA	86.9	7.1	84.1	78.2
Z angle	75.0	2.0	90.6	89.9

ANB, A point nasion B point; *FH*, Frankfurt horizontal; *FMA*, Frankfurt mandibular plane angle; *FMIA*, Frankfurt mandibular incisal angle; *IMPA*, incisor mandibular plane angle; *Occ. pl. a.*, occlusal plane angle; *Post*, post-treatment; *Pre*, pre-treatment; *SD*, standard deviation; *U1*, upper incisor.

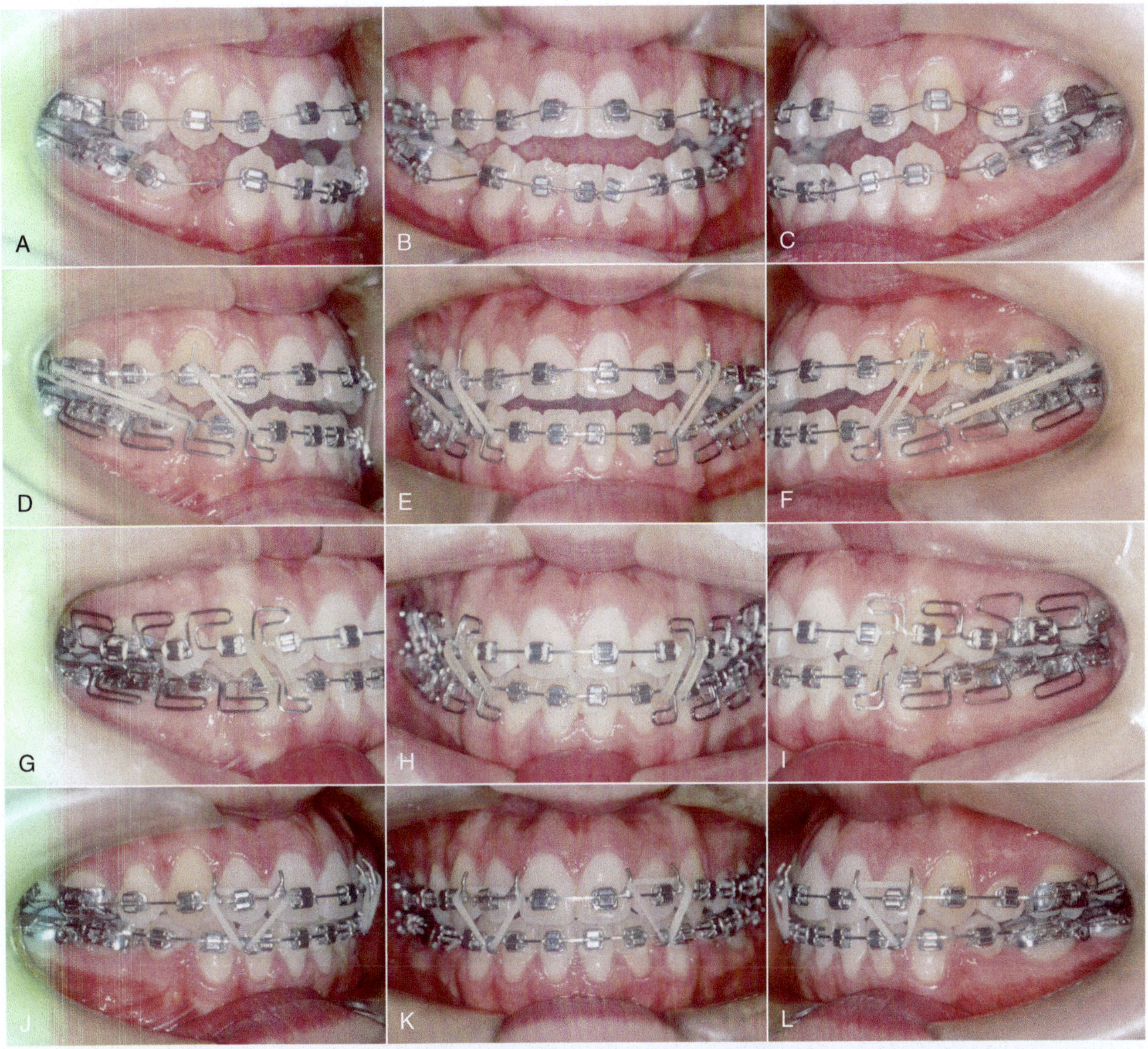

Figure 14-39 Treatment progress photographs of KG. **A–C,** Initial archwire was placed after fixed appliance was bonded and banded on upper and lower dentition. **D–F,** Stabilizing archwire was placed in upper arch and MEAW was placed in lower arch. **G–I,** Upper MEAW was placed to control upper molar tip and produce good interdigitation. **J–L,** Finishing of the ideal arch with intermaxillary elastics.

Problems. It is difficult to control the force direction to go above CR, because placing the head of the micro-implant close to the cervical area is challenging. If force can be directed below CR with low placement of micro-implant, then one can increase the occlusal plane angle due to the vertical force vector.

Upper Micro-Implant Anchorage

This option is our treatment protocol for high angle skeletal Class III malocclusion with open bite. Before development of the micro-implants, we had been using the MEAW technique for the treatment of high angle Class III cases with open bite. However, it had two problems. The MEAW technique requires complicated wire bending and very good patient compliance with full-time wearing of heavy elastics. As well, the treatment results in high angle cases showed some unfavorable effects, such as longer face with clockwise rotation of the mandible and too much extrusion of the upper and lower incisors due to Class III and vertical elastics (see Fig. 14-41, C). We had been thinking about simple options without using the MEAW technique and heavy intermaxillary elastics. First, we tried to place lower reverse-curved wires in the lower dentition instead of MEAW and applied Class III elastics and vertical elastics as in the MEAW technique. The results were almost the same as with the MEAW technique. However, there was extrusion of the first molar and slight flaring of upper incisors due to Class III elastics. Finally, we tried to use two upper maxillary

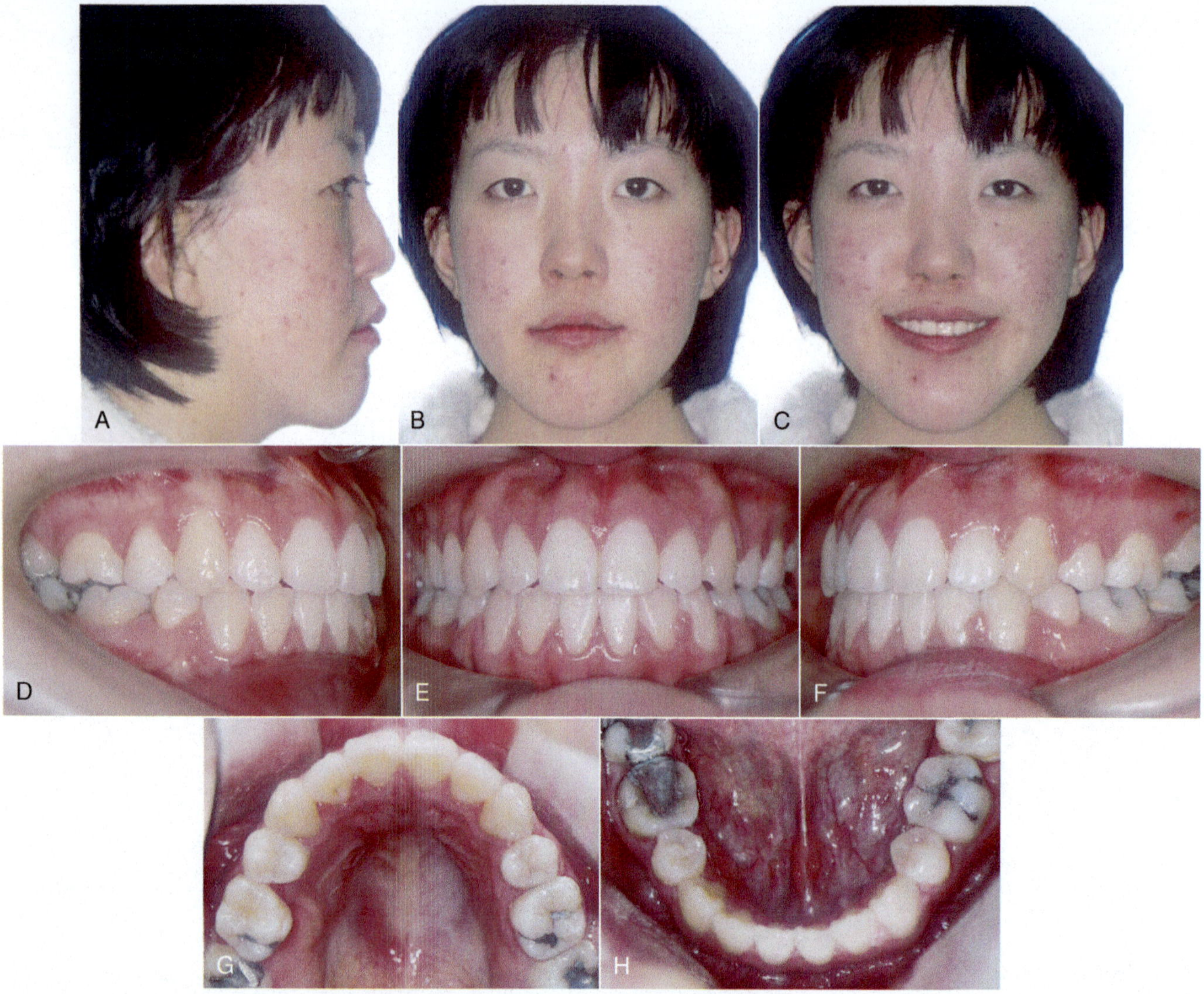

Figure 14-40 Post-treatment (**A–C**) facial and (**D–H**) intraoral photographs of KG.

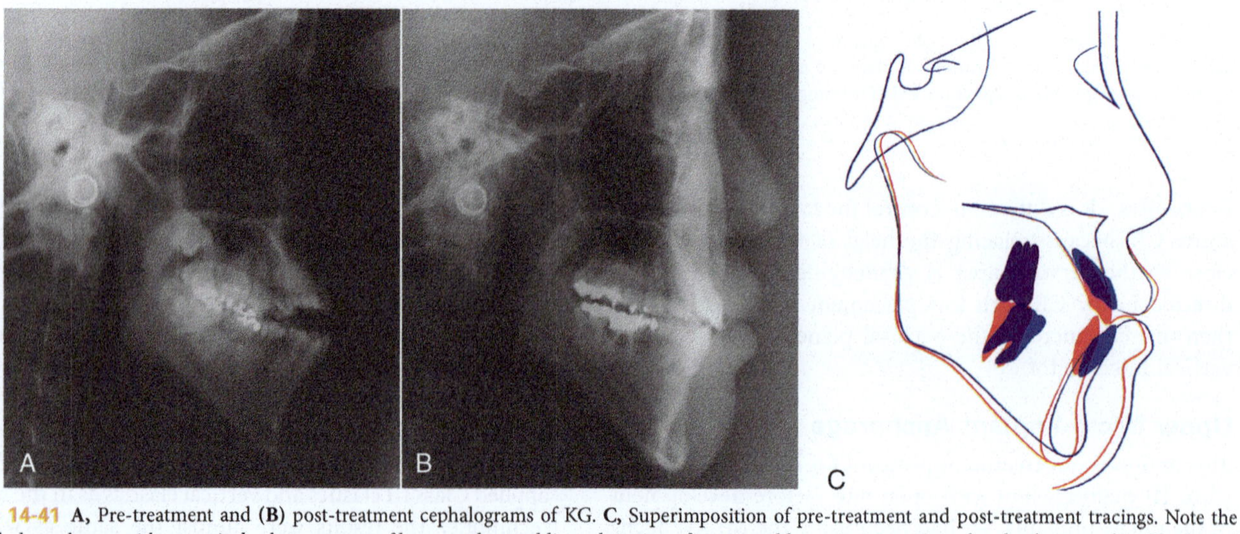

Figure 14-41 **A,** Pre-treatment and (**B**) post-treatment cephalograms of KG. **C,** Superimposition of pre-treatment and post-treatment tracings. Note the occlusal plane change with great tip-back movement of lower molars and lingual tipping of upper and lower incisors. Note also the downward and backward rotation of the mandible with elongated lower face.

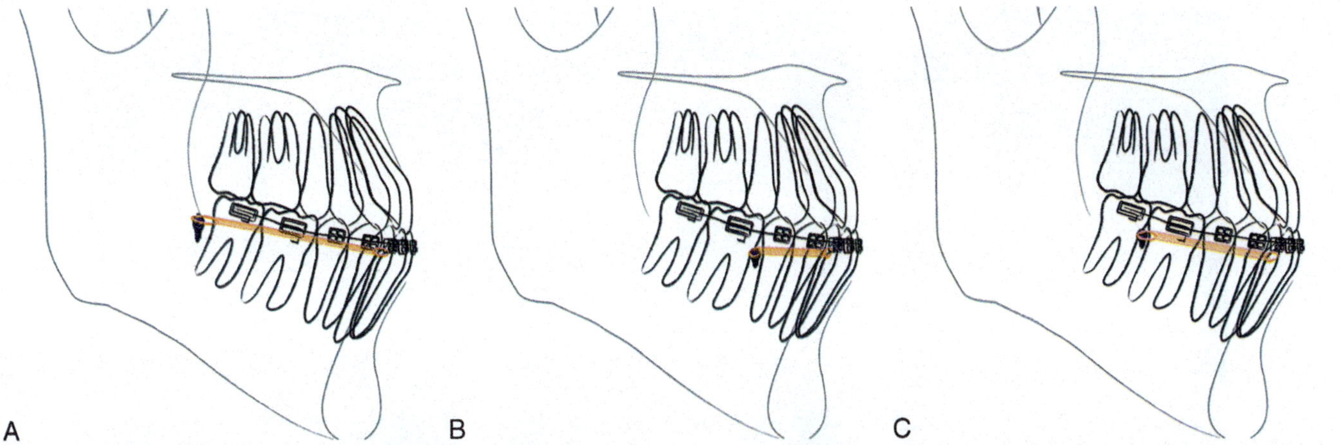

Figure 14-42 Various sites of lower micro-implant placement. **A,** Micro-implant in the retromolar area. **B,** Micro-implant in the interradicular space between first molars and second premolars. **C,** Implant in the interradicular space between the second and first molars.

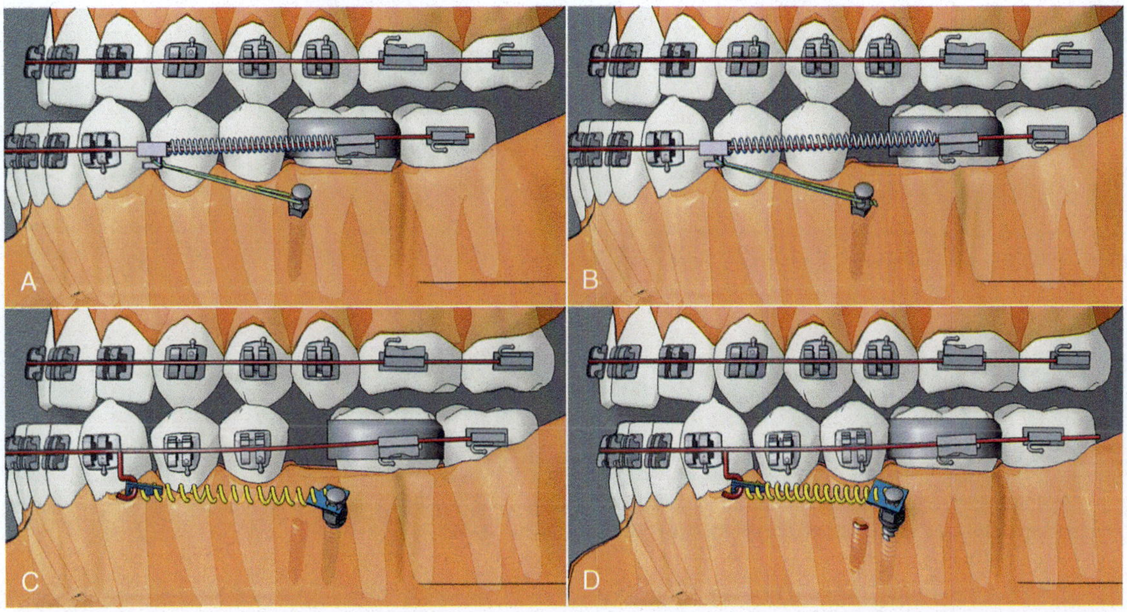

Figure 14-43 Sequential retraction. **A,** Distal movement of posterior teeth using open coil springs that are compressed with ligature tied from MIA to the sliding hook. **B,** Posterior teeth were moved distally to gain Class I molar relationship. **C,** MIA was relocated distally to retract anterior teeth. **D,** Final stage.

micro-implants instead of the first molars as anchorage for Class III elastics and place a very flexible Ni-Ti wire in the lower dentition instead of a MEAW. The results were very satisfactory.

The indications for upper MIA are mild skeletal Class III with high angle and open-bite cases that have mesially inclined lower posterior teeth.

Treatment Protocol (Figs. 14-19 to 14-48)

1. Place brackets on upper and lower arches by bonding or banding and insert an initial light archwire such as a 0.014-inch or 0.016-inch NiTi.
2. Place micro-implants with a 1.5-mm diameter and 7.0-mm length, Circular Head type (CH 1514-07, Dentos Inc., Daegu, Korea; Fig. 14-49, A) or Double Head type (DH 1514-07, Dentos Inc., Daegu, Korea; Fig. 14-49, B), between the upper second premolars and first molars.
3. Apply Class III elastics—3/8 inch, 5 oz. to 1/4-inch, 5 oz., depending on the teeth involved (canines or first premolars)—for 24 hours per day except at mealtimes.
4. Following the leveling stage, increase the archwire size from 0.014-inch Ni-Ti to 0.016-inch or 0.016-inch × 0.022-inch Ni-Ti or stainless steel.

Through uprighting of the posterior teeth with Class III elastics, some space between the lower incisor and canine might be created, which can be used for correction of anterior crossbite and arch length discrepancy.

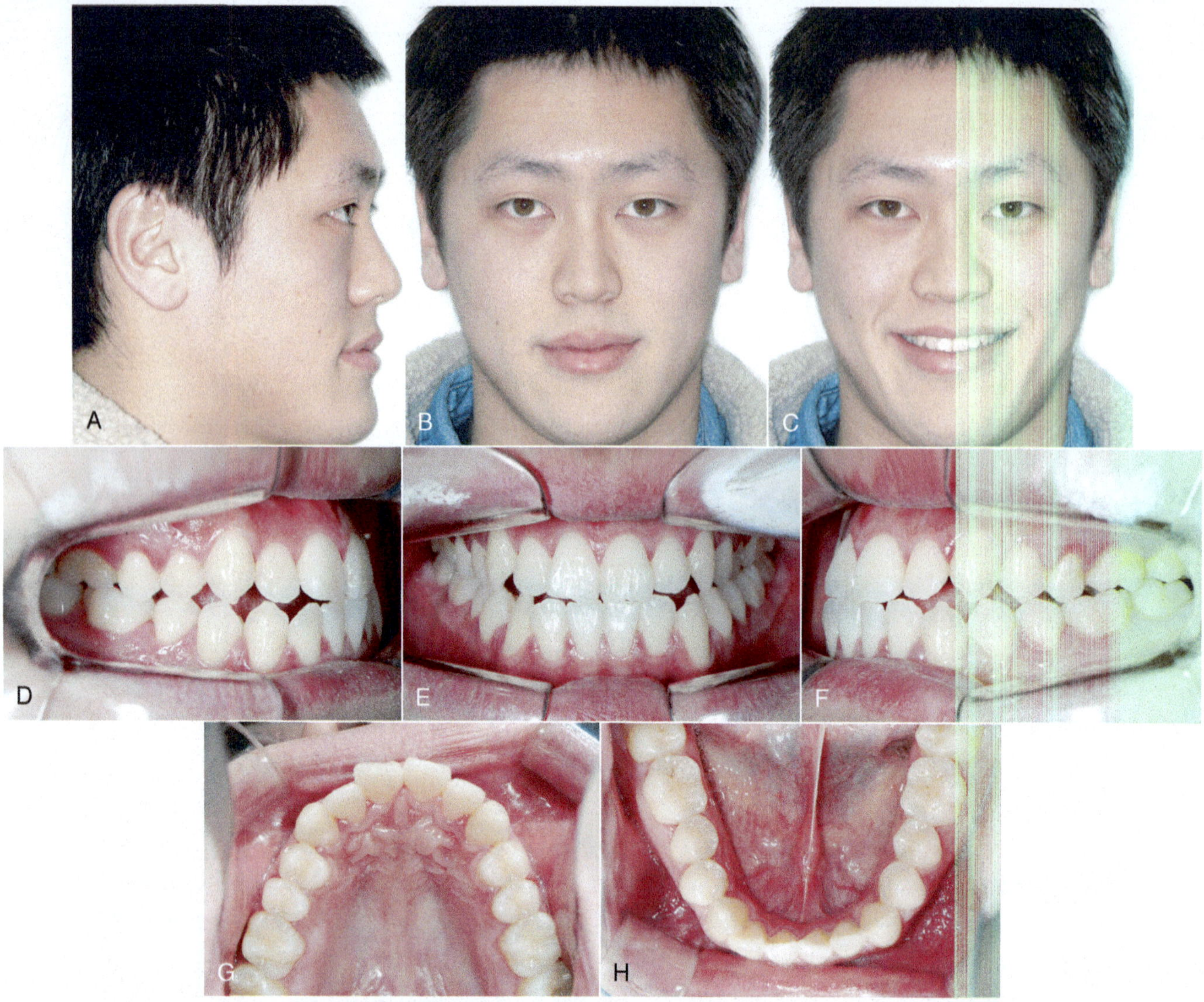

Figure 14-44 Pre-treatment facial photographs of patient PJ showing only chin prominence (**A-C**) of patient PJ. Intraoral photographs showing mild Class III canine and molar relationships and slight crowding in the upper and lower arches (**D-H**).

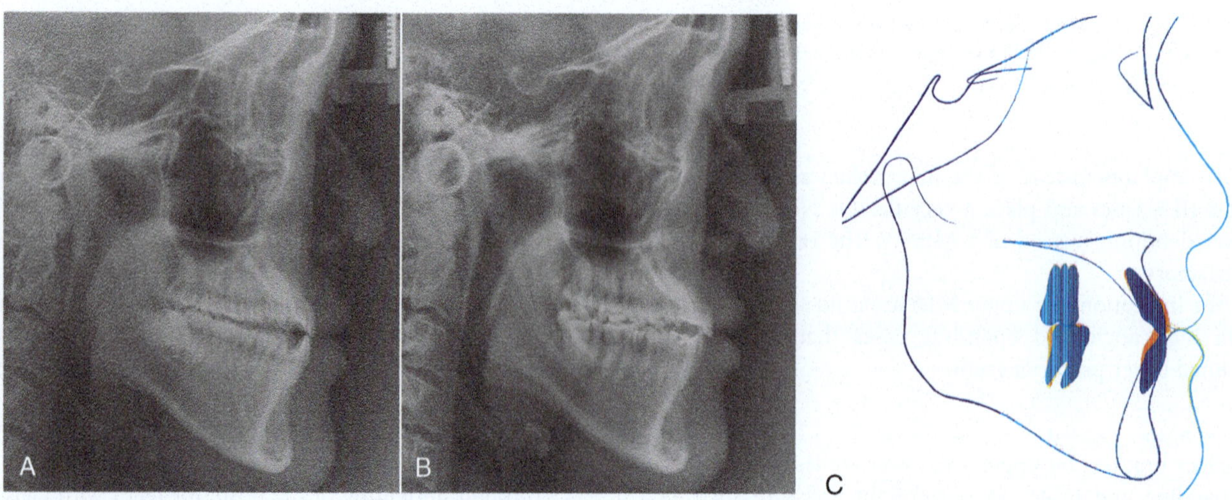

Figure 14-45 **A,** Pre-treatment and (**B**) post-treatment cephalograms of patient PJ. **C,** Superimposition of the pre- and post-treatment radiographs of patient PJ.

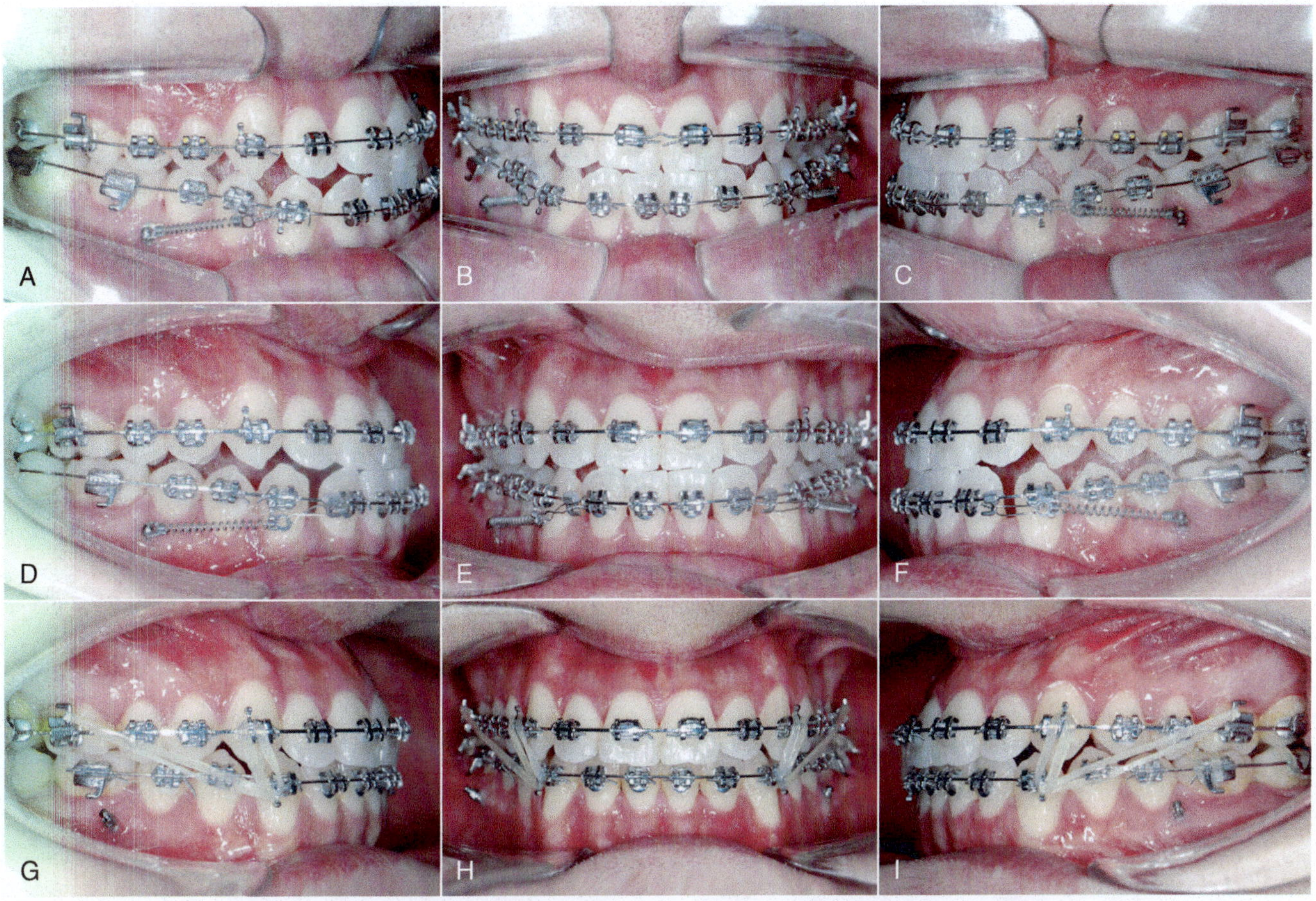

Figure 14-46 Treatment progress photographs of patient PJ. **A–C,** A nickel-titanium (Ni-Ti) coil spring applied from the micro-implant to canine in order to first move the posterior teeth distally. **D–F,** The lower incisor is retracted using a coil spring from the micro-implant to hook between the lateral incisor and canine. **G–I,** Lower occlusal plane closed with vertical and Class III elastics.

Biomechanics

The biomechanics involved in upper MIA is a simple tip-back mechanism produced by Class III elastics from micro-implant anchorage to the canine or premolar of the lower dentition.

Figure 14-50, A, shows a force system where a resilient wire of small dimension is placed within the brackets of mesially inclined lower posterior teeth. The force should be analyzed in each pair of teeth based on Burstone's geometry.[56] It can be classified as Class I or Class II of Burstone's six basic two-tooth movement geometries. The moment and force of each pair of posterior teeth can be analyzed sequentially in the following order: the second and first molars, the first molar and second premolar, the second and first premolars, and the first premolar and canine. In each pair of teeth the posterior tooth will show an extrusive force and tip-back moment while the mesial tooth will show intrusive force and tip-back moment.[56,57] The same force and moment will be shown in all pairs of teeth. As a result, all teeth except the terminal molar and canine will have tip-back moment without force due to canceling each other out. Finally, the second molar will have an extrusive force and tip-back moment while the canine will have intrusive force and tip-back moment. Therefore, without any other force involved, the lower occlusal plane will tip down anteriorly.

However, if an upward and backward force is applied to the canine or first premolar as in Figure 14-50, B, all posterior teeth will be uprighted and retracted and the lower occlusal plane will be flattened upward; therefore the lower occlusal plane will become parallel with the upper occlusal plane. This mechanism can be very effective in the correction of Class III cases with open bite.

After leveling and placement of a heavy rectangular archwire, the lower arch will act as one body. If the Class III elastic force is applied continuously, the lower dentition will rotate counterclockwise around the center of resistance (Fig. 14-50, C). As a result, the lower occlusal plane will be flattened and sometimes posterior disclusion is created. In addition, Class III force might give some retraction force to the whole mandible.

CASE REPORTS

For a better understanding of the use of micro-implants to treat Class III malocclusion, three cases are presented here.

Text continued on p. 292

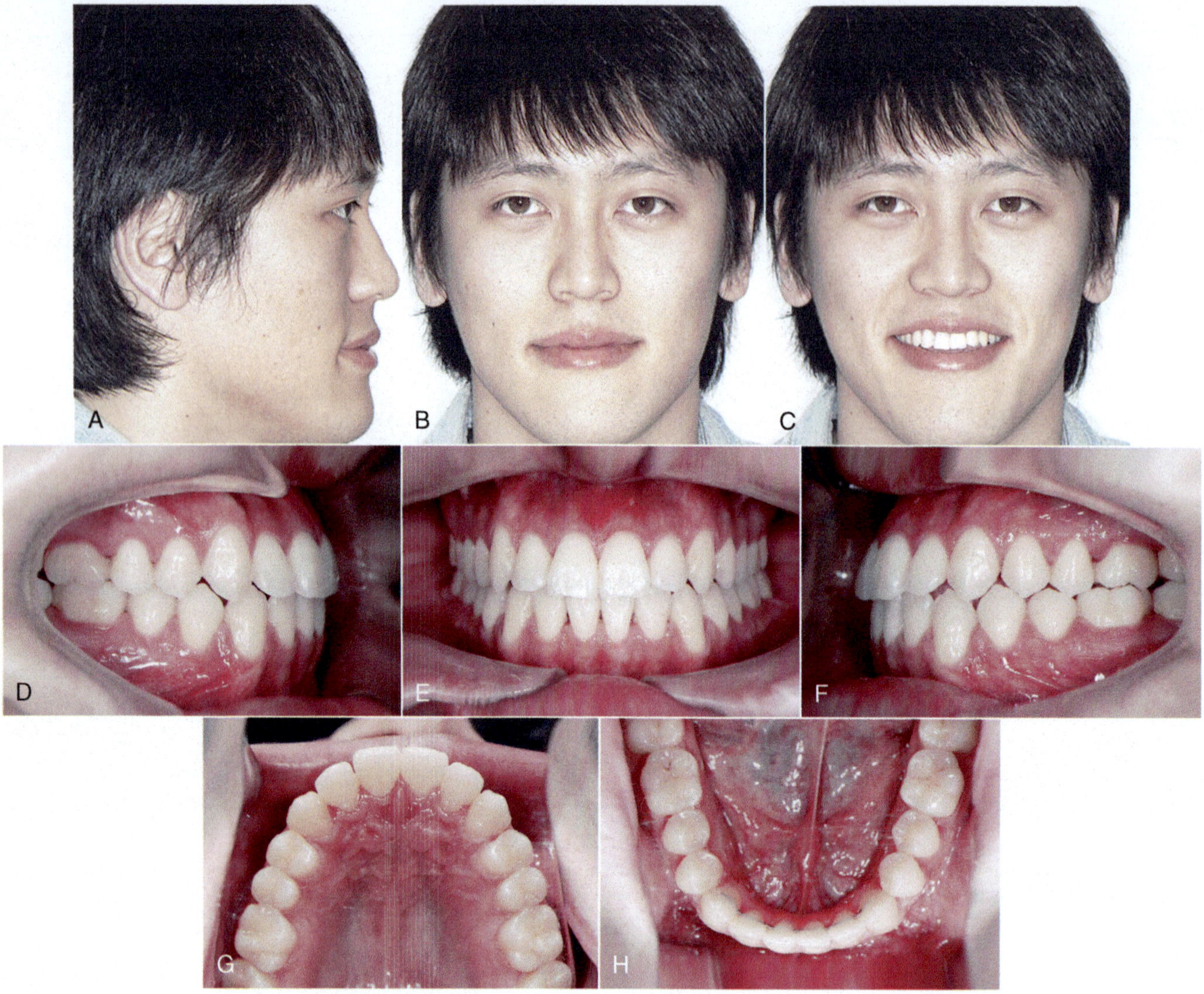

Figure 14-47 Post-treatment (**A–C**) facial and (**D–H**) intraoral photographs of patient PJ.

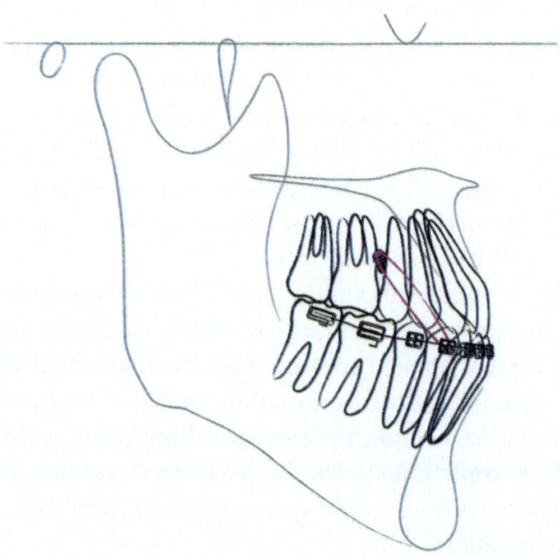

Figure 14-48 Treatment protocol for upper micro-implant anchorage (MIA). Brackets are placed on the upper and lower arches by bonding or banding and then a 0.014-inch nickel-titanium (Ni-Ti) wire is placed. Two micro-implants are placed between upper second premolars and first molars. Class III elastics (3/8 inch, 5 oz. or 5/16 inch, 5 oz.) are run from the micro-implants to the lower canines or first premolars (depending on the case).

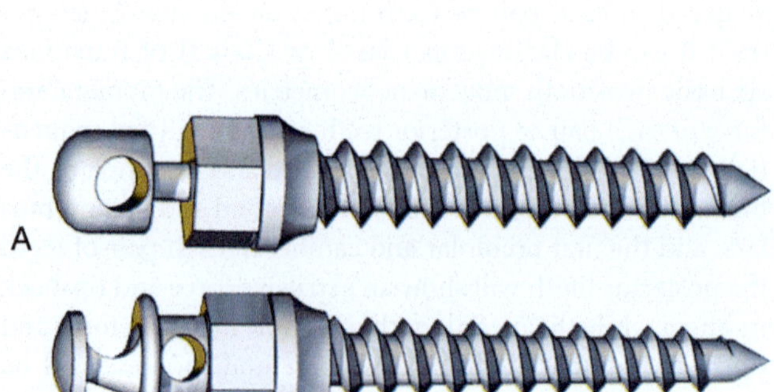

Figure 14-49 Micro-implants with a diameter of 15 mm at the neck of the micro-implant and a 7-mm length of the screw part are recommended. **A,** Circular Head type (CH 1514-07, Dentos Inc., Daegu, Korea). **B,** Double Head type (DH 1514-07, Dentos Inc., Daegu, Korea).

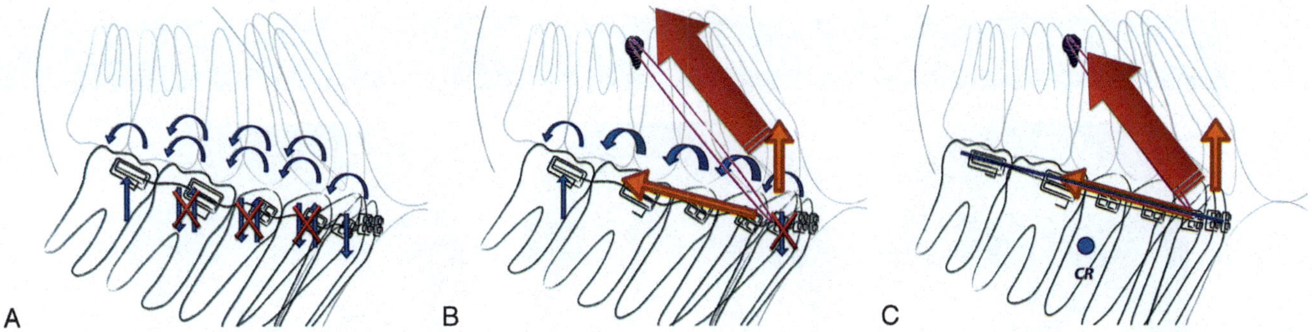

Figure 14-50 **A,** Force system in which the initial archwire is placed in brackets of mesially inclined lower posterior teeth. **B,** Class III elastics are applied on the canines; all posterior teeth will have distal tip-back moments and incisors will have extrusion force. **C,** When the archwire size is increased after leveling, the lower dentition will act as one body. The lower occlusal plane will rotate counterclockwise around the center of resistance (CR) if Class III elastics are used continuously.

CASE REPORT 1

A 35-year-old female patient, PK, presented with a soft tissue profile that was esthetically acceptable according to Korean standards. The frontal view showed slight deviation of the chin to the right. However, her dentition showed many problems, such as Class III molar and canine relationship, edge-to-edge bite with anterior open bite, and mesially tipped lower posterior teeth. The upper dentition had a very slight discrepancy and the lower dentition had 4.3-mm of crowding (Fig. 14-51). Cephalometric measurements before treatment were an ANB angle of 0.2, an FMA of 29.3, Frankfurt Horizontal (FH) to upper incisors of 122.7, incisor mandibular plane angle (IMPA) of 96.5, and Frankfurt Mandibular Incisal Angle (FMIA) of 54.2. The diagnosis was mild skeletal Class III with open bite (Fig. 14-52; Table 14-8).

TABLE 14-8 Cephalometric Measurements of Patient PK

	Mean	SD	Pre	Post
ANB	2.8	2.3	0.2	1.6
FMA	25.4	6.1	29.4	29.7
Occ. pl. a.	5.9	4.6	12.6	11.4
U1 to FH	116.6	5.7	122.6	118.6
FMIA	64.8	7.2	54.2	64.3
IMPA	87.3	6.8	96.5	86.0
Z angle	77.0	2.0	79.1	78.9

ANB, A point nasion B point; *FH,* Frankfurt horizontal; *FMA,* Frankfurt mandibular plane angle; *FMIA,* Frankfurt mandibular incisal angle; *IMPA,* incisor mandibular plane angle; *Occ. pl. a.,* occlusal plane angle; *Post,* post-treatment; *Pre,* pre-treatment; *SD,* standard deviation; *U1,* upper incisor.

All teeth were bonded and a 0.014-inch Ni-Ti archwire was placed as an initial archwire. Two micro-implants were placed on the maxilla between the second premolars and first molars. Then Class III elastics were applied immediately from the micro-implants to the lower first premolars. The patient was directed to wear the elastics 24 hours per day except at mealtimes (Fig. 14-53, A–C). The patient was checked every 4 weeks for changes in the dentition. After the leveling stage and achieving the uprighting of the posterior teeth, the archwire size was increased to 0.016-inch × 0.022-inch stainless steel in the lower arch. After 6 months of treatment the patient showed a good occlusion, corrected overbite, good interdigitation, and a Class I molar and canine relationship (Fig. 14-53, D–E). However, the patient complained that her dental midline did not coincide with her facial midline. She wanted her dental midline shifted slightly to the left in order to coincide with her facial midline. Therefore an effort was made to move the upper dentition to the left with Ni-Ti closed coil springs from the left micro-implant to the hook of the archwire; the lower dentition was moved simultaneously to the left with Class III elastics (Fig. 14-53, G–I). The patient was satisfied with the results after an additional 6 months of treatment (Fig. 14-54). The case was finished after 15 months of active treatment.

The superimposition of cephalometric radiographs before and after treatment (Fig. 14-55) showed tremendous molar distal movement and tip back along with lingual tipping and extrusion of lower incisors due to Class III elastic force. The occlusal plane angle was decreased. Slight retraction of the mandible was shown, which might be a result of the Class III elastics. Stable results were shown after 27 months of retention (Fig. 14-56).

Continued

CASE REPORT 1—cont'd

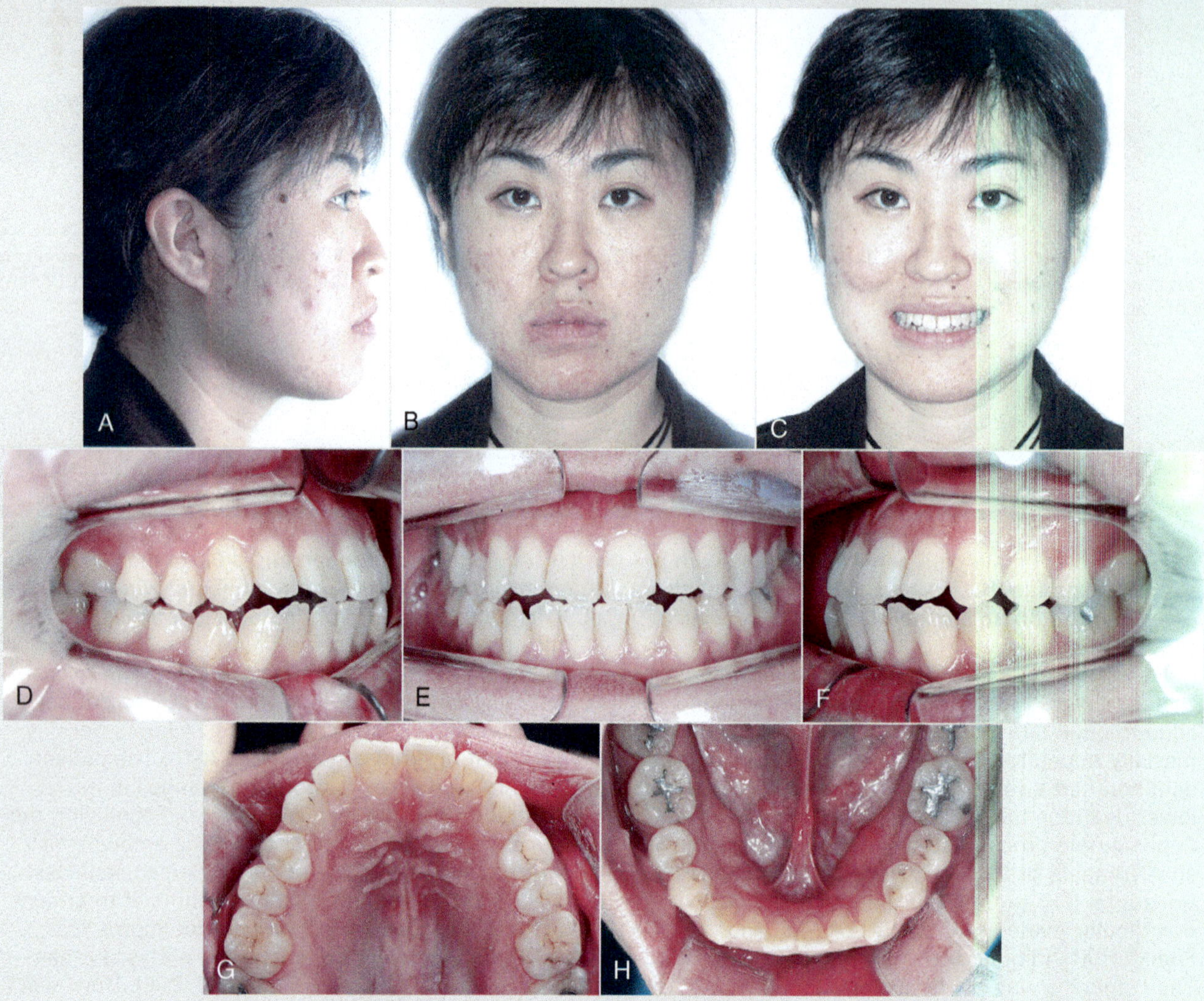

Figure 14-51 Pre-treatment (A–C) facial and (D–H) intraoral photographs of patient PK.

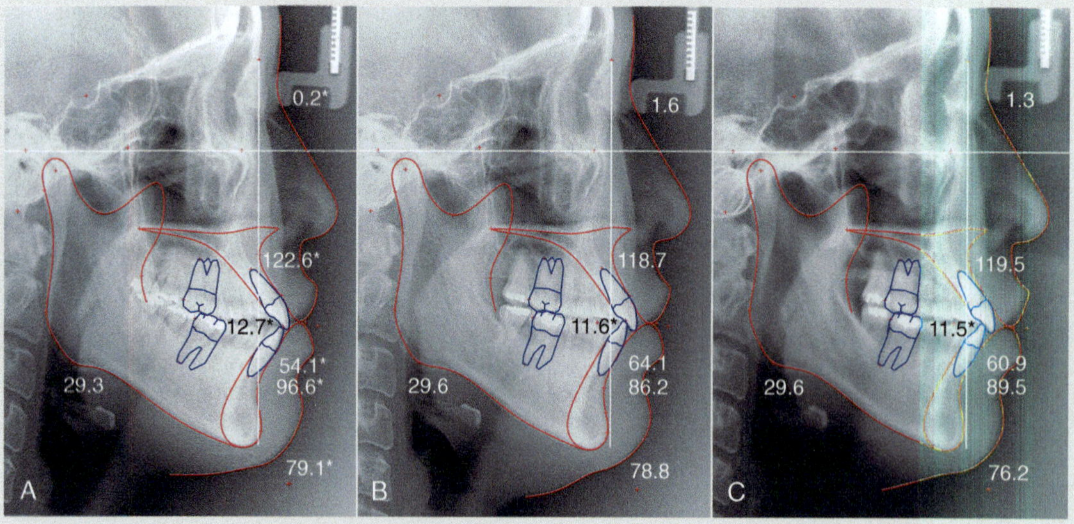

Figure 14-52 A, Pre-treatment and (B) post-treatment cephalometric radiographs and tracings of PK. C, Retention. Note the difference in the occlusal plane and molar inclination between pre-treatment and post-treatment images.

CASE REPORT 1—cont'd

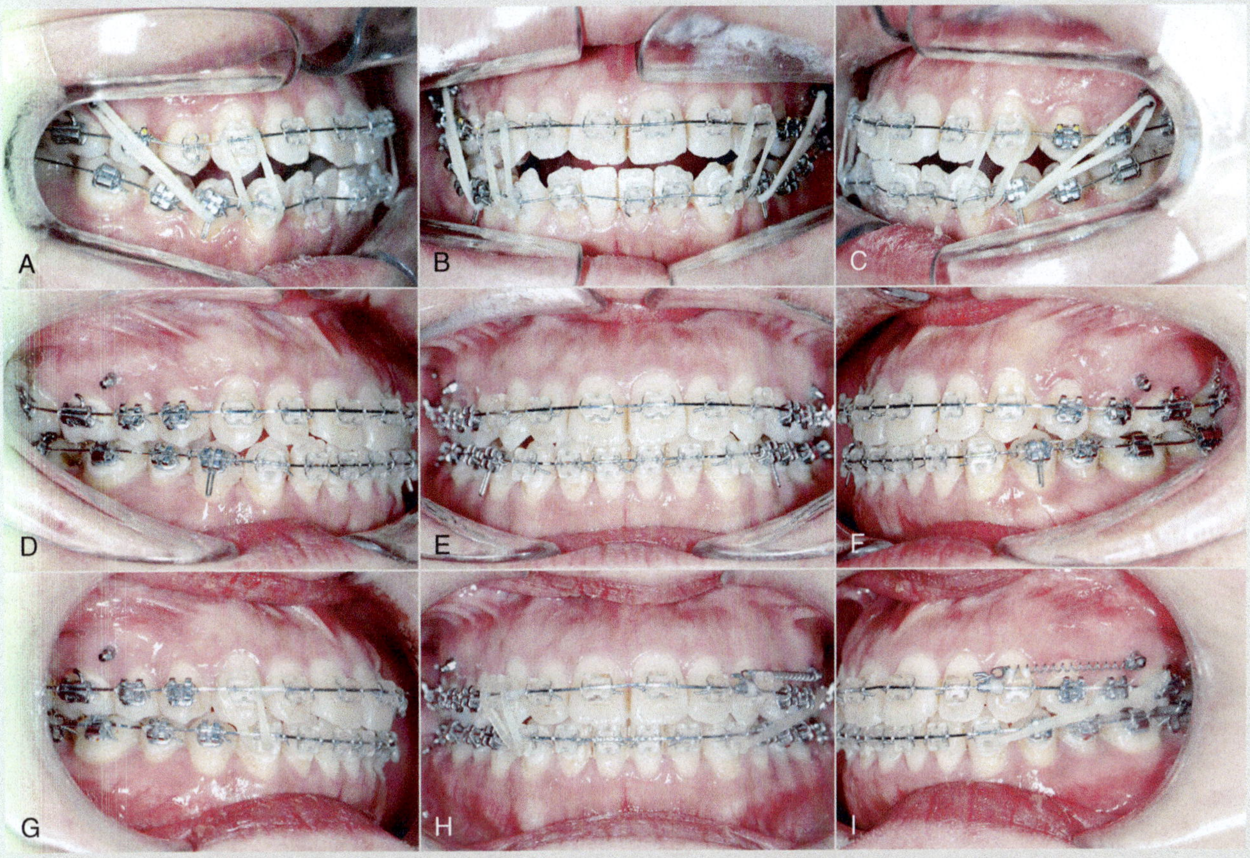

Figure 14-53 Treatment progress photographs of PK. **A–C,** Initial stage: 0.014-inch nickel-titanium (Ni-Ti) archwire, Class III elastics (3/8 inch, 5 oz.), and vertical elastics (3/16 inch, 5 oz.). **D–F,** After 6 months of treatment. **G–I,** The upper midline was shifted to the left using a Ni-Ti closed coil spring, which ran from the micro-implant to hooks placed on upper arch. The lower midline was shifted to the left simultaneously using Class III elastics.

Continued

CASE REPORT 1—cont'd

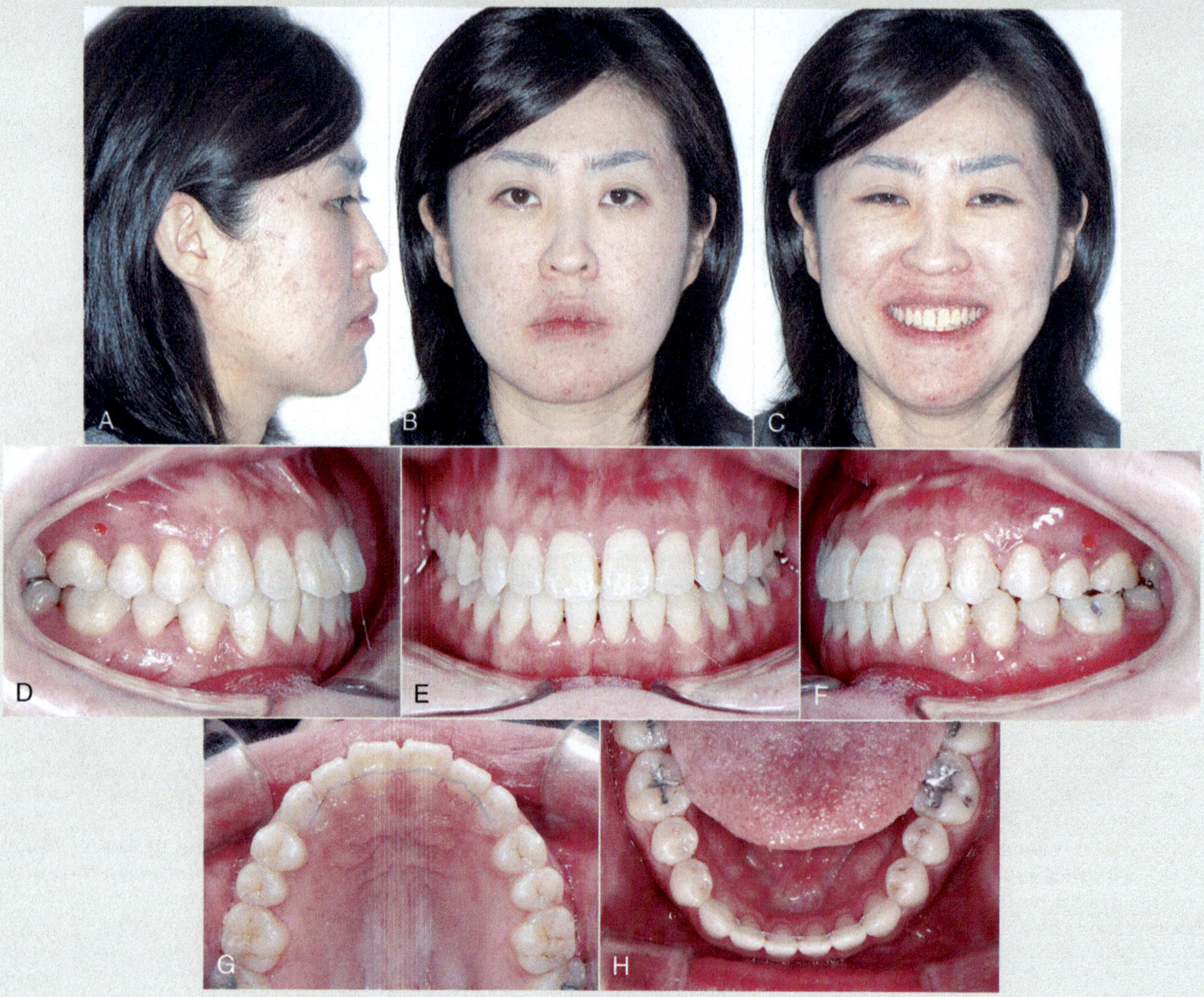

Figure 14-54 Post-treatment **(A–C)** facial and **(D–H)** intraoral photographs of PK.

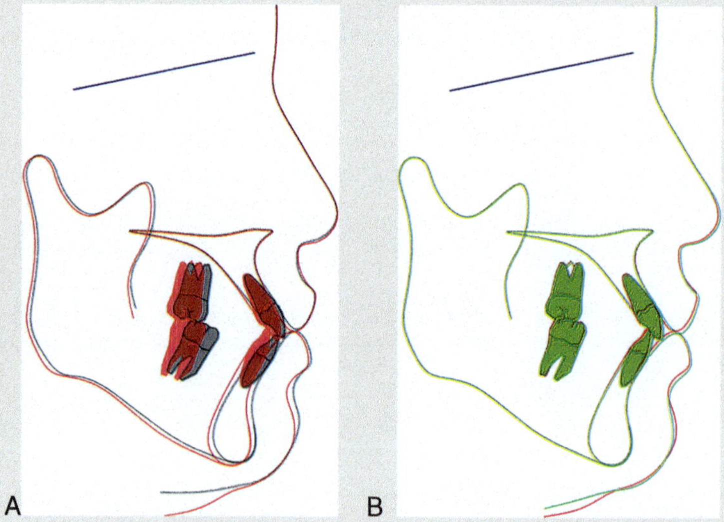

Figure 14-55 A, Superimposition of pre-treatment and post-treatment findings for PK. Note the distal movement of the lower molars, with uprighting and lingual movement of the lower incisors. The upper dentition was retracted through reaction force to correct the midline. There was a little retraction of mandible. **B,** Superimposition of post-treatment and 2-year post-treatment findings. Note that there have been no significant changes during the 2-year retention period.

CASE REPORT 1—cont'd

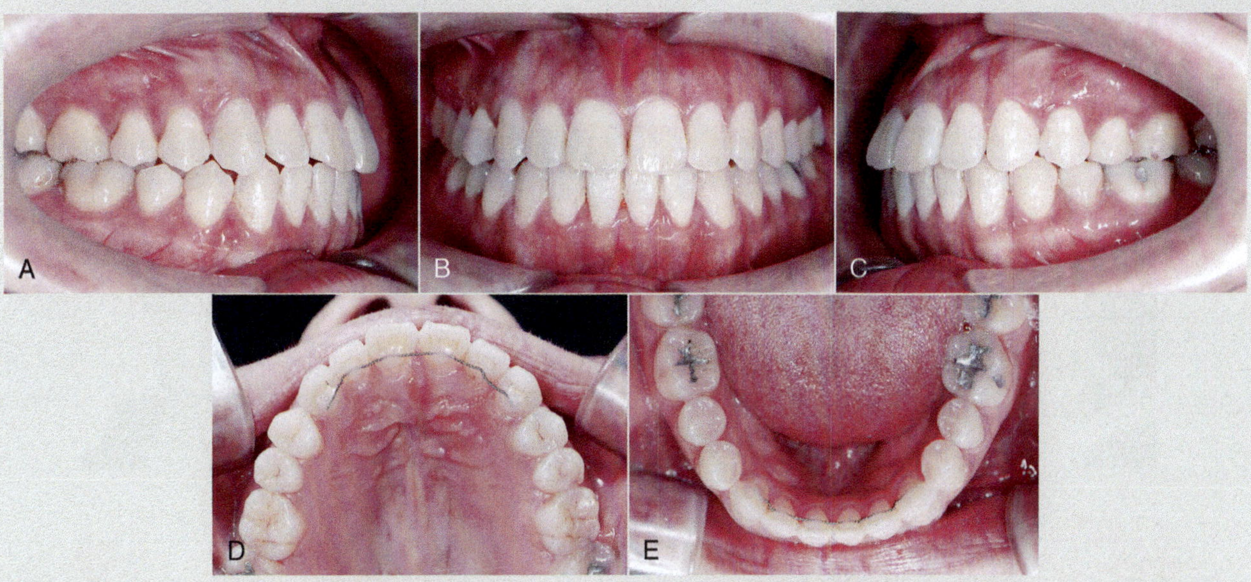

Figure 14-56 **A–E,** Two-year post-treatment intraoral photographs of PK.

CASE REPORT 2

A 23-year-old male patient, CW, presented with a profile that showed slight lower lip protrusion and a long face. The frontal view showed facial asymmetry and canting of occlusion. The intraoral photographs showed a Class III molar and canine relationship, anterior crossbite and open bite, lower midline shift to the right of 2.5-mm, and slight crowding of both arches (Fig. 14-57). The diagnosis was skeletal Class III with open bite (ANB angle −2.0, FMA 26.8, U1 to FH 121.7, IMPA 76.5, FMIA 77.2; Fig. 14-58 and Table 14-9). The occlusion showed that all posterior teeth in the lower arch were mesially tipped including the canines. Class III elastics were applied from the upper posterior teeth to the lower canine. The mechanics in Case Report I were used for this patient (Figs. 14-59 to 14-62). Total treatment took 15 months.

TABLE 14-9 Cephalometric Measurements of Patient CW

	Mean	SD	Pre	Post
ANB	1.5	1.8	−1.9	−1.2
FMA	23.8	5.3	26.3	26.8
Occ. pl. a.	4.6	4.1	5.1	2.4
U1 to FH	119.0	4.6	121.7	125.7
FMIA	65.8	7.0	77.3	78.0
IMPA	86.9	7.1	76.5	75.2
Z angle	75.0	2.0	77.9	82.5

ANB, A point nasion B point; *FH,* Frankfurt horizontal; *FMA,* Frankfurt mandibular plane angle; *FMIA,* Frankfurt mandibular incisal angle; *IMPA,* incisor mandibular plane angle; *Occ. pl. a.,* occlusal plane angle; *Post,* post-treatment; *Pre,* pre-treatment; *SD,* standard deviation; *U1,* upper incisor.

Continued

CASE REPORT 2—cont'd

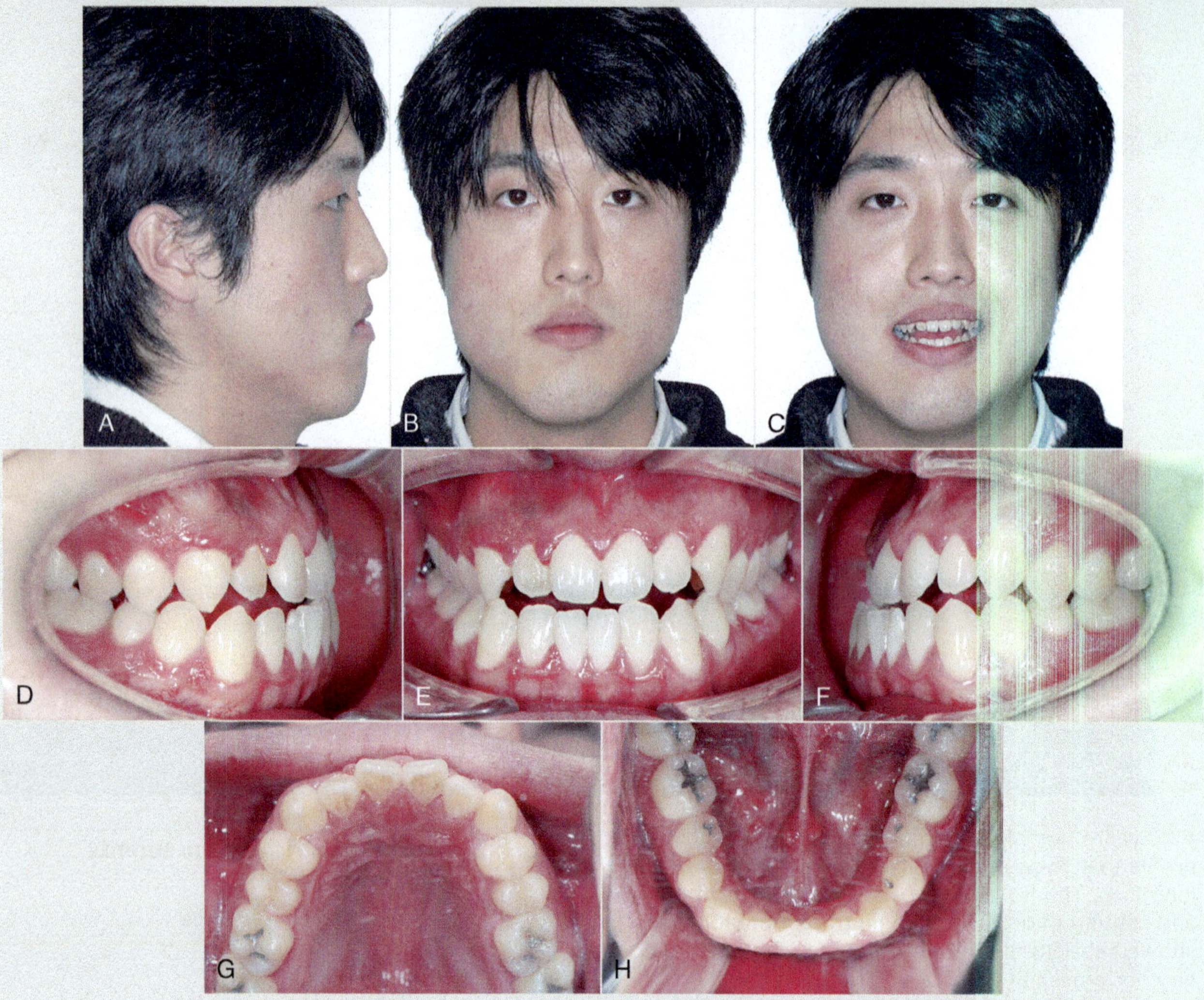

Figure 14-57 Pre-treatment (**A–C**) facial and (**D–H**) intraoral photographs of patient CW.

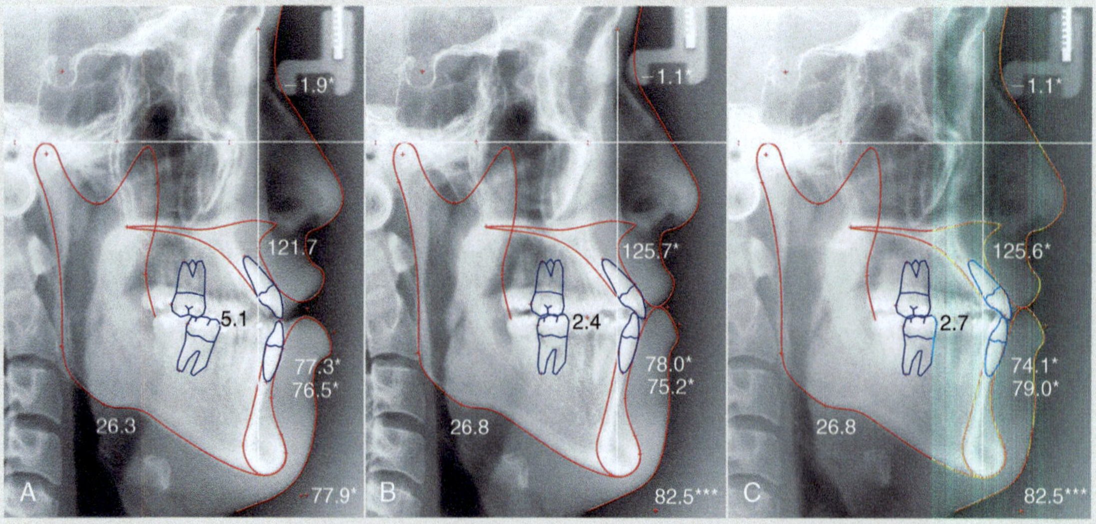

Figure 14-58 **A,** Pre-treatment and (**B**) post-treatment cephalometric radiographs and tracings of CW. **C,** Case retention showing good skeletal, dental, and soft tissue changes.

CASE REPORT 2—cont'd

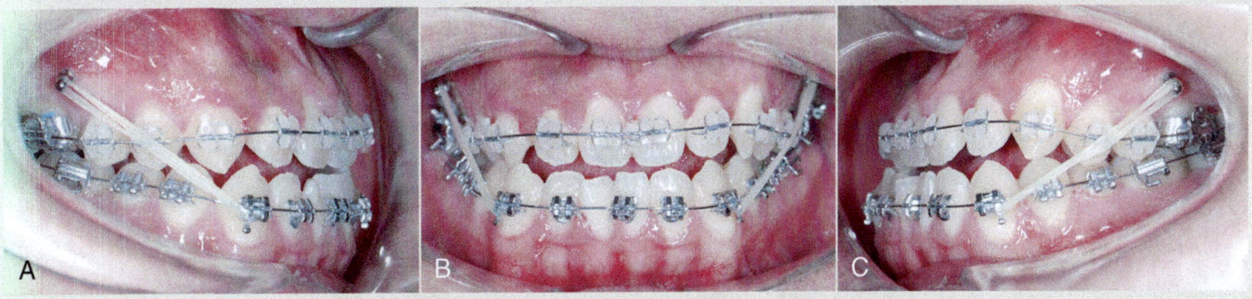

Figure 14-59 **A–C,** Treatment progress intraoral photographs of CW.

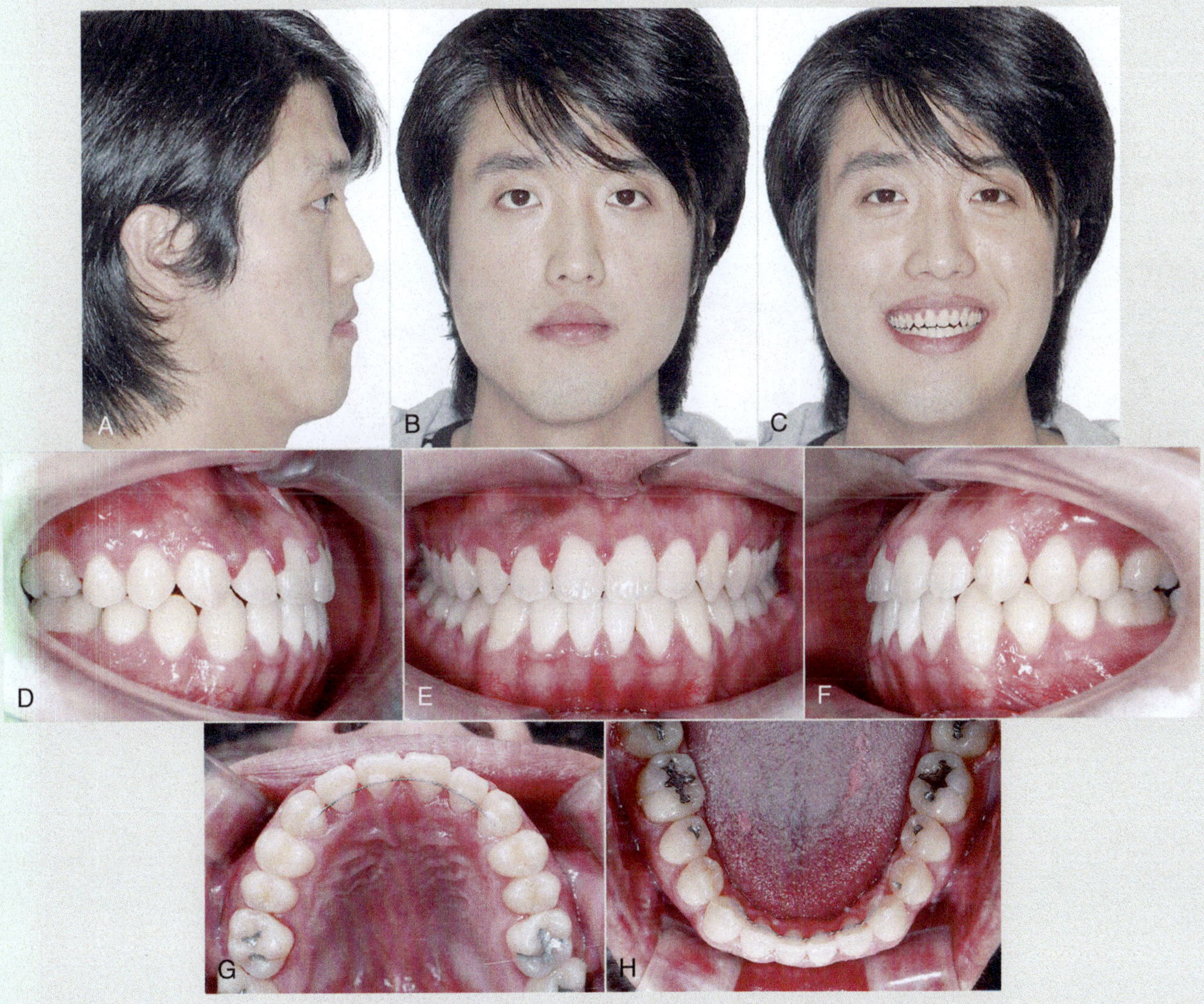

Figure 14-60 Post-treatment **(A–C)** facial and **(D–H)** intraoral photographs of CW.

Continued

CASE REPORT 2—cont'd

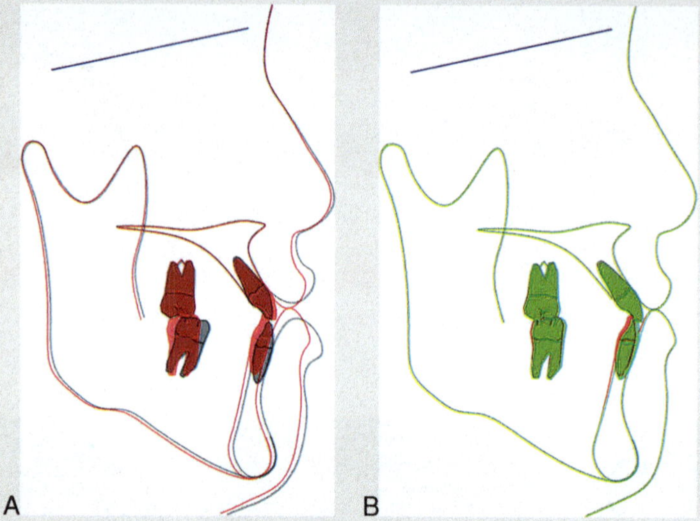

Figure 14-61 **A,** Superimposition of pre-treatment and post-treatment findings for CW. Note the great uprighting of the molars, the changes in the occlusal plane, and the retraction of the mandible after treatment. **B,** Superimposition of post-treatment and 2-year post-treatment findings. No significant changes are noted during retention.

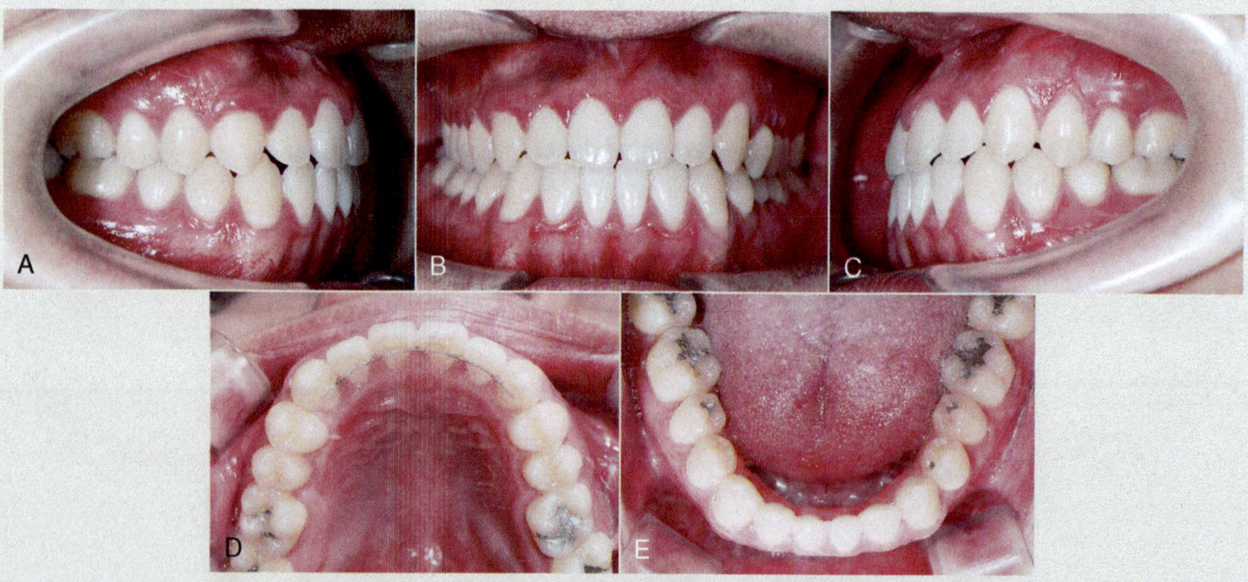

Figure 14-62 **A–E,** Two-year post-treatment intraoral photographs of CW.

CASE REPORT 3

A 24-year-old female patient, PY, presented with chief complaints of a protruded lower lip and an anterior open bite with severe crossbite (Fig. 14-63). The patient rejected surgical correction and wanted camouflage treatment. Mechanics similar to those used in Case Reports 1 and 2 were applied for this patient (Figs. 14-64 to 14-68 and Table 14-10). After 29 months of treatment, final results were achieved (see Fig. 14-66).

TABLE 14-10 Cephalometric Measurements of Patient PY

	Mean	SD	Pre	Post
ANB	2.8	2.3	0.4	1.3
FMA	25.4	6.1	32.9	33.7
Occ. pl. a.	5.9	4.6	11.9	5.7
U1 to FH	116.6	5.7	108.6	121.0
FMIA	64.8	7.2	60.1	75.3
IMPA	87.3	6.8	87.0	71.0
Z angle	77.0	2.0	60.7	65.0

ANB, A point nasion B point; *FH,* Frankfurt horizontal; *FMA,* Frankfurt mandibular plane angle; *FMIA,* Frankfurt mandibular incisal angle; *IMPA,* incisor mandibular plane angle; *Occ. pl. a.,* occlusal plane angle; *Post,* post-treatment; *Pre,* pre-treatment; *SD,* standard deviation; *U1,* upper incisor.

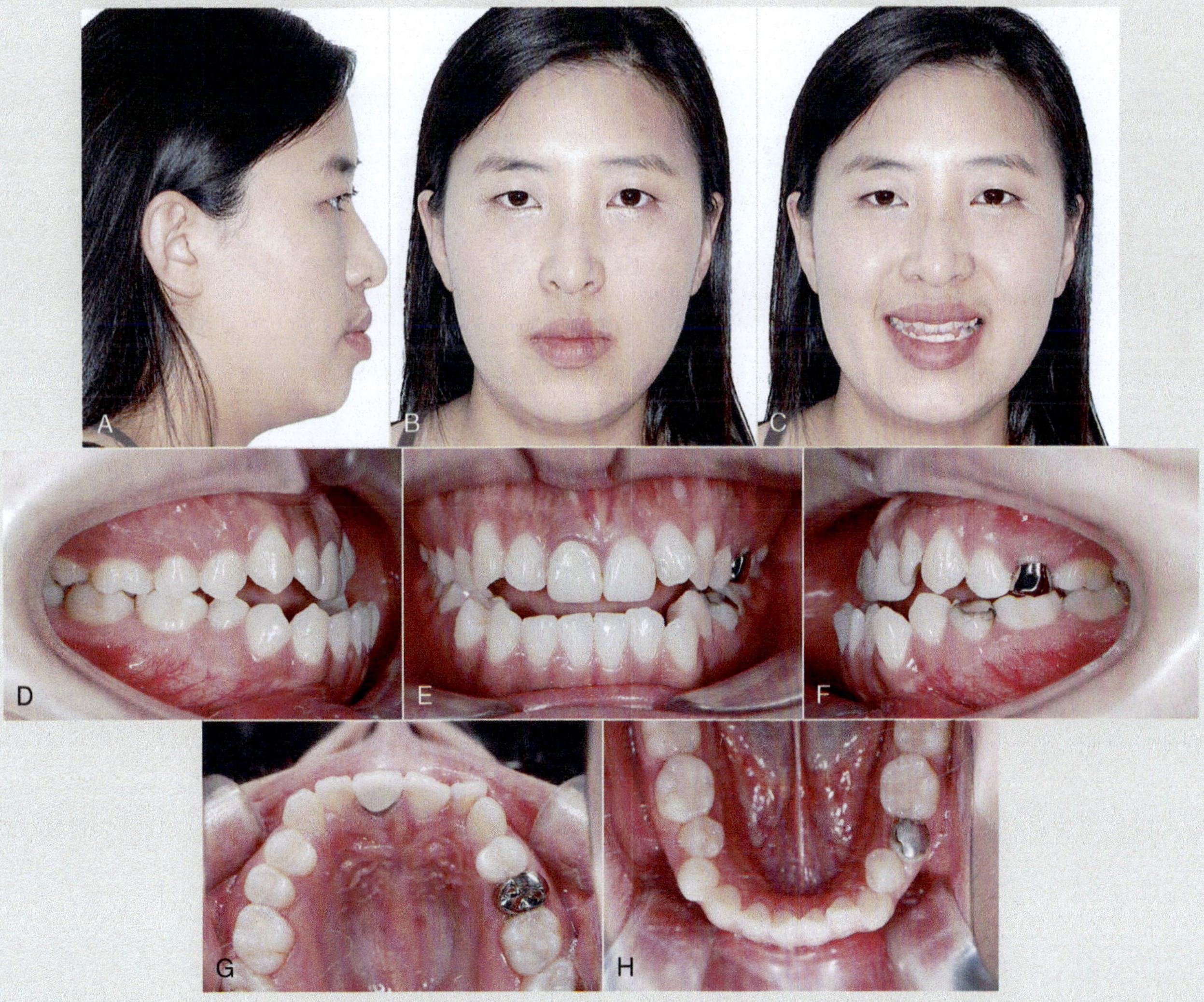

Figure 14-63 Pre-treatment **(A–C)** facial and **(D–H)** intraoral photographs of patient PY.

Continued

CASE REPORT 3—cont'd

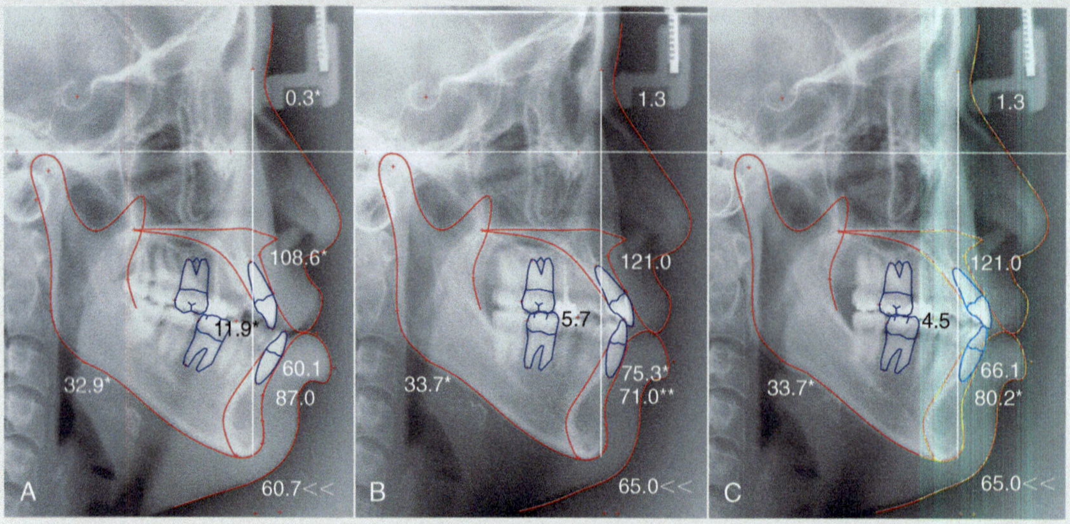

Figure 14-64 **A,** Pre-treatment and **(B)** post-treatment cephalometric radiographs and tracings of PY. **C,** Retention. Note the changes in the occlusal plane and the inclination of posterior teeth in the post-treatment cephalometric radiograph.

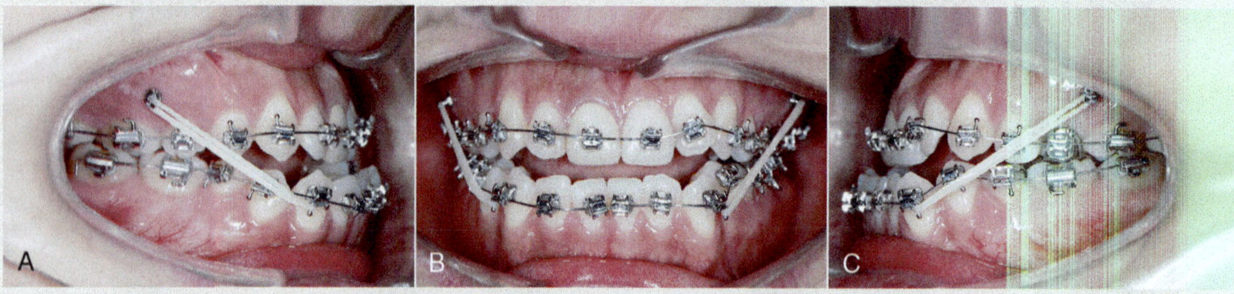

Figure 14-65 **A–C,** Treatment progress photographs of PY.

CASE REPORT 3—cont'd

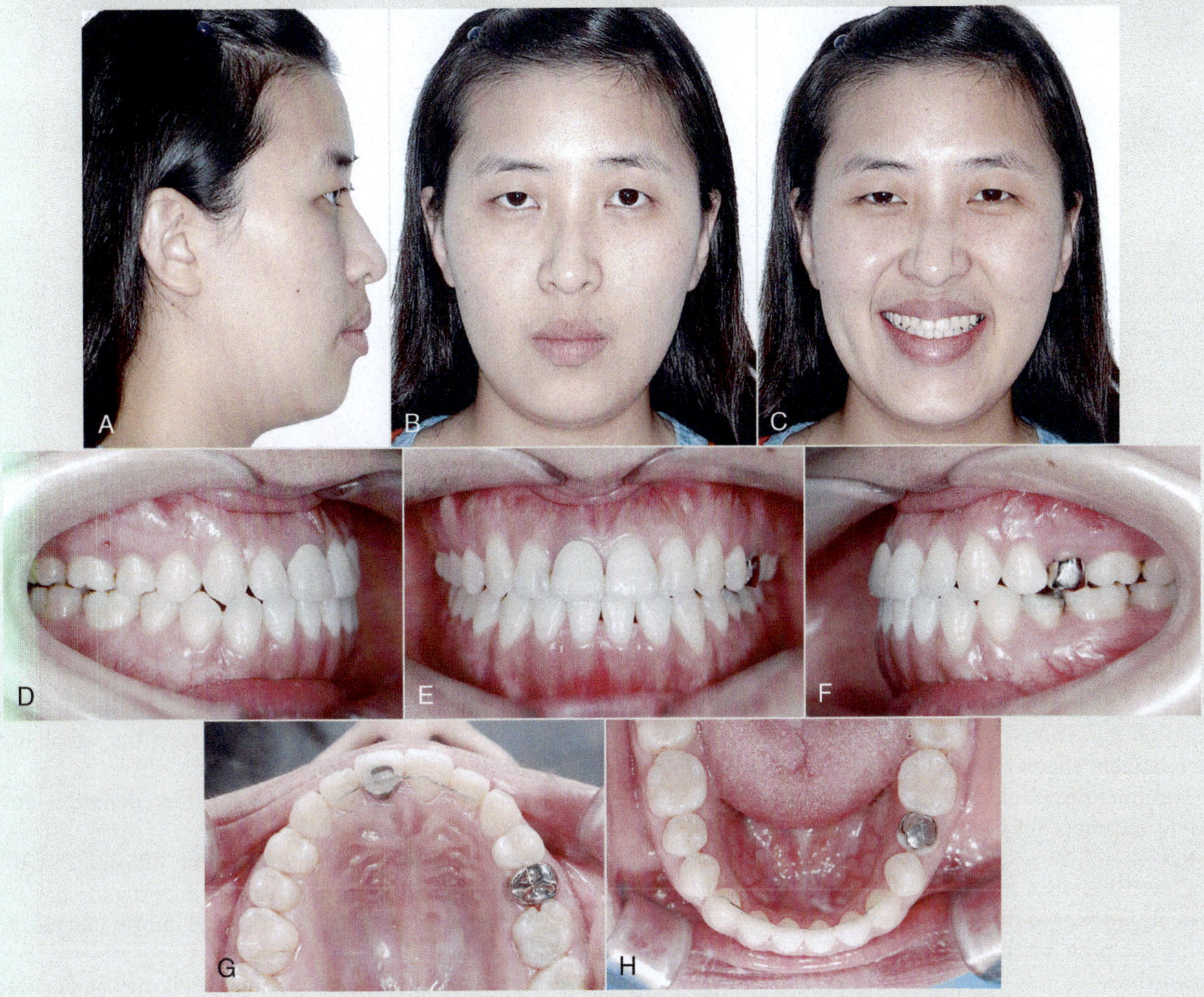

Figure 14-66 Post-treatment (**A–C**) facial and (**D–H**) intraoral photographs of PY.

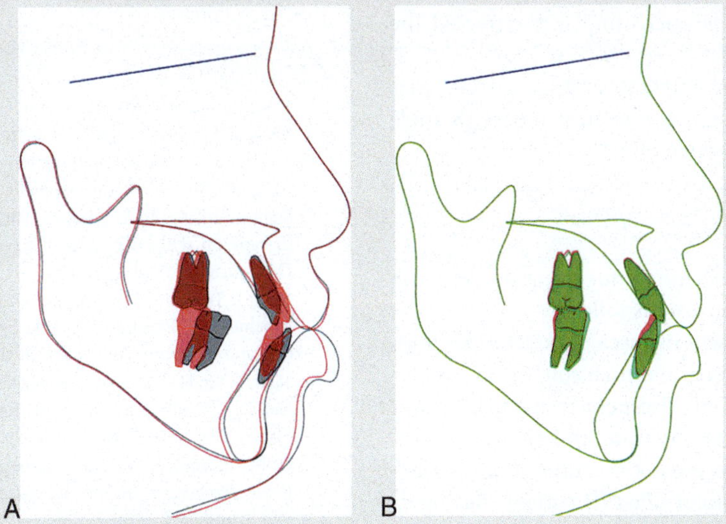

Figure 14-67 **A,** Superimposition of pre-treatment and post-treatment findings for PY. Note the great distal movement of lower molars, with tip-back movement and a decreased occlusal plane after treatment. **B,** Superimposition of post-treatment and 2-year post-treatment findings. No significant changes are noted during retention.

Continued

CASE REPORT 3—cont'd

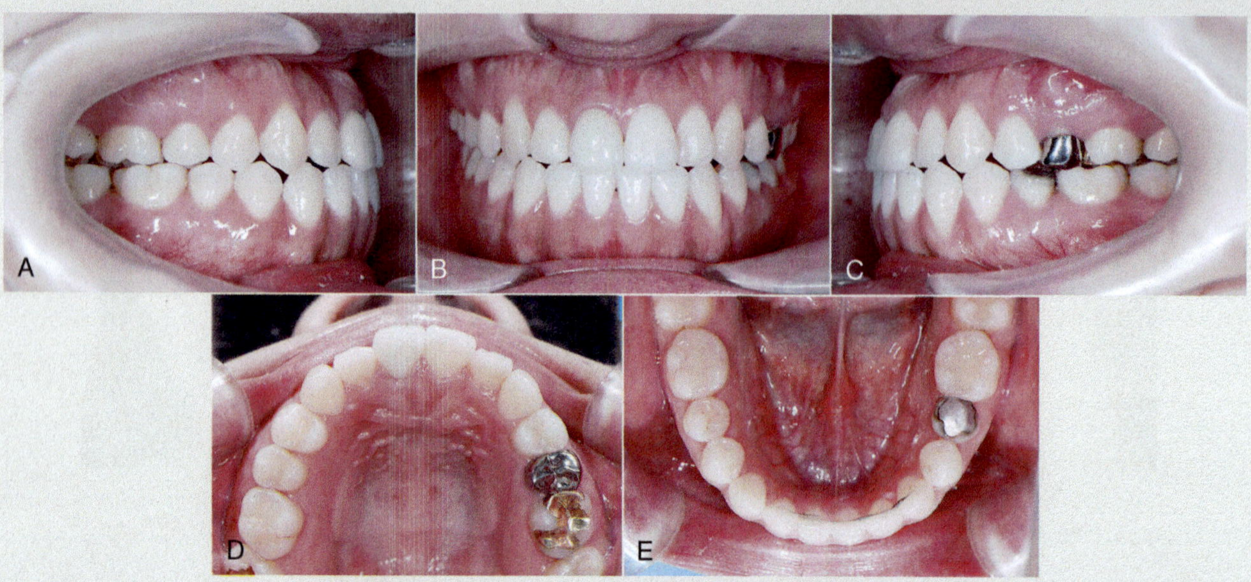

Figure 14-68 **A–E,** Two-year post-treatment photographs of PY.

Treatment Effects

Based on numerous cases treated with the above protocol, the treatment effects can be summarized as follows:

- Two micro-implants in the maxillary arch provide absolute anchorage for Class III elastics along with additional forces.
- Class III elastics from the micro-implants to the lower dentition moved the lower dentition distally by uprighting the posterior teeth to make space for correction of crossbite.
- Class III elastics from the micro-implants decreased the steep occlusal plane angle to correct open bite.
- Class III elastics from the micro-implants retracted the mandible slightly.

Thus two maxillary micro-implants and Class III elastics can be an effective technique in the treatment of high angle Class III malocclusion with open bite.

SUMMARY

A summary of recommendations for treating growing patients with class III malocclusions follows:

- Avoid orthopedic treatment in cases of skeletal developing Class III with high vertical dimension.
- Avoid entering phase II of treatment immediately after phase I is complete. It is best to wait until growth is completed. It is impossible to predict the amount and direction of mandibular growth of Class III patients during or after puberty. Not only the amount but also the direction of mandibular growth causes a change in maxillomandibular relationship during and after puberty. Remarkable mandibular growth is continued after the pubertal growth spurt. Therefore it is critical to keep the variability of growth of the mandible in mind.
- Avoid extracting premolars in lower dentition during phase I (this is critical).
- Even though favorable treatment outcomes may be achieved in growing patients, it is important to pay attention to late mandibular growth and inform parents of the possibility of relapse.
- By following these basic principles, it may be possible to avoid many of the problems that often develop in Class III malocclusion cases.

REFERENCES

1. Sakamoto T. Effective timing for the application of orthopedic force in the skeletal Class III malocclusion. *Am J Orthod*. 1981;80:411–416.
2. Mermigos J, Full CA, Andreasen G. Protraction of the maxillofacial complex. *Am J Orthod Dentofacial Orthop*. 1990;98:47–55.
3. Sugawara J, Asano T, Endo N, Mitani H. Long-term effects of chincap therapy on skeletal profile in mandibular prognathism. *Am J Orthod Dentofacial Orthop*. 1990;98:127–133.
4. Ngan P, Tremont T. Treatment of Class III malocclusions. In: Miles PG, Rinchuse DJ, Rinchuse DJ, eds. *Evidence-Based Clinical Orthodontics*. Chicago, IL: Quintessence Publishing Co, Inc.; 2012:61–87.
5. Ngan P, He H. Effective maxillary protraction for Class III patients. In: Nanda R, Kapila S, eds. *Current Therapy in Orthodontics*. St. Louis, MO: Mosby Elsevier; 2010:143–158.
6. Uribe F, Nanda R. Skeletal anchorage based on biomechanics. In: Nanda R, ed. *Temporary Anchorage Devices in Orthodontics*. Philadelphia, PA: WB Saunders; 2008:145–163.
7. Emrich RE, Brodie AG, Blayney JR. Prevalence of Class I, Class II, and Class III malocclusions (Angle) in an urban population: an epidemiological study. *J Dent Res*. 1965;44:947–1014.

8. Thilander B, Myrberg N. The prevalence of malocclusion in Swedish school children. *Scan J Dent Res.* 1973;81:12–20.
9. Magnusson TE. An epidemiologic study of occlusal anomalies in relation to the development of the dentition in Icelandic children. *Community Dent Oral Epidemiol.* 1976;4:121–128.
10. Tschill P, Bacon W, Sonko A. Malocclusion in the deciduous dentition of Caucasian children. *Eur J Orthod.* 1997;19:361–367.
11. Chan GK. Class III malocclusion in Chinese: etiology and treatment. *Am J Orthod.* 1974;65:152–156.
12. Lew KKK, Foong WC, Loh E. Malocclusion status in Singapore school children. Cited in: Lew KKK, Foong WC. Horizontal skeletal typing in an ethnic Chinese population with true Class III malocclusion. *Br J Orthod.* 1993;20:19–23.
13. Allwright WC, Burndred WH. A survey of handicapping dentofacial anomalies among Chinese in Hong Kong. *Int Dent J.* 1964;14:505–519.
14. Lin JJ. Prevalence of malocclusion in Chinese children age 9–15. *Clin Dent (Chinese).* 1985;5:57–65.
15. Endo T. An epidemiological study of reversed occlusion: part 1: incidence of reversed occlusion in children 6 to 14 years old. *J Jpn Orthod Soc.* 1971;30:73–77.
16. Susami R, Asai Y, Hirose K, et al. The prevalence of malocclusion in Japanese school children. *J Jpn Orthod Soc.* 1972;31:319–324.
17. Baik HS, Han HK, Kim DJ, et al. Cephalometric characteristics of Korean Class III surgical patients and their relationship to plans for surgical treatment. *Int J Adult Orthod Orthognath Surg.* 2000;15:119–128.
18. Toms AP. Class III malocclusion: a cephalometric study of Saudi Arabians. *Br J Orthod.* 1989;16:201–206.
19. Ingervall B, Mohlin B, Thilander B. Prevalence and awareness of malocclusion in Swedish men. *Community Dent Oral Epidemiol.* 1979;6:308–314.
20. Altemus LA. Frequency of the incidence of malocclusion in American Negro children aged 12–16. *Angle Orthod.* 1959;29:189–200.
21. Kim JH, Viana MAG, Graber TM, Omerza FF, BeGole EA. The effectiveness of protraction face mask therapy: a meta-analysis. *Am J Orthod Dentofacial Orthop.* 1999;115:675–685.
22. Ngan P. Treatment of Class III malocclusion in the primary and mixed dentitions. In: Bishara SE. *Textbook of Orthodontics.* Philadelphia, PA: WB Saunders; 2001:375–414.
23. Kambara T. Dentofacial changes produced by extraoral forward force in *Macaca irus. Am J Orthod.* 1977;71:249–277.
24. Hata S, Itoh T, Nakagawa M, et al. Biomechanical effects of maxillary protraction on the craniofacial complex. *Am J Orthod Dentofacial Orthop.* 1987;91:305–311.
25. Droshl H. The effect of heavy orthopaedic forces on the sutures of the facial bones. *Angle Orthod.* 1975;45:26–33.
26. Engstrom C, Thilander B. Premature facial synostosis: the influence of biomechanical factors in normal and hypocalcemic young rats. *Eur J Orthod.* 1985;785:35–47.
27. Linge L. Tissue reactions incident to widening of facial sutures: an experimental study in the *Macaca mulatta. Trans Eur Orthod Soc.* 1972;48:487–497.
28. Liou EJW. Effective maxillary orthopedic protraction for growing Class III patients: a clinical application simulates distraction osteogenesis. *Prog Orthod.* 2005;6:36–53.
29. Yen SL. Protocols for late maxillary protraction in cleft lip and palate patients at Children's Hospital, Los Angeles. *Sem Orthod.* 2011;17:138–148.
30. Melsen B, Melsen F. The postnatal development of the palato-maxillary region studied on human autopsy material. *Am J Orthod.* 1983;82:329–342.
31. Ngan PW, Hägg U, Yiu C, et al. Treatment response and long-term dentofacial adaptations to maxillary expansion and protraction. *Semin Orthod.* 1997;3:255–264.
32. Franchi L, Baccetti T, McNamara JA. Postpubertal assessment of treatment timing of maxillary expansion and protraction therapy followed by fixed appliances. *Am J Orthod Dentofacial Orthop.* 2004;126:555–568.
33. Sung JH. A clinical consideration on treatment of anterior cross-bite in growing children (the effect of chin cap). *Korean J Orthod.* 1982;12:117–126.
34. Mitani H, Sakamoto T. Chin cap force to a growing mandible: long-term clinical reports. *Angle Orthod.* 1984;54:93–122.
35. Sugawara J, Asano T, Endo N, Mitani H. Long-term effects of chincap therapy on skeletal profile in mandibular prognathism. *Am J Orthod Dentofacial Orthop.* 1990;98:127–133.
36. Deguchi T, Kuroda T, Hunt NP, Graber TM. Long-term application of chincup force alters the morphology of the dolichofacial Class III mandible. *Am J Orthod Dentofacial Orthop.* 1999;116:610–615.
37. Deguchi T, Kuroda T, Minoshima Y, Graber TM. Craniofacial features of patients with Class III abnormalities: growth-related changes and effects of short-term and long-term chincup therapy. *Am J Orthod Dentofacial Orthop.* 2002;121:84–92.
38. Loh MK, Kerr WJ. The function regulator III: effects and indications for use. *Br J Orthod.* 1985;12:153–157.
39. McNamara JA Jr, Huge SA. The functional regulator (FR-3) of Fränkel. *Am J Orthod.* 1985;88:409–424.
40. Song K, Sung JH. A clinical consideration on the effect of FR III in growing patients with anterior cross-bite. *Korean J Orthod.* 1989;19:130–143.
41. Yang KH. Fränkel appliance type III: correct fabrication and case report of skeletal Class III malocclusion. *J Clin Pediatr Dent.* 1996;20:281–292.
42. Eganhouse GR. Two piece corrector for Class III skeletal and dental malocclusions. *J Clin Orthod.* 1997;31:246–251.
43. Yang KH. Treatment of Class III malocclusion with the horseshoe appliance: case reports in growing patients. *J Clin Pediatr Dent.* 1997;22:1–8.
44. Isaacson RJ, Rebellato J. Two-couple orthodontic appliance systems: torquing arches. *Semin Orthod.* 1995;1:31–36.
45. Kim YH. Anterior openbite and its treatment with multiloop edgewise archwire. *Angle Orthod.* 1987;57:290–321.
46. Protacio C, Sato S. The role of posterior discrepancy in the development of skeletal Class III malocclusion: its clinical importance. *Int J MEAW Tech Res Found.* 1995;2:5–18.
47. Oh SS. Nonsurgical correction of severe skeletal Class III maloclussion. *Int J MEAW Tech Res Found.* 1995;2:51–68.
48. Sung JH, Kyung HM, Bae SM, Kwon OH, McNamara JA. *Microimplants in Orthodontics.* Daegu, Korea: Dentos Inc.; 2006.
49. Sung JH. Nonsurgical orthodontic treatment of skeletal Class III with high angle and open bite by using two maxillary microimplants and Class III elastics. *Tweed Profile.* 2011;10:24–27.
50. Sanborn RT. Differences between the facial skeletal patterns of Class III malocclusion and normal occlusion. *Angle Orthod.* 1955;25:208–222.
51. Sassouni V. A classification of skeletal facial types. *Am J Orthod.* 1969;55:109–123.
52. Park HS, Bae SM, Kyung HM, Sung JH. Micro-implant anchorage for treatment of skeletal Class I bialveolar protrusion. *J Clin Orthod.* 2001;35:417–422.
53. Park HS, Kwon TG, Sung JH. Nonextraction treatment with microscrew implants. *Angle Orthod.* 2004;74:539–549.
54. Park HS, Jeong SH, Kwon OW. Factors affecting the clinical success of screw implants used as orthodontic anchorage. *Am J Orthod Dentofacial Orthop.* 2006;130:18–25.
55. Sugawara J, Daimaruya T, Umemori M, et al. Distal movement of mandibular molars in adult patients with the skeletal anchorage system. *Am J Orthod Dentofacial Orthop.* 2004;125:130–138.
56. Burstone CJ, Koenig H. Force systems from an ideal arch. *Am J Orthod.* 1974;65:270–289.
57. Burstone CJ, Koenig H. Creative wire bending: the force system from step and V bends. *Am J Orthod Dentofacial Orthop.* 1988;93:59–67.

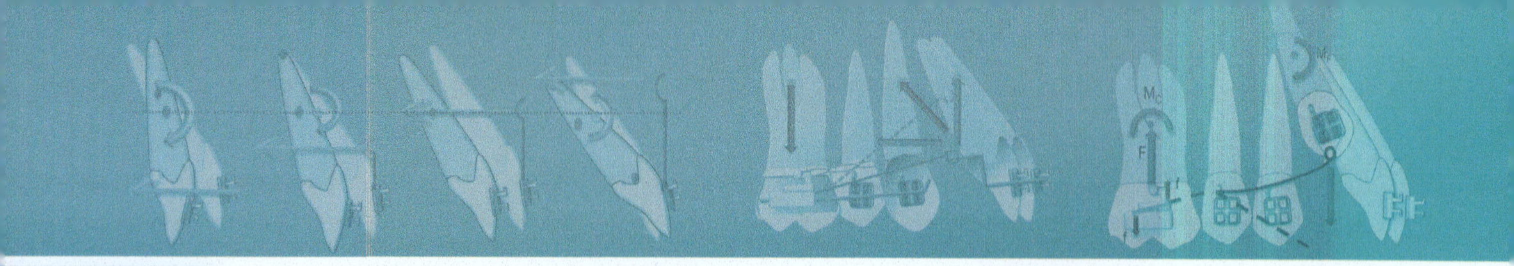

CHAPTER 15

Clinical Practice Guidelines for Developing Class III Malocclusion

Junji Sugawara

Class III malocclusion can be defined as a skeletal facial deformity characterized by a forward mandibular position with respect to the cranial base and/or maxilla (Fig. 15-1). This facial dysplasia can be classified as mandibular prognathism, maxillary retrognathism, or a combination of both, depending on the variation of the anteroposterior jaw relationships. Vertically, it can also be divided into three basic types depending on the vertical disproportions: long, average, and short face (see Fig. 15-1). In this chapter, Class III malocclusion will refer only to anteroposterior dysplasia. Class III malocclusion represents patients with anterior crossbite and a skeletal Class III jaw disharmony (Fig. 15-2). Pseudo–Class III malocclusion, which is characterized by an anterior crossbite and a skeletal Class I relationship, is excluded from this category.

It has been believed that Class III malocclusion may be caused by excessive growth of the mandible with respect to the maxilla and/or cranial base. However, the results of our longitudinal studies show similar maxillary and mandibular incremental changes during the prepubertal, pubertal, and postpubertal periods when compared to Class I subjects. Therefore it would be rational to assume that the skeletal framework of Class III malocclusion must have been established early before the prepubertal growth period. In addition, the manner of mandibular growth during the postpubertal period seems to be quite critical in Class III treatment, because the maxillary growth changes are almost negligible and only the mandible is displaced in a downward–forward direction according to its growth potential.

Concerning mandibular growth control that can possibly alter the skeletal framework of Class III patients, our aforementioned studies on the short-term and long-term effects of chin cap force indicate that the skeletal framework is greatly improved during the initial stages of chin cap therapy. However, such changes are rarely maintained during the pubertal growth period and, when growth is complete, results suggest that treatment with chin cap force seldom alters the inherited prognathic characteristics of Class III profiles.

Considering the scientific evidence, we have produced a clinical practice guideline for managing Class III patients and practiced in accordance with this guideline for more than 10 years. The principal role of the guideline is to make provisions so that almost all patients achieve functional occlusion and esthetic dentition until adulthood and lifelong stability thereafter. In addition, it aims to assure the quality of orthodontic treatment and to provide risk management strategies for unexpected situations occurring during treatment and management.

The clinical practice guideline for the correction of developing Class III malocclusion is outlined below, with particular consideration given to Class III facial growth and the long-term effects of chin cap orthopedic force for controlling Class III mandibular growth. In addition, treatment progress and the results of representative Class III patients who were managed in accordance with the clinical practice guideline are reported. Figure 15-3 shows the clinical practice guideline for growing and developing Class III patients and represents our present concept of their treatment and management.[1]

At the initial diagnosis in the deciduous dentition or early mixed dentition, patients receive a differential diagnosis and are divided into two groups according to the extent of their three-dimensional jaw disharmonies. Long-term management is usually recommended for patients diagnosed with mild or moderate skeletal Class III and this management is clearly separated into two treatment phases (see Fig. 15-3). The early mixed dentition is the most desirable time for the first phase of orthodontic treatment (although not all patients seek consultation early enough for this) and the second phase of treatment is generally applied during or after the postpubertal period. The growth observation period runs from the end of the first phase of treatment to the beginning of the second phase.

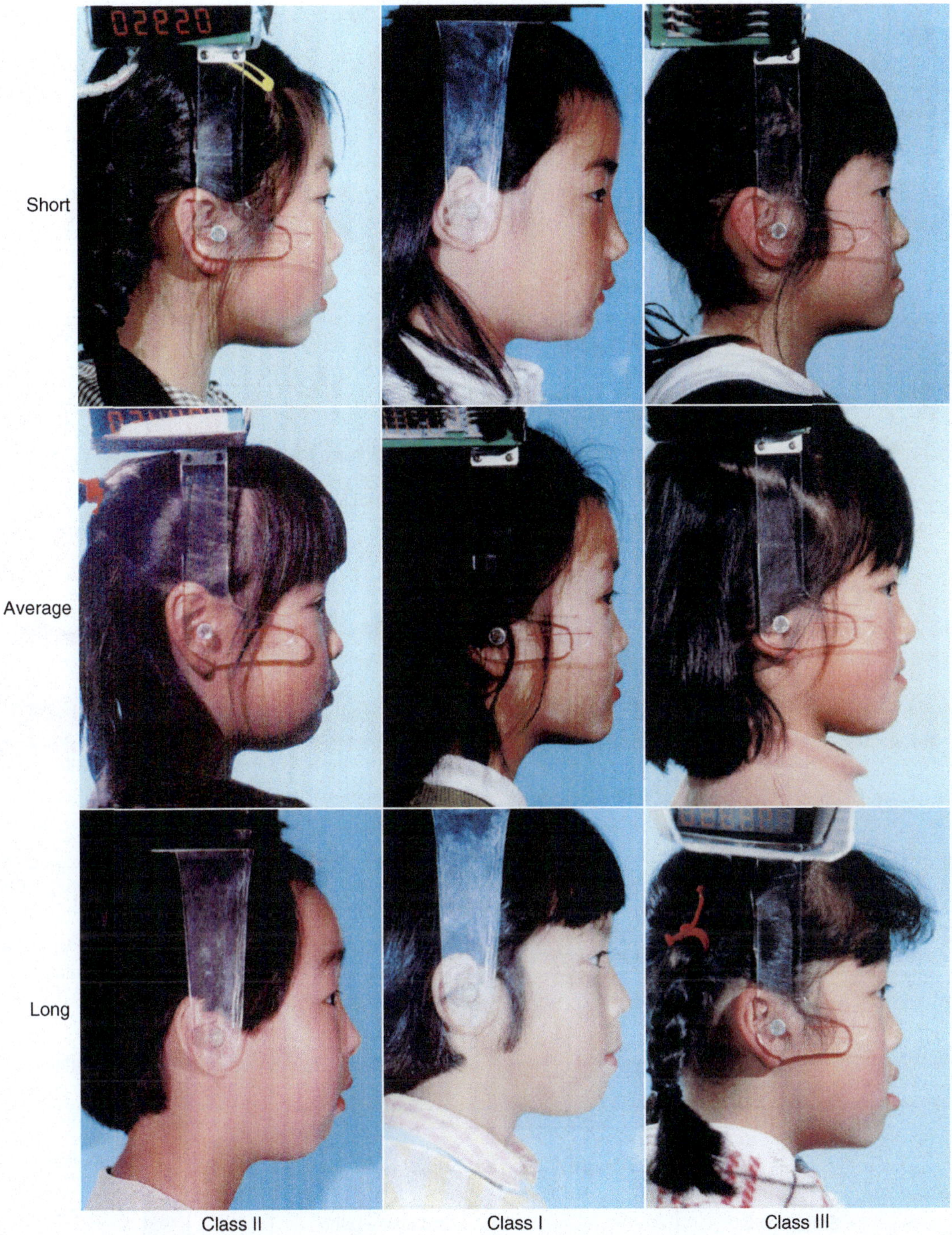

Figure 15-1 Classification of facial types.

The treatment objectives of the first phase are:

1. To maintain good oral hygiene with the help of dental caries risk tests
2. To correct functional deviation of the mandible and to stabilize the jaw position
3. To improve the three-dimensional jaw deformity as much as possible
4. To correct and control the deviation of the dental midline
5. To accomplish desirable anterior occlusion for establishing anterior guidance in the future
6. To establish bilateral posterior support
7. To gain enough space for the buccal teeth
8. To normalize and enhance orofacial functions

In contrast, the treatment objectives of the second phase of treatment are:

1. To achieve a balanced soft tissue profile
2. To establish final functional occlusion
3. To regulate temporomandibular joint (TMJ) and oral functions
4. To prevent periodontal disease and promote oral health

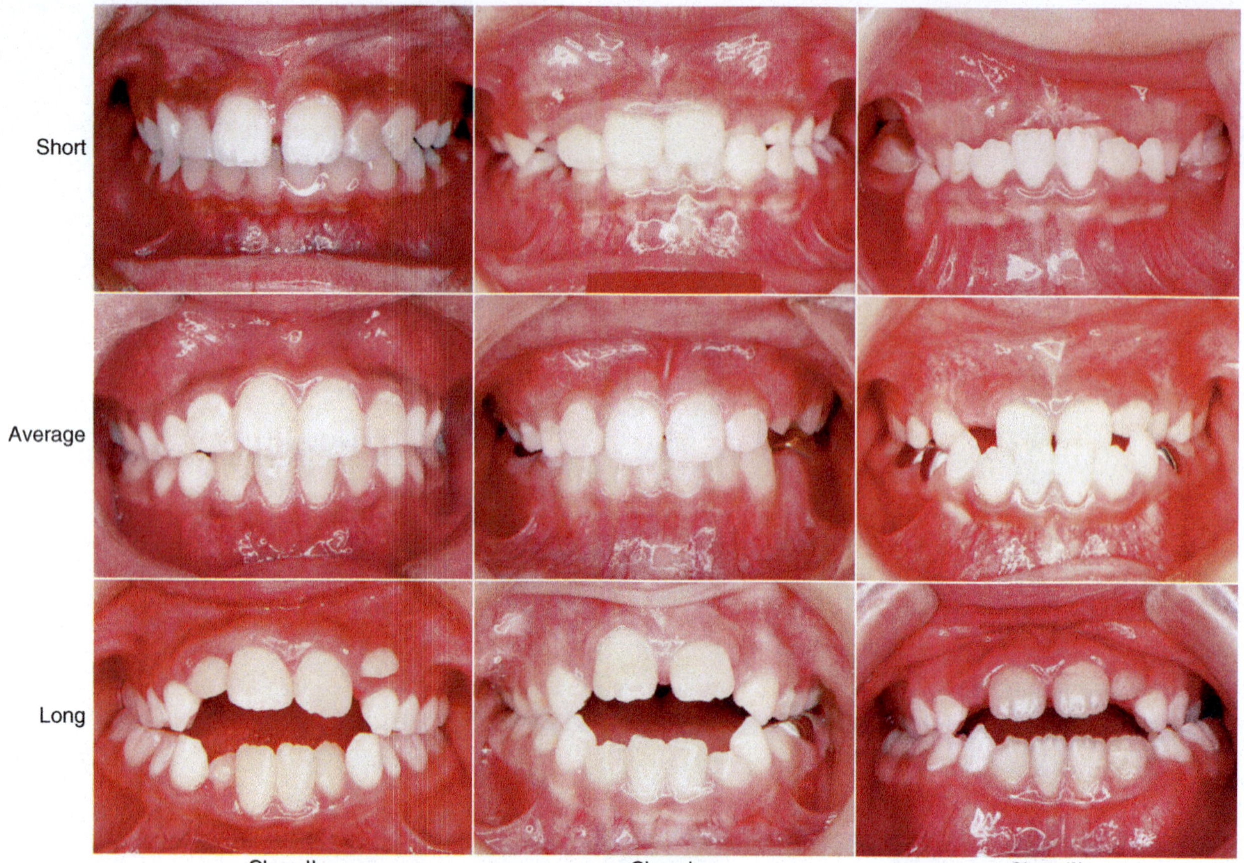

Figure 15-2 Occlusion of each skeletal facial type.

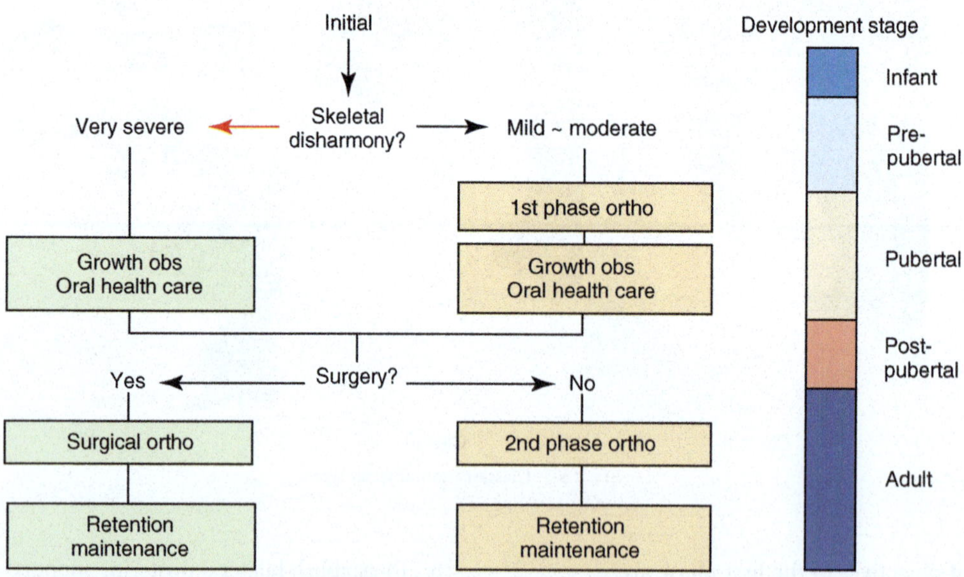

Figure 15-3 Clinical practice guidelines for developing Class III malocclusion.

During the observation period, growth data are collected from the patient and his or her oral hygiene is professionally controlled. A very important point is that the quick completion of each phase will motivate the patient to comply throughout the long-term management period.

Patients with extremely severe skeletal Class III malocclusion, in whom orthognathic surgery is indicated, usually skip the first phase of treatment and their orthodontic problems cannot be addressed until the postpubertal period. It is important to collect growth data from these patients to establish an individual growth database that can be used to determine the timing of orthognathic surgery and to professionally control oral hygiene during the observation period.

Most Class III patients are managed according to one of the two pathways described above but occasionally a patient is managed in a modified manner. For instance, it is possible that patients diagnosed as requiring jaw surgery at the initial examination can be camouflaged with usual second-phase orthodontic treatment. Conversely, some patients may need to change from the right to the left side of the clinical practice guideline (see Fig. 15-3) if they experience abnormal jaw growth.

The reasons for proposing this clinical practice guideline for the correction of growing Class III malocclusion can be narrowed down to two points: Class III facial growth and chin cap orthopedic effects.

CLASS III FACIAL GROWTH

Most malocclusions and dentofacial deformities do not result from some pathological process but rather from a moderate distortion of normal development. Class III malocclusion appears to develop from an interaction between environmental and innate factors. An understanding of craniofacial growth behavior in Class III patients will help in determining the treatment timing and biomechanics. However, little is known about the craniofacial growth pattern of Class III malocclusion in comparison to normal patients. Early studies were largely based either on cross-sectional[2] and semilongitudinal samples[3] or on longitudinal data[4,5] that encompassed too few subjects to be statistically valid.

In 1981 Mitani[6] published a longitudinal study on Class III growth during the prepubertal period. Since then, our research group has conducted several longitudinal studies[7-12] using the growth records of patients who were waiting for orthognathic surgery. The craniofacial growth of skeletal Class III Japanese female subjects during the prepubertal, pubertal, and postpubertal periods, which was one of the sources that informed the development of the clinical practice guideline, is shown in Figure 15-4.

Prepubertal Growth Period

Mitani[6] compared growth changes between Class III and Class I patients during the prepubertal growth period. The investigation was based on two groups of Japanese girls: an experimental group of 18 girls (Class III group) and a control group of 22 girls (Class I group). Each set of serial lateral cephalometric head films consisted of a 4-year series from ages 7 to 10 years. All Class III subjects exhibited Class III malocclusion and all Class I subjects showed excellent or mild Class I malocclusion. None of the Class III subjects underwent any growth-related orthopedic treatment before or during the study period.

Table 15-1 shows mean and standard deviations of linear and angular measurements at the ages of 7 and 10 years and the overall changes during this period. No significant difference was found between the two groups with regard to the size of the maxilla (Ptm-A). However, the maxilla, as measured from basion to Ptm (Ba-Ptm), was more retruded among the Class III group ($p < 0.01$). The incremental changes in both groups for these two measurements were relatively similar.

Comparison of the annual size increase in the mandible showed that the total mandibular length (Ar-Pog) of the Class III group maintained greater values than the Class I group until the age of 10 years. There was no significant difference between the means of the two groups for the total incremental changes in any measurements.

The ANPog angle showed a significant difference in facial convexity between the two groups. The amount of reduction in convexity was slightly greater in the Class I group than in the Class III group with age but there was no significant difference between the two groups.

In conclusion, skeletal Class III malocclusion showed an incremental growth change similar to the Class I group during the prepubertal period. These results suggest that the morphological pattern of the prognathic face associated with

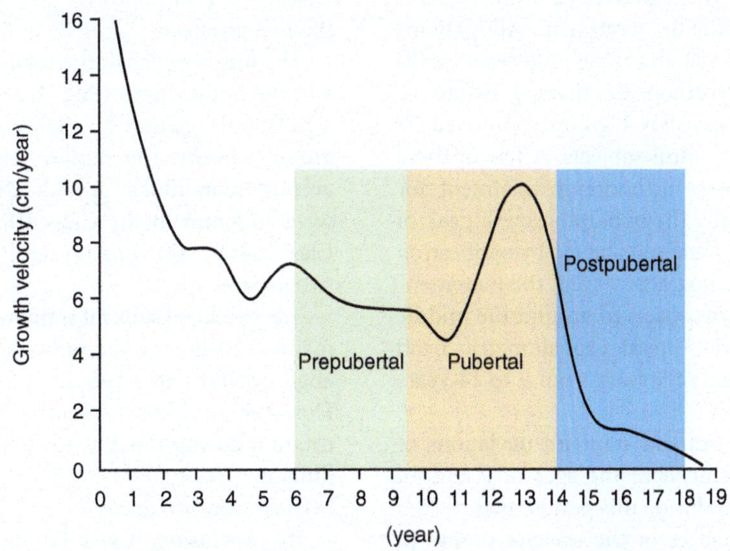

Figure 15-4 Growth curve showing the development stages.

TABLE 15-1 Results of Measurements for Class III (n = 18) and Class I (n = 22) Groups During Prepubertal Growth Period in Japanese Females

	7 Years Old					10 Years Old					Total Change				
	Class III		Class I			Class III		Class I			Class III		Class I		
	x	SD	x	SD	Sig.	x	SD	x	SD	Sig.	x	SD	x	SD	Sig.
Maxilla															
Ptm-A (mm)	42.6	1.5	43.1	1.7	NS	44.0	1.9	44.7	1.8	NS	1.7	0.8	1.6	1.0	NS
Ba-A (mm)	83.3	2.7	85.7	2.3	**	86.1	2.9	89.4	2.3	**	3.0	1.4	3.7	1.7	NS
Ba-Ptm (mm)	40.5	2.0	42.5	2.4	**	42.1	2.4	44.6	2.5	**	1.5	1.0	2.1	1.4	NS
Mandible															
Ar-Pog (mm)	96.6	2.8	92.5	3.6	**	101.6	4.3	99.4	3.9	NS	7.0	1.5	7.1	1.5	NS
Go-Pog (mm)	68.8	2.5	66.6	3.0	*	73.1	3.4	71.7	3.5	NS	5.2	1.5	5.3	1.5	NS
Ar-Go (mm)	38.9	2.2	38.0	2.5	NS	41.7	2.7	41.5	2.9	NS	3.4	1.3	3.4	1.4	NS
Ba-Pog (mm)	79.0	3.3	76.5	3.0	*	83.2	3.7	81.9	3.8	NS	3.7	2.3	5.5	2.7	NS
Gonial angle (degree)	126.5	3.8	128.4	5.3	NS	124.8	4.1	127.8	6.5	NS	−1.6	1.4	−0.6	2.5	NS
Mand. pl. (degree)	28.2	3.6	32.5	3.2	**	28.1	3.3	31.0	3.6	*	0.1	0.9	−1.5	2.3	NS
Intermaxillary															
ANPog (degree)	1.0	1.2	6.3	1.8	**	0.6	0.9	4.9	1.8	**	−0.5	0.9	−1.4	0.9	NS

Reprinted with permission from Mitani H. Prepubertal growth of mandibular prognathism. *Am J Orthod.* 1981;80:546–553.
A, A point; *Ar,* articulare; *Ba,* basion; *Go,* gonion; *Mand. pl.,* mandibular plane; *NS,* not significant; *Pog,* pogonion; *Ptm,* pterygomaxillary fissure; *SD,* standard deviation; *Sig.,* significance.
*p <0.05.
**p <0.01.

mandibular excess is probably established in early life. Once established, the annual growth increment is quite similar to that in an individual with a normal or Class I face before puberty.

Pubertal Growth Period

Bandai et al.[12] reported on the craniofacial growth pattern of skeletal Class III malocclusion during the pubertal growth period (9 to 14 years) in Japanese girls. The Class III group comprised 16 Class III girls selected from patients waiting for surgical orthodontic treatment. All patients exhibited a large reverse overjet and none underwent orthodontic or growth-related orthopedic therapy before or during the study period. The Class I group comprised 18 Class I girls who served as control subjects. A few of these patients underwent first-phase orthodontic treatment for the alignment of incisors only. The pubertal growth peak of all subjects, which was individually evaluated by ossification events of hand-wrist roentgenograms[12,13] and the incremental curve of body height,[14] was observed around the middle of the period studied. Serial lateral cephalometric head films were used over a period of 5 years from 9 to 14 years of age.

Table 15-2 shows the mean and standard deviations of linear and angular measurements at the ages of 9 and 14 years and the overall changes during this period. Figure 15-5 depicts the longitudinal changes of the skeletal profile in each group. These skeletal profiles were constructed with 13 cephalometric landmarks measured in terms of the x–y coordinates.

No significant difference between the two groups was found in the total increase of any cephalometric measurements or in any measurements regarding the maxilla at ages 9 and 14 years. Although the midfacial length (Cd-A) and upper facial height (N-ANS) of the Class III patients were significantly smaller ($p < 0.05$) than those of the Class I group, the average incremental changes in the maxillary length (A′-Ptm′) showed no significant difference between the two groups.

The mean values of the total mandibular length (Gn-Cd) and the body length (Pog′-Go) of the Class III group were significantly greater ($p < 0.001$) than those of the Class I group, whereas the ramus height (Cd-Go) was not. The average mandibular growth changes measured at Gn-Cd were 14.9 mm in the Class III group and 13.1 mm in the Class I group, showing no significant difference between the two groups.

The principal skeletal frameworks of the two groups were maintained during the pubertal period. The occlusal plane angle (SNOP) of Class III subjects remained unchanged. However, in Class I subjects it showed counterclockwise rotation during this growth period. There was a significant difference ($p < 0.001$) in the total change of Wits appraisal between the two groups.

In conclusion, Class III malocclusion showed neither excessive mandibular growth nor deficient maxillary growth

TABLE 15-2 Measurements for Class III (n = 16) and Class I (n = 18) Groups During Pubertal Growth Period in Japanese Females

	9 Years Old					14 Years Old					Total Change				
	Class III		Class I			Class III		Class I			Class III		Class I		
	x	SD	x	SD	Sig.	x	SD	x	SD	Sig.	x	SD	x	SD	Sig.
Cranial Base															
S-N (mm)	61.6	1.8	62.3	2.2	NS	64.3	2.2	65.3	2.3	NS	2.7	0.9	3.0	0.9	NS
S-Ba (mm)	42.9	2.6	43.0	2.2	NS	45.9	2.2	47.0	2.6	NS	3.0	1.5	3.9	1.5	NS
Ba-S/FH angle (degree)	123.8	4.0	124.2	3.3	NS	123.2	4.0	123.7	3.0	NS	−0.6	1.4	−0.4	1.3	NS
Maxilla															
A′-Ptm′ (mm)	43.1	2.1	43.6	1.5	NS	46.0	2.3	47.3	2.1	NS	2.9	1.3	3.8	1.3	NS
Cd-A (mm)	77.4	3.3	77.4	2.5	NS	83.2	3.4	84.7	2.6	NS	5.8	1.9	7.2	1.8	*
N-ANS (mm)	49.4	2.3	49.5	2.1	NS	54.5	2.3	55.7	2.4	NS	5.1	0.8	6.2	1.0	*
SNA (degree)	80.2	1.5	80.1	3.2	NS	81.1	1.5	81.0	2.7	NS	0.9	1.3	0.9	0.9	NS
Mandible															
Gn-Cd (mm)	106.8	3.9	101.0	4.1	***	121.7	4.8	114.1	5.1	***	14.9	2.5	13.1	2.6	NS
Pog′-Go (mm)	70.7	2.4	67.5	3.2	**	79.3	3.0	75.6	3.5	**	8.6	1.8	8.1	1.3	NS
Cd-Go (mm)	49.2	2.3	48.2	3.2	NS	57.7	2.4	56.2	4.3	NS	8.6	2.1	8.0	2.1	NS
SNB (degree)	81.3	1.7	77.4	2.6	***	83.8	1.8	78.6	2.5	***	2.0	1.8	1.4	1.4	NS
SNPog (degree)	80.1	2.0	77.0	2.7	***	82.4	2.2	77.8	3.3	***	2.2	1.5	0.8	2.9	NS
Gonial angle (degree)	128.6	7.0	124.6	5.3	NS	127.9	6.8	122.5	5.8	*	−0.7	2.3	−2.1	3.0	NS
Mand. pl. (degree)	38.0	5.5	37.0	3.3	NS	37.8	5.9	36.1	4.1	NS	−0.1	2.0	−0.9	2.4	NS
Intermaxillary															
Wits appraisal (mm)	−8.6	2.0	−3.0	1.4	***	−12.4	2.7	−3.0	1.3	***	−3.8	2.4	0.0	1.5	***
ANS-Me (mm)	61.1	3.9	61.2	4.3	NS	69.2	5.5	67.4	5.2	NS	8.1	2.5	6.2	1.6	*
ANB (degree)	−1.1	1.7	2.7	1.6	***	−2.2	1.9	2.4	1.7	***	−1.1	1.6	−0.2	1.4	NS
SN to Occlusal (degree)	20.2	3.3	22.2	2.5	NS	20.3	2.6	18.9	3.0	NS	0.2	2.7	−3.3	2.5	*

Reprinted with permission from Bandai (Sakamoto) E, Sugawara J, Umemori M, et al. Craniofacial growth of mandibular prognathism in Japanese girls during pubertal growth period: longitudinal study from 9 to 14 years of age. *Orthod Waves*. 2000;59:77–89.

A, A point; *ANB*, A point nasion B point; *ANS*, anterior nasal spine; *Ba*, basion; *Gn*, gnathion; *Go*, gonion; *Mand. pl.*, mandibular plane; *Me*, menton; *N*, nasion; *NS*, not significant; *Pog*, pogonion; *Ptm*, pterygomaxillary fissure; *S*, sella; *SD*, standard deviation; *Sig.*, significance; *SN*, sella-nasion; *SNA*, sella-nasion A point; *SNB*, sella-nasion B point.

*$p < 0.05$.

**$p < 0.01$.

***$p < 0.001$.

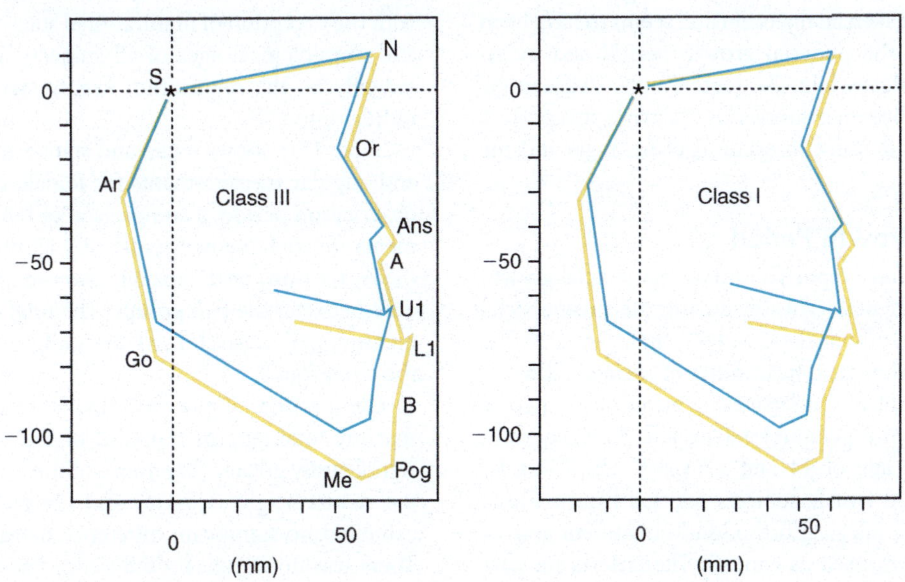

Figure 15-5 Longitudinal changes in the skeletal profiles of Class III and Class I groups. *A*, A point; *Ans*, anterior nasal spine; *Ar*, articulare; *B*, B point; *Go*, gonion; *L1*, lower incisor; *Me*, menton; *N*, nasion; *Or*, orbitale; *Pog*, pogonion; *S*, sella; *U1*, upper incisor.

TABLE 15-3 Results of Measurements for Class III (n = 20) and Class I (n = 20) Groups During Postpubertal Growth Period in Japanese Females

	14 Years Old					17 Years Old					Total Change				
	Class III		Class I			Class III		Class I			Class III		Class I		
	x	SD	x	SD	Sig.	x	SD	x	SD	Sig.	x	SD	x	SD	Sig.
Cranial Base															
S-N (mm)	63.7	3.2	65.0	2.8	NS	64.4	3.0	65.3	2.9	NS	0.7	0.5	0.3	0.4	*
S-Ba (mm)	45.6	2.2	45.4	1.9	NS	46.0	2.3	45.9	1.9	NS	0.4	0.5	0.5	0.5	NS
Ba-S/FH angle (degree)	120.7	4.0	129.9	3.4	**	120.0	3.8	123.8	3.6	**	−0.3	1.5	−0.1	1.0	NS
Maxilla															
Ptm-A (mm)	44.8	3.1	46.7	3.1	NS	45.2	2.9	47.2	3.3	NS	0.4	0.8	0.5	1.2	NS
Ba-A (mm)	86.5	4.3	90.7	5.4	**	86.9	4.2	91.3	5.5	**	0.4	0.8	0.6	1.3	NS
Ba-Ptm (mm)	41.7	3.4	44.0	3.2	*	41.7	3.5	44.1	3.2	*	0.1	0.8	0.1	0.7	NS
N′-ANS (mm)	54.9	3.3	53.8	2.4	NS	55.5	3.6	54.6	2.6	NS	0.6	1.0	0.9	1.2	NS
SNA (degree)	81.5	4.3	81.9	4.0	NS	81.3	4.3	82.0	4.2	NS	−0.1	0.9	0.1	1.0	NS
Mandible															
Gn-Cd (mm)	120.1	7.8	113.4	4.9	**	123.0	8.6	116.2	5.0	**	2.9	1.9	2.8	1.8	NS
Go-Pog (mm)	76.3	6.0	73.4	3.5	NS	77.9	6.0	74.9	3.7	NS	1.6	0.9	1.5	1.4	NS
Cd-Go (mm)	56.0	3.6	55.3	5.3	NS	57.9	4.0	57.4	5.1	NS	1.9	1.8	2.1	1.0	NS
SNPog (degree)	83.6	5.4	77.9	4.3	**	84.5	5.9	78.7	4.1	**	0.9	1.4	0.8	0.8	NS
Gonial angle (degree)	132.3	6.2	125.0	6.5	**	132.2	5.8	124.7	6.4	**	0	1.6	−0.3	0.8	NS
Mand. pl. (degree)	31.2	5.7	30.0	4.9	NS	30.7	6.1	29.8	4.8	NS	−0.5	1.8	−0.3	1.5	NS
Intermaxillary															
Wits appraisal (mm)	−11.4	4.3	−0.6	2.6	**	−12.7	4.9	−1.3	2.1	**	−1.6	1.9	−1.3	1.7	NS
ANS-Me (mm)	75.0	5.8	70.4	4.6	*	77.3	6.2	72.2	4.3	**	2.3	1.5	1.8	1.5	NS
ANB (degree)	−2.9	2.7	3.0	1.8	**	−3.8	3.3	2.5	2.1	**	−1.3	2.0	−0.7	1.3	NS

Reprinted with permission from Mitani H, Sato K, Sugawara J. Growth of mandibular prognathism after pubertal growth peak. *Am J Orthod Dentofacial Orthop.* 1993;104:330–336.

A, A point; *ANB*, A point nasion B point; *ANS*, anterior nasal spine; *Ba*, basion; *Gn*, gnathion; *Go*, gonion; *Mand. pl.*, mandibular plane; *Me*, menton; *N*, nasion; *NS*, not significant; *Pog*, pogonion; *Ptm*, pterygomaxillary fissure; *S*, sella; *SD*, standard deviation; *Sig.*, significance; *SNA*, sella-nasion A point.

*p <0.05.

**p <0.01.

when compared to Class I subjects during the pubertal growth period. The skeletal malocclusion seems to have been established before the pubertal growth period and maintained thereafter. Meanwhile, the dentoalveolar disharmony is aggravated and becomes more severe during this period, as shown by the difference in occlusal plane angle and the Wits appraisal.

Postpubertal Growth Period

Several studies[7–10] have reported on the craniofacial growth pattern of Class III malocclusion during the postpubertal period using longitudinal data. Mitani et al.[10] studied the serial lateral cephalometric head films of skeletal Class III and Class I malocclusion in Japanese females over a period of 3 years during the postpubertal period. Cephalograms were taken at the age of 14 and 17 years. The Class III group comprised 20 female subjects selected from a file of patients waiting for surgical orthodontic treatment and 20 female subjects were used as control. The criteria for case selection were the same as in the studies described above, with the exception of maturational stage. Maturational stages and physiological ages of all subjects were evaluated individually by the ossification events taken from hand-wrist radiographs.[13–17]

Table 15-3 shows mean and standard deviations of linear and angular measurements for female subjects. During the observation period, a comparison of the maxillary measurements showed that neither the size (Ptm-A) nor the position (SNA, Ba-Ptm) of the maxilla showed any significant difference between the two groups. The total change in maxillary measurements also showed no significant difference between the two groups.

Comparison of the mandibular measurements showed that the total lengths (Gn-Cd) of the Class III group were significantly greater than those of the Class I group, whereas the ramus height (Cd-Go) and the body length (Go-Pog) exhibited no significant difference between the two groups. There was no significant difference between the two groups in any of the changes in mandibular measurements during the time periods studied.

No significant difference was observed between the two groups in the total changes in A point nasion B point (ANB) angle and Wits appraisal. Differential growth between the maxilla and the mandible was observed in each group but the changes were minimal. The skeletal frameworks of the two groups were maintained during the postpubertal period.

In conclusion, the Class III group showed an incremental growth change similar to the Class I group. The morphological characteristics of the skeletal Class III malocclusion are maintained during the postpubertal period.

Clinical Implications

The results of our longitudinal studies[6–12] on Class III facial growth suggest that Class III malocclusion is established early and before the prepubertal growth period. The authors[11,12] speculated the reason why Class I subjects with growth changes similar to those of Class III subjects could maintain a normal occlusion. This phenomenon may be attributed to the rotational change of the occlusal plane (Fig. 15-6). Namely, in the Class I group the occlusal plane is displaced in a downward-forward direction with counterclockwise rotation. Therefore the anteroposterior relationship between the bimaxillary apical bases evaluated on the occlusal plane (Wits appraisal) is harmoniously maintained despite differential jaw growth. However, in Class III subjects the amount of maxillomandibular differential growth is not compensated for by the counterclockwise rotational change of the occlusal plane. The dentoalveolar disharmony evaluated by Wits appraisal is significantly aggravated due to lack of homeostasis of the neuromuscular system, which functions to maintain a stable intercuspal position in normal occlusion. These results may point to the benefit of early orthodontic intervention that may minimize the amount of apical base discrepancy that seems to be aggravated with growth.

ORTHOPEDIC EFFECTS OF CHIN CAP THERAPY

The orthopedic effects of chin cap appliances, which were thought to improve facial growth in Class III patients with mandibular excess, became the object of orthodontists' attention in the 1960s. Since then, chin cap therapy has been widely recognized as a method for treating developing Class III malocclusion in young patients. A number of clinical and experimental studies[2,17–26] have reported that chin cap force has several short-term orthopedic effects: (1) redirection of mandibular growth, (2) backward repositioning of the mandible, (3) retardation of mandibular growth, and (4) remodeling of the mandible and the TMJ.

Sugawara et al.[27] reported long-term growth changes in patients treated with chin cap therapy at different ages and with various treatment schedules. The possibility that these effects may induce permanent skeletal changes and alter the prognathic skeletal profile, particularly when applied at an early age,[20,28] has kept attention on chin cap therapy. However, little is known about whether the improved skeletal profile can be maintained until craniofacial growth is complete. Most studies have been based on either relatively short-term results that are of too short a duration to determine the final result or long-term results that encompass too few subjects to be statistically valid. The short-term and long-term results of chin cap therapy on the developing Class III malocclusion are reviewed below.

In this study it was hypothesized that (1) early application of chin cap force is more effective for correction of skeletal discrepancies and (2) the short-term effects of chin cap therapy are maintained after complete growth. This study involved 63 Japanese girls who showed anterior crossbite and Class III skeletal pattern before treatment and who were divided into three groups according to their age at the start of chin cap therapy: age 7 (before the pubertal growth spurt),

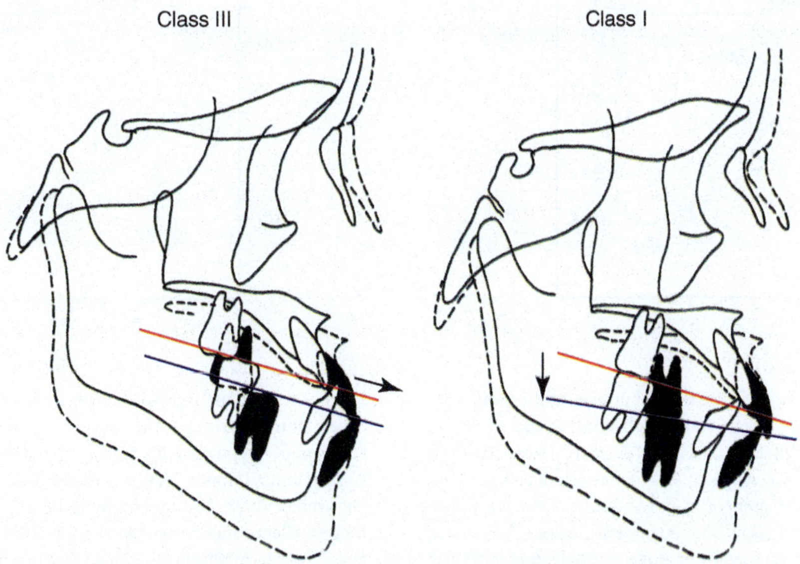

Figure 15-6 Differences in facial growth changes between Class III and Class I groups.

age 9 (at the beginning of the growth spurt), and age 11 (around the peak of the growth spurt). The data were derived from lateral cephalometric head films taken serially at the ages of 7, 9, 11, 14, and 17 years for analysis of intercuspal position. All patients underwent chin cap therapy at the beginning of the treatment but the length of time the chin cap was worn varied. Half of the patients in the total sample were also treated with a multibracket system at a later stage. Basically the same type of chin cap was worn by all patients. The force applied on the chin was oriented along a line from the gnathion to the sella turcica and ranged from 250 to 300 g per side of the chin. Patients were instructed to wear the chin cap for at least 14 hours daily. All subjects attained a normal anterior bite with the initial chin cap treatment but two cases showed anterior crossbite. Seven subjects had edge-to-edge bites at the final observation.

The average skeletal profile diagram for each group was constructed from x–y coordinates of 14 representative cephalometric landmarks using the same method as in the study by Bandai et al.[12] The results are summarized by the superimposition of the skeletal profile diagrams. Figures 15-7 to 15-9 show the longitudinal changes of the skeletal profiles in the groups that began chin cap therapy at ages 7, 9 and 11 years, respectively. Figures 15-10 and 15-11 represent the short-term and long-term effects of chin cap therapy on the skeletal profiles, respectively.

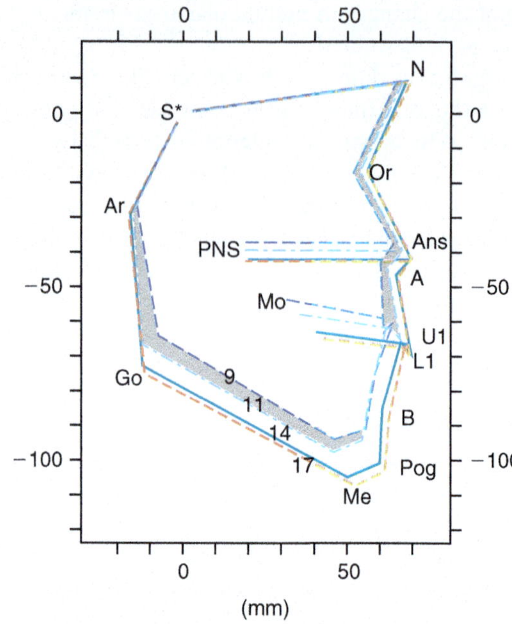

Figure 15-8 Longitudinal changes in the skeletal profiles of the group that began chin strap treatment at age 9 years and was observed at ages 11, 14, and 17 years. *A*, A point; *Ans*, anterior nasal spine; *Ar*, articulare; *B*, B point; *Go*, gonion; *L1*, lower incisor; *Me*, menton; *Mo*, medio-orbitale; *N*, nasion; *Or*, orbitale; *PNS*, posterior nasal spine; *Pog*, pogonion; *S**, sella; *U1*, upper incisor. (Reproduced with permission from Sugawara J, Asano T, Endo N, et al. Long-term effects of chincap therapy on skeletal profile in mandibular prognathism. *Am J Orthod Dentofacial Orthop.* 1990;98:127–133.)

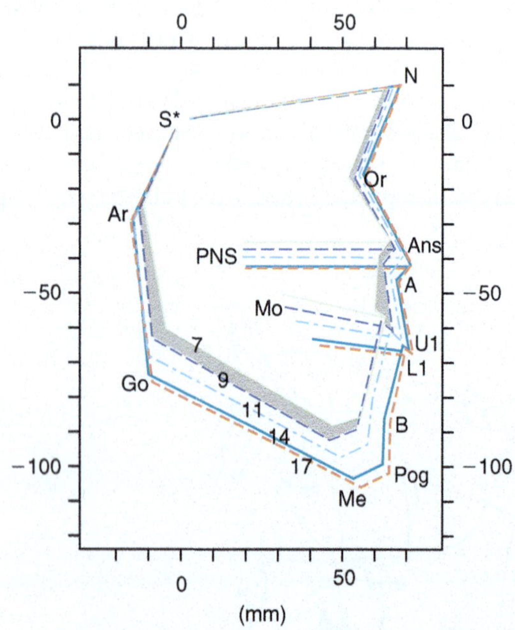

Figure 15-7 Longitudinal changes in the skeletal profiles of the group that began chin cap treatment at age 7 years and was observed at ages 9, 11, 14, and 17 years. *A*, A point; *Ans*, anterior nasal spine; *Ar*, articulare; *B*, B point; *Go*, gonion; *L1*, lower incisor; *Me*, menton; *Mo*, medio-orbitale; *N*, nasion; *Or*, orbitale; *PNS*, posterior nasal spine; *Pog*, pogonion; *S**, sella; *U1*, upper incisor. (Reproduced with permission from Sugawara J, Asano T, Endo N, et al. Long-term effects of chincap therapy on skeletal profile in mandibular prognathism. *Am J Orthod Dentofacial Orthop.* 1990;98:127–133.)

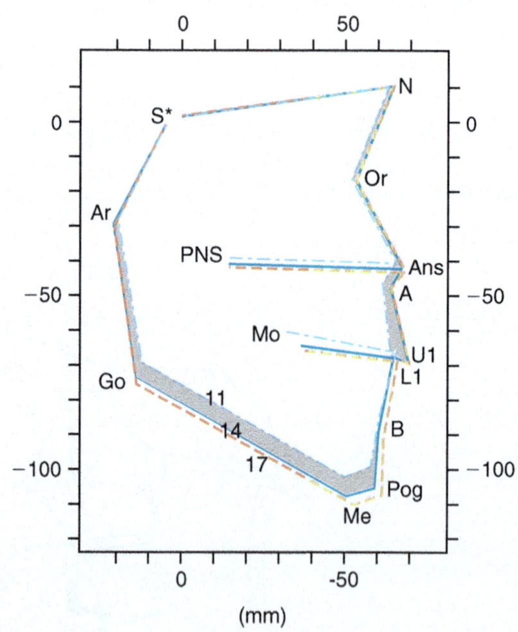

Figure 15-9 Longitudinal changes in the skeletal profiles of the group that began chin cap treatment at age 11 years and was observed at ages 14 and 17 years. *A*, A point; *Ans*, anterior nasal spine; *Ar*, articulare; *B*, B point; *Go*, gonion; *L1*, lower incisor; *Me*, menton; *Mo*, medio-orbitale; *N*, nasion; *Or*, orbitale; *PNS*, posterior nasal spine; *Pog*, pogonion; *S**, sella; *U1*, upper incisor. (Reproduced with permission from Sugawara J, Asano T, Endo N, et al. Long-term effects of chincap therapy on skeletal profile in mandibular prognathism. *Am J Orthod Dentofacial Orthop.* 1990;98:127–133.)

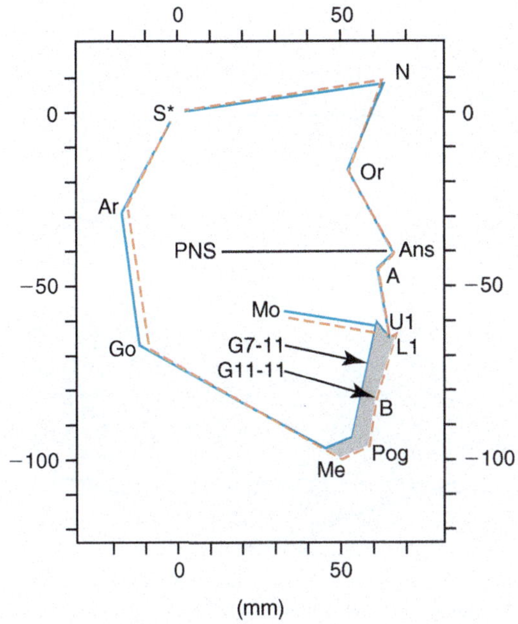

Figure 15-10 Comparison of skeletal profiles at age 11 years between a group of patients who began chin cap treatment at age 7 years and a control group of patients who had no prior treatment. *A*, A point; *Ans*, anterior nasal spine; *Ar*, articulare; *B*, B point; *Go*, gonion; *L1*, lower incisor; *Me*, menton; *Mo*, medio-orbitale; *N*, nasion; *Or*, orbitale; *PNS*, posterior nasal spine; *Pog*, pogonion; *S**, sella; *U1*, upper incisor. (Reproduced with permission from Sugawara J, Asano T, Endo N, et al. Long-term effects of chincap therapy on skeletal profile in mandibular prognathism. *Am J Orthod Dentofacial Orthop*. 1990;98:127–133.)

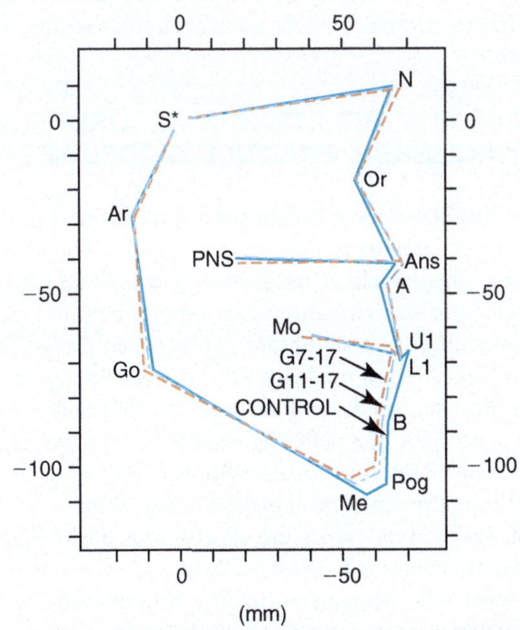

Figure 15-11 Comparison of skeletal profiles at age 17 years between a group of patients who began chin cap treatment at age 7 years, a group of patients who began chin cap treatment at age 11 years, and a control group of patients who had no prior treatment. *A*, A point; *Ans*, anterior nasal spine; *Ar*, articulare; *B*, B point; *Go*, gonion; *L1*, lower incisor; *Me*, menton; *Mo*, medio-orbitale; *N*, nasion; *Or*, orbitale; *PNS*, posterior nasal spine; *Pog*, pogonion; *S**, sella; *U1*, upper incisor. (Reproduced with permission from Sugawara J, Asano T, Endo N, et al. Long-term effects of chincap therapy on skeletal profile in mandibular prognathism. *Am J Orthod Dentofacial Orthop*. 1990;98:127–133.)

Short-Term Effects

The skeletal profiles of patients were significantly improved and there was retrusion of the mandible during the initial stage of chin cap therapy for every group (see Figs. 15-7 to 15-9). In response to the orthopedic force, the skeletal profiles of patients who began treatment at age 7 years changed more than those who began treatment at a later age. In addition, patients who began treatment at age 7 years showed a more posterior positioning of the mandible than those who entered treatment at age 11 years. These results indicate that chin cap treatment is more effective before the pubertal growth spurt. In other words, it appears that the effects of chin cap force may be offset by rapid mandibular growth during puberty, if all patients receive treatment under the same conditions. These data support the hypothesis that "the early application of chin cap force is more effective for correction of skeletal discrepancies."

Long-Term Effects

Figure 15-10 shows the differences in skeletal profiles at age 11 years for patients who had begun treatment at age 7 years and those who were just entering treatment at age 11 years. The latter group had received no treatment up to this age. When comparing these two groups, significant differences were observed in the anteroposterior position of the mandible but no significant difference in the maxillary region was apparent. The mandible of the first group had apparently been displaced in a backward direction during the 3 years of treatment. Moreover, a significant reduction in the gonial angle was observed during this period. Figure 15-10 shows that chin cap treatment had significant orthopedic effects (short-term) on the mandible in patients who began treatment at age 7 years.

Figure 15-11 shows the differences in skeletal profiles at age 17 years between patients who began treatment at age 7 years and at age 11 years, compared with the control group of 19-year-olds. For the group that began treatment at age 11 years, the position of the mandible was relatively more forward than the group who began treatment at age 7 years. Statistically, there was no significant difference between these two groups with respect to any of the landmarks. Although a great difference was observed in the position of the mandible at age 11 years, these differences decreased gradually up to age 17 years. The control Class III group, which received no treatment, showed the mandible in a relatively more forward position than the other two groups but anteroposteriorly there was no significant difference in any specific landmark. The changes in skeletal profile, although they represent significant improvement in the younger children, are not maintained in most cases. This finding suggests that skeletal profiles have a tendency to return to their original shapes, which may have been predetermined morphogenetically.[29,30] It has been speculated that some skeletal rebound may occur during or after the pubertal growth period. The significant rebound observed in this study indicates that the hypothesis that "the short-term

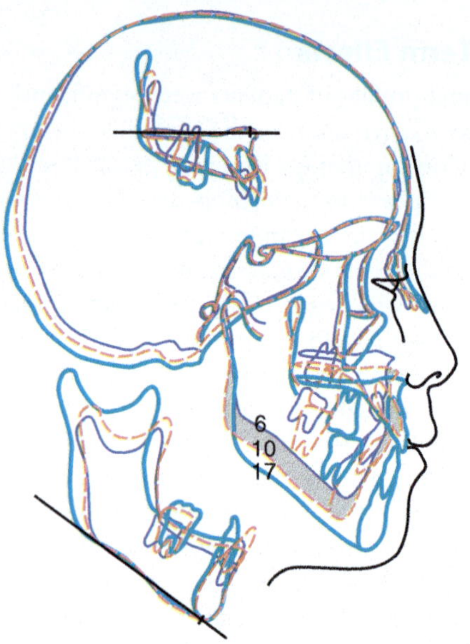

Figure 15-12 Cephalometric superimpositions for patient MS from the group that began chin cap therapy at age 7 years; observed at ages 10 and 17 years.

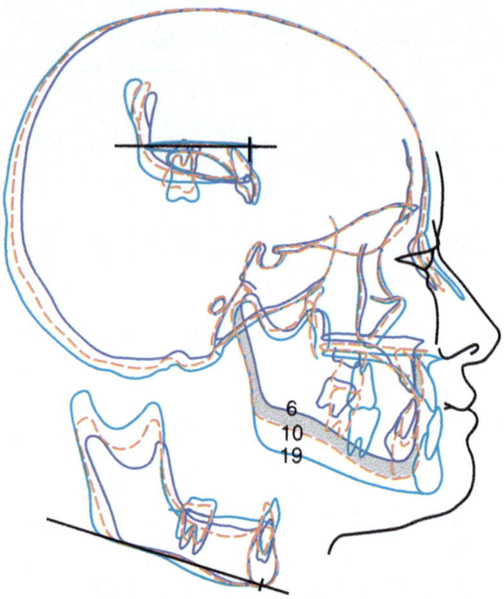

Figure 15-13 Cephalometric superimpositions for patient TS from the group that began chin cap therapy at age 7 years; observed at ages 10 and 19 years.

effects of chin cap therapy are maintained after complete growth" should be rejected.

Two cases manifest the effects and the limitations of chin cap orthopedic force. Figure 15-12 shows the changes with treatment of a patient from the group that began chin cap therapy at age 7 years. She received chin cap treatment for 3 years and at age 10 years her prognathic profile was drastically altered into a rather retrognathic profile by the short-term effects of the chin cap orthopedic force. At age 17 years, after the second phase of treatment with a multibracket system, her profile changed from retrognathic to a straight type, mainly due to skeletal rebound during the pubertal and postpubertal growth period. Despite orthopedic relapse, recurrence of anterior crossbite was avoided by dentoalveolar compensation in the second phase of orthodontic treatment.

The patient shown in Figure 15-13 also belonged to the group that began chin cap therapy at age 7 years. By age 10 years her skeletal profile had changed into a straight type. However, at age 19 years recurrence of anterior crossbite was observed, probably due to skeletal rebound and postpubertal differential growth.

Clinical Implications

Short-term and long-term studies on the effects of chin cap force indicate that the skeletal profile is greatly improved during the initial stages of chin cap therapy but such changes are often not maintained thereafter. In other words, chin cap force seldom alters the inherited prognathic characteristics of Class III profiles after growth.

Based on these findings, the following recommendations can be made on the use of chin cap therapy. First, the chin cap appliance should be considered only as an option to correct anterior crossbite in the first phase of treatment for Class III patients who are still growing. Second, indications for chin cap therapy should be limited to mild-to-moderate skeletal Class III malocclusions that can be camouflaged by dentoalveolar compensation in the second phase of orthodontic treatment, even if anterior crossbite recurs after the first phase of treatment. Third, chin cap therapy is contraindicated in Class III patients with apparent mandibular excess. For such cases, surgical orthodontic treatment is recommended to construct stable and functional occlusion after growth.

CLASS III CORRECTION IN ACCORDANCE WITH CLINICAL PRACTICE GUIDELINES

The clinical practice guidelines help practitioners to decide on the best treatment options in consultation with their patients. The guidelines for growing Class III patients were derived from studying numerous reported clinical studies. However, there is a significant gap between the guidelines and evidence-based medicine (EBM), because almost all of the clinical studies did not undergo critical examination by EBM specialists. The deficit of evidence in the guidelines is supplemented by empirical knowledge that was accumulated over a long time in clinical orthodontic practice.

The only way to verify the effectiveness of the proposed clinical guidelines is to statistically evaluate the outcome in long-term follow-up cases, because orthodontic treatment mostly targets symptoms rather than causes.

We have been managing Class III patients in accordance with the clinical practice guidelines and practicing post-treatment evaluation for more than 10 years. No fundamental problems with the guidelines have been identified.

The treatment progress and results of three subjects who have undergone orthodontic management in accordance with the guidelines are reported below.

Text continued on p. 322

CASE REPORT 1

This patient was a 7-year-old girl. Although she did not complain about her profile and occlusion, her mother seriously worried about her anterior crossbite and prognathic profile. Figure 15-14 shows her facial and oral photographs at the initial examination.

Problem List

The patient's principal problems identified from various analyses were:

- Forward position of the mandible
- Mild Class III jaw relationship
- Short face tendency
- Occlusal interference at incisors
- Gingival recession at lower left central incisor
- Anterior crossbite
- Deep bite
- Class III denture
- Excessive interaction between the upper and lower lips at the intercuspal position

She was diagnosed as having a good prognosis because her mild anteroposterior jaw disharmony would allow downward–backward rotation of the mandible to correct the anterior crossbite and deep

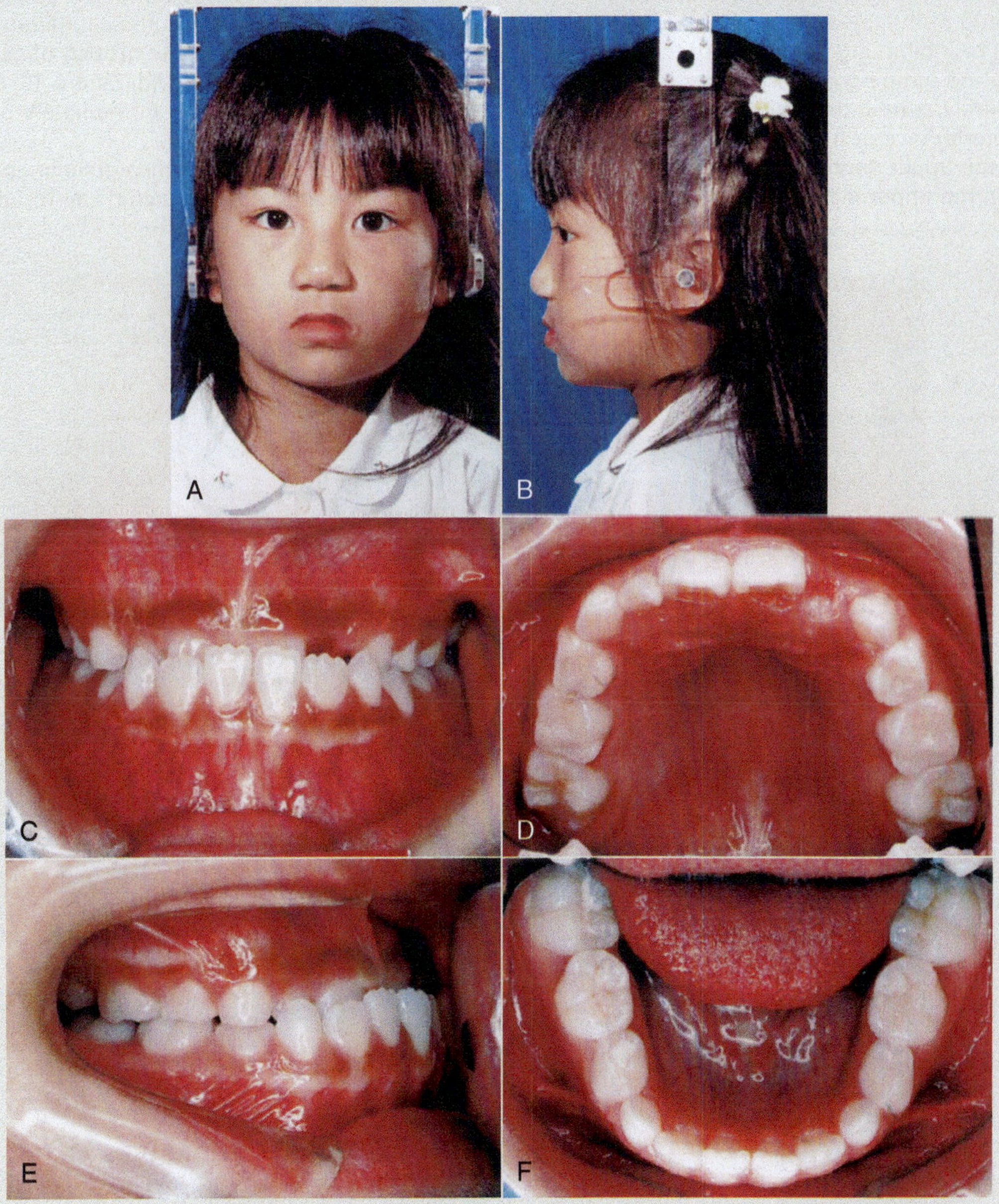

Figure 15-14 Facial (**A and B**) and intraoral (**C–F**) photographs at initial examination (age 7 years, 3 months).

Continued

CASE REPORT 1—cont'd

bite. Her treatment plan was established by following the right-hand pathway in the clinical practice guidelines (see Fig. 15-3).

First Phase of Treatment

Figure 15-15 shows the progress of the patient's first phase of orthodontic treatment. A jumping plate was applied to the lower dentition and a partial bracket system was applied to the upper dentition. The roles of the jumping plate were (1) to stabilize her mandibular position, (2) to raise her bite to allow the placement of brackets at the upper incisors, (3) to promote the eruption of the first molars by cutting the jumping plate off at the distal end of the lower second deciduous molars, (4) to inhibit lingual tipping of the lower incisors during jumping of the anterior bite, and (5) to smoothly correct the anterior crossbite without occlusal interference at the incisors. A partial bracket system in the upper dentition was applied to expand and intrude the upper incisors.

Figure 15-16 shows the patient at age 8 years, immediately after the first phase of treatment. The cephalometric superimpositions during the first phase of treatment show that her anterior crossbite was corrected by labial movement of the upper incisors and a clockwise rotation of the mandible (Fig. 15-17). In addition, the short face tendency and excessive interaction of the lips were simultaneously improved.

Growth Observation Period

After the first phase of treatment, growth observation and control of oral hygiene were performed every 6 months until the postpubertal period. Figure 15-18 shows the cephalometric superimpositions during the growth observation period from 8 to 16 years old. Figure 15-19 shows the patient at age 16 years immediately before the second phase of treatment.

The current clinical practice guidelines do not recommend applying a chin cap to inhibit

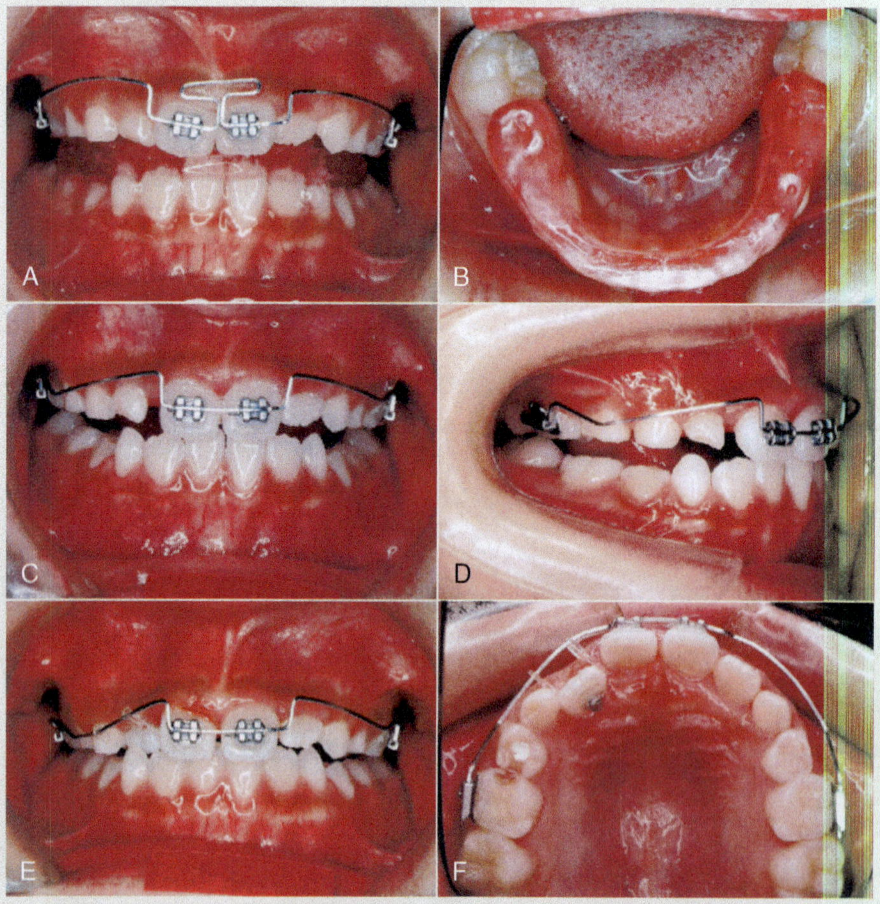

Figure 15-15 Biomechanics for the first phase of treatment. **A and B,** Partial brackets and jumping plate. **C and D,** Jumped with upper utility arch and vertical stop at first molars. **E and F,** Utility arch and labial movement of the upper right lateral incisor.

CASE REPORT 1—cont'd

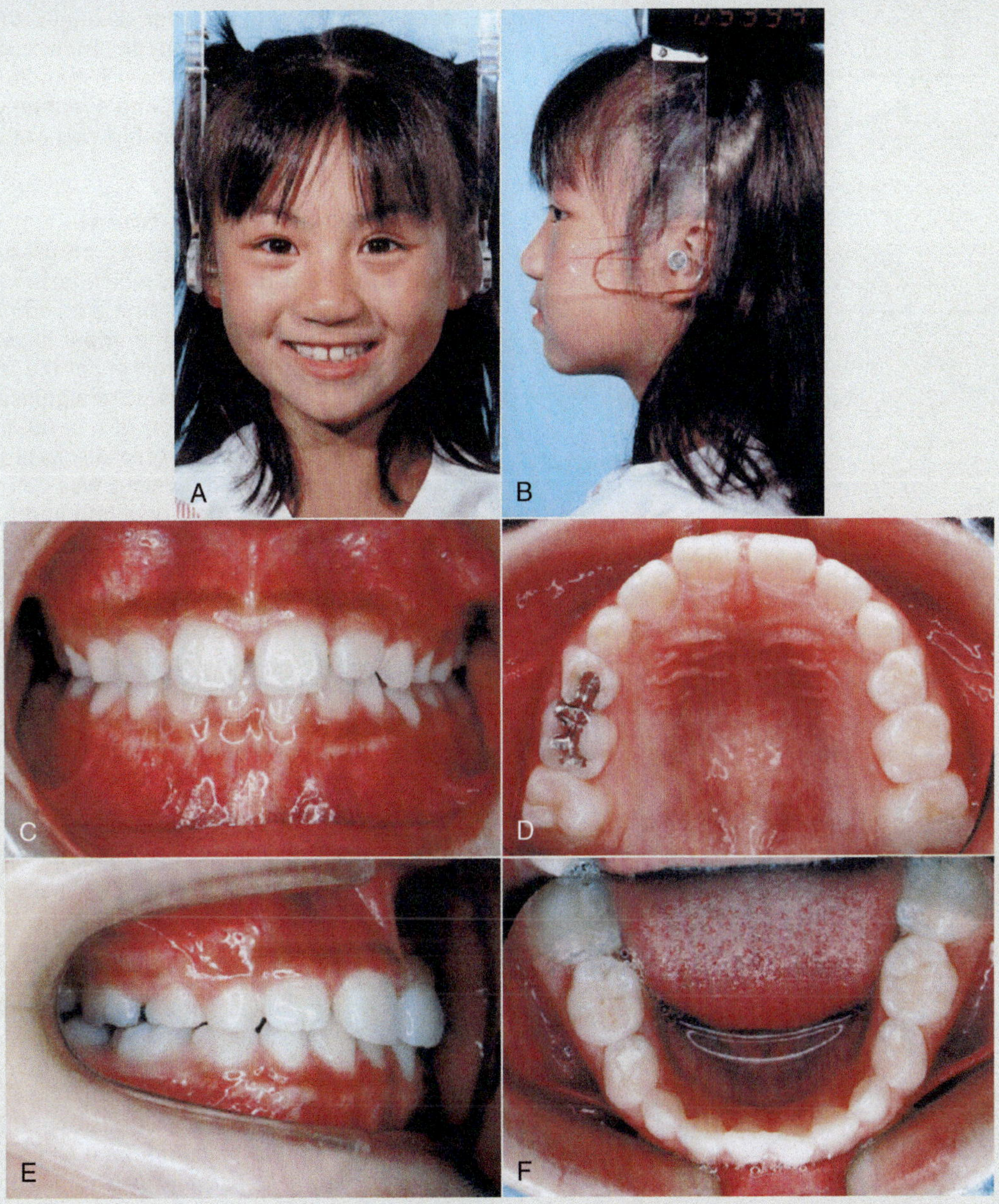

Figure 15-16 Facial (**A and B**) and intraoral (**C–F**) photographs after the first phase of treatment (age 8 years, 3 months).

Continued

CASE REPORT 1—cont'd

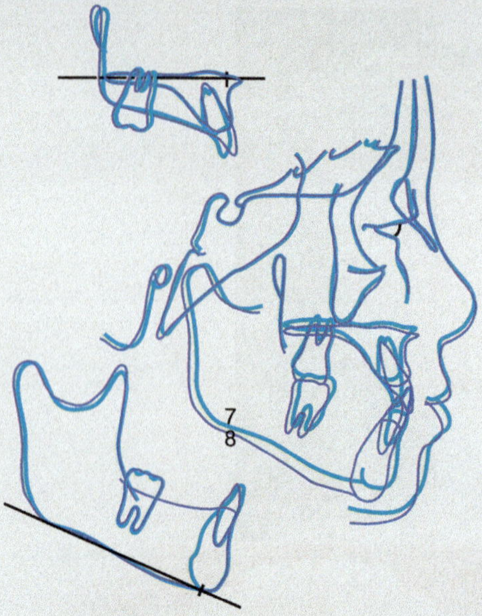

Figure 15-17 Cephalometric superimpositions show the dentofacial changes during the first phase of treatment. Thick solid line is age 7 years, 3 months (initial); thin solid line is age 8 years, 3 months (immediately after the first phase of treatment).

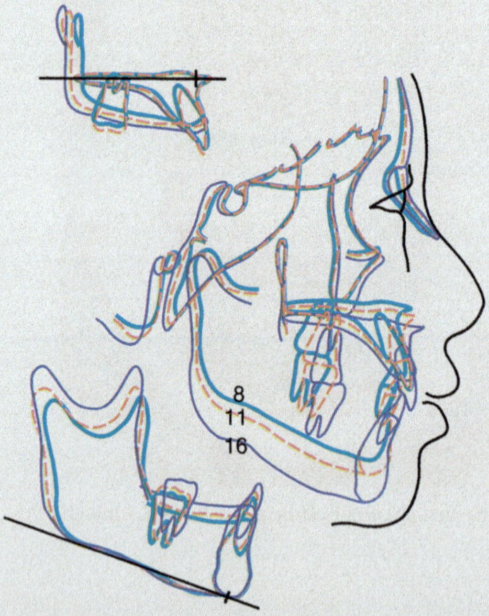

Figure 15-18 Cephalometric superimpositions show the dentofacial changes during the growth observation period. Thick solid line is age 8 years, 3 months (immediately after the first phase of treatment); dotted line is age 11 years, 3 months (during growth observation); thin solid line is age 16 years, 3 months (immediately prior to the second phase of treatment).

mandibular growth and alter skeletal profile. Although a chin cap orthopedic force was not applied in this case, the patient's mandible mostly showed downward growth and eventually her anteroposterior jaw relationship was not aggravated (see Fig. 15-18).

Second Phase of Treatment

Figure 15-20 shows the patient's progress during the second phase of treatment, which lasted just a year. A multibracket system was first applied only to the upper dentition to intrude the upper incisors and to enable the placement of brackets at the lower incisors. The upper incisors were significantly intruded with the application of a basal arch (see Fig. 15-20, A and B). Then brackets were bonded to the lower dentition and leveling was performed (see Fig. 15-20, C and D). After detailing and finishing, all brackets were debonded and a wrap-around type of retainer and lingual bonded retainer were applied to the upper and lower dentition, respectively (see Fig. 15-20, E and F). The cephalometric superimpositions indicate dentofacial changes during the second phase of treatment (Fig. 15-21). Figure 15-22 shows the patient 1 year after debonding. She has maintained a balanced profile, function, and occlusion and a caries-free status. Regarding skeletal changes, her mandible showed slight downward growth but the maxilla did not change at all. It is obvious that her orthodontic problems were improved by intrusion of the upper incisors and proclination of the bimaxillary incisors.

Summary

This patient exhibited anterior crossbite with short face and overclosured bite. However, as her anteroposterior jaw disharmony was quite mild, she could be diagnosed as skeletal Class I. In cases with good prognosis, such as this one, therapeutic intervention should be as minimal as possible. In this case the total treatment period (first and second phases) was only 1 year, 5 months. "The minimum intervention and the maximum profit for each patient" is one of the important mottos in the clinical practice guidelines. In keeping with this, the length of time that orthodontic appliances, which can injure teeth and periodontal tissue, are worn should be shortened.

CASE REPORT 1—cont'd

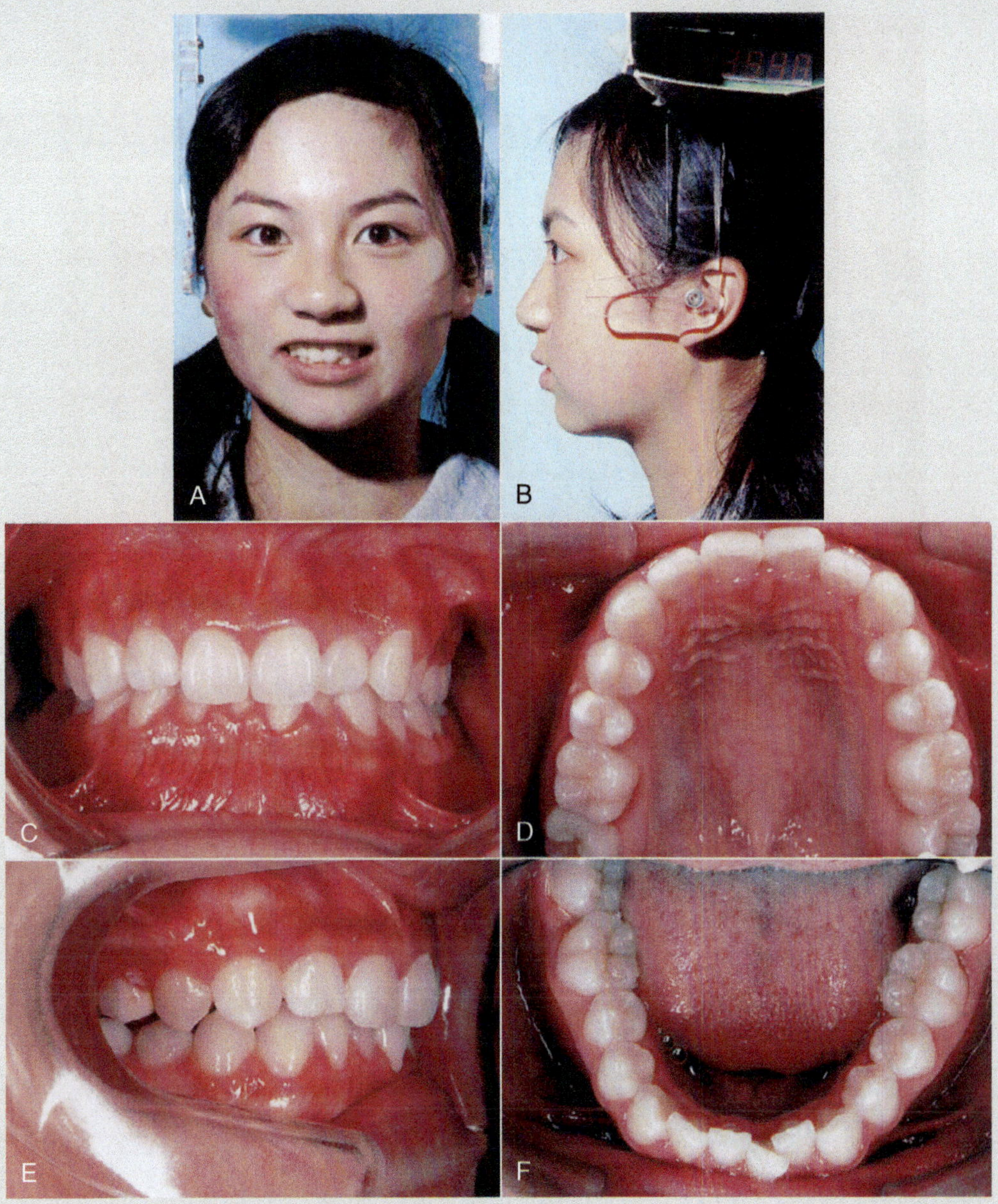

Figure 15-19 Facial (**A and B**) and intraoral (**C–F**) photographs before the second phase of treatment (age 16 years, 3 months).

Continued

CASE REPORT 1—cont'd

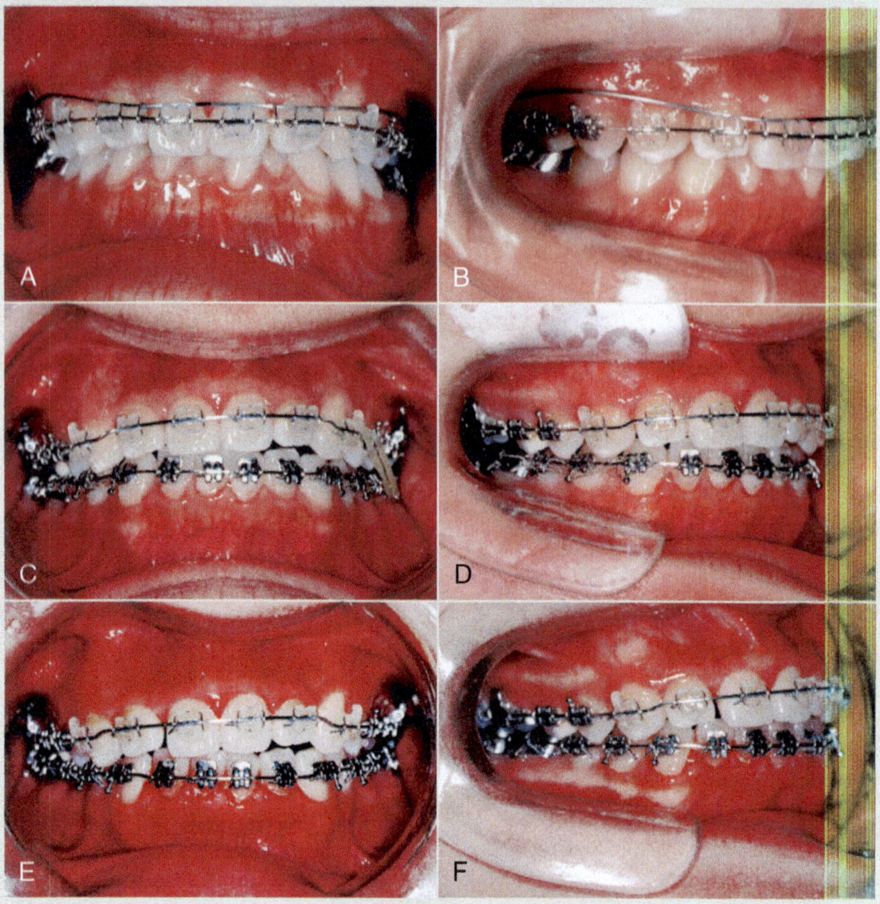

Figure 15-20 Biomechanics for the second phase of treatment. **A and B,** Upper multibracket system and a basal arch for incisor intrusion. **C and D,** Lower multibracket system. **E and F,** Overcorrection for deep bite.

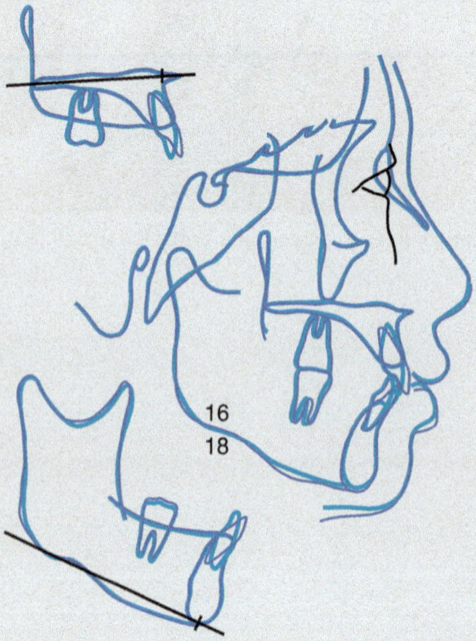

Figure 15-21 Cephalometric superimpositions show the dentofacial changes during the second phase of treatment. Thick solid line is age 16 years, 3 months (immediately prior to the second phase of treatment); thin solid line is 18 years, 4 months (at debonding).

CASE REPORT 1—cont'd

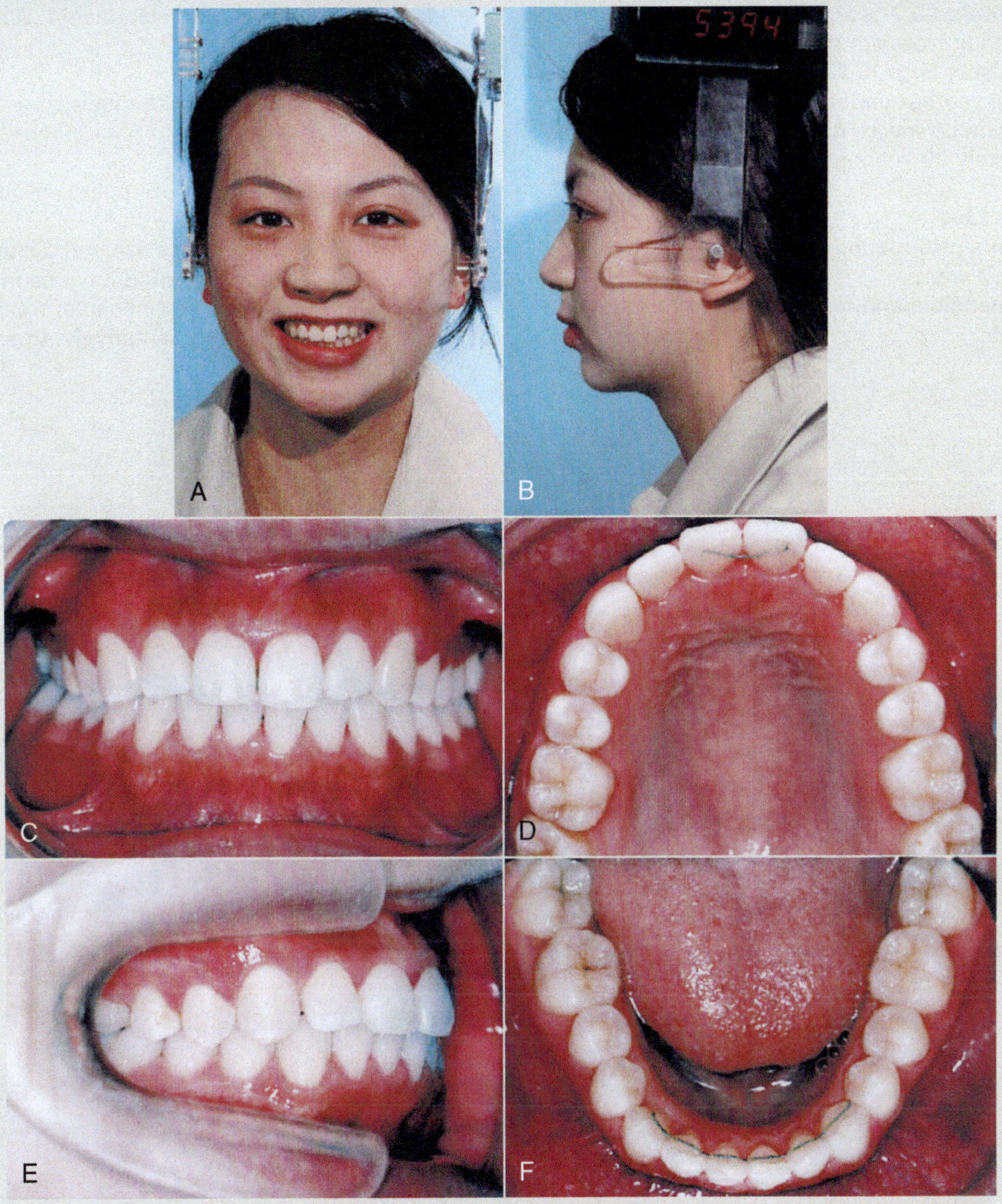

Figure 15-22 Facial (**A and B**) and intraoral (**C–F**) photographs 2 years after completion of the second phase of treatment (age 19 years, 4 months).

CASE REPORT 2

This patient was a 7-year-old girl who complained about anterior crossbite and winging of the upper central incisors (Fig. 15-23). Regarding family history, her mother underwent orthognathic surgery for correction of severe mandibular prognathism approximately 30 years earlier.

Problem List

The patient's orthodontic problems at the initial examination were:

- Large mandible and forward position of the mandible
- Moderate Class III jaw relationship (Wits appraisal: –8.5 mm)
- Long face tendency
- Occlusal interference at the incisors
- Anterior crossbite
- Class III denture
- Diastema and winging of upper central incisors

Considering the patient's skeletal disharmony and genetic background, she could have been managed surgically, skipping the first phase of treatment. However, it was decided, tentatively, to apply

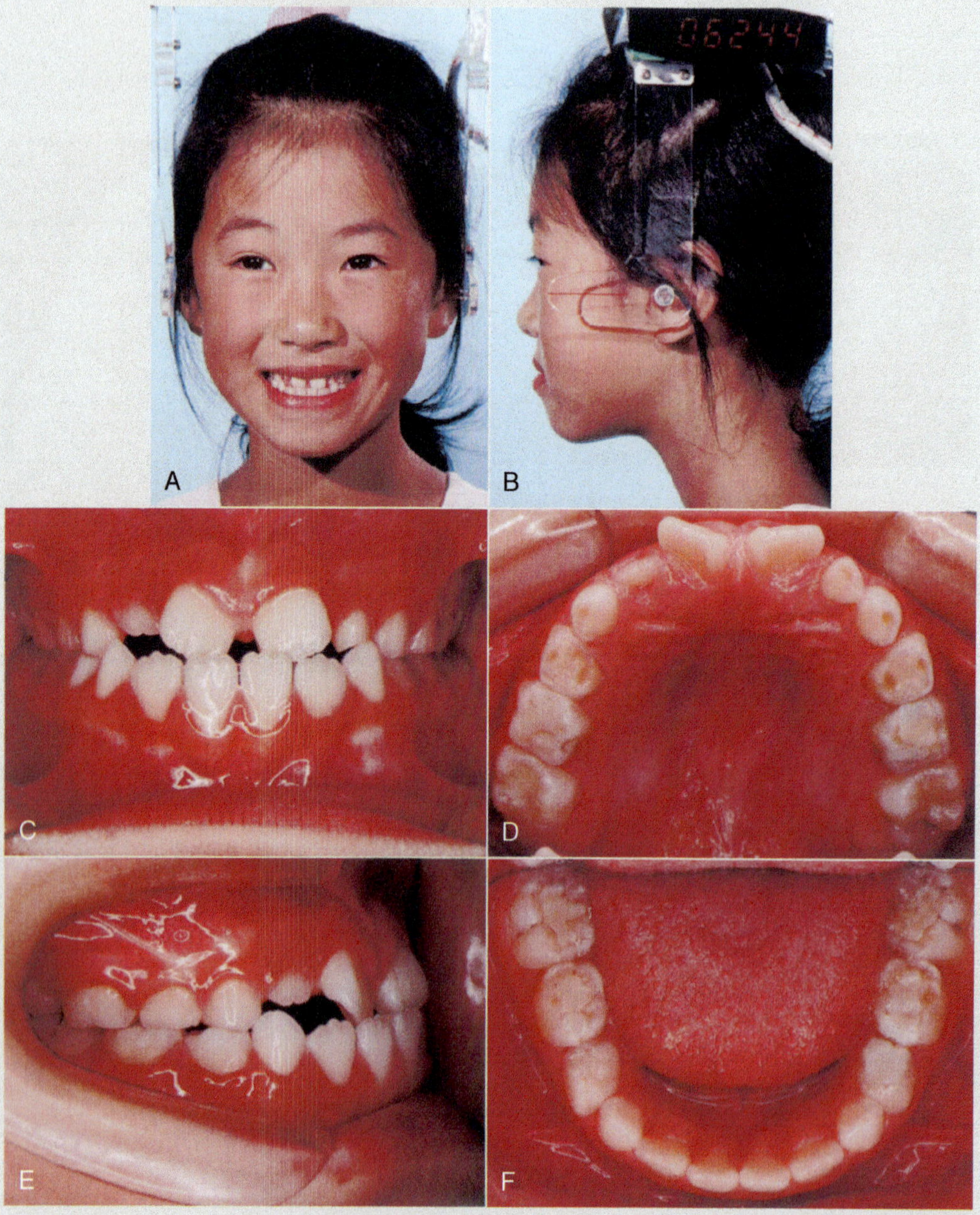

Figure 15-23 Facial (**A and B**) and intraoral (**C–F**) photographs at initial examination (age 7 years, 10 months).

CASE REPORT 2—cont'd

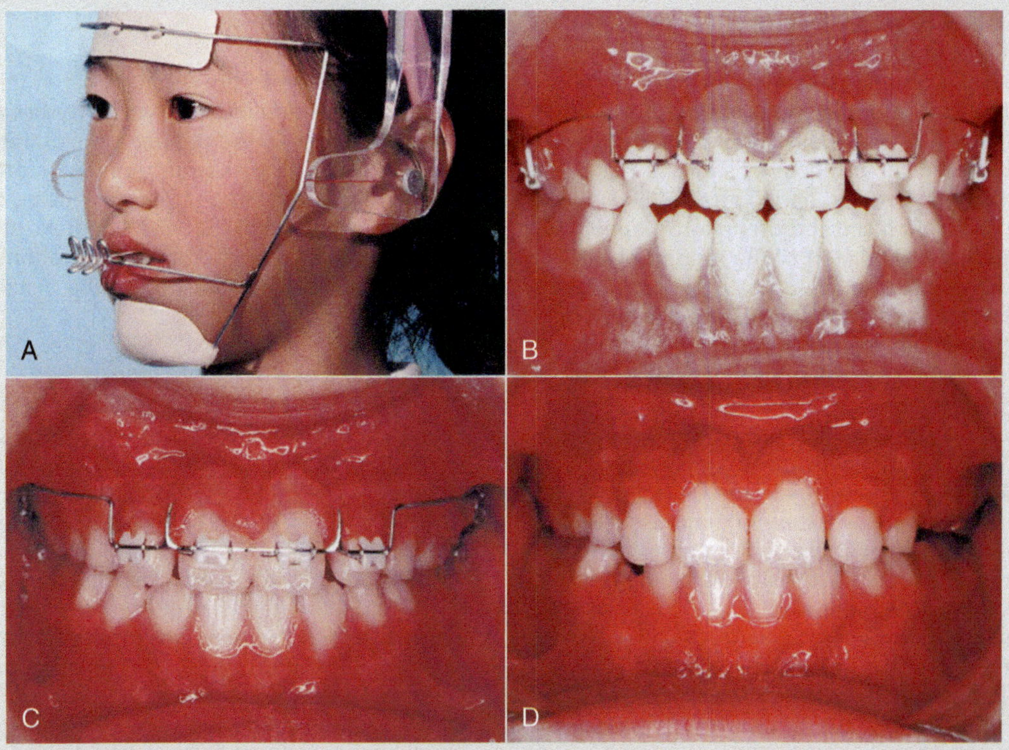

Figure 15-24 Biomechanics for the first phase of treatment. **A,** Face mask (maxillary incisors protraction [MIP]). **B,** Oral appliance (upper utility arch). **C,** Correction of anterior crossbite. **D,** Immediately after the first phase of treatment (age 9 years, 4 months).

first-phase mechanics, because she was not a clear case for surgery at that time.

First Phase of Treatment

After eruption of the upper lateral incisors, the first phase of treatment began at the age of 8 years and the progress is shown in Figure 15-24. Because the long-term effects of chin cap orthopedic force for alteration of skeletal profile were already being questioned at that time, protraction of the upper incisors using a face mask (referred to as maxillary incisors protraction [MIP])[31] was applied (see Fig. 15-24, A). A 2 × 4 partial bracket system was used as an oral appliance (see Fig. 15-24, B and C). Her anterior crossbite was corrected within 1 month with the application of these first-phase mechanics (see Fig. 15-24, C). After stabilizing the occlusion, all appliances were removed (see Fig. 15-24, D). The first phase of treatment lasted just 5 months.

The cephalometric superimpositions show the dentofacial changes during the first phase of treatment (Fig. 15-25). Her anterior crossbite was corrected by labial movement of the upper incisors and retroclination of the lower incisors; following these dental changes the mandible showed downward growth and displacement.

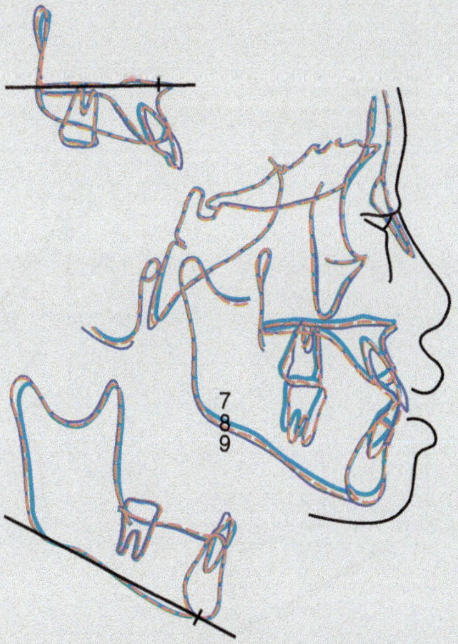

Figure 15-25 Cephalometric superimpositions show the dentofacial changes during the first phase of treatment. Thick solid line is age 7 years, 10 months (initial); dotted line is age 8 years, 10 months (during the first phase of treatment); thin solid line is age 9 years, 4 months (immediately after the first phase of treatment).

Continued

CASE REPORT 2—cont'd

Growth Observation Period

Between the ages of 9 and 16 years, growth observation and oral hygiene management were performed every 6 months and no orthodontic appliances needed to be worn. Figure 15-26 shows the cephalometric superimpositions during the growth observation period and Figure 15-27 shows the patient's facial and oral photographs immediately before the start of the second phase of treatment at 16 years old. Since a chin cap orthopedic force for controlling mandibular growth was not applied, her mandible appeared to grow excessively in a downward and forward direction. However, the amount of mandibular growth measured at Cd-Gn was 13.0 mm during the growth observation period, which is the same average mandibular growth change as in the Class I girls (13.1 mm) and less growth than in the Class III girls (14.9 mm) described in Table 15-2.

The patient's problem list immediately before the second phase of treatment was:

- Mandibular asymmetry
- Large mandible and forward displacement
- Skeletal Class III jaw relation (Wits appraisal: –9.0 mm)
- Deviation of lower dental midline
- Anterior crossbite
- Open bite tendency
- Class III denture

In comparison to the problem list at initial examination, mandibular asymmetry became obvious. However, the patient's skeletal disharmony was still not severe enough to indicate orthognathic surgery and camouflage treatment using the skeletal anchorage system (SAS) (see Chapter 20)[31,32] was chosen for the second phase of orthodontic mechanics without extraction of the bicuspids (Fig. 15-28).

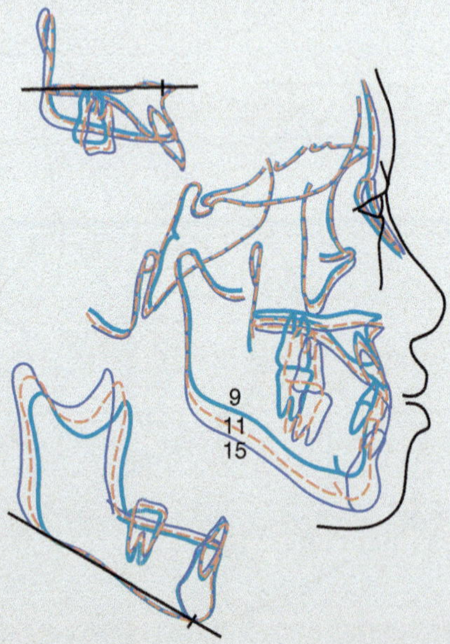

Figure 15-26 Cephalometric superimpositions show the dentofacial changes during the growth observation period. Thick solid line is age 9 years, 4 months (immediately after the first phase of treatment); dotted line is age 11 years, 10 months (during the growth observation period); thin solid line is age 15 years, 10 months (immediately prior to the second phase of treatment).

Second Phase of Treatment

Figure 15-29 shows the treatment progress during the second phase. Subsequent to extraction of the bilateral mandibular third molars, leveling and aligning of the upper and lower dentition began (see Fig. 15-29, A). Four months later, orthodontic anchor plates were bilaterally implanted beneath the apices of the molars at the mandibular body. Then the lower molars were distalized using SAS,[32–34] in which the anchor plates are implanted as absolute anchorage (see Fig. 15-29, B). Deviation of the mandibular dental midline was improved within 1 month and the major problems with occlusion were mostly corrected within 2 months (see Fig. 15-29, C and D).

Figure 15-30 shows the facial and oral photographs 1 year after debonding. The patient's skeletal problems were successfully camouflaged with the application of SAS mechanics. As shown in the cephalometric superimpositions (Fig. 15-31), the entire mandibular dentition was distalized asymmetrically. Therefore the post-treatment evaluation of this case suggested that SAS is very effective as second-phase mechanics and will be widely used for Class III correction and revision.

Summary

Throughout the treatment it was difficult to determine whether orthognathic surgery was indicated. It appears that the first phase of treatment made almost no significant difference to the final result. However, it is easy to be wise after the event; therefore in borderline cases such as this, the decision as to which management pathway to follow should be left to the patient's choice and the doctor's discretion. It is very important to recognize that the second phase of orthodontic treatment after the postpubertal growth period places a great deal of weight on such a borderline Class III case. The first phase of treatment must be completed quickly and not allowed to continue aimlessly, so that the effective and reliable camouflage biomechanics of SAS can be applied.

CASE REPORT 2—cont'd

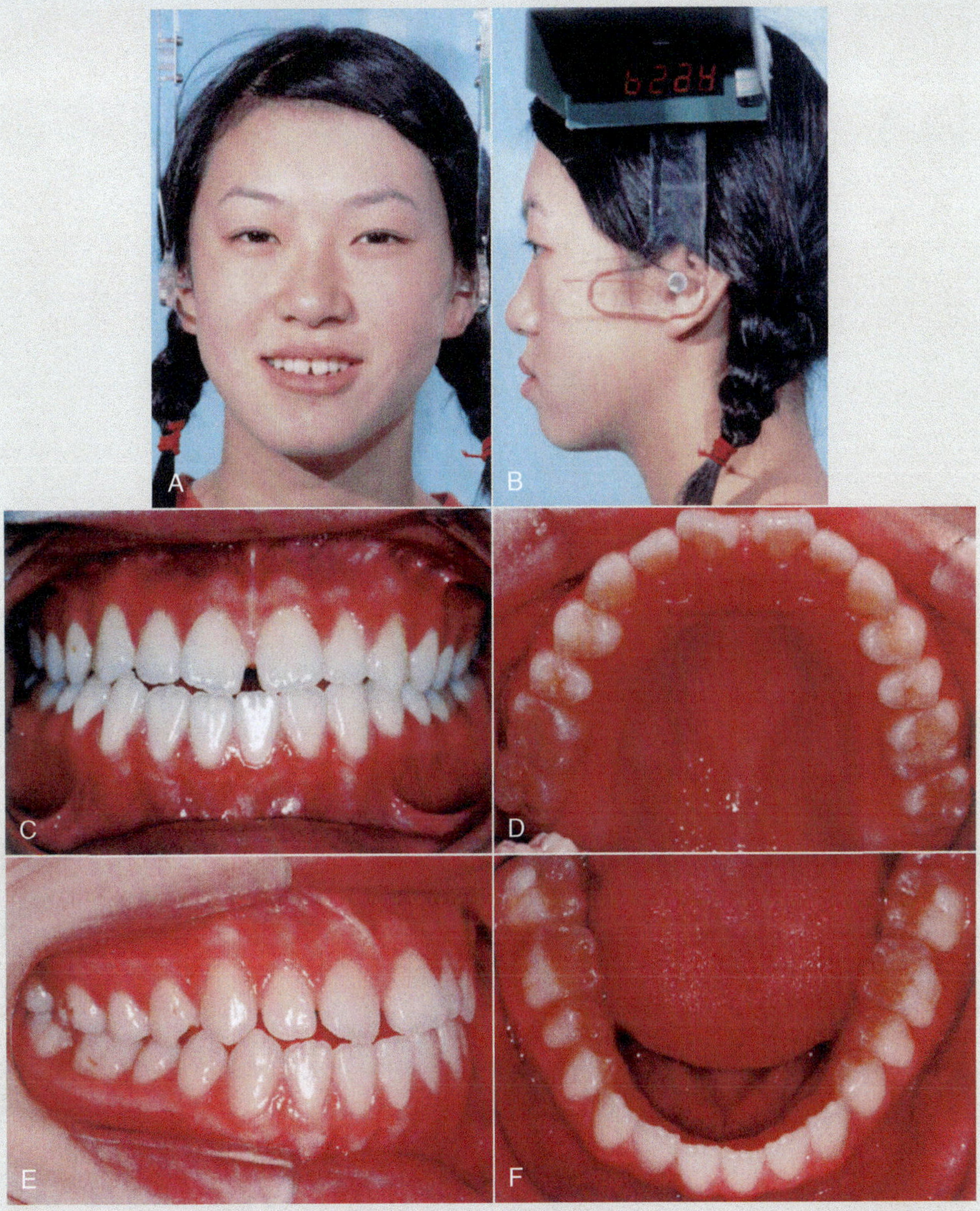

Figure 15-27 Facial (**A and B**) and intraoral (**C–F**) photographs before the second phase of treatment (age 15 years, 11 months).

Continued

CASE REPORT 2—cont'd

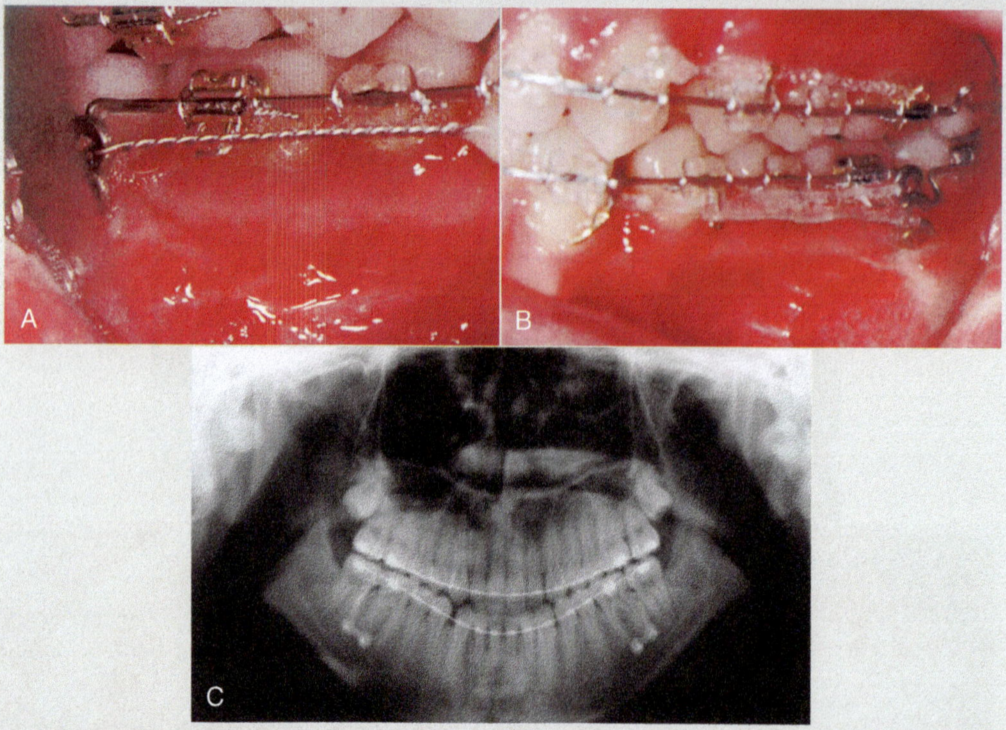

Figure 15-28 Skeletal anchorage system (SAS). Anterior crossbite and asymmetrical mandibular dentition were corrected by asymmetrical distalization of the lower molars with titanium anchor plates.

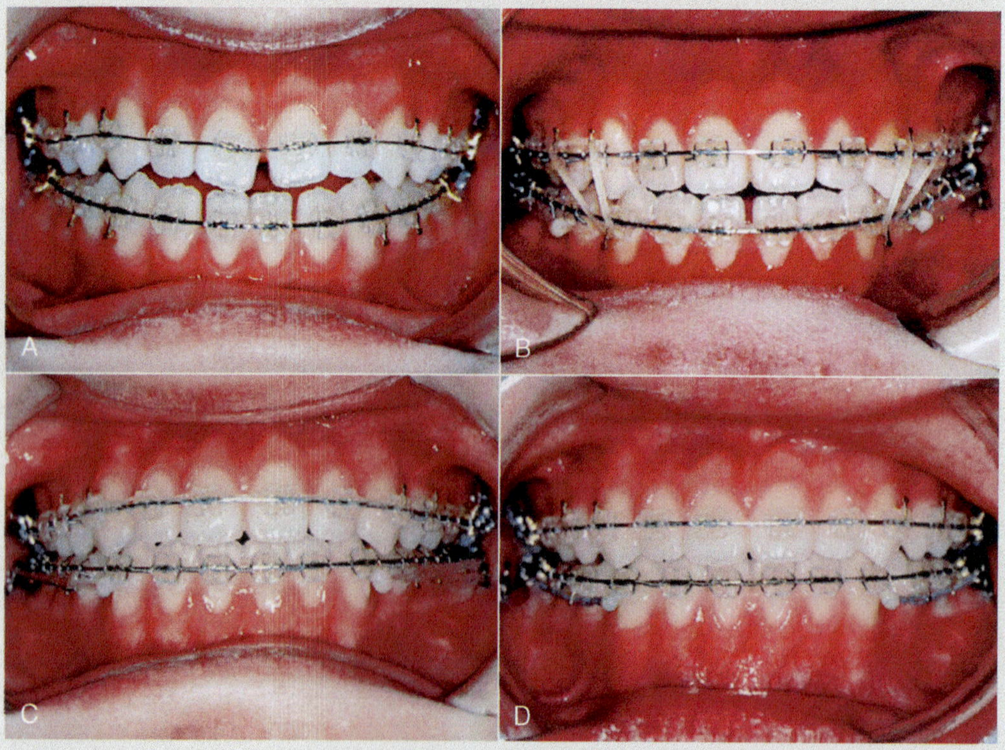

Figure 15-29 Treatment progress of the second phase of treatment. **A,** Leveling and aligning of the upper and lower arches. **B,** Distalization of the lower molars. **C,** Anterior crossbite and asymmetrical dentition were corrected. **D,** Immediately prior to debonding.

CASE REPORT 2—cont'd

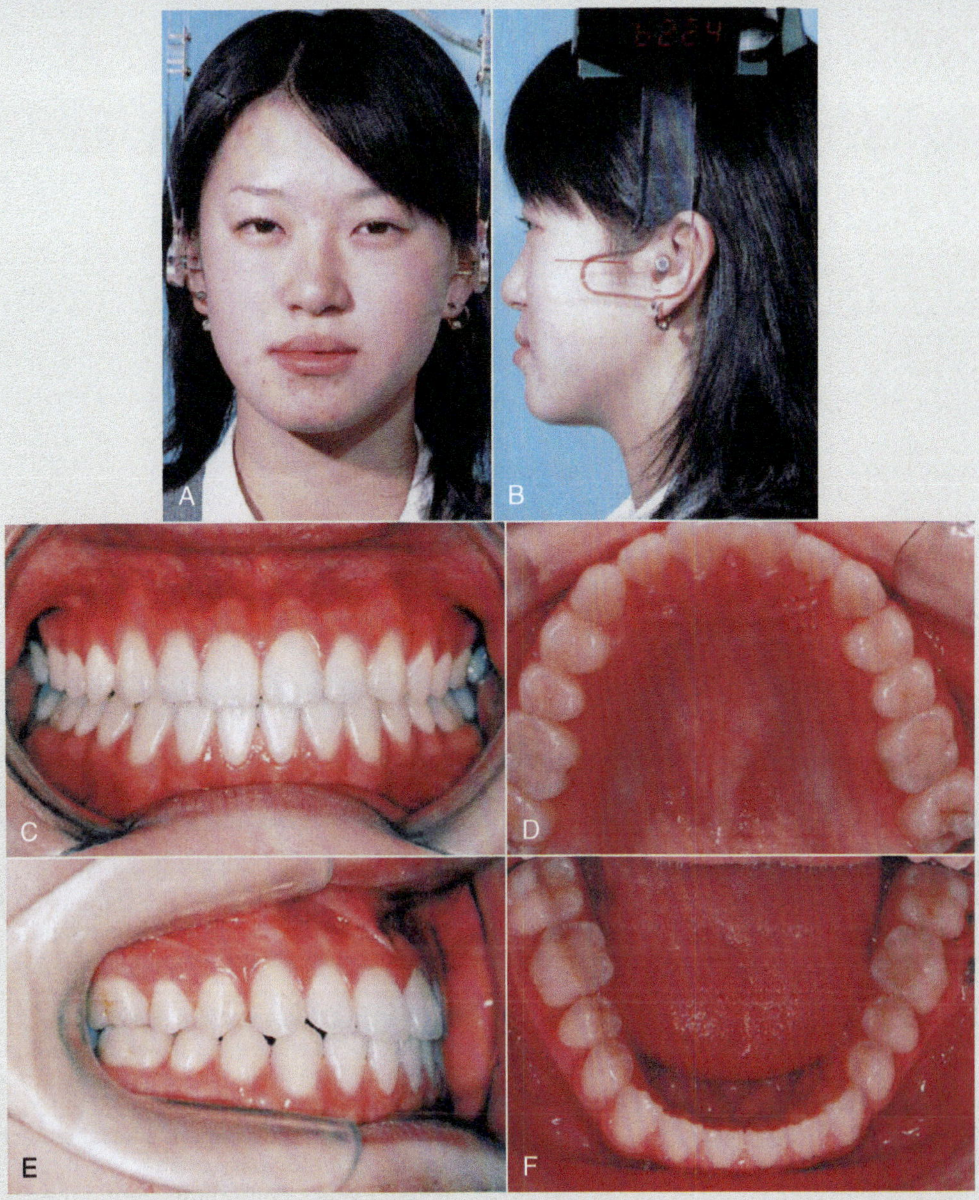

Figure 15-30 Facial (**A and B**) and intraoral (**C–F**) photographs 1 year after completion of the second phase of treatment (age 18 years, 1 month).

Continued

CASE REPORT 2—cont'd

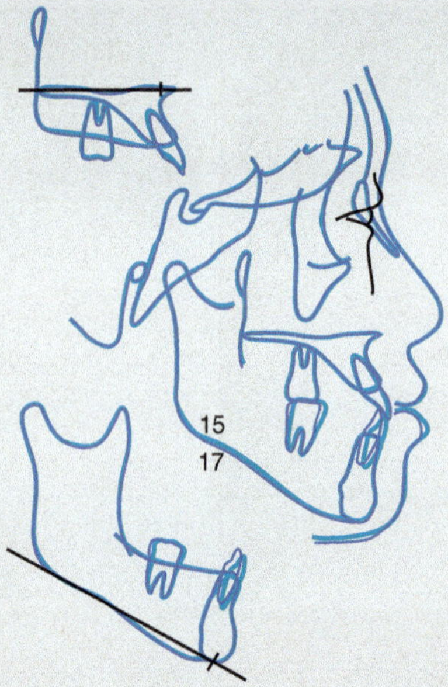

Figure 15-31 Cephalometric superimpositions show dentofacial changes during the second phase of treatment. Thick solid line is age 15 years, 10 months (immediately prior to the second phase of treatment); thin solid line is age 17 years, 1 month (at debonding).

CASE REPORT 3

This patient is a 6-year-old girl who complained of anterior crossbite at the initial consultation (Fig. 15-32). Regarding her family history, her father had anterior crossbite.

Problem List

The patient's problem list at the initial examination was:

- Extremely large mandible and forward position of the mandible
- Severe Class III jaw relationship (Wits appraisal: −13.5 mm)
- Hypodontia
- Total crossbite
- Deviation of maxillary dental midline
- Class III denture
- High risk of dental caries

Considering the patient's severe skeletal disharmony, genetic background, hypodontia, and high risk of caries, following the left-hand pathway of the clinical practice guidelines (see Fig. 15-3) was proposed to her parents, because it was thought to be very difficult to control her mandibular excess even by means of chin cap orthopedic force. After a growth observation period without having received any first-phase treatment, surgical orthodontic treatment was to be undertaken depending on the final differential diagnosis. However, it was important to inform her parents of the possibility of a nonsurgical approach. Her parents understood the meaning of the clinical guidelines and accepted the comprehensive treatment plan.

Growth Observation Period

Figure 15-33 shows the facial and oral photographs at age 15 years and immediately before presurgical orthodontic treatment. It was cephalometrically confirmed that the patient's facial growth almost ceased after 15 years of age. The observation period lasted 9 years. During this period the maxilla showed a downward growth tendency but the mandible showed downward–forward growth. Consequently, anteroposterior jaw disharmony seemed to become more severe (Fig. 15-34). Her problem list at that time was:

- Mild facial asymmetry
- Severe Class III jaw relationship (Wits appraisal: −14.5 mm)
- Deviation of the mandibular dental midline (2 mm to the right)
- Total crossbite
- Dental compensation of the upper and lower incisors
- Class III denture
- Hypodontia (#22, #25, #27)

CASE REPORT 3—cont'd

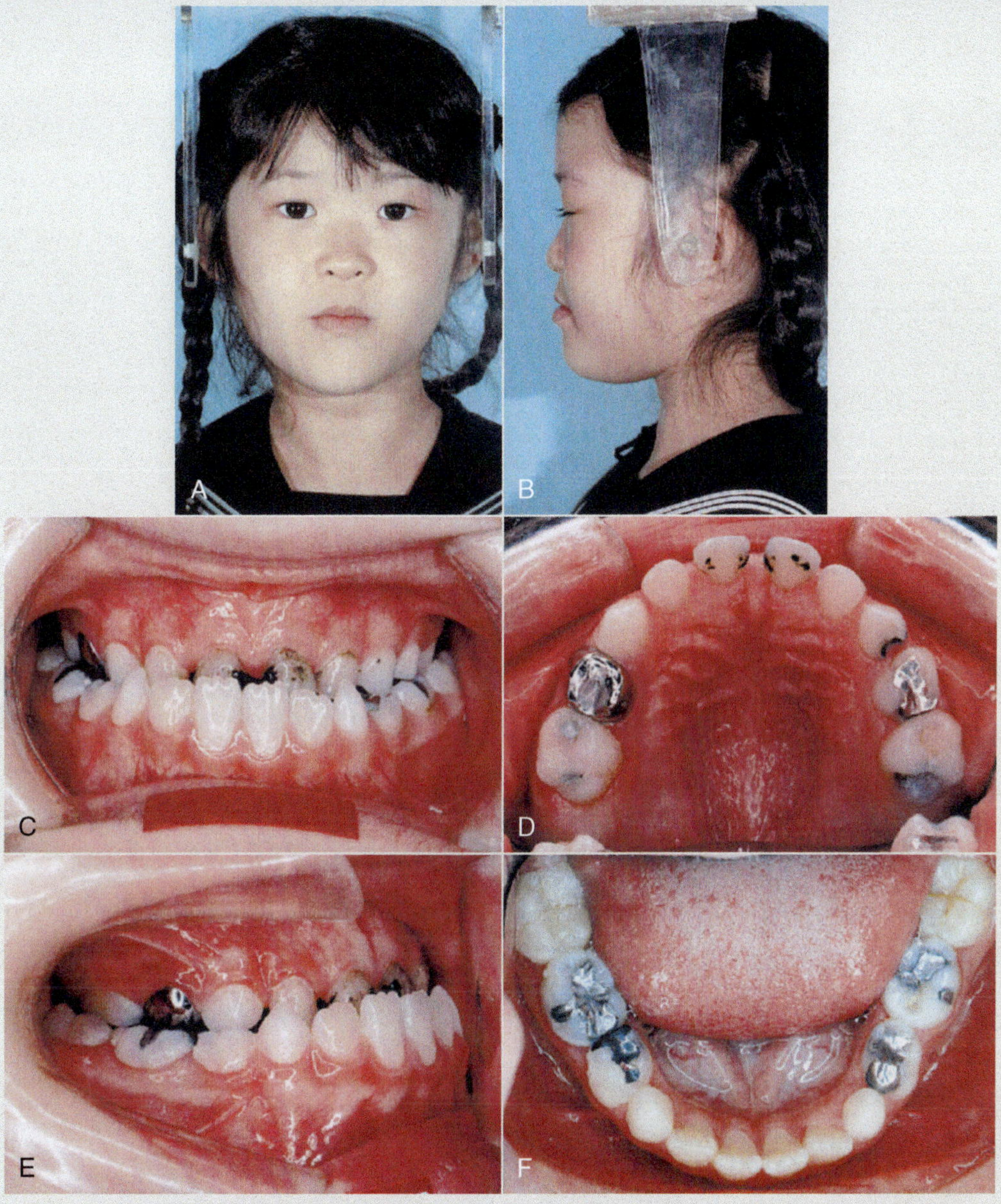

Figure 15-32 Facial **(A and B)** and intraoral **(C–F)** photographs at initial examination (age 6 years, 5 months).

Given the patient's problems, especially considering her severe skeletal disharmony, it was finally decided that she needed surgical orthodontics.

Surgical Orthodontics

Figure 15-35 shows the dentofacial changes with cephalometric superimpositions before presurgical orthodontics (15 years, 4 months) and debonding (18 years, 5 months). It can be seen that her orthodontic problems were mostly improved with the application of surgical orthodontics. In addition, her awareness of oral health was significantly promoted during a long-term management period and good oral health conditions have been maintained.

Figure 15-36 shows the treatment progress with surgical orthodontics. First, leveling and aligning began using a multibracket system (see Fig. 15-36, A). Then space regaining for the upper left lateral incisor that was congenitally missing, decompensation of the lower incisors, and coordination of upper and lower arches were performed as presurgical orthodontic treatment

Continued

CASE REPORT 3—cont'd

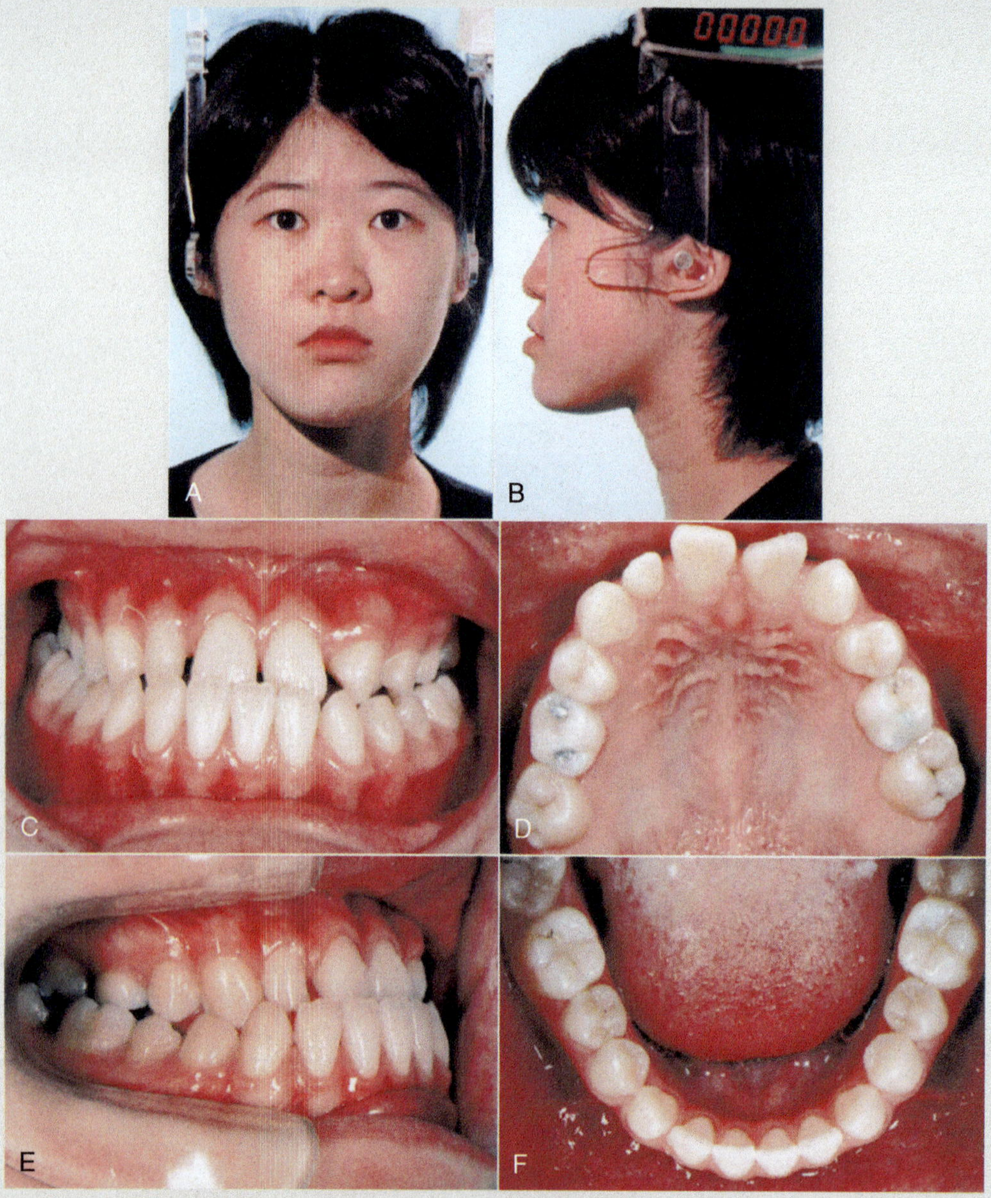

Figure 15-33 Facial (**A and B**) and intraoral (**C–F**) photographs before presurgical orthodontic treatment (age 15 years, 4 months).

(see Fig. 15-36, B). Figure 15-36, C shows the occlusion immediately after orthognathic surgery. Bilateral sagittal split ramus osteotomy (BSSO) was bilaterally applied and proximal and distal segments were semirigidly fixed with titanium bone plates and screws. Following orthognathic surgery, rehabilitation and postsurgical orthodontics were carried out (see Fig. 15-36, D). Brackets were debonded 5 months after surgery. A wrap-around retainer in the upper dentition and lingual bonded retainer in the lower dentition were placed for retention. The total length of the active treatment was 1 year, 9 months.

Figure 15-37 shows the patient's facial and oral photographs at age 19 years, 1 year after debonding.

CASE REPORT 3—cont'd

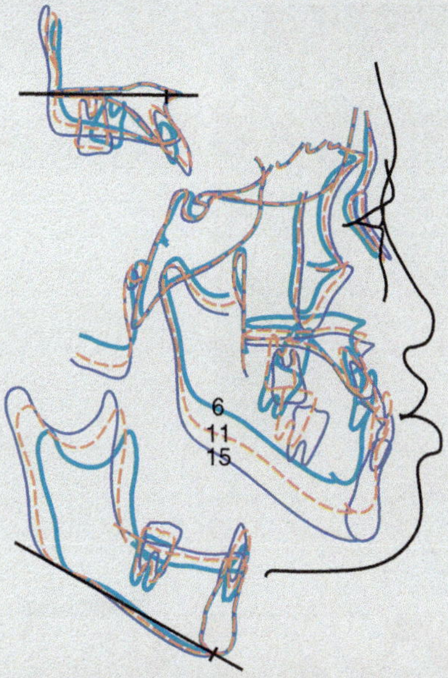

Figure 15-34 Cephalometric superimpositions show the dentofacial changes during the growth observation period. Thick solid line is 6 years, 5 months (initial examination); dotted line is age 11 years, 7 months (during the growth observation period); thin solid line is age 15 years, 4 months (immediately prior to the presurgical orthodontics).

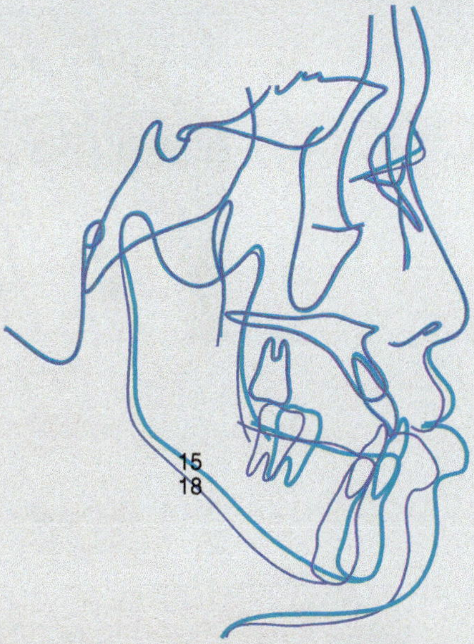

Figure 15-35 Cephalometric superimpositions show dentofacial changes during the surgical orthodontic treatment. Thick solid line is age 15 years, 4 months (immediately prior to the presurgical orthodontics); thin solid line is age 18 years, 5 months (at debonding).

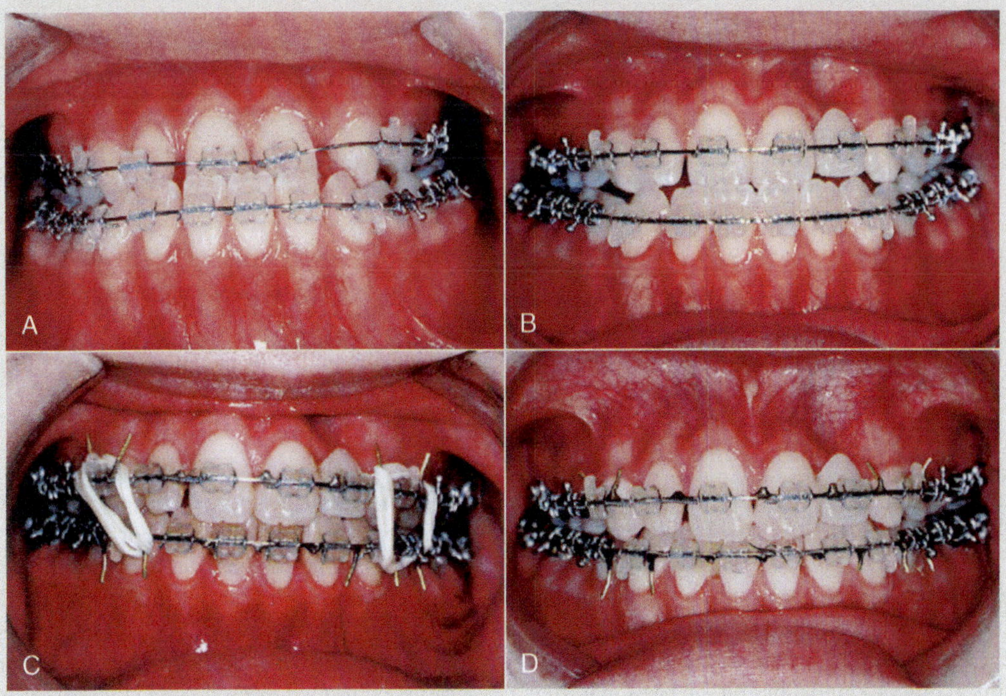

Figure 15-36 Treatment progress of surgical orthodontic treatment. **A,** Leveling and aligning of the upper and lower arches. **B,** Immediately prior to jaw surgery. **C,** Immediately following sagittal split ramus osteotomy (SSRO). **D,** Immediately prior to debonding.

Continued

CASE REPORT 3—cont'd

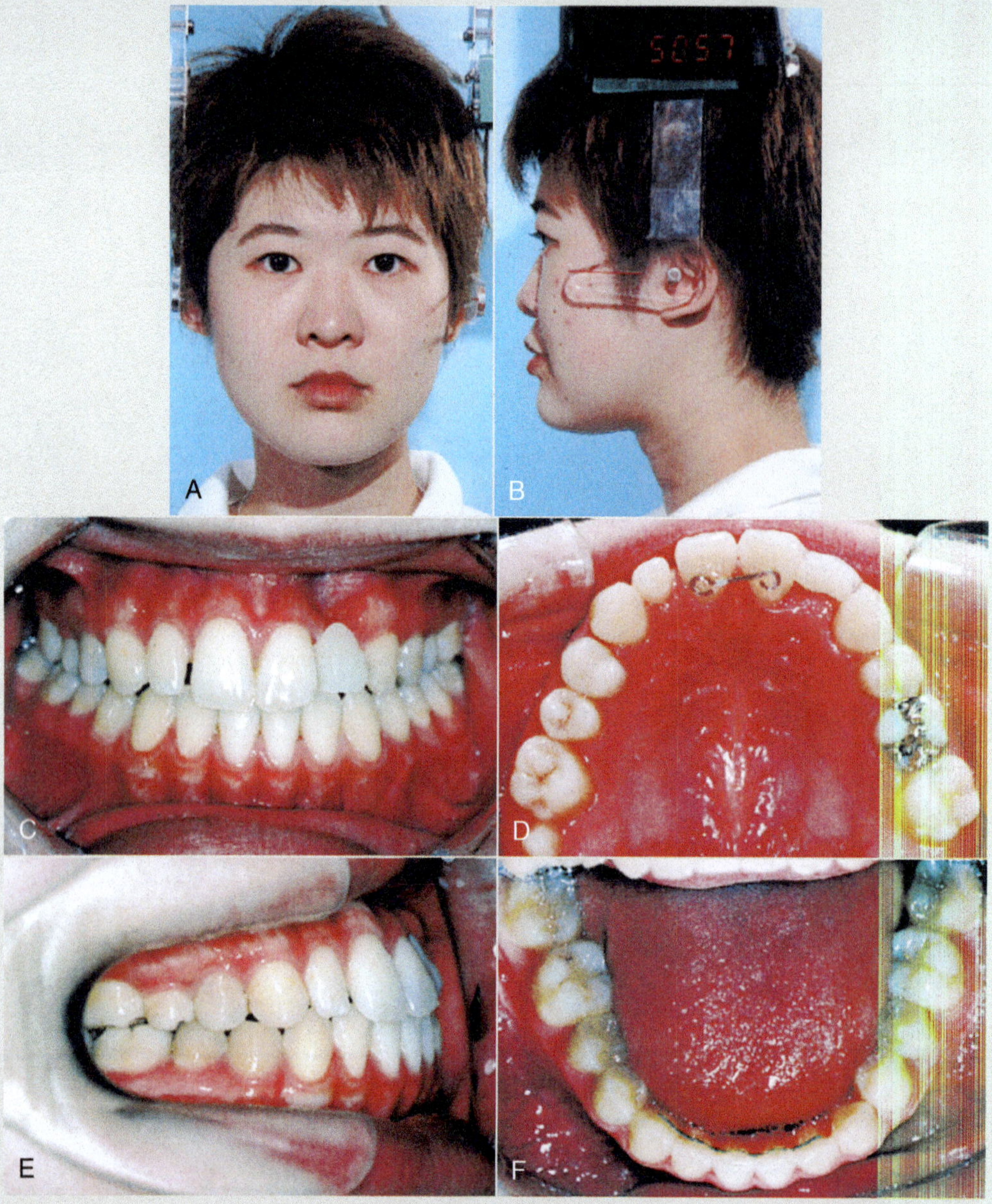

Figure 15-37 Facial (**A and B**) and intraoral (**C–F**) photographs 1 year after debonding (age 19 years, 1 month).

SUMMARY

Generally, the prognathic profile and anterior crossbite in patients with very severe skeletal disharmony are not corrected until the postpubertal period. Some orthodontists criticize the clinical practice guidelines on the basis that they do not allow all orthodontic problems to be addressed during the growth period and psychosocial disorders may occur as a result. However, in our clinical survey,[35] on interview after surgical orthodontic treatment, most patients said that they had not worried about their profiles and occlusions during the observation period because they believed that surgical orthodontics would solve their orthodontic problems in the future. As mentioned above, the long-term effects of orthopedic force are quite limited and surgical orthodontics must be the first treatment option for patients with very severe Class III malocclusion. Orthodontists should be cautioned against continued unpredictable therapy with a multibracket system because of the risk of dental cavities and iatrogenic side effects. The left-hand pathway shown in Figure 15-3 for severe Class III patients seems to be a relatively passive strategy but it is the most realistic alternative considering the cost and the need to eliminate iatrogenic factors and maintain the masticatory system through the lifespan. Of course, this pathway should not be forced on patients by practitioners but chosen by informed patients.

REFERENCES

1. Sugawara J, Asano T. The clinical practice guideline for treatment of developing Class III malocclusion. In: Sugawara J, Asano T, eds. *Seeking a Consensus for Class III Treatment.* Osaka, Japan: Tokyo Rinsho Shuppan; 2002:21–30.
2. Susami R. A cephalometric study of dentofacial growth in mandibular prognathism. *J Jpn Orthod Soc.* 1967;26:1–34.
3. Sawa S. Roentgeno-cephalometric study on the dentocraniofacial growth of the individuals with reversed occlusion. *J Jpn Orthod Soc.* 1978;37:237–268.
4. Yamazaki O, Sawa S, Hayashi M, et al. Studies on the longitudinal and individual growth of children with anterior reversed occlusion. *J Jpn Orthod Soc.* 1979;38:8–13.
5. Takeuchi U, Genba Y, Suzuki S, et al. Longitudinal growth study of untreated cases with reversed occlusion. *J Jpn Orthod Soc.* 1979;38: 14–29.
6. Mitani H. Prepubertal growth of mandibular prognathism. *Am J Orthod.* 1981;80:546–553.
7. Sugawara J, Tsuchikawa T, Soya T, et al. Late adolescent growth of skeletal Class III craniofacies in Japanese girls: average growth from 14 to 17 years of age based on longitudinal data. *J Jpn Orthod Soc.* 1983; 42:399–408.
8. Sato K, Sugawara J, Mitani H. Longitudinal study on average craniofacial growth of skeletal Class III girls in the late adolescent period: possibility of early orthognathic surgery. *J Jpn Orthod Soc.* 1989;48: 21–28.
9. Sato K, Sugawara J, Mitani H. Longitudinal study on average craniofacial growth of skeletal Class III males in late adolescent period: possibility of early orthognathic surgery. *J Jpn Orthod Soc.* 1992;51:25–30.
10. Mitani H, Sato K, Sugawara J. Growth of mandibular prognathism after pubertal growth peak. *Am J Orthod Dentofacial Orthop.* 1993;104: 330–336.
11. Sakamoto M, Sugawara J, Umemori M, et al. Craniofacial growth of mandibular prognathism during pubertal growth period in Japanese boys: longitudinal study from 10 to 15 years of age. *J Jpn Orthod Soc.* 1996;55:372–386.
12. Bandai (Sakamoto) M, Sugawara J, Umemori M, et al. Craniofacial growth of mandibular prognathism in Japanese girls during pubertal growth period: longitudinal study from 9 to 14 years of age. *Orthod Waves.* 2000;59:77–89.
13. Houston WJB, Miller JC, Tanner JM. Prediction of the timing of the adolescent growth spurt from ossification events in hand-wrist films. *Br J Orthod.* 1979;6:142–152.
14. Houston WJB. Relationship between skeletal maturity estimated from hand-wrist radiographs and the timing of the adolescent growth spurt. *Eur J Orthod.* 1980;2:81–93.
15. Sato K. A study on growth timing of mandibular length, body height, hand bones and cervical vertebrae during puberty. *J Jpn Orthod Soc.* 1987;46:517–533.
16. Grave KC. Timing of facial growth: a study of relations with stature and ossification in the hand around puberty. *Aust J Orthod.* 1973;3: 117–122.
17. Hägg U, Taranger J. Skeletal stages of the hand and wrist as indicators of the pubertal growth spurt. *Acta Odontol Scand.* 1980;38:187–200.
18. Suzuki N. A cephalometric observation on the effect of the chin cap. *J Jpn Orthod Soc.* 1972;31:64–74.
19. Irie M, Nakamura S. Orthopedic approach to severe skeletal Class III malocclusion. *Am J Orthod.* 1975;67:377–392.
20. Graber LW. Chin cup therapy for mandibular prognathism. *Am J Orthod.* 1977;72:23–41.
21. Nukatsuka S. The longitudinal study of orthopedic effect caused by chin cap treatment. *Tohoku Univ Dent J.* 1982;1:1–17.
22. Janzen EK, Bluher JA. The cephalometric, anatomic, and histologic changes in *Macaca nulatta* after application of a continuous-acting retraction force on the mandible. *Am J Orthod.* 1965;51:823–855.
23. Matsui Y. Effect of chin cap on the growing mandible. *J Jpn Orthod Soc.* 1965;24:165–181.
24. Joho JP. The effects of extraoral low-pull traction to the mandibular dentition of *Macaca nulatta. Am J Orthod.* 1973;64:555–577.
25. Petrovic AG, Stutzman JJ, Oudet CL. Control processes in the postnatal growth of the condylar cartilage of the mandible: effect of orthopedic therapy on condylar growth. In: McNamara JA Jr, ed. *Determinants of Mandibular Form and Growth.* Ann Arbor, MI: University of Michigan; 1975:101–153.
26. Asano T. The effects of mandibular retractive force on the growing rat. *Am J Orthod Dentofacial Orthop.* 1986;90:464–474.
27. Sugawara J, Asano T, Endo N, Mitani H. Long-term effects of chincap therapy on skeletal profile in mandibular prognathism. *Am J Orthod Dentofacial Orthop.* 1990;98:127–133.
28. Wendell PD, Nanda R. The effects of chin cap therapy on the mandible: a longitudinal study. *Am J Orthod.* 1985;87:265–274.
29. Tsuchikawa T, Sugawara J, Nakamura H, et al. Long-term results of skeletal profile changes occurred in the chin cap therapy of Japanese male skeletal Class III cases. *J Jpn Orthod Soc.* 1985;44:644–659.
30. Endo N. A study on the variation and formation of vertical skeletal facial patterns in skeletal Class III cases. *J Jpn Orthod Soc.* 1987;46: 50–70.
31. Oyama A, Sugawara J. Maxillary incisors protraction (MIP). In: Sugawara J, Asano T, eds. *Seeking a Consensus for Class III Treatment.* Osaka, Japan: Tokyo Rinsho Shuppan; 2002:148–155.
32. Umemori M, Sugawara J, Mitani H, Nagasaka H, Kawamura H. Skeletal anchorage system for open-bite. *Am J Orthod Dentofacial Orthop.* 1999;115:166–174.
33. Sugawara J. JCO interviews: Dr Junji Sugawara on the skeletal anchorage system. *J Clin Orthod.* 2000;33:689–696.
34. Sugawara J, Baik UB, Umemori M, et al. Treatment and posttreatment dentoalveolar changes following intrusion of mandibular molars with application of a skeletal anchorage system (SAS) for open bite correction. *Int J Adult Orthod Orthognath Surg.* 2002;17:1–11.
35. Kawauchi M. Evaluation for psycho-social problems in patients who have possibility to undergo orthognathic surgery after completion of jaw growth. In: Sugawara J, Asano T, eds. *Seeking a Consensus for Class III Treatment.* Osaka, Japan: Tokyo Rinsho Shuppan; 2002:368–375.

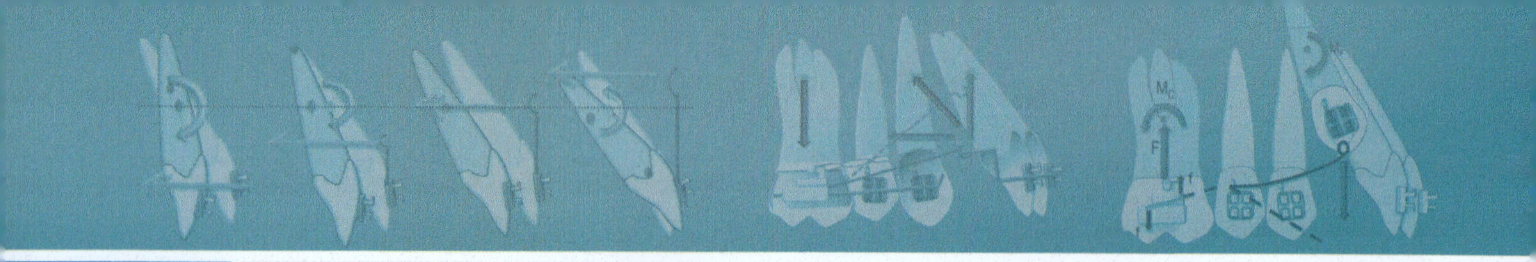

CHAPTER 16

Biomechanical Aspects of a Modified Protraction Headgear

Ravindra Nanda

A routine dilemma in the treatment of children with developing Class III malocclusions is the choice of treatment strategy and whether early intervention will be successful in the long-term. Early treatment decisions should be based on several considerations, including genetics and family history; severity of the problem; whether the problem is diagnosed in the midface, mandible, or both; the age of the patient; patient compliance; and growth status of the patient.

The prevalence of children with Class III malocclusion in the United States is relatively small compared to Japan, Korea, and Taiwan. Two studies evaluating the incisor relationship in children have reported an anterior crossbite incidence of 0.8% to 1.0%.[1,2] One study reported a Class III molar relationship incidence of 3.8% in high school children.[3] However, a Class III malocclusion in a child deserves special attention due to the esthetic, occlusion, function, and psychosocial concerns it raises.

Treatment of developing Class III patients is often based on the orthodontist's expectations of treatment. The parents should be fully informed about the variability of results that can be expected. It is likely wishful thinking to aim to always convert a Class III growth pattern to a Class I growth pattern. The reality is that treatment results range from 100% success to no change at all in the long-term. The degree of success is based on the etiology of the Class III pattern, severity of malocclusion, age and growth status, choice of appliance used, and degree of patient cooperation. Other short-term goals should not be overlooked (i.e., to provide young Class III patients with a functioning occlusion, reduction in severity, and some esthetic improvement during their formative years).

RATIONALE FOR USING PROTRACTION HEADGEAR

Delaire et al.[4–8] are credited with introducing the concept of protraction headgear to treat Class III malocclusions. Nanda introduced a modified protraction headgear in 1980,[9] based on biomechanical concepts.

The rationale for protraction headgear is to apply heavy forces on the midface in order to advance the maxilla anteriorly. In patients with a normal sized mandible and retrusive maxilla, forward displacement of the maxilla is conceptually good. Several studies in the past 3 decades have shown that 25% to 41% of Class III problems in children are primarily the result of a retrognathic maxilla.[10–12]

The efficacy of protraction headgear is also supported by several studies in primates in the 1970s and 1980s.[13–17] These studies, using cephalometrics and histological techniques, showed that treatment with an anterior force on the maxilla is capable of causing disassociation of sutural articulations by a resorption and apposition process at the sutural interfaces. Our own experience has also shown that the direction of midface protraction can be altered by changing the direction and point of delivery of the force.

In recent years noteworthy clinical studies have been reported regarding the use of protraction headgear.[18–25] The majority of these studies show an anterior movement of the maxillary dentition, a significant extrusion of the upper molars, anterior displacement of the maxillary dentition, 1- to 3-mm anterior displacement of the maxilla, and a significant rotation of the mandible downward and backward.

A conventional protraction headgear, as described by Delaire et al.,[4–8] and its variations use elastics from the molars (or other points at the occlusal plane level) to the facial mask. The interlabial gap and lips limit the ability to change the point of force application to attain predictable movement of the maxilla in the anterior direction.

Nanda[9] introduced a modified protraction headgear in 1980, which allowed changes in the direction of force and point of force application on the maxilla as well as the chin. The study showed that use of a modified protraction headgear for 4 to 8 months can displace the maxilla 1- to 3-mm and maxillary dentition 1- to 4-mm. These changes were accompanied by remodeling at the B point, lingual tipping of the mandibular incisors, and downward rotation of the mandible. The cumulative effect of these changes was the correction of the Class III malocclusion. This chapter describes the biomechanical aspects of this headgear, which allows modification of forces in Class III patients to achieve the desired changes, such as in long face and short face Class III patients.

COMPONENTS OF MODIFIED PROTRACTION HEADGEAR

There are two main components of a protraction headgear: intraoral setup and extraoral setup.

Intraoral Components

The protraction headgear force is applied via elastics to teeth or other devices supported by teeth and/or the palate. The primary aim is to transmit the force to the midface sutural interfaces. To achieve this, it is important to stabilize the maxilla as one unit (Fig. 16-1). In the primary dentition, it is advisable to use a cemented acrylic occlusal bite block or a removable acrylic plate with occlusal coverage (see Chapter 12). In patients with the mixed dentition and early permanent dentition, a removable acrylic plate (Fig. 16-2) should be used, supported by bands with headgear tubes on the molars or a rigid archwire with a palatal arch. Probably the best stabilization in patients with maxillary first molars is provided by a fixed rapid palatal expansion (RPE) device (Fig. 16-3). We prefer a Hyrax type of nonbonded device, as bonded RPEs (Fig. 16-4) interfere with the primary exfoliating teeth or teeth in the eruptive phase. Studies have also indicated that a simultaneous sutural expansion with an RPE at the start of protraction headgear treatment facilitates the anterior movement of the maxilla.[19,20,26,27]

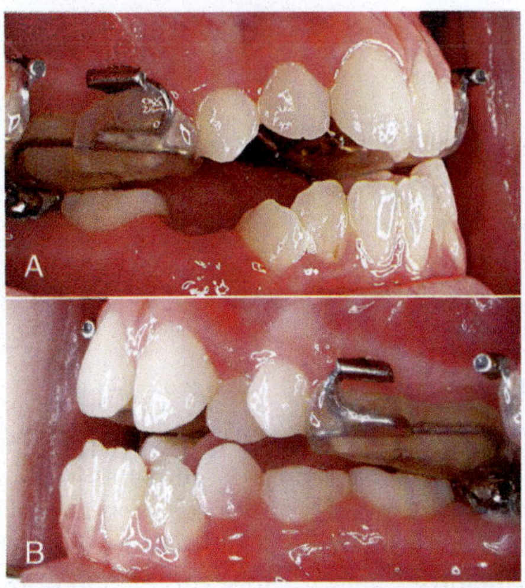

Figure 16-1 **A,** Left and (**B**) right lateral views of an intraoral stabilization appliance. An acrylic bite block includes a heavy archwire to which a headgear tube is soldered. The bite block provides disocclusion to facilitate forward displacement of the maxilla and is cemented to posterior maxillary teeth.

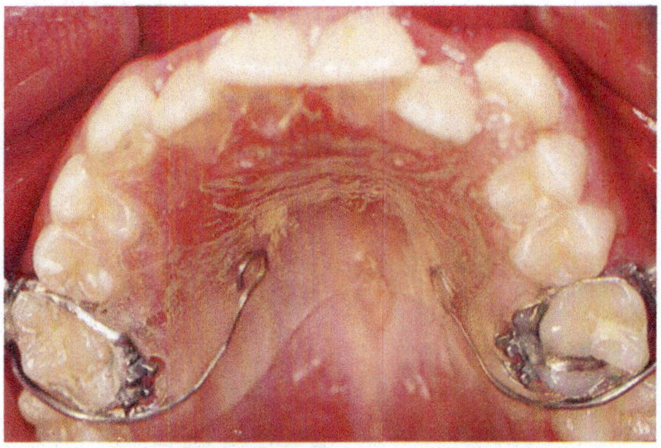
Figure 16-2 Occlusal view of a removable intraoral stabilization appliance. The acrylic plate has a clasp that fits on a molar tube of a cemented band. This plate must be worn when the protraction appliance is in use.

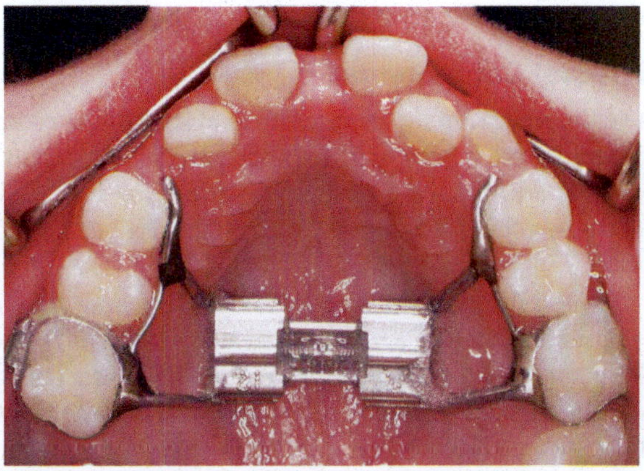
Figure 16-3 Occlusal view of a rapid palatal expansion (RPE) device used as a stabilization appliance. This is an ideal stabilization device if the first molars are fully erupted.

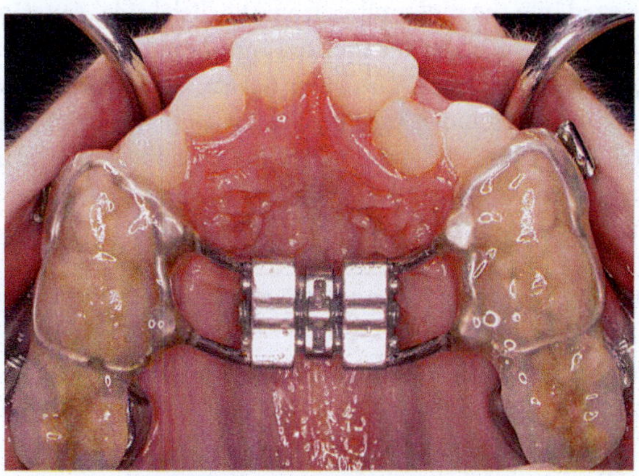
Figure 16-4 Occlusal view of a bonded rapid palatal expansion (RPE) device. In mixed dentition patients its use may interfere with the exfoliation of primary teeth and eruption of permanent teeth.

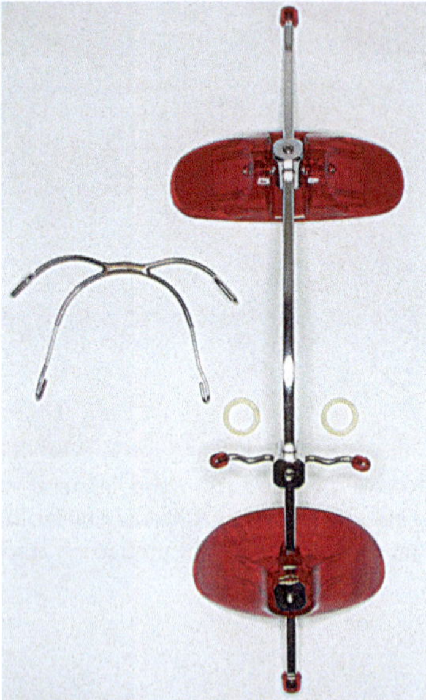

Figure 16-5 Complete modified protraction headgear device. It includes a facemask, a modified inner bow of a headgear, and elastics.

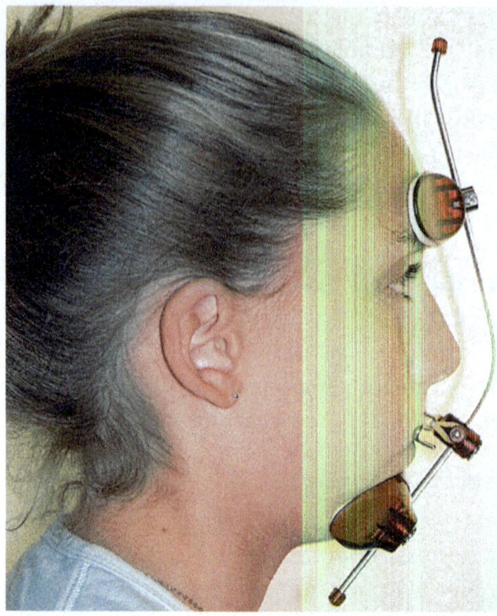

Figure 16-6 Lateral view of a patient with the appliance shown in Figure 16-5 in place. The outer bow of the headgear is attached to the center bar of the facemask. The point of attachment on the mask can be moved up or down and the outer bow can be similarly positioned to achieve the desirable line of force.

Extraoral Components

The extraoral components (Fig. 16-5) of a modified protraction headgear have two parts. The first is a facemask and the second is an intraoral-to-extraoral connecting force device that uses a modified headgear bow instead of intraoral elastics.

Commonly used facemasks have chin and forehead support connected by a heavy metal arch that has a horizontal bar for attachment of a force module. The forehead and chin supports are adjustable. The horizontal bar also must be adjustable vertically to vary the point of force attachment (Figs. 16-6 and 16-7).

A conventional headgear bow with a standard outer and inner bow without loops can be easily converted into a modified bow for use with the facemask. It is important that the molar band has a headgear tube. In cemented acrylic stabilization devices, a headgear tube can be embedded in acrylic.

To construct a reverse headgear bow (Fig. 16-8), a U-shaped horizontal bend is made in such a way that it can be inserted into the molar tubes from the distal side. Anteriorly, the bow should clear the incisors and should be between the upper and lower lips. The outer bow is modified to make a hook in the premolar area in such a way that elastics can be attached to the horizontal bar of the facemask. The vertical position of the outer bow is adjusted to deliver the necessary force for a predictable maxillary displacement.

PROTRACTION HEADGEAR FORCE SYSTEM

The following four components of force systems are important for proper adjustments of the protraction headgear.

1. Magnitude of force
2. Direction and point of force application
3. Duration of force
4. Force constancy

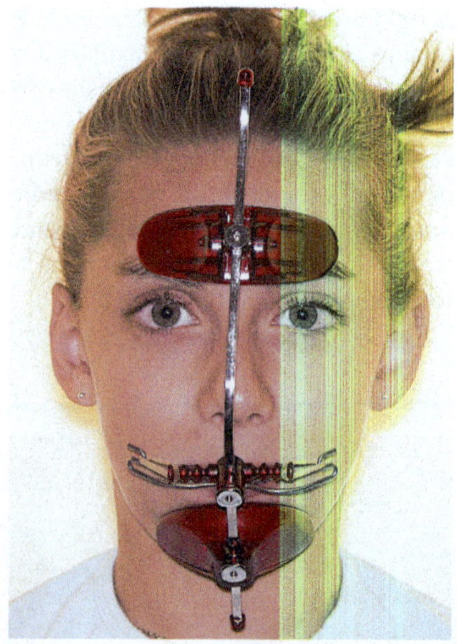

Figure 16-7 Frontal view of the modified protraction headgear device.

Magnitude of Force

Hickory and Nanda[28] showed in an in vitro study of 2-day-old rat cranial sutures that very small forces (0.2 to 0.6 g) applied with wire springs are capable of generating cellular activity along with an increase in the suture width. In human studies, the force values used for protraction of the maxilla have ranged from 200 to 800 g. Most of the studies give no rationale for the magnitude of the force selected and in clinical practice the force used is often based on anecdotal experience.

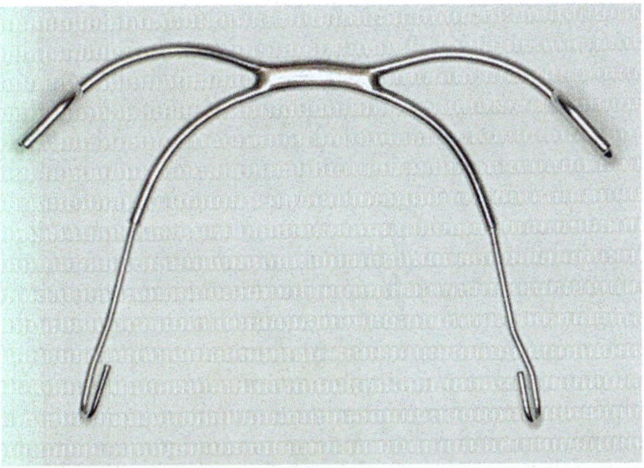

Figure 16-8 Close-up view of a modified headgear bow. The distal ends of the inner bow can be bent to achieve distal insertion of the appliance.

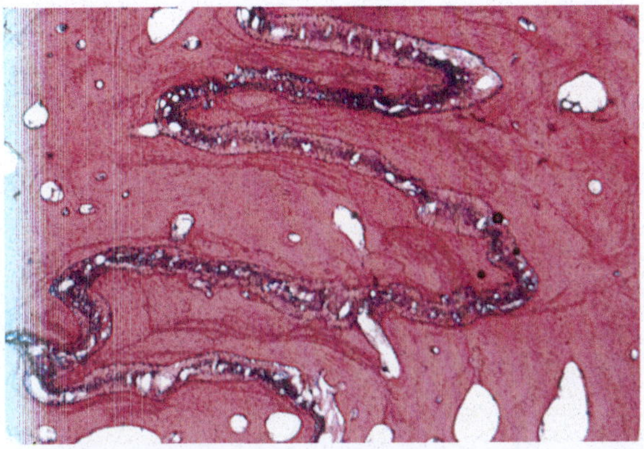

Figure 16-9 Histological photograph of an area of zygomaticomaxillary suture of a *Macaca nemestrina* monkey subjected to an anterior protraction force. Note the tortuous nature of the suture with areas of stress and strain and resting lines.

Indeed, there have been no prospective studies to determine the optimal force to protract the maxilla. However, based on clinical experience, studies in the literature, and sutural morphology changes related to age progression, certain observations regarding the desirable magnitude of force can be made.

The sutural articulations in children are simple; interdigitations interlock more with age. A clear example is the midpalatal suture. The suture remains patent long after growth is complete but it becomes difficult to open with an RPE after the age of 15 to 16 years due to the complex interlocking of sutures. Conversely, in adolescents, midpalatal suture opening is very simple and can be accomplished with minimal tipping of the posterior teeth. A protraction force on the maxilla needs "disarticulation" at numerous sutures (Fig. 16-9), most notably zygomaticomaxillary, pterygopalatine, and nasomaxillary sutures of the midface. With age, these sutures become not only more mechanically intertwined, but also more tortuous in their orientation. Also, for the maxilla to advance forward in each affected suture, numerous areas of resorption and apposition must take place due to their tortuous nature, quite unlike the midpalatal suture.

Thus the sutural anatomy and age of the patient play a major role in determining the amount of force needed to bring the maxilla forward with protraction forces. For preadolescent patients (5 to 8 years), a force of 200 to 250 g on each side is adequate and for early adolescent patients (8 to 11 years), a force of 300 to 450 g on each side may be desirable. In late adolescent patients (12 years and up), higher forces (450 to 600 g) can be used but, in our experience, protraction of the midface in the latter group is minimal. It is advisable to start with lower force values that can be increased if needed, especially in late adolescent patients.

Direction and Point of Force Application

Direction of the applied force is one of the most important force components for anterior displacement of the maxilla. Nanda[17] varied the point of force application in primates and showed that by changing the line of force on the midface, the center of rotation of the maxilla could be altered. Later, Nanda and Hickory[16] speculated, based on different centers of rotation created by varying the line of protraction force, that the center of resistance of the midface is probably 5- to 10-mm below the orbitale on the zygomatic bone. Later, Tanne et al.[29,30] reported that the center of resistance of the maxilla was located between the root tip of the maxilla first and second premolars. Miki[31] agreed with the previous two authors but added that, in the vertical direction, the center of resistance of the midface was between the orbitale and the distal root apex of the first maxillary molars. Hata et al.[32] and Lee et al.[33] studied the effects of changing the level of force application on dried skulls and confirmed the findings of Nanda[17] in primates. They reported that a line of force 5-mm above the palatal plane and 15-mm above the occlusal plane did not result in counterclockwise movement of the maxilla and dentition.

Keles et al.[34] studied the effects of varying the force direction on maxillary orthopedic protraction in two groups of patients. The first group received protraction headgear with a force applied by intraoral elastics and the second group received a force applied with a modified protraction headgear as described above.[9] The authors reported that in the first group the maxilla rotated counterclockwise (Fig. 16-10), resulting in downward and backward rotation of the mandible, while in the second group an anterior translation of the maxilla with no to minimal mandibular rotation occurred. This important study showed that predictable changes can be achieved in the direction of maxillary advancement with desired or without undesirable mandibular changes.

By changing the point of force attachment on the facemask or outer bow of the headgear, the vertical dimension of the face can be very nicely controlled. This is especially important in Class III patients with a long vertical dimension and a steep mandibular plane. Similarly, in Class III patients with a flat mandibular plane and a deep bite, a force below the level of the occlusal plane may be more desirable to rotate the mandible downward and backward (see Fig. 16-10). A line of force closer to the center of resistance of the midface will deliver a translatory force (Fig. 16-11) and

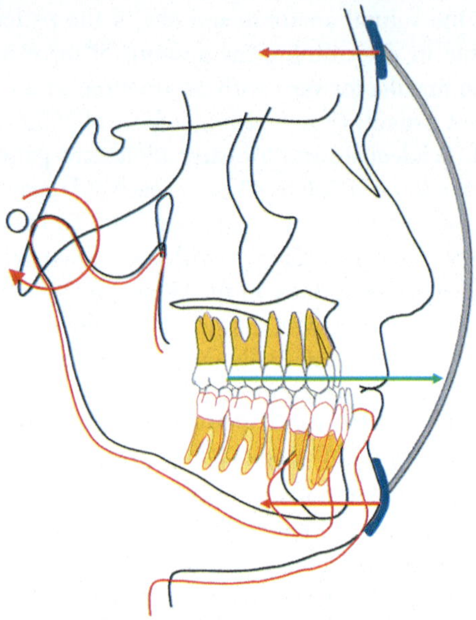

Figure 16-10 Force diagram of a protraction headgear device using intraoral elastics to deliver force. Note the clockwise moment on the midface and dentition resulting in a downward and backward rotation of the mandible.

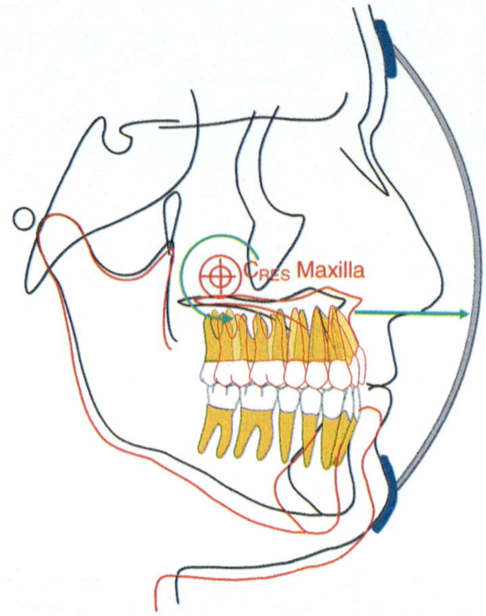

Figure 16-12 Force diagram showing the nature of the maxillary and mandibular change when the point of force application is at the level of the root apices of the maxillary teeth. C_{RES}, Center of resistance.

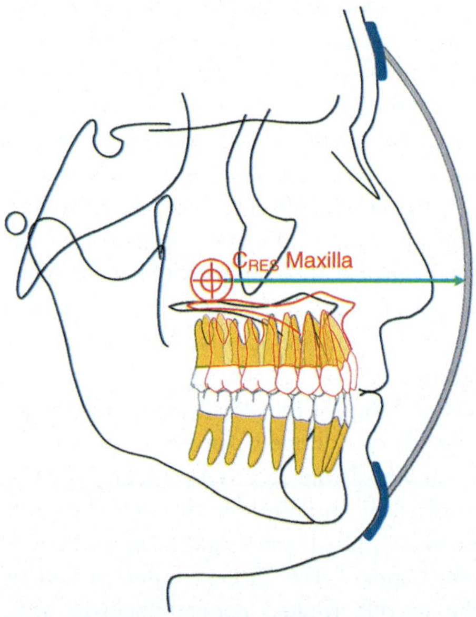

Figure 16-11 Schematic representation of a line of force through the center of resistance (C_{RES}) of the maxilla, which will result in a translatory movement of the maxilla. The precise location of the C_{RES} of the midfacial bones is difficult to locate but most studies point to the area 5- to 10-mm below the orbitale.

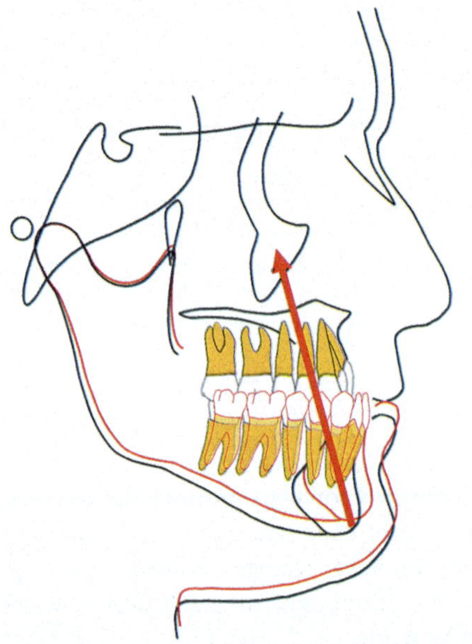

Figure 16-13 Force diagram showing the line of force of an added chin cap. In the long vertical dimension of Class III patients, it is advisable to use a vertical pull chin cap to prevent downward rotation of the mandible.

a line of force closer to the occlusal plane has a rotational force (Fig. 16-12).

The force delivered by the protraction facemask on the chin is almost a "forgotten" force and is very rarely mentioned in the literature. An anterior force on the midface applies equal and opposite force on the forehead and chin (see Fig. 16-10). The direction of the force on the chin is distal and almost in a straight line, which can also cause a rotation of the mandible downward and backward. In Class III long faced patients, a vertical pull chin cap (Fig. 16-13) can be added to minimize the undesirable forces on the chin. A chin cap is especially desirable in Class III patients with a long vertical dimension and open-bite tendency (Fig. 16-14).

Duration of Force

The majority of clinical studies recommend use of a protraction headgear for anywhere from 3 to 12 months. Patient compliance beyond 6 months is difficult. Also, the older the patient, the less cooperative he or she will be. In our clinic, use of a protraction headgear is stopped after 6 months. In some cases, if necessary after an observation period, patients are asked to use the headgear again for 3 to 4 months.

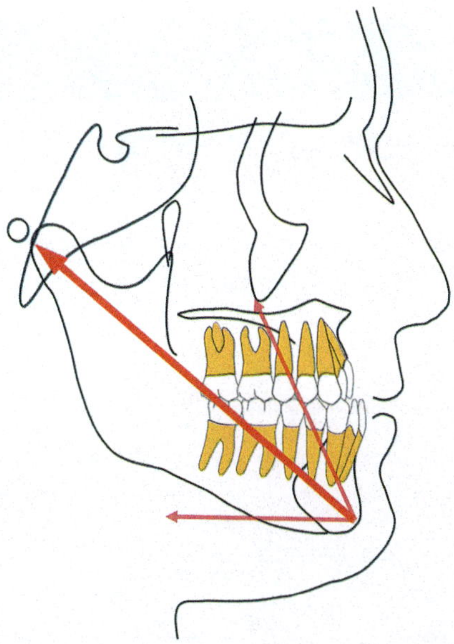

Figure 16-14 Addition of a cervical strap or a vertical pull chin cap will change the resultant force vector of a chin cap.

The daily wear time also depends on the age of the patient. In preadolescent patients, 10 to 12 hours of use per day is sufficient. In adolescent patients, it may be necessary to increase the wear time from 12 to 16 hours per day. The latter group may have problems with compliance.

Force Constancy

The force is applied with elastics from the outer bow of the headgear to the facemask. The elastic force should be measured at the beginning to determine the desired force level. Patients should be instructed to use fresh elastics as much as possible.

SUMMARY

This chapter illustrated the biomechanical principles to consider when utilizing the modified protraction facemask in the treatment of Class III patients. Intraoral and extraoral components of the appliance, point of force application, force magnitude, and duration were discussed.

CASE REPORTS 1 AND 2

Two patient examples are presented. The first patient is unique because a decision was made to extract four premolars after protraction headgear use (Fig. 16-15). Clinical photographs are shown for the second patient 6 years after protraction (Fig. 16-16). In both patients a modified protraction headgear was used and the point of attachment and line of force were changed at various times during the protraction period.

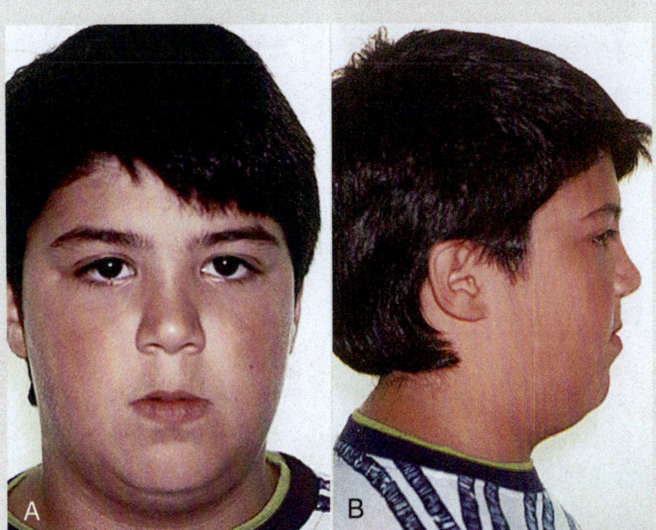

Figure 16-15 **A–F**, Frontal and lateral facial and intraoral views of an adolescent patient determined to have a developing Class III malocclusion after a careful examination of dental, facial, and family history findings and a cephalometric analysis.

Continued

CASE REPORT 1 AND 2—cont'd

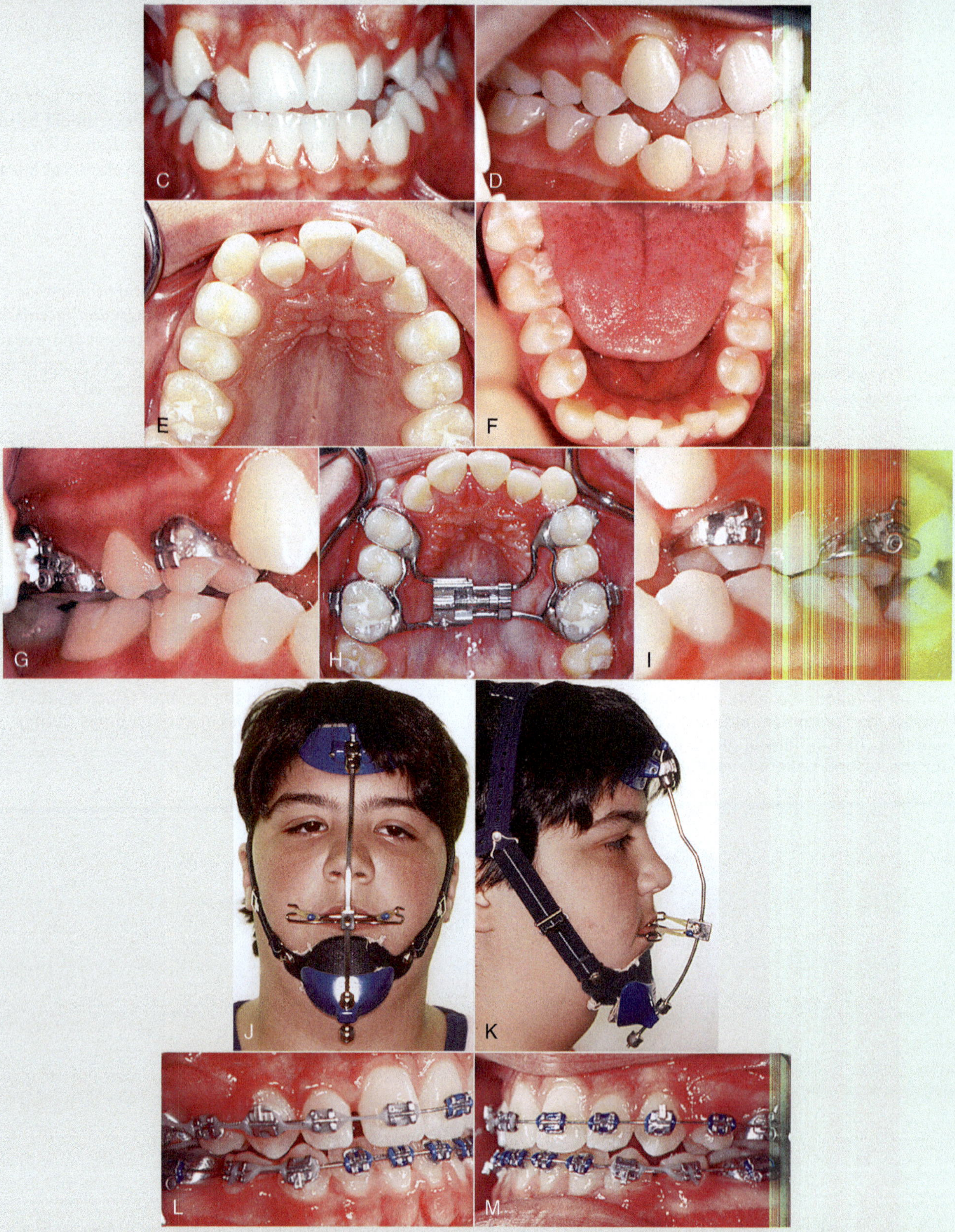

Figure 16-15, cont'd **C and D,** Edge-to-edge anterior bite and skeletal maxillary constriction. **E and F,** Intraoral view of upper and lower arches. **G–I,** Intraoral view showing a rapid palatal expansion (RPE) appliance at the end of the maxillary expansion. **J and K,** Frontal and lateral extraoral views with the protraction headgear in place. The chin cap component is added during the active RPE phase to prevent any extrusion of the maxillary posterior teeth. **L and M,** Lateral intraoral views and **(N)** frontal view with smile after extraction of the four first premolars and completion of the space closure. Protraction headgear was used for 6 months prior to the extractions.

CASE REPORT 1 AND 2—cont'd

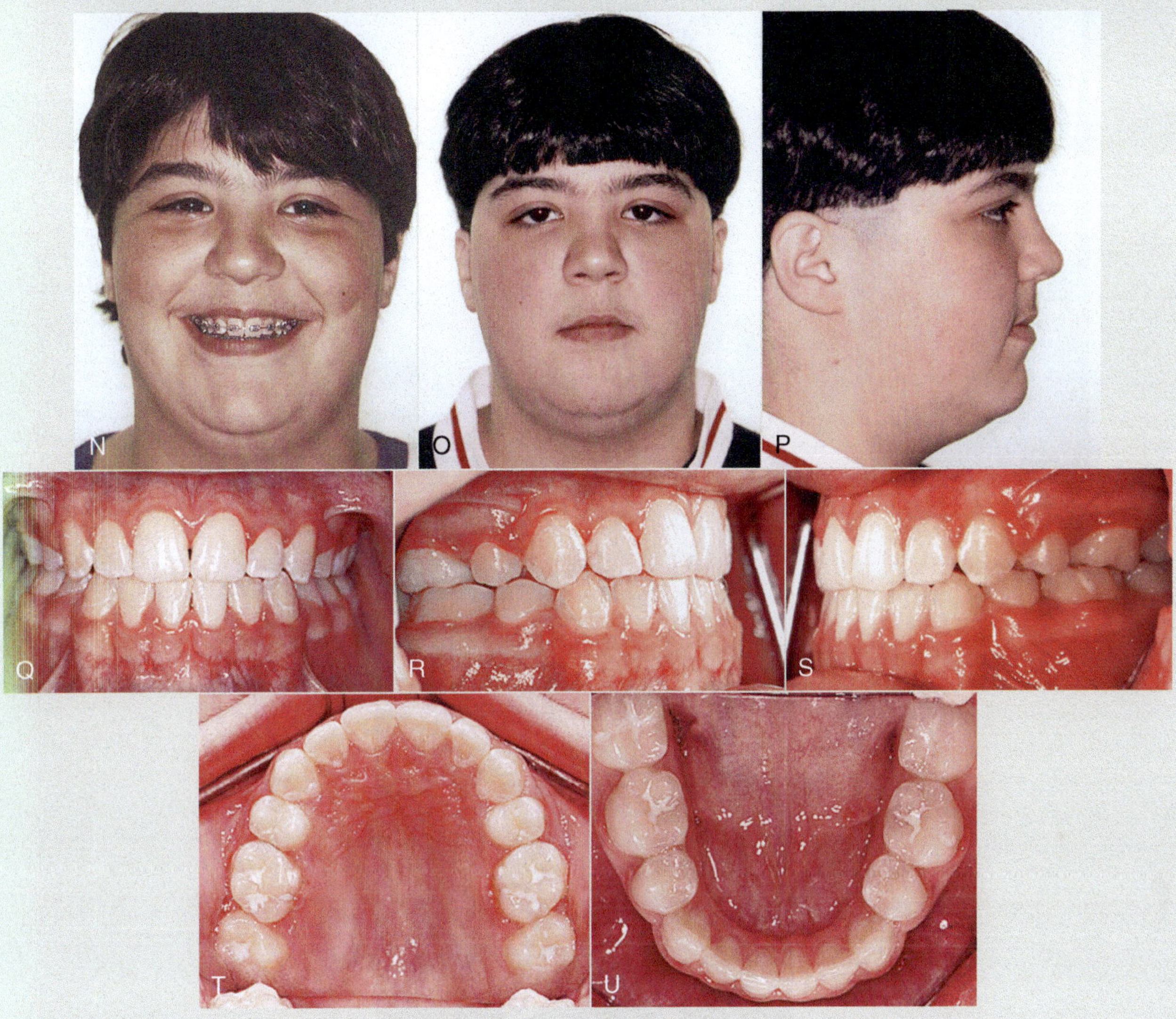

Figure 16-15, cont'd **O–U,** Facial and intraoral views at the end of the treatment.

Continued

CASE REPORT 1 AND 2—cont'd

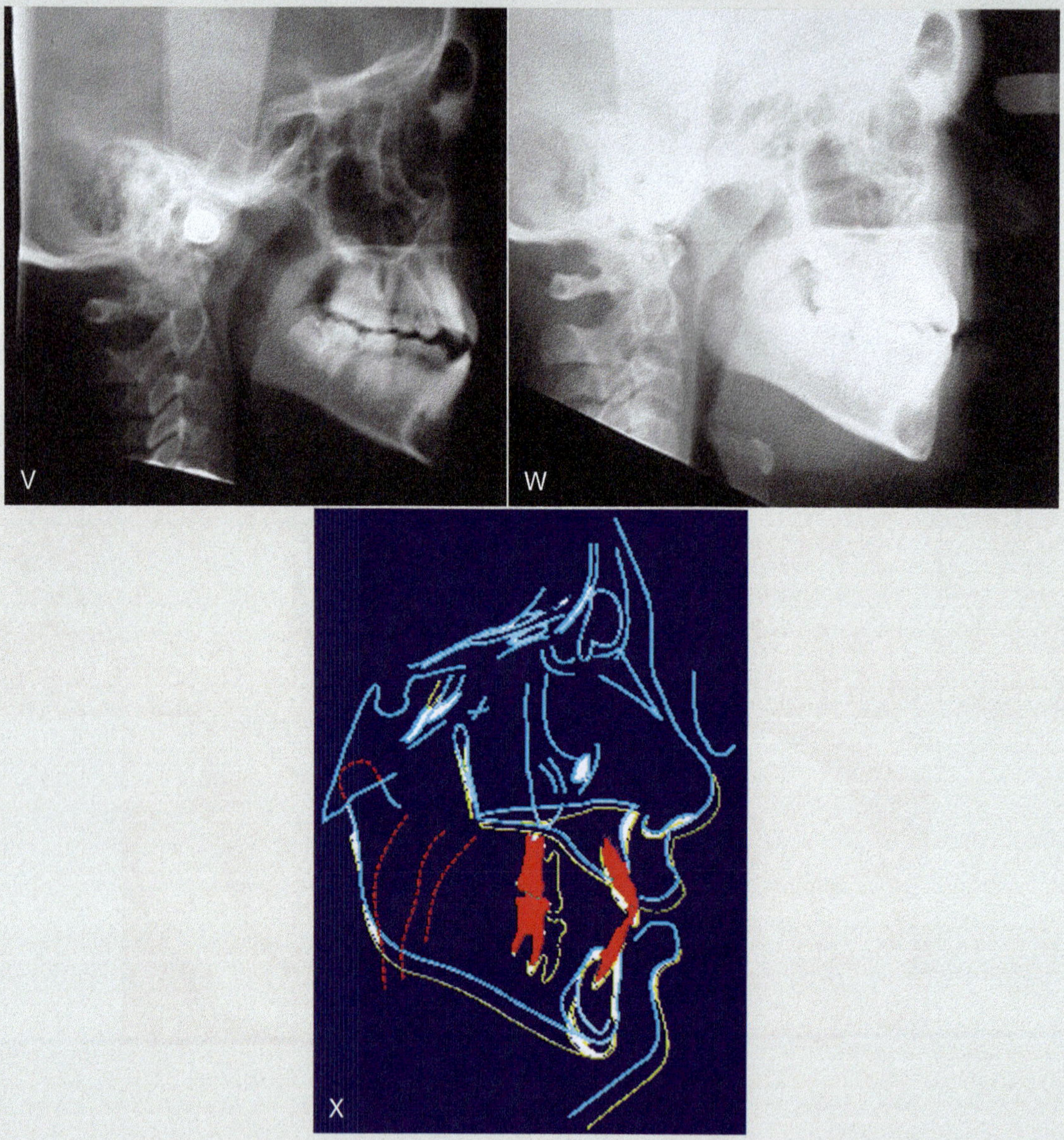

Figure 16-15, cont'd **V,** Before and (**W**) after cephalograms and (**X**) superimposition tracings showing cumulative changes over a 3-year treatment period.

CASE REPORT 1 AND 2—cont'd

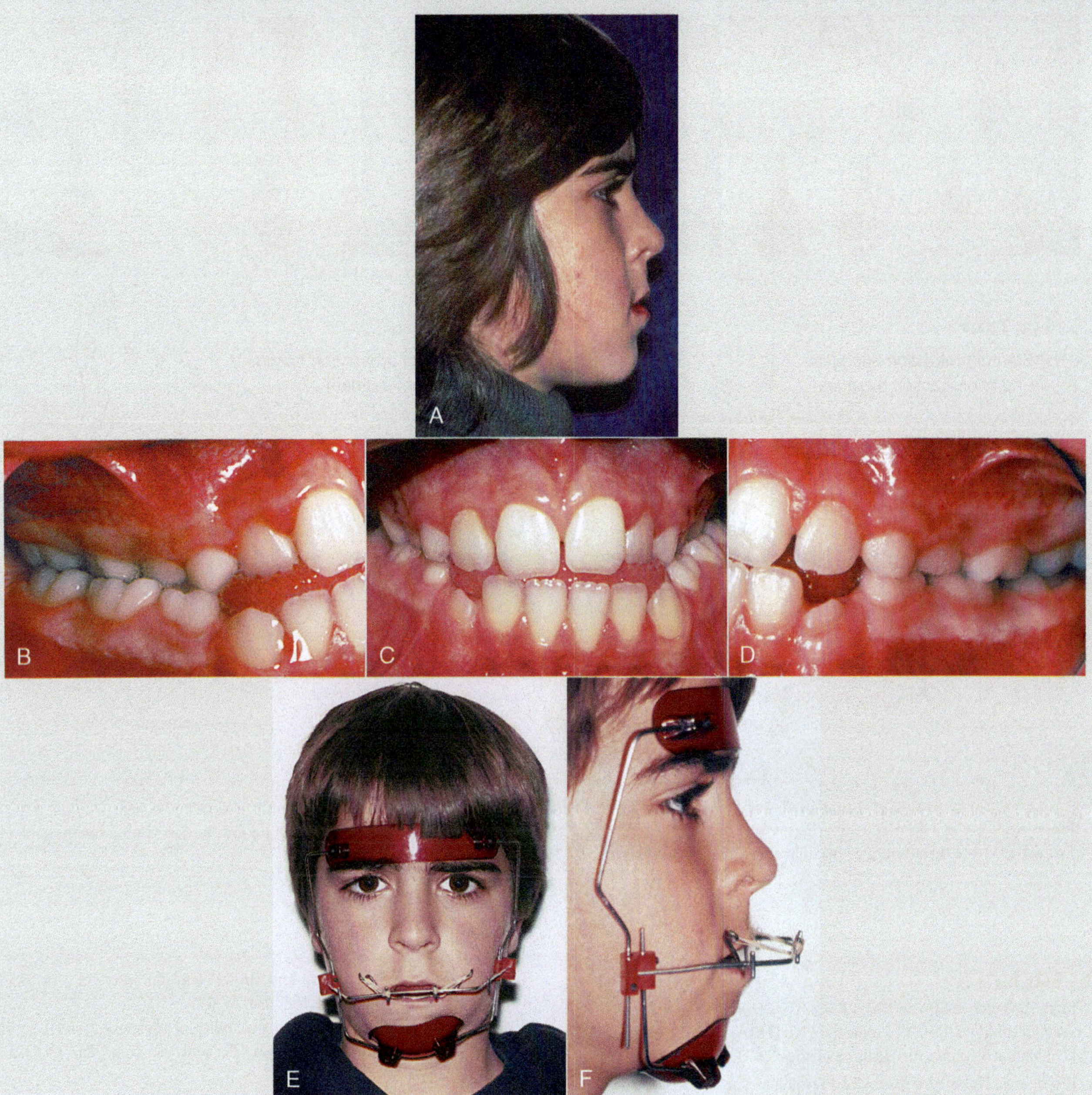

Figure 16-16 **A–D,** Extraoral and intraoral views of a developing Class III malocclusion in an early adolescent patient. **E and F,** Extraoral frontal and lateral views of the protraction headgear appliance in place. Note that the line of force in this patient is at the level of the root apices of the maxillary teeth. The line of force was adjusted at various times during the 6-month protraction headgear application to achieve the desired results.

Continued

CASE REPORT 1 AND 2—cont'd

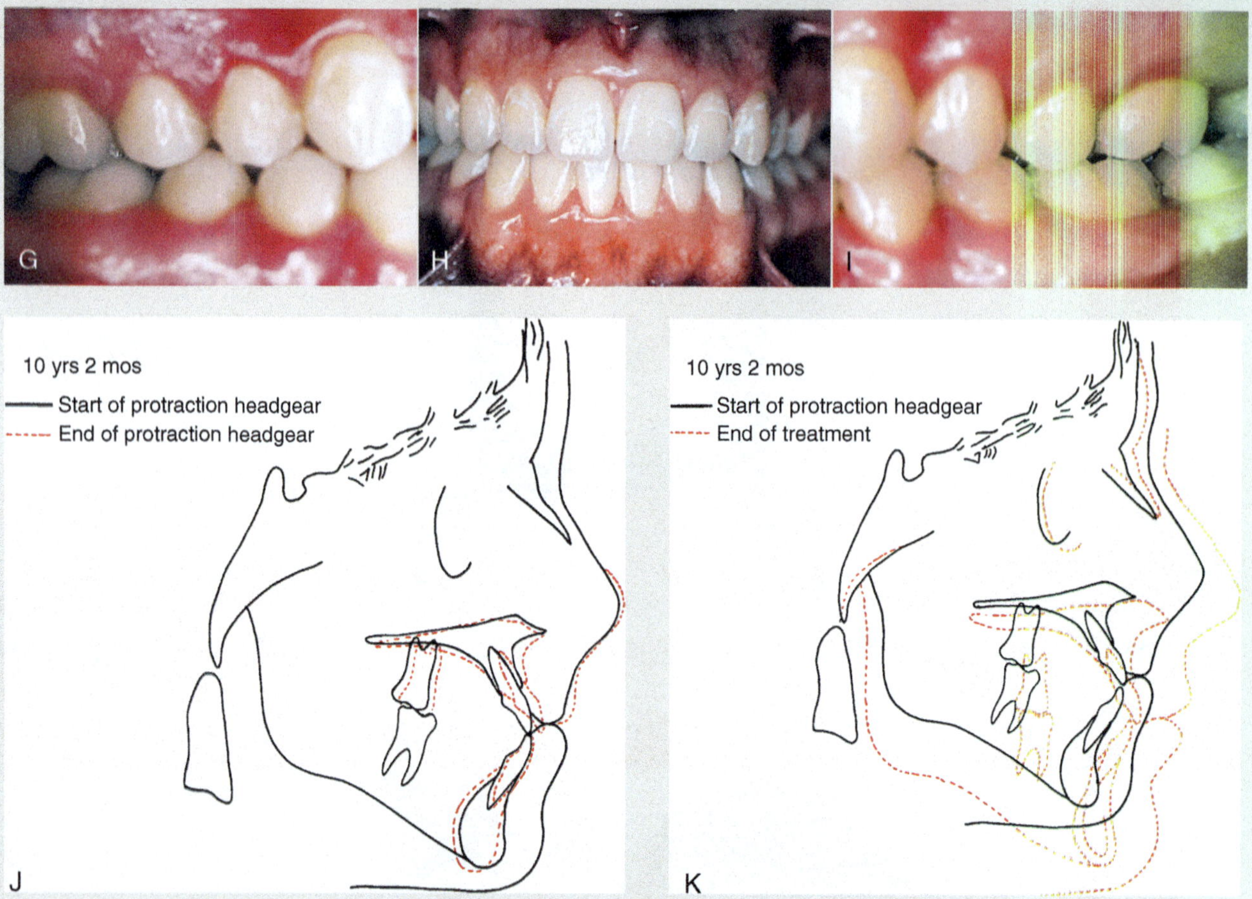

Figure 16-16, cont'd **G-I,** Intraoral views of the dentition 6 years following the application of the protraction headgear and 3 years into the retention period. **J,** Cephalometric superimposition tracings of the patient at the end of the protraction headgear period. **K,** Six years after the end of protraction. Note the amount of maxillary and mandibular growth.

REFERENCES

1. Kelly JE, Sanchez M, Van Kirk LE. *An Assessment of the Occlusion of the Teeth of Children.* DHEW Publication No (HRA) 74-1612. Washington, DC: National Center for Health Statistics; 1973.
2. Proffit WR, Fields HW, Moray LJ. Prevalence of malocclusion and orthodontic treatment need in the United States: estimates from the N-HANES III survey. *Int J Adult Orthod Orthogn Surg.* 1998;13:97–106.
3. Mills LF. Epidemiologic studies of occlusion IV: the prevalence of malocclusion in a population of 1,455 school children. *J Dent Res.* 1966; 45:332–336.
4. Delaire J. Confection du masque orthopedique. *Rev Stomat Paris.* 1971;72:579–584.
5. Delaire J. La croissance maxillaire. *Trans Eur Orthod Soc.* 1971:81–102.
6. Delaire J. L'articulation fronto-maxillaire: bases theoretiques et principles generaux d'application de forces extra-orales postero-anterieures sur masque orthopedique. *Rev Stomat Paris.* 1976;77:921–930.
7. Delaire J, Verdon P, Lumineau JP, Cherga-Negrea A, Talmant J, Boisson M. Note de tecnique. *Rev Stomatol.* 1972;73:633–642.
8. Delaire VJ, Verdon P, Floor J. Moglichkeiten und Grenzen Extraoraler Kratie in Postereo-anterior Richtung unter Verwandung der Orthopadischen Maske. *Forsch Keiferorthop.* 1978;39:27–45.
9. Nanda R. Biomechanical and clinical considerations of a protraction headgear. *Am J Orthod.* 1980;78:125–139.
10. Dietrich UC. Morphological variability of skeletal Class III relationships as revealed by cephalometric analysis. *Trans Eur Orthod Soc.* 1970;46:131–140.
11. Guyer EC, Ellis E, McNamara JA Jr, Behrents RG. Components of Class III malocclusion in juveniles and adolescents. *Angle Orthod.* 1986;56: 7–30.
12. Williams S, Andersen CE. The morphology of the potential Class III skeletal pattern in the growing child. *Am J Orthod.* 1986;89:302–311.
13. Dellinger EL. A preliminary study of anterior maxillary displacement. *Am J Orthod.* 1973;63:509–516.
14. Jackson GW, Kokich VG, Shapiro PA. Experimental and postexperimental response to anteriorly directed extraoral force in young *Macaca nemestrina. Am J Orthod.* 1979;75:318–333.
15. Kambara T. Dentofacial changes produced by extraoral forward force in the *Macaca irus. Am J Orthod.* 1977;71:249–277.
16. Nanda R, Hickory W. Zygomaticomaxillary suture adaptations incident to anteriorly-directed forces in rhesus monkeys. *Angle Orthod.* 1984;54: 199–210.
17. Nanda R. Protraction of maxilla in rhesus monkeys by controlled extraoral forces. *Am J Orthod.* 1978;74:121–141.

18. Baccetti T, Franchi L, McNamara JA Jr. Treatment and post-treatment craniofacial changes following rapid maxillary expansion and facial mask therapy. *Am J Orthod Dentofacial Orthop*. 2000;118:404–411.
19. Baccetti T, McGill JS, Franchi L, McNamara JA Jr, Tollaro I. Skeletal effects of early treatment of Class III malocclusion with maxillary expansion and face-mask therapy. *Am J Orthod Dentofacial Orthop*. 1998;113:333–343.
20. MacDonald KE, Kapust AJ, Turley PK. Cephalometric changes after correction of Class III malocclusion with maxillary expansion/facemask therapy. *Am J Orthod Dentofacial Orthop*. 1999;116:13–24.
21. McGill JS, McNamara JA Jr. Treatment and post-treatment effects of rapid maxillary expansion and facial mask therapy. In: McNamara JA Jr, ed. *Growth Modification: What Works, What Doesn't and Why*. Monograph 36, Craniofacial Growth Series. Ann Arbor, MI: Center for Human Growth and Development, University of Michigan, 1999.
22. Ngan P, Hägg U, Yiu C, Merwin D, Wei SH. Treatment response to maxillary expansion and protraction. *Eur J Orthod*. 1996;18:151–168.
23. Ngan P, Yiu C, Hu A, Hägg U, Wei SH, Gunel E. Cephalometric and occlusal changes following maxillary expansion and protraction. *Eur J Orthod*. 1998;20:237–254.
24. Pangrazio-Kulbersh V, Berger J, Kersten G. Effects of protraction mechanics on the midface. *Am J Orthod Dentofacial Orthop*. 1998;114:484–491.
25. Turley PK. Orthopedic correction of Class III malocclusion with palatal expansion and custom protraction headgear. *J Clin Orthod*. 1988;22:314–325.
26. Ngan P, Hägg U, Yiu C, Wei H. Treatment response and long-term dentofacial adaptations to maxillary expansion and protraction. *Semin Orthod*. 1997;3:255–264.
27. Shanker S, Ngan P, Wade D, et al. Cephalometric A point changes during and after maxillary protraction and expansion. *Am J Orthod Dentofacial Orthop*. 1996;110:423–430.
28. Hickory WB, Nanda R. Effect of tensile force magnitude on release of cranial suture cells into S phase. *Am J Orthod Dentofacial Orthop*. 1987;91:328–334.
29. Tanne K, Hiraga J, Kakiuchi K, Yamagata Y, Sakuda M. Biomechanical effect of anteriorly directed extraoral forces on the craniofacial complex: a study using the finite element method. *Am J Orthod Dentofacial Orthop*. 1989;95:200–207.
30. Tanne K, Sakuda M. Biomechanical and clinical changes of the craniofacial complex from orthopedic maxillary protraction. *Angle Orthod*. 1991;61:145–152.
31. Miki M. An experimental research on the directional of the complex by means of the external force: two dimensional analysis on the sagittal plane of the craniofacial skeleton. *J Tokyo Dent Coll*. 1979;79:1563–1597.
32. Hata S, Itoh T, Nakagawa M, et al. Biomechanical effects of maxillary protraction on the craniofacial complex. *Am J Orthod*. 1987;91:305–311.
33. Lee K, Ryu Y, Park Y, Rudolph D. A study of holographic interferometry on the initial reaction of maxillofacial complex during protraction. *Am J Orthod*. 1997;111:623–632.
34. Keles A, Erverdi N, Sezen S. Bodily distalization of molars with absolute anchorage. *Angle Orthod*. 2003;73:471–482.

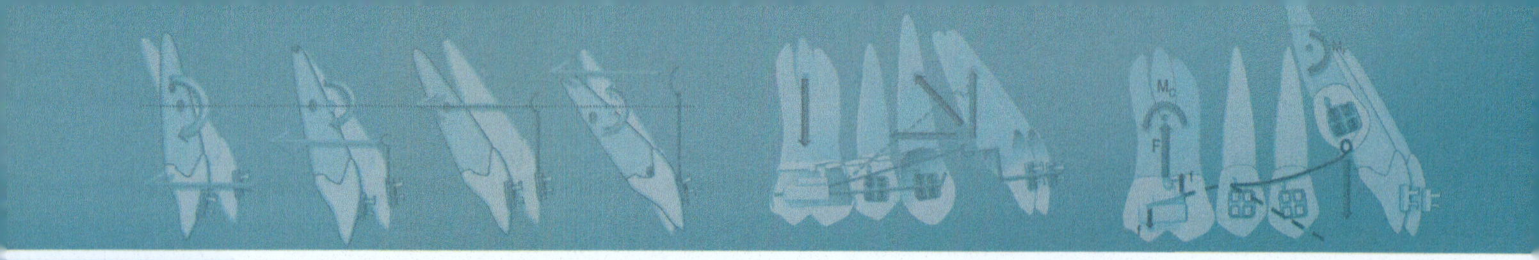

CHAPTER 17

New Treatment Modalities for Class III Malocclusion

Nazan Küçükkeleş, Hanife Nuray Yılmaz, and Şirin Nevzatoğlu

Patients with Class III malocclusion comprise a relatively small percentage of the average orthodontic practice but these cases are among the most difficult to treat effectively and efficiently.[1] Until the 1970s, skeletal Class III malocclusions were thought to be caused solely by a large and/or protrusive mandible. Now we know that they can be a result of various factors: (1) prognathic mandible with a normally positioned maxilla, (2) retrognathic maxilla with a normal mandible, (3) combination maxillary retrognathism and mandibular prognathism, and (4) normal skeletal relationship of maxilla and mandible with reverse overjet in the presence of centric relation–centric occlusion (CR-CO) discrepancy, also known as a "pseudo" Class III relationship.

According to studies by Ellis and McNamara[2] and Guyer et al.,[3] 40% to 60% of skeletal Class III patients have maxillary deficiency or retrusion, suggesting that maxillary deficiency does play a role in most skeletal Class III malocclusions. Therefore the appropriate treatment option for growing patients with Class III malocclusions should include maxillary protraction. For more than 40 years, protraction facemask therapy has been the most popular method of protracting the maxilla and the effects are well documented. This chapter discusses the effects of protraction facemask therapy as well as the timing of its application for maximum efficiency.

TIMING OF TREATMENT FOR CLASS III MALOCCLUSION

The timing of treatment for Class III malocclusion has always been a matter of debate among orthodontists. Should treatment start early in the patient's childhood or should clinicians wait until growth is completed and then proceed with orthognathic surgery? Some authors support the benefits of early treatment and point to the disadvantages of a long treatment time while waiting for the skeletal maturation of a child before sending him or her for orthognathic surgery. Others choose early orthognathic surgery because of concerns about dental compensation and/or mistiming of the cessation of mandibular growth during orthopedic treatment.

Proffit[4] contended that treatment should start as soon as possible after Class III malocclusion is diagnosed. He pointed to an ideal age of 8 years. Baccetti et al.[5] studied a sample of 46 subjects in mixed dentition and compared them with a control sample of 32 subjects with untreated Class III malocclusion. Treated and untreated samples were divided into early and late mixed dentition groups for identification of the optimum treatment timing. The younger group showed significantly greater advancement of maxillary structures and significantly more upward and forward direction of condylar growth after treatment.

Kapust et al.[6] examined patients divided into three different age groups and suggested that earlier treatment produces a more favorable result; however, the older children did have significant treatment outcomes, indicating that orthopedic changes can be obtained in the 10- to 14-year-old age group as well.

In 2000 Saadia and Torres[7] examined the sagittal response of Class III patients in the primary, mixed, and late mixed dentition phases who were treated with expansion followed by facemask therapy. They found that greater significant changes were seen in patients treated in the primary and mixed dentition phases, even with fewer hours of appliance wear per day.

In 2004 Ochoa and Nanda[8] examined the growth pattern of maxilla and mandible with ages ranging from 6 to 20 years and reported that maximum maxillary growth was observed between the ages of 6 and 8 years. The maxillary complex was still growing after the age of 8 years but at a decreasing pace until the age of 14 years. Moreover, in girls there was a significant decrease in maxillary growth after the age of 12 years while in some male patients even little maxillary growth was seen until the age of 20 years.

In the same year, Franchi et al.[9] treated 50 patients who were in late deciduous/early mixed or late mixed dentition with an initial phase of rapid palatal expansion (RPE) and facemask therapy followed by a second phase of preadjusted edgewise therapy. They reported that orthopedic treatment of Class III malocclusion was more effective when it was initiated at an early developmental phase rather than at later stages with respect to untreated Class III control groups. However, patients treated with RPE and facemask therapy in the late mixed dentition did exhibit improvement with the treatment but to a lesser degree.

Baik[10] examined 47 Korean children who were divided into three groups according to their ages and found no statistically significant difference among the groups.

Sung and Baik[11] subsequently evaluated the effect of maxillary protraction in patients who were divided into six age groups from ages 7 to 12 years and found that the amount of skeletal change among the groups was not statistically significant.

Merwin et al.[12] examined 30 patients who were divided into two age groups of 5 to 8 years and 9 to 12 years and reported that cephalometric changes were similar between the two groups, suggesting that a similar skeletal response can be expected in patients in either the early or the late mixed dentition.

Looking at all of these results, it seems favorable to apply maxillary protraction before the age of 12 years. Nevertheless, the treatment results are more effective when maxillary protraction is initiated at an early developmental phase of the dentition rather than at later stages.

TREATMENT APPROACHES IN CLASS III MALOCCLUSION

There are three main approaches for the treatment of a skeletal Class III malocclusion:

1. Camouflage of the skeletal jaw discrepancy by orthodontic tooth movement so that the dental occlusion is corrected although the skeletal discrepancy remains
2. Growth modification consisting of maxillary protraction together with restriction of mandibular growth
3. Surgical correction of the jaw discrepancy

Because this chapter is concerned with the new orthopedic treatment modalities, the first and third treatment options will not be discussed and we will focus on the treatment option of growth modification.

EFFECTS OF FACEMASK THERAPY

Since most skeletal Class III patients have maxillary deficiency or retrusion, the appropriate treatment option for growing patients is protraction of the maxilla. The literature reports a series of approaches regarding orthopedic treatment of Class III malocclusions.[13] Facemask treatment is the most frequently used treatment protocol for this anomaly. The treatment effects of facemask therapy are a combination of skeletal and dental changes of the maxilla and the mandible.[9] The maxilla moves downward and forward with a slight upward movement in the anterior and downward movement in the posterior palatal plane as a result of protraction force together with the extrusion of posterior teeth. Consequently, downward and backward rotation of the mandible improves the maxillomandibular skeletal relationship in the sagittal dimension. This rotation is a major contributing factor in establishing positive overjet. Currently there seems to be general agreement on applying a downward and forward force with 30 degrees to occlusal plane in order to achieve anterior displacement of maxilla with minimal downward and forward rotation.[14–16] There are also some dentoalveolar changes, such as increase in upper incisor inclinations due to mesial movement of upper dental arch and decrease in lower incisor inclinations due to the pressure applied by the chin cup of the facemask.

In clinical studies the duration of facemask use ranges from 12 to 24 hours per day with a force amount of 300 to 600 g per side, with most studies showing an average of 2 mm maxillary advancement.[5,9,17–21]

In a prospective clinical trial,[22] after facemask treatment in 20 patients, overjet correction was found to be the result of forward maxillary movement (31%), backward movement of the mandible (21%), labial movement of the maxillary incisors (28%), and lingual movement of the mandibular incisors (20%).

In 2003 Cha[23] evaluated skeletal and dentoalveolar changes produced by RPE and facemask therapy in 85 subjects who were divided into three groups: prepubertal growth group (Group 1; n = 34), pubertal growth group (Group 2; n = 32), and postpubertal growth group (Group 3; n = 19). The Delaire type facemask was used for 12 hours with 500 g of force. Negative overjet was corrected by 80.1% skeletal and 19.9% dentoalveolar changes in Group 1, 84.0% skeletal and 16.0% dentoalveolar changes in Group 2, and 63.6% skeletal and 36.4% dentoalveolar changes in Group 3. The maxillary anterior movement in Groups 1, 2, and 3 was 2.69, 2.69, and 0.97 mm, respectively.

CHALLENGES OF USING FACEMASK THERAPY

Although the main target of the treatment is forward movement of the maxilla, the values for maxillary advancement reported in the literature[5,9,17–19] are not more than 2-mm with 6 to 12 months of treatment. Also, there are some limitations of this method, such as insufficient skeletal correction in severe Class III malocclusions and undesired dentoalveolar effects due to application of high forces to the teeth.

In 2003 Hägg et al.[24] reported that 7 of 21 patients who were treated by facemask had negative overjet after an average of 8 years recall. Of these patients, 29% were considered for orthognathic surgery. Baccetti et al.[25] reported that 12 of 41 patients (28%), all of whom had comprehensive orthodontics after facemask therapy, had negative overjet and Class III molar relationships after an average of 6.5 years recall at a mean age of 15 years. In 2006 Wells et al.[26]

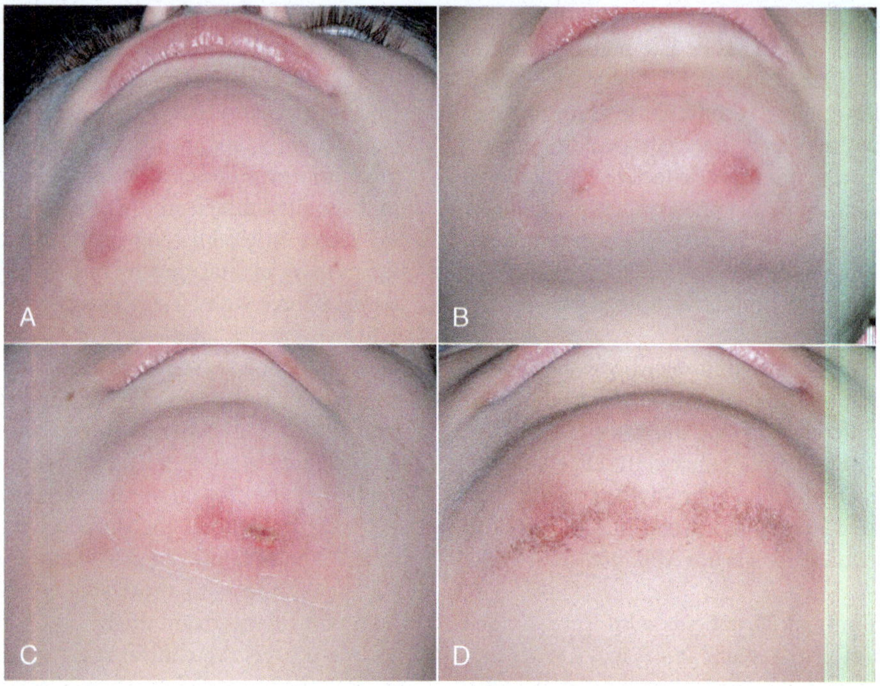

Figure 17-1 **A–D,** Examples of chin irritation due to facemask therapy.

examined 41 Class III patients 10 years after the treatment of facemask therapy and reported 30% relapse into reverse overjet, mainly because of increased horizontally directed and often late mandibular growth. Due to the unpredictable long-term relapse potential, it was recommended by the authors to overcorrect the overjet in anticipation of some relapse. Furthermore, using various types of retention appliances was also proposed to improve stability.[26] Since dentoalveolar changes are the most prone to relapse, it would be advantageous to eliminate or at least minimize dentoalveolar effects and maximize orthopedic effects of the treatment.[24-26]

Another problem encountered with extraoral appliances is the need for patient compliance and parental support.[27] These appliances are bulky yet need to be worn for at least 12 to 16 hours per day for a total duration of 9 to 12 months. Also, high forces usually cause irritation of the skin in the chin area (Fig. 17-1). All of these factors lead to compliance problems and impair the treatment results. In 2006 Brandao et al.[28] examined the duration of extraoral appliance use using an electronic recording device. Interestingly, they found that the electronic recording device reported 6 to 7 hours of use whereas the patient reported 13 to 14 hours of use of the extraoral device.

PERCEPTIONS OF FACIAL ESTHETICS AND PSYCHOLOGICAL DEVELOPMENT

The perception of facial esthetics influences one's psychological development from early childhood to adulthood. In the literature it has been reported that laypersons evaluate prognathic profiles more negatively than retrognathic profiles.[29-31] Therefore early intervention in cases of orthodontic malocclusion is important from the standpoint of the patient's psychological development. Some clinicians prefer orthognathic surgery for the correction of Class III malocclusion and wait until age 20 years because of the potential relapse seen with late mandibular growth. However, delaying the treatment time results in patients coping with all of the problems mentioned above during adolescence. At the end of this challenging stage patients will then have orthognatic surgery under general anesthesia in addition to an extensive period of orthodontic treatment.

PROBLEMS RELATED TO SURGERY

Sometimes surgery requires blood transfusion and bone grafts at the time of operation, which make the surgery even more difficult. It was reported that 51% of maxillary advancement and extrusion surgery requires bone grafts. Sixty-five percent of bone grafts are taken from the iliac bone whereas 8.5% are taken from the rib area.[32] During or after maxillary osteotomy the complication rate is reported to be approximately 4.2%. In addition, damage to the roots of teeth due to the internal rigid fixation screws, hemorrhage, morbidity, and hearing and vision loss are reported as other complications of orthognathic surgery.

Regarding the stability of the maxillary advancement surgery, relapse of less than 2-mm is found in 80% of cases and relapse of 2- to 4-mm is reported in the remaining 20% of cases. However, the relapse rate increases when maxillary advancement and extrusion are both performed. Although the maxillary advancement is found to be stable, 40% to 50% of extrusion is prone to relapse, indicating the instability of this intervention. Stable results are obtained when the rigid internal fixation is used in maxillary advancement plus mandibular setback surgery. However, 40% to 50% of relapse is also seen when the mandibular setback surgery is performed alone.[33–36]

IMPROVED TREATMENT MODALITIES FOR CLASS III MALOCCLUSIONS

Based on the information discussed above, new treatment protocols that are effective, efficient, and applicable at any age are needed for the treatment of Class III malocclusions. A new focus is the use of skeletal anchorage devices to achieve protraction of the maxillary complex, with some using these devices in conjunction with corticotomies. In 1999 Rachmiel et al.[37] presented 14 cleft lip and palate patients (8 to 10 years old) treated by an incomplete Le Fort I osteotomy followed by protraction of the maxilla with facemask. The results showed a mean maxillary forward movement of 7.2-mm after 3 weeks of protraction, which was followed by a retention period of 9 weeks for callus maturation. In 2001 Molina[38] also applied a facemask in conjunction with incomplete Le Fort I osteotomy in 43 patients who were divided into two groups according to the severity of the maxillary retrusion. He reported a mean maxillary forward movement of 9-mm in the severe group and of 5-mm in the moderately retrusive group. Unfortunately, neither study reported long-term results of the corticotomy-assisted maxillary protraction protocol. In the similar time period, Singer et al.[39] achieved 4-mm of advancement with the facemask applied from Brånemark implants on the zygomatic buttress region. It was the first report in which temporary anchorage devices (TADs) were used for the orthopedic protraction of maxilla in growing patients. Currently, in the field of orthodontics, a dramatic increase in the use of TADs, such as palatal implants, onplants, mini-screws, and mini-plates, has been observed. Currently, mini-plates are commonly used in maxillofacial surgery for rigid fixation of the bony segments. Most of the literature reports that the mini-plates are quite stable, even with the high forces.[40] In 2008 Kircelli and Pektas[41] applied the Delaire type facemask from mini-plates, which were placed on the lateral nasal walls of the maxilla. The elastic force was 300 g per side and they reported 4.8-mm maxillary advancement together with 3.3-mm forward movement of the infraorbital region in six patients.

In 2010 Heymann et al.[42] applied Class III elastics between mini-plates on the zygomatic region in the maxilla and the canine region in the mandible. They reported that forward movement of the maxilla ranged from 0.4- to 4.7-mm in 12 months for six patients with a mean age of 11.8 years. In the same year, De Clerck et al.[43] reported on a group of 21 patients (mean age of 11.10 years) consecutively treated with the same protocol. The results were compared with a matched control group of 18 untreated Class III patients and revealed that A point showed an average of 4-mm forward movement in the treated subjects compared to the control subjects. Orbital and pterygomaxillary points advanced almost 3-mm and 2-mm, respectively, with more advancement in the treated group. A significant restraining effect on mandibular growth (–2-mm) was also recorded in the treated group.

ORTHOPEDIC EFFECTS OF RAPID PALATAL EXPANSION VERSUS CORTICOTOMY-ASSISTED MAXILLARY PROTRACTION (STUDY I)

In 2007 our team[44] designed a study to compare corticotomy-assisted maxillary protraction with conventional rapid palatal expansion (RPE)–assisted facemask therapy. Subjects with comparatively mild maxillary retrognathism were treated by conventional RPE plus facemask. This group included 18 patients with a mean age of 12.9 ± 1.1 years. Another 16 patients with a mean age of 13.1 ± 2.1 years who had moderate to severe maxillary retrognathism were treated by surgery plus facemask. In the latter group, Le Fort I osteotomy was performed for each patient under general anesthesia by the same surgeon and facemask was applied on the fifth to seventh day postsurgery with a total force value ranging from 1700 to 2000 g (Figs. 17-2 to 17-4). The elastics were oriented with a 30-degree angle to the occlusal plane as in the other study group. Facemasks were worn 24 hours per day (except during meals) until the achievement of Class II dental relationships, after which patients were told to switch to nighttime wear for another 3 months for retention purposes. In both groups maxillary splints were debonded following retention periods.

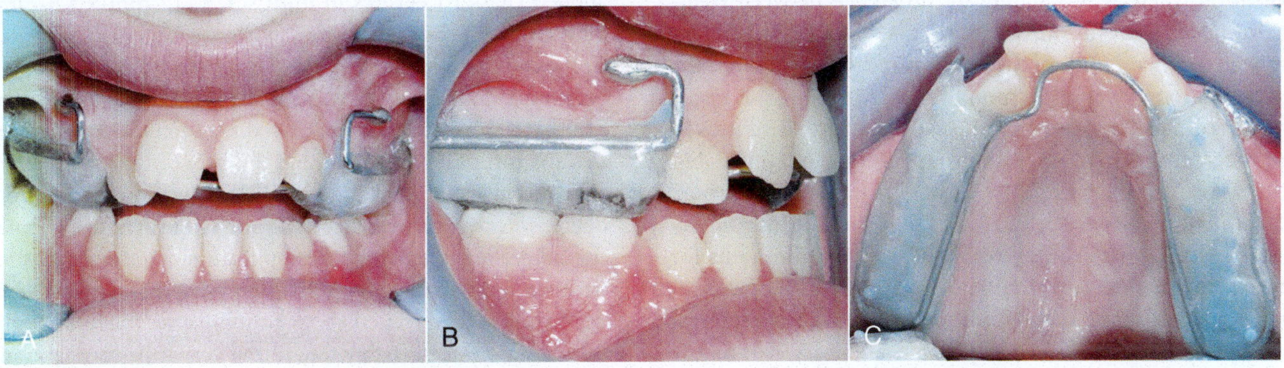

Figure 17-2 Study I. Intraoral views (A-C) of the appliance in the surgery-assisted group.

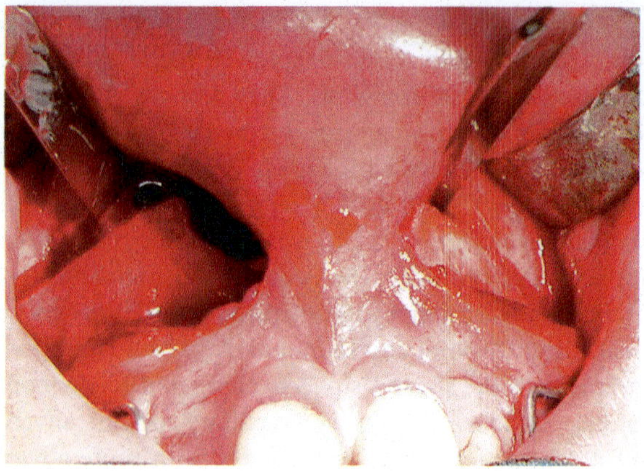

Figure 17-3 Study I. Corticotomy line.

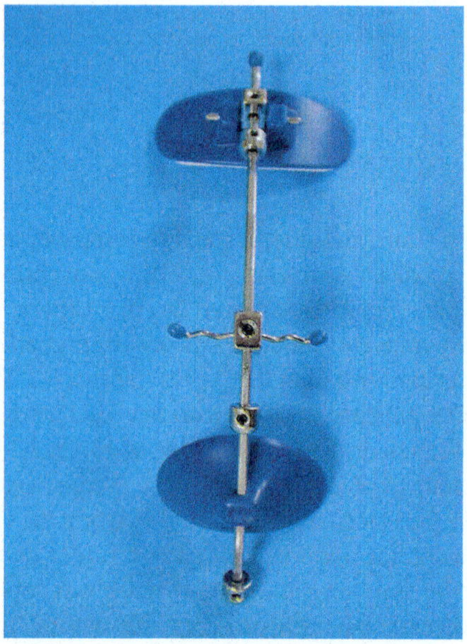

Figure 17-4 Petit type facemask appliance.

After the protraction phase, sella-nasion A point (SNA) and A point nasion B point (ANB) angles increased and sella-nasion B point (SNB) angle decreased significantly in both groups and sagittal maxillomandibular relationships were normalized (Table 17-1). The cephalometric findings demonstrated significant maxillary advancement in both groups together with mandibular backward rotation. However, there was a significant difference between treatment groups from the point of maxillary advancement reflected on hard and soft tissues (4-mm advancement in the surgery group versus 1.3-mm in the RPE group). Soft tissue results revealed that the upper lip and upper lip sulcus moved significantly forward in both groups during treatment but the values were significantly higher in the surgery group. Treatment duration was also found to be significantly different between groups. Total treatment time was 5 months for the corticotomy group and 9 months for the RPE plus facemask group. Therefore the surgically assisted facemask treatment was found to be more efficient and effective for the correction of Class III malocclusion when compared to the RPE-assisted facemask treatment. A patient treated with corticotomy-assisted facemask therapy is presented in Case Report 1.

LONG-TERM EVALUATION OF CORTICOTOMY-ASSISTED FACEMASK THERAPY (STUDY II)

We decided to evaluate the long-term stability of the surgery-assisted protraction group in 2012. Sixteen patients were recalled 5 years following the surgically assisted protraction. Only nine patients presented for the follow-up study and records were renewed. The study was carried out using lateral cephalometric films taken before treatment (T_0), immediately after maxillary protraction (T_1), and after 5 years (T_2). Although the cases maintained normal overjet and overbite and the Class I relationship, significant relapse of maxillary advancement was noted in the follow-up period (Table 17-2). On the other hand, the statistically significant decrease of the SNB angle obtained during treatment remained unchanged after treatment. During maxillary protraction upper incisors moved bodily without proclination whereas in the follow-up period significant increase in the upper incisor inclination was observed, probably to compensate for the relapse of maxillary position. During treatment the upper molars moved forward and they maintained their position throughout the follow-up period. There were no significant changes in the lower incisor inclination at all stages. Skeletal and dental extrusion achieved during protraction was preserved. It was interesting that even though some soft tissue improvements were lost, forward movement of the maxilla and the upper lip was partially maintained. This led to a well-maintained facial appearance in the follow-up period. Clinical examination of the recall period showed well-preserved dental relationships. There were no discrepancies between the final and recall occlusions and the residual changes were still significant compared to the pre-treatment values.[45]

Class III Elastic Application Between Upper and Lower Mini-Screws

Taking into consideration all of the problems noted in the previous studies, such as undesired dentoalveolar movements and poor cooperation with facemask, we decided to modify the treatment protocol to an intraoral design. We applied Class III elastics to mini-screws (7-mm × 1.6-mm) between the upper posterior and lower anterior region of two growing patients as a preliminary study (Fig. 17-5). An acrylic-cap Hyrax device was constructed for the upper dentition and mini-screws were placed between the first premolars and canines in the mandible and between the first molars and second premolars in the maxilla. Activation of the Hyrax device was performed twice a day for 10 days for disarticulation of the maxilla before the application of Class III elastics between mini-screws. The elastic force was 200 g per side but upper mini-screws failed about 1 month after the force application. This was probably due to the very thin cortical bone in the upper posterior region in young patients.[46,47] We then

TABLE 17-1 Means and SD Values Before and After Treatment in Study I

		Surgery + Facemask	RPE + Facemask	p
SNA (degree)	Before	75.44 ± 4.92	78.78 ± 3.28	0.025
	After	78.91 ± 3.62	80.42 ± 3.18	*NS*
	p	0.0001	0.001	
SNB (degree)	Before	78.84 ± 3.56	79.44 ± 3.66	*NS*
	After	77.22 ± 3.07	78.33 ± 3.68	*NS*
	p	0.002	0.001	
ANB (degree)	Before	−2.91 ± 2.52	−0.89 ± 1.84	0.011
	After	1.66 ± 2.35	2.31 ± 1.59	*NS*
	p	0.0001	0.0001	
Max depth (degree)	Before	83.25 ± 6	86.75 ± 3.21	0.039
	After	87 ± 4.45	88.47 ± 3.25	*NS*
	p	0.0001	0.0001	
N⊥A	Before	−6.84 ± 5.2	−3.83 ± 2.97	0.043
	After	−3.38 ± 4.76	−1.67 ± 3.45	*NS*
	p	0.0001	0.0001	
SN-PP (degree)	Before	10.16 ± 4.93	9.83 ± 3.2	*NS*
	After	8.44 ± 3.81	8.64 ± 3.18	*NS*
	p	*NS*	*NS*	
SN-UOP (degree)	Before	20.5 ± 5.38	20.94 ± 3.73	*NS*
	After	17.06 ± 6.93	19.5 ± 4.13	*NS*
	p	0.011	0.038	
SN-MP (degree)	Before	36.03 ± 4.34	35.92 ± 4.23	*NS*
	After	38.44 ± 4.08	37.53 ± 4.58	*NS*
	p	0.001	0.0001	
N-ANS	Before	54.38 ± 2.52	54.75 ± 3.52	*NS*
	After	54.94 ± 2.76	55.67 ± 3.25	*NS*
	p	*NS*	0.002	
ANS-Me	Before	64.63 ± 7.56	63.89 ± 4.09	*NS*
	After	68.97 ± 7.46	67.5 ± 4.41	*NS*
	p	0.0001	0.0001	
I-SN (degree)	Before	98 ± 11.78	100.39 ± 5.91	*NS*
	After	99.38 ± 11.66	102.25 ± 5.3	*NS*
	p	*NS*	0.05	
IMPA (degree)	Before	80.25 ± 5.99	83.11 ± 4.85	*NS*
	After	78.41 ± 6.87	82.19 ± 6.47	*NS*
	p	*NS*	*NS*	
Nasolabial angle (degree)	Before	99.59 ± 24.12	110.11 ± 12.39	*NS*
	After	111.25 ± 18.71	109.75 ± 11.53	*NS*
	p	0.015	*NS*	
RP2-L_S	Before	77.91 ± 6.89	82.81 ± 5.99	0.034
	After	82.34 ± 6.83	85.17 ± 6.23	*NS*
	p	0.0001	0.0001	
RP2-L_i	Before	65.41 ± 4.87	68.56 ± 6.56	*NS*
	After	63.28 ± 4.94	66.72 ± 5.79	*NS*
	p	0.007	0.044	

Student t test (statistical analysis used in this study).

ANB, A point nasion B point; *ANS,* anterior nasal spine; *ANS-Me,* Distance of ANS to Menton; *I-SN,* upper incisors sella-nasion; *IMPA,* incisor mandibular plane angle; *MP,* mandibular plane; *N,* nasion; *N⊥A,* distance of A point to a line drawn from nasion perpendicular to Frankfort horizontal plane; *NS,* not significant; *RP2-L_i,* distance of vertical reference plane to labrale inferior; *RP2-L_s,* distance of vertical reference plane to labrale superior; *RPE,* rapid palatal expansion; *SN,* sella-nasion; *SN-PP,* sella-nasion palatal plane; *SN-UOP,* sella-nasion upper occlusal plane; *SNA,* sella-nasion A point; *SNB,* sella-nasion B point.

TABLE 17-2 Dental, Skeletal, and Soft Tissue Sagittal and Vertical Changes in Study II: Initial, Postprotraction, and Recall Means and SD Values (n = 9)

			Post Hoc		
Changes		**Mean ± SD**	**T_0-T_1**	**T_0-T_2**	**T_1-T_2**
SNA (degree)	T_0	74.11 ± 5.28	**	*NS*	*
	T_1	79.05 ± 3.47			
	T_2	74.28 ± 4.44			
	p	**			
SNB (degree)	T_0	78.55 ± 3.00	*	*NS*	*NS*
	T_1	77.11 ± 3.34			
	T_2	76.28 ± 4.94			
	p	*			
ANB (degree)	T_0	−3.55 ± 2.30	**	*NS*	*
	T_1	1.94 ± 2.28			
	T_2	−2.00 ± 3.58			
	p	**			
Max depth (degree)	T_0	82.39 ± 7.56	*	*NS*	**
	T_1	87.39 ± 5.38			
	T_2	83.67 ± 6.30			
	p	**			
N┴A	T_0	−7.39 ± 6.52	*	*NS*	*
	T_1	−2.83 ± 5.54			
	T_2	−7.22 ± 7.26			
	p	**			
SN-PP (degree)	T_0	10.61 ± 6.08	*NS*	*NS*	*NS*
	T_1	8.78 ± 3.80			
	T_2	10.89 ± 4.67			
	p	*NS*			
SN-UOP (degree)	T_0	22.05 ± 5.11	*	*	*NS*
	T_1	17.67 ± 7.55			
	T_2	19.67 ± 4.41			
	p	*			
SN-MP (degree)	T_0	36.67 ± 3.00	*NS*	*NS*	*NS*
	T_1	38.55 ± 2.96			
	T_2	39.83 ± 5.64			
	p	*NS*			

			Post Hoc		
Changes		**Mean ± SD**	**T_0-T_1**	**T_0-T_2**	**T_1-T_2**
N-ANS	T_0	54.33 ± 2.83	*NS*	*NS*	*
	T_1	54.72 ± 2.95			
	T_2	56.44 ± 2.45			
	p	*			
ANS-Me	T_0	63.55 ± 7.08	*	**	*NS*
	T_1	67.83 ± 7.38			
	T_2	69.78 ± 7.33			
	p	**			
I-SN (Degree)	T_0	99.83 ± 8.46	*NS*	**	*
	T_1	102.66 ± 6.38			
	T_2	106.22 ± 6.32			
	p	**			
IMPA (Degree)	T_0	79.22 ± 7.64	*NS*	*NS*	*NS*
	T_1	78.00 ± 7.90			
	T_2	82.22 ± 8.56			
	p	*NS*			
Nasolabial angle (Degree)	T_0	95.61 ± 15.95	*NS*	*NS*	*NS*
	T_1	106.55 ± 9.12			
	T_2	98.11 ± 6.95			
	p	*NS*			
RP2-L_s	T_0	77.55 ± 6.59	**	*	*
	T_1	83.78 ± 6.66			
	T_2	80.67 ± 7.16			
	p	**			
RP2-L_i	T_0	65.78 ± 4.11	*NS*	*NS*	*NS*
	T_1	63.61 ± 5.05			
	T_2	65.05 ± 6.67			
	p	*NS*			

ANB, A point nasion B point; *ANS*, anterior nasal spine; *ANS-Me*, Distance of ANS to Menton; *I*-SN, upper incisors sella-nasion; *IMPA*, incisor mandibular plane angle; *MP*, mandibular plane; *N*, nasion; *N┴A*, distance of A point to a line drawn from nasion perpendicular to Frankfort horizontal plane; *NS*, not significant; *RP2-L_i*, distance of vertical reference plane to labrale inferior; *RP2-L_s*, distance of vertical reference plane to labrale superior; *SD*, standard deviation; *SN*, sella-nasion; *SNS*, not significant; *SN-PP*, sella-nasion palatal plane; *SN-UOP*, sella-nasion upper occlusal plane; *SNA*, sella-nasion A point; *SNB*, sella-nasion B point; *T_0*, initial; *T_1*, postprotraction; *T_2*; recall.

*p <0.05.

**p <0.01.

Note: Wilcoxon signed-rank test was used in comparing Friedman test and post-hoc analysis.

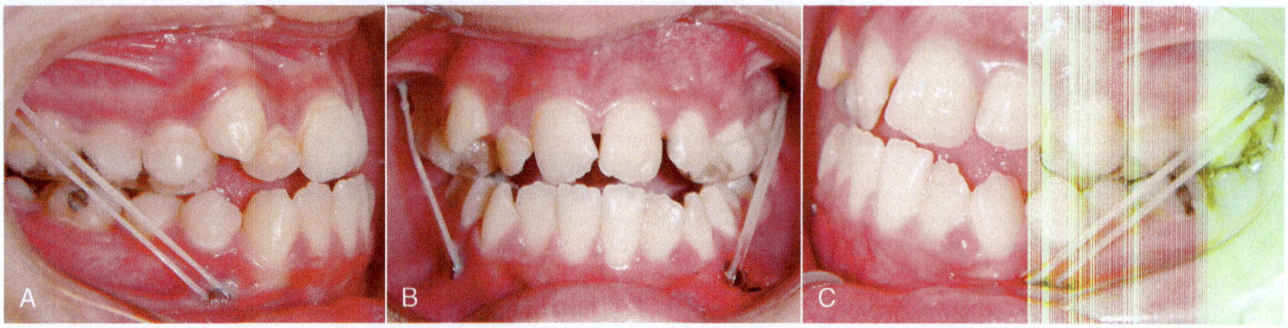

Figure 17-5 Class III elastic application **(A-C)** between mini-screws in the upper and lower jaws.

decided to modify the protocol and apply Class III elastics between mini-plates in the lower anterior region and the maxillary splint and the protraction was supported by Le Fort I osteotomy (see Case Report 2).

CORTICOTOMY-ASSISTED MAXILLARY PROTRACTION USING SKELETAL ANCHORAGE DEVICE (STUDY III)

The study group consisted of 19 patients (9 female, 10 male) with a mean age of 13.12 ± 1.28 years. They all had skeletal Class III malocclusion characterized by maxillary retrognathism, normal or low angle vertical pattern, and permanent dentition. A customized acrylic splint with the hooks in the molar region was constructed for each patient and bonded on maxillary dentition. All patients were operated on under general anesthesia and were treated by the protocol described earlier in the chapter. Maxillary protraction was continued until the achievement of Class II canine relationship in all cases.

Cephalometric radiographs were taken just before bonding of the upper splint and after protraction. To determine the sagittal and vertical changes, two reference planes were used. The horizontal reference plane (RP1) was drawn with a 7-degree angle below the sella-nasion (SN) plane at sella point and a perpendicular line was drawn to the first plane through the sella point (RP2). Perpendicular lines were drawn to these reference planes from selected anatomic points (Fig. 17-6). The data were evaluated statistically by means of t-tests (Table 17-3).

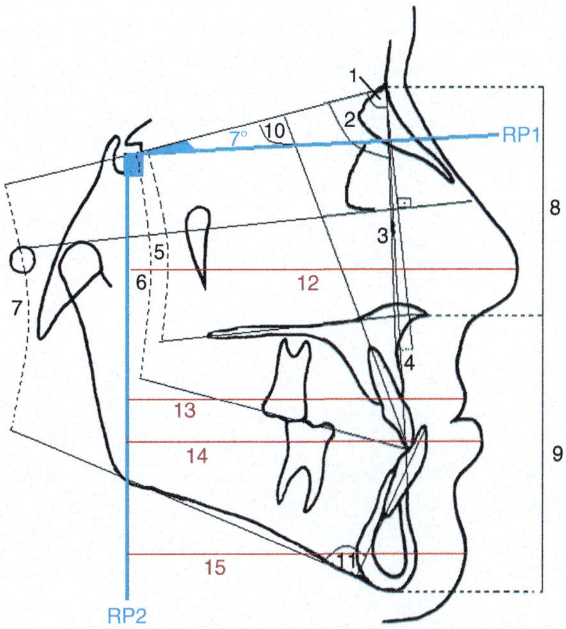

Figure 17-6 Cephalometric parameters used in study III and case report 2. *1,* Sella-nasion A point (SNA); *2,* sella-nasion B point (SNB); *3,* A point nasion B point (ANB); *4,* N⊥A (distance of A point to a line drawn from nasion perpendicular to Frankfort horizontal plane); *5,* SN-PP sella-nasion palatal plane (SN-PP); *6,* sella-nasion upper occlusal plane (SN-UOP); *7,* sella-nasion to Gonion-Menton (mandibular plane) (SN-MP); *8,* distance of nasion to anterior nasal spine (N-ANS); *9,* distance of anterior nasal spine to menton (ANS-Me); *10,* upper incisors sella-nasion (UI-SN); *11,* incisor mandibular plane angle (IMPA); *12,* distance of vertical reference plane to nose tip (RP2⊥NT); *13,* distance of vertical reference plane to Labrale superior (RP2⊥L_S); *14,* distance of vertical reference plane to labrale inferior (RP2⊥L_I); *15,* distance of vertical reference plane to pogonion (RP2⊥Pog′); *RP1,* horizontal reference plane.

Short-Term Results of Corticotomy-Assisted Maxillary Protraction Using Skeletal Anchorage

Class II canine relationships were achieved successfully in all cases at the end of the protraction period, which lasted 3.85 ± 1.12 months. Mini-plates were stable and the soft tissue around the hooks was healthy throughout the treatment period. Surgical removal of the mini-plates was uneventful and new bone formation was observed around the mini-plates during removal.

During protraction, A point moved forward (3.50 ± 0.35 mm), SNA (2.76 ± 0.26 degrees) and ANB (4.18 ± 0.34 degrees) increased and SNB (−1.45 ± 0.21 degrees) decreased significantly, which led to Class I skeletal relationship in 3.85 months. Kircelli and Pektas[41] reported 4.8-mm maxillary advancement in 10.8 months whereas Sar et al.[48] reported 2.3-mm advancement in 6.78 months by using a facemask through mini-plates on the lateral nasal wall of the maxilla. These values were similar to our results but the speed of protraction in our study was dramatically faster. On the other hand, in the studies of corticotomy-assisted facemask therapy Molina[38] reported 4- to 12-mm change of A point in 3 to 4 weeks whereas Rachmiel et al.[37] and Küçükkeleş et al.[44] reported 6.8-mm advancement in 3 weeks and 4-mm advancement in 2 months. These protraction rates were faster than ours but they were based on full-time facemask wear and so on patient cooperation. In the study by De Clerck et al.,[43] maxilla was protracted through Class III elastics between mini-plates on both maxilla and mandible, which was called bone-anchored maxillary protraction (BAMP) protocol. The authors reported 4-mm forward movement of A point in 12 months, a longer protraction period that requires a lot of patient cooperation.

Palatal and occlusal planes rotated anteriorly during protraction in our study. This can be explained by the force vector, which was located below the center of resistance of maxilla and the corticotomy line. It was not possible to avoid the vertical force vector of the Class III elastics, although the hooks were located as occlusally as possible on both jaws. This rotation led to an anterior open bite clinically but was spontaneously corrected by occlusal forces after the removal of the appliance as observed in the initial few patients. Sometimes it was beneficial to have the patients chew gum (hard sugar-free gum chewed three times daily for 30 minutes after meals) to aid in open-bite correction. Small increases were found in vertical parameters, though these were not clinically significant. The mandibular plane rotated posteriorly during protraction and B point was carried backward, decreasing the projection of the mandible. This was similar to the findings of many other studies in the literature.[44,48] This result occurred due to the chin cup effect of facemask and anterior rotation of the maxilla.

TABLE 17-3 Dental, Skeletal and Soft Tissue Changes Before and After Protraction in Study III

	Preprotraction (n = 19) Mean ± SD	Postprotraction (n = 19) Mean ± SD	Difference (n = 19) Mean ± SD	p
SNA	78.11 ± 3.45	80.87 ± 3.74	2.76 ± 0.26	**
SNB	82.03 ± 3.61	80.58 ± 3.62	−1.45 ± 0.21	**
ANB	−3.92 ± 2.43	0.26 ± 2.77	4.18 ± 0.34	**
N⊥A	−3.18 ± 2.88	0.32 ± 3.55	3.50 ± 0.35	**
SN-PP	9.79 ± 3.16	8.89 ± 3.75	−0.90 ± 0.37	*
SN-UOP	18.21 ± 5.95	9.93 ± 6.57	−8.28 ± 1.01	**
SN-MP	34.34 ± 6.64	35.68 ± 6.53	1.34 ± 0.18	**
N-ANS	57.20 ± 3.49	57.13 ± 4.05	−0.07 ± 0.26	NS
ANS-Me	68.42 ± 5.78	70.92 ± 5.83	2.50 ± 0.42	**
UI-SN	105.84 ± 6.20	115.50 ± 7.44	9.66 ± 1.21	**
IMPA	82.47 ± 5.99	86.11 ± 6.72	3.63 ± 0.72	**
RP2⊥NT	102.98 ± 6.60	105.54 ± 6.99	2.56 ± 0.27	**
RP2⊥L_S	89.28 ± 7.11	92.61 ± 7.70	3.33 ± 0.48	**
RP2⊥L_i	90.08 ± 8.49	90.00 ± 8.16	−0.08 ± 0.37	NS
RP2⊥Pog′	85.26 ± 9.99	108.82 ± 8.34	−1.71 ± 0.42	**

Student t-test (statistical analysis used in this study).

ANB, A point nasion B point; *ANS,* anterior nasal spine; *ANS-Me,* distance of ANS to Menton; *IMPA,* incisor mandibular plane angle; *MP,* mandibular plane; *N,* nasion; *N⊥A,* distance of A point to a line drawn from nasion perpendicular to Frankfort horizontal plane; *NS,* not significant; *RP2⊥L_i,* distance of vertical reference plane to labrale inferior; *RP2⊥L_s,* distance of vertical reference plane to labrale superior; *RP2⊥NT,* distance of vertical reference plane to nose tip; *RP2⊥Pog,* distance of vertical reference plane to pogonion; *RPE,* rapid palatal expansion; *SD,* standard deviation; *SN,* sella-nasion; *SN-PP,* sella-nasion palatal plane; *SN-UOP,* sella-nasion upper occlusal plane; *SNA,* sella-nasion A point; *SNB,* sella-nasion B point; *UI-SN,* upper incisors sella-nasion.

*p <0.05.

**p <0.01.

Similar to the findings of previous studies, upper incisors were proclined in our study. However, this effect was due to two factors: the counterclockwise rotation of the upper occlusal plane due to force vector and the use of a tooth-borne device (acrylic cap splint). Interestingly, lower incisors were also proclined, which was reported in the study of De Clerck et al.[43] It has been well documented that facemask treatment results in retroclination of lower incisors.[6,44,48,49] Lower incisor proclination in this new protocol could be due to the new posture of the tongue acting on the lower incisors following the correction of anterior crossbite, similarly reported by De Clerck et al.[43]

Conclusion for Study III

Changes in skeletal and dental structures following protraction with this method were significant. The treatment results were fast and effective. This treatment protocol can be a treatment alternative for subjects with Class III malocclusion characterized by maxillary retrognathism and normal mandible with normal or low angle pattern of growth.

THE FUTURE OF CLASS III MALOCCLUSION TREATMENT

In the future, our focus should be finding ways to decrease the amount of surgery performed while also finding ways to increase patient comfort by simplifying the intraoral appliance. To achieve these goals we must use mini-screws and minimize the use of mini-plates, which require added surgical procedures. We hope that new screw designs will be developed that can withstand the high orthopedic forces needed for maxillary protraction. Meanwhile, we work on finding optimum forces for different ages and force vectors to carry maxilla forward without undesired rotations (see Case Report 3).

Text continued on p. 358

CASE REPORT 1

Le Fort I Osteotomy and Facemask Therapy

An 11-year-old female patient with Class III malocclusion characterized by maxillary retrognathia was treated by corticotomy-assisted facemask therapy (Fig. 17-7). According to cephalometric analysis, she had a normal vertical growth pattern and moderate skeletal Class III malocclusion characterized by maxillary retrognathism (Fig. 17-8 and Table 17-4). Upper incisors were proclined and

CASE REPORT 1—cont'd

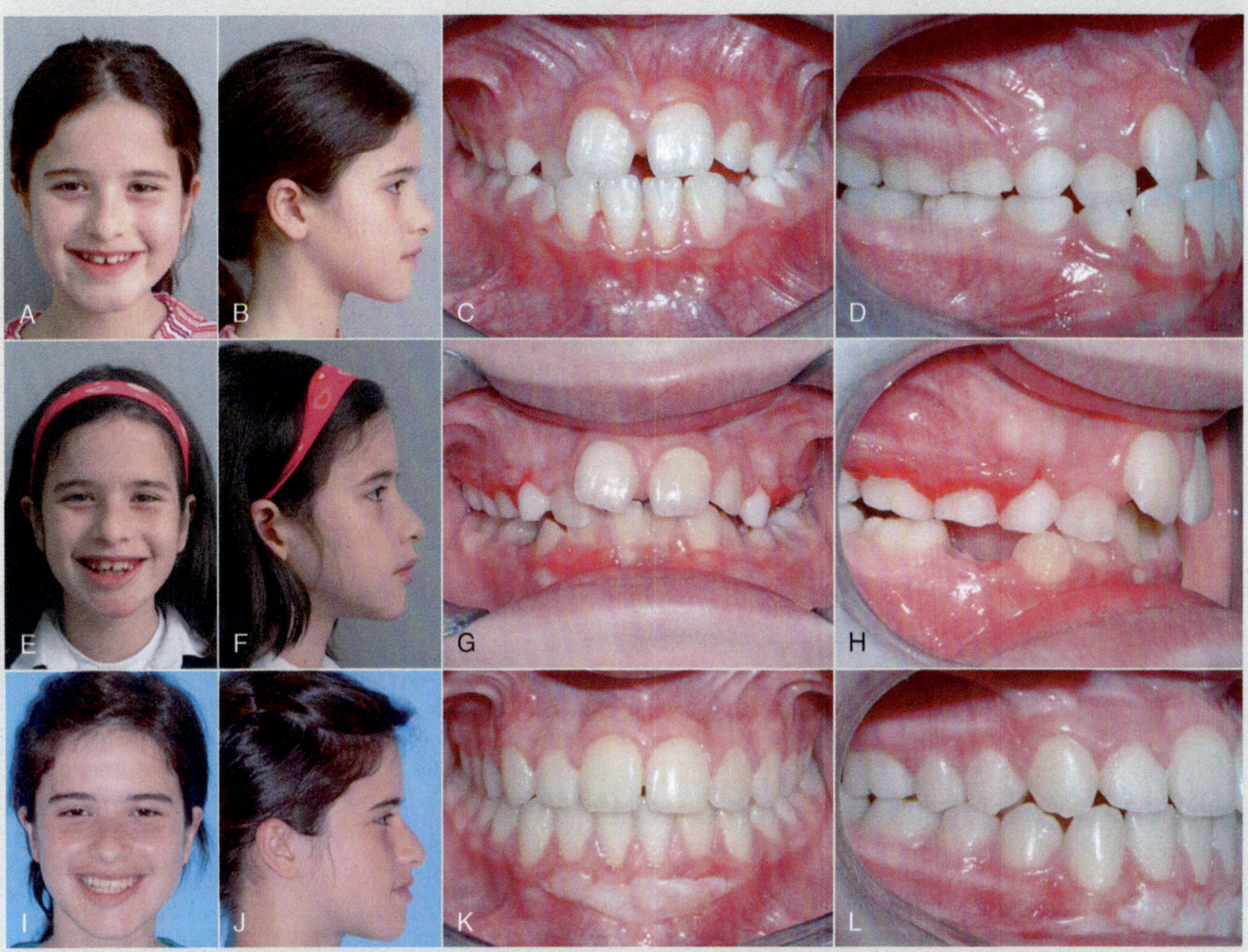

Figure 17-7 **A–D,** Initial photographs of the patient treated by corticotomy-assisted maxillary protraction. **E–H,** After protraction. **I–L,** After fixed orthodontic treatment.

TABLE 17-4 Cephalometric Measurements of Patient in Case Report 1 Before Treatment, After Protraction, After Fixed Treatment, and at Follow-Up

Evaluation	Initial	Postprotraction	Final	Recall
Σ (°)	397	399	398	397
GoMe-SN (°)	39	39	39	39
Maxillary height (°)	62	60	62	62
SNA (°)	78	82	82	82
SNB (°)	80	80	81	82.5
ANB (°)	−2	2	1	−0.5
RP2⊥A (mm)	65	69	69	70
ACB/corpus	69/67	69/67	69/70	69.5/72
I-SN (°)	110	106	110	113
IMPA (°)	83	80	87	79

Σ, Sum of inner (saddle + articulare + gonial) angles; *ACB/corpus,* ratio of anterior cranial base to corpus; *ANB,* A point nasion B point; *GoMe-SN,* gonion-menton (mandibular plane) to sella-nasion; *I-SN,* upper incisors sella-nasion; *IMPA,* incisor mandibular plane angle; *RP2⊥A,* distance of vertical reference plane to A point; *SNA,* sella-nasion A point; *SNB,* sella-nasion B point.

Continued

CASE REPORT 1—cont'd

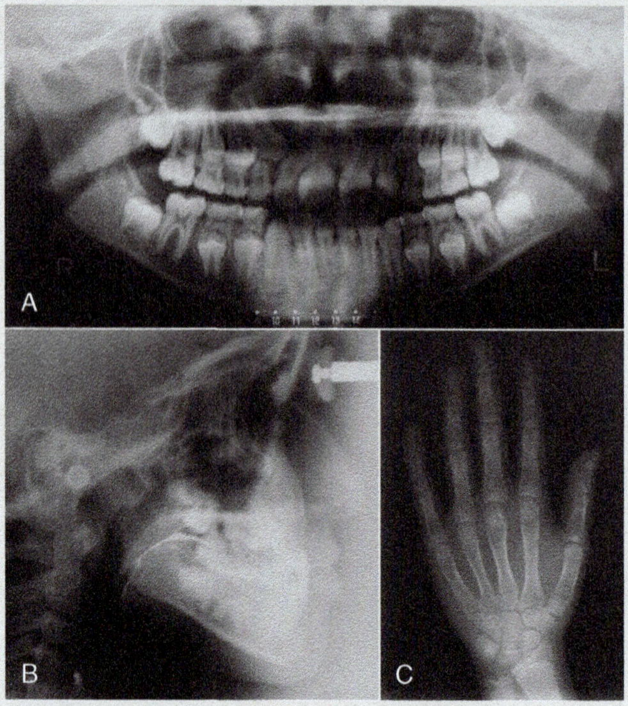

Figure 17-8 Initial radiographs (**A-C**) of the patient.

lower incisors were retroclined. Two treatment options were discussed with the patient and her parents. The first option was to apply the conventional facemask therapy, which required long-term compliance. The second option was surgery-assisted facemask therapy by which the effect of the appliance could be achieved more rapidly. The patient and parents chose the second option.

Preparation of Intraoral Appliance

Wire framework from 1.1-mm stainless steel wire was bent on the upper plaster model. The wire was adapted to the palatal surfaces of all upper teeth, bent buccally from the distal surface of the last molar, and adapted to the buccal surfaces of the teeth until the canine. At the canine level, two ends of the wire were shaped as hooks to permit attachment of elastics on the facemask. The palatal component of the metal framework was sandblasted and covered with acrylic. The intraoral device was bonded with glass ionomer cement on the day before surgery.

Surgical Procedure and Facemask Application

Under general anesthesia, a plastic surgeon performed an incomplete Le Fort I osteotomy on the patient. The osteotomy involved the lateral walls of the maxilla, starting from the apertura piriformis and extending to the tuberosity, without separation of the pterygomaxillary suture. The facemask was applied on the fifth day following surgery with 1000 g of force per side. The patient was instructed to wear the facemask 24 hours per day, except during meals, and was recalled on the tenth day following application of the facemask. It was observed that crossbite had been eliminated and the overjet had increased from −1-mm to +4-mm. Seven weeks later, Class II canine and molar relationships were achieved and overjet increased to 6-mm. Facemask wear was decreased to 14 hours per day with a force value of 700 g per side (Fig. 17-9). The patient continued to wear the facemask only at nighttime for 3 retention months. Following removal of the appliance, the treatment continued with the fixed appliances (see Fig. 17-7, E-H). Total treatment time was 5 months for protraction and 2.5 years for fixed treatment (see Fig. 17-7, I-L). Three years after completion of the fixed treatment, the patient was recalled and all records were renewed (Fig. 17-10). Despite minor relapse of the Class III correction during retention, the overall treatment result was satisfactory to both the clinician and the patient.

At the end of the protraction period a Class II dental relationship was achieved, anterior crossbite was eliminated, and profile was improved. SNA angle increased from 78 to 82 degrees and maxillary depth angle increased from 90 to 95.5 degrees. Upper and lower incisors were retroclined 4 and 3 degrees, respectively. At the end of the fixed treatment, the maxillary advancement achieved was maintained while the mandible continued to grow. In the long-term, the attained maxillary advancement was stable for this patient while growth of the mandible continued (see Table 17-4). Superimposition of all cephalometric radiographs is presented in Figure 17-11.

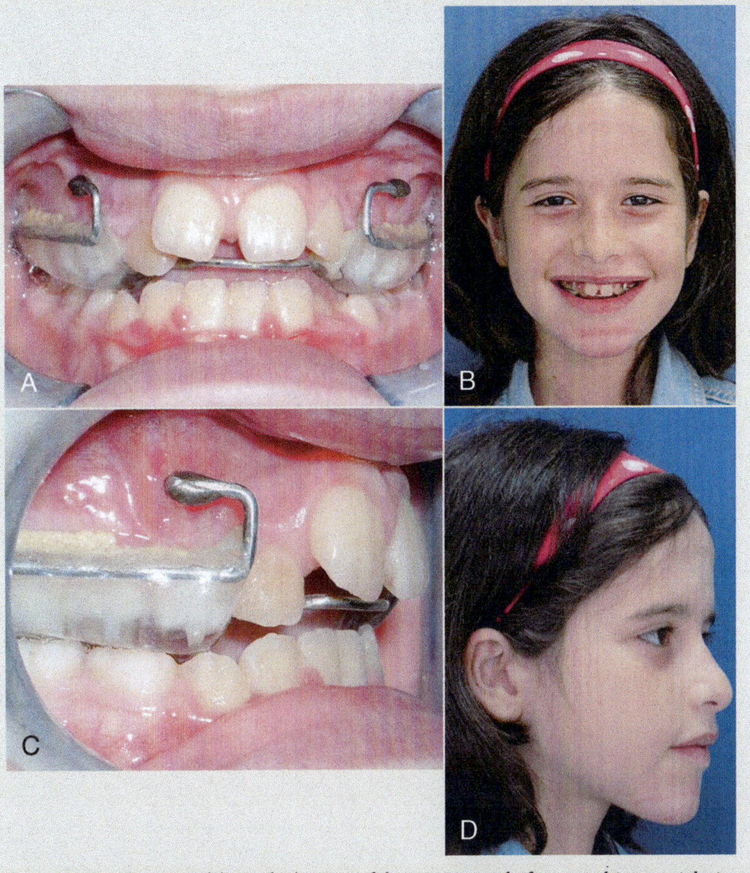

Figure 17-9 Intraoral (**A and C**) and extraoral (**B and D**) views of the patient just before switching to nighttime wear of the facemask.

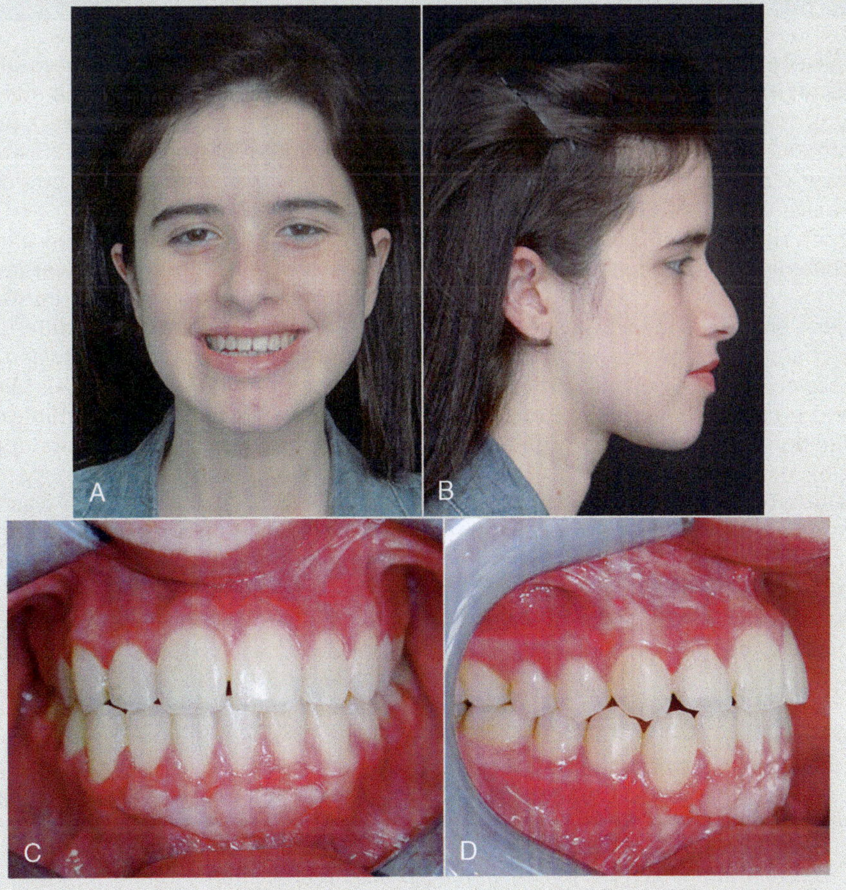

Figure 17-10 Extraoral (**A and B**) and intraoral (**C and D**) photographs taken 3 years after treatment with fixed orthodontic appliance (recall records).

Continued

CASE REPORT 1—cont'd

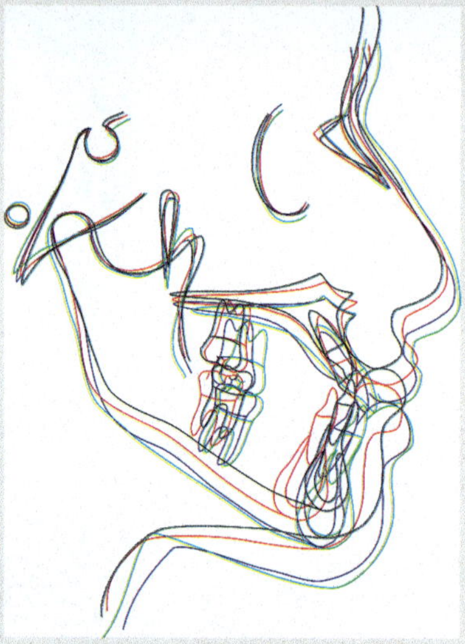

Figure 17-11 Superimposition of the cephalometric radiographs taken at preprotraction, postprotraction, final, and recall periods.

CASE REPORT 2

Corticotomy, Skeletal Anchorage, and Class III Elastics

A 13-year-old boy presented with chief complaints of mandibular prominence, an unaesthetic smile, and upper and lower crowding. He had a straight profile with a retrusive upper lip, Class III molar relationships on both right and left posterior sides, 2-mm overbite, and 2-mm negative overjet (Fig. 17-12).

The cephalometric analysis showed Class III skeletal problems characterized by retrognathic maxilla, concave skeletal profile, normal vertical growth pattern, and proclined upper and retroclined lower incisor inclinations. The soft tissue profile was straight (Table 17-5).

The skeletal deformity of this patient was too severe to be treated by dentoalveolar compensation alone. Therefore growth modification using a facemask was planned for the treatment but the patient refused to use an extraoral device. It was then decided to protract the maxilla using intraoral mechanics.

Treatment Protocol

The maxillary device was an acrylic splint made of of 1.1-mm stainless steel wire, which was adjusted to the palatal surfaces of the upper teeth and bent toward the distobuccal surfaces of the upper first molars to form a hook for the attachment of elastics. After adjustment the framework was covered with acrylic material from the canines to the last molars. The splint was then bonded one day before the surgery (Fig. 17-13).

The surgery was performed under general anesthesia starting in the lower jaw. Two mini-plates (Multipurpose Implant, Tasarimmed, Istanbul, Turkey) were placed on the anterior wall of the symphysis on both sides between the canines and the first premolars (Fig. 17-14). Mini-screws (2-mm × 7-mm) were used to fix the mini-plates (Fig. 17-15). Then surgery continued on the upper jaw to perform incomplete Le Fort I corticotomy to release the maxilla. A horizontal incision was made through the mucoperiosteum above the mucogingival junction in the depth of the buccal vestibular fold, extending from the canine region to the first molars area. Nasal mucosa was elevated gently from the lateral nasal wall. A horizontal low-level osteotomy was made through the lateral wall of the maxilla 5-mm superior to the apices of the anterior and posterior teeth, first with tiny rounded burrs and then with a microsaw. The corticotomy line was extended from the inferolateral aspect of the piriform rim posteriorly to the inferior aspect of the junction of

CASE REPORT 2—cont'd

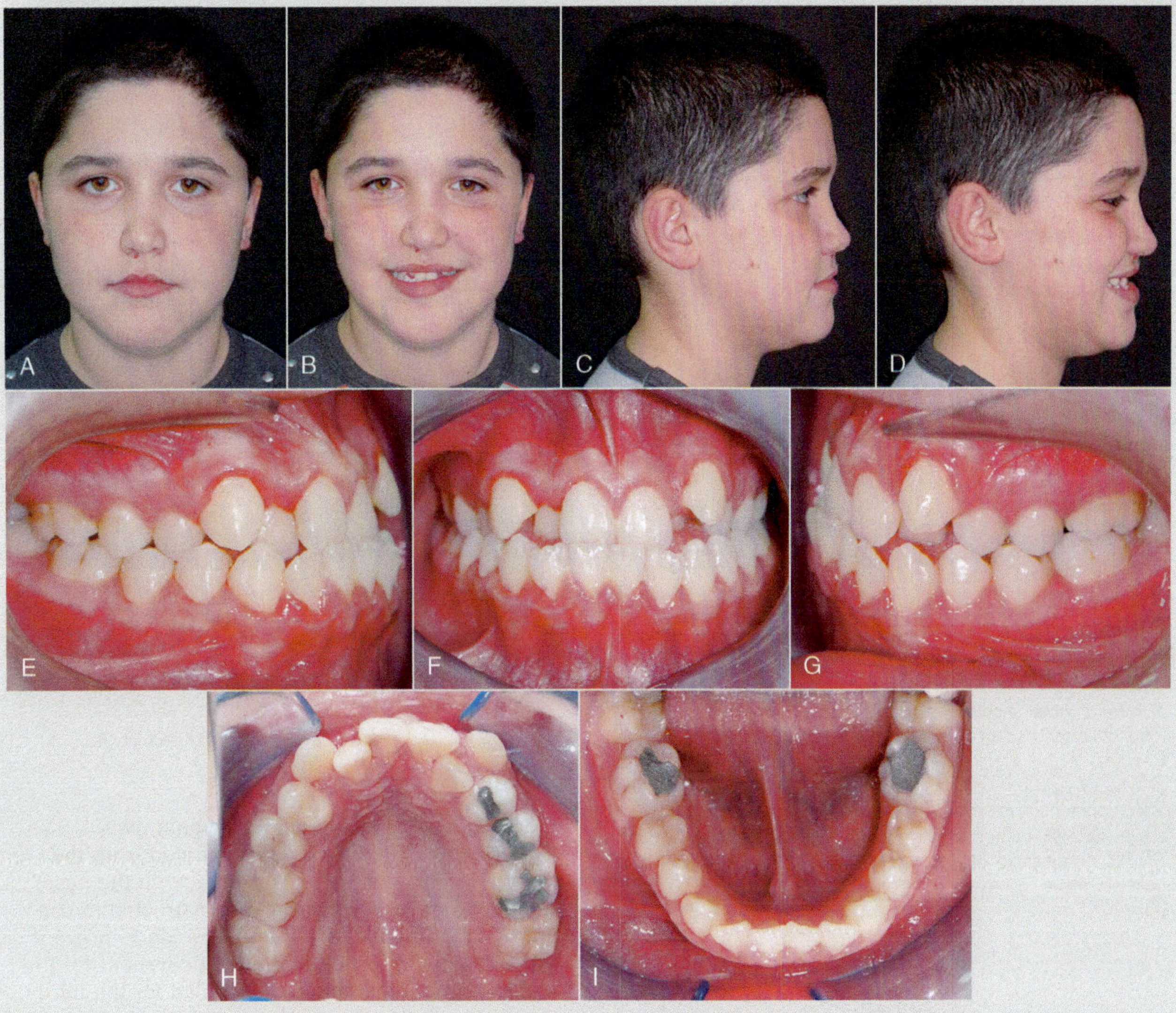

Figure 17-12 Initial extraoral (**A-D**) and intraoral (**E-I**) photographs of the patient.

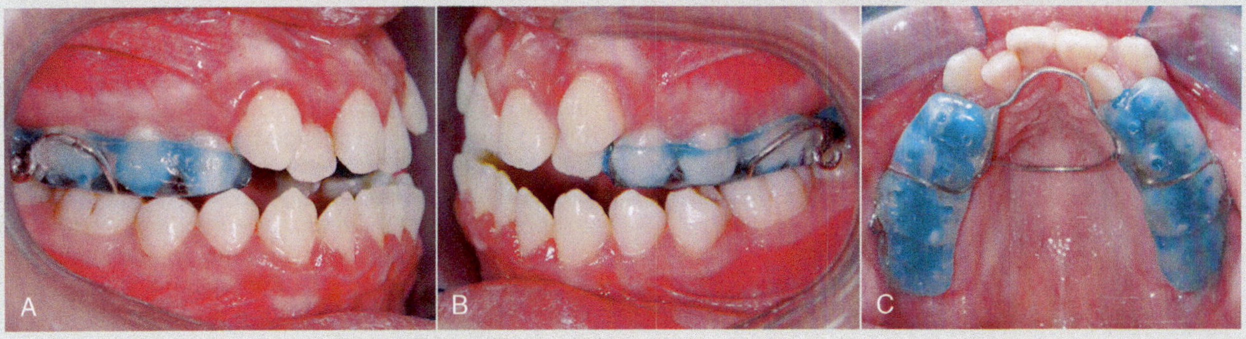

Figure 17-13 **A-C,** Upper acrylic splint.

Continued

CASE REPORT 2—cont'd

TABLE 17-5 Cephalometric Measurements of Patient in Case Report 2 Before Protraction, After Protraction, and After Fixed Treatment

Evaluation	Initial	Postprotraction	Final
Σ (degree)	398	399.5	400
GoMe-SN (degree)	36	38	39
Maxillary height (degree)	59	55.5	58
FMA (degree)	30	31.5	32
SNA (degree)	78	82	82
SNB (degree)	81	80.5	79.5
ANB (degree)	−3	1.5	2.5
RP2⊥A (mm)	70	75	75.5
Maxillary depth (degree)	85	88.5	88
ACB/corpus	75/82	75/83	75/85
SN-PP (degree)	8	7.5	9
SN-UOP (degree)	19	12	15
I-SN (degree)	105	109.5	105
IMPA (degree)	84	88	85
Holdaway	6/1	7.5/1	7.5/2
Nasolabial angle (degree)	103	97.5	98

Σ, Sum of inner (saddle + articulare + gonial) angles; *ACB/corpus,* ratio of anterior cranial base to corpus; *ANB,* A point nasion B point; *FMA,* Frankfort horizontal plane mandibular plane; *GoMe-SN,* gonion-menton (mandibular plane) to sella-nasion; *I-SN,* upper incisors sella-nasion; *IMPA,* incisor mandibular plane angle; *RP2⊥A,* distance of vertical reference plane to A point; *SN-PP,* sella-nasion palatal plane; *SN-UOP,* sella-nasion upper occlusal plane; *SNA,* sella-nasion A point; *SNB,* sella-nasion B point.

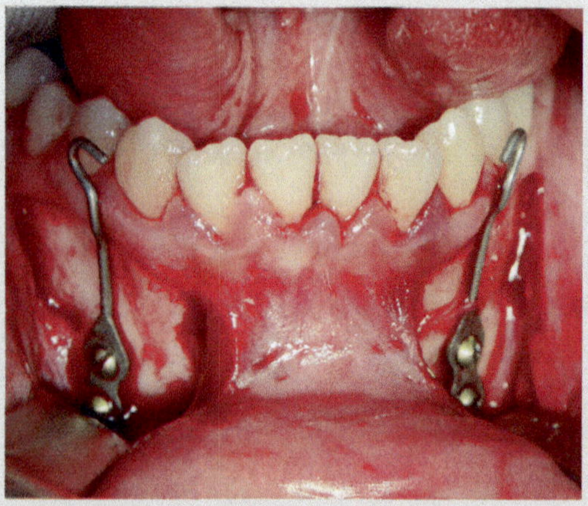

Figure 17-14 Mini-plates placed on the anterior wall of the symphysis.

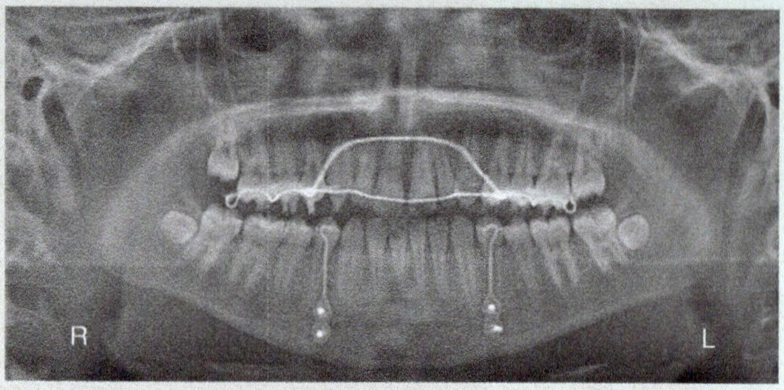

Figure 17-15 Orientation of the mini-plates.

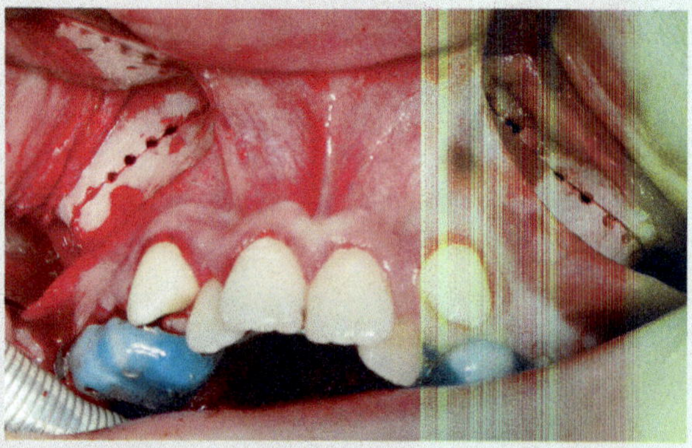

Figure 17-16 Incomplete Le Fort I osteotomy line.

the maxillary tuberosity and pterygoid plate (Fig. 17-16). The maxilla was separated from the pterygoid plate with an osteotome, with the nasal walls left intact. The patient was instructed to use antibiotics, analgesics, and mouthwash to prevent postoperative infection and an appointment for the application of elastics was scheduled for the third day after surgery.

The elastics were attached between maxillary hooks and the mandibular mini-plates with an initial force of 300 g per side; the force was then increased to 600 g per side at the end of the tenth day after surgery (Fig. 17-17). Total force was almost similar with previous facemask studies. The patient was instructed to use Class III elastics full-time, except during meals, and to change the elastics twice per day. He was monitored every 2 weeks until Class II dental relationships were achieved. The splint was debonded after 2.5 months when 2.5-mm positive overjet and Class II canine and molar relationships were obtained (Fig. 17-18). Bite opening was observed during the protraction protocol due to the vertical component of the applied force vector (Fig. 17-19). Because there was no space for upper

CASE REPORT 2—cont'd

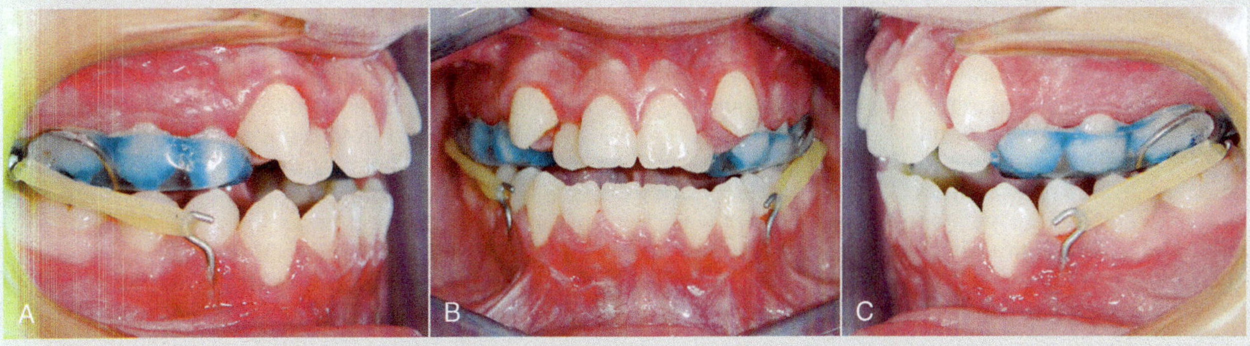

Figure 17-17 Force application (**A-C**) between the upper splint and lower mini-plates.

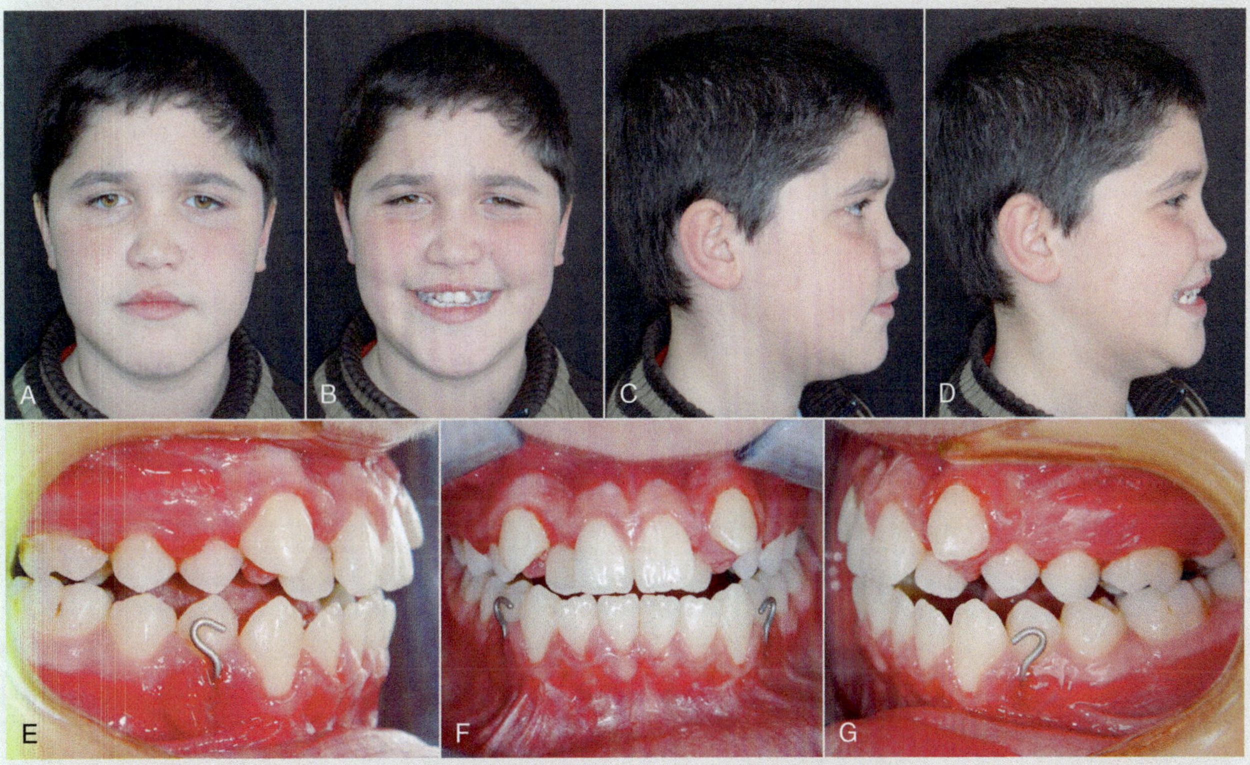

Figure 17-18 Extraoral (**A-D**) and intraoral (**E-G**) photographs taken after maxillary protraction and removal of the upper splint (Class II molar and canine relationships).

Continued

CASE REPORT 2—cont'd

canines and the crowding was too much to resolve without extraction, upper first premolars were extracted (Fig. 17-20). Before lower brackets were placed, the mini-plates were removed under local anesthesia without any problems.

Class I canine relationship with normal overbite and overjet was achieved. Brackets were debonded and lingual retainers were bonded for both arches (Fig. 17-21). The entire treatment time was 24 months.

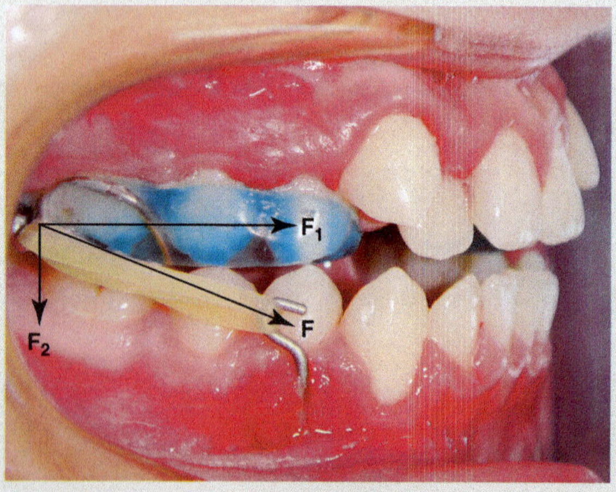

Figure 17-19 Horizontal (F_1) and vertical (F_2) force vectors of the Class III elastics.

Treatment Outcome

Clinically, a significant amount of maxillary protraction and midfacial advancement were achieved. Changes in the dentofacial structures were determined through the evaluation of cephalometric radiographs that were taken just before the surgery, after protraction, and at the end of fixed orthodontic treatment (Fig. 17-22). At the end of 2.5 months of protraction, maxilla was displaced 5-mm anteriorly with a 4-degree increase in SNA angle and a 3.5-degree increase in maxillary depth angles while SNB angle decreased by 0.5 degree. These changes resulted in a 4.5-degree decrease in ANB angle, thereby resulting in a skeletal Class I relationship. Upper occlusal plane angle decreased 7 degrees due to counterclockwise rotation. These changes improved the soft tissue profile and led to a 5.5-degree decrease in nasolabial angle (Fig. 17-23; see Table 17-5). During protraction, upper and lower incisors proclined by 4.5 and 4 degrees, respectively, but they corrected spontaneously after the removal of the acrylic cap appliance. The overbite also decreased during protraction due to the counterclockwise rotation of palatal and occlusal planes.

After the treatment of a few cases, this method was found to be effective and reliable. Based on the initial successful results with this protocol, we decided to evaluate the effectiveness of this treatment philosophy prospectively.

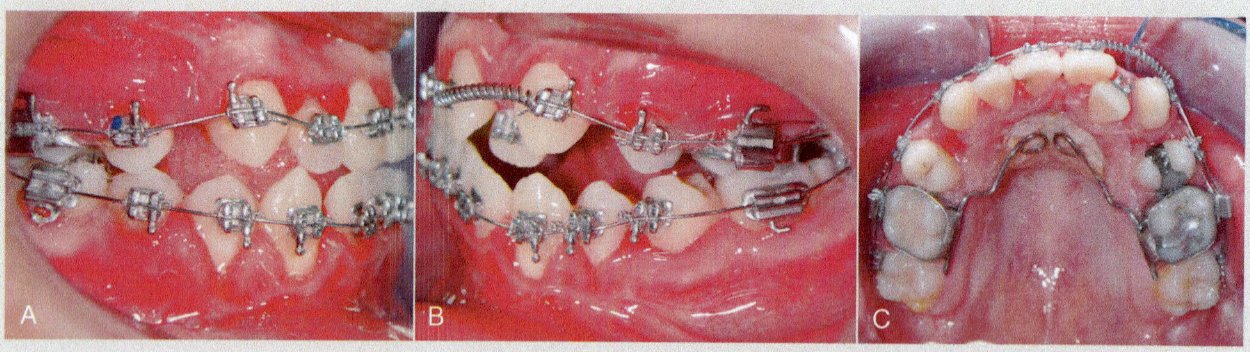

Figure 17-20 **A-C,** Fixed treatment after extraction of upper first premolars.

CASE REPORT 2—cont'd

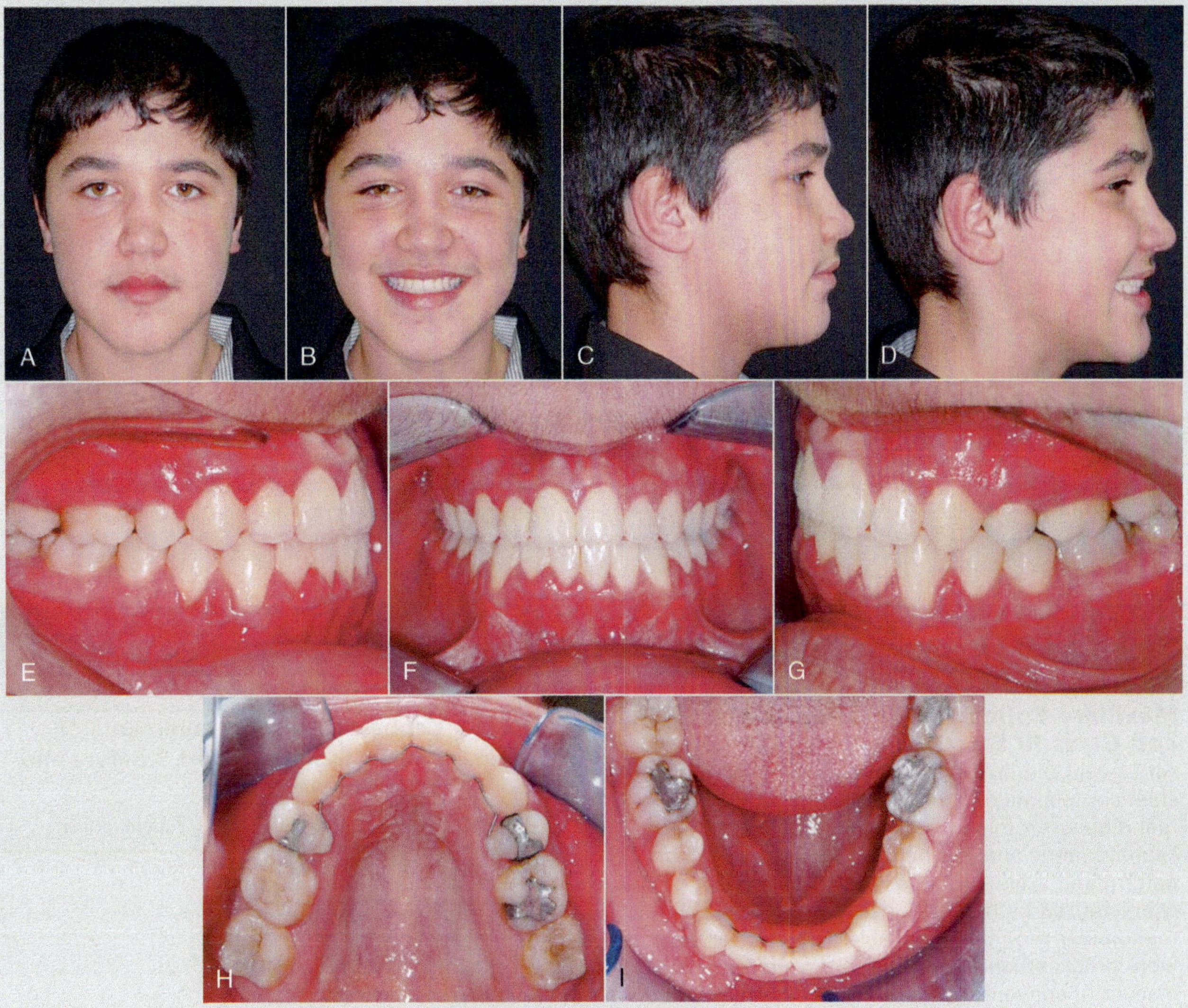

Figure 17-21 Final (**A–D**) extraoral and (**E–I**) intraoral photographs.

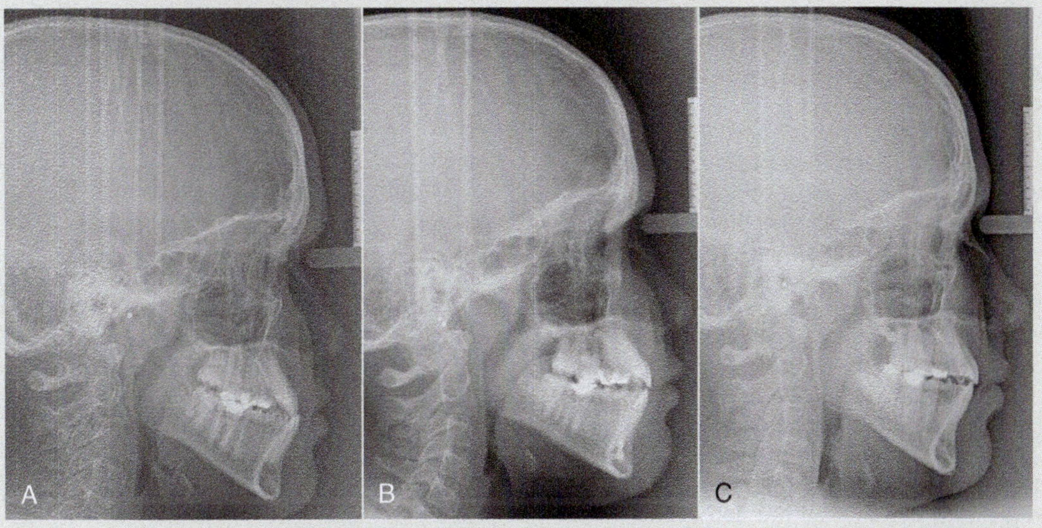

Figure 17-22 Cephalometric radiographs (**A**) before protraction, (**B**) after protraction, and (**C**) after fixed orthodontic treatment.

Continued

CASE REPORT 2—cont'd

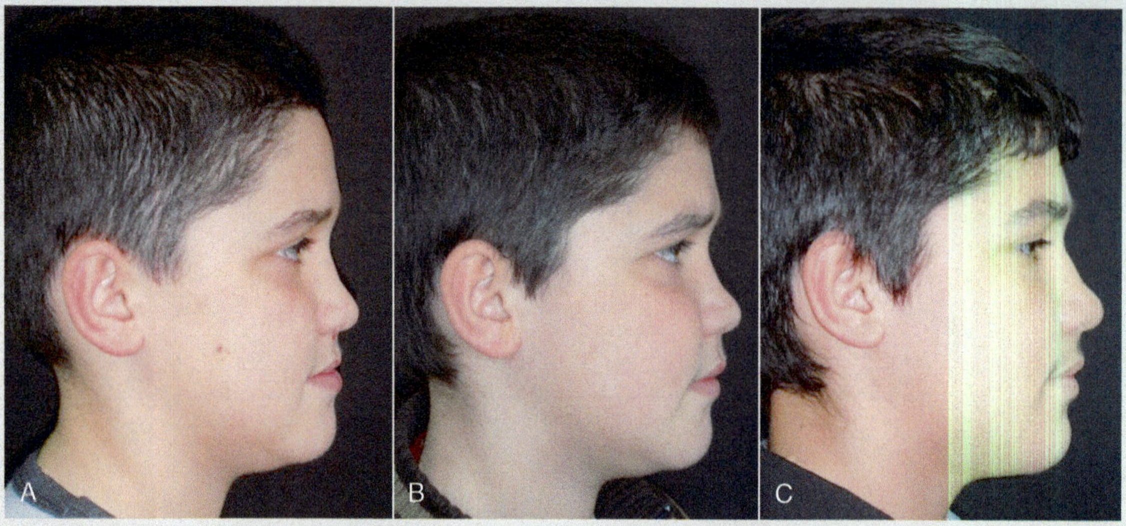

Figure 17-23 Profile comparison of the patient (**A**) before protraction, (**B**) after protraction, and (**C**) after fixed orthodontic treatment.

CASE REPORT 3

Maxillary Splint, Mini-Screws in Mandible, and Class III Elastics

An 11-year-old boy reported to the clinic with the chief complaints of anterior crossbite and mandibular prominence (Fig. 17-24). According to cephalometric analysis he had low vertical growth pattern and skeletal Class III malocclusion characterized by maxillary retrognathism and slight mandibular prognathism (Table 17-6). Upper incisors were proclined and lower incisors were retroclined. Instead of conventional facemask application, the decision was made to apply Class III elastics between the maxillary acrylic splint and the mini-screws inserted in the lower anterior region. The patient approved highly of this decision.

Preparation of Intraoral Appliance and Progress

An acrylic-cap Hyrax device was prepared for the upper dentition and hooks were placed buccally inside the acrylic on the level of upper first premolars in order to attach Class III elastics. After bonding the upper splint, two mini-screws (7-mm × 1.6-mm) were placed between the lower first premolars and the canines on both sides (Fig. 17-25). Afterward the patient was instructed to turn the screw twice a day for 10 days in order to achieve disarticulation of maxilla and to use Class III elastics between the upper hooks and lower mini-screws except during meals (Fig. 17-26). Elastics were changed once a day and the force value of the elastics was 110 g per side. At the end of the tenth

TABLE 17-6 Cephalometric Measurements of Patient in Case Report 3 Before and After Protraction

Evaluation	Initial	Postprotraction
Σ (degree)	380.7	380.7
GoMe-SN (degree)	25	25
Maxillary height (degree)	61	57
FMA (degree)	21	21
SNA (degree)	80	83
SNB (degree)	85	84
ANB (degree)	−5	−1
N⊥A (mm)	−6	−3
Maxillary depth (degree)	83	86
ACB/corpus	72/83	72/85
SN-PP (degree)	6	6
SN-UOP (degree)	13	6
I-SN (degree)	110	115
IMPA (degree)	78	82
Holdaway	2.8/0	4.7/0
Nasolabial angle (degree)	111	102

Σ, Sum of inner (saddle + articulare + gonial) angles; *ACB/corpus,* ratio of anterior cranial base to corpus; *ANB,* A point nasion B point; *FMA,* Frankfort horizontal plane mandibular plane; *GoMe-SN,* gonion-menton (mandibular plane) to sella-nasion; *I-SN,* upper incisor sella-nasion; *IMPA,* incisor mandibular plane angle; *N⊥A,* distance of A point to a line drawn from nasion perpendicular to Frankfort horizontal plane; *SN-PP,* sella-nasion palatal plane; *SN-UOP,* sella-nasion upper occlusal plane; *SNA,* sella-nasion A point; *SNB,* sella-nasion B point.

CASE REPORT 3—cont'd

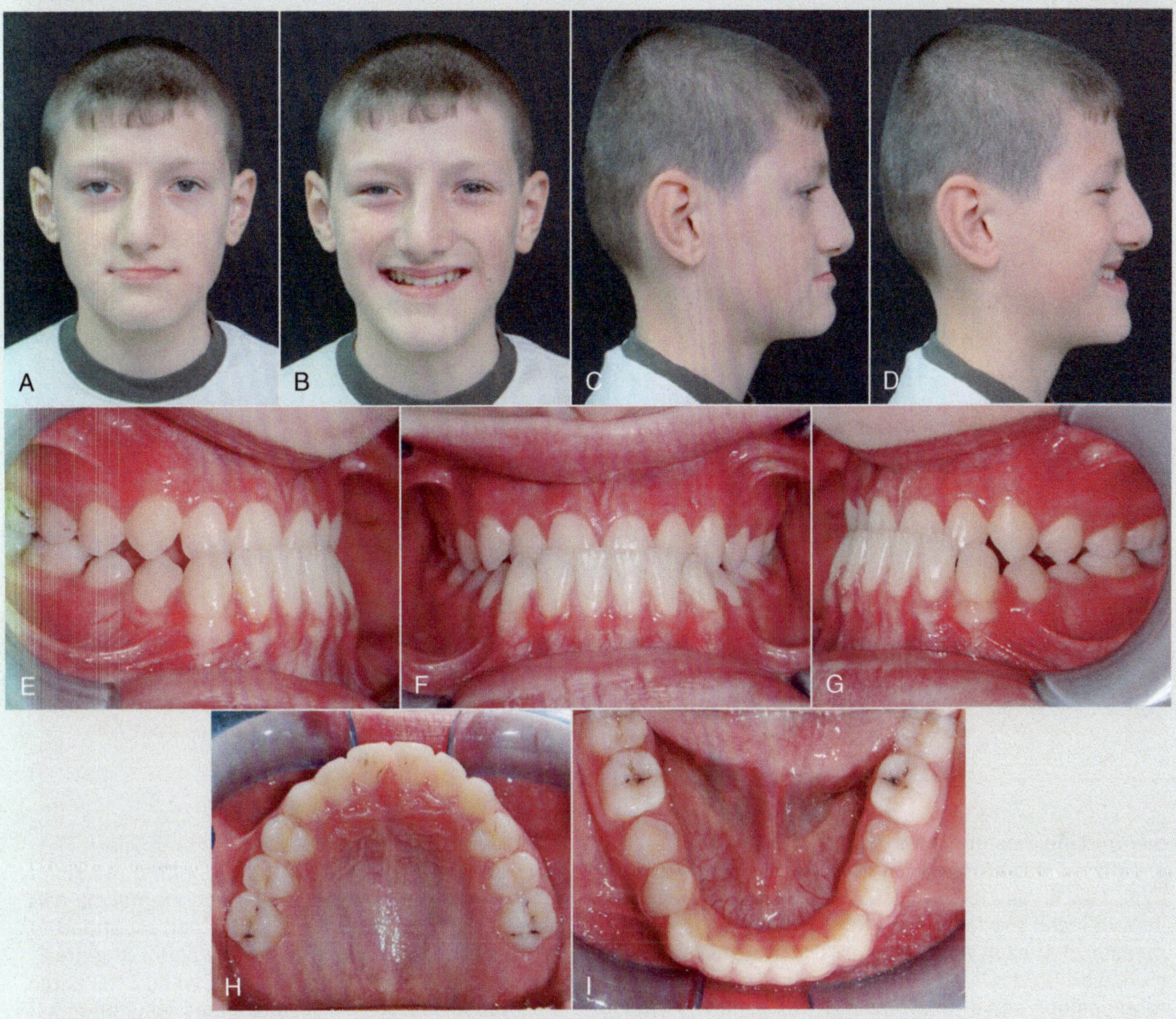

Figure 17-24 Initial **(A–D)** extraoral and **(E–I)** intraoral views of the patient.

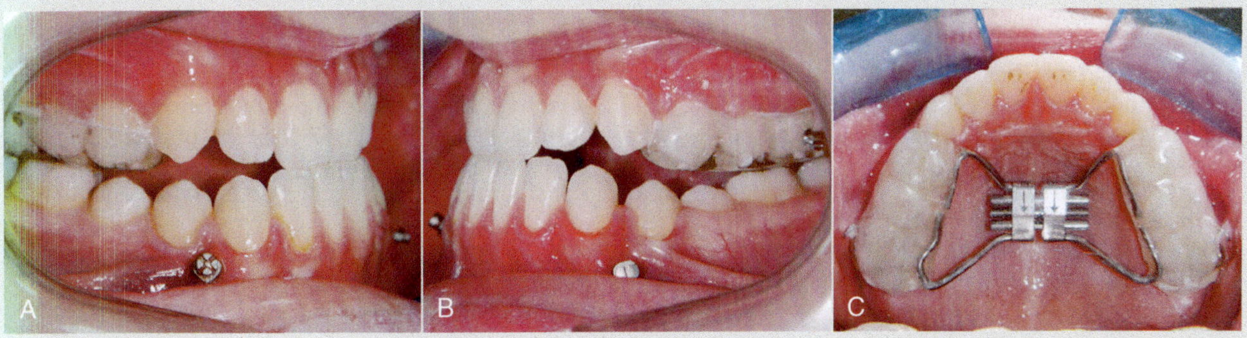

Figure 17-25 Intraoral **(A-C)** views of the appliance showing the position of the mini-screws.

Continued

CASE REPORT 3—cont'd

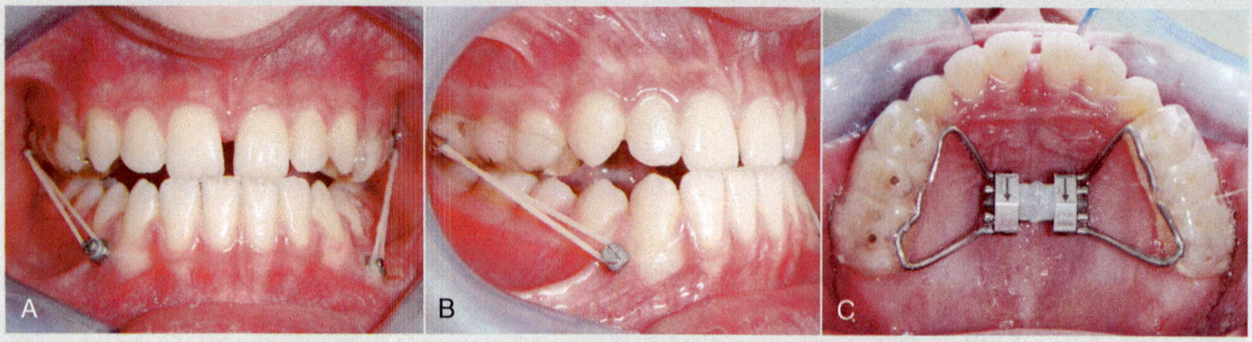

Figure 17-26 A-C, Force application between upper hooks and lower mini-screws following the appearance of midline diastema.

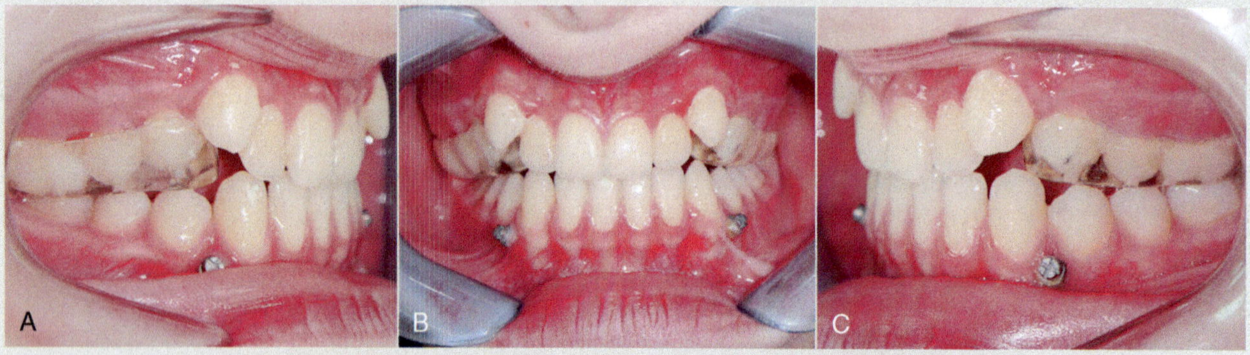

Figure 17-27 A-C, After protraction, just before removal of the upper splint.

day midline diastema was seen and maxillary expansion was stopped but the patient continued to use Class III elastics. He was monitored at 4 week intervals and the force value of the elastics was measured at each appointment. The force value was increased gradually to 200 g per side. Class II canine relationships and 1.5-mm overjet was achieved after 8 months. Proclination of upper incisors together with mesialization of posterior dentition, which led to a constriction of the upper canine area, were recorded at the end of the elastic wear (Fig. 17-27). Straight-wire brackets were bonded on the upper arch following debonding of the upper splint and the treatment continued with straight-wire mechanics (Fig. 17-28).

Treatment Results

Changes in the dentofacial structures were determined through evaluation of cephalometric radiographs, which were taken just before the acrylic splint cementation and after maxillary protraction immediately after debonding the splint. At the end of 8 months of protraction, maxilla was displaced 3-mm anteriorly, which corresponded to a 3-degree increase in SNA angle and a 3-degree increase in maxillary depth angle while SNB angle decreased 1 degree. These changes resulted in a 4-degree decrease in ANB angle. A 7-degree counterclockwise rotation of the maxillary occlusal plane angle was seen. Superimposition of the pretreatment and postprotraction cephalograms (Fig. 17-29) showed that the upper dental arch moved forward, which resulted in a more protrusive upper lip, and the nose tip moved upward as in surgical cases (see Table 17-6). All of these changes decreased the concavity of the patient's profile. Considering that the technique is simple and less invasive, this method seems to be promising but we need to document the treatment effects on a larger group.

CASE REPORT 3—cont'd

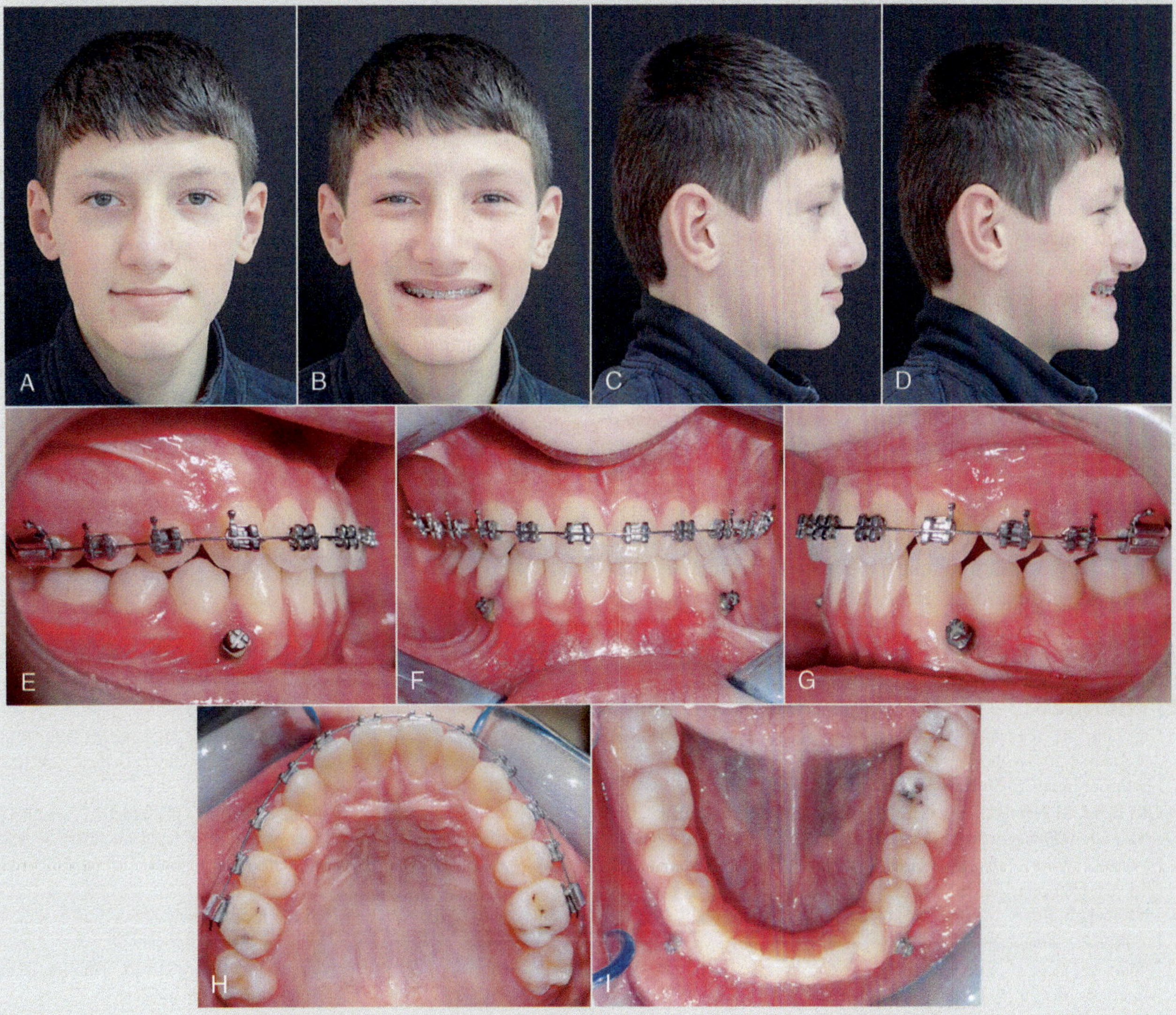

Figure 17-28 (A–D) Extraoral and (E–I) intraoral views of fixed treatment in progress.

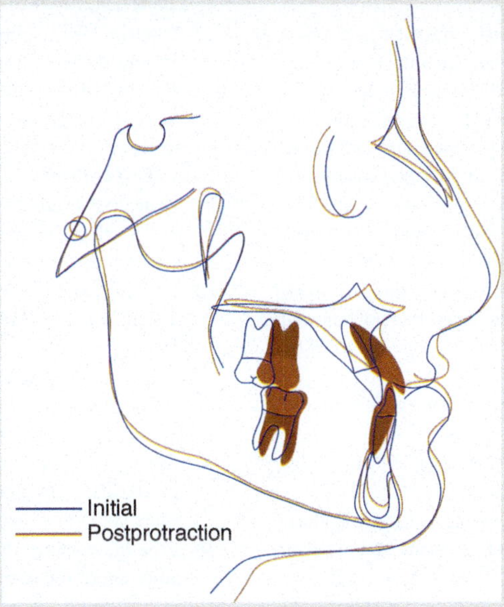

Figure 17-29 Superimposition of the cephalometric radiographs taken before and after maxillary protraction.

SUMMARY

In the light of all research discussed in this chapter, we can formulate basic guidelines for the method and timing of Class III treatment in particular cases. In mild Class III cases diagnosed before age 10 years, conventional maxillary protraction protocol (RPE plus facemask) seems to be sufficient. In such mild cases after age 10 years until the completion of growth, orthopedic protraction via skeletal anchorage (maxillary mini-plates plus facemask or Class III elastics between upper and lower mini-plates) can be selected considering that the maxillary sutures become highly interdigitated with increasing age. However, we should keep in mind that both protocols need good patient cooperation for about 1 year or more. In more severe cases when it is too late for orthopedic protraction but too early for orthognathic surgery, corticotomy-assisted protraction protocol, with either facemask or Class III elastics, can be selected as fast and effective options. Clinicians should be careful when selecting the appropriate protocol for each particular case. It is necessary to monitor the long-term results of all treatment approaches mentioned above and to make necessary changes in the protocols regarding both patient selection and mode of intervention.

REFERENCES

1. Heymann GC. *Temporary Anchorage Devices for Maxillary Protraction: 3D Analysis of Treatment Outcomes* [master's thesis]. (Chapel Hill/North Carolina/US) University of North Carolina, 2008.
2. Ellis E 3rd, McNamara JA Jr. Components of adult Class III malocclusion. *J Oral Maxillofac Surg*. 1984;42(5):295–305.
3. Guyer EC, Ellis EE 3rd, McNamara JA Jr, Behrents RG. Components of class III malocclusion in juveniles and adolescents. *Angle Orthod*. 1986;56(1):7–30.
4. Proffit WR. *Contemporary Orthodontics*. 3rd ed. St Louis, MO: Mosby; 2000.
5. Baccetti T, McGill JS, Franchi L, McNamara JA Jr, Tollaro I. Skeletal effects of early treatment of Class III malocclusion with maxillary expansion and face-mask therapy. *Am J Orthod Dentofacial Orthop*. 1998;113:333–343.
6. Kapust A, Sinclair M, Turley P. Cephalometric effects of face mask/expansion therapy in Class III children: a comparison of three age groups. *Am J Orthod Dentofacial Orthop*. 1998;113(2):204–212.
7. Saadia M, Torres E. Sagittal changes after maxillary protraction with expansion in class III patients in the primary, mixed, and late mixed dentitions: a longitudinal retrospective study. *Am J Orthod Dentofacial Orthop*. 2000;117(6):669–680.
8. Ochoa BK, Nanda RS. Comparison of maxillary and mandibular growth. *Am J Orthod Dentofacial Orthop*. 2004;125(2):148–159.
9. Franchi L, Baccetti T, McNamara JA. Postpubertal assessment of treatment timing for maxillary expansion and protraction therapy followed by fixed appliances. *Am J Orthod Dentofacial Orthop*. 2004;126(5):555–568.
10. Baik HS. Clinical results of the maxillary protraction in Korean children. *Am J Orthod Dentofacial Orthop*. 1995;108(6):583–592.
11. Sung SJ, Baik HS. Assesment of skeletal and dental changes by maxillary protraction. *Am J Orthod Dentofacial Orthop*. 1998;114(5):492–502.
12. Merwin D, Ngan P, Hagg U, Yiu C, Wei SH. Timing for effective application of anteriorly directed orthopedic force to the maxilla. *Am J Orthod Dentofacial Orthop*. 1997;112(3):292–299.
13. Toffol LD, Pavoni C, Baccetti T, Franchi L, Cozza P. Orthopedic treatment outcomes in Class III malocclusion: a systematic review. *Angle Orthod*. 2008;78(3):561–573.
14. Itoh T, Chaconas SJ, Caputo AA, Matyas J. Photoelastic effects of maxillary protraction on the craniofacial complex. *Am J Orthod*. 1985;88(2):117–124.
15. Tanne K, Hiraga J, Kakiuchi K, Yamaqata Y, Sakuda M. Biomechanical effect of anteriorly directed extraoral forces on the craniofacial complex: a study using the finite element method. *Am J Orthod Dentofacial Orthop*. 1989;95(3):200–207.
16. Lee KG, Ryu YK, Park YC, Rudolph DJ. A study of holographic interferometry on the initial reaction of maxillofacial complex during protraction. *Am J Orthod Dentofacial Orthop*. 1997;111(6):623–632.
17. Tortop T, Keykubat A, Yuksel S. Facemask therapy with and without expansion. *Am J Orthod Dentofacial Orthop*. 2007;132(4):467–474.
18. Ngan P, Cheung E, Wei SHY. Comparison of protraction facemask response using banded and bonded expansion appliances as anchorage. *Semin Orthod*. 2007;13:175–185.
19. Vaughn GA, Mason B, Moon HB, Turley PK. The effects of maxillary protraction therapy with or without rapid palatal expansion: a prospective, randomized clinical trial. *Am J Orthod Dentofacial Orthop*. 2005;128(3):299–309.
20. Nanda R. Protraction of maxilla in rhesus monkeys by controlled extraoral forces. *Am J Orthod*. 1978;74(2):121–141.
21. Nanda R. Biomechanical and clinical considerations of a modified protraction headgear. *Am J Orthod*. 1980;78(2):125–139.
22. Ngan PW, Hägg U, Yiu C, Wei SH. Treatment response and long-term dentofacial adaptations to maxillary expansion and protraction. *Semin Orthod*. 1997;3(4):255–264.
23. Cha KS. Skeletal changes of maxillary protraction in patients exhibiting skeletal Class III malocclusion: a comparison of three skeletal maturation groups. *Angle Orthod*. 2003;73(1):26–35.
24. Hägg U, Tse A, Bendeus M, Rabie AB. Long-term follow-up of early treatment with reverse headgear. *Eur J Orthod*. 2003;25(1):95–102.
25. Baccetti T, Franchi L, McNamara JA Jr. Cephalometric variables predicting the long-term success or failure of rapid maxillary expansion and facemask therapy. *Am J Orthod Dentofacial Orthop*. 2004;126(1):16–22.
26. Wells AP, Sarver DM, Proffit WR. Long-term efficacy of reverse pull headgear therapy. *Angle Orthod*. 2006;76(6):915–922.
27. Nanda RS, Kierl MJ. Prediction of cooperation in orthodontic treatment. *Am J Orthod Dentofacial Orthop*. 1992;102(1):15–21.
28. Brandao M, Pinho HS, Urias D. Clinical and quantitative assessment of headgear compliance: a pilot study. *Am J Orthod Dentofacial Orthop*. 2006;129(2):239–244.
29. Demellweek C, Humphris GM, Hare M, Brown J. Children's perception of, and attitude towards, unfamiliar peers with facial port-wine stains. *J Pediatr Psychol*. 1997;22(4):471–485.
30. Shaw WC, Meek SC, Jones DS. Nicknames, teasing, harassment and the salience of dental features among school children. *Br J Orthod*. 1980;7(2):75–80.
31. Kenealy P, Frude N, Shaw W. An evaluation of the psychological and social effects of malocclusion: some implications for dental policy making. *Soc Sci Med*. 1989;28(6):583–591.
32. Cheung LK, Chua HD. A meta-analysis of cleft maxillary osteotomy and distraction osteogenesis. *Int J Oral Maxillofac Surg*. 2005;35(1):14–24.
33. Bailey L, Cevidanes LH, Proffit WR. Stability and predictability of orthognathic surgery. *Am J Orthod Dentofacial Orthop*. 2004;126(3):273–277.
34. Cheung LK, Samman N, Hiu E, Tideman H. The 3-dimensional stability of maxillary osteotomies in cleft palate patients with residual alveolar clefts. *Br J Oral Maxillofac Surg*. 1994;32(1):6–12.
35. Erbe M, Stoelinga PJ, Leenen RJ. Long-term results of segmental repositioning of the maxilla in the cleft palate patients without previously

grafted alveolo-palatal clefts. *J Craniomaxillofac Surg.* 1996;24(2): 109–117.

36. da Motta AT, de Assis Ribeiro Carvalho F, Oliveira AE, Cevidanes LH, de Oliveira Almeida MA. Superimposition of 3D cone-beam CT models in orthognathic surgery. *Dental Press J Orthod.* 2010;15(2): 39–41.
37. Rachmiel A, Aizenbud D, Ardekian L, Peled M, Laufer D. Surgically-assisted orthopedic protraction of the maxilla in cleft lip and palate patients. *Int J Oral Maxillofac Surg.* 1999;28(1):9–14.
38. Molina F. Maxillary distraction osteogenesis. In: Samchukov ML, Cope JB, Cherkashin AM, eds. *Craniofacial Distraction Osteogenesis, Maxillary and Midface Distraction.* St. Louis, MO: Mosby; 2001: 494-500.
39. Singer SL, Henry PJ, Rosenberg I. Osseointegrated implants as an adjunct to facemask therapy: a case report. *Angle Orthod.* 2000;70(3): 253–262.
40. Cornelis MA, Scheffler NR, De Clerck HJ, Tulloch JF, Behets CN. Systematic review of the experimental use of temporary skeletal anchorage devices in orthodontics. *Am J Orthod Dentofacial Orthop.* 2007; 131(4):52–58.
41. Kircelli BH, Pektas ZO. Midfacial protraction with skeletally anchored face mask therapy: a novel approach and preliminary results. *Am J Orthod Dentofacial Orthop.* 2008;133(3):440–449.
42. Heymann GC, Cevidanes L, Cornelis M, Clerck HD, Tulloch JF. Three-dimensional analysis of maxillary protraction with intermaxillary elastics to miniplates. *Am J Orthod Dentofacial Orthop.* 2010;137(2): 274–284.
43. De Clerck H, Cevidanes L, Baccetti T. Dentofacial effects of bone-anchored maxillary protraction: a controlled study of consecutively treated Class III patients. *Am J Orthod Dentofacial Orthop.* 2010;138(5): 577–581.
44. Küçükkeleş N, Nevzatoğlu Ş, Koldaş T. Rapid maxillary expansion compared to surgery for assistance in maxillary facemask protraction. *Angle Orthod.* 2011;81(1):42–49.
45. Nevzatoğlu Ş, Küçükkeleş N. Long term treatment results in surgery assisted facemask therapy. Paper presented at: 88th Congress of the European Orthodontic Society; June 18–23, 2012; Santiago de Compostela, Spain.
46. Erverdi N, Acar A. Zygomatic anchorage for en masse retraction in the treatment of severe Class II division 1. *Angle Orthod.* 2005;75(3): 483–490.
47. Ludwig B, Glasl B, Kinzinger GS, Lietz T, Lisson JA. Anatomical guidelines for miniscrew insertion: vestibular interradicular sites. *J Clin Orthod.* 2011;45(3):165–173.
48. Sar C, Arman-Özçırpıcı A, Uçkan S, Yazıcı AC. Comparative evaluation of maxillary protraction with or without skeletal anchorage. *Am J Orthod Dentofacial Orthop.* 2011;139(5):636–649.
49. Ngan P. Treatment of Class III malocclusion in the primary and mixed dentitions. In: Bishara SE, ed. *Textbook of Orthodontics.* Philadelphia, PA: WB Saunders; 2001:375–411.

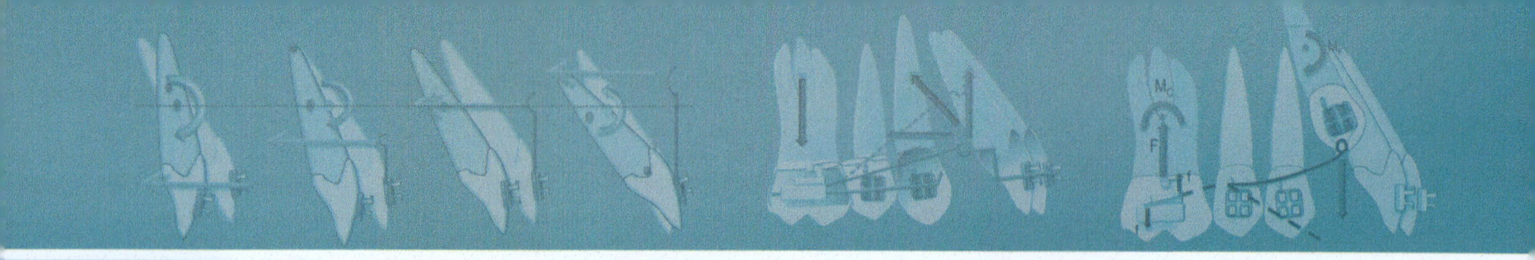

CHAPTER 18

Achieving Optimal Esthetics with Palatal Mini-Implants: The Benefit Technique

Benedict Wilmes

The advent of mini-implant technology continues to broaden the spectrum of what is achievable by orthodontics. The challenges associated with certain types of tooth movement can now be overcome by applying sound biomechanical principles to skeletal anchorage with even more potential for ideal esthetic outcomes. This chapter discusses the use of different forms of skeletal anchorage and considerations to achieve optimal esthetic goals.

STABLE ANCHORAGE

Orthodontic mini-implants have become increasingly popular in recent years because of their versatility, minimal invasiveness, and low cost.[1-5] Their small size allows them to be inserted in a variety of sites. Currently, the alveolar process is the most preferred insertion site. However, due to varying bone quality and the risk of root contact, the survival rate of implants inserted in the alveolar ridge still needs improvement, with current failure rates at approximately 10% to 30%.[6-11] The following factors seem to be relevant for the premature loss or tipping of a mini-implant:

1. Insufficient bone quality and/or inadequate bone quantity at the insertion site.[12-14]
2. Employment of mini-implants with a small diameter and/or length.[9,15-17]
3. Inappropriate intraosseous design.[17-19]
4. Root contact at the time of insertion.[20]
5. Manipulation with the fingers or tongue.[15]
6. Insufficient oral hygiene.
7. Application of high forces or moments.[16,21]
8. Use of a large lever arm. This occurs if the mini-implant is inserted in a region where the gingiva or mucosa is too thick.[16,21,22]
9. Insertion in the region of the movable mucosa.[8,15]
10. Insufficient primary stability.[2,22-24]
11. Bone damage at insertion due to high stress or bone overheating.[8,25] This phenomenon is well known in dental implantology.[26]

Other regions, such as the anterior palate and the mental region, provide much better conditions for temporary anchorage device (TAD) insertion since the amount and quality of the available bone is superior.[27] Using TADs in the anterior palate and the mental region eliminates the risk of root injury and takes the TADs out of the path of tooth movement.

Benefit Mini-Implants with Exchangeable Abutments

The Benefit mini-implant has an inner thread on its top (Fig. 18-1; PSM, Tuttlingen, Germany; PSM North America, Indio, CA). It is made of titanium alloy (Grade 5: Ti-6Al-4V) and due to its self-drilling thread design, insertion can be done without predrilling with a handpiece. Available dimensions are diameter of 2 or 2.3 mm and length of 7, 9, 11, 13, or 15 mm. On the top of the mini-implant four different types of stainless steel abutments can be fixed with a tiny fixing screw that is integrated into the abutment (Fig. 18-2). This small fixing screw can be turned within the abutment but cannot fall out of it. Different types of abutments allow the construction of versatile appliances for a large variety of clinical applications. The Benefit mini-implants are inserted primarily in the anterior palate and in edentulous areas of the alveolar process.

The Beneplate: A Mini-Plate for the Easy Coupling of Two Mini-Implants

To improve their stability and to prevent mini-implant tipping, two Benefit mini-implants can easily be coupled with the Beneplate (Fig. 18-3; PSM). The Beneplate is a stainless steel plate with a thickness of 1.2 mm. To cover multiple distances of two mini-implants, it has a round hole and a long hole. As well, it is available in two different lengths, resulting in possible distances of 3.5 to 14 mm measured from the center of one mini-implant to the center of the other. To enable a stable connection to the orthodontic appliance, Beneplates with a 1.1-mm-diameter stainless steel

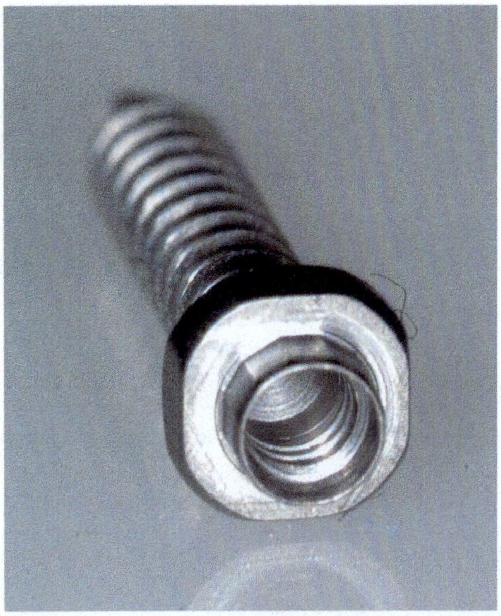

Figure 18-1 Benefit mini-implant with an inner thread.

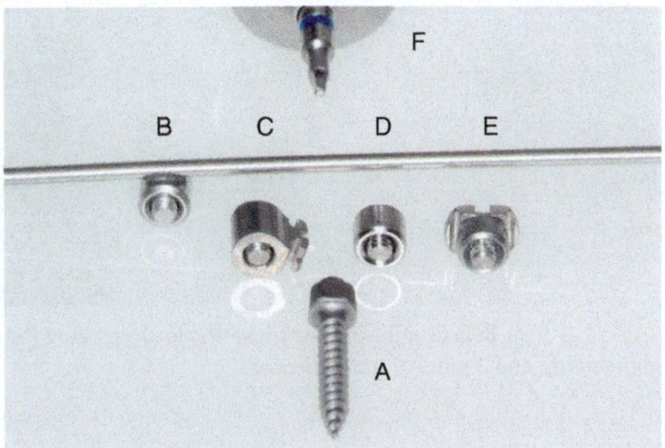

Figure 18-2 Benefit system. **A,** Mini-implant. **B,** Abutment with wire in place. **C,** Bracket abutment. **D,** Standard abutment. **E,** Slot abutment. **F,** Screwdriver.

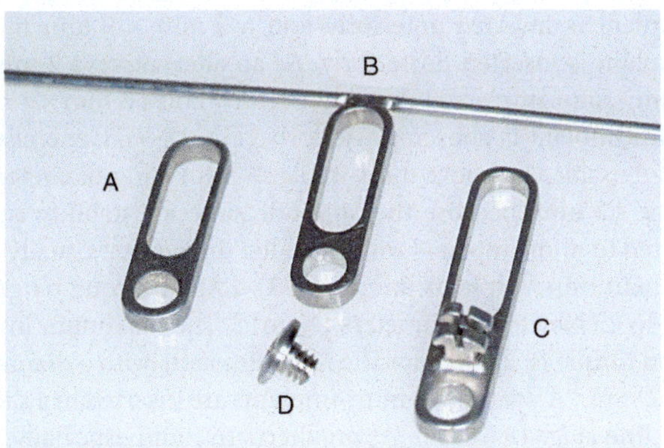

Figure 18-3 Beneplate system. **A,** Short Beneplate. **B,** Short Beneplate with wire in place. **C,** Long Beneplate with bracket in place. **D,** Fixation screw.

wire (for a Beneslider, Mesialslider, Mesial-Distal-Slider), a 0.8-mm-diameter stainless steel wire (for a Pendulum B or molar intrusion with the Mousetrap mechanics), and a stainless steel bracket (to ligate in lever arms) are available (see Fig. 18-3). The Beneplate can be adapted to the Benefit

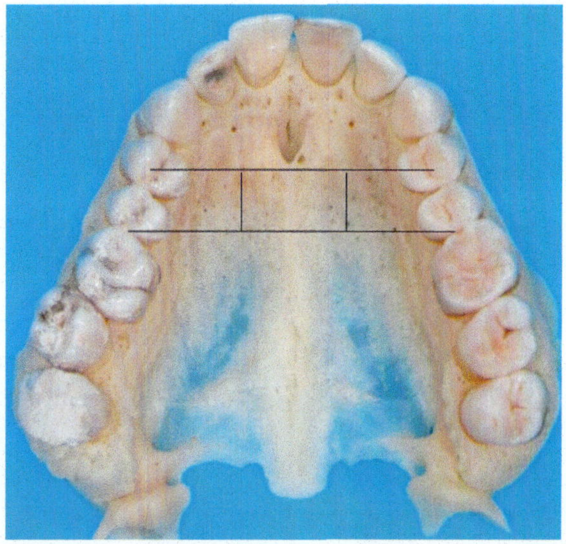

Figure 18-4 Prepared maxilla with two lines showing the optimal insertion site between the premolars. Less bone is available in the areas that are more lateral and posterior.

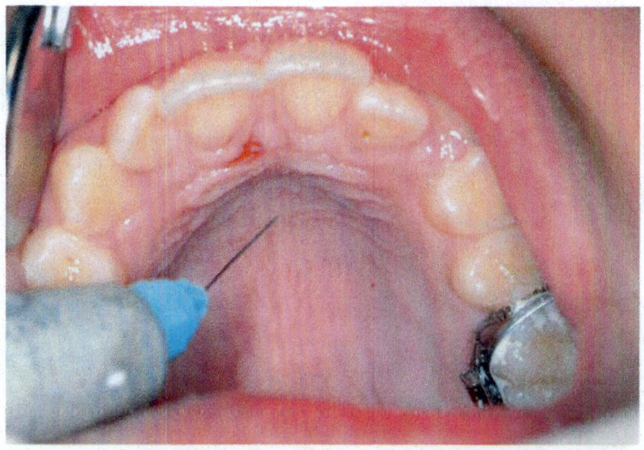

Figure 18-5 Local anesthesia administered directly into the insertion site using a SOPIRA Citoject syringe (Heraeus Kulzer GmbH, Hanau, Germany).

mini-implants by bending the plate body as well as the wire. Small fixing screws are used to fix the Beneplate on top of the mini-implants (see Fig. 18-3).

STEP-BY-STEP CLINICAL PROCEDURE

The optimum insertion site in the maxilla is located in the anterior palate distally from the palatal rugae on a line between the premolars. Advantages of this region are a thin soft tissue layer and sufficient bone height. Less bone is available in the areas that are more lateral and posterior (Fig. 18-4).[28,29] The first step is local anesthesia administered directly in the insertion site (Fig. 18-5). If the patient is afraid of a syringe, only topical anesthesia can be used. The second step is predrilling (to 3 mm depth) with a 1.4-mm drill for the 2-mm mini-implants and a 1.7-mm drill for the 2.3-mm mini-implants. This can be done manually using a special handpiece equipped with a 1:1 contra angle (Fig. 18-6; PSM). Due to the low speed there is no need for cooling. In very young patients (i.e., less than 12 years of age) predrilling

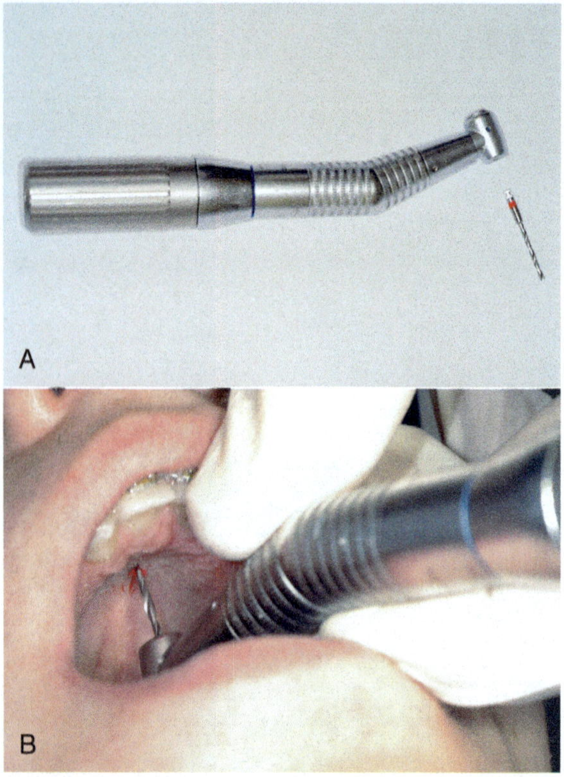

Figure 18-6 **A,** Preparation for predrilling using a contra angle equipped with a special handpiece. **B,** Predrilling with the contra angle and the handpiece.

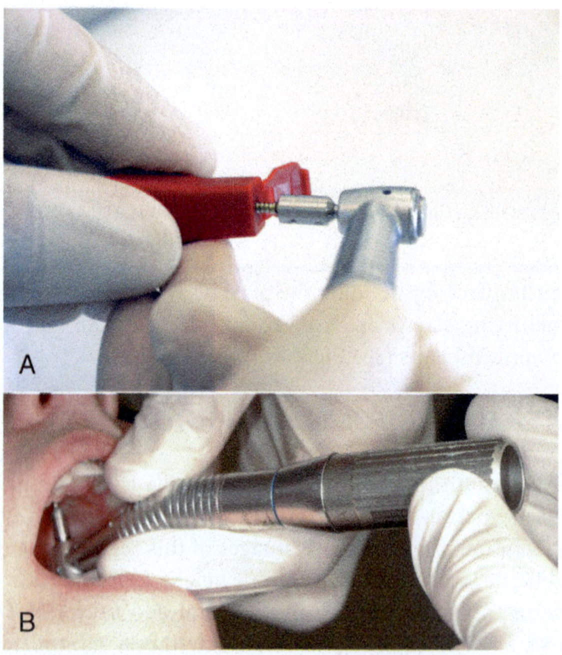

Figure 18-7 **A,** Preparing a Benefit mini-implant before insertion. **B,** Insertion of a Benefit mini-implant using the contra-angle screwdriver.

is not necessary due to the low mineralization rate of the bone.

Once the sites have been prepared, one or two Benefit mini-implants are inserted near the midpalatal suture, again using the contra-angle screwdriver (Fig. 18-7). If just one

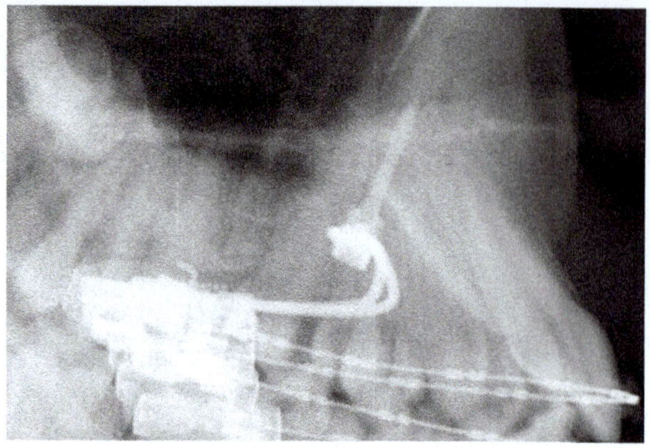

Figure 18-8 One Benefit mini-implant in the palate (2.3 mm × 11 mm).

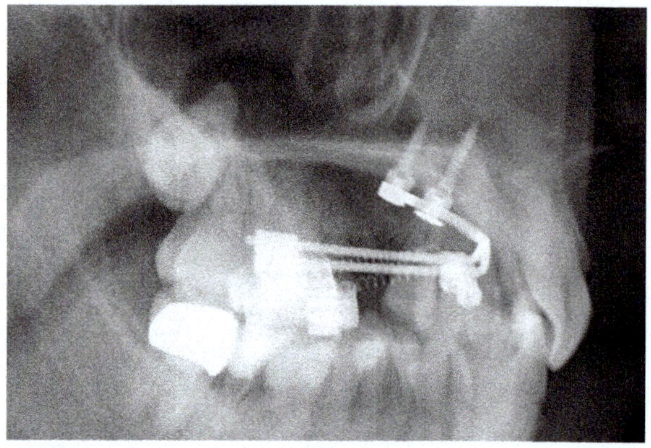

Figure 18-9 Two Benefit mini-implants inserted in the palate (2 mm × 11 mm anterior and 2 mm × 9 mm posterior).

mini-implant is employed (e.g., for molar anchorage), the dimension 2.3 mm × 11 mm is chosen (Fig. 18-8); if two mini-implants are employed, usually a 2 mm × 11 mm mini-implant is inserted anteriorly and a 2 mm × 9 mm mini-implant is inserted posteriorly. As an alternative, a 2 mm × 9 mm mini-implant is chosen anteriorly and a 2 mm × 7 mm mini-implant is chosen posteriorly (Fig. 18-9). Generally, it is advisable to choose mini-implants with a big diameter of 2 or 2.3 mm, because they provide superior stability compared to mini-implants with a smaller diameter.[22] Usually the Benefit mini-implants are inserted within a torque range of 10 to 25 Newton centimeters (Ncm).[30] The maximum insertion torque is 35 Ncm for the mini-implants with a diameter of 2 mm.[31] Usually, two mini-implants are inserted in a sagittal line (Fig. 18-10, A). As an alternative and especially if a rapid palatal expansion with the Hybrid Hyrax is planned, the mini-implants are inserted in a transversal lineup (Fig. 18-10, B). The distance between the two mini-implants should be at least 4 mm to enable enough space for the supraconstruction (two abutments or one Beneplate). Additionally, if an impression is planned, there must be enough space for two impression caps. The Benefit mini-implants are self-drilling and can be inserted without predrilling. However, there is very high bone density in the anterior

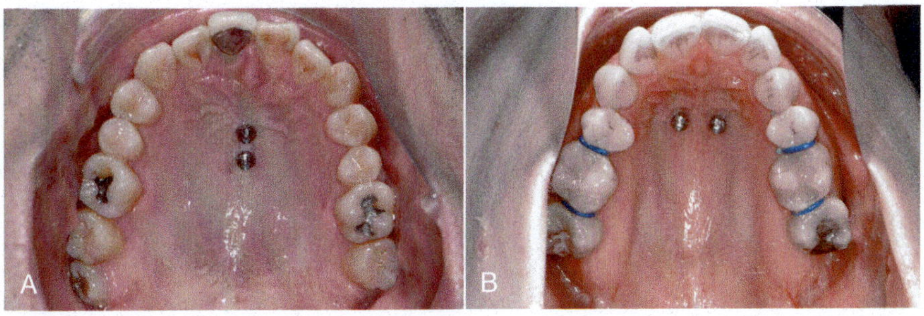

Figure 18-10 **A,** In most cases, two mini-implants are inserted in a sagittal line. **B,** If a rapid palatal expansion with the Hybrid Hyrax is planned, the mini-implants are inserted in a transversal lineup.

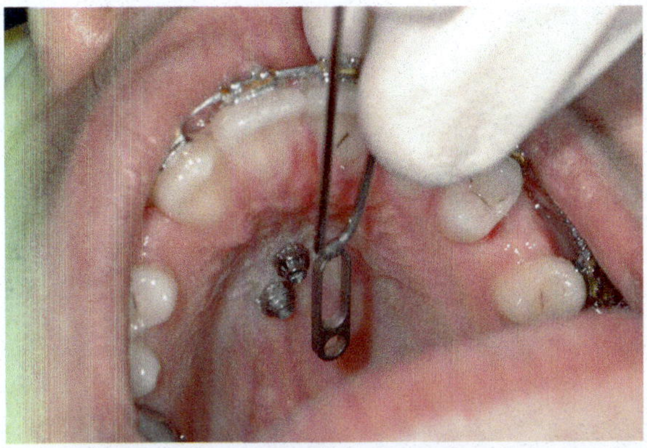

Figure 18-11 Chairside adaption of the T-bow for front anchorage during molar mesialization in the upper arch.

palate, especially in older patients. Soft tissue thickness can be measured using a dental probe from anterior to posterior to identify a region with thin mucosa. This is important in order to achieve a sufficient primary stability and to avoid large lever arms.[21,22] The soft tissue in the anterior region nearby the first and second rugae is very thick.[29]

Depending on the mechanics, bands with lingual sheaths are fixed to the upper molars. The appliance can be bent either directly chairside (Fig. 18-11) or after impression taking in the laboratory. In the latter case, impression caps (Fig. 18-12, A) are placed on top of the mini-implant (Fig. 18-12, B and C) and a silicone impression is taken (Fig. 18-12, D). If desired, the impression caps can be secured by dental floss. Subsequently, laboratory analogs are inserted in the impression caps and fixed by wax (Fig. 18-12, E). At the end, a plaster model is manufactured. The only appliance that has to be manufactured in the laboratory is the Hybrid Hyrax since it requires soldering or welding connections. Bands should be adapted on the teeth and later in the impression if they will be integrated in the appliance (Fig. 18-12, F).

The mini-implants are loaded immediately after insertion; in the case of a laboratory procedure, they are loaded a maximum of 1 week after insertion of the TADs. It is recommended that the appliance be inserted as soon as possible. If there is a long period until the appliance is fixed, the patient has time to jiggle the mini-implants with the tongue or fingers and as a consequence they may become loose.

DISTALIZATION IN THE UPPER ARCH

Principle: Direct versus Indirect Anchorage

Class II malocclusions are very common. For patients with a dental Class II malocclusion with increased overjet and/or anterior crowding, upper molar distalization is a frequently chosen treatment alternative. Molar distalization with a headgear is unpleasant for many patients for esthetic reasons and because of the length of time the headgear needs to be worn.[32,33]

These factors resulted in a tendency to prefer purely intraoral appliances that require minimal patient cooperation. Unfortunately, most conventional devices for noncompliance upper molar distalization produce unwanted side effects such as anchorage loss.[34] One possible method to reduce unwanted orthodontic effects of reciprocal forces is the use of palatal acrylic pads (Nance buttons). However, the anchorage stability of this soft tissue–borne element is not always certain. Moreover, oral hygiene is impaired due to the partial coverage of the palatal area. If the anchorage unit includes teeth, mesial migration and/or protrusion of the anterior dentition must be considered as a major drawback.[34–36] Anchorage loss of conventional intraoral distalization devices ranges from 24% to 55%.[34]

To minimize or eliminate anchorage loss of the anterior dentition, skeletal anchorage devices have been integrated into distalization appliances.[37–46] Although indirect anchorage can be used to support the premolars during maxillary molar distalization, mini-screw tipping and wire deformation may result in anchorage loss and mesial premolar migration. Moreover, after molar distalization the appliance must be reconstructed in order to distalize the premolars and anterior teeth. Therefore direct anchorage is preferable (Fig. 18-13).

Direct Anchorage with the Beneslider

The Beneslider[3,30,47,48] is a distalization appliance that uses direct anchorage and is based on one (Fig. 18-14, A) or two (Fig. 18-14, B) mini-implants in the anterior palate. Through the use of the Benefit mini-implants with exchangeable abutments, a stable and safe connection between the mini-implants and the distalization mechanics is achieved. To couple the Beneslider with the molars, bands with lingual sheaths are fixed to the upper molars. Directly thereafter,

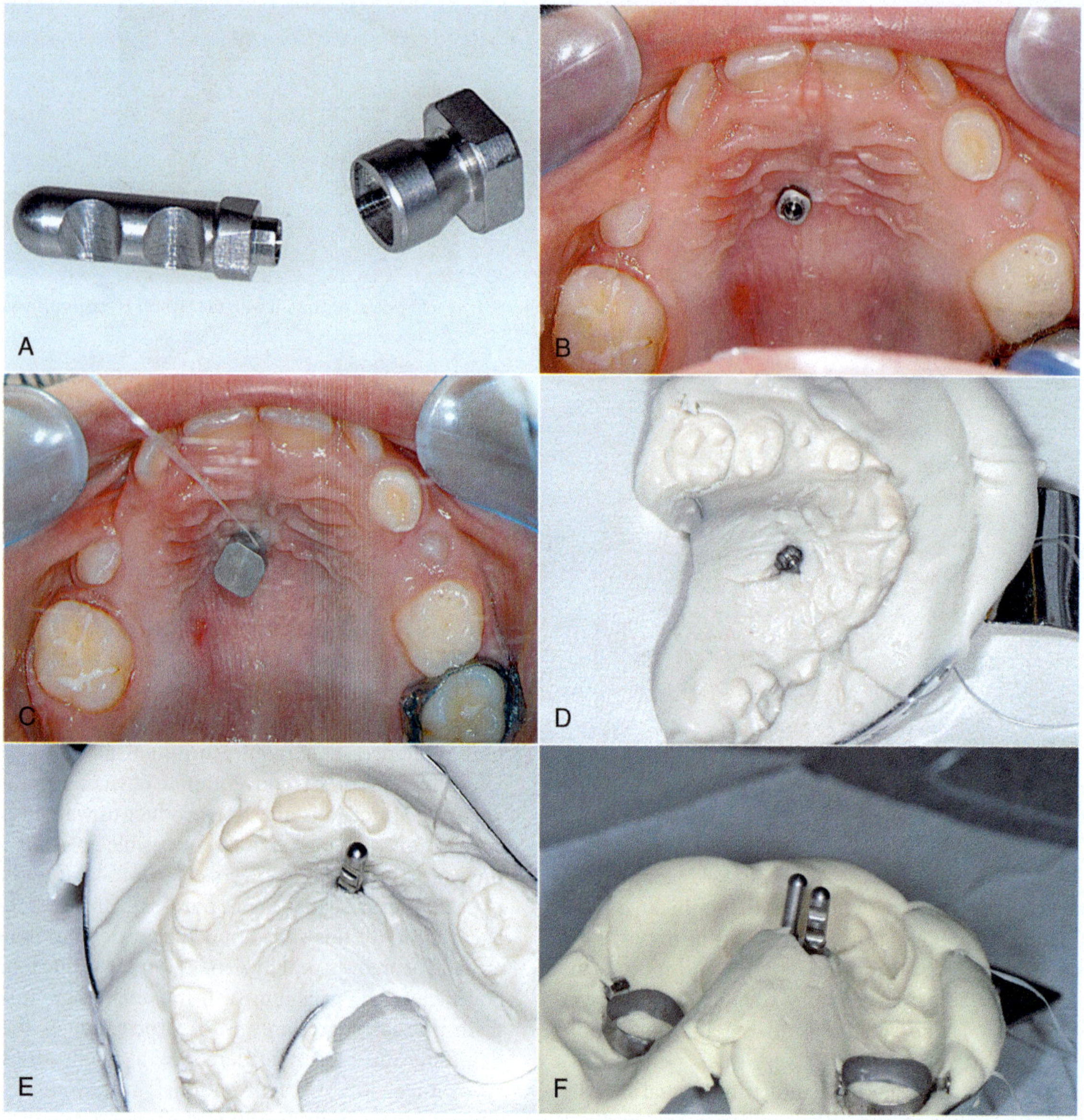

Figure 18-12 **A,** Laboratory analog *(left)* and impression cap *(right)*. **B,** One Benefit mini-implant after insertion. **C,** An impression cap is placed on top of the mini-implant. **D,** Impression tray. Note that the impression cap is visible. **E,** A laboratory analog is inserted in the impression cap. **F,** Impression for a Hybrid Hyrax with replaced bands and laboratory analogs.

Benetubes are plugged into the sheaths from the mesial side (Fig. 18-15). To avoid irritation of the soft tissues, the Benetube must be bent slightly in most cases. If one mini-implant was inserted, an abutment with a wire in place (see Fig. 18-2) is adapted to the curvature of the palate. If two mini-implants were inserted, a Beneplate with a 1.1-mm stainless steel wire in place (see Fig. 18-3) is now adapted (see Fig. 18-15, B). Depending on the axis and the location of the two mini-implants, the Beneplate body must be bent (Fig. 18-16). By changing the angulation of the 1.1-mm stainless steel wire, it is possible to achieve a simultaneous intrusion or extrusion of the molars (Fig. 18-17). The adapted abutment is now fixed on the mini-implant by the inner fixing screw. If two mini-implants were inserted, the Beneplate is fixed by two fixing screws (see Fig. 18-3, D). This can be performed with the screwdriver or with the contra angle and the handpiece (Fig. 18-18). Finally, the distalization force is applied by springs that are activated by pushing the activation locks distally (Fig. 18-19). The author recommends the use of nickel-titanium (Ni-Ti) springs (240 g in children and 500 g in adults). It seems advantageous that the Beneslider mechanics can be installed without need for any laboratory work in terms of welding or soldering. In other words, the Beneslider mechanics can be applied directly in the oral cavity without taking an impression. To save chair time, however, the Beneslider can also be adapted on a plaster model (see Fig. 18-12).

Follow-up should be scheduled every 4 to 6 weeks. Usually the premolars and canines migrate distally toward the molars due to stretching of the interdental fibers. After distalization of the molars with the Beneslider, the Beneslider stays in place as an anchorage device during retraction of the

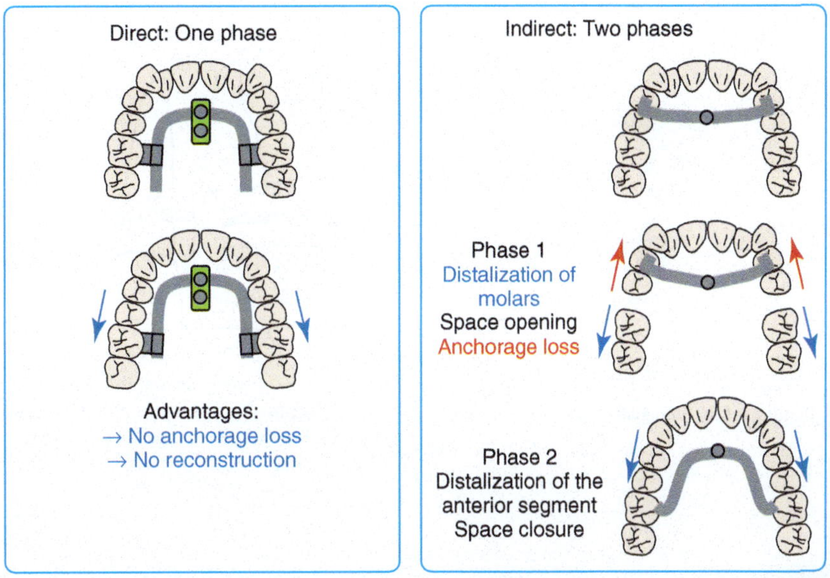

Figure 18-13 Direct anchorage (one phase) versus indirect anchorage (two phases) for upper molar distalization.

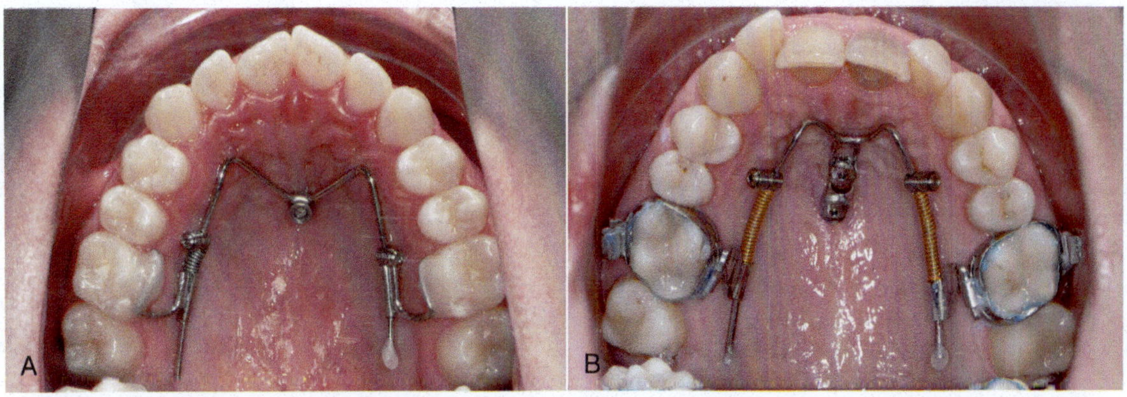

Figure 18-14 **A,** Beneslider based on one mini-implant (2.3 mm × 11 mm). **B,** Beneslider based on two mini-implants (2 × 11 mm anterior and 2 × 9 mm posterior).

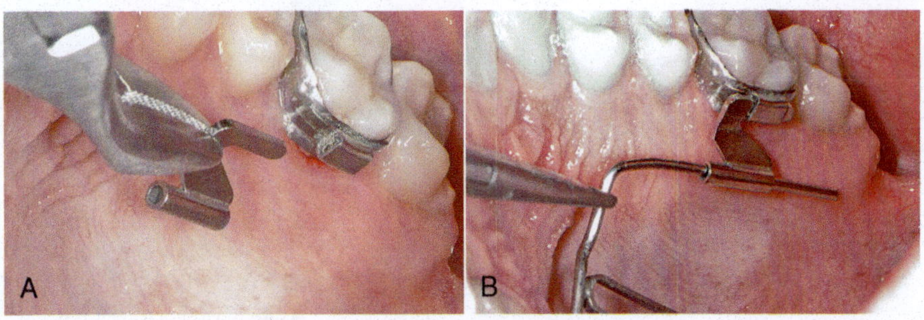

Figure 18-15 **A,** Benetube is plugged into the sheaths from the mesial side. **B,** Afterwards, the wire of the Beneplate must be adapted to the curvature of the palate.

anterior dentition. The treatment can be finished with buccal brackets, lingual brackets, or aligners.

Clinical Example Using the Beneslider

The patient was a 13-year-old male with a Class II relationship and severe bialveolar protrusion. In the canine region, half of a Class II occlusion was found (Figs. 18-20 and 18-21). The treatment plan was distalization and correction of the protrusion in the upper arch with a Beneslider and distalization with a lip bumper and retrusion of the incisors in the lower arch. After insertion of two Benefit mini-implants in the anterior palate, the Beneslider mechanics were applied and activated (Fig. 18-22, A). After 6.5 months the upper molars were distalized approximately 4 mm and brackets were bonded (Fig. 18-22, B). The radiographs show a bodily distalization of the molars (Fig. 18-23). Steel ligatures were

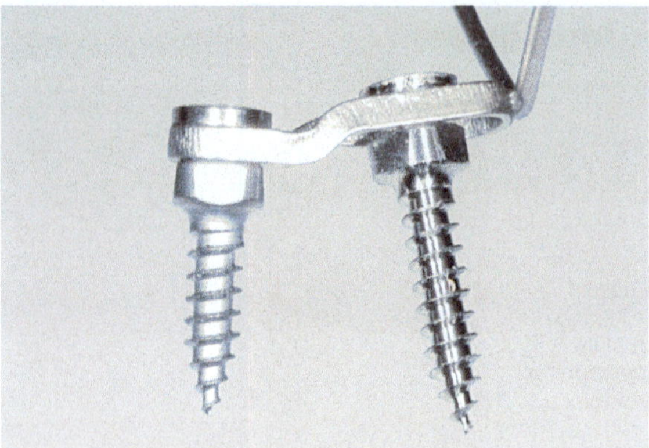

Figure 18-16 Bending of the Beneplate body.

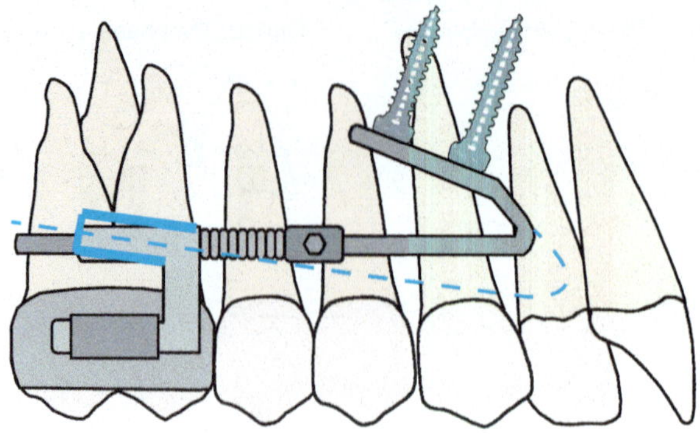

Figure 18-17 By changing the angulation of the 1.1-mm stainless steel wire, it is possible to achieve a simultaneous intrusion or extrusion of the molars. The dashed blue line represents the mechanics for intrusion during distalization.

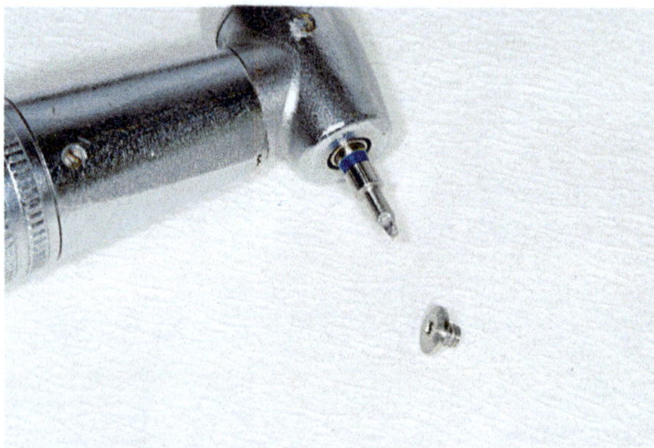

Figure 18-18 Tiny screw used to fix the Beneplate on top of the mini-implant. This can be performed with the screwdriver or the contra angle (shown).

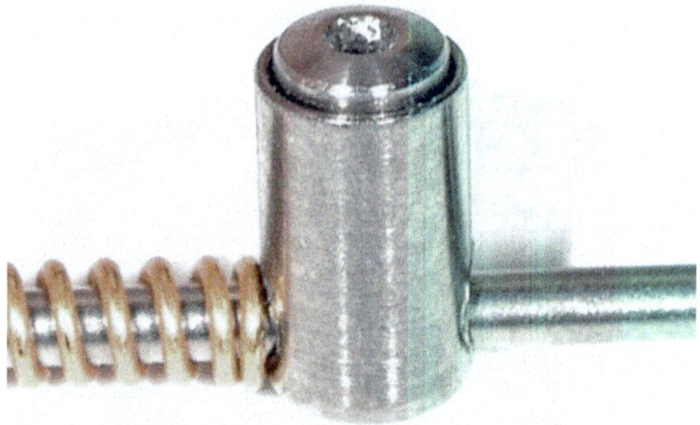

Figure 18-19 Activation lock and a spring on a 1.1-mm stainless steel wire.

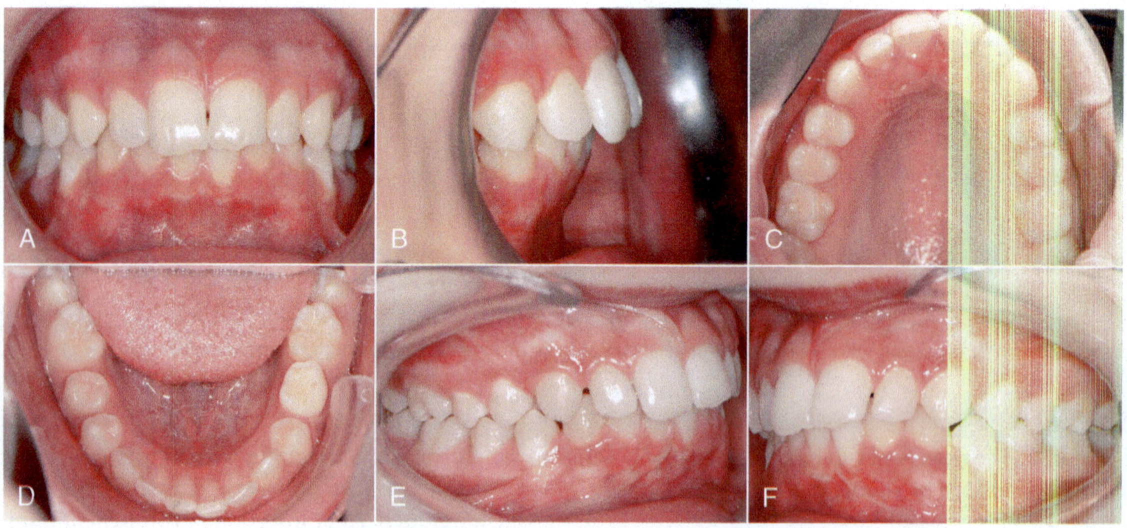

Figure 18-20 **A–F,** Intraoral photographs of 13-year-old male patient with Class II malocclusion and severe bialveolar protrusion.

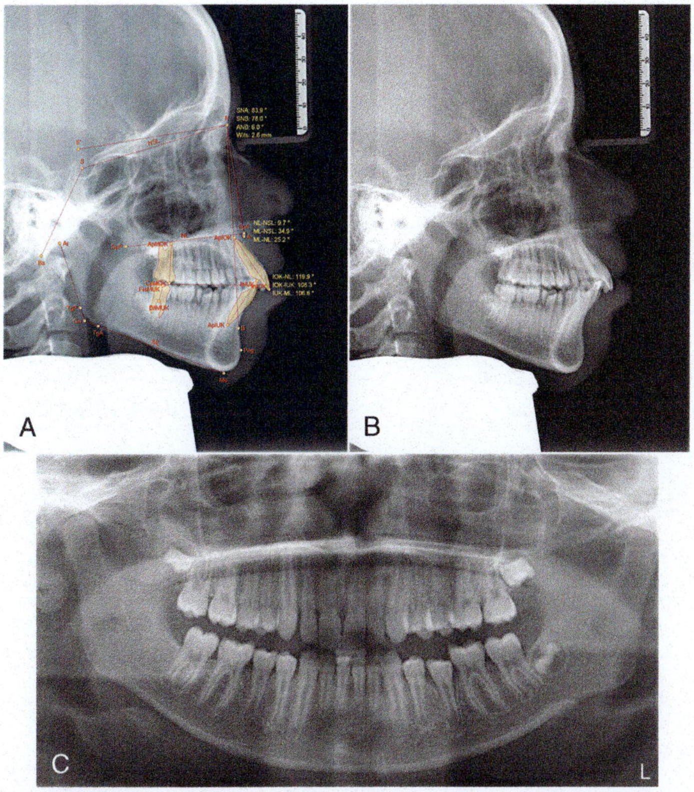

Figure 18-21 **A and B,** Cephalometric and **(C)** panoramic radiographs showing a dentoalveolar class II and a front protrusion.

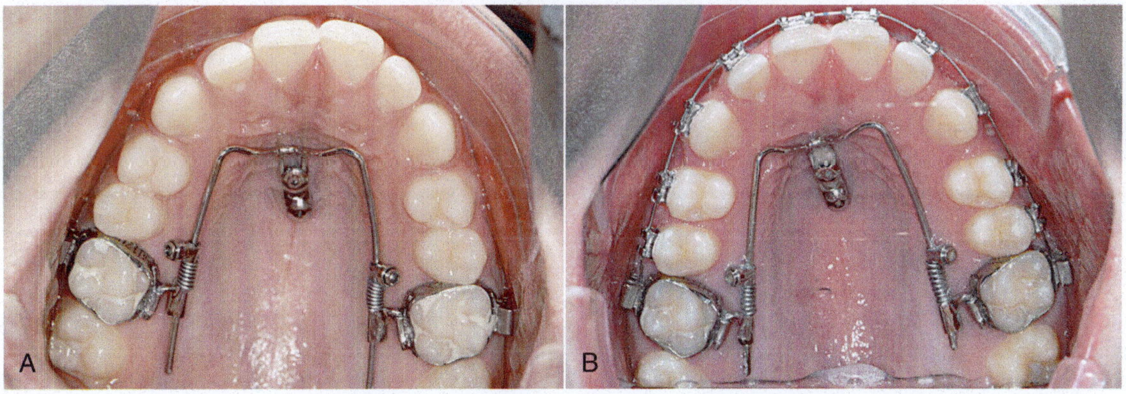

Figure 18-22 **A,** The Beneslider in situ. **B,** After 6.5 months the upper molars were distalized approximately 4 mm and brackets were bonded.

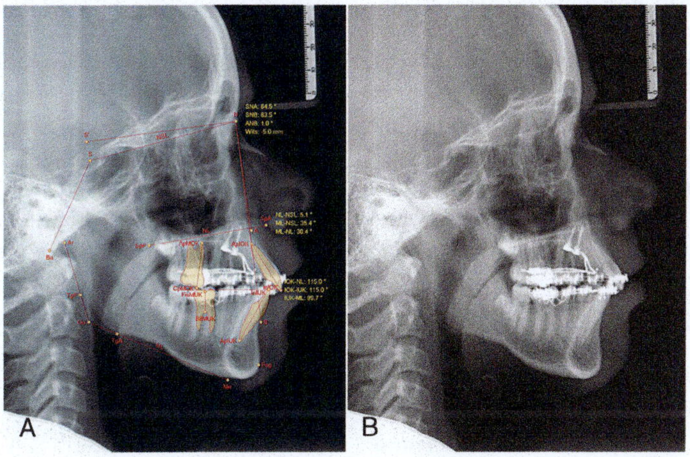

Figure 18-23 **A and B,** Radiographs show a bodily distalization of the molars.

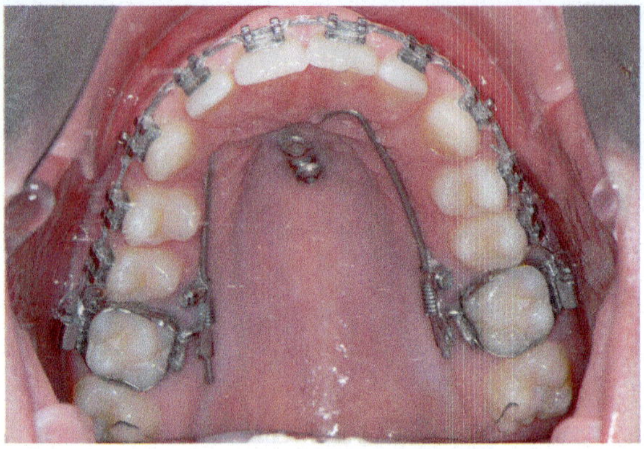

Figure 18-24 Continuation of front retraction.

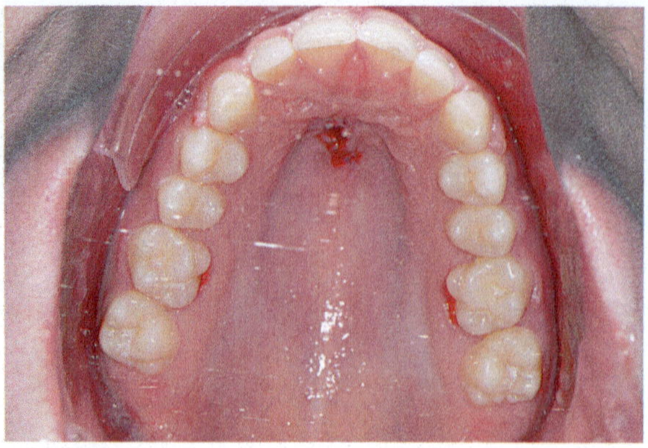

Figure 18-25 The Beneslider and the Benefit mini-implants are removed.

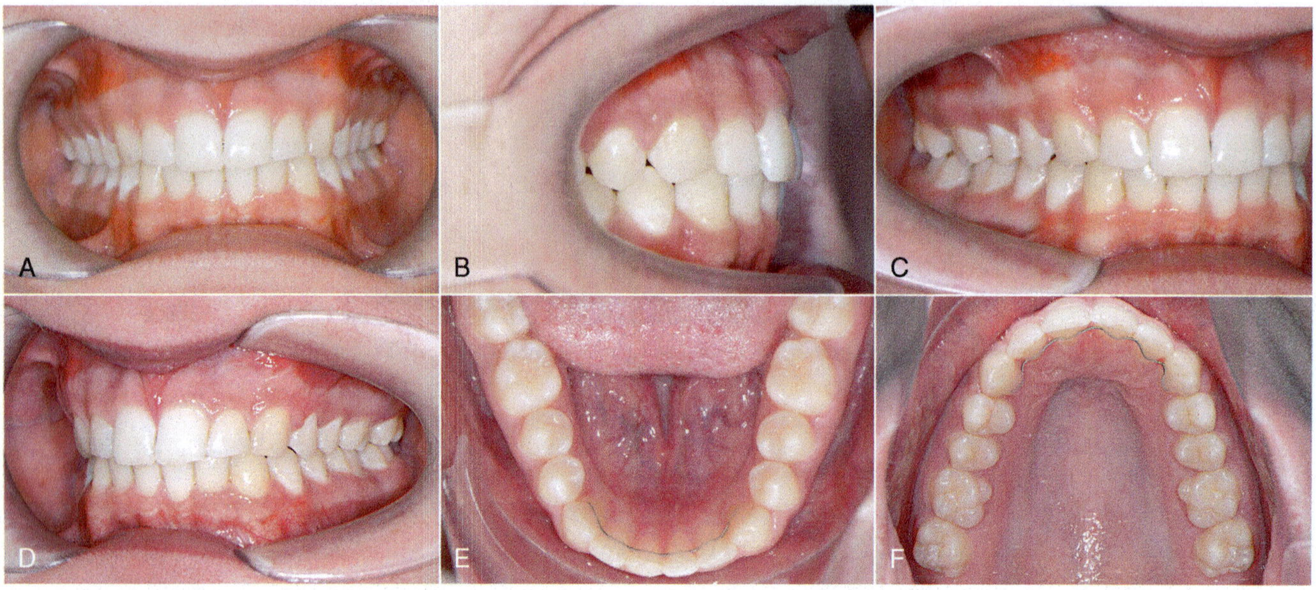

Figure 18-26 **A–F,** Intraoral photographs taken at the end of the treatment (18 months) showing a class I occlusion and successfully retracted upper front teeth.

inserted between the Benetubes and the activation locks to deactivate the Beneslider. As an alternative, the Ni-Ti springs can be removed. In other words, the Beneslider was modified from a distalization device to a molar anchorage device. An elastic chain was inserted from the first molar to the contralateral first molar to retract the anterior dentition. After 5 months of retraction the spaces were almost closed to the distal. To avoid contact of the Beneplate wire and the soft tissues it is important to anticipate the amount of front retraction at the time of bending the wire; in this case, this issue was not properly addressed (Fig. 18-24). After the finishing phase the brackets were debonded. The Beneslider and the Benefit mini-implants were removed without anesthesia (Fig. 18-25). End of treatment was reached after 18 months (Figs. 18-26 and 18-27).

MESIALIZATION IN THE UPPER ARCH

Principle: Direct versus Indirect Anchorage

Congenitally missing lateral incisors or second premolars, extremely displaced canines, or a severe trauma of a central incisor are potential complaints that result in a reduced upper dentition. The two major treatment approaches are space closure or space opening to allow prosthodontic replacements with either a fixed prosthesis or a single-tooth implant. Both of these treatment approaches can potentially compromise esthetics, periodontal health, and function.[49] In many cases space closure to the mesial (front teeth should stay where they are, when posterior teeth are moving mesially) seems to be the favorable treatment goal, since treatment can be completed as soon as the dentition is complete.[50] Canine substitutions can be accomplished with good esthetic outcomes by tooth reshaping and positioning, bleaching, and porcelain veneers.[51,52]

The more mesial the missing tooth is, the higher will be the demands for anchorage quality, especially in asymmetrical cases with a midline deviation. If the central incisors are in the correct position (midline, torque, and angulation is correct), a T-bow[3,30,49,53] can be bonded to the lingual surfaces of the central incisors to apply an *indirect anchorage*, with the goal being to avoid lingual tipping of the central incisors during space closure.[30,47,53] As an alternative to the T-bow

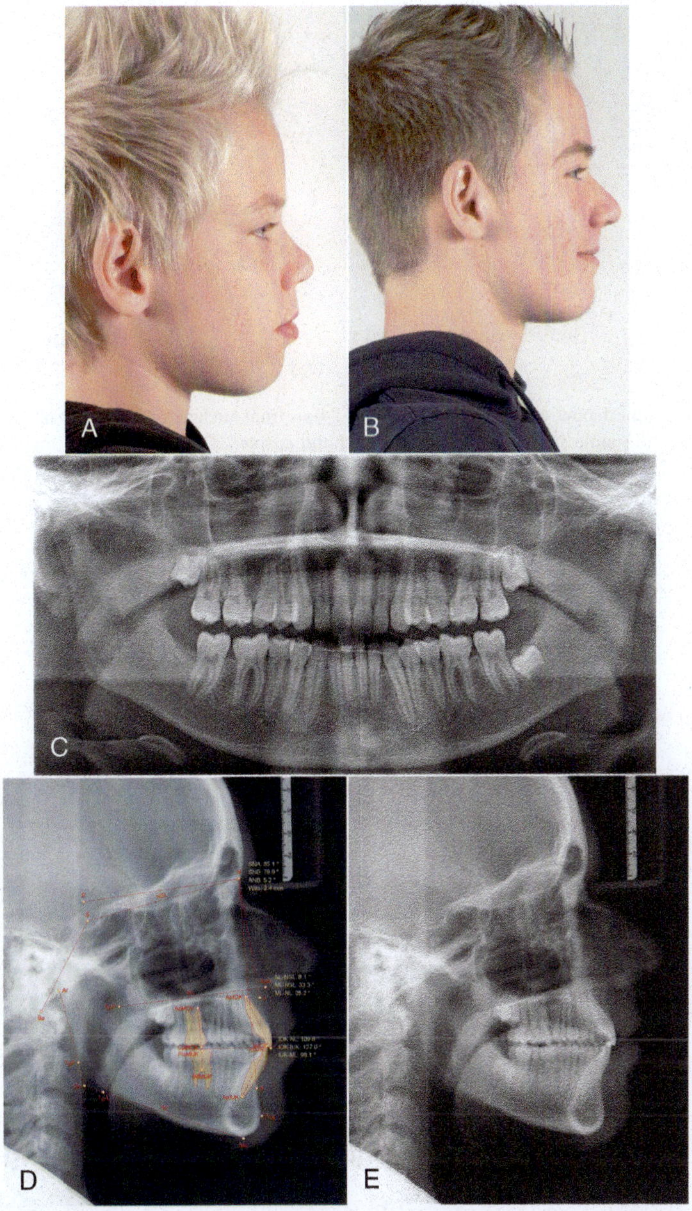

Figure 18-27 Profile views (**A**) before and (**B**) after treatment. **C–E,** Radiographs obtained at the end of treatment showing the achieved improvement of the overjet and the upper front inclination.

(indirect anchorage), the Mesialslider[30,47,54] can be used as a *direct anchorage* device. The Mesialslider enables clinicians to mesialize upper molars unilaterally or bilaterally. Since the incisors are not fixed, a midline deviation can be corrected at the same time. The Mesialslider can also be used for protrusion of the whole upper dentition to compensate a mild Class III occlusion.

Clinical Application of the T-Bow

The T-bow[3,30,49,53] is an archwire that is connected from one (Fig. 18-28, A) or two (Fig. 18-28, B) mini-implants in the anterior palate to the lingual surfaces of the upper central incisors. Using the T-bow avoids an undesired lingual tipping of the incisors during mesialization in the upper arch. Typical indications are unilateral or bilateral agenesis of the lateral incisors or missing canines. The incisors should already be well aligned and in the correct position when the T-bow is applied. After insertion of the mini-implants, a Beneplate with a 1.1-mm stainless steel wire in place is bent and adapted to fit between the mini-implants and the central incisors. Depending on the insertion axis and the position of the mini-implants, the Beneplate body must be adapted as well. After fixation of the Beneplate on top of the mini-implants by tiny fixing screws, the wire is bonded to the lingual surfaces of the central incisors (see Fig. 18-28, B).

Clinical Example Using the T-Bow

The patient was a 14-year-old female with missing upper lateral incisors and second molars. The treatment plan was mesialization in the upper arch without anchorage loss of the incisors by using a T-bow. After leveling, one Benefit mini-implant was inserted in the anterior palate (Fig. 18-29, A).

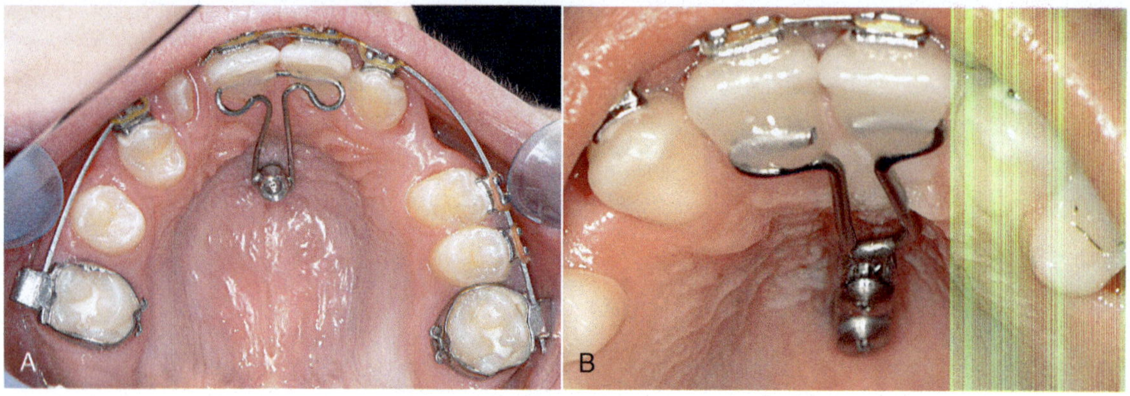

Figure 18-28 **A,** T-bow front anchorage mechanics on one mini-implant. **B,** T-bow front anchorage mechanics on two mini-implants. After insertion of the mini-implants, a Beneplate with a 1.1-mm stainless steel wire in place is bent and adapted. Depending on the insertion axis and the position of the mini-implants, the Beneplate body may need to be adapted as well. After fixation of the Beneplate on top of the mini-implants by tiny fixing screws, the wire is bonded to the lingual surfaces of the central incisors.

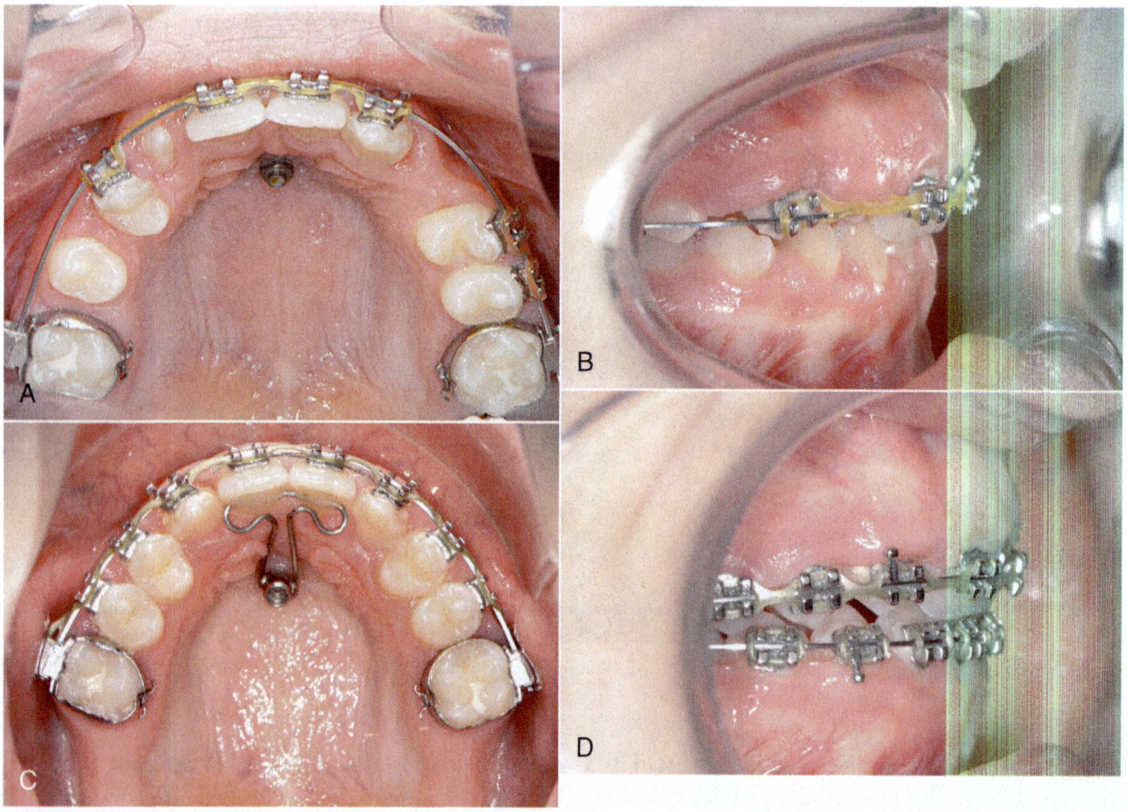

Figure 18-29 Pre-treatment **(A and B)** intraoral photographs of a 14-year-old female patient with missing upper lateral incisors and second molars. After 17 months the upper dentition was mesialized **(C)**, and the overjet was maintained **(D)**.

An abutment with a 1.1-mm stainless steel wire in place (see Fig. 18-2, B) was adapted to fit between the mini-implant and the incisors (see Fig. 18-28, A). Following bonding of the T-bow an elastic chain was used to apply mesialization forces to the lateral dentition. After 17 months the upper dentition was mesialized (Fig. 18-29, C, D). The treatment result showed a well-preserved overjet and a proper occlusion. However, it seems recommendable to use two mini-implants (see Fig. 18-28, B) to achieve a high anchorage quality.

Clinical Application of the Mesialslider

After insertion of two Benefit mini-implants, bands with lingual sheaths are fixed to the upper molars. Subsequently, two Benetubes and a Beneplate with a 1.1-mm stainless steel wire in place are adapted to the curvature of the palate. To avoid irritation of the soft tissues, the Benetubes must be bent in most cases. Depending on the axis and the location of the two mini-implants, the Beneplate body also must be bent. The mesialization force is delivered by two Ni-Ti closing springs (200 g) that are attached to the activation

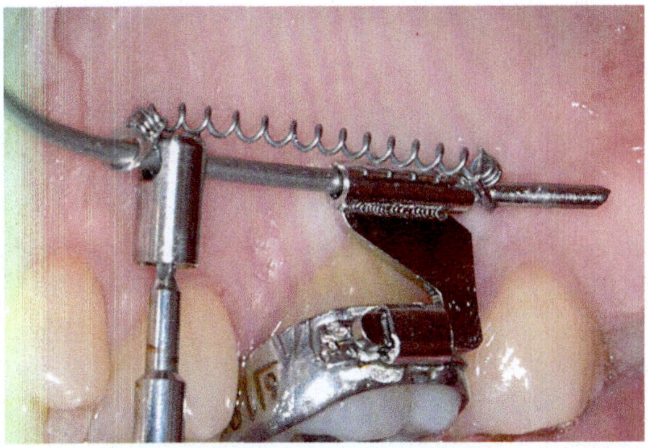

Figure 18-30 Benetubes and a Beneplate are adapted to the curvature of the palate; the activation lock is pushed mesially.

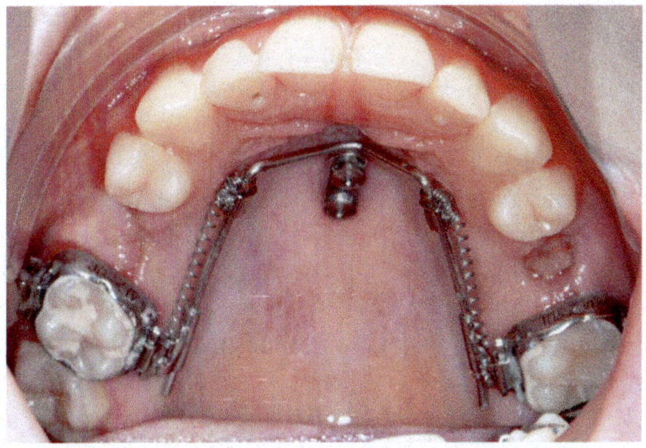

Figure 18-31 Mesialslider inserted.

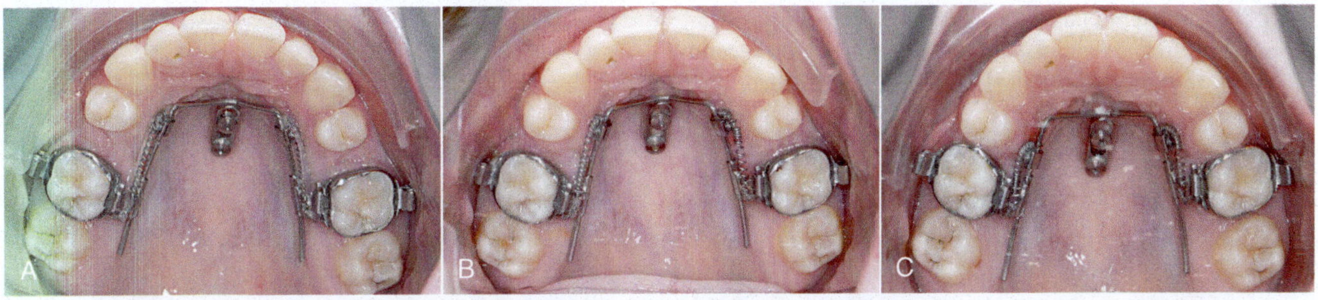

Figure 18-32 **A–C,** The spaces were closed mesially after 12 months.

locks. The Beneplate is fixed by two fixing screws using a screwdriver or the contra angle and the handpiece, which is more comfortable. Finally, the Mesialslider is activated by pushing the activation locks mesially (Fig. 18-30). In cases with missing second premolars or first molars, the Mesialslider can be inserted without putting brackets on the other teeth. Similar to the Beneslider, the Mesialslider can be installed without the need for laboratory work in terms of welding or soldering. In other words, the Mesialslider device can be applied directly in the oral cavity without an impression but can also be fabricated indirectly to save chair time.

Clinical Example Using the Mesialslider

A 13-year-old female patient with missing upper second premolars was treated with a Mesialslider (Fig. 18-31). The spaces were closed in the mesial direction after 12 months (Fig. 18-32).

Additional Tips for Using the Mesialslider

When second premolars or first molars are missing, the Mesialslider can be installed without brackets on the other teeth. If a more anterior tooth is missing, such as a lateral incisor or a canine, it is recommended to apply an additional mesialization force anterior by using:

1. An additional lever arm that is soldered to the Mesialslider. Using this lever arm, buccal and lingual forces can be applied (Fig. 18-33).
2. An additional Benetube that is bonded to a canine or bicuspid (Fig. 18-34).

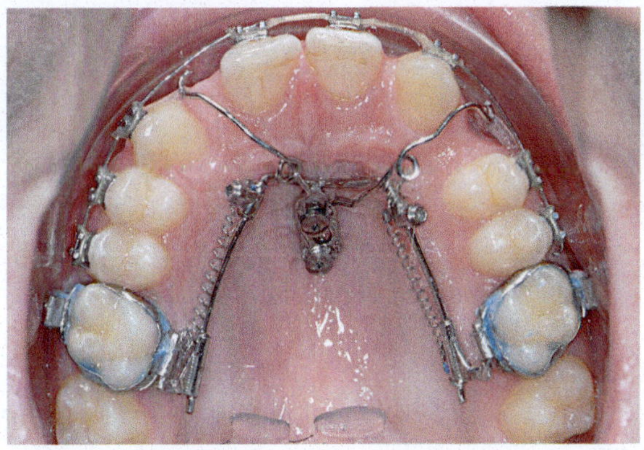

Figure 18-33 Mesialslider with additional lever arms, enabling application of buccal and lingual forces.

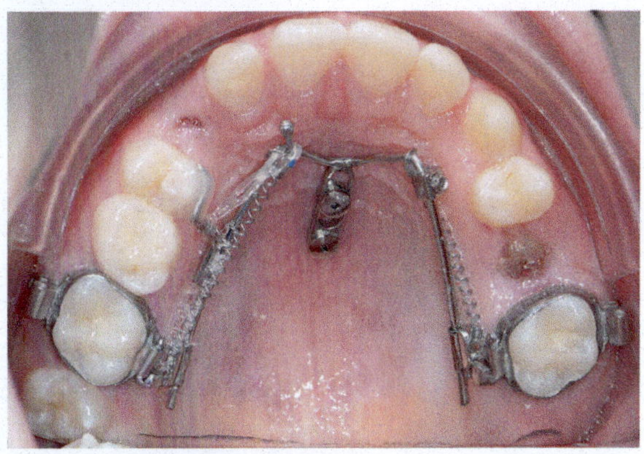

Figure 18-34 An additional Benetube (according to Dr. Banach, who invented the tubes) bonded to a bicuspid.

3. A combination of the Mesialslider and a T-bow: the T-Mesialslider. Forces can be applied buccally and lingually (Fig. 18-35).

Clinical Application of the Mesial-Distal-Slider

The Mesial-Distal-Slider is a combination device of the Beneslider (distalization) on one side and the Mesialslider (mesialization) on the contralateral side. As described, the Benetube is inserted mesially on the distalization side (see Fig. 18-15) and distally on the mesialization side (see Fig. 18-30).

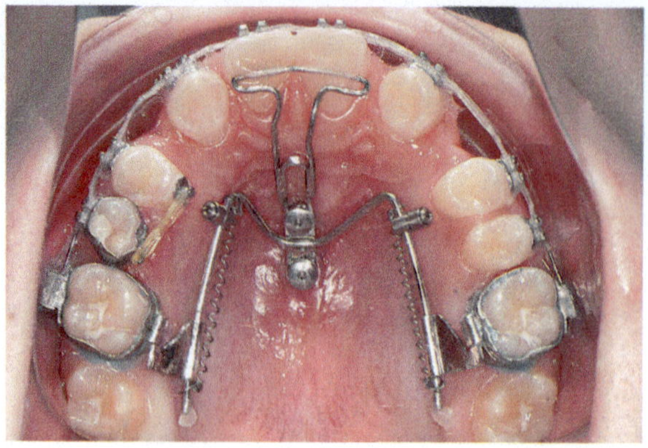

Figure 18-35 A combination of the Mesialslider and the T-bow. The T-Mesialslider allows forces to be applied buccally (elastic chain) and lingually (Ni-Ti spring). The T-Mesialslider/Beneplate has two wires in place, so there is no need for welding or soldering.

Clinical Example Using the Mesial-Distal-Slider

The treatment protocol for a 14-year-old female patient with a missing upper right lateral incisor is shown (Figs. 18-36 and 18-37). The canine erupted palatally, resulting in a crossbite. The treatment plan was canine substitution, mesialization in the first quadrant, and distalization in the second quadrant to correct the shifted midline. After extraction of

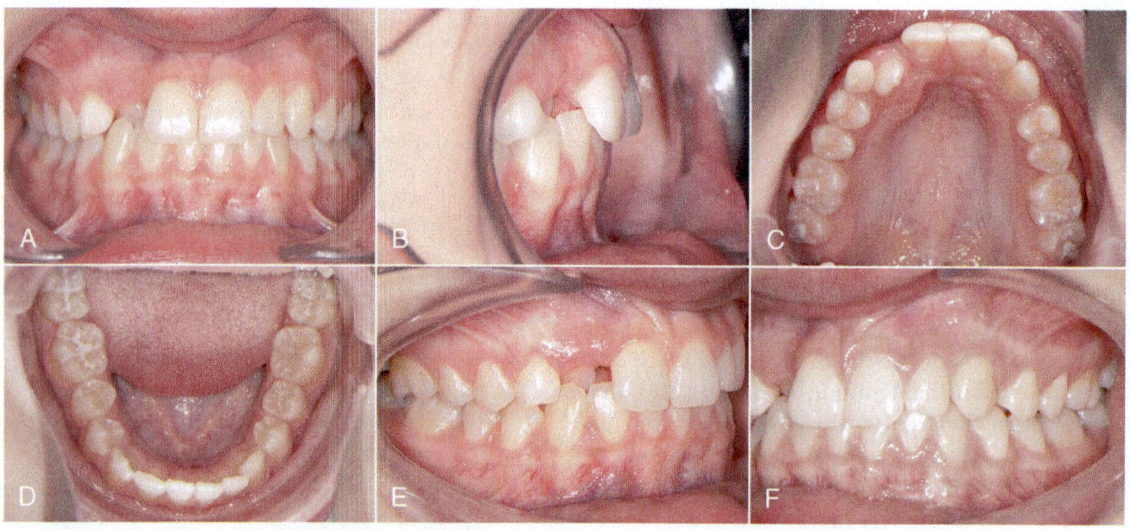

Figure 18-36 **A–F,** Intraoral photos of a 14-year-old female patient with a missing upper right lateral incisor.

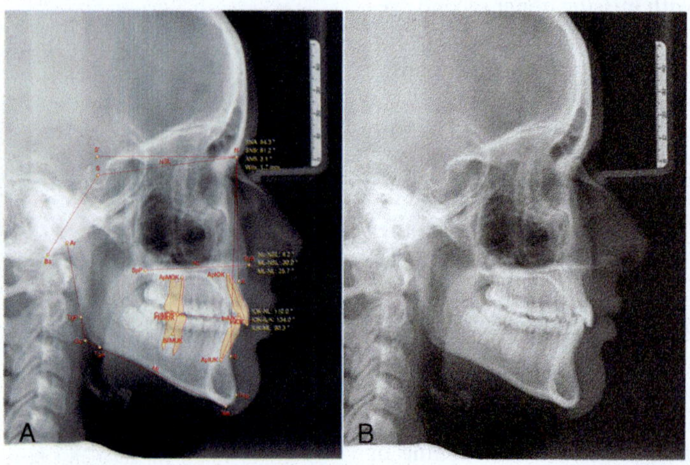

Figure 18-37 **A and B,** Radiographs of the patient with the missing upper lateral incisor.

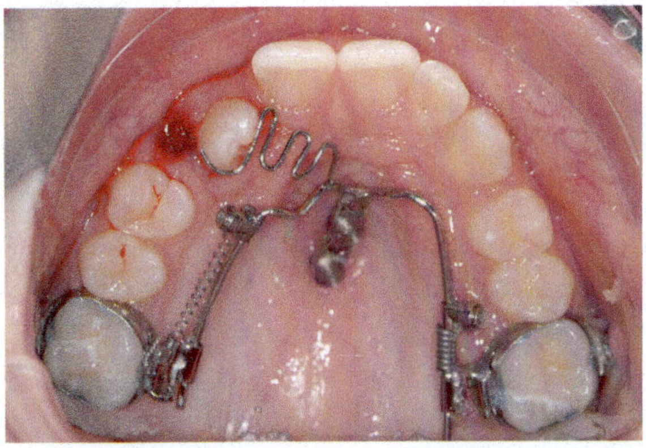

Figure 18-38 Mesialslider, with an additional spring, is used to move the upper right canine buccally.

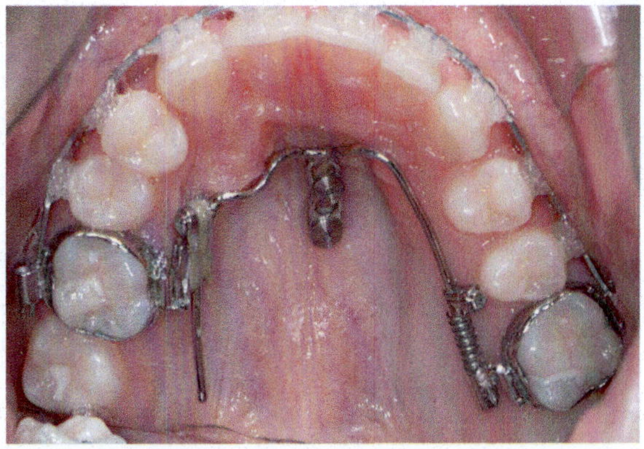

Figure 18-39 The intraoral situation after 16 months. The spaces in the first quadrant are closed on the mesialization side. Many small spaces were established on the distalization side.

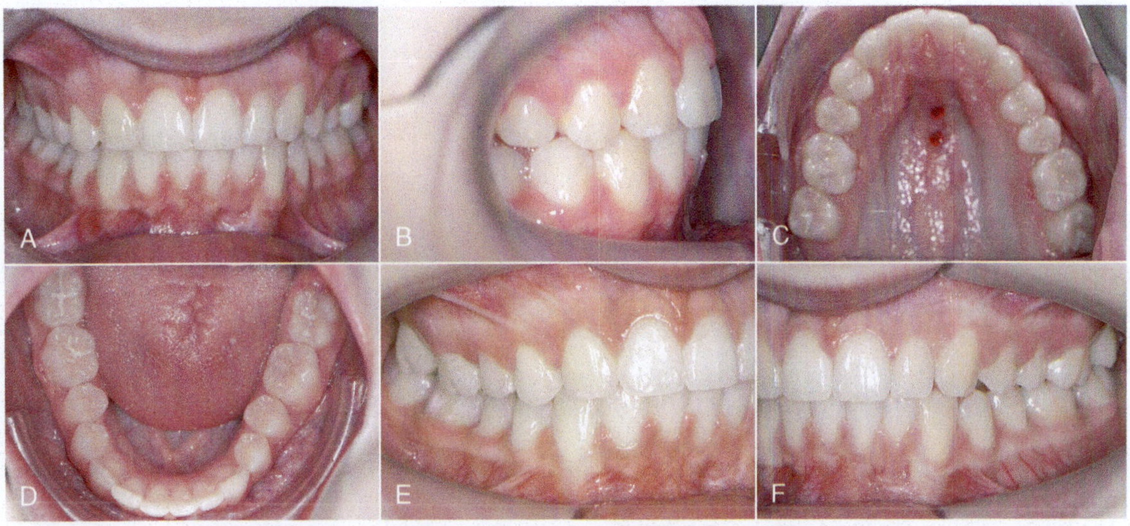

Figure 18-40 **A–F,** Debonding and reshaping of the canine were performed after a total treatment time of 24 months.

the deciduous canine a Mesial-Distal-Slider was installed and activated. To reduce the time in full braces, an additional spring was soldered to push the canine buccally (Fig. 18-38). After 8 months, brackets were bonded. The spaces in the first quadrant were closed on the mesialization side after 16 months and many small spaces were established on the distalization side (Fig. 18-39). Debonding and reshaping of the canine was performed after a total treatment time of 24 months (Fig. 18-40).

EN MASSE RETRACTION

Clinical Considerations for Maximum Anchorage of the Molars

Conventional appliances designed to provide molar anchorage are the headgear, Class II elastics, the transpalatal arch (TPA), the Nance button, and the incorporation of additional bends in the archwire such as tip-back and buccal root torque. However, these anchorage mechanics are limited in their efficiency, which depends in part on patient compliance.[55,56] A mean of 1.6 to 4 mm anchorage loss can be anticipated during conventional anchorage.[57,58] As a consequence, mini-implants prove to be very useful if the molar mesial migration should be avoided during en masse retraction.[57] To avoid the risk of root damage and mini-implant fracture and the high failure rate of mini-implants in the alveolar process, bigger mini-implants in the anterior palate instead of small mini-implants between the second bicuspids and the first molars seems advantageous.[59] It is feasible to anchor the molars with a Beneslider appliance (Fig. 18-41). To establish this posterior anchorage, the Beneslider is left in place and deactivated by two steel ligatures after distalization for molar anchorage during anterior retraction.

The second alternative is to adapt a Beneplate or similar abutment with a 1.1-mm stainless steel wire in place and bond it to the lingual surfaces of the molars (Fig. 18-42). However, these two mechanics tend to expand the molars if they are loaded with the force delivered for the en masse retraction. To avoid side effects in the transverse dimension, the author found it advisable to carry out corresponding additional posterior transversal reinforcement, resulting in the Triangle-TPA.

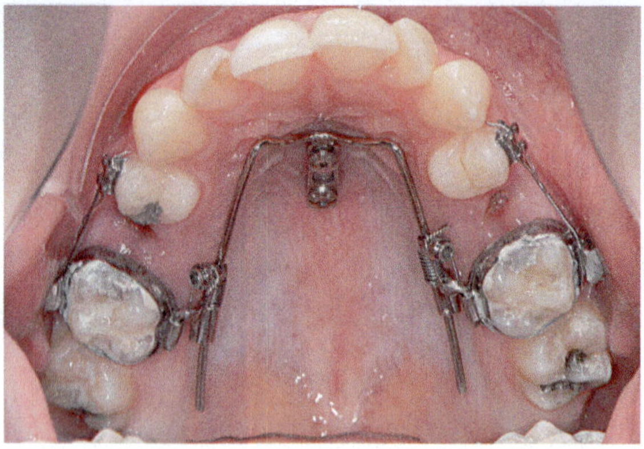

Figure 18-41 Beneslider is deactivated by two steel ligatures. This procedure allows it to serve as a molar anchorage device during front retraction. If indicated, the mechanics could be easily transformed into distalization mechanics by cutting the steel ligatures unilaterally or bilaterally.

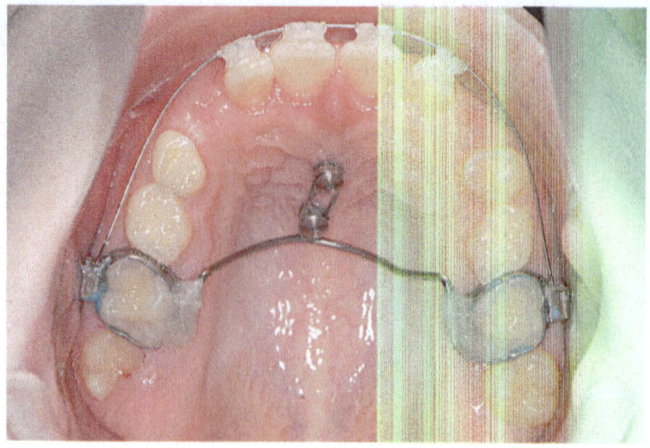

Figure 18-42 Molar anchorage via a Beneplate with a 1.1-mm stainless steel wire in place. The wire is bonded to the lingual surfaces of the molars.

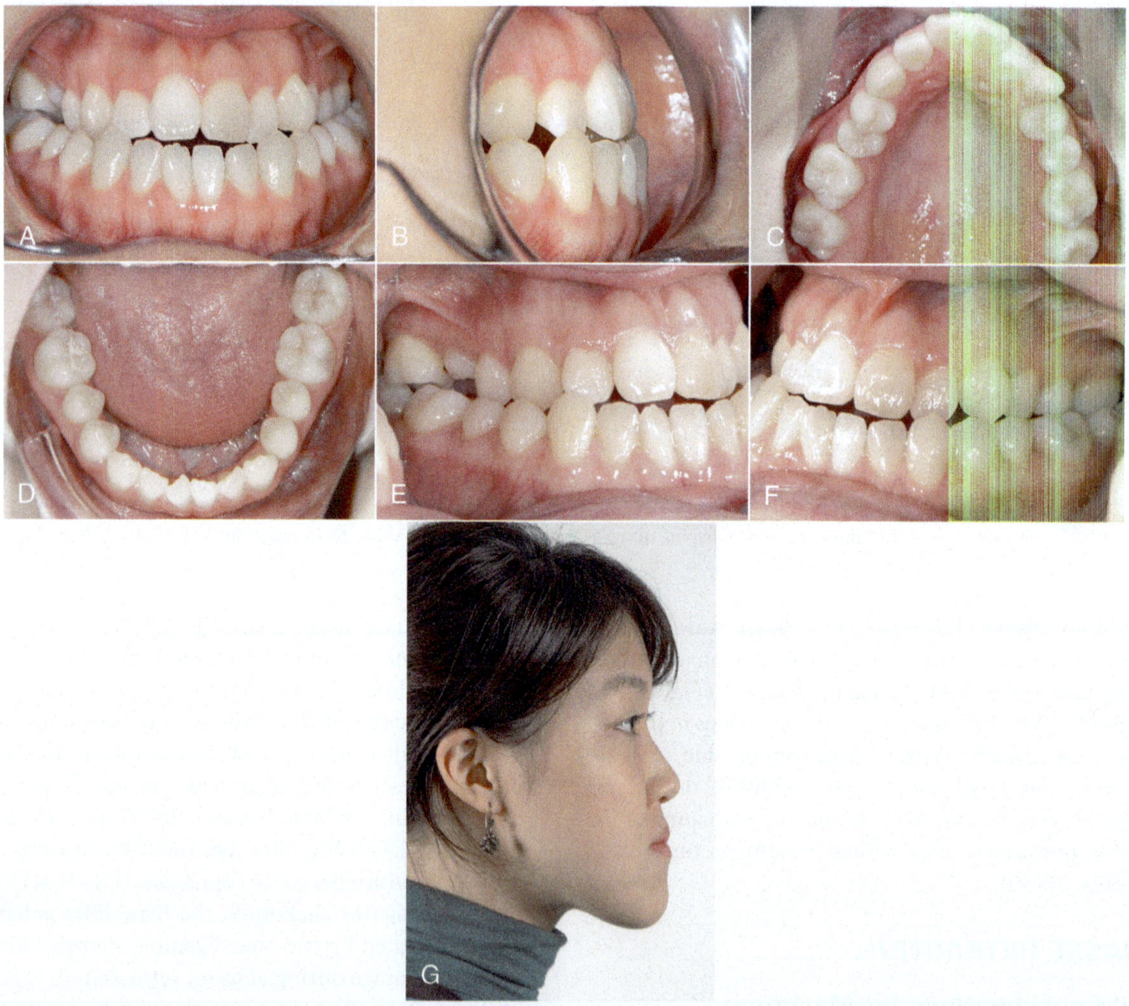

Figure 18-43 **A–F**, Intraoral photographs and (**G**) a profile view of an 18-year-old female patient with a severe skeletal Class III malocclusion.

Clinical Example Using the Triangle-TPA for Upper Molar Anchorage

The treatment protocol for an 18-year-old female patient with a severe skeletal Class III malocclusion is shown (Figs. 18-43 and 18-44). The goal was dentoalveolar decompensation in terms of retrusion of the upper incisors and protrusion of the lower incisors ahead of bimaxillary osteotomy. To facilitate upper front retrusion, distalization of the molars or extraction must be done. In this case, two premolars were extracted due to a dysplastic upper right second bicuspid. After insertion of one Benefit mini-implant (2.3 mm × 11 mm) the Triangle-TPA was manufactured on a plaster

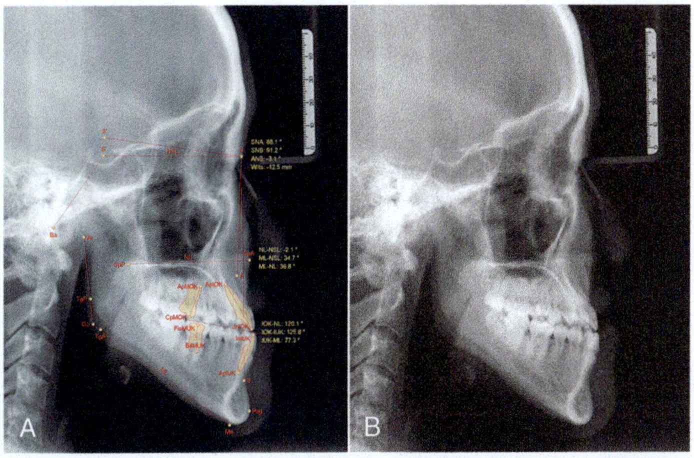

Figure 18-44 **A and B,** The cephalograms show a severe skeletal class III with much compensation (protrusion of the upper front teeth, retrusion of the lower front teeth).

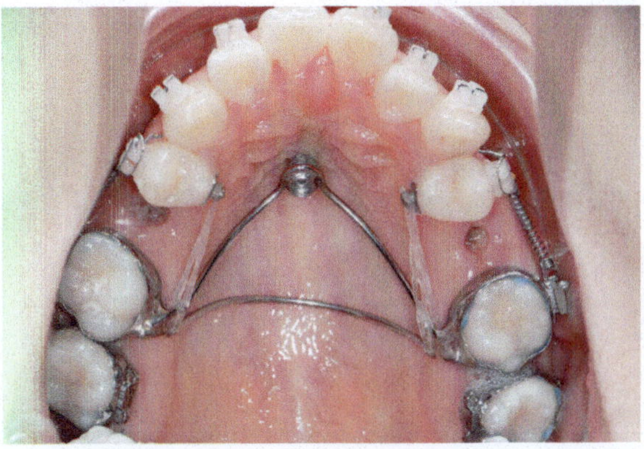

Figure 18-45 The start of front retraction, after fixation of the Triangle-TPA and extraction of the second premolars.

model. The abutment with a wire in place and an additional posterior stainless steel wire were soldered to the molar bands. After fixation of the Triangle-TPA the second premolars were extracted and retraction of the first premolars was initiated (Fig. 18-45). A cephalogram was made after closure of half of the extraction space (Fig. 18-46). After 14 months the en masse retraction was achieved without mesial migration of the molars, resulting in a sufficient negative overjet (Fig. 18-47). After bimaxillary osteotomy (Fig. 18-48), the last steps in terms of finishing of the occlusion and debonding were conducted (Fig. 18-49). Due to the large amount of decompensation that was enabled by the skeletal anchorage, an enormous improvement of the profile was obtained (see Fig. 18-49, G).

ALIGNMENT OF IMPACTED TEETH

Principle: Direct versus Indirect Anchorage

Dystopic and impacted teeth are frequent clinical findings. Epidemiological studies report an incidence of impacted teeth of up to 39% for the lower third molars, 0.92% to 3% for the upper canines, and 0.2% for the upper central incisors.[60,61] The treatment of impacted teeth usually comprises three phases: (1) surgical exposure and bonding of an attachment, (2) eruption of the impacted tooth by application of an extrusive force, and (3) three-dimensional orthodontic alignment.[62] The force needed to extrude an impacted tooth very often produces side effects on the dentition.[63] Intrusion of the adjacent teeth or even a cant of the occlusal plane may be encountered. Consequently, stable anchorage is essential to minimize the stated side effects. Adjustment of the line of force during the extrusion phase is crucial to prevent root damage. Depending on the anchorage needed, standard constructions providing either direct or indirect anchorage are indicated. In indirect anchorage mechanics the TAD immobilizes one tooth or some teeth to prevent side effects during extrusion of an impacted tooth, while in direct anchorage mechanics the force is applied on the TAD only.[64] Clinically, we notice a slightly lower failure rate when employing the indirect anchorage mechanics due to its higher resistance against jiggling by the tongue and fingers.

Indirect Anchorage Mechanics for Alignment of Impacted Teeth

By employing indirect anchorage mechanics, unwanted side effects such as tipping of teeth used for anchorage for extrusion of impacted teeth should be avoided. Depending on the requirements of the particular situation, the mechanics for distalization, mesialization, and molar anchorage described earlier can be used to avoid unwanted side effects on the molars. This principle can be applied when the molars are being used as an anchorage unit for extrusion of incisors or canines. Figure 18-50 shows a 10-year-old female patient with a horizontally impacted upper left central incisor. After surgical exposure, a Beneslider with an additional soldered tube was installed and a 0.016-inch × 0.022-inch β-Titanium segmental archwire was inserted in the tube. After 3 months the incisor erupted successfully (Fig. 18-51). After 6 months the incisor was almost fully erupted and the bracket was removed (Fig. 18-52). After 8 months the incisor was at its final position; the molars were distalized to gain enough space in the upper arch (Fig. 18-53).

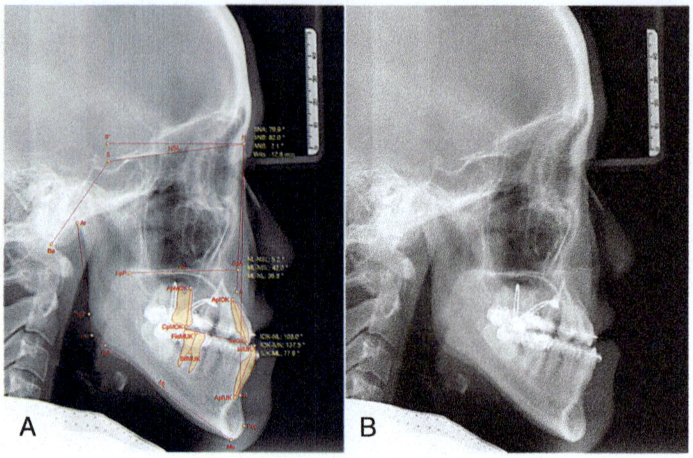

Figure 18-46 **A and B,** Radiographs after half of the retraction of the front teeth.

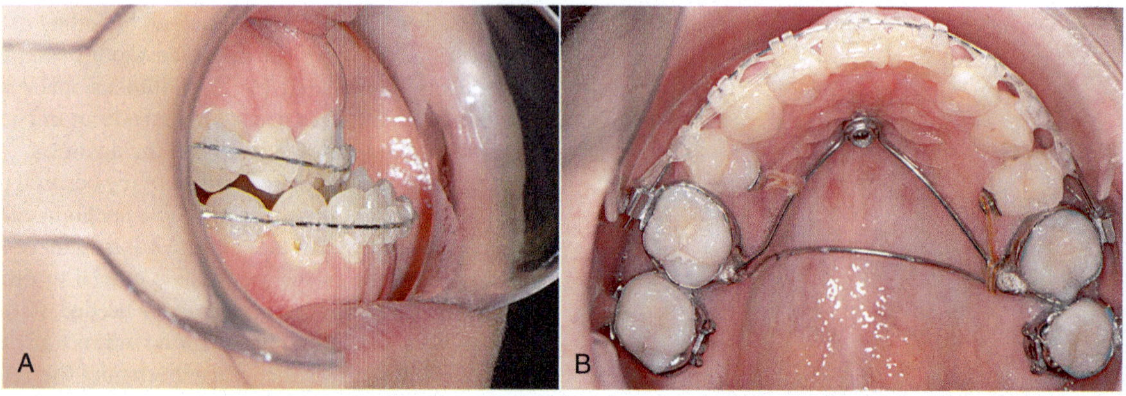

Figure 18-47 **A and B,** After 14 months, en masse retraction was achieved without mesial migration of the molars, resulting in a sufficient negative overjet.

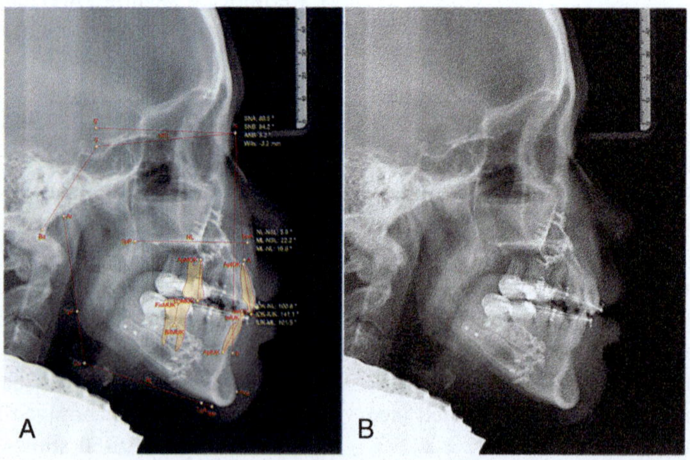

Figure 18-48 **A and B,** Radiographs obtained after bimaxillary osteotomy.

Direct Anchorage Mechanics for Alignment of Impacted Teeth

Especially if molars are impacted, direct anchorage mechanics is appropriate to extrude them. In this case, the alignment of an impacted upper second left molar is shown (Fig. 18-54). After insertion of two Benefit mini-implants (Fig. 18-55, A) and bonding of an attachment to the second molar, a Beneplate with a 0.8-mm stainless steel wire in place is adapted to the curvature of the palate. One side of the wire is activated as an extrusion lever arm; the other side

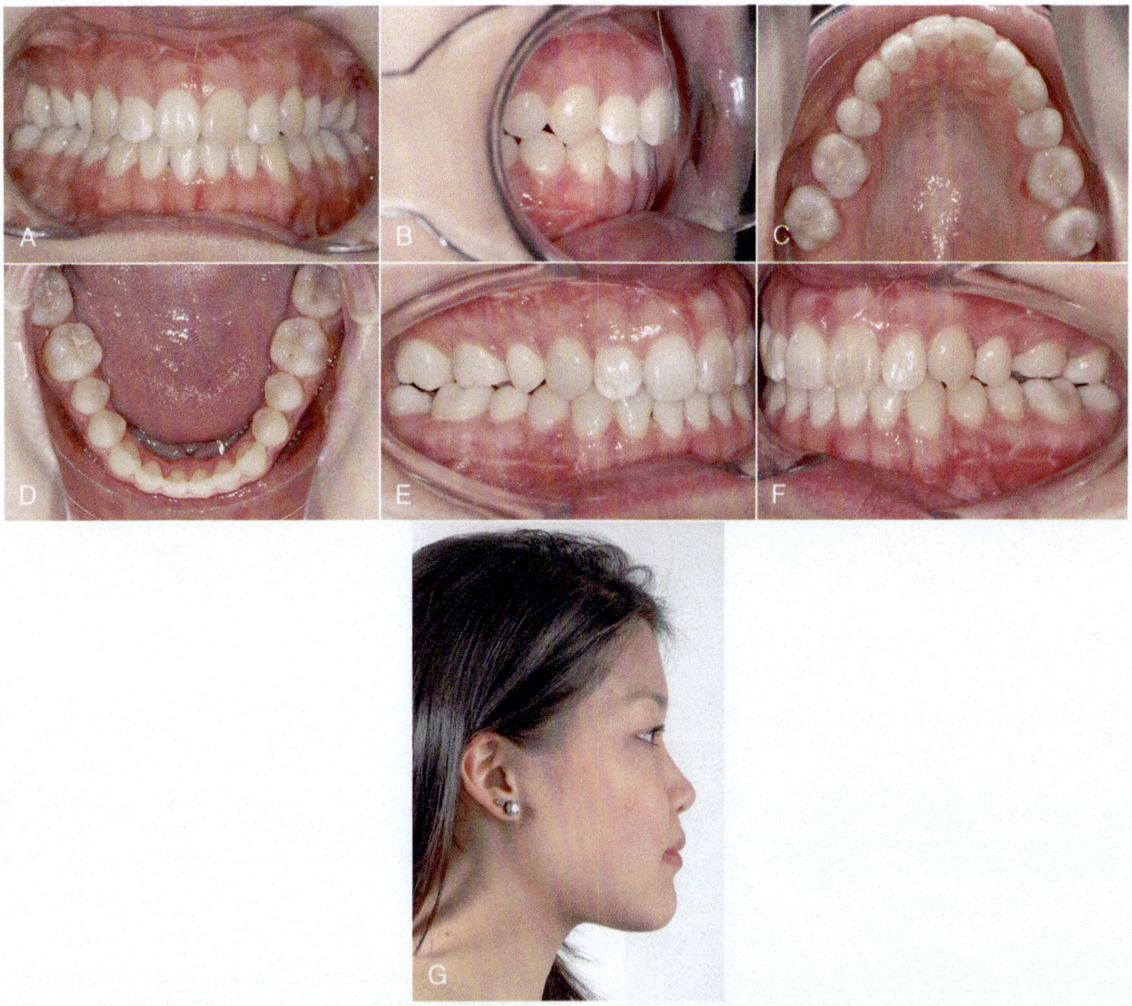

Figure 18-49 **A–F,** Intraoral views and **(G)** a profile view of the patient after debonding. Note the significant improvement in the patient's profile.

of the wire is cut (Fig. 18-55, B). The molar was fully erupted after 4 months (Fig. 18-55, C) and the attachment was removed (Fig. 18-55, D).

PREPROSTHODONTIC MECHANICS FOR MOLAR INTRUSION

Molar Intrusion with the Mousetrap Mechanics

Overerupted upper molars due to missing lower antagonists are a common finding, especially in adult patients. To facilitate prosthodontic restoration in the mandible, these overerupted molars must be intruded. However, molar intrusion is a difficult orthodontic treatment task, since there is a tendency of the teeth adjacent to the molars to be extruded when using conventional appliances. In recent years TADs have been integrated into various molar intrusion mechanics to overcome these side effects and to avoid an unesthetic full-appliance therapy.[3,65–69] To avoid tipping of the molars that are to be intruded, forces must be applied both buccally and lingually. If the intrusive force is applied only at one side, a TPA can be inserted to avoid buccal or palatal tipping. Mini-plates inserted in the area of the zygomatic buttress can be employed to apply a buccal intrusive force for upper molar intrusion.[67,68,70–72] However, surgical placement of the titanium plate requires a surgical flap and full exposure of the bone. Insertion of mini-implants with greater dimensions in the zygomatic buttress is a second but less recommended alternative since the insertion site is covered by movable mucosa. Drawbacks of mini-implant insertion in movable mucosa are the higher failure rate of the screws and soft tissue irritations causing discomfort and pain.[8,15]

A third alternative is to insert a couple of mini-implants in the alveolar process.[65,66,69,73] However, there are some disadvantages regarding the insertion between the roots of the upper molars:

- In many cases there is not enough space on the buccal side to insert a mini-implant safely between the roots, especially in the region of the upper molars.[74–76]
- On the palatal side of the alveolar process the soft tissue often happens to be very thick.[29] This results in a long lever arm and a very high risk of mini-implant tipping and failure.[16]
- If the mini-implant comes into contact with a root, periodontal structures may be damaged and the risk of failure of the mini-implant will be higher.[10,20]

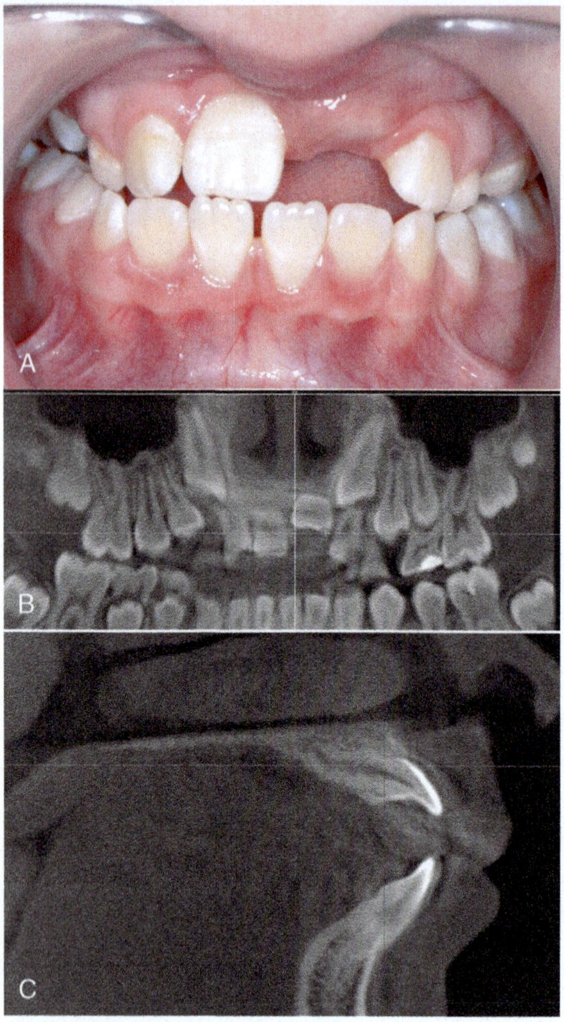

Figure 18-50 **A,** Intraoral view and **(B and C)** radiographs of a 10-year-old female patient with a horizontally impacted upper left central incisor.

- Since on the buccal side the available space between the roots of the upper molars is usually very small, only mini-implants with a small diameter can be inserted in the alveolar process. However, small implant diameters also mean a higher risk of fracture[77] and a higher risk of failure.[9,15,16]
- The intrusion may be stopped and the root surface may be damaged when the molar is moved against a mini-implant during intrusion.[78,79]
- There is a risk of penetration of the maxillary sinus when a mini-implant is inserted in the posterior area of the upper alveolar process.[80]

As a consequence, it seems to be a good strategy to insert the mini-implants away from the roots. With the anterior palate as the insertion site, mini-implants with larger dimensions and a higher stability[17,81] can be inserted in this region, which has high bone quality, thin soft tissues, and minimal risk of interference with teeth or root damage.[29]

The Mousetrap appliance[82] comprises one or two lever arms connected to two Benefit mini-implants inserted in the

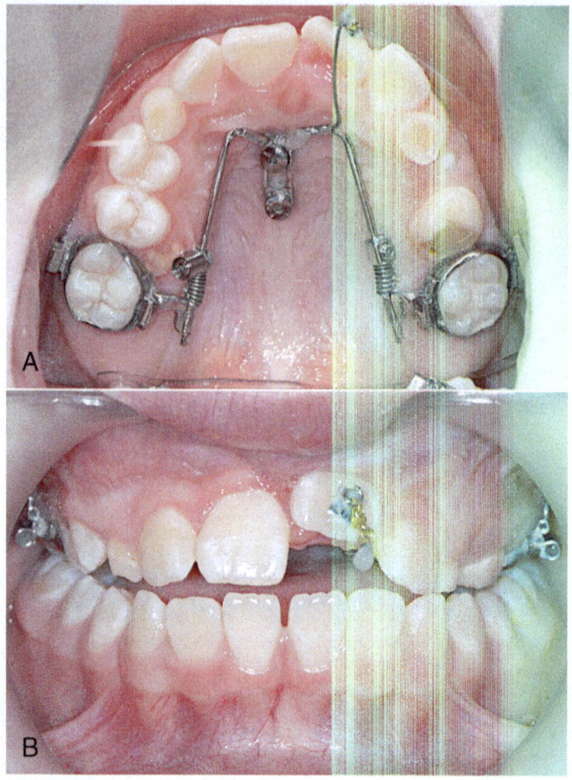

Figure 18-51 **A,** The situation after 3 months; the Beneslider in place with an additional soldered tube and a 0.016-inch × 0.022-inch β-Titanium segmental lever arm for extrusion of the incisor. **B,** The incisor after eruption.

anterior palate, depending on the need for either unilateral or bilateral molar intrusion. In the deactivated state the distal ends of the lever arms are located apically to the center of resistance of the molars. Activation of the lever arms occlusally and engaging them to the molars produces a significant, constant intrusive force. By using a skeletally anchored lever arm, an intrusive force of approximately 100 g is applied palatally to the molar. Due to the point of force application, palatal tipping can be significant and should be controlled with the use of a TPA.

There are two different options to construct the palatal lever arm for molar intrusion:

1. A Beneplate with a bracket in place is used (see Fig. 18-3, C). Afterwards, a 0.017-inch × 0.025-inch stainless steel lever arm is bent and ligated to the bracket of the Beneplate.
2. A Beneplate with a 0.8-mm stainless steel wire in place (see Fig. 18-3, B) is adapted to the curvature of the palate.

In the posterior region, the intrusive force can be applied using two different approaches:

1. Using a steel ligature
2. Soldering a hook on the TPA that is used as a stop for the lever arm

The Mousetrap is a reliable appliance for the intrusion of overerupted molars. At first glance its sophisticated design appears to be more complex and a bit more bulky compared

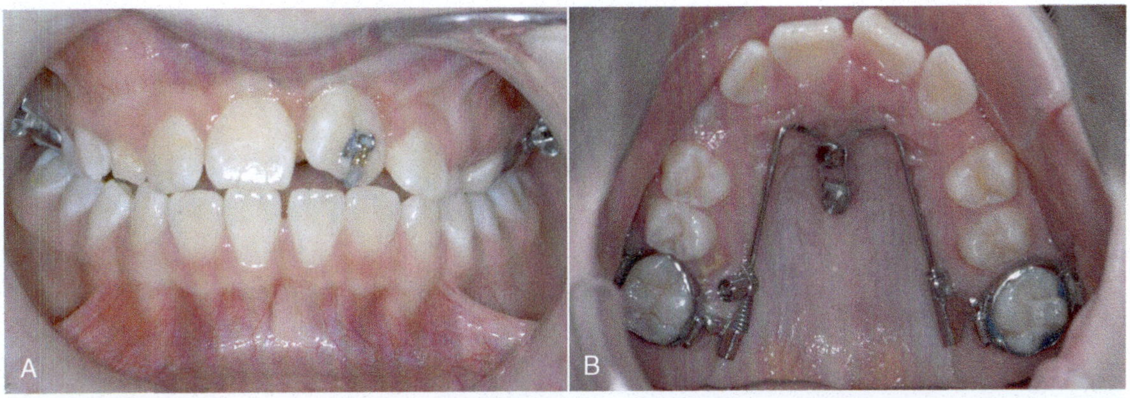

Figure 18-52 **A,** After 6 months the incisor was almost fully erupted and (**B**) the bracket was removed.

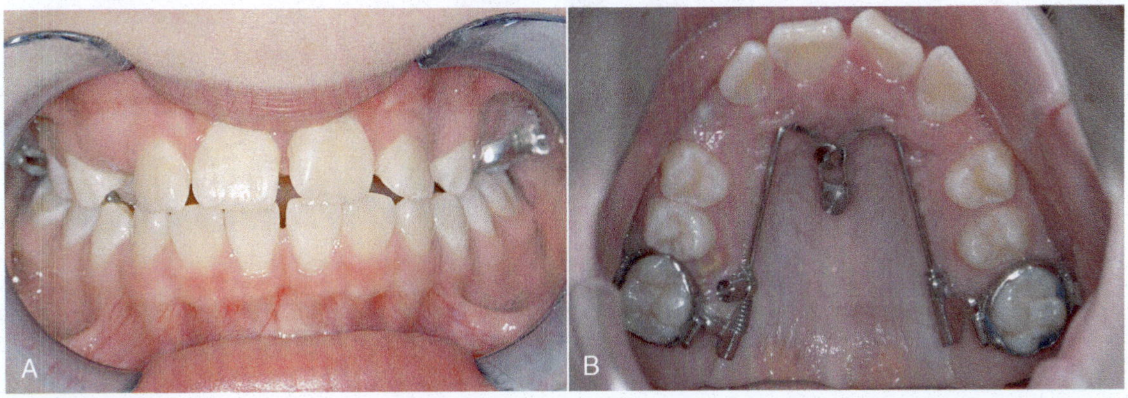

Figure 18-53 **A and B,** After 8 months the incisor was at its final position. The molars were distalized to gain enough space in the upper arch.

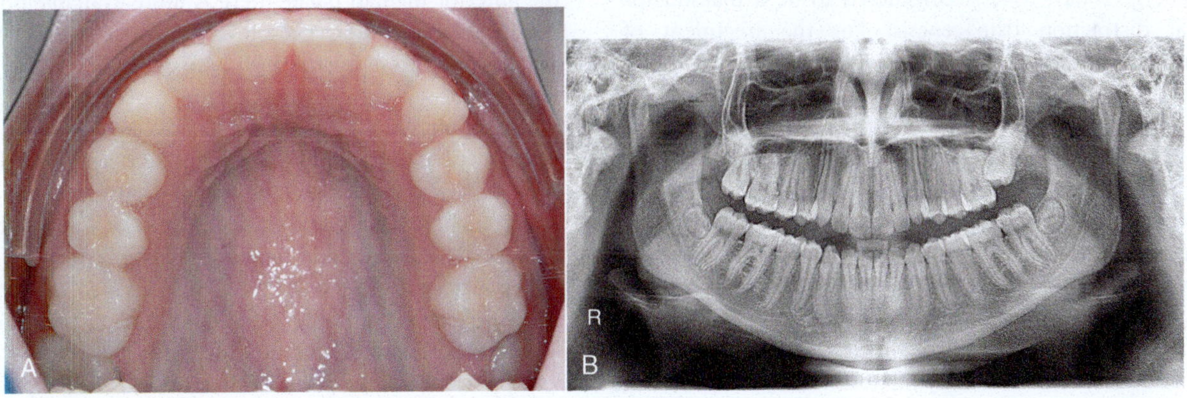

Figure 18-54 **A,** Intraoral view and (**B**) orthopantomogram of a 14-year-old female patient with an impacted upper left second molar.

to other TAD-based appliances. Nevertheless, it provides the following advantages:

- Low surgical invasiveness
- No risk of penetration of the maxillary sinus
- No risk of root damage at the time of insertion of the mini-implant or during molar intrusion
- TADs can be inserted in an optimum insertion site; the anterior palate ensures low failure rates and no risk of mini-implant fracture
- Constant force delivery that is easy to measure and adjust intraorally

RAPID PALATAL EXPANSION AND EARLY CLASS III TREATMENT

Rationale for Using Mini-Implant–Supported Rapid Palatal Expansion

Rapid palatal expansion (RPE) is considered the first orthodontic procedure to achieve skeletal widening of the maxilla. However, Angell's[83] first description in 1860 received comprehensive disapproval at that time due to the lack of radiological confirmation, which was achieved in 1908 by

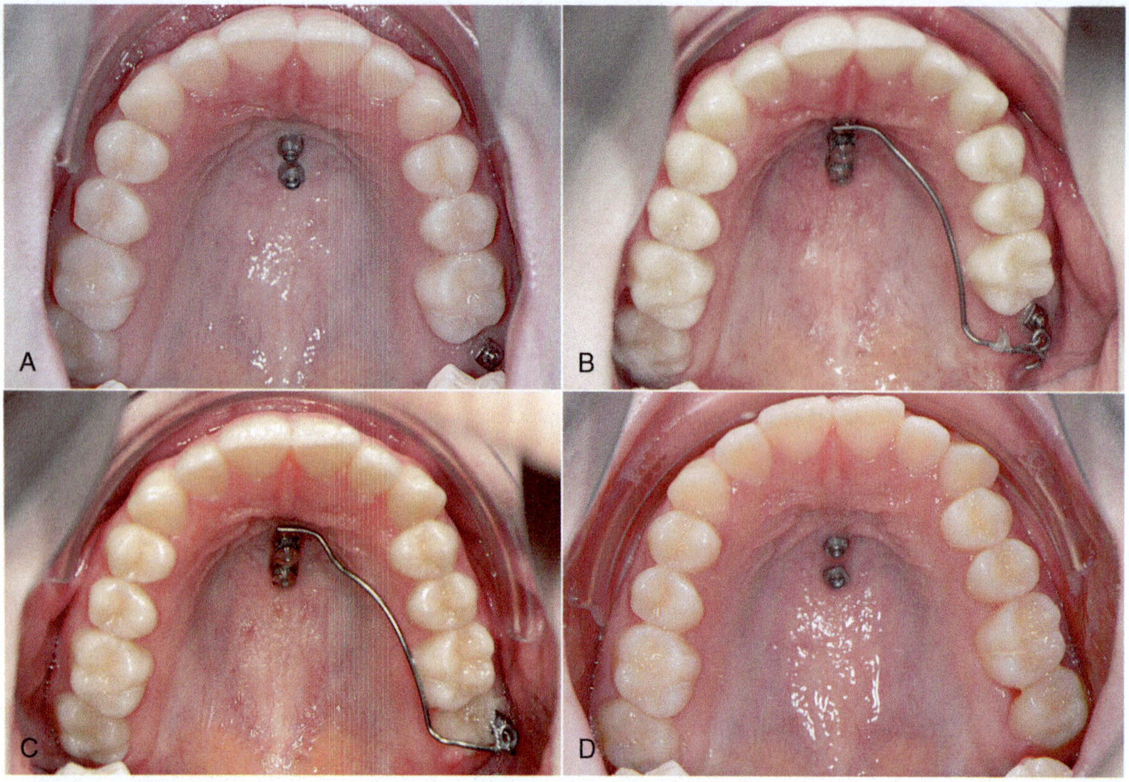

Figure 18-55 **A,** Insertion of two Benefit mini-implants. **B,** A Beneplate with a 0.8-mm stainless steel wire in place that has been adapted to the curvature of the palate. One side of the wire is activated as an extrusion lever arm and the other side of the wire is cut. **C,** Eruption of the molar after 4 months. **D,** After removal of the attachment.

Landsberg. Today, RPE is considered to be a method for sutural distraction osteogenesis. For the treatment of patients with a Class III malocclusion caused by a retrognathic maxilla, RPE is combined with a facemask for protraction of the maxilla. Since the orthopedic forces are transmitted to the skeletal structures via the anchor teeth, distribution of the forces to as many teeth as possible as well as completion of root formation are considered essential. However, in addition to the therapeutically intended skeletal expansion, side effects such as buccal tipping of the anchor teeth, fenestration of the buccal bone, root resorptions, and gingiva recessions were reported in some cases.[84,85] To avoid these complications caused by the tooth-borne character of the conventional appliances, some authors reported about pure bone-borne RPE devices. Several palatal distractors have been presented over the last decade.[86,87] However, insertion and removal of these mini-plate–borne distractors can require invasive surgical procedures with the need for a flap preparation and risk of root lesions and infections.[86,88] As a consequence, distractors of this type could not establish themselves as standard devices for RPE. To minimize the surgical procedure, Harzer introduced the Dresden Distractor, which is borne solely on an implant and a mini-implant.[89–91] Due to the risk of a root lesion at insertion of implants in the lateral posterior alveolar process and lack of available bone in the posterior palate (see Fig. 18-4), the author used the first molars as a posterior anchorage unit. In the anterior median palate there is more available bone for mini-implants[92] and the resulting appliance is a half tooth-borne, half bone-borne RPE device called the Hybrid Hyrax.[3,47,49,93–95]

The application of the Hybrid Hyrax is minimally surgically invasive compared with pure bone-borne RPE devices such as distractors.[86,87,94] Employing the first molars as a posterior anchorage unit and mini-implants as a skeletal anterior anchorage unit provides several advantages:[93–95]

- Applicable in cases with limited anterior dental anchorage quality due to missing deciduous molars or deciduous molar with short roots.
- Applicable in cases with immature root development of the premolars.
- No risk of impairment of root development (curved roots).
- Reduction of the dental side effects (i.e., premolar tipping).[94]
- Anterior dentition is not bonded during the retention phase and thus regular orthodontic treatment can be started earlier.
- Advantageous in cases with a need for early Class III treatment, where the RPE supports maxillary advancement by weakening the midface sutures.
- Avoidance of mesial migration of the upper dentition during application of a facemask or the Mentoplate,[93] thus enhancing the skeletal effects.[94]

Hybrid Hyrax in Early Class III Treatment

Skeletal Class III malocclusions are relatively infrequent and their genesis is usually associated with genetic factors.[96,97] The Class III relationship may be caused by a retrognathic maxilla, a prognathic mandible, or both.[96,97] Treatment of young Class III patients with maxillary deficiency is mostly conducted with a facemask. Since the force is applied to the teeth, mesial migration of the dentition is inevitable and may result in severe anterior crowding.[98] On the other hand, the desired skeletal effect of this commonly used approach often turns out to be less than expected.[98] To overcome these drawbacks and to minimize mesial migration of the molars, sagittal skeletal support by the Hybrid Hyrax is very useful. Second, to facilitate the advancement of the maxilla, opening of the midface sutures by RPE is recommended.[99] With the goal being to avoid an extraoral device (facemask) and to apply the forces directly to the skeletal structures, De Clerck introduced the use of four mini-plates (two anterior in the lower jaw and two posterior in the upper jaw) in combination with Class III elastics.[100] This represents a new purely skeletal approach to correct the skeletal discrepancy. To enhance the skeletal effect by opening the midface sutures, the author employs the Hybrid Hyrax appliance in the upper jaw, allowing simultaneous rapid maxillary expansion and skeletally borne maxillary protraction. In the lower jaw the Bollard mini-plates by De Clerck are usually inserted after eruption of the canines. To allow earlier insertion of the mini-plate in the mandible, Dr. Drescher developed the Mentoplate.[93] Since the Mentoplate is inserted subapically to the lower incisors, it typically can be used as early as age 8 to 9 years. By means of the Hybrid Hyrax in combination with a facemask or a Mentoplate, forces are applied to skeletal structures only with the goal of achieving an optimum skeletal effect (Figs. 18-56 and 18-57).

Clinical Procedure Using the Hybrid Hyrax

After topical anesthesia, two Benefit mini-implants (2 mm × 9 mm or 2 mm × 7 mm) are inserted in transversal orientation (see Fig. 18-10, B). At the same appointment, bands are fitted to the upper first molars or second deciduous molar. After application of impression caps (see Fig. 18-12), an impression is taken using silicone. In cases where the distance between the mini-implants is too small, the impression caps are cut to fit side-by-side. After the impression is taken, the laboratory analogs are placed on the transfer caps (see Fig. 18-12, F). Positioning the bands in the impression results in a plaster model with the two bands and the two laboratory analogs in place. Afterwards, two standard abutments (see Fig. 18-2, D) are screwed on top of the laboratory analogs. Subsequently, a regular palatal spilt screw is connected by laser welding or soldering anteriorly with the two abutments and posteriorly with the molar bands (see Fig. 18-56, A). If maxillary protraction is desired, lateral hooks can be added (Fig. 18-58, A). Parallelism of the two mini-implants is advisable but even if the two mini-implants are not absolutely parallel, the appliance can be fitted on the implants.

The Hybrid Hyrax is inserted as soon as possible after insertion of the mini-implants by alternating screwing of the two abutments on the mini-implants followed by the final adjustment of the molar bands. During screwing the Hybrid Hyrax should be gently pressed to the mini-implants to facilitate the fixation. To allow enough time to install the Hybrid Hyrax, use of a light curing cement (Band-Lok,

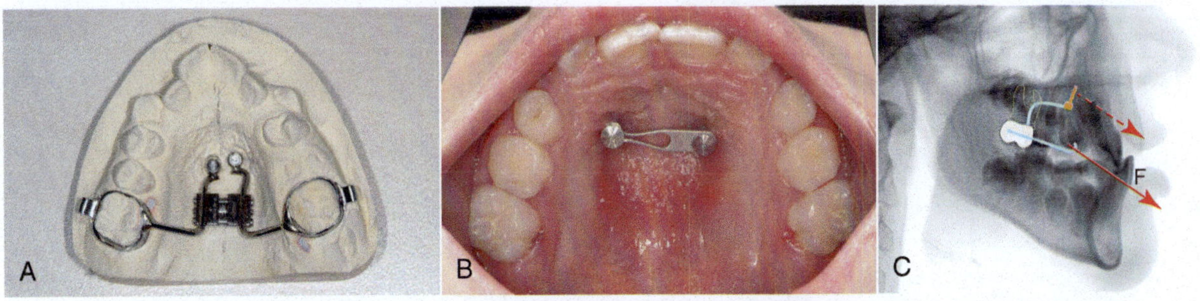

Figure 18-56 **A,** Plaster model with a Hybrid Hyrax. A regular palatal split screw is connected by laser welding with the two abutments anteriorly and with the molar bands posteriorly. **B,** A Beneplate used to establish skeletal retention after rapid palatal expansion. **C,** The rationale for using the Hybrid Hyrax-Facemask combination is that forces are transferred to the maxillary bone to avoid dental side effects.

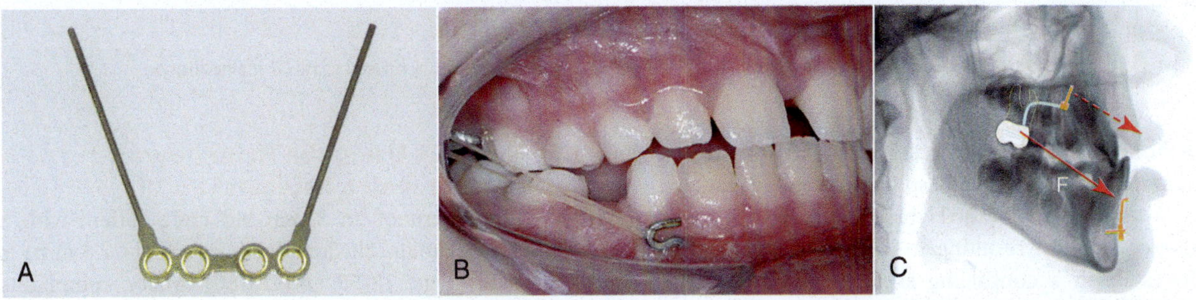

Figure 18-57 **A,** Mentoplate, which would be installed in the mental region. **B,** The extensions should penetrate the soft tissue in the region of attached mucosa. **C,** The rationale for using the Hybrid Hyrax–Mentoplate combination is that forces are transferred to skeletal structures to avoid dental side effects.

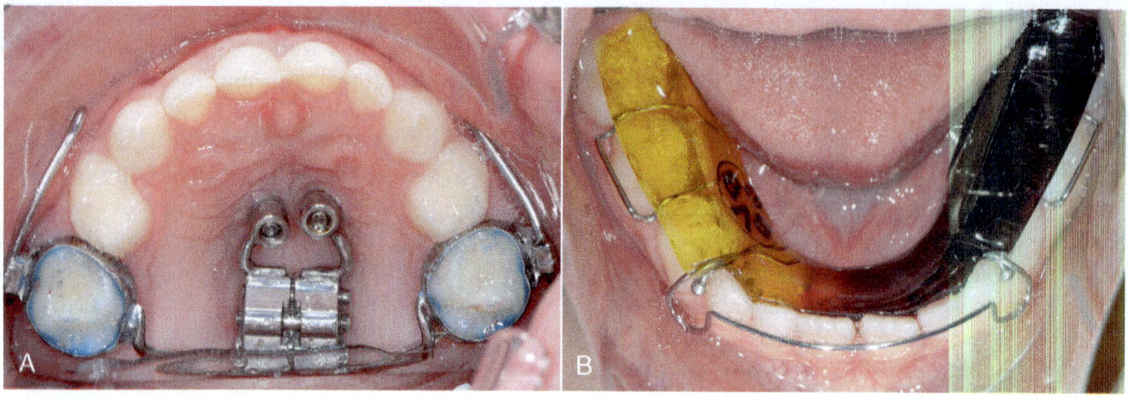

Figure 18-58 **A,** Hybrid Hyrax with two additional lateral wires for protraction with a facemask. **B,** A removable plate was made for the lower arch to facilitate the correction of the negative overjet.

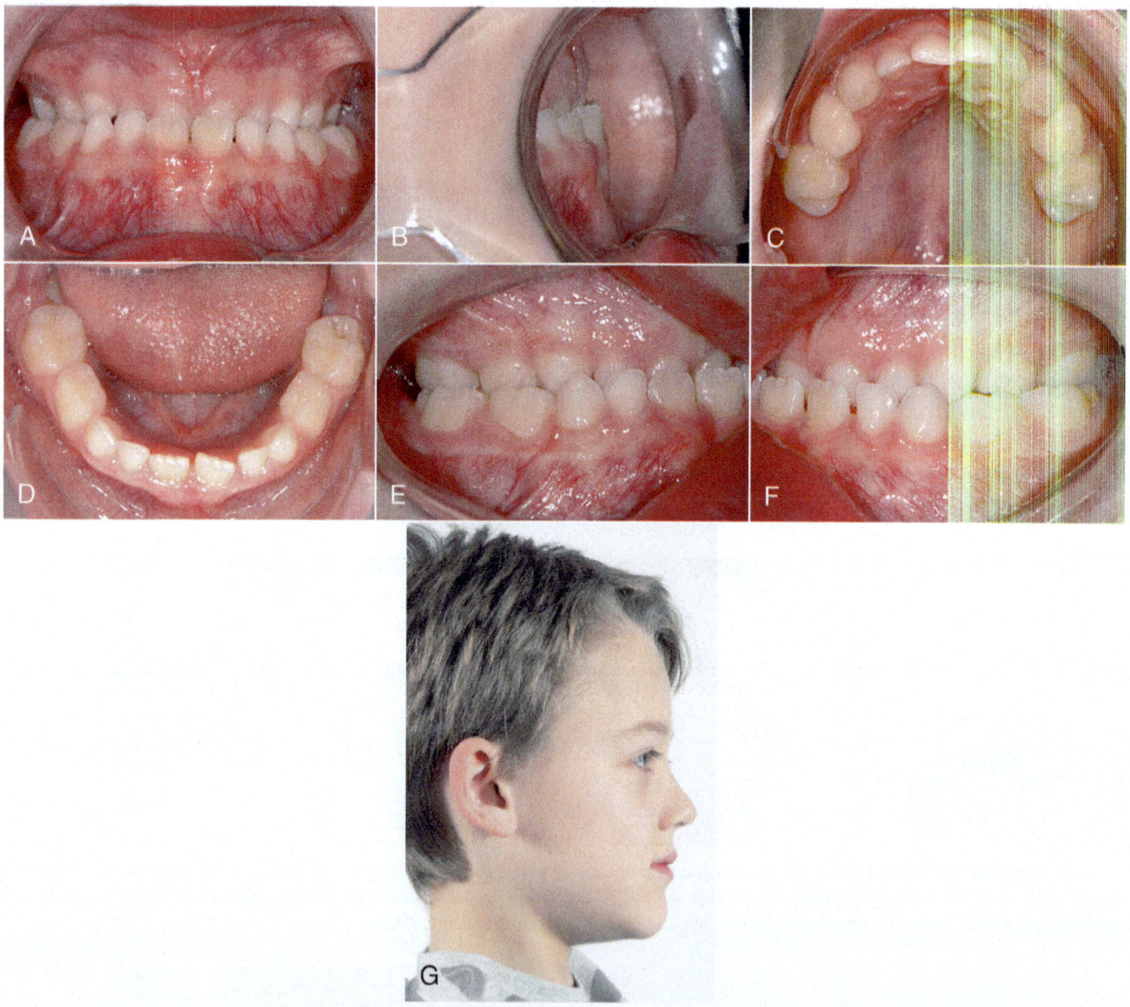

Figure 18-59 **A–F,** Intraoral and **(G)** profile views of an 8-year-old male patient with a skeletal Class III malocclusion.

Reliance Orthodontic Products, Itasca, IL.) is recommended for the molar bands. The sagittal split screw is activated immediately after insertion of the Hybrid Hyrax twice a day by a 180-degree rotation resulting in a daily activation of 0.8 mm. To establish a continuing skeletal retention, the insertion of a Beneplate preserving the distance between the two mini-implants seems advisable (Fig. 18-56, B).

Clinical Example Using the Hybrid Hyrax in Combination with a Facemask

The early treatment of an 8-year-old male patient with a skeletal Class III malocclusion (Wits appraisal −7.6 mm) is demonstrated (Figs. 18-59 and 18-60). Major complaints were the sagittal and transversal deficiency of the maxilla. Two Benefit mini-implants (2 mm × 7 mm) were inserted

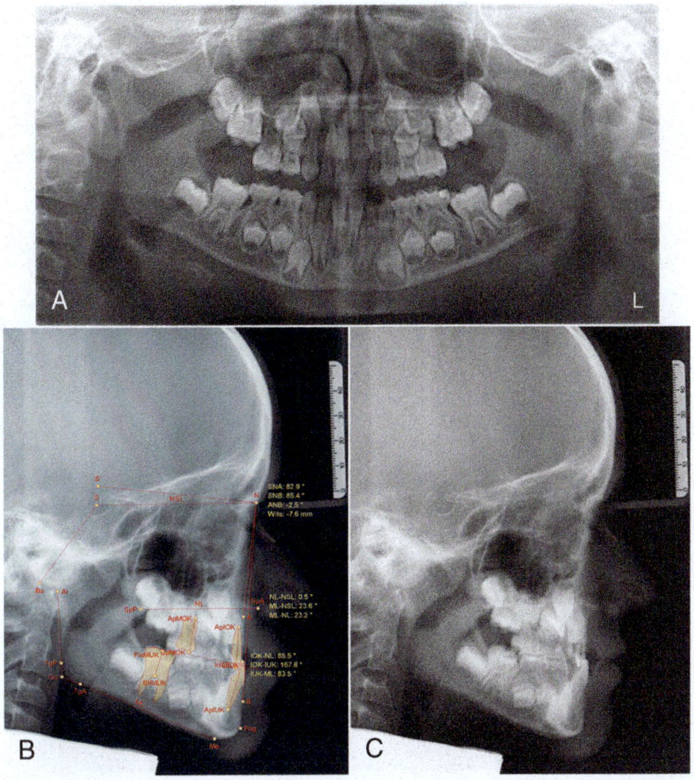

Figure 18-60 **A,** Panoramic and **(B and C)** cephalometric radiographs showing the patient's Class III malocclusion. The Wits appraisal is –7.6 mm.

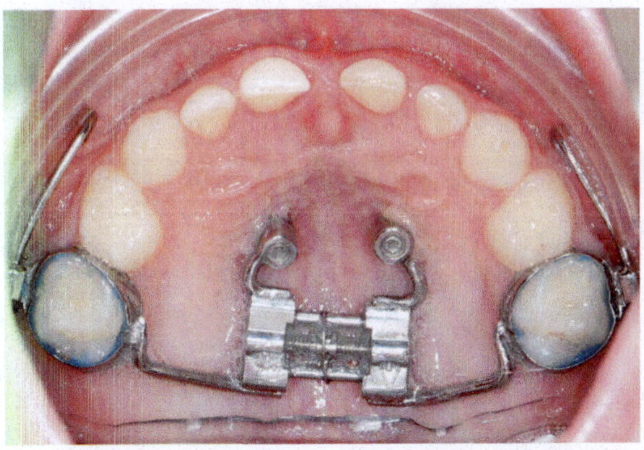

Figure 18-61 Intraoral view showing the situation after rapid palatal expansion.

after topical anesthesia. Predrilling was not performed due to the low mineralization of the bone in young patients. The Hybrid Hyrax with two additional lateral wires was manufactured in a laboratory and inserted after 4 days (see Fig. 18-58, A). RPE was started immediately in combination with application of a facemask. To facilitate the correction of the negative overjet, a removable plate was made for the lower arch (see Fig. 18-58, B). RPE was finished after 10 days (Fig. 18-61). After 5 months the Wits appraisal improved significantly to 0.1 mm (Fig. 18-62). This early treatment was finished after 11 months (Fig. 18-63).

As an alternative to the facemask, a purely intraoral treatment approach can be offered to patients by using the Mentoplate.

Introduction of the Mentoplate

The Mentoplate[93] is a titanium mini-plate (see Fig. 18-57, A) that is inserted in the mental region. After preparation of a mucoperiosteal flap, the two extensions are shortened and adapted. The extensions should penetrate the soft tissue in the region of attached mucosa (see Fig. 18-57, B). After fixation of the Mentoplate by four screws, the flap is flipped back and fixed by stitches. The Class III elastics (3.5 oz, 3/16 inch) are worn immediately after expansion of the maxilla for 24 hours per day.

Advantages of the Hybrid Hyrax–Mentoplate approach for early Class III treatment are:

1. Forces are applied directly to (Mentoplate) or are transferred to (Hybrid Hyrax) skeletal structures (see Fig. 18-57, C)
2. Almost invisible mechanics with no extraoral devices
3. The "RPE effect" with opening of midface sutures for easier maxillary protraction
4. Stable anchorage with a high reliability
5. Insertion before complete eruption of the lower canines is possible
6. Low surgical invasiveness
7. Upper and lower arches remain fully accessible for orthodontic corrections

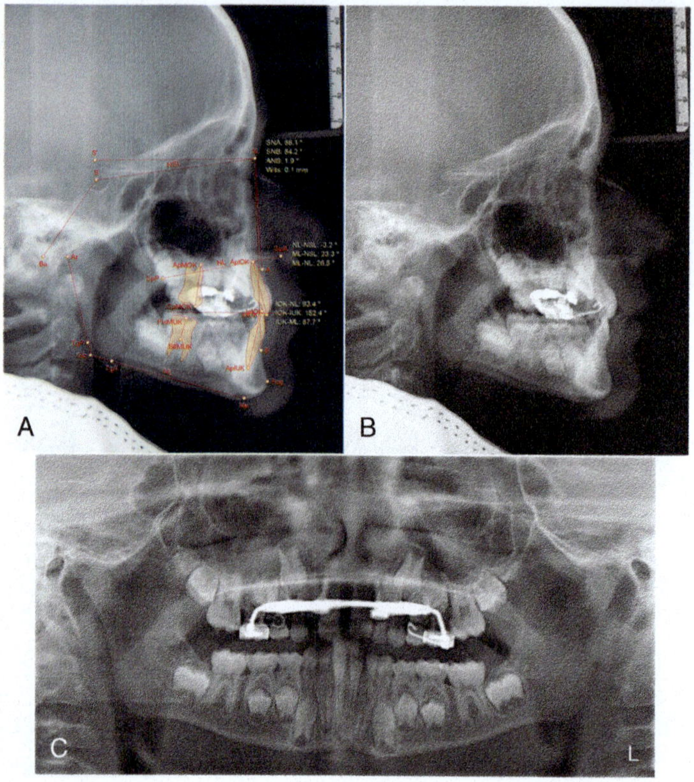

Figure 18-62 **A and B,** Cephalometric and **(C)** panoramic radiographs obtained after 5 months. The Wits appraisal improved significantly to 0.1 mm.

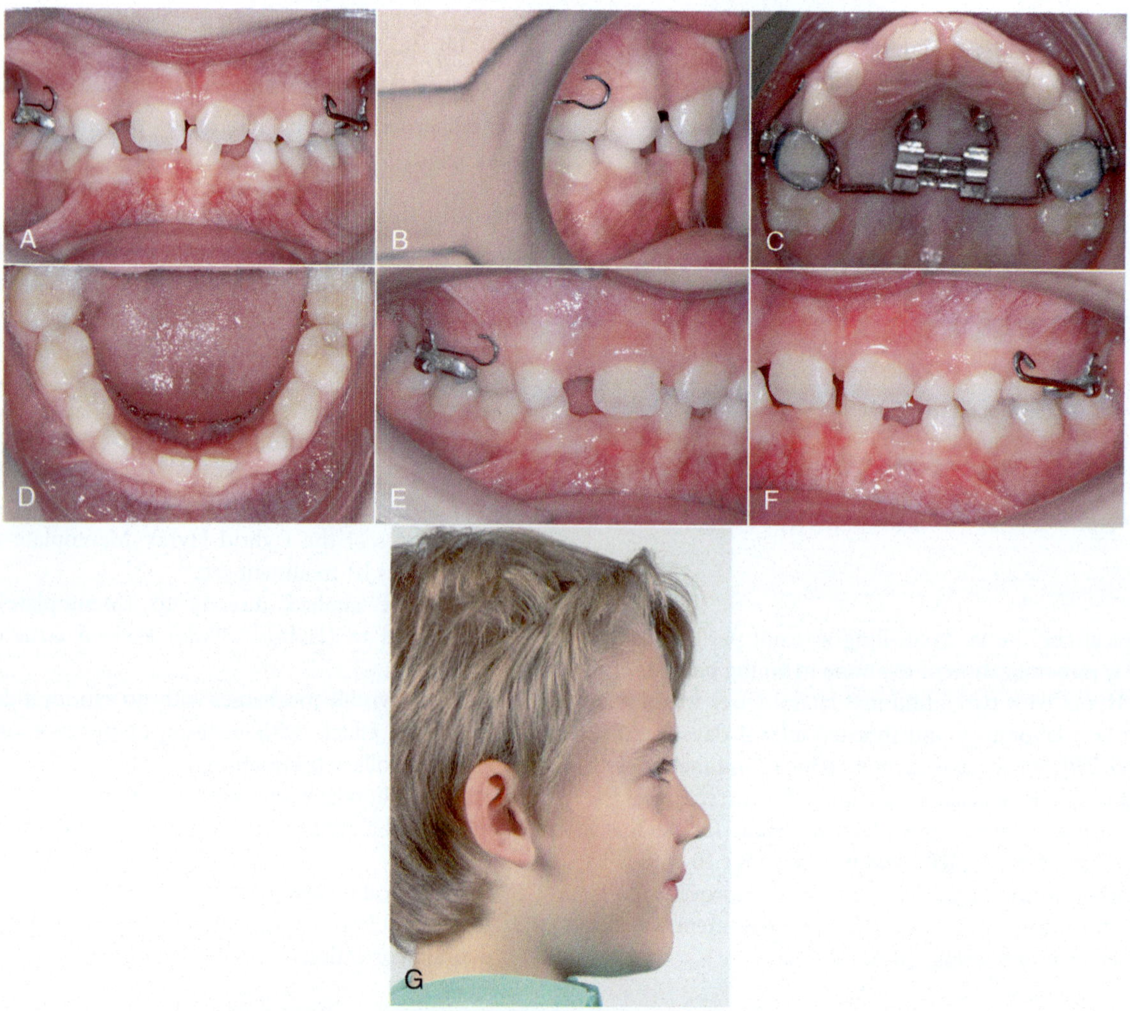

Figure 18-63 **A–F,** Intraoral and **(G)** profile views at the end of the early Class III treatment. Treatment time was 11 months.

The combination of the Hybrid Hyrax and the Mentoplate seems to be a very promising approach for early treatment of Class III patients.

Based on the author's clinical experiences, the Mentoplate has the potential to be used not only for orthopedic but also for orthodontics purposes (e.g., lower molar protraction), since the mini-implant failure rates in the alveolar process are still too high. As a consequence, the mental region seems to be the best site for skeletal anchorage in the mandible; it is the "anterior palate of the lower jaw."

Clinical Example Using the Hybrid Hyrax in Combination with a Mentoplate

The clinical example presents a 9-year-old girl with a skeletal class III malocclusion (Wits appraisal –6.7 mm; Figs. 18-64 and 18-65). Two Benefit mini-implants (2 mm × 7 mm) were inserted and an impression was taken to manufacture the Hybrid Hyrax (Fig. 18-66). Since the patient preferred an intraoral approach, the Hybrid Hyrax was combined with a Mentoplate instead of a facemask (Fig. 18-67). Afterwards, Class III elastics were applied. Due to a lack of space for the canines, the Hybrid Hyrax was removed after the early class III treatment (7 months) and a Beneslider was inserted for molar distalization in the upper arch. For this purpose the same mini-implants were used and a Beneplate with a wire at the long site was employed (Fig. 18-68, A). This multipurpose use is one of the advantages when mini-implants with exchangeable abutments are used.[101] Six months later a bodily distalization of the molars was recognizable (Fig. 18-68, B and C). At the end of the phase I treatment, the Class III dysgnathia has been improved (Wits appraisal –2.6 mm) and space has been generated by distalization of the molars (Fig. 18-69).

SUMMARY

The Benefit mini-implant in combination with the Beneplate expands skeletal anchorage options in orthodontic treatment and reduces the failure rate significantly. Insertion and removal are minimally invasive procedures. Orthodontists can place the screws and load them immediately. Usually the screws can be removed without anesthesia. The anterior palate is the preferred insertion region because of its superior bone quality and relatively low rates of mini-screw instability

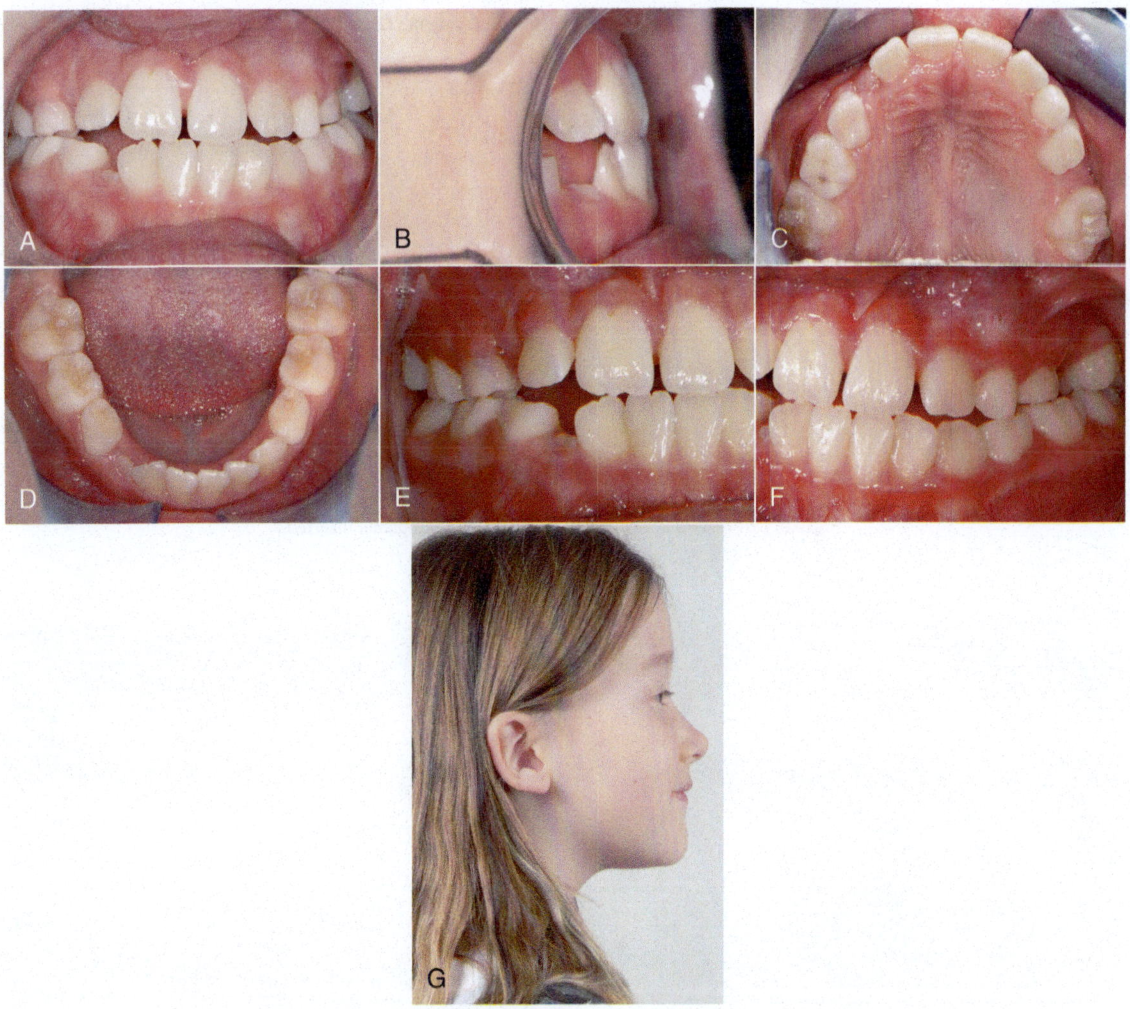

Figure 18-64 **A–F,** Intraoral and **(G)** profile views of a 9-year-old girl with a skeletal Class III malocclusion.

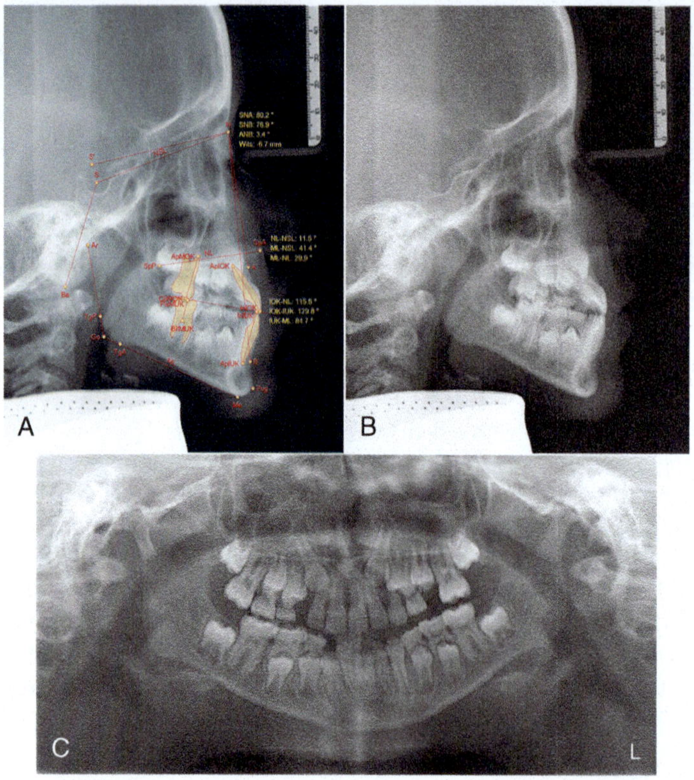

Figure 18-65 **A and B,** Cephalometric and **(C)** panoramic radiographs showing the patient's Class III malocclusion. The Wits appraisal is –6.7 mm.

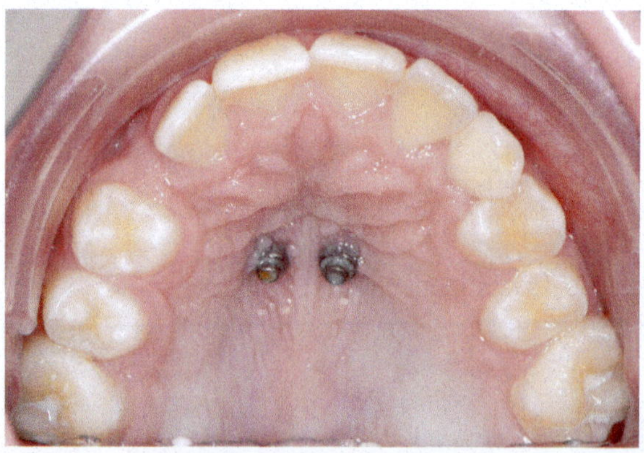

Figure 18-66 Two 2 mm × 7 mm Benefit mini-implants inserted.

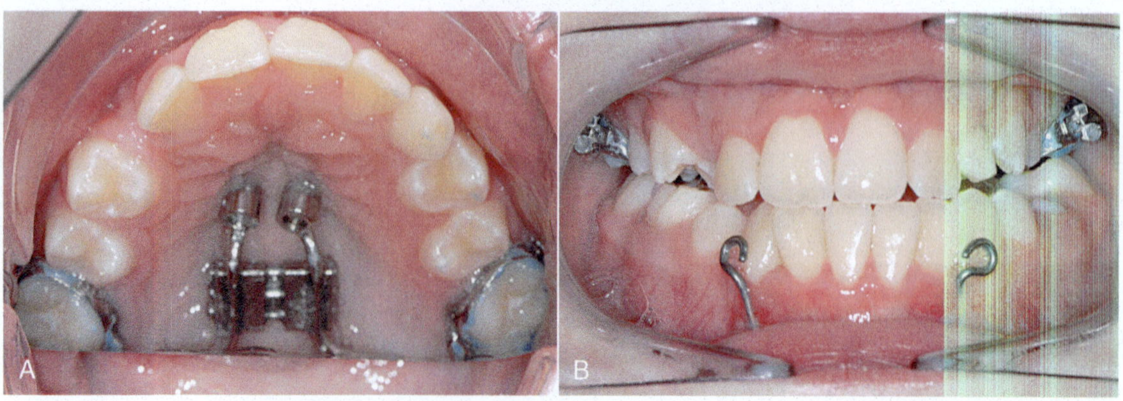

Figure 18-67 The Hybrid Hyrax–Mentoplate combination using Class III elastics for an intraoral-only approach.

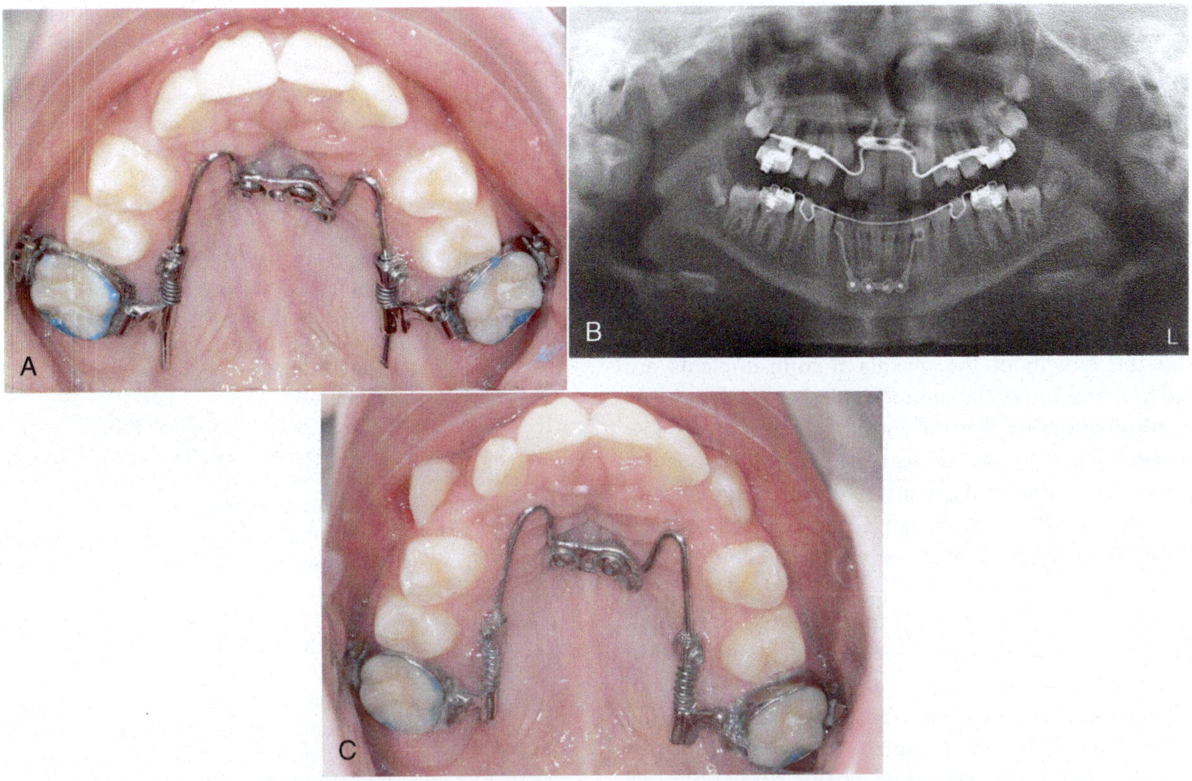

Figure 18-68 **A,** Beneslider used for molar distalization in the upper arch. The same mini-implants were used. **B,** Six months later a bodily distalization of the molars is recognizable in the orthopantomogram. **C,** Intraoral situation after 6 months of distalization.

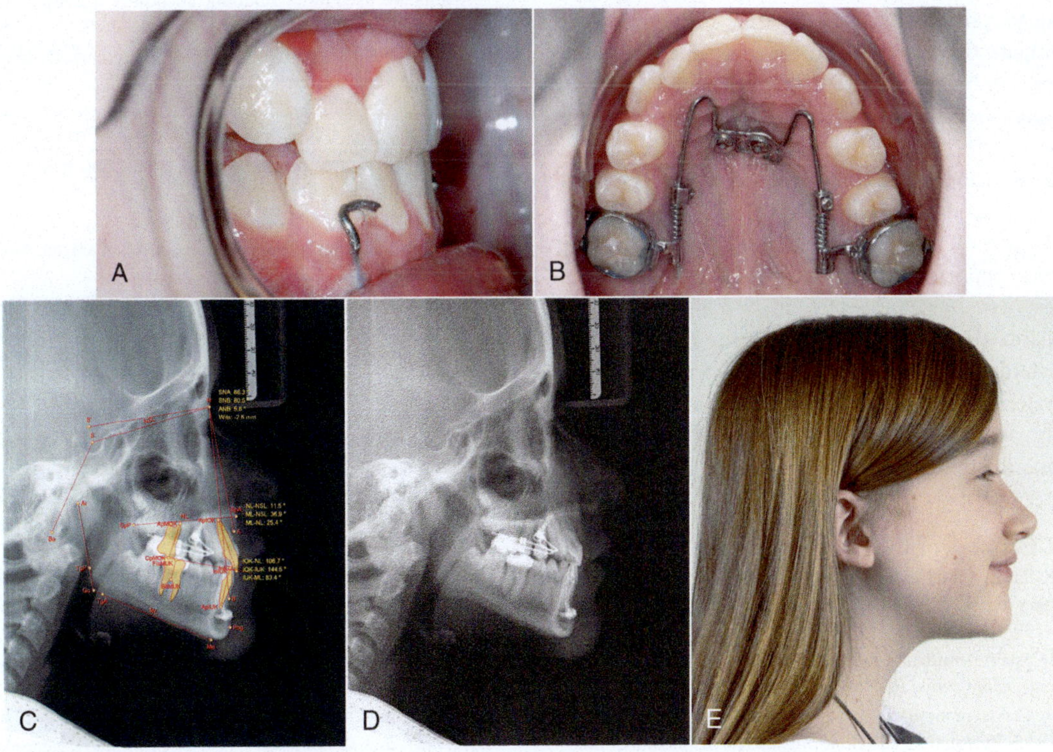

Figure 18-69 **A and B,** Intraoral views, **(C and D)** radiographs, and **(E)** profile view at the end of the phase I treatment. The Class III dysgnathia has been improved (Wits appraisal −2.6 mm) and space has been generated by distalization of the molars.

and failure. The attached mucosa leads to a better prognosis for the implants compared with other areas. In addition, there is no risk of tooth damage. By coupling two mini-implants in the line of force the author was able to minimize the failure rate very distinctively. This coupling can be accomplished very easily by the Beneplate.

The mini-implants were inserted in the region of the mid-palatal suture in the presented cases, including in adolescents. This is a procedure worth discussing, with two questions arising: (1) Is mini-implant stability sufficient if they are inserted near the suture? and (2) Is there any influence on the growth of the maxilla if mini-implants are inserted in the region of the suture? Regarding the first issue, it is worth mentioning that the author achieved a very low failure rate. As well, the measured maximum insertion moments of the mini-implants inserted in the anterior and median regions of the suture ranged from 8 to 25 Ncm, which can be considered adequate values to achieve sufficient primary stability.[30,48,59,64,101]

The question of whether there might be an impairment of transversal maxillary growth due to implants inserted in the midpalatal suture was investigated by Asscherickx et al.,[102] who inserted two Orthosystem implants into the suture of beagle dogs and recognized a transversal growth inhibition of the maxilla. However, in this study only one control animal was available and only one parameter was found to be different.[103] As well, the transferability to mini-implants is questionable due to the larger diameter and the rough surface of the Orthosystem implants. Also, the author's clinical observation did not reveal any signs of impaired transversal growth of the maxilla. Further studies should investigate this issue in more detail. If desired, the mini-implants can be inserted laterally to the suture as well, since a sufficient bone quantity can be found up to 3 mm lateral to the suture.[104] If the patient has a minimal bone height in the anterior palate, long mini-implants (11 mm) may penetrate the nasal cavity. Complications are very unlikely and did not occur in the author's patients. Only some patients reported nose itching at the time of insertion.

In conclusion, the advanced design of the exchangeable abutment system provides the orthodontist with a skeletal anchorage system that is easy to integrate in clinical practice and allows the orthodontist to solve problems that were difficult or impossible to address before.

REFERENCES

1. Costa A, Raffainl M, Melsen B. Miniscrews as orthodontic anchorage: a preliminary report. *Int J Adult Orthodon Orthognath Surg*. 1998; 13(3):201–209.
2. Melsen B, Costa A. Immediate loading of implants used for orthodontic anchorage. *Clin Orthod Res*. 2000;3(1):23–28.
3. Wilmes B. Fields of application of mini-implants. In: Ludwig B, Baumgaertel S, Bowman SJ, eds. *Mini-Implants in Orthodontics: Innovative Anchorage Concepts*. New York, NY: Quintessence Publishing Co; 2008:91–122.
4. Kanomi R. Mini-implant for orthodontic anchorage. *J Clin Orthod*. 1997;31(11):763–767.
5. Wilmes B, Drescher D. Vertical periodontal ligament distraction: a new method for aligning ankylosed and displaced canines. *J Orofac Orthop*. 2009;70(3):213–223.
6. Papageorgiou SN, Zogakis IP, Papadopoulos MA. Failure rates and associated risk factors of orthodontic miniscrew implants: a meta-analysis. *Am J Orthod Dentofacial Orthop*. 2012;142(5):577–595.e7.
7. Berens A, Wiechmann D, Dempf R. Mini- and micro-screws for temporary skeletal anchorage in orthodontic therapy. *J Orofac Orthop*. 2006;67(6):450–458.
8. Cheng SJ, Tseng IY, Lee JJ, Kok SH. A prospective study of the risk factors associated with failure of mini-implants used for orthodontic anchorage. *Int J Oral Maxillofac Implants*. 2004;19(1):100–106.
9. Fritz U, Ehmer A, Diedrich P. Clinical suitability of titanium microscrews for orthodontic anchorage: preliminary experiences. *J Orofac Orthop*. 2004;65(5):410–418.
10. Miyawaki S, Koyama I, Inoue M, Mishima K, Sugahara T, Takano-Yamamoto T. Factors associated with the stability of titanium screws placed in the posterior region for orthodontic anchorage. *Am J Orthod Dentofacial Orthop*. 2003;124(4):373–378.
11. Janson G, Gigliotti MP, Estelita S, Chiqueto K. Influence of miniscrew dental root proximity on its degree of late stability. *Int J Oral Maxillofac Surg*. 2013;42(4):527–534.
12. Wilmes B, Rademacher C, Olthoff G, Drescher D. Parameters affecting primary stability of orthodontic mini-implants. *J Orofac Orthop*. 2006;67(3):162–174.
13. Huja SS, Litsky AS, Beck FM, Johnson KA, Larsen PE. Pull-out strength of monocortical screws placed in the maxillae and mandibles of dogs. *Am J Orthod Dentofacial Orthop*. 2005;127(3):307–313.
14. Huja SS, Rao J, Struckhoff JA, Beck FM, Litsky AS. Biomechanical and histomorphometric analyses of monocortical screws at placement and 6 weeks postinsertion. *J Oral Implantol*. 2006;32(3):110–116.
15. Tsaousidis G, Bauss O. Influence of insertion site on the failure rates of orthodontic miniscrews. *J Orofac Orthop*. 2008;69(5):349–356.
16. Wiechmann D, Meyer U, Buchter A. Success rate of mini- and micro-implants used for orthodontic anchorage: a prospective clinical study. *Clin Oral Implants Res*. 2007;18(2):263–267.
17. Wilmes B, Ottenstreuer S, Su YY, Drescher D. Impact of implant design on primary stability of orthodontic mini-implants. *J Orofac Orthop*. 2008;69(1):42–50.
18. Kim JW, Baek SH, Kim TW, Chang YI. Comparison of stability between cylindrical and conical type mini-implants. *Angle Orthod*. 2008;78(4):692–698.
19. Lim SA, Cha JY, Hwang CJ. Insertion torque of orthodontic miniscrews according to changes in shape, diameter and length. *Angle Orthod*. 2008;78(2):234–240.
20. Chen YH, Chang HH, Chen YJ, Lee D, Chiang HH, Yao CC. Root contact during insertion of miniscrews for orthodontic anchorage increases the failure rate: an animal study. *Clin Oral Implants Res*. 2008; 19(1):99–106.
21. Buchter A, Wiechmann D, Koerdt S, Wiesmann HP, Piffko J, Meyer U. Load-related implant reaction of mini-implants used for orthodontic anchorage. *Clin Oral Implants Res*. 2005;16(4):473–479.
22. Wilmes B, Drescher D. Impact of insertion depth and predrilling diameter on primary stability of orthodontic mini-implants. *Angle Orthod*. 2009;79(4):609–614.
23. Motoyoshi M, Hirabayashi M, Uemura M, Shimizu N. Recommended placement torque when tightening an orthodontic mini-implant. *Clin Oral Implants Res*. 2006;17(1):109–114.
24. Motoyoshi M, Yoshida T, Ono A, Shimizu N. Effect of cortical bone thickness and implant placement torque on stability of orthodontic mini-implants. *Int J Oral Maxillofac Implants*. 2007;22(5):779–784.
25. Wawrzinek C, Sommer T, Fischer-Brandies H. Microdamage in cortical bone due to the overtightening of orthodontic microscrews. *J Orofac Orthop*. 2008;69(2):121–134.
26. Buchter A, Kleinheinz J, Wiesmann HP, et al. Biological and biomechanical evaluation of bone remodelling and implant stability after

using an osteotome technique. *Clin Oral Implants Res.* 2005;16(1): 1–8.
27. Ludwig B, Glasl B, Walde K. Miniscrews in the anterior palate. *Orthod Products.* August 31, 2011:91–94.
28. Kang S, Lee SJ, Ahn SJ, Heo MS, Kim TW. Bone thickness of the palate for orthodontic mini-implant anchorage in adults. *Am J Orthod Dentofacial Orthop.* 2007;131(4 suppl):S74–S81.
29. Ludwig B, Glasl B, Bowman SJ, Wilmes B, Kinzinger GS, Lisson JA. Anatomical guidelines for miniscrew insertion: palatal sites. *J Clin Orthod.* 2011;45(8):433–441.
30. Wilmes B, Drescher D, Nienkemper M. A miniplate system for improved stability of skeletal anchorage. *J Clin Orthod.* 2009;43(8): 494–501.
31. Wilmes B, Panayotidis A, Drescher D. Fracture resistance of orthodontic mini-implants: a biomechanical in vitro study. *Eur J Orthod.* 2011; 33(4):396–401.
32. Clemmer EJ, Hayes EW. Patient cooperation in wearing orthodontic headgear. *Am J Orthod.* 1979;75(5):517–524.
33. Egolf RJ, BeGole EA, Upshaw HS. Factors associated with orthodontic patient compliance with intraoral elastic and headgear wear. *Am J Orthod Dentofacial Orthop.* 1990;97(4):336–348.
34. Fortini A, Lupoli M, Giuntoli F, Franchi L. Dentoskeletal effects induced by rapid molar distalization with the first class appliance. *Am J Orthod Dentofacial Orthop.* 2004;125(6):697–704.
35. Bussick TJ, McNamara JA Jr. Dentoalveolar and skeletal changes associated with the pendulum appliance. *Am J Orthod Dentofacial Orthop.* 2000;117(3):333–343.
36. Ghosh J, Nanda RS. Evaluation of an intraoral maxillary molar distalization technique. *Am J Orthod Dentofacial Orthop.* 1996;110(6): 639–646.
37. Byloff FK, Karcher H, Clar E, Stoff F. An implant to eliminate anchorage loss during molar distalization: a case report involving the Graz implant-supported pendulum. *Int J Adult Orthodon Orthognath Surg.* 2000;15(2):129–137.
38. Gelgor IE, Buyukyilmaz T, Karaman AI, Dolanmaz D, Kalayci A. Intraosseous screw-supported upper molar distalization. *Angle Orthod.* 2004;74(6):838–850.
39. Karaman AI, Basciftci FA, Polat O. Unilateral distal molar movement with an implant-supported distal jet appliance. *Angle Orthod.* 2002; 72(2):167–174.
40. Kyung SH, Hong SG, Park YC. Distalization of maxillary molars with a midpalatal miniscrew. *J Clin Orthod.* 2003;37(1):22–26.
41. Sugawara J, Kanzaki R, Takahashi I, Nagasaka H, Nanda R. Distal movement of maxillary molars in nongrowing patients with the skeletal anchorage system. *Am J Orthod Dentofacial Orthop.* 2006;129(6): 723–733.
42. Kircelli BH, Pektas ZO, Kircelli C. Maxillary molar distalization with a bone-anchored pendulum appliance. *Angle Orthod.* 2006;76(4): 650–659.
43. Escobar SA, Tellez PA, Moncada CA, Villegas CA, Latorre CM, Oberti G. Distalization of maxillary molars with the bone-supported pendulum: a clinical study. *Am J Orthod Dentofacial Orthop.* 2007;131(4): 545–549.
44. Kinzinger G, Gulden N, Yildizhan F, Hermanns-Sachweh B, Diedrich P. Anchorage efficacy of palatally-inserted miniscrews in molar distalization with a periodontally/miniscrew-anchored distal jet. *J Orofac Orthop.* 2008;69(2):110–120.
45. Velo S, Rotunno E, Cozzani M. The implant distal jet. *J Clin Orthod.* 2007;41(2):88–93.
46. Kinzinger GS, Diedrich PR, Bowman SJ. Upper molar distalization with a miniscrew-supported distal jet. *J Clin Orthod.* 2006;40(11): 672–678.
47. Wilmes B, Drescher D. A miniscrew system with interchangeable abutments. *J Clin Orthod.* 2008;42(10):574–580.
48. Wilmes B, Drescher D. Application and effectiveness of the Beneslider molar distalization device. *World J Orthod.* 2010;11:331–340.
49. Robertsson S, Mohlin B. The congenitally missing upper lateral incisor: a retrospective study of orthodontic space closure versus restorative treatment. *Eur J Orthod.* 2000;22(6):697–710.
50. Zachrisson BU, Rosa M, Toreskog S. Congenitally missing maxillary lateral incisors: canine substitution: point. *Am J Orthod Dentofacial Orthop.* 2011;139(4):434, 436, 438, passim.
51. Zachrisson BU, Mjor IA. Remodeling of teeth by grinding. *Am J Orthod.* 1975;68(5):545–553.
52. Thordarson A, Zachrisson BU, Mjor IA. Remodeling of canines to the shape of lateral incisors by grinding: a long-term clinical and radiographic evaluation. *Am J Orthod Dentofacial Orthop.* 1991;100(2): 123–132.
53. Baumgaertel S. Maxillary molar movement with a new treatment auxiliary and palatal miniscrew anchorage. *J Clin Orthod.* 2008;42(10): 587–589.
54. Wilmes B, Nienkemper M, Nanda R, Lübberink G, Drescher D. Palatally anchored maxillary molar mesialization using the mesialslider. *J Clin Orthod.* 2013;47(3):172–179.
55. Feldmann I, Bondemark L. Orthodontic anchorage: a systematic review. *Angle Orthod.* 2006;76(3):493–501.
56. Guray E, Orhan M. "En masse" retraction of maxillary anterior teeth with anterior headgear. *Am J Orthod Dentofacial Orthop.* 1997;112(5): 473–479.
57. Thiruvenkatachari B, Pavithranand A, Rajasigamani K, Kyung HM. Comparison and measurement of the amount of anchorage loss of the molars with and without the use of implant anchorage during canine retraction. *Am J Orthod Dentofacial Orthop.* 2006;129(4):551–554.
58. Ziegler P, Ingervall B. A clinical study of maxillary canine retraction with a retraction spring and with sliding mechanics. *Am J Orthod Dentofacial Orthop.* 1989;95(2):99–106.
59. Wilmes B, Olthoff G, Drescher D. Comparison of skeletal and conventional anchorage methods in conjunction with pre-operative decompensation of a skeletal class III malocclusion. *J Orofac Orthop.* 2009;70(4):297–305.
60. Hattab FN, Rawashdeh MA, Fahmy MS. Impaction status of third molars in Jordanian students. *Oral Surg Oral Med Oral Pathol Oral Radiol Endod.* 1995;79(1):24–29.
61. Bishara SE. Clinical management of impacted maxillary canines. *Semin Orthod.* 1998;4(2):87–98.
62. Becker A. *The Orthodontic Treatment of Impacted Teeth.* London, England: Martin Dunitz Ltd; 1998.
63. Kokich VG, Mathews DP. Surgical and orthodontic management of impacted teeth. *Dent Clin North Am.* 1993;37(2):181–204.
64. Nienkemper M, Wilmes B, Lubberink G, Ludwig B, Drescher D. Extrusion of impacted teeth using mini-implant mechanics. *J Clin Orthod.* 2012;46(3):150–155.
65. Kravitz ND, Kusnoto B, Tsay PT, Hohlt WF. Intrusion of overerupted upper first molar using two orthodontic miniscrews: a case report. *Angle Orthod.* 2007;77(5):915–922.
66. Kravitz ND, Kusnoto B, Tsay TP, Hohlt WF. The use of temporary anchorage devices for molar intrusion. *J Am Dent Assoc.* 2007;138(1): 56–64.
67. Yao CC, Lee JJ, Chen HY, Chang ZC, Chang HF, Chen YJ. Maxillary molar intrusion with fixed appliances and mini-implant anchorage studied in three dimensions. *Angle Orthod.* 2005;75(5):754–760.
68. Sherwood KH, Burch JG, Thompson WJ. Closing anterior open bites by intruding molars with titanium miniplate anchorage. *Am J Orthod Dentofacial Orthop.* 2002;122(6):593–600.
69. Lin JC, Liou EJ, Yeh CL. Intrusion of overerupted maxillary molars with miniscrew anchorage. *J Clin Orthod.* 2006;40(6):378–383.
70. Erverdi N, Keles A, Nanda R. The use of skeletal anchorage in open bite treatment: a cephalometric evaluation. *Angle Orthod.* 2004;74(3): 381–390.
71. Umemori M, Sugawara J, Mitani H, Nagasaka H, Kawamura H. Skeletal anchorage system for open-bite correction. *Am J Orthod Dentofacial Orthop.* 1999;115(2):166–174.

72. Moon CH, Wee JU, Lee HS. Intrusion of overerupted molars by corticotomy and orthodontic skeletal anchorage. *Angle Orthod.* 2007; 77(6):1119–1125.
73. Lee M, Shuman J. Maxillary molar intrusion with a single miniscrew and a transpalatal arch. *J Clin Orthod.* 2012;46(1):48–51.
74. Ludwig B, Glasl B, Kinzinger GS, Lietz T, Lisson JA. Anatomical guidelines for miniscrew insertion: vestibular interradicular sites. *J Clin Orthod.* 2011;45(3):165–173.
75. Poggio PM, Incorvati C, Velo S, Carano A. "Safe zones": a guide for miniscrew positioning in the maxillary and mandibular arch. *Angle Orthod.* 2006;76(2):191–197.
76. Kim SH, Yoon HG, Choi YS, Hwang EH, Kook YA, Nelson G. Evaluation of interdental space of the maxillary posterior area for orthodontic mini-implants with cone-beam computed tomography. *Am J Orthod Dentofacial Orthop.* 2009;135(5):635–641.
77. Wilmes B, Panayotidis A, Drescher D. Fracture resistance of orthodontic mini-implants: a biomechanical in vitro study. *Eur J Orthod.* 2011; 33(4):396–401.
78. Kadioglu O, Buyukyilmaz T, Zachrisson BU, Maino BG. Contact damage to root surfaces of premolars touching miniscrews during orthodontic treatment. *Am J Orthod Dentofacial Orthop.* 2008;134(3): 353–360.
79. Maino BG, Weiland F, Attanasi A, Zachrisson BU, Buyukyilmaz T. Root damage and repair after contact with miniscrews. *J Clin Orthod.* 2007;41(12):762–766.
80. Gracco A, Tracey S, Baciliero U. Miniscrew insertion and the maxillary sinus: an endoscopic evaluation. *J Clin Orthod.* 2010;44(7):439–443.
81. Wilmes B, Drescher D. Impact of bone quality, implant type, and implantation site preparation on insertion torques of mini-implants used for orthodontic anchorage. *Int J Oral Maxillofac Surg.* 2011;40(7): 697–703.
82. Wilmes B, Nienkemper M, Ludwig B, Nanda R, Drescher D. The "mousetrap": a new molar intrusion mechanics using mini-implants in the anterior palate. *J Clin Orthod.* 2013;47(5):314–320, quiz 328.
83. Angell E. Treatment of irregularities of permanent or adult teeth. *Dent Cosmos.* 1860;1:540–544, 599–600.
84. Garib DG, Henriques JF, Janson G, de Freitas MR, Fernandes AY. Periodontal effects of rapid maxillary expansion with tooth-tissue-borne and tooth-borne expanders: a computed tomography evaluation. *Am J Orthod Dentofacial Orthop.* 2006;129(6):749–758.
85. Schuster G, Borel-Scherf I, Schopf PM. Frequency of and complications in the use of RPE appliances: results of a survey in the Federal State of Hesse, Germany. *J Orofac Orthop.* 2005;66(2):148–161.
86. Mommaerts MY. Transpalatal distraction as a method of maxillary expansion. *Br J Oral Maxillofac Surg.* 1999;37(4):268–272.
87. Koudstaal MJ, van der Wal KG, Wolvius EB, Schulten AJ. The Rotterdam Palatal Distractor: introduction of the new bone-borne device and report of the pilot study. *Int J Oral Maxillofac Surg.* 2006;35(1): 31–35.
88. Fuck L, Wilmes B, Drescher D. Rapid palatal expansion with a transpalatal distractor [in German]. *Kieferorthopädie.* 2008;22(4): 251–258.
89. Hansen L, Tausche E, Hietschold V, Hotan T, Lagravere M, Harzer W. Skeletally-anchored rapid maxillary expansion using the Dresden Distractor. *J Orofac Orthop.* 2007;68(2):148–158.
90. Harzer W, Schneider M, Gedrange T. Rapid maxillary expansion with palatal anchorage of the hyrax expansion screw: pilot study with case presentation. *J Orofac Orthop.* 2004;65(5):419–424.
91. Harzer W, Schneider M, Gedrange T, Tausche E. Direct bone placement of the hyrax fixation screw for surgically assisted rapid palatal expansion (SARPE). *J Oral Maxillofac Surg.* 2006;64(8):1313–1317.
92. Kang S, Lee SJ, Ahn SJ, Heo MS, Kim TW. Bone thickness of the palate for orthodontic mini-implant anchorage in adults. *Am J Orthod Dentofacial Orthop.* 2007;131(4 suppl):S74–S81.
93. Wilmes B, Nienkemper M, Ludwig B, Kau CH, Drescher D. Early Class III treatment with a hybrid hyrax-mentoplate combination. *J Clin Orthod.* 2011;45(1):1–7.
94. Wilmes B, Nienkemper M, Drescher D. Application and effectiveness of a mini-implant- and tooth-borne rapid palatal expansion device: the Hybrid Hyrax. *World J Orthod.* 2010;11(4):323–330.
95. Ludwig B, Glas B, Bowman SJ, Drescher D, Wilmes B. Miniscrew-supported Class III treatment with the Hybrid RPE Advancer. *J Clin Orthod.* 2010;44(9):533–539.
96. Litton SF, Ackermann LV, Isaacson RJ, Shapiro BL. A genetic study of Class 3 malocclusion. *Am J Orthod.* 1970;58(6):565–577.
97. Proffit WR, Fields HW Jr, Moray LJ. Prevalence of malocclusion and orthodontic treatment need in the United States: estimates from the NHANES III survey. *Int J Adult Orthodon Orthognath Surg.* 1998;13(2): 97–106.
98. Williams MD, Sarver DM, Sadowsky PL, Bradley E. Combined rapid maxillary expansion and protraction facemask in the treatment of Class III malocclusions in growing children: a prospective long-term study. *Semin Orthod.* 1997;3(4):265–274.
99. Baccetti T, McGill JS, Franchi L, McNamara JA Jr, Tollaro I. Skeletal effects of early treatment of Class III malocclusion with maxillary expansion and face-mask therapy. *Am J Orthod Dentofacial Orthop.* 1998;113(3):333–343.
100. De Clerck HJ, Cornelis MA, Cevidanes LH, Heymann GC, Tulloch CJ. Orthopedic traction of the maxilla with miniplates: a new perspective for treatment of midface deficiency. *J Oral Maxillofac Surg.* 2009; 67(10):2123–2129.
101. Nienkemper M, Wilmes B, Pauls A, Drescher D. Multipurpose use of orthodontic mini-implants to achieve different treatment goals. *J Orofac Orthop.* 2012;73(6):467–476.
102. Asscherickx K, Hanssens JL, Wehrbein H, Sabzevar MM. Orthodontic anchorage implants inserted in the median palatal suture and normal transverse maxillary growth in growing dogs: a biometric and radiographic study. *Angle Orthod.* 2005;75(5):826–831.
103. Borsos G, Rudzki-Janson I, Stockmann P, Schlegel KA, Vegh A. Immediate loading of palatal implants in still-growing patients: a prospective, comparative, clinical pilot study. *J Orofac Orthop.* 2008;69(4): 297–308.
104. Bernhart T, Freudenthaler J, Dortbudak O, Bantleon HP, Watzek G. Short epithetic implants for orthodontic anchorage in the paramedian region of the palate: a clinical study. *Clin Oral Implants Res.* 2001;12(6): 624–631.

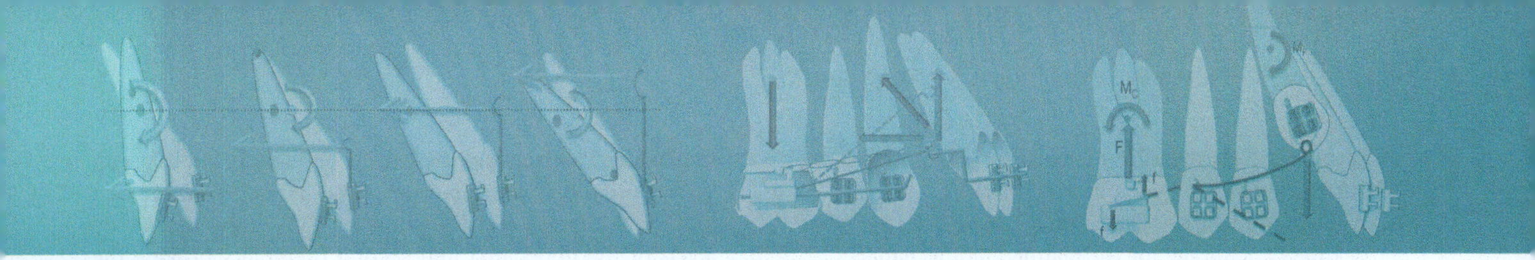

CHAPTER 19

Expanding the Limits for Esthetic Strategies by Skeletal Anchorage

Nejat Erverdi, Mustafa Burhan Ateş, and Melih Motro

The importance of anchorage in orthodontics can best be described by the famous quote from the Greek philosopher Archimedes: "Give me a place to stand and I will move the earth." Orthodontic anchorage can also be explained by Newton's Third Law of Motion, which states that every action creates a reaction, which is equal in size and opposite in direction. The anatomic unit that antagonizes the active force is called anchorage in orthodontics.

Anchorage preparation is a very important part of orthodontic treatment. The success of orthodontic treatment generally relies on the anchorage protocol planned for a particular case. When preparing anchorage, the clinician must be realistic enough to foresee the possibility of losing some anchorage. Anchorage loss can result from unrealistic anchorage construction as well as lack of patient cooperation. The type of anchorage is based on the desired type of tooth movement. Maximum anchorage is frequently required in the treatment of orthodontic cases and is usually obtained by extraoral appliances. Adults and teenagers are prone to reject extraoral appliances because of esthetic problems and the discomfort they cause.[1–3] Thus different intraoral mechanics to gain maximum anchorage have been designed by various investigators.

The term *stationary anchorage* means that the anchorage unit does not move in reaction to the applied orthodontic forces and moments.[4] Recent developments in implantology now allow stationary anchorage without extraoral appliances or complex biomechanical procedures. Implants used for orthodontic anchorage are generally classified as osseointegrated or nonosseointegrated implants. Conventional dental implants and palatal implants are considered osseointegrated implants and mini-screws, micro-screws, and various surgical plates are considered nonosseointegrated implants. However, these two concepts are sometimes confused in orthodontics and need to be clarified.

Orthodontic patients usually have an intact dentition with no available sites for implant placements. Therefore various methods for bone anchorage have been tested recently: cobalt-chromium (Vitallium) screws, vitreous carbon, bioglass-coated aluminium oxide implants, stainless steel plates and screws,[5–13] Brånemark implants,[14,15] retromolar implants,[14] onplants,[16] zygomatic wires,[17] ankylosed teeth,[18] palatal implants,[19] mini-plates,[20,21] and mini-screws.[9,13,22] Among these, zygomatic and symphyseal mini-plates have particular importance because they have been widely used and tested in recent years.[8]

This chapter discusses clinical use of different orthodontic implants to correct different malocclusions. Although orthodontic implants can be used in any case, their use should be limited to cases in which treatment results will be improved when compared with conventional biomechanical procedures or radical surgery, which always carries a risk of morbidity. Otherwise, serious ethical concerns may arise. Therefore the treatment methods presented in this chapter are compared with the conventional methods and advantages, disadvantages, and long-term treatment outcomes are clarified.

ANATOMIC SITES FOR ORTHODONTIC IMPLANT PLACEMENT

In cases with multiple lost teeth in the dental arch, placement of implants at the beginning of treatment is a useful procedure.[23] These implants will serve first as anchor units during orthodontic treatment and then as abutments for the restorations after orthodontic treatment. In such cases the implants must be positioned accurately prior to orthodontics so they can be used as restorative abutments following tooth movement. The overall treatment in these cases must be planned by a team that includes a prosthodontist, orthodontist, and oral surgeon.

In cases without previous tooth loss in the dental arch, orthodontic implants are used only as anchorage units. These are nonroot-form onplants and implants that can be placed in nonalveolar bone and explanted after treatment.[19,24,25–30]

Several criteria must be evaluated prior to the selection of the implant site for nonalveolar implants:

1. A location must be selected that can be used as indirect or direct anchorage for the planned biomechanics.
2. Care must be taken not to create any root, nerve, or artery injury.
3. The implant site must contain enough depth and thickness of bone material.
4. Areas rich in cortical bone are preferred, as they improve the primary stability of the implant.

The hard palate, mandibular retromolar area, inferior border of the zygomatic buttress, symphysis region, and labial or buccal interradicular bone are usually the sites of choice for orthodontic implant placement.

PALATAL IMPLANTS

The hard palate has long been used as an anchorage site in conventional orthodontics. The Nance button, which is a common anchorage appliance used in the hard palate, is a suitable choice in moderate anchorage situations but it is not sufficient in maximum anchorage requirement. The hard palate is easily accessible to the surgeon and offers excellent peri-implant conditions due to the presence of abundant attached mucosa. Osseointegrated implants placed in the hard palate can be used for anchorage reinforcement in many demanding orthodontic applications.[31–33]

ANATOMIC RESTRICTIONS IN PALATAL IMPLANT PLACEMENT

Bone Thickness for Implant Placement

The midpalatal suture, the area adjacent to the midpalatal suture, and the incisor region are the areas with maximal bone height in the hard palate. In a computed tomography (CT) study carried out by Gahleitner et al.,[34] the overall mean palatal bone height was found to be 5.01-mm, ranging from 0 to 16.9-mm. The maximum palatal height was 6.17-mm, measured 6-mm dorsally from the incisive canal. Henriksen et al.[35] reported that the actual bone available for midsagittal implants was 4.3 ± 1.6-mm. The minimum bone thickness necessary for palatal implant placement is 4-mm. These findings indicate that there is sufficient bone for complete osseointegration of 4-mm implants; 6-mm implants should be used with caution.

Incisive Canal Perforation

Implants placed in an anterior location along the midpalatal suture area can create incisive nerve injury. Bernhard et al.[36] conducted a study of 22 patients using CT scans and reported that in order not to perforate the incisive canal, the implant must be placed 6- to 9-mm distal to it.

Root Injuries

Palatal implants placed in the anterior slope of the hard palate can cause incisor root injuries. In some cases the implant and incisor root may not be in contact but they can be in close proximity; if incisor retraction is performed as a part of the treatment, root injuries can easily result. The levels of the upper first and second premolars provide the most appropriate anteroposterior site for implant entry.

Placing the Palatal Implant Paramedially

Melsen et al.[37] concluded that ossification in the midpalatal suture was variable and was completed after age 27 years in males and even later in females. More recently, Schlegel et al.[38] conducted a study on cadavers and reported that complete ossification of the suture was rare before age 23 years. They also stated that since the anterior part of the midpalatal suture was often less ossified than the posterior region, a bone bed more favorable for osseointegration might be found posterior to the interconnecting line of the first premolars.

Both median[19,39] and paramedian[32,33,40] placements of palatal implants have been reported in the literature. In subjects with complete suture ossification, a median location would not create any problem; however, in subjects with unossified sutures, the implant would be in contact with the fibrous tissue in the suture and therefore the chances of total osseointegration would be less compared to the implants with paramedian implantation. On the other hand, Schlegel et al.[38] reported that the connective tissue band in the midpalatal suture area was only 0.03 cm. Considering that the palatal implant has a diameter of 3.3-mm in Orthosystem (Institute Strauman, Waldenburg, Switzerland) and 4.5-mm in the Frialit system (Friadent GmbH, Mannheim, Germany), only a very small portion of the implant would be in contact with the connective tissue when it is placed in the midpalatal suture area, minimizing the concerns about poor osseointegration.

Another critical issue is the possible effect of an implant placed in the midpalatal suture on transverse growth of the maxilla. Growth in the midpalatal suture increases the width of the palate and is considered to be more important than appositional remodeling of the alveolar processes in the development of maxillary width.[41] Björk and Skieller[42] found an average increase in maxillary width of 3-mm between ages 10 and 18 years, as measured between posterior implants on the radiographs of nine boys. Asscherickx et al.[43] evaluated the influence of orthodontic anchorage implants on transverse maxillary growth when inserted in the median palatal suture of growing dogs and reported restricted transversal growth of hard palate in the canine region. Because of ethical considerations, such investigations can be carried out only in animals. In light of these findings, paramedian placement of palatal implants may be recommended in growing individuals.

Palatal Artery Injury

There is always a risk of causing an arterial injury in punch burr application. To prevent bleeding during the operation, infusion of an anesthetic with a vasoconstricter agent is recommended around the area where the implant will be placed. In cases where there is aggressive bleeding, suturing of the artery is recommended.

To avoid the complications described above, an implant must be placed with special care. An acrylic resin template, including a cylindrical metal housing (similar to the stents that are used in implantology for prosthetic purposes), must be used. A method that was developed for precise placement of palatal implants is explained next.

METHOD FOR PALATAL IMPLANT PLACEMENT

Preparation of Acrylic Resin Template

A spherical metal marker is embedded in an acrylic resin template, which covers the occlusal surfaces of the maxillary teeth. The metal marker is placed at the highest point of the palate in the midline. The purpose of placing a metal marker is to calculate the magnification of the radiograph when assessing the exact bony dimensions of the area where the implant will be placed. At least 4-mm of bone thickness is required in this area. Moreover, the metal marker creates a reference point in the sagittal direction for identifying the location of the drilling site for implant placement.

Radiographic Evaluation

A lateral cephalogram with the patient wearing the maxillary acrylic template is obtained (Fig. 19-1). Bone depth in the area where the implant will be placed is measured in relation to the metal marker, which has a diameter of 5-mm. Cases having at least 4-mm of bone height are considered suitable for palatal implant placement and cases without enough bone thickness are candidates for onplant placement.

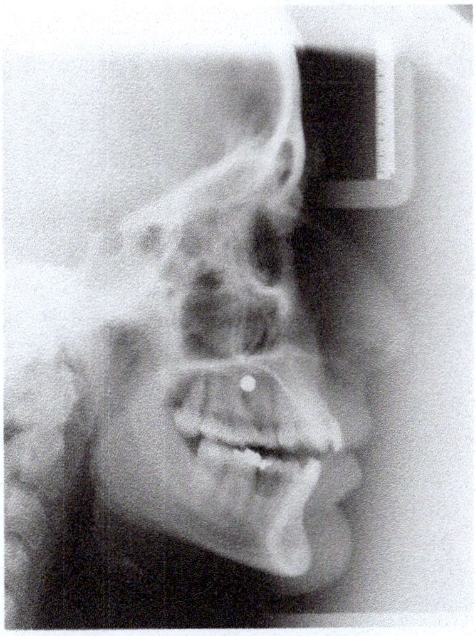

Figure 19-1 A lateral cephalogram of the patient with the template inserted in the mouth is obtained. The spherical marker is useful in measuring the actual bone height at the implant site.

Preparation of the Surgical Template for Positioning the Implant

The plaster cast used for template preparation is cut along the paramedian line, passing through the mesial aspect of the central incisor. On the lateral cephalogram, radiographic views of the maxilla and central incisor are traced on tracing paper and then a cut is made along the pencil line and carried to the paramedian section of the plaster cast. A drill insertion hole is prepared in the acrylic resin template, using a 2.5-mm-diameter stainless steel burr. A cylindrical metal housing, 7-mm in length and 2.1-mm in diameter, which contains a pilot drill, is placed in the implant access hole. The extension of the implant drill is adjusted to 8-mm from the metal housing. In the sagittal plane the desired implant inclination in relation to the incisor roots and the nasal cavity is defined. The implant axis is adjusted between 45 and 60 degrees to the occlusal plane, pointing to the anterior nasal spine (ANS). Care is taken to place the implant at least 3- to 4-mm above the apices of the incisor roots. The metal housing is fixed to the acrylic plate by some cold curing acrylic. In the transverse plane the metal housing should have a lateral orientation with 2-mm of distance from the palatine suture. Thus a three-dimensional surgical template for accurate implant angulation is obtained (Fig. 19-2).

Surgical Method

Before the surgical procedure the patient is asked to rinse his or her mouth with 0.2% chlorhexidine gluconate for 1 minute. After this rinsing the palatal region is locally anesthetized with an agent that has a vasoconstrictive effect. The three-dimensional surgical template is placed in the mouth to mark the implant position. A pilot drill is applied through the metal housing in the template. Then mucosa is removed using a punch drill and the standard surgical protocol for placing the chosen implant system is followed. Drilling is carried out at 1000 revolutions per minute (rpm) under internal and external sterile saline cooling. Drills with 8-mm-long stoppers are used in the following order: a pilot drill of 2-mm diameter, a twist drill of 3-mm diameter, and a spade drill of 4.5-mm diameter (Fig. 19-3, A–E).

In the standard surgical protocols for almost all implant systems, the implant carrier is removed after the initial placement of the implant in the cavity before screwing. The implant is placed transmucosally so that 4-mm of the implant will stay in the bone and 4-mm will stay in the palatal mucosa and serve as an extension to reach the oral cavity (Fig. 19-3, F–I). Transmucosal placement of the implant has the advantage of avoiding the need for secondary surgery. To avoid postoperative pain an analgesic agent is recommended and the patient is instructed to use an antiseptic mouthwash twice a day for 2 weeks. The osseointegration of the palatal implants takes about 3 months and during this period the implant should not be loaded. After waiting 3 months for osseointegration, a gingiva former of proper size is screwed to the implant. One week is usually enough time for shaping of the palatal mucosa (Fig. 19-4).

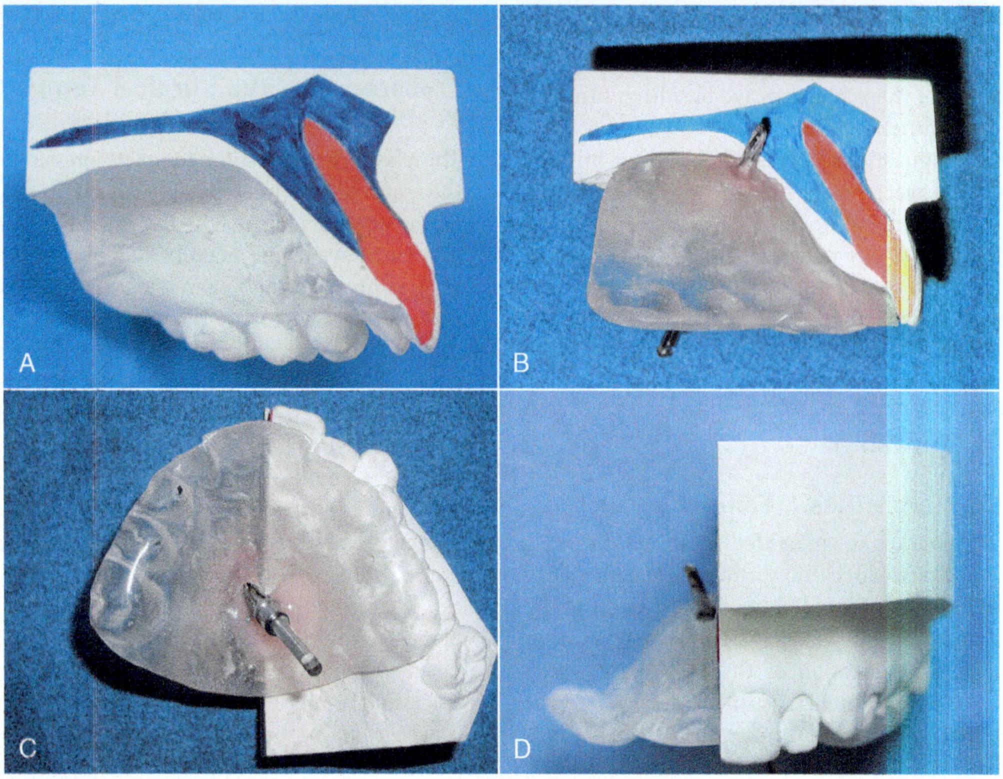

Figure 19-2 **A,** Maxillary tracing is superimposed on the model. **B,** The pilot drill should be oriented between 45 and 60 degrees to the occlusal plane. The drill axis should pass at least 3- to 4-mm above the apices of the incisors. **C,** The metal housing is fixed to the template with cold curing acrylic. **D,** In the frontal plane the pilot drill should be laterally oriented about 2-mm from the median line.

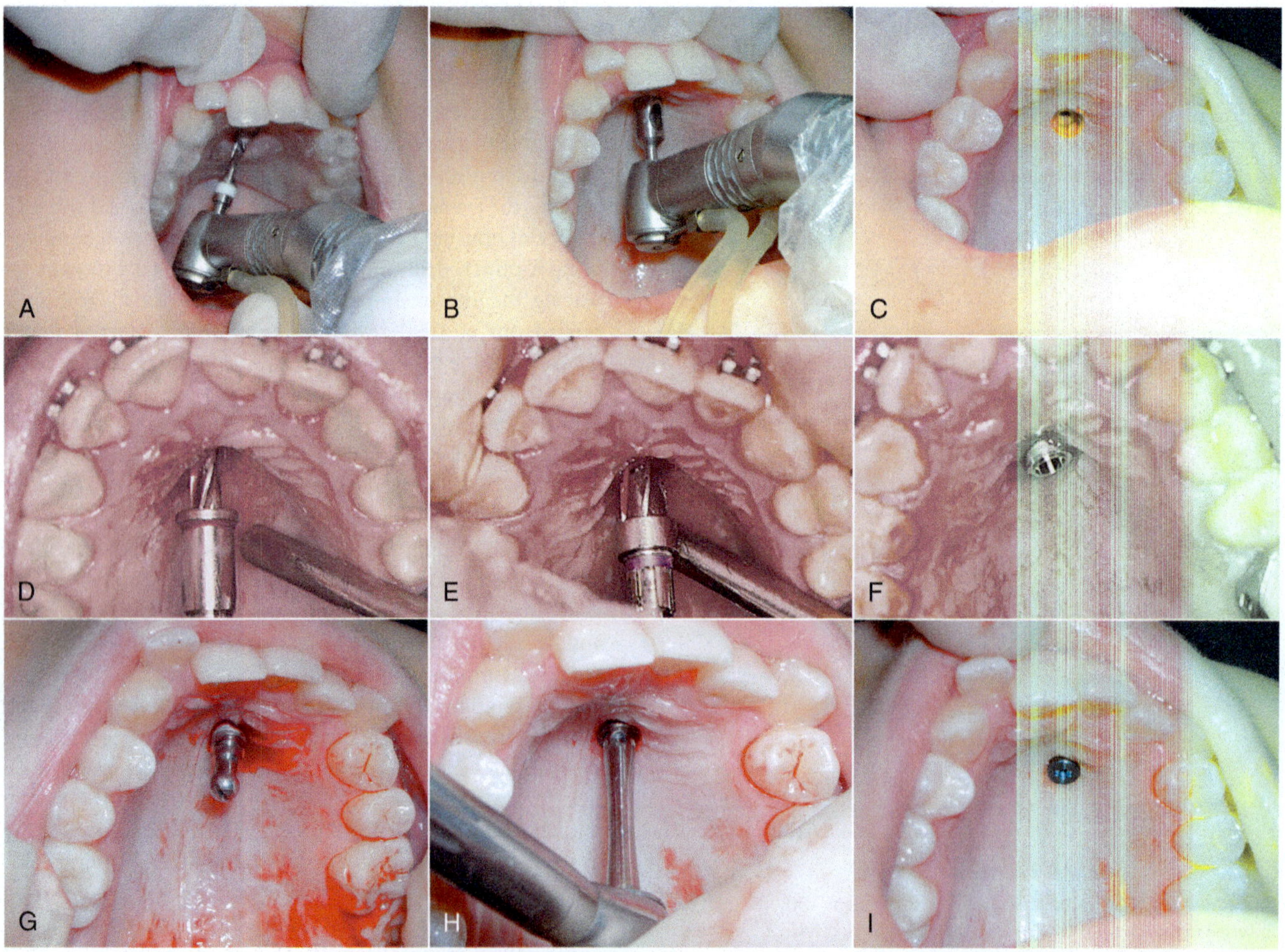

Figure 19-3 **A,** Pilot drill application through the metal housing in the template. **B,** The template is removed from the mouth and a punch drill is applied to the implant site to remove the mucosa. **C,** Implant site after removal of the mucosa. **D and E,** Preparation of the implant bed. **F,** Placement of the palatal implant. **G,** Removal of the implant carrier. **H and I,** The implant is screwed into place.

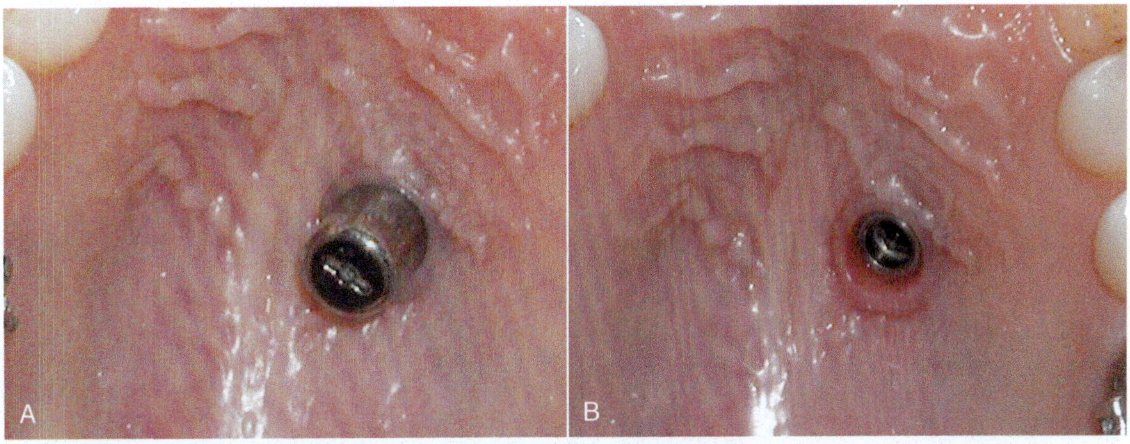

Figure 19-4 **A,** Healing cap applied after 3 months. **B,** Appearance of the palatal mucosa after removal of the healing cap.

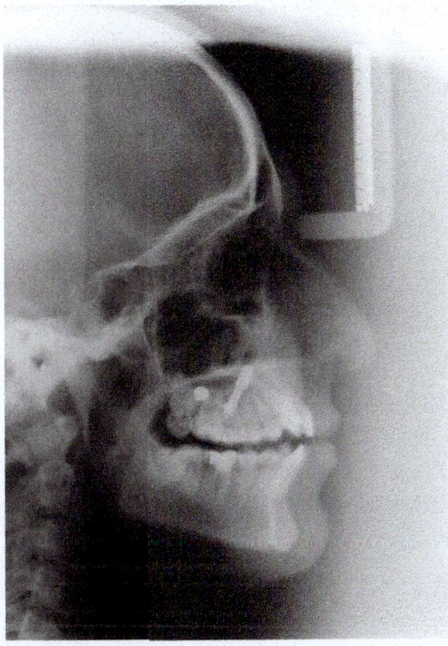

Figure 19-5 Superimposition of the presurgical and postsurgical lateral cephalograms taken with the template in the mouth. The implant is located on the same axis as the metal housing, indicating the accuracy of implant positioning.

Evaluation of Implant Placement Method

The accuracy of the implant placement method was tested by superimposing the presurgical lateral cephalogram with the template and the postsurgical lateral cephalogram with the implant (Fig. 19-5).

The method seems to be successful and practical, with only a few complications such as slight bleeding, which can be easily controlled. Patient comfort during and after the operation is excellent and the procedure does not last more than 10 minutes. The only risk related to this procedure is the possibility of the implant carrier being swallowed by the patient while it is being removed in the conventional way. The location of the implant and possible vomiting reflex during removal of the implant carrier are the two factors that create this risk. To avoid this risk a safe method was developed especially for the removal of the implant carrier.

To avoid the risk of the implant carrier being swallowed, it is recommended that it be removed outside the mouth and that the implant be carried to the cavity while it is seated on the screwing instrument. Care must be taken to hold the implant with Weingart pliers at the polished band, which is designed normally for gingival attachment. The implant holder is removed while the implant is held by Weingart pliers and seated on the screwing instrument. Then the implant is carried to the cavity by the screwing instrument and screwed on directly (Fig. 19-6).

Laboratory Procedures

After completion of the healing period, a transfer kit is screwed to the implant and a plastic cap is mounted. Molar bands and an impression post are transferred to the plaster cast by a conventional impression technique. If needed, premolar bands are transferred as well. An orthodontic abutment (Friadent, Mannheim, Germany) is fixed to the implant analog on the plaster (Fig. 19-7).

STATIONARY ANCHORAGE

On the stone model, a transpalatal arch made of 1.2-mm-thick stainless steel wire is adjusted to connect the anchor teeth to the orthodontic abutment and then is soldered to the bands (Fig. 19-8). Care should be taken not to overheat the wire and not to create dead wire, which can be a cause of anchorage loss.

Orthodontic Mechanics with Palatal Implants

Using this stationary anchorage supported by a palatal implant, various procedures such as en masse retraction of six anterior teeth, canine distalization, and correction of excessive crowding can be carried out without any anchorage loss.

Molar Distalization with Palatal Mechanics

Molar bands and implant abutment are transferred to the plaster cast as explained above. Molar distalizations were made by using mini expansion screws against palatal

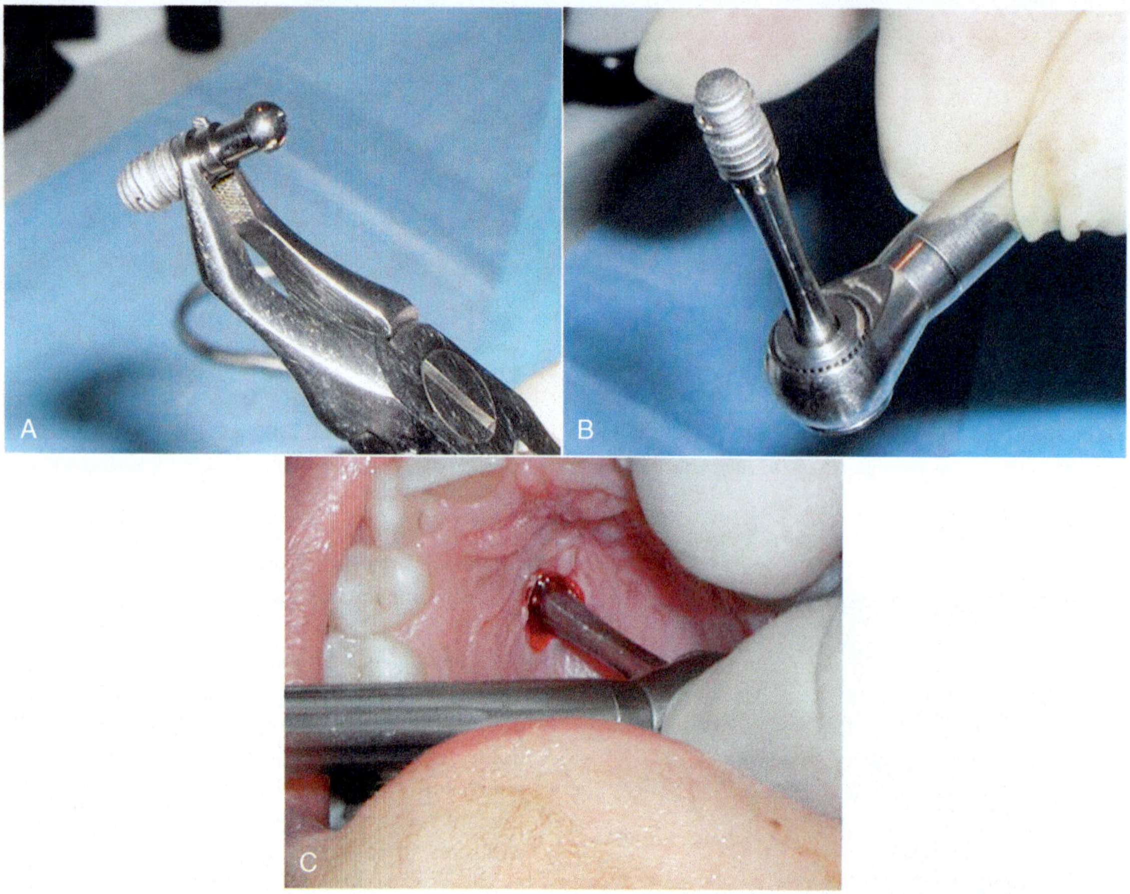

Figure 19-6 Safe method for removing the implant carrier. **A,** Implant is held by its polished neck section with Weingart pliers. **B,** Implant is seated on the screwing instrument. **C,** Implant is carried to the cavity with the screwing instrument.

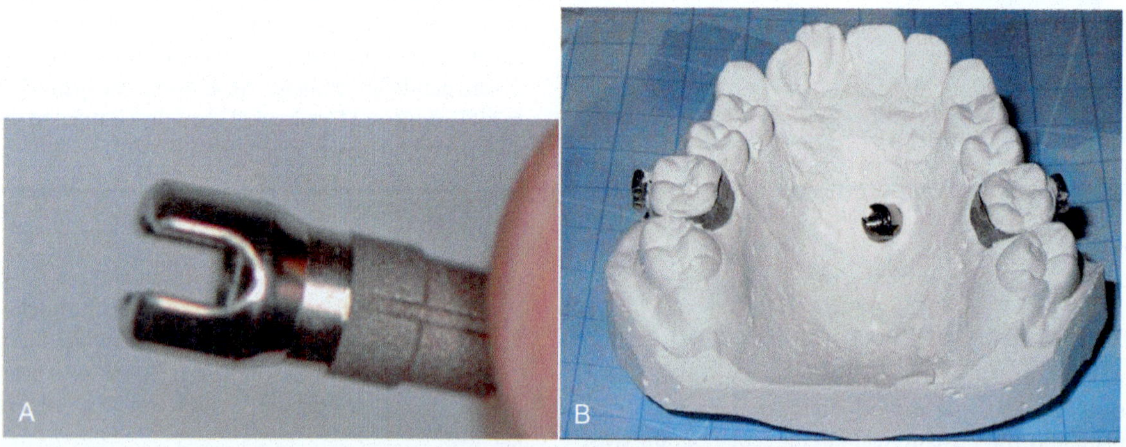

Figure 19-7 Impression procedure. **A,** Orthodontic abutment. **B,** Orthodontic abutment is fixed to the implant analog.

implants. Patients were instructed to turn the screw twice each week (½ turn) and activation was continued until the achievement of super Class I occlusal relationships. Figure 19-9 shows a patient treated using an appliance with the expansion screw for molar distalization supported by the palatal implant.

Explantation

The palatal implant is removed easily by first loosening the implant with the help of a hollow drill and then unscrewing it with a screwing instrument in the counterclockwise direction. The implant site heals rapidly, within approximately 5 days (Fig. 19-10).

ZYGOMATIC ANCHORAGE

The maxilla is made up of thin cortical bone in its buccal and labial aspects. Bone thickness is not >2-mm except in the three buttress areas: the posterior buttress close to the tuber area, the zygomatic buttress, and the nasal buttress close to

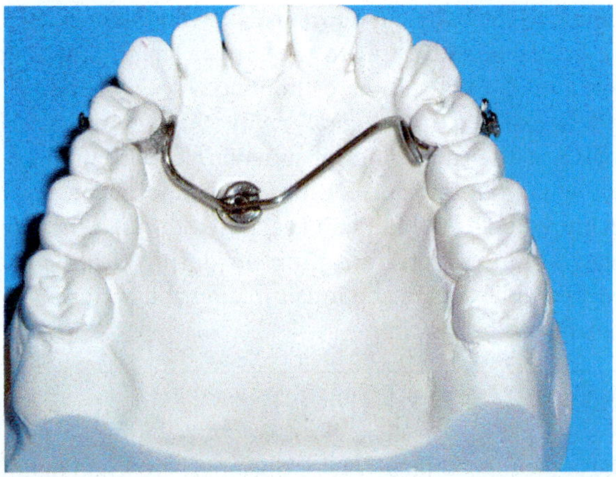

Figure 19-8 Stationary anchorage. Transpalatal bar for reinforcement of premolar anchorage.

the nasal area. All of these areas contain a thick and solid bony structure, which makes implant placement possible. The anatomic location of the posterior buttress prevents easy access to this area. The nasal buttress area is not suitable because of its close location to the infraorbital foramen and nasal cavity. The inferior border of the zygomaticomaxillary buttress is therefore the most suitable area for implant placement because of its anatomic location, which provides an opportunity for easy and direct access (Fig. 19-11). A second advantage of the zygomatic area is that it is distant from critical anatomic structures such as nerves and blood vessels. Owing to its close location to the first molar, the zygomatic buttress can be used directly as anchorage or as indirect anchorage to support maxillary molar anchorage. Zygomatic buttress anchorage can also be used for the intrusion of

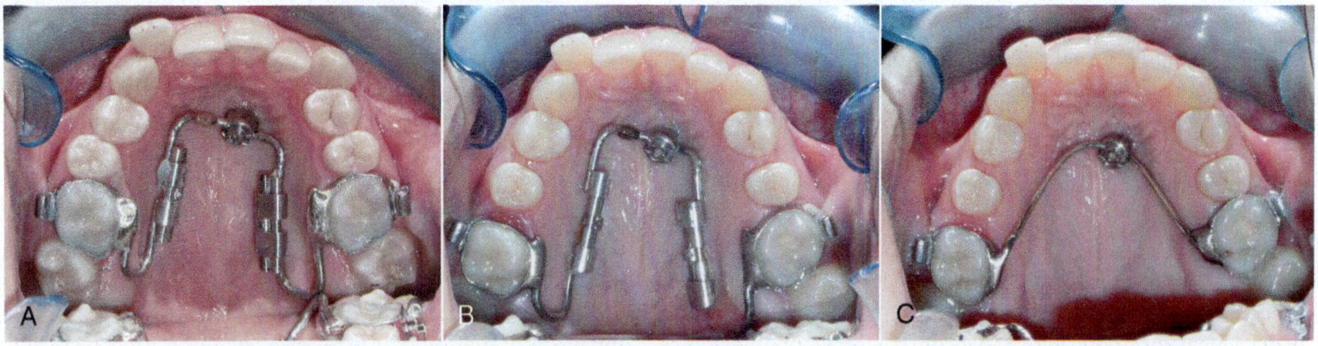

Figure 19-9 **A and B,** Progress photographs of the molar distalization by expansion screw. **C,** After removal of the distalization screws, a transpalatal arch, which was connected to the palatal implant, was constructed to maintain the position of the first molars and to reinforce anchorage during the remaining treatment.

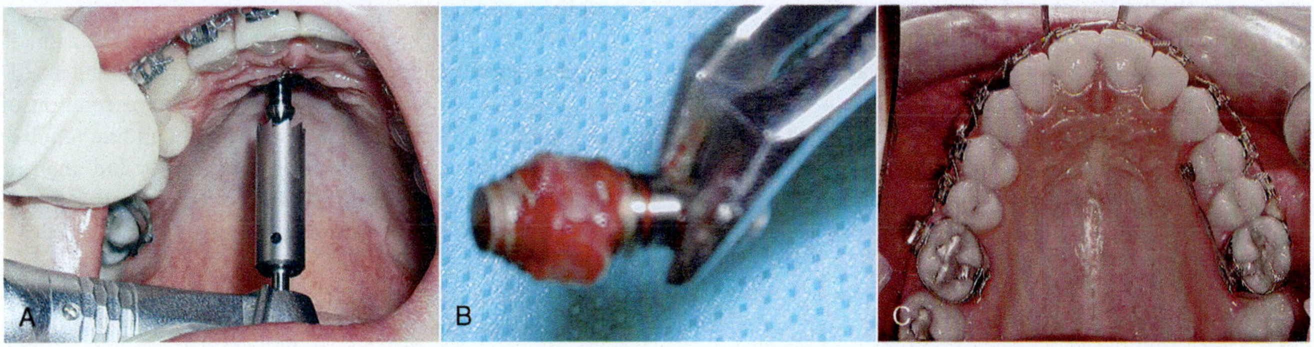

Figure 19-10 **A,** Palatal implant removal. **B,** The appearance of the implant site immediately after removal of the implant. **C,** Healing occurs rapidly and with no complications.

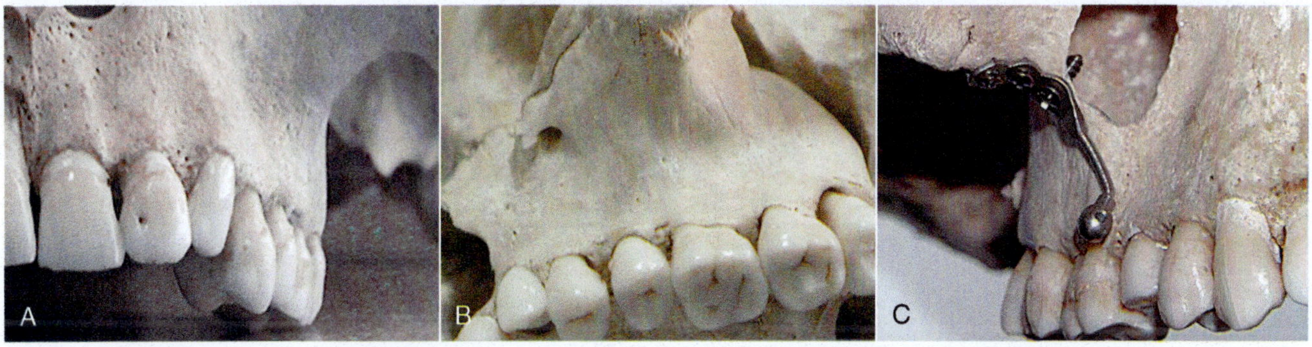

Figure 19-11 Location of **(A and B)** the zygomaticomaxillary buttress on a dry skull where **(C)** the implants can be securely placed.

maxillary dentoalveolar segments, which can otherwise be achieved only by orthognathic surgery.[44]

Since the zygomatic anchorage is located approximately in the middle of the maxillary half, it is possible to carry the anchor to any area where it is needed simply by bending the extension of the implant in the distal or mesial direction. A multipurpose implant (MPI) has been developed for use as an orthodontic anchorage unit.

MULTIPURPOSE IMPLANT

An implant in the form of a surgical mini-plate with a round bar extension has been developed from pure titanium for general use as an orthodontic anchorage unit (patented to Erverdi by Tasarim Med, Istanbul, Turkey) (Fig. 19-12). The MPI has two parts: a retentive part in the form of a surgical mini-plate with three holes for mini-screws and a round bar extension that is 20-mm in length and bendable. Formability of the extension bar makes it possible to carry the anchor to the area where it is required. Screws that are 5-mm in length and 2.2-mm in diameter are advised for low-positioned holes to avoid perforation of sinus mucosa. For the hole in a higher position, screws that are 7- or 9-mm in length can be used.

Surgical Procedure

After rinsing the mouth for 1 minute with 0.2% chlorhexidine gluconate, the zygomatic buttress region is anesthetized using a local anesthetic with a vasoconstrictor agent. Incision is the most important part of the surgical procedure. The correct location of the incision is decided by digital palpation. The zygomatic buttress is palpated using the index finger and the incision is made along the buttress in a vertical direction. The lower border of the incision is at the intersection of the attached and the mobile gingiva; the total length of the incision is no longer than 1 cm. Care is taken to cut the periosteum completely during the incision, to prevent penetration of the buccal fat pad into the area. The mucoperiosteum is elevated and the upper part of the MPI is adapted to the bony curvature using orthodontic pliers. The free bendable end is cut to the proper length and bent to form a hook to attach the orthodontic mechanic units. The MPI is exposed in the oral cavity through the attached gingiva at the mucogingival junction. The location of the area where the implant is exposed is important to prevent inflammation. If the implant is exposed through the mobile gingiva, this will create a problem during treatment; the patient will have pain and inflammation and accordingly the implant will be lost.

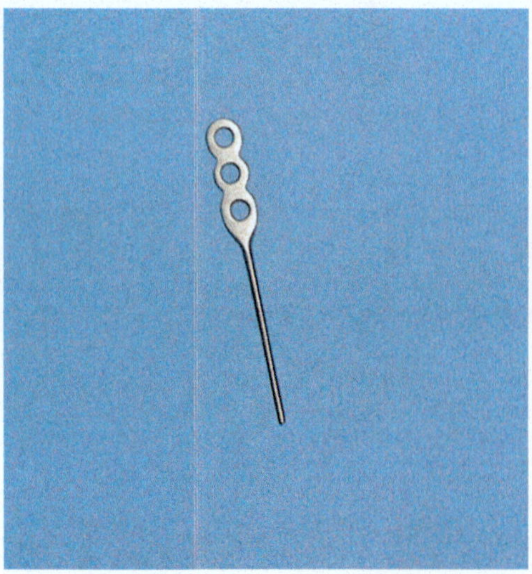

Figure 19-12 Multipurpose implant (Tasarim Med, Istanbul, Turkey).

OPEN-BITE TREATMENT

One of the most difficult malocclusions to treat and maintain in orthodontics is the anterior open bite. Several approaches for the treatment of open bite have been reported. Some investigators used fixed appliances with multiloop archwires and intermaxillary elastics[45,46] while others used preformed reverse-curved nickel-titanium (Ni-Ti) arches and intermaxillary elastics.[47] Some investigators used posterior bite blocks with and without magnets[48–51] and others applied functional appliances[52] for the treatment of anterior open bite. In all of these procedures anterior open bite was treated by the extrusion of anterior teeth rather than the intrusion of posterior dentition. Ohmae et al.,[53] in an animal model, and Umemori et al.,[20] in humans, applied titanium mini-plates to the mandibular corpus area and used them as anchorage for the intrusion of mandibular posterior segments. They were able to intrude the mandibular posterior dentoalveolar segments and correct the anterior open bite. This can be an effective method of anterior open-bite treatment in cases with overerupted mandibular molars.

In most anterior open-bite cases, the malocclusion is morphologically characterized by overeruption of the maxillary posterior teeth and the resultant posterior rotation of the mandible. True treatment of anterior open bite requires intrusion of the maxillary posterior segments and anterior rotation of the mandible. The only treatment modality in which this goal can be achieved effectively is orthognathic surgery.[44]

Since the zygomatic anchor is located in a superior position to the maxillary posterior dentition, by using its support it is possible to achieve maxillary posterior dentoalveolar intrusion and mandibular anterior rotation for the correction of anterior open bite.[54,55]

Before the development of MPIs, surgical mini-plates were used as zygomatic anchors. A patient treated with this approach is shown in Figure 19-13. Mini-plates were adapted and fixed with three mini-screws to the inferior border of the zygomatic buttress. The free end of the plate was extended to the oral cavity and exposed through the line of horizontal incision. Closed Ni-Ti coil springs were applied between the free end of the mini-plate and the maxillary posterior dentition (see Fig. 19-13, F–H). To prevent buccal tipping of the molars during intrusion, a transpalatal arch constructed from 1.5-mm stainless steel round wire was used (see Fig. 19-13, I). The transpalatal arch passed at least

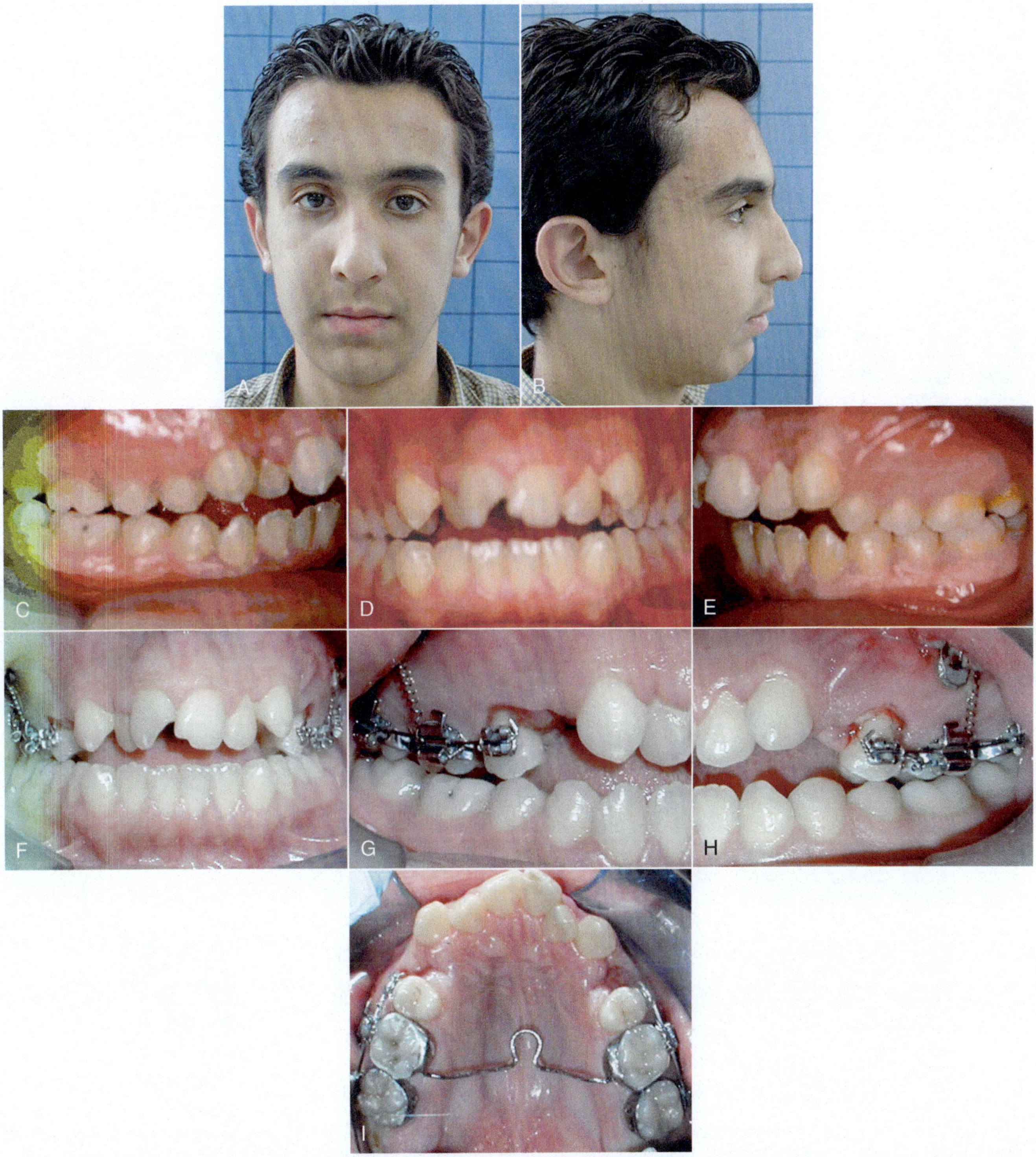

Figure 19-13 A 21-year-old male patient with high angle growth pattern, Class II molar and canine relationship, anterior crowding, and open bite. The treatment plan involved extraction of the upper first premolars to resolve crowding and intrusion of the upper posterior segments to close the open bite. Pretreatment **(A and B)** facial and **(C–E)** intraoral views. **F–H,** Following upper first premolar extraction, intrusion of the right and left posterior segments was initiated using nickel-titanium (Ni-Ti) closed coil springs, which were placed between the free ends of the mini-plates and the first molar tubes. **I,** Transpalatal arch was placed to prevent buccal tipping of the molars.

Continued

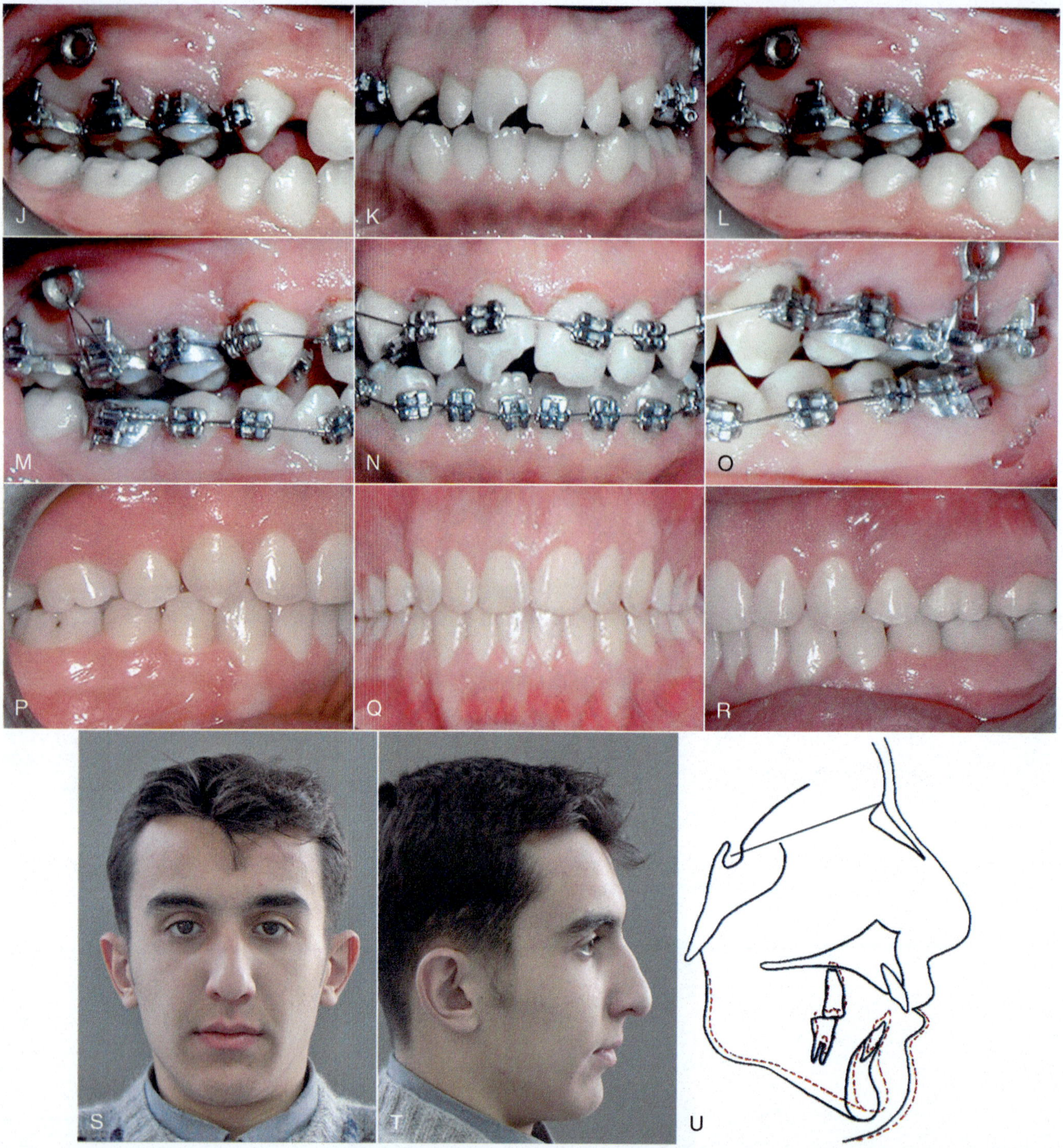

Figure 19-13, cont'd **J–L,** After 5 months of posterior intrusion. **M–O,** After 8 months of treatment. **P–R,** After orthodontic treatment was completed. **S and T,** Facial views of the patient after treatment. **U,** Schematic illustration of the dental and skeletal changes related to treatment. Note the counterclockwise rotation of the mandible.

3-mm from the palatal mucosa so as not to hinder molar intrusion.

Evaluation of the Treatment Modality

This treatment method was found to be effective but some problems arose during the procedure:

- Surgical mini-plates were bulky and created some hygiene problems and discomfort.
- It is difficult to control all premature contacts in the posterior region by means of fixed mechanics. Occlusal interferences prevented anterior rotation of the mandible.
- The transpalatal arch was not enough to prevent buccal tipping of the molars during intrusion.

OPEN-BITE APPLIANCE

The open-bite appliance (OBA) was developed specifically for open-bite correction and has undergone various modifications with clinical experience.

Fabrication of Open-Bite Appliance

Wire Bending

The OBA has three palatal bars made of 1.5-mm round stainless steel wire. Palatal bars are 4-mm apart from the palatal mucosa. Palatal arches are bent on two layers of wax to avoid impingement to palatal mucosa during intrusion.

Buccal bars are constructed using 0.8-mm round stainless steel wire. They are adjusted to be parallel to the maxillary dental arch and are placed at least 5-mm buccal from the labial faces of the molars. Ni-Ti coil springs with required force magnitude are engaged on the buccal bars. Buccal bars extend from the second molar to the second premolar. In the coronal section the angulation of the buccal bars must be made according to the width of the attached gingiva. In patients with insufficient gingival band width the vertical height also is insufficient for activation of Ni-Ti coil springs. In these patients, buccal bars are angled downward to gain more vertical distance, which is necessary for activation of the coil springs.

Acrylic Cap

The intrusion appliance consists of two shallow acrylic bite blocks connected with palatal arches and wire attachments on each buccal side, used for force application. An acrylic cap splint is used for the retention of the appliance. It must cover whole occlusal surfaces of the posterior teeth and end at the level of the widest crown diameter. Occlusal thickness must be about 3-mm (Fig. 19-14).

Clinical Application

After 7 to 10 days of wound healing and removal of the sutures, the OBA is tried in the mouth to check for even occlusal contact bilaterally. The cusp tips of the appliance segments are trimmed flat to control bite opening during expansion and generation of eccentric and unilateral contact points. This step is especially important; occlusal interference is the main threat to the stability of the appliance.

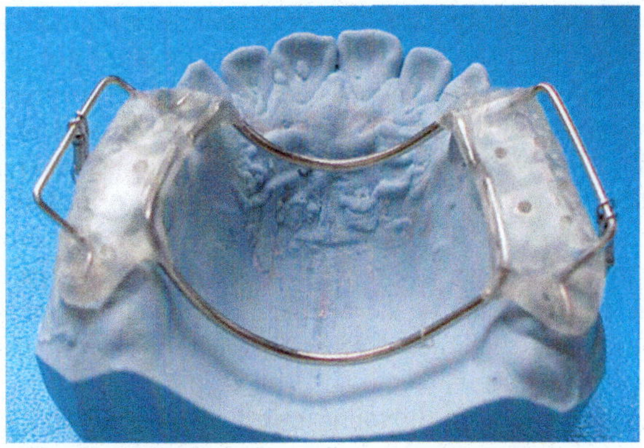

Figure 19-14 An acrylic cap covers the occlusal surfaces and extends about 1.5- to 2-mm away from the gingival margin.

The bonding material is glass ionomer cement, which provides adequate appliance retention. After cleaning the residual adhesive material, coils are engaged to the implants and treatment begins. Two 9-mm Ni-Ti coil springs (Masel, Bristol, PA.) placed bilaterally between the tip of the implant and the outer wire create an intrusive force of 400 g.

Mode of Action

In OBA treatment, the intrusive force has three components functioning in the same favorable way to intrude the maxillary dentoalveolar segment:

- *Coil springs:* Ni-Ti coil springs providing bilateral intrusive force are the main intrusive component. The individual force is calculated for each case, as explained below. Because of the buccal bars, it is possible to exert a perpendicular force with this method. This means that there will be no force loss.
- *Acrylic cap:* An acrylic cap with 3-mm of thickness is very effective in transferring forces from muscle tonus and occlusal function to the dentition as an intrusive vector.
- *Palatal bars:* Palatal bars are in contact with the corpus of the tongue, transferring this intrusive force to the dentition.

Force Calculation

The chart developed by Ricketts for "bioprogressive therapy" is used for the calculation of the force magnitude. In this system, force is calculated according to the maximum cross-section of the root area, using 100 g and 150 g of force per square centimeter (cm^2).

Clinical Experience

In the OBA treatment philosophy, upper third molars are extracted before treatment. Patient selection is important and patients with very good oral hygiene are good candidates for orthodontic implants. Patients must be instructed about oral hygiene requirements and special care in cleaning the areas where the implant is exposed in the oral cavity.

Treatment is divided into two phases. In the first phase, open-bite correction is achieved with the OBA; this takes approximately 5 months. The appliance is then removed and the open bite is reduced by the autorotation of the mandible. If posterior crossbite and maxillary constriction are present, the acrylic cap Hyrax should be preferred instead of the OBA. However, when the case needs surgically assisted rapid palatal expansion, corticotomy could be performed at the same time as MPI placement. The osteotomy line should be below the zygomatic buttress where the MPI was placed. The bar extension of the MPI should be bended buccally considering the amount of expansion to avoid soft tissue impingement.

Conventional orthodontic treatment of a Class I case resumes, as the underlying malocclusion has been corrected with the OBA. In some patients the incisor position will not allow completion of the anterior rotation of the mandible after removal of the OBA. In these patients, upper incisor leveling and proclination must be started during the intrusion phase of the OBA treatment. For this action, the acrylic in the buccal aspect of the premolar is removed and brackets are placed, including on the canines and incisors (Fig. 19-15).

In the second phase of treatment, fixed appliances are placed completely and the first molar is kept ligated to the implant until the end of treatment. In this way vertical position of the posterior teeth is maintained.

Risk of Root Resorption

The only investigation on the risk of root resorption reported in the literature found no clinically significant root resorption with OBA treatment.[56]

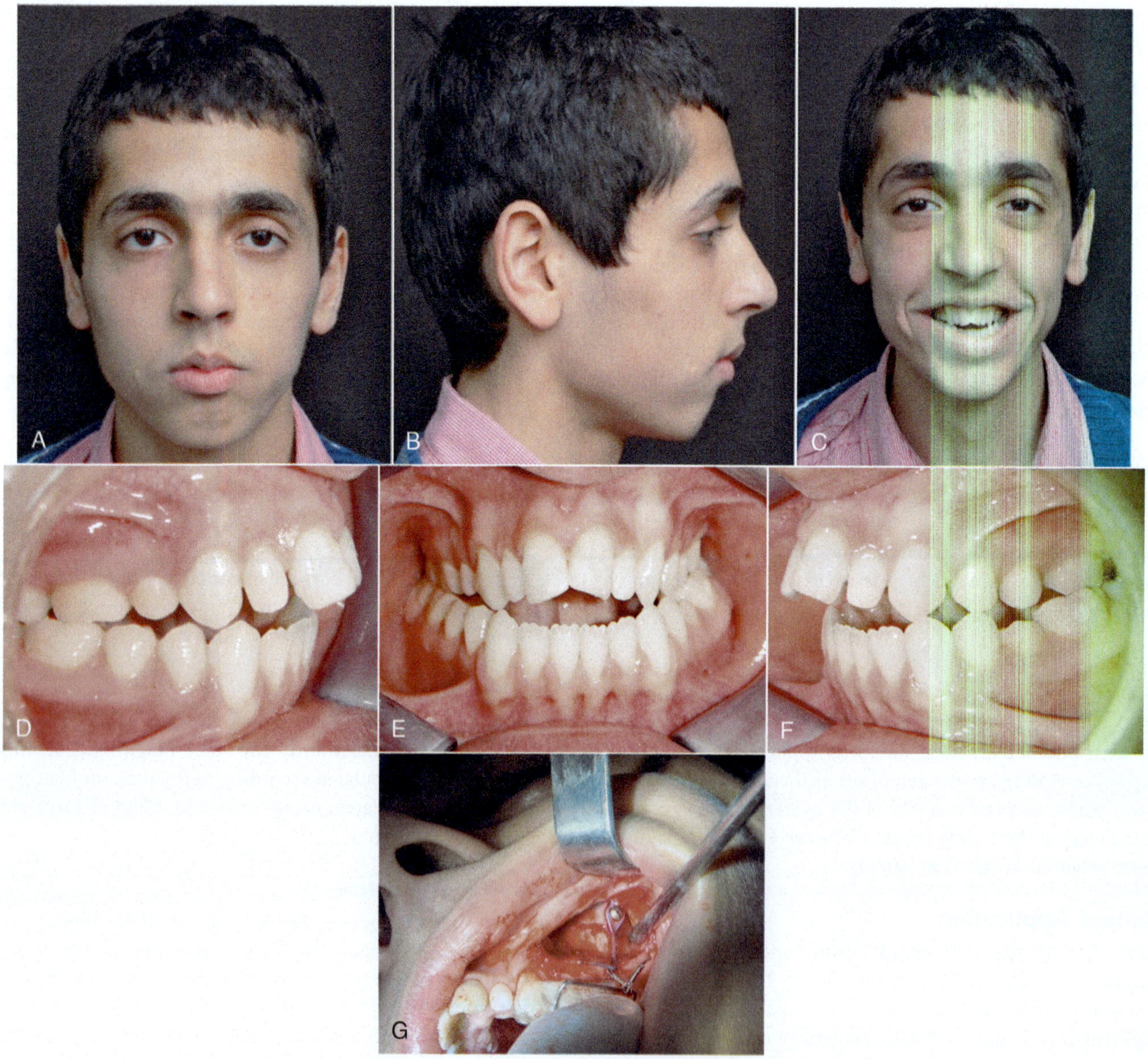

Figure 19-15 A 19-year-old male patient with high angle growth pattern, Class II molar and canine relationship, posterior crossbite, and open bite. The treatment plan involved surgically assisted rapid palatal expansion followed by posterior intrusion. Pre-treatment **(A–C)** facial and **(D–F)** intraoral views. **G,** Corticotomy applied during multipurpose implant (MPI) placement surgery.

MOLAR DISTALIZATION USING MULTIPURPOSE IMPLANT ANCHORAGE

For molar distalization, an MPI with 0.9-mm bar thickness is used. The upper part of the MPI is adapted to the bony curvature, 5-mm mesial to the line passing from the mesial edge of the first molar tube. The round bar is extended in the downward direction to the level of the first molar tube and then bent in the mesial direction along the sulcus depth 3-mm apart from the vestibular mucosa (Fig. 19-16). A 1-mm-thick stainless steel round wire is soldered to the lower surface of the custom fabricated metal sliding lock (Dentaurum), extending toward the archwire. A horizontal U-bend is made in the wire to be used in adjusting the force vector. A segmental round tube is soldered to the lower edge of the round wire at the same level as the main archwire, to be used for compressing the open coil spring. The metal sliding lock is engaged on the mesial extension of the zygomatic implant.

First molars are banded and first premolars are bonded. A 0.016-inch × 0.022-inch rectangular stainless steel archwire is engaged passing through the segmental tube, a segmental Ni-Ti open coil spring is placed on the archwire after the segmental tube, and the archwire is engaged in the main tube of the molar band. A metal sliding lock is engaged in the distal direction so that sufficient activation of the compressed open coil spring to distalize the molars is provided and is fixed in that position.

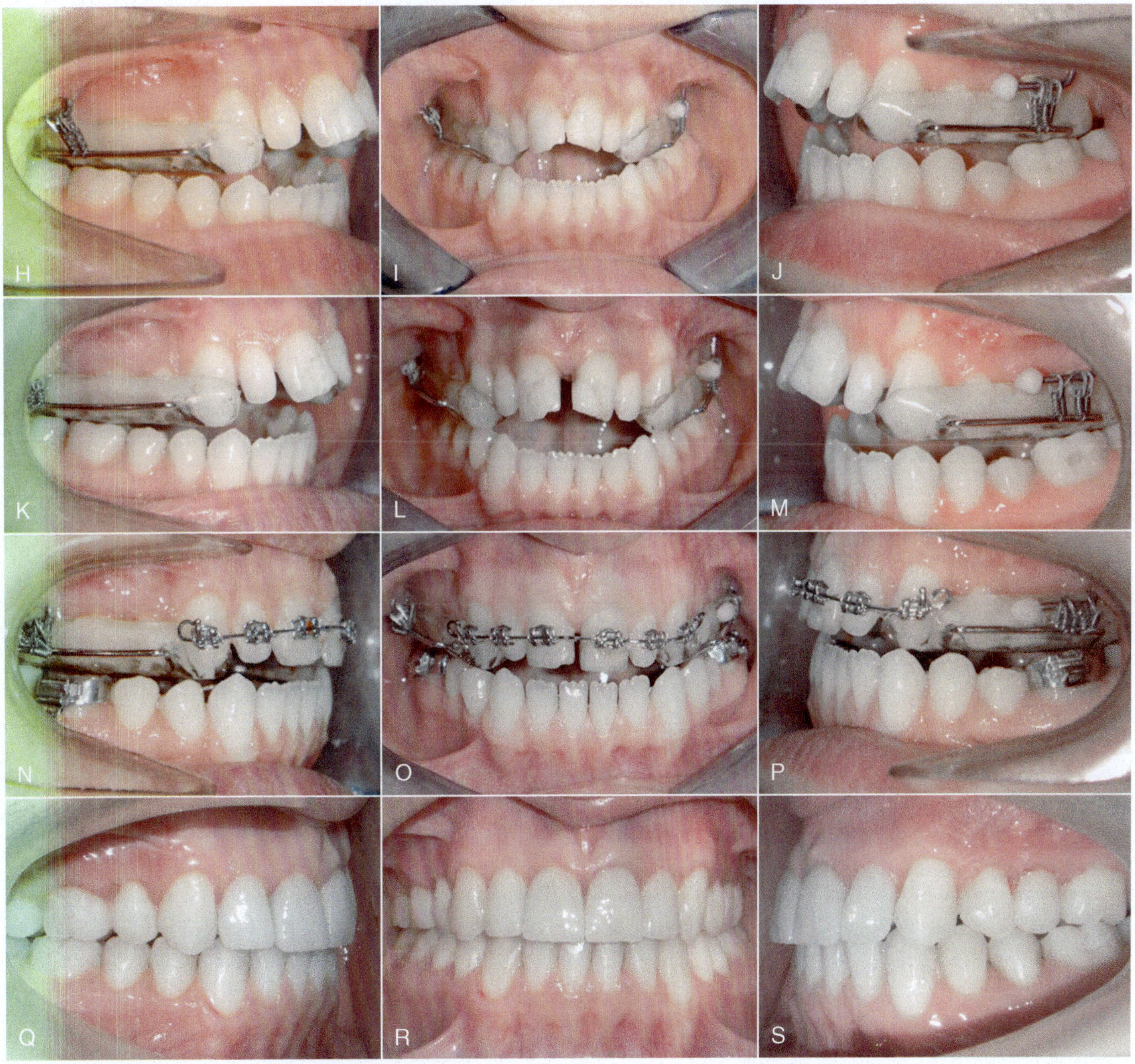

Figure 19-15, cont'd **H–J,** Nickel-titanium (Ni-Ti) closed coil springs were placed at the free ends of the mini-plates. **K–M,** After surgically assisted rapid maxillary expansion. **N–P,** After 8 months of treatment. **Q–S,** After prosthetic restoration. *Continued*

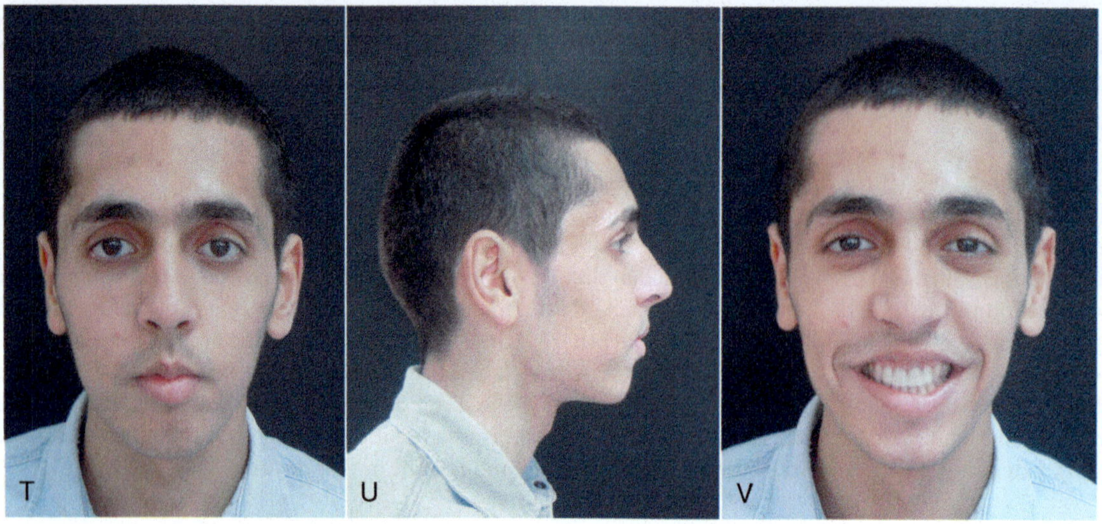

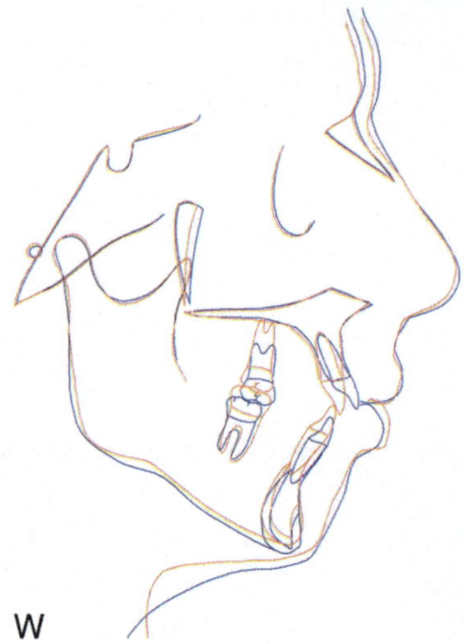

Figure 19-15, cont'd **T–V,** Facial views of the patient after treatment. **W,** Cephalometric superimposition. Autorotation of the mandible is due to significant posterior intrusion.

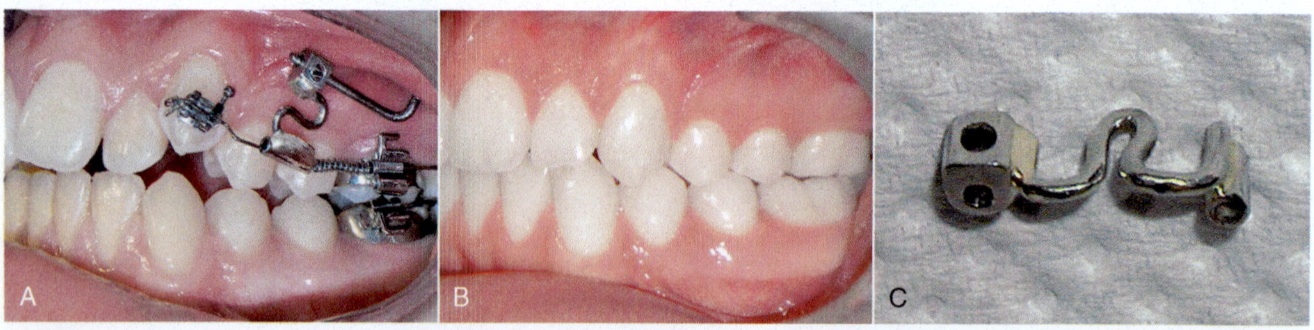

Figure 19-16 Clinical examination of a 17-year-old male patient revealed unilateral Class II molar relationship on the left side. Tooth 26 was distalized using zygomatic anchorage followed by fixed appliance. **A,** Molar distalization mechanics with zygomatic implant. **B,** Post-treatment results. **C,** Sliding bar extension and segmental tube.

CLASS III TREATMENT APPROACHES USING MULTIPURPOSE IMPLANT ANCHORAGE

Class III malocclusions are considered to be among the most challenging orthodontic problems to treat. The prevalence of Class III malocclusions is approximately 1% to 5% in white populations.[57,58] The Class III malocclusion might be due to mandibular prognathism, maxillary retrognathism, protrusive mandibular dentition or retrusive maxillary dentition, or a combination of these components. It has been reported that two-thirds of skeletal Class III malocclusions are due to either maxillary retrognathism or a combination of maxillary retrognathism and mandibular prognathism.[59–63]

Early treatment is commonly indicated to obtain a more normal jaw relationship. A facemask is thought to be an effective treatment approach for skeletal Class III patients with maxillary deficiency. The results of previous clinical studies have indicated that the application of an orthopedic force with a protraction facemask to the craniofacial complex during the early phase of growth can contribute to the correction of Class III malocclusion.[64–68]

Facemask therapy is usually managed with tooth-borne anchorage devices such as lingual arches and expansion appliances. Orthopedic force on the nasomaxillary complex is directed along the occlusal plane rather than at the center of resistance of the maxilla. As a result, bone remodeling occurs not only at the circumaxillary sutures, but also within the periodontal ligament. Another side effect of protracting along the occlusal plane is the loss of arch length due to mesial movement of the posterior teeth, especially in the mixed dentition or in patients with missing teeth.[69] To eliminate the undesirable dental effects and to achieve more skeletal effects, it is recommended to have a stable anchorage to transfer the force directly to the circumaxillary sutures. Ankylosed teeth, osseointegrated implants, titanium screws, onplants, and mini-plates have been used as stable anchorage for maxillary protraction.[70–74]

Although these studies showed encouraging results, they still relied on facemask wear and thus on patient compliance. Wearing maxillomandibular elastics is, without doubt, socially less constraining than wearing a facemask. The cooperation needed by these patients was limited to replacement of the elastics once a day and maintenance of good oral hygiene. By contrast, with facemask forces, these elastics could easily be maintained 24 hours per day. The direction of force application between the acrylic cap and mandibular mini-plates was located below the center of resistance of the maxilla.

Clinical results obtained by different applications of MPIs with malleable extension are presented in the case reports.

CASE REPORTS

Two case reports are presented to illustrate different applications of skeletal anchorage.

CASE REPORT 1

A 14-year-old female patient presented with a Class III malocclusion. Her chief complaint was underbite. The patient was characterized by a slightly concave facial profile resulting from a retrognathic maxilla (Fig. 19-17, A). She presented with a Class III molar and canine relationship on both sides along with a 3-mm negative overjet and a slight amount of spacing in the lower anterior region (Fig. 19-17, B–D).

Treatment Objectives

The treatment objectives were to improve the facial esthetics by advancing the midface anteriorly and to coordinate the arches sagittally. The treatment plan consisted of protraction of the maxilla by facemask using zygomatic anchorage and surgical assistance.

Treatment Progress

Le Fort I osteotomy was performed during MPI placement surgery. The multipurpose mini-plates were contoured and placed horizontally in the zygomatic region under the corticotomy borders (Fig. 19-17, E and F) and straight extensions were bent in a hook shape and projected into the oral cavity on the inferior attached gingiva to retain the facemask elastics. Maxilla was mobilized but down fracture was not carried out. Surgery was done under local anesthesia and intravenous sedation.

After adaptation of a facemask, an elastic force of 400 g per side was applied to the MPI extensions (Fig. 19-17, G). The direction of force was adjusted approximately 30 degrees downward to the occlusal plane. Throughout the active treatment period, the patient was asked to wear the facemask full-time except during meals until positive overjet and a satisfying profile were achieved.

Normal overjet was achieved in 3 months and the overall treatment lasted 15 months (Fig. 19-17, H–K).

Continued

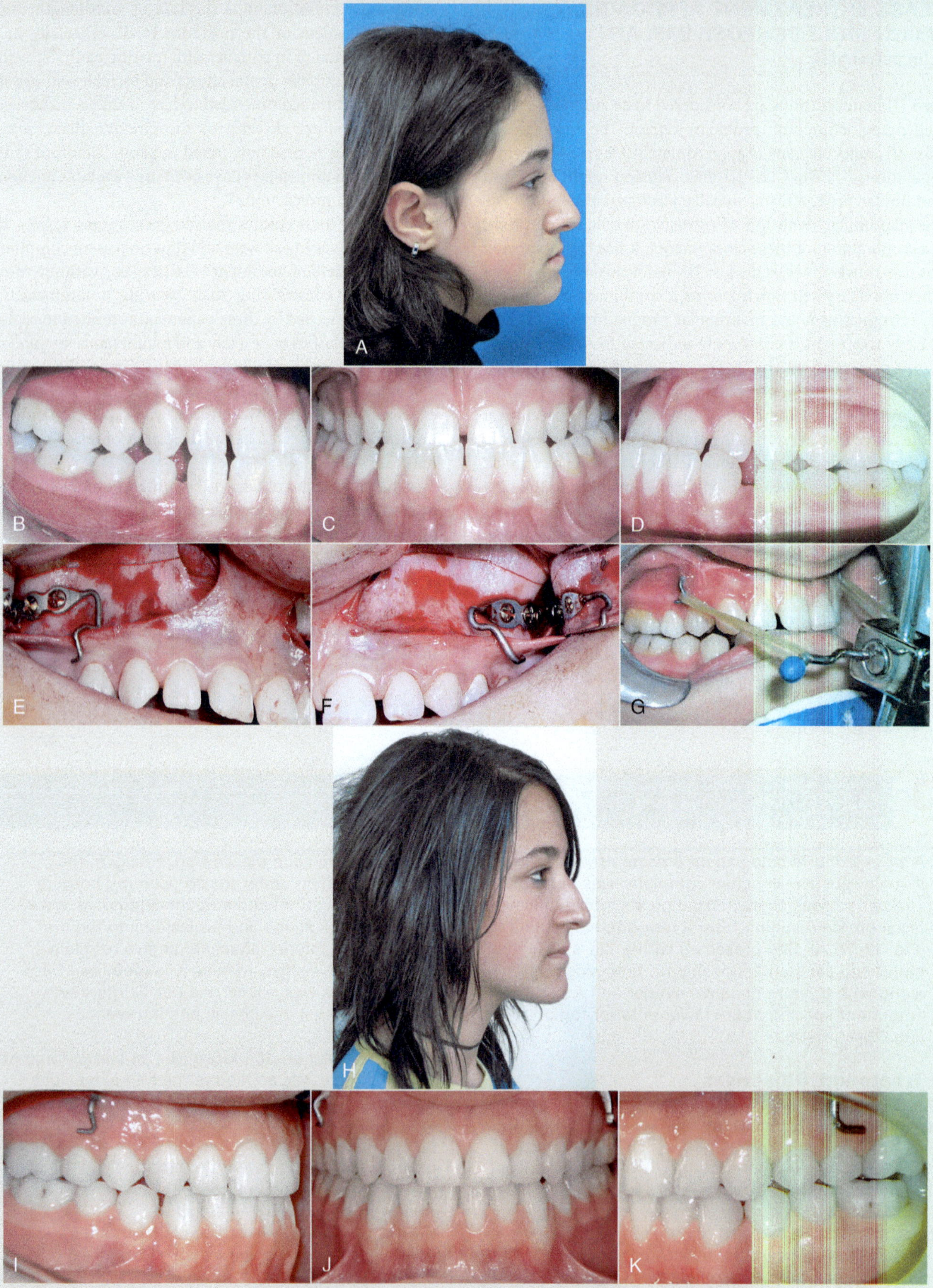

Figure 19-17 A 14-year-old female patient presented with a Class III malocclusion with maxillary deficiency. The treatment plan was to use Class III elastics by chinplate to achieve normal overjet and to correct the molar and canine relationship. Pre-treatment **(A)** facial and **(B–D)** intraoral views. **E and F,** Corticotomy line. **G,** Class III elastics were placed between the facemask and multipurpose implant (MPI). Post-treatment **(H)** facial and **(I–K)** intraoral views.

CASE REPORT 2

A 12-year-old female patient presented with a skeletal and dental Class III relationship due to retrognathic maxilla. Her chief complaint was smile esthetics due to anterior crossbite. The patient was characterized by a straight profile and had a 3-mm negative overjet and 2-mm overbite. She presented with a Class III canine relationship on both sides but Class II molar relationship on the right side due to early loss of a deciduous molar. She had a low smile line and the lower midline was shifted to the left by 2-mm (Fig. 19-18, A–C).

Treatment Objectives

Since the patient was in her pubertal growth spurt, the treatment objectives were to improve the skeletal jaw relationship as much as possible by growth modification and to correct the occlusal discrepancies by dentoalveolar compensation. An upper second premolar extraction treatment plan was adopted, which involved protraction of the maxilla by intermaxillary elastics using the MPIs placed in the mandibular symphysial region.

Treatment Progress

An acrylic bite block that included a 1-mm thick heavy wire to which intermaxillary elastics were attached was bonded on the upper arch for intraoral stabilization. The multipurpose mini-plates were contoured and placed in the symphysial region and then the straight extensions were bent in a hook shape and projected into the oral cavity on the inferior attached gingiva to retain the Class III elastics with a force of 300 g per side (Fig. 19-18, D and E). After achieving positive overjet, the upper arch was leveled and aligned by the extraction of teeth 14 and 25. Class III elastics were applied to the MPI extensions to close the extraction spaces.

The ideal overjet and overbite was achieved to normal limits (Fig. 19-18, F–L). The overall treatment lasted 18 months.

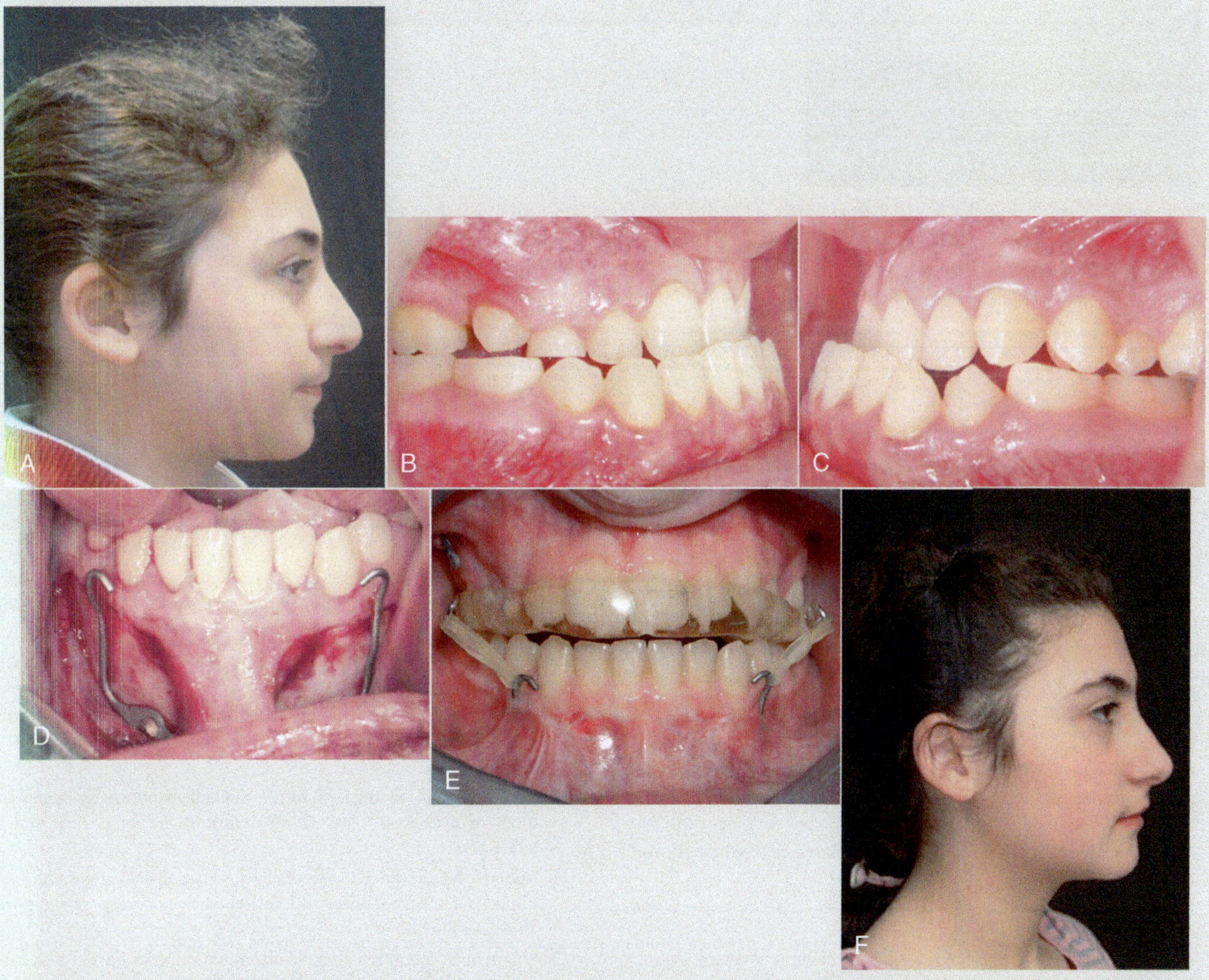

Figure 19-18 A 12-year-old female patient presented with a Class III malocclusion with maxillary deficiency. The treatment plan was to use Class III elastics by chinplate to achieve normal overjet and to correct the molar and canine relationship. Pre-treatment (**A**) facial and (**B and C**) intraoral views. **D,** Placement of chinplates. **E,** Class III elastics were placed between the acrylic cap and chinplate. **F,** Improvement in profile and overjet after 6 months.

Continued

CASE REPORT 2—cont'd

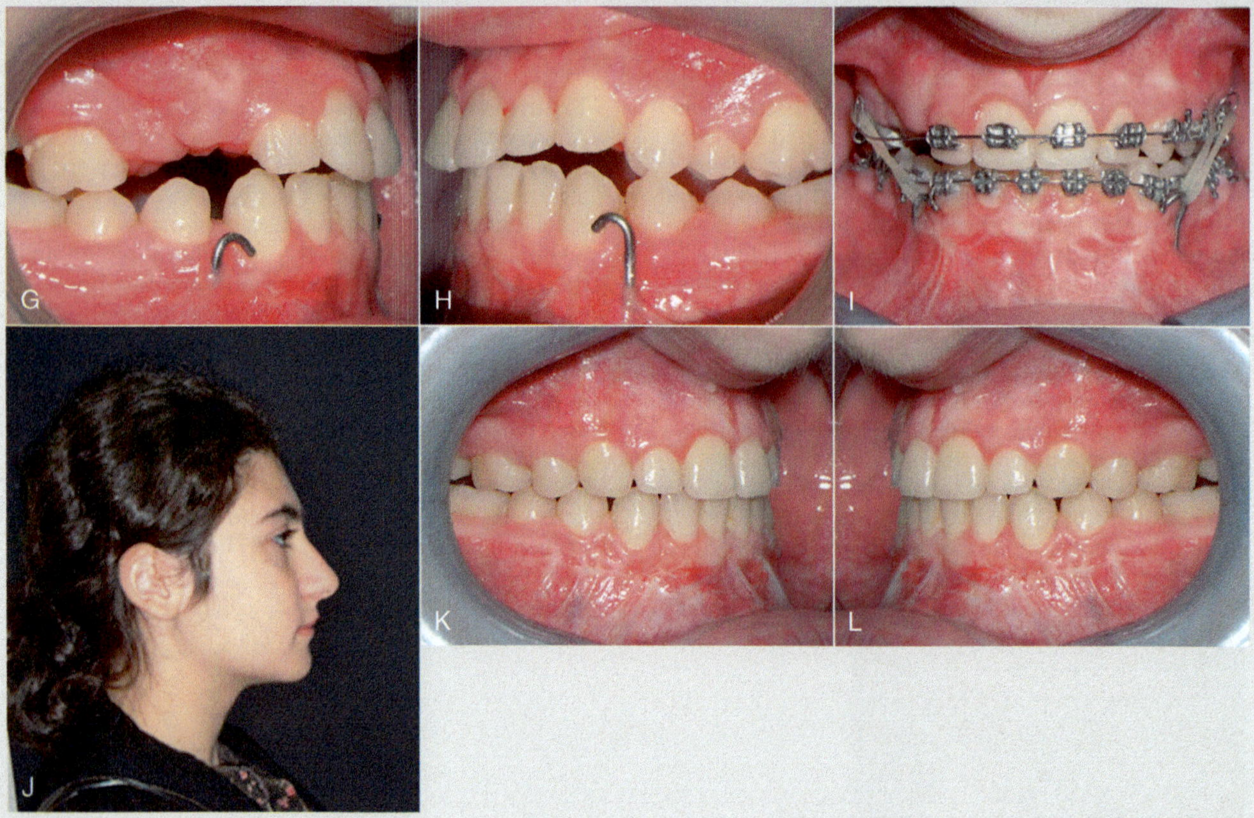

Figure 19-18, cont'd **G–I,** Class III elastics were used during fixed orthodontic treatment. Post-treatment **(J)** facial and **(K and L)** intraoral views.

SUMMARY

Skeletal anchorage has expanded the orthodontic treatment limits, and skeletal anchorage devices provide an excellent solution in critical anchorage situations. These skeletal anchorage devices do not show clinically significant movement in reaction to orthodontic forces, and they eliminate the need for patient compliance during anchorage maintenance. The number of extraction and orthognathic surgical cases can significantly be decreased with the aid of skeletal anchorage.

REFERENCES

1. Egolf RJ, Begole EA, Upshaw HS. Factors associated with orthodontic patient compliance with intraoral elastic and headgear wear. *Am J Orthod*. 1990;97:336–348.
2. AAO issues special bulletin on extraoral appliance care [editorial]. *Am J Orthod*. 1975;68(4):457.
3. Preliminary results of headgear survey. *Bulletin (American Association of Orthodontists)*. 1982;1:1.
4. Diedrich P. Different orthodontic anchorage systems: a critical examination [in German]. *Fortschr Kieferorthop*. 1993;54:156–171.
5. Gainsforth BL. A study of orthodontic anchorage possibilities in basal bone. *Am J Orthod Oral Surg*. 1945;31:406–417.
6. Linkow LI. Implanto-orthodontics. *Clin J Orthod*. 1970;4(12):685–705.
7. Schlegel KA, Schweizer C, Janson IR, Wiltfang J. A new anchorage concept for orthodontic treatment in the mandible. *World J Orthod*. 2002;3:353–357.
8. Clerck H, Geerinckx V, Siciliano S. The zygoma anchorage system. *J Clin Orthod*. 2002;36:455–459.
9. Kanomi R. Mini-implant for orthodontic anchorage. *J Clin Orthod*. 1997;31:763–767.
10. Costa A, Raffling M, Millstone B. Miniscrews as orthodontic anchorage: a preliminary report. *Int J Adult Orthod Orthogn Surg*. 1998;13: 201–209.
11. Bousquet F, Bousquet P, Mauran G, Parguel P. Use of an impacted post for anchorage. *J Clin Orthod*. 1996;30:261–265.
12. Park H, Bae S, Kyung H, Sung J. Micro-implant anchorage for treatment of skeletal Class I bialveolar protrusion. *J Clin Orthod*. 2001;35: 417–422.
13. Lee JS, Park HS, Kyung HM. Micro-implant anchorage for lingual treatment of a skeletal Class II malocclusion. *J Clin Orthod*. 2001;35: 643–647.
14. Roberts WE, Helm FR, Marshall KJ, Gongloff RK. Rigid endosseous implants for orthodontic and orthopedic anchorage. *Angle Orthod*. 1989;59:247–255.
15. Sherman A. Bone reaction to orthodontic forces on vitreous carbon dental implants. *Am J Orthod*. 1978;74:79–87.
16. Block MS, Hoffman DR. A new device for absolute anchorage for orthodontics. *Am J Orthod*. 1995;107:251–258.

17. Melsen B, Petersen JK, Costa A. Zygoma ligatures: an alternative form of maxillary anchorage. *J Clin Orthod.* 1998;32:154–158.
18. Kokich VG, Shapiro PA, Oswald R, Koskinen-Moffett L, Clarren SK. Ankylosed teeth as abutments for maxillary protraction: a case report. *Am J Orthod.* 1985;88(4):303–307.
19. Wehrbein H, Glatzmaier J, Mundwiller U, Diedrich P. The Orthosystem: a new implant system for orthodontic anchorage in the palate. *J Orofac Orthop.* 1996;57(3):142–153.
20. Umemori M, Sugawara J, Nagasaka H, Kawamura H. Skeletal anchorage system for open-bite correction. *Am J Orthop.* 1999;115:166–174.
21. Chung KR, Kim YS, Linton JL, Lee YJ. The miniplate with tube for skeletal anchorage. *J Clin Orthod.* 2002;36:407–412.
22. Maino BG, Bednar J, Pagin P, Mura P. The spider screw for skeletal anchorage. *J Clin Orthod.* 2003;37:90–97.
23. Higuchi KW. Ortho-integration: the alliance between orthodontics and osseointegration. In: Higuchi KJ, ed. *Orthodontic Applications of Osseointegrated Implants.* Chicago, IL: Quintessence Publishing Co; 2000: 1–19.
24. Roberts WE, Marshall KJ, Mozsary PG. Rigid endosseous implant utilized as anchorage to protract molars and close an atrophic extraction site. *Angle Orthod.* 1990;60:135–152.
25. Higuchi KW, Slack JM. The use of titanium fixtures for intraoral anchorage to facilitate orthodontic tooth movement. *Int J Oral Maxillofac Implants.* 1991;6(3):338–344.
26. Abels N, Schiel HJ, Hery-Langer G, Neugebauer J, Engel M. Bone condensing in the placement of endosteal palatal implants: a case report. *Int J Oral Maxillofac Implants.* 1999;14(6):849–852.
27. Glatzmaier J, Wehrbein H, Diedrich P. Die Entwicklung eines resorbierbaren Implantatsystems zur orthodontischen Verankerung [The development of a resorbable implant system for orthodontic anchorage: the BIOS implant system: bioresorbable implant anchor for orthodontic systems]. *Fortschr Kieferorthop.* 1995;56(3):175–181.
28. Triaca A, Antonini M, Wintermantel E. Ein neues Titan-Flachschraubenimplantat zur Verankerung am anterioren Gaumen. *Inf Orthod Orthop.* 1992;24:251–257.
29. Turley PK, Shapiro PA, Moffett BC. The loading of bioglass-coated aluminum oxide implants to produce sutural expansion of the maxillary complex in the pigtail monkey *(Macaca nemestrina). Arch Oral Biol.* 1980;25:459–469.
30. Wehrbein H. Enossale Titanimplantate als orthodontische Verankerungselemente. Experimentelle Untersuchungen und klinische Anwendung [Endosseous titanium implants as orthodontic anchoring elements: experimental studies and clinical application]. *Fortschr Kieferorthop.* 1994;55(5):236–250.
31. Wehrbein H, Feifel H, Diedrich P. Palatal implant anchorage reinforcement of posterior teeth: a prospective study. *Am J Orthod Dentofacial Orthop.* 1999;116:678–686.
32. Bantleon H, Bernhart T, Crismani AG, Zachrisson U. Stable orthodontic anchorage with palatal osseointegrated implants. *World J Orthod.* 2002;3:109–116.
33. Keles A, Erverdi N, Sezen S. Bodily molar distalization with absolute anchorage. *Angle Orthod.* 2003;73:471–482.
34. Gahleitner A, Podesser B, Schick S, Watzek G, Imhof H. Dental CT and orthodontic implants: imaging technique and assessment of available bone volume in the hard palate. *Eur J Radiol.* 2004;51(3):257–262.
35. Henriksen B, Bavitz B, Kelly B, Harn SD. Evaluation of bone thickness in the anterior hard palate relative to midsagittal orthodontic implants. *Int J Oral Maxillofac Implants.* 2003;18:578–581.
36. Bernhard T, Vollgruber A, Gahleitner A, Dortbudak O, Haas R. Alternative to median region of the palate for placement of an orthodontic implant. *Clin Oral Implant Res.* 2000;11:595–601.
37. Melsen B. Palatal growth studied on human autopsy material. *Am J Orthod.* 1975;68:42–54.
38. Schlegel KA, Kinner F, Schlegel KD. The anatomic basis for palatal implants in orthodontics. *Int J Adult Orthod Orthognath Surg.* 2002;17: 133–139.
39. Wehrbein H, Merz BR, Diedrich P, Glatzmaier J. The use of palatal implants for orthodontic anchorage: design and clinical application of the Orthosystem. *Clin Oral Implants Res.* 1996;7:410–416.
40. Wehrbein H, Glatzmaier J, Yildirim M. Orthodontic anchorage capacity of short titanium screw implants in the maxilla: an experimental study in the dog. *Clin Oral Implants Res.* 1997;8:131–141.
41. Björk A, Skieller V. Postnatal growth and development of the maxillary complex. In: McNamara JA Jr, ed. *Factors Affecting the Growth of the Midface.* Craniofacial Growth Series; monograph 6. Ann Arbor, MI: Center For Human Growth and Development, University of Michigan; 1976:61–69.
42. Björk A, Skieller V. Growth of the maxilla in three dimensions as revealed radiographically by the implant method. *Br J Orthod.* 1977;4: 53–64.
43. Asscherickx K, Hanssens JL, Wehrbein H, Sabzevar MM. Orthodontic anchorage implants inserted in the median palatal suture and normal transverse growth in growing dogs: a biometric and radiographic study. *Angle Orthod.* 2005;75:826–831.
44. Lawry DM, Heggie AA, Crawford EC, Ruljancich MK. A review of the management of anterior open bite malocclusion. *Aust Orthod J.* 1990; 11:147–160.
45. Rinchuse DJ. Vertical elastics for correction of anterior openbite. *J Clin Orthod.* 1994;28(5):284.
46. Kim YH. Anterior openbite and its treatment with multi loop edgewise archwire. *Angle Orthod.* 1997;57:171–178.
47. Kucukkeleş N, Acar A, Demirkaya A, Evrenol B, Enacar A. Cephalometric evaluation of open bite treatment with NiTi archwires and anterior elastics. *Am J Orthod Dentofacial Orthop.* 1999;116:555–562.
48. Dellinger EL. A clinical assessment of the active vertical corrector: a nonsurgical alternative for skeletal open bite treatment. *Am J Orthod Dentofacial Orthop.* 1986;89:428–436.
49. Kaira V, Burstone CJ, Nanda R. Effects of a fixed magnetic appliance on the dentofacial complex. *Am J Orthod Dentofacial Orthop.* 1989;95: 467–478.
50. Kiliaridis S, Egermark B, Thilander B. Anterior open bite treatment with magnets. *Eur J Orthod.* 1990;12(4):447–457.
51. İşcan HN, Sansoy L. Comparison of the effects of passive bite blocks with different construction bites on the craniofacial and dentoalveolar structures. *Am J Orthod Dentofacial Orthop.* 1997;112:171–178.
52. Stellzig A, Steegmayer-Gilde G, Basdra EK. Elastic activator for treatment of open bite. *Br J Orthod.* 1999;26(2):89–92.
53. Ohmae M, Saito S, Morohashi T, et al. A clinical and histological evaluation of titanium mini-implants as anchors for orthodontic intrusion in the beagle dog. *Am J Orthod Dentofacial Orthop.* 2001;119(5): 489–497.
54. Erverdi N, Tosun T, Keles A. A new anchorage site for the treatment of anterior open bite: zygomatic anchorage: case report. *Orthodontics (Chic).* 2002;3(2):147–153.
55. Sherwood K, Burch J, Thompson W. Closing anterior open bites by intruding molars with titanium miniplate anchorage. *Am J Orthod Dentofacial Orthop.* 2002;122:593–600.
56. Ari-Demirkaya A, Al Masry M, Erverdi N. Apical root resorption of maxillary first molars after intrusion with zygomatic skeletal anchorage. *Angle Orthod.* 2005;75:761–767.
57. Haynes S. The prevalence of malocclusion in English school children aged 11–12 years. *Trans Eur Orthod Soc.* 1970;89–98.
58. Thilander B, Myberg N. The prevalence of malocclusion in Swedish school children. *Scand J Dent Res.* 1973;81:12–20.
59. Ellis EE, McNamara JA Jr. Components of adult Class III malocclusion. *Am J Orthod.* 1984;85:277–290.
60. Nanda R. Biomechanical and clinical considerations of a modified protraction headgear. *Am J Orthod.* 1980;78:125–139.
61. Sanborn RT. Differences between the facial skeletal patterns of Class III malocclusion and normal occlusion. *Angle Orthod.* 1955;25:208–222.
62. McNamara JA, Brudon WL. *Orthodontic and Orthopedic Treatment in the Mixed Dentition.* Ann Arbor, MI: Needham Press; 1993:285–293.

63. Guyer EC, Ellis EE, McNamara JA Jr, Behrents RG. Components of Class III malocclusion in juveniles and adolescents. *Angle Orthod.* 1986;56:7–30.
64. Kajiyama K, Murakami T, Suzuki A. Evaluation of the modified maxillary protractor applied to Class III malocclusion with retruded maxilla in early mixed dentition. *Am J Orthod Dentofacial Orthop.* 2000;118:549–559.
65. Baccetti T, Franchi L, McNamara JA Jr. Treatment and posttreatment craniofacial changes after rapid maxillary expansion and facemask therapy. *Am J Orthod Dentofacial Orthop.* 2000;118:404–413.
66. Chong YH, Ive JC, Artun J. Changes following the use of protraction headgear for early correction of Class III malocclusion. *Angle Orthod.* 1996;66:351–362.
67. Kapust AJ, Sinclair PM, Turley PK. Cephalometric effects of face mask/expansion therapy in Class III children: a comparison of three age groups. *Am J Orthod Dentofacial Orthop.* 1998;113:204–212.
68. Franchi L, Baccetti T, McNamara JA. Postpubertal assessment of treatment timing for maxillary expansion and protraction therapy followed by fixed appliances. *Am J Orthod Dentofacial Orthop.* 2004;126:555–568.
69. Cha BK, Choi DS, Ngan P. Maxillary protraction with miniplates providing skeletal anchorage in a growing Class III patient. *Am J Orthod Dentofacial Orthop.* 2011;139:99–112.
70. Kokich VG, Shapiro PA, Oswald R, Koskinen-Moffett L, Clarren SK. Ankylosed teeth as abutments for maxillary protraction: a case report. *J Orthod.* 1985;88:303–307.
71. Singer SL, Henry PJ, Rosenberg I. Osseointegrated implants as an adjunct to facemask therapy: a case report. *Angle Orthod.* 2000;70:253–262.
72. Enacar A, Giray B, Pehlivanoglu M, Iplikcioglu H. Facemask therapy with rigid anchorage in a patient with maxillary hypoplasia and severe oligodontia. *Am J Orthod Dentofacial Orthop.* 2003;123(5):571–577.
73. Hong H, Ngan P, Han G, Qi LG, Wei SH. Use of onplants as stable anchorage for facemask treatment: a case report. *Angle Orthod.* 2005;75:453–460.
74. Kircelli BH, Pektas ZÖ. Midfacial protraction with skeletally anchored face mask therapy: a novel approach and preliminary results. *Am J Orthod Dentofacial Orthop.* 2008;133(3):440–449.

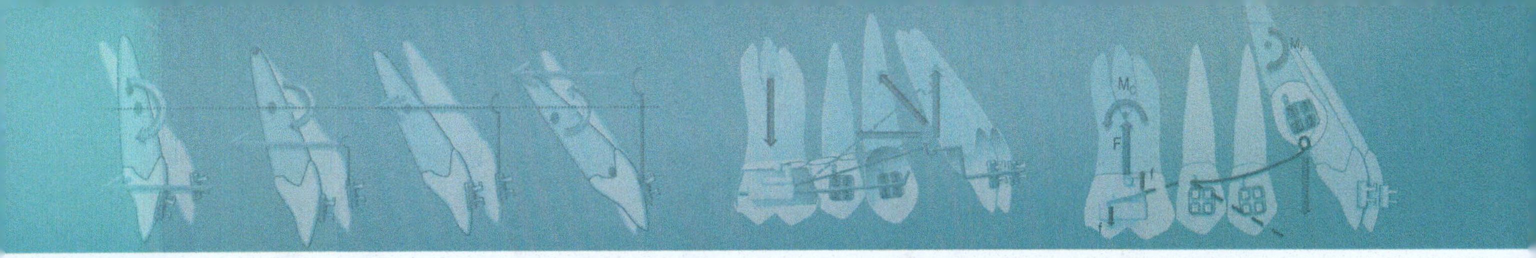

CHAPTER 20

A Bioefficient Skeletal Anchorage System

Junji Sugawara

Anchorage has long been one of the greatest problems in the field of orthodontics because teeth, even molars, move in response to orthodontic forces. Therefore, in maximal anchorage cases, patients have needed to wear headgear. Thus reinforced anchorage with extraoral appliances has severe limitations because it requires excellent patient compliance.

In the intermaxillary fixation after jaw surgery, maxillofacial surgeons have also found that teeth do not make reliable anchor units. To solve this problem, surgeons proposed "skeletal anchorage" as an adjunct to tooth-borne anchorage. The maxillary teeth and bone were fixed with wires from the anterior nasal spine (ANS), infraorbital rim, or zygomatic arch. The mandibular teeth were anchored to the mandible with wires that circled the mandibular body in the anterior and posterior regions.

In 1983 Creekmore and Eklund[1] reported a severe deep bite case that was successfully treated with a surgical vitallium bone screw inserted just below the ANS to intrude the upper incisors. This was the first clinical report of "skeletal anchorage" for orthodontic tooth movement. A second case was reported by Jenner and Fitzpatrick[2] in 1985. They applied a large bone plate in the ramus to tip the mandibular molar distally with a leading wire and elastics.

Our research group noted that the osteosynthesis titanium mini-plate had been thoroughly evaluated as an excellent biocompatible material in the field of maxillofacial surgery. In 1992 we developed the skeletal anchorage system (SAS) using titanium mini-plates[3] and, since then, SAS mechanics have been applied to various types of malocclusions in daily orthodontic practice.

The advantages and disadvantages of the SAS are listed in Boxes 20-1 and 20-2.

This chapter outlines the SAS and describes a typical case in which the patient was treated with the application of SAS.

NEW ORTHODONTIC ANCHOR PLATES

Because osteosynthesis titanium mini-plates were not designed as orthodontic anchor plates and are not necessarily suitable for orthodontic treatment, they were noted to have the following shortcomings:

- The shape of the mini-plate is not suitable for the application of orthodontic force.
- The surface of the arm portion that penetrates the mucoperiosteum is roughly sandblasted and difficult to clean.
- The size of the mini-plate is relatively thick and large.

To solve those problems, our research group developed the new orthodontic anchor plates.[4]

Features

Figure 20-1 shows the newly developed anchor plates, which are called SMAP (Super Mini Anchor Plate®, Dentsply-Sankin, Tokyo, Japan). These plates are made of pure titanium, which is suitable for osseointegration and also tissue integration. In addition, Class II pure titanium is used, which is strong enough to withstand the usual orthodontic forces but can also be bent with ease for fitting into the bone contour of the implantation site.

Figure 20-2 shows an example of the T-type anchor plate. The anchor plate consists of three portions: head, arm, and body. The head portion is intraorally exposed and positioned outside the dentition so that it never disturbs any kind of tooth movement. Each head portion has three continuous hooks for easier application of orthodontic forces. As the need arises, it is possible to cut off the first and second hooks. There are two types of head portion, which differ with regard to the direction of hooks, and which type is used depends on the manner of tooth movement.

The arm portion is transmucosal and has three graduated lengths—short (10.5-mm), medium (13.5-mm), and long (16.5-mm)—to compensate for individual morphological differences and to accommodate the manner of tooth movement (Fig. 20-3).

The body portion is positioned subperiosteally. There are three basic types: T, Y, and I. The T-type plates are frequently used as L-type plates by cutting off one of the circles. The variations in shape mean that the surgeon can select the most appropriate anchor plate according to the bone contour of the implantation site.

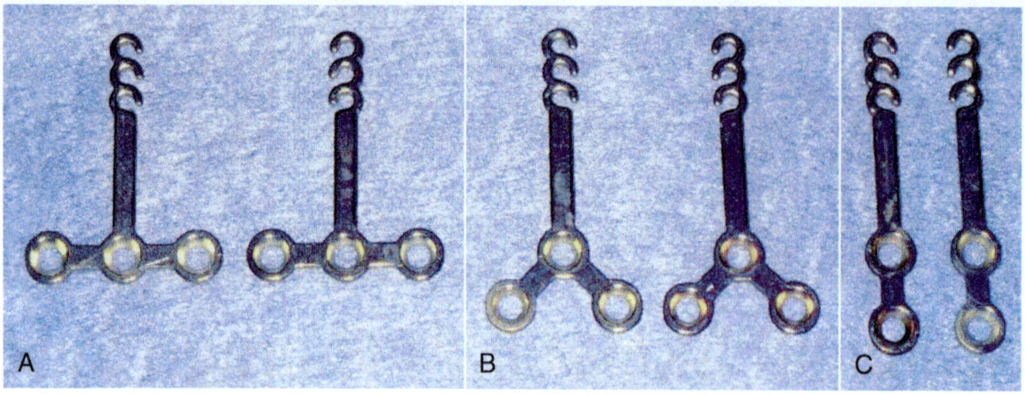

Figure 20-1 Orthodontic anchor plates. **A,** T-type. **B,** Y-type. **C,** I-type.

BOX 20-1 Advantages of Skeletal Anchorage System Treatment

Anchor plates are made of pure titanium, making them very stable and safe.
Anchor plates do not disturb any kind of tooth movement because they are placed outside the dentition. This is the most distinctive feature of the SAS in comparison with the other implant systems currently being used in orthodontics.
Molars can be moved as easily as teeth in the anterior dentition can be moved. It is now possible to easily control the occlusal plane and even the level of this plane.
Patients are no longer required to wear uncomfortable extraoral appliances (i.e., the SAS can function like an invisible headgear).
Patient compliance is not necessary, except with regard to oral hygiene.
Orthodontic therapy based on treatment goals can go ahead with a very predictable outcome.
The quality of orthodontic treatment is raised with the SAS.
The number of nonextraction cases can be significantly increased.
The number of orthognathic surgery cases can be significantly decreased.

BOX 20-2 Problems with Skeletal Anchorage System Treatment

Infection can be associated with anchor plate implantation. Better methods need to be established to prevent infection.
There are limitations to the shapes and sizes of the anchor plates.
Improvement in orthodontic anchor plate design is ongoing.
SAS treatment is a symptomatic, not a causative, treatment and therefore long-term evaluation is the only way to confirm its effectiveness.
Guidelines for the differential diagnosis of the indications for SAS treatment must be established.
SAS mechanics has yet to become an established technique. The mechanics need to be continually refined and improved.

In addition, the surface attached to the bone is sandblasted (Fig. 20-4) so that it is osseointegrated more readily. The other surfaces are polished with a mirrorlike surface so that they safely penetrate soft tissue and are effective in plaque control for preventing infection.

Positioning

The implantation site for the anchor plate must have sufficient depth of cortical bone (at least 2- to 3-mm) to allow it to be fixed with monocortical mini-screws. The screws are also made of pure titanium. Each screw has a head with a tapered inside square and self-tapping thread. The diameter of the screw is 2-mm and the available lengths are 5- and 7-mm. If the screw becomes loose or bent, an emergency screw with a diameter of 2.2-mm is used.

Figure 20-5 shows the positioning of the orthodontic anchor plates. The Y-type plates are placed in the maxilla at the zygomatic buttress to either intrude or distalize the upper molars. Although the lateral wall of the maxilla is too thin to carry the screws for the anchor plates, the bone of the zygomatic buttress is thick enough. The I-type plates are mostly placed at the anterior ridge of the pyriform opening for intrusion of the upper anterior teeth and protraction of the upper molars. In fact, the areas where titanium screws can be implanted in the maxilla are limited to the zygomatic buttress and the pyriform rim.

The T- and L-type plates are usually placed with titanium mini-screws in the mandibular body to intrude, protract, and distalize the lower molars or at the anterior border of the mandibular ramus to distalize the molars and tract the impacted second molars. The bone thickness of the lateral cortex in the mandible is sufficient to secure titanium screws at any point except around the foramen mentalis.

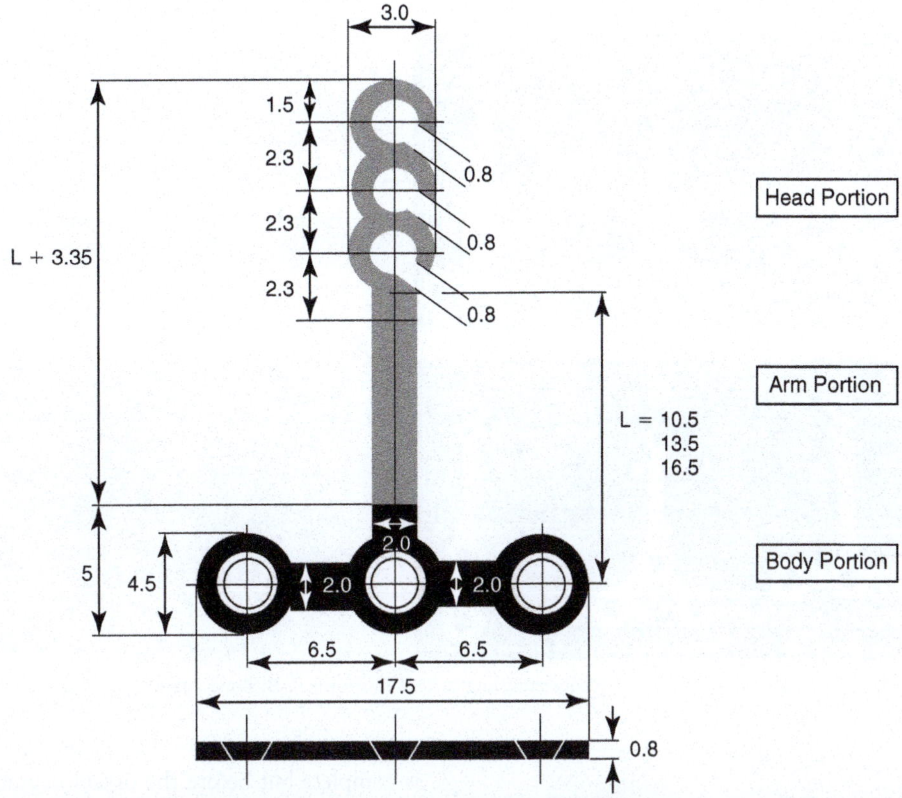

Figure 20-2 Design of a T-type anchor plate.

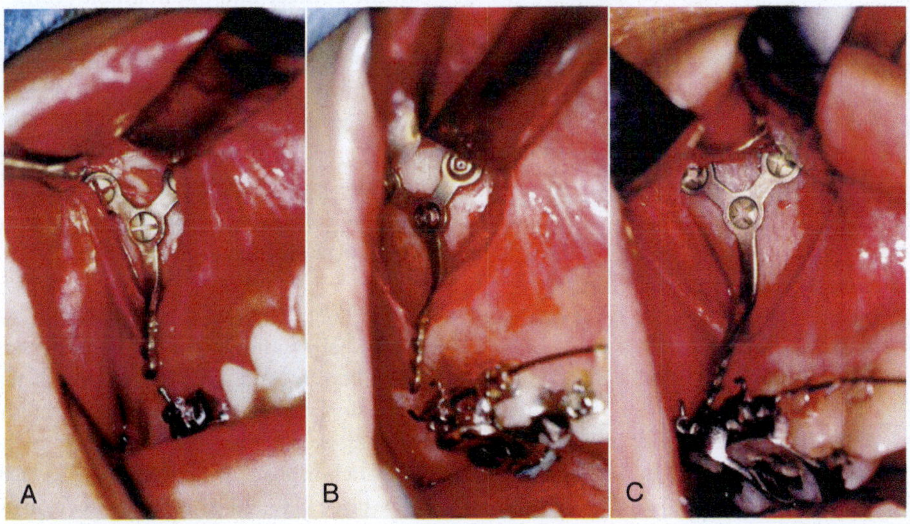

Figure 20-3 Variation in arm portion (length). **A,** Short type (10.5-mm). **B,** Medium type (13.5-mm). **C,** Long type (16.5-mm).

Surgical Procedures

The surgery is carried out under local anesthesia administered with intravenous sedation. First, a mucoperiosteal incision is made at the buccal vestibular of the implantation site. A vertical incision is usually made in the maxilla and a horizontal one is made in the mandible (Fig. 20-6, A and E). The mucoperiosteal flap is elevated following the subperiosteal ablation and the surface of the cortical bone at the implantation site is exposed (Fig. 20-6, B and F). Then the appropriate type of anchor plate is selected according to the distance between the implantation site and the dentition. This should be quite clear from the panoramic x-ray film taken prior to surgery. The selected plate is contoured to fit the bone surface.

A pilot hole is drilled and one self-tapping and monocortical screw is inserted. With the insertion of the remaining screws, the anchor plate is firmly placed on the bone surface (Fig. 20-6, C and G). At this moment it is important to ensure that the anchor plate does not disturb mandibular movement or adjacent soft tissues. The wound is finally

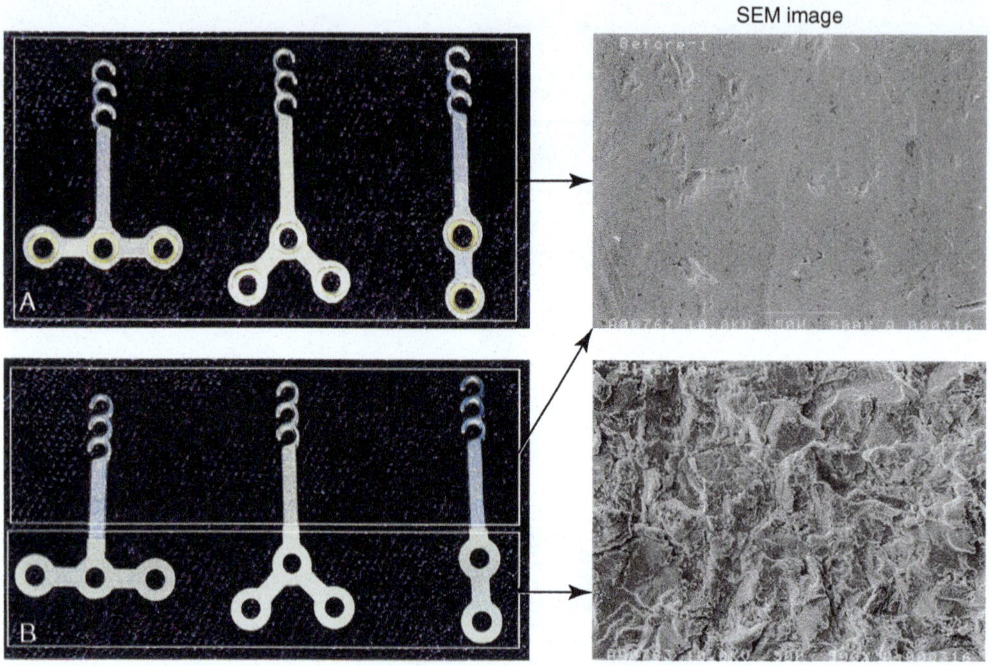

Figure 20-4 Surface property of each anchor plate. **A,** Mucous-attaching surface (mirrorlike). **B,** Bone-attaching surface (sandblasted). *SEM,* Scanning electron microscope.

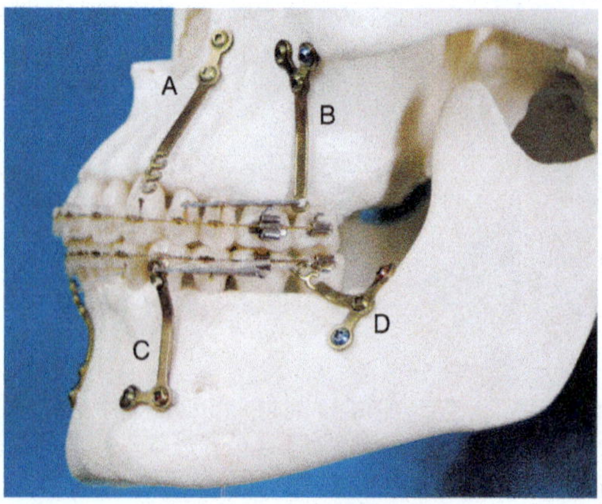

Figure 20-5 Positioning of anchor plates. **A,** I-type. **B,** Y-type. **C,** L-type (modified T-type). **D,** T-type.

closed and sutured with absorbable thread (Fig. 20-6, D and H). The surgery takes about 10 to 15 minutes for each anchor plate.

Timing of Orthodontic Treatment

Most patients who undergo implantation surgery for SAS show mild to moderate facial swelling for a week after the operation. This is almost inevitable. In addition, infection occurs in about 10% of patients. Mild infections can be controlled with antiseptic mouth rinses and careful brushing. In more severe cases, antibiotics are needed. Practitioners must thoroughly instruct patients in home care and professionally clean the plates every 3 to 4 weeks at routine appointments. This regimen has greatly reduced postsurgical infections.

Orthodontic force is usually applied about 3 weeks after implantation surgery (i.e., once postsurgical management is complete but before the osseointegration of the titanium screws and plates). Figure 20-7 shows the osseointegration of titanium screws in SAS in an animal model.[5] As shown on the contact microradiograph (CMR) images, the thread of the bone screws is attached directly to the bone because of osseointegration. Loaded bone screws show a higher level of osseointegration than unloaded screws. The loaded bone screw is surrounded by smaller but much more numerous Haversian system units and the remodeling of this bone is more significant. This phenomenon suggests that orthodontic force application to the implants promotes higher levels of osseointegration.

Removal

Immediately after orthodontic treatment, all anchor plates must be removed. First, a mucoperiosteal incision and subperiosteal ablation are performed at the implantation site (Fig. 20-8, A). Then the implanted anchor plate is exposed. The anchor plates are often observed to be covered with thin new bone (Fig. 20-8, B). As shown in Figure 20-8, C, even though the monocortical bone screws have been removed, the anchor plate is still firmly attached to the bone surface because of enhanced osseointegration. After removing the anchor plate, new bone formation can usually be observed surrounding the plate (Fig. 20-8, D).

SKELETAL ANCHORAGE SYSTEM BIOMECHANICS FOR MOLAR MOVEMENT

Figure 20-9 shows the SAS mechanics for intrusion and distalization of the molars. The SAS has been applied to more than 400 patients in our clinic, of whom about 85% needed one of these types of tooth movement.

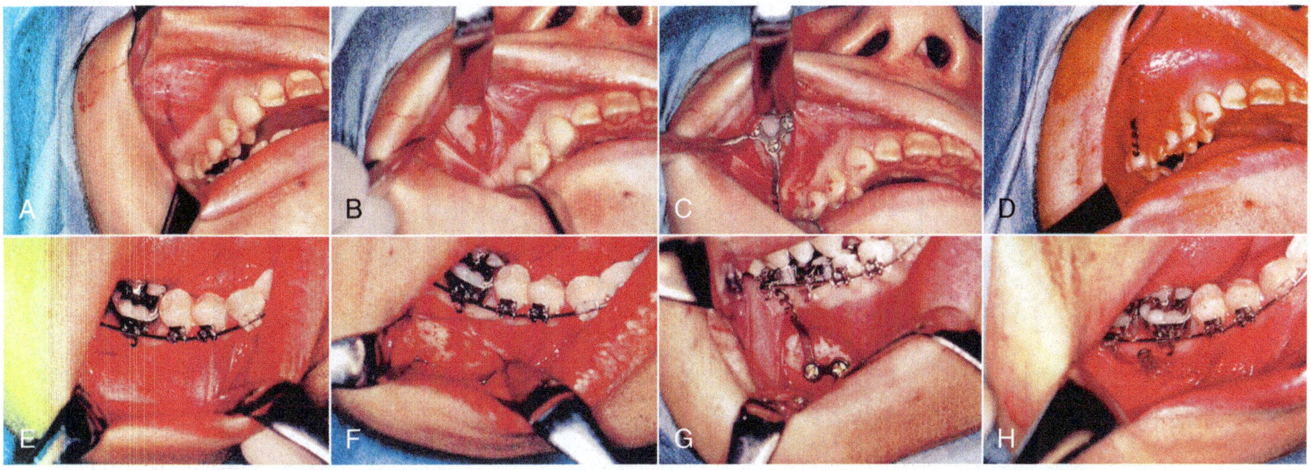

Figure 20-6 Surgical procedures for implantation of anchor plates. *Maxilla:* **A,** Incision line. **B,** Incision and exposure of the implantation site. **C,** Placement of anchor plates. **D,** Suture. *Mandible:* **E,** Incision line. **F,** Incision and exposure of the implantation site. **G,** Placement of anchor plates. **H,** Suture.

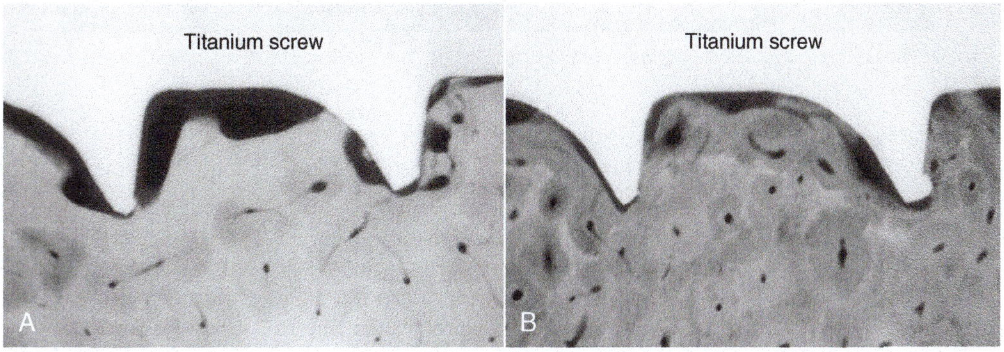

Figure 20-7 Contact microradiograph (CMR) images showing osseointegration of titanium. **A,** Unloaded sample. **B,** Loaded sample (orthodontic force was applied for 7 months). (Reproduced with permission from Daimaruya T, Nagasaka H, Umemori M, Sugawara J, Mitani H. The influences of molar intrusion on the inferior alveolar neurovascular bundle and root resorption by using anchorage system in dogs. *Angle Orthod.* 2001;71:60–70.)

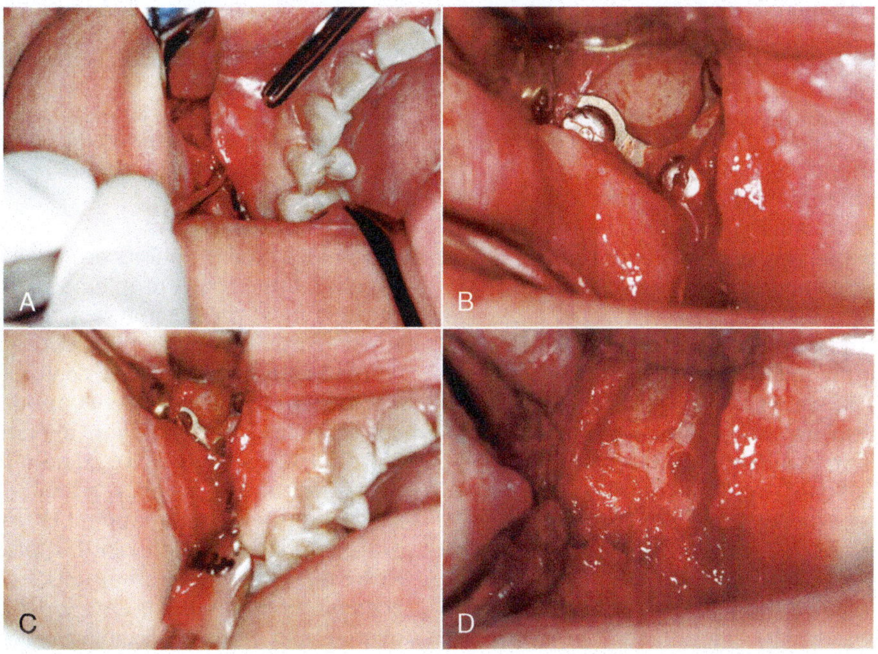

Figure 20-8 Anchor plate removal. **A,** Ablation. **B,** Exposure. **C,** Removal of screws. **D,** Immediately before suture.

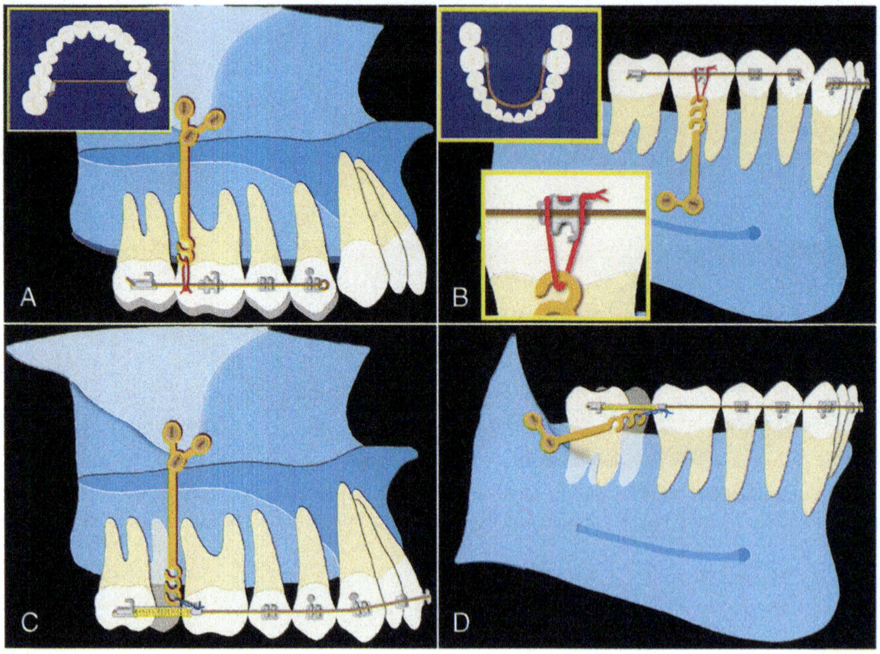

Figure 20-9 Biomechanics for molar movement. Intrusion of (**A**) upper and (**B**) lower molars. Distalization of (**C**) upper and (**D**) lower molars.

It has been extremely difficult, if not impossible, to intrude the upper and lower molars with traditional orthodontic mechanotherapies. Impacting the lower molar region especially, even with orthognathic surgery, has posed real problems because of the risk of injuring the inferior alveolar nerve. SAS mechanics, however, can accomplish the intrusion of molars, making it possible to correct even severe open-bite cases without orthognathic surgery and without iatrogenic side effects (see Fig. 20-9, A and B).[5–8]

Distalization of the upper or lower molars has long been considered a very difficult tooth movement even using headgear, and this is especially so in adult patients. However, using SAS mechanics to achieve distalization of the molars, it is now possible to correct even severe crowding, upper protrusion, anterior crossbite, and asymmetrical dentition without premolar extraction and without the need for constant patient cooperation (see Fig. 20-9, C and D).[9,10]

Text continued on p. 422

CASE REPORT

Problem List

The patient was a 19-year-old Japanese girl who complained of anterior open bite, difficulty in incising, and temporomandibular joint disorder (TMD). She had mild facial asymmetry, a long face, and a large interlabial gap (Fig. 20-10). Intraorally, she showed severe anterior open bite, crowding of the upper and lower incisors, a narrow upper arch, and large overjet (Fig. 20-11). In addition, ankylosis was suspected in the lower left first molar (Fig. 20-12). Figure 20-13 shows the results of her cephalometric template analysis, referred to as a craniofacial drawing standards (CDS) analysis,[11] compared to the Japanese norm. The major problems of her skeletal and soft tissue profiles were (1) a large interlabial gap, (2) a short ramus, and (3) a vertical maxillary excess. It was obvious that these problems were closely associated with her excessive lower facial height. In addition to the orthodontic problems, she also exhibited TMD (pain and noise) and gingivitis in the lower incisors and had a low lying tongue.

Treatment Options

Several treatment options are available to solve the patient's orthodontic problems. The common and perhaps most predictable response would be to advise surgical orthodontics. Orthognathic surgery would be an excellent treatment option because it would be the most effective modality for the correction of her vertical jaw disharmony. In fact, all of her orthodontic problems could have been fixed with surgical orthodontics. It can be safely said that surgical orthodontic treatment is the strategy most orthodontists would choose for this patient.[12] However, what about other options? It may be possible to improve her anterior open bite, large overjet, and anterior crowding using a multibracket

CASE REPORT—cont'd

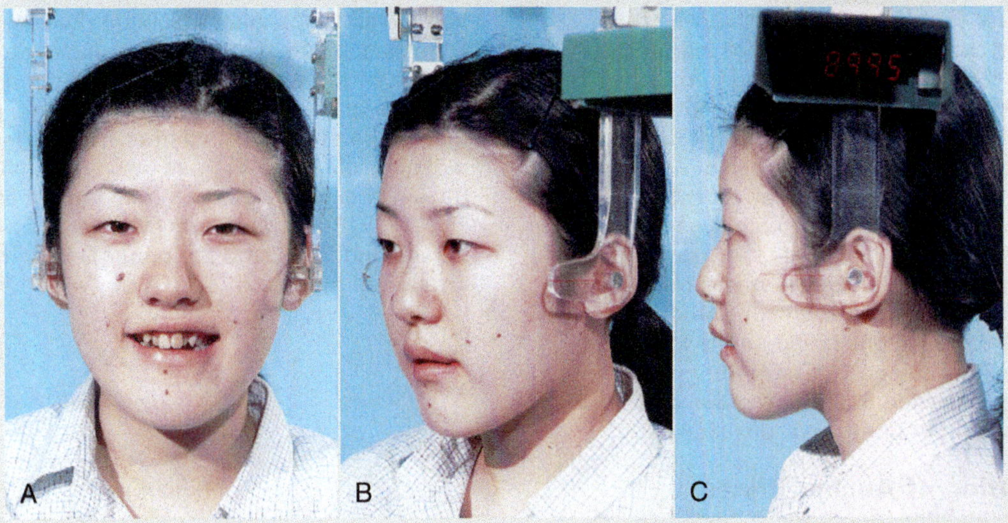

Figure 20-10 Facial photographs at the initial examination. **A,** Frontal view. **B,** Forty-five–degree view. **C,** Side profile.

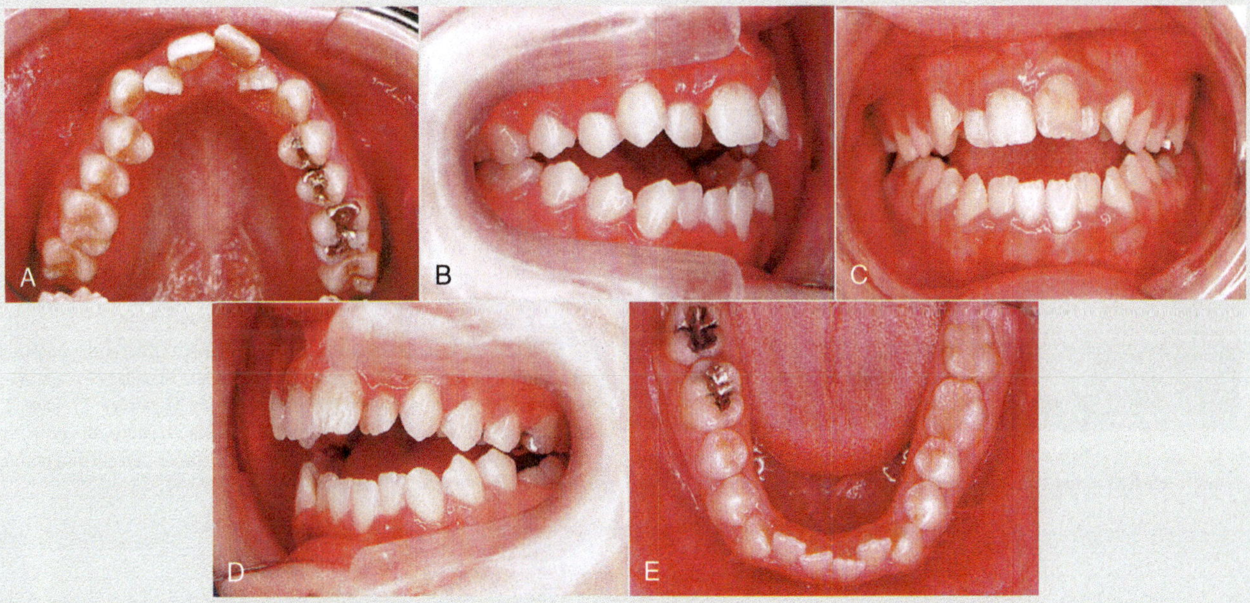

Figure 20-11 **A–E,** Intraoral photographs at the initial examination show a severe anterior open bite, crowding of the upper and lower incisors, a narrow upper arch, and a large overjet.

system but clearly it would be very difficult to improve her skeletal profile using this approach. Therefore the conventional multibracket system should probably be discarded as an option in this case. Multiloop edgewise archwire (MEAW) therapy[13] has been recognized as a viable modality for open-bite correction. However, MEAW has almost no impact on jaw disharmony and the patient's severe vertical disharmony means that MEAW is not the best option either.

SAS can solve most of this patient's orthodontic problems with the exception of her mild facial asymmetry. SAS makes it possible to voluntarily intrude the molars and significantly improve her vertical facial disproportion. In this case, SAS can address problems that are almost equivalent to those addressed by surgical orthodontic treatment. SAS was recommended to the patient as the first option based on a risk–benefit analysis.

Continued

CASE REPORT—cont'd

Treatment Goal

The patient chose SAS treatment to intrude her upper and lower molars. Following intrusion of the molars, a counterclockwise rotation (autorotation) of the mandible will occur automatically (Fig. 20-14, A). Then her excessive lower facial height and anterior open bite will simultaneously correct themselves. In addition, the upper and lower arches needed to be slightly expanded to coordinate her upper and lower dental arches. The intercuspation was checked with setup models made from the cephalometric and occlusogram predictions based on the treatment goals (Fig. 20-14, B and C). The lower left first molar, which was suspected of ankylosis, was coincidently required to neither intrude nor distalize.

Implantation of Anchor Plates

To intrude the upper and lower molars, two orthodontic anchor plates were placed in the maxilla at the zygomatic buttress and another two plates were implanted in the mandible at the mandibular body (Fig. 20-15). After placing a rigid rectangular wire, elastic intrusive force was applied to the upper molars with Y-type anchor plates and the lower molars were tightly ligatured with L-type plates. The magnitude of the elastic intrusive force in the upper molars could be as high as 500 g on each side. A transpalatal arch was used in the upper molars (see Fig. 20-15, B and C) to prevent buccal flaring of the molars and to expand the upper arch with the distal rotation of the first molars.

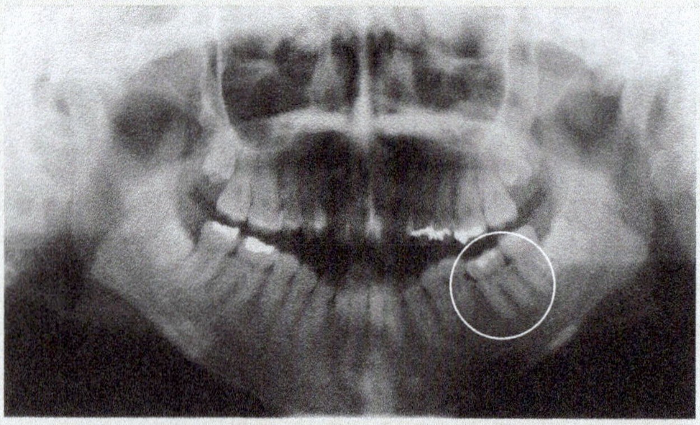

Figure 20-12 Panoramic radiograph at the initial examination. The lower left first molar (*circled*) was suspected of ankylosis.

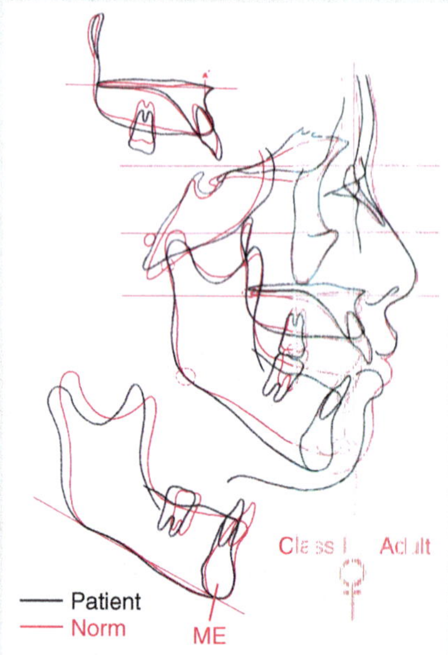

Figure 20-13 Craniofacial drawing standards (CDS) analysis. This case shows a long face, short ramus, and vertical maxillary excess. *Me,* menton. (Reproduced with permission from Sugawara J, Soya T, Kawamura H, Kanamori Y. Analysis of craniofacial morphology using craniofacial drawing standards [CDS]: application for orthognathic surgery. *J Jpn Orthod Soc.* 1988;47:394–408.)

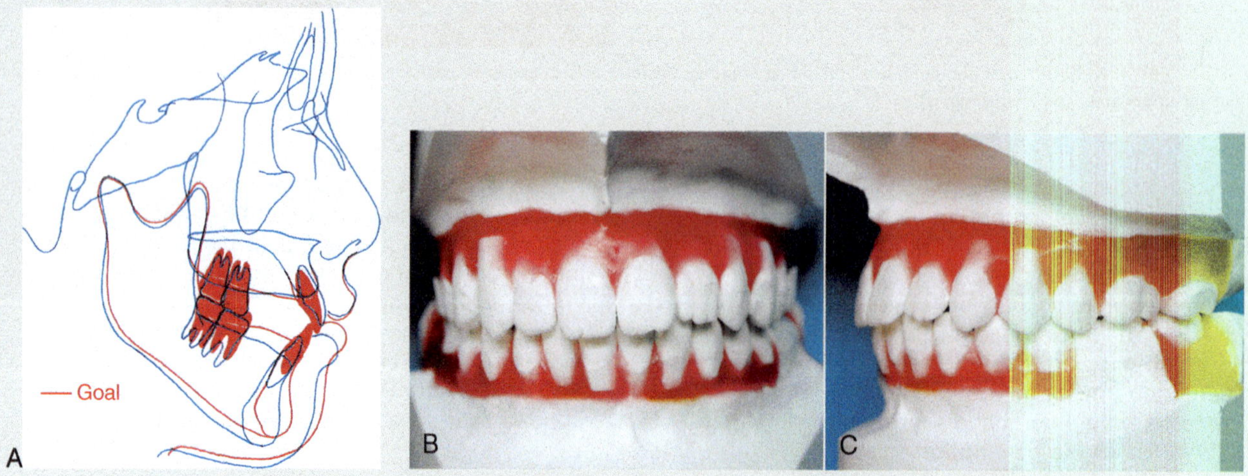

Figure 20-14 Treatment goals. **A,** Cephalometric prediction. **B and C,** Setup model.

CASE REPORT—cont'd

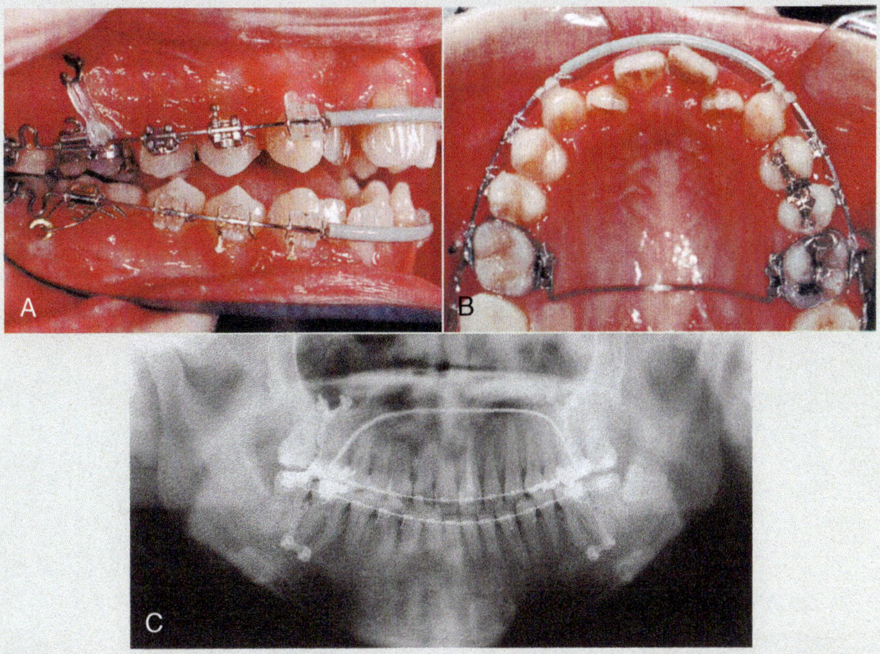

Figure 20-15 Implantation of orthodontic anchor plates. **A,** Intrusion of the upper and lower molars. **B,** Transpalatal arch. **C,** Y-type (zygomatic buttress) and L-type (mandibular body).

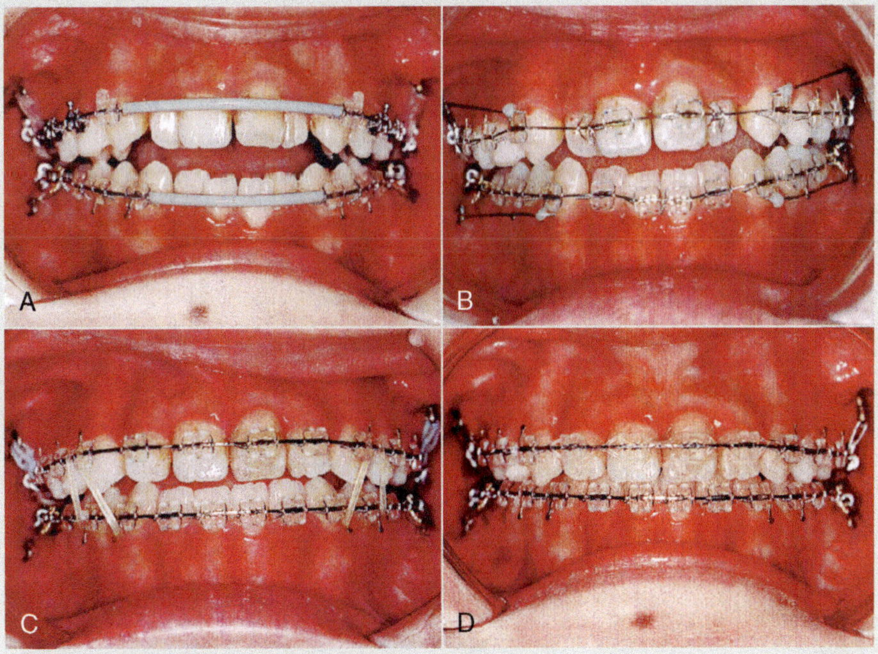

Figure 20-16 Treatment progress. **A,** Intrusion of the upper molars and expansion of the upper arch. **B,** Leveling of the upper anteriors. **C,** Intrusion of the upper molars. **D,** Detailing and finishing.

Treatment Progress

Figure 20-16 shows the treatment progress of the patient. After completion of the expansion of the upper and lower arches, the brackets were bonded at the incisors and leveling with continuous archwires was initiated (see Fig. 20-16, B). Leveling and aligning of the entire dentition was completed but the intrusion of the upper molars was still in progress (see Fig. 20-16, C). Even at this early stage (7 months since SAS had been applied) the anterior

Continued

CASE REPORT—cont'd

open bite had significantly improved (see Fig. 20-16, D). At this detailing and finishing step, occlusal equilibrium was applied to stabilize the intercuspation.

Outcome

Figures 20-17 and 20-18 show the facial and oral photographs, respectively, taken at debonding after 11 months of treatment. The patient had a balanced profile and a functional occlusion. Her orthodontic problems at the initial diagnosis had been drastically corrected with the application of SAS treatment. After debonding, lingual bonded retainers from canine to canine were placed in the upper and lower dentitions. Judging from the panoramic x-ray film that was taken immediately after debonding

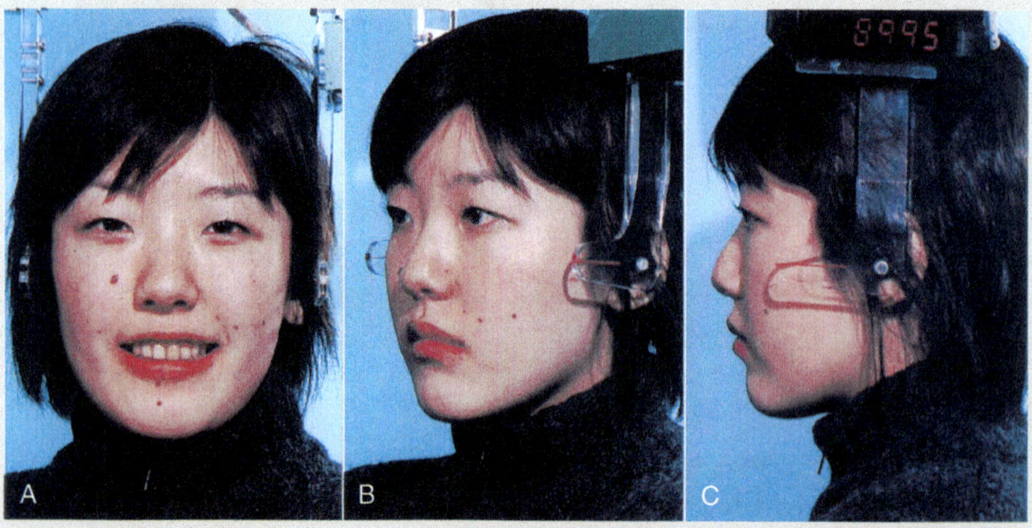

Figure 20-17 Facial photographs immediately after debonding. **A,** Frontal view. **B,** Forty-five–degree view. **C,** Side profile.

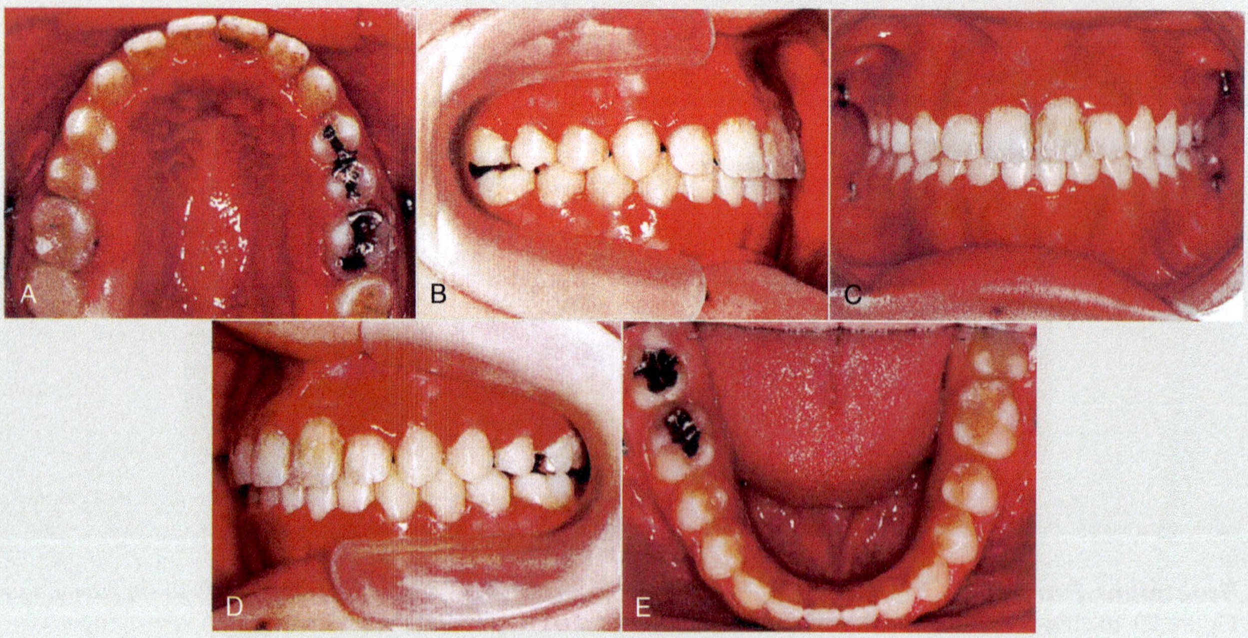

Figure 20-18 **A–E,** Intraoral photographs immediately after debonding show a balanced profile and a functional occlusion.

CASE REPORT—cont'd

(Fig. 20-19), root parallelism was accomplished and no significant root resorption of the upper and lower molars was observed following intrusion. In addition, no sinusitis was observed following significant intrusion of the upper molars. The orthodontic anchor plates were removed a month after debonding and the lower left third molar was extracted at the same time. According to the pre- and post-treatment cephalometric superimpositions, her anterior open bite was drastically corrected thanks to the radical intrusion of her upper and lower molars and eventually her long face and large interlabial gap improved because of the counterclockwise rotation of the mandible (Fig. 20-20). In fact, the amount of intrusion in the upper and lower second molars was 3.0- and 2.0-mm, respectively. Moreover, no significant change was observed in the clinical crown length. In other words, there was a significant decrease in the alveolar bone height, especially following intrusion of the upper molars. In addition, her large overjet was significantly improved following the distalization of the upper molars (4.0 mm) with the application of SAS. Figure 20-21 shows her oral photographs taken 1 year after debonding. She has maintained esthetic and functional occlusion.

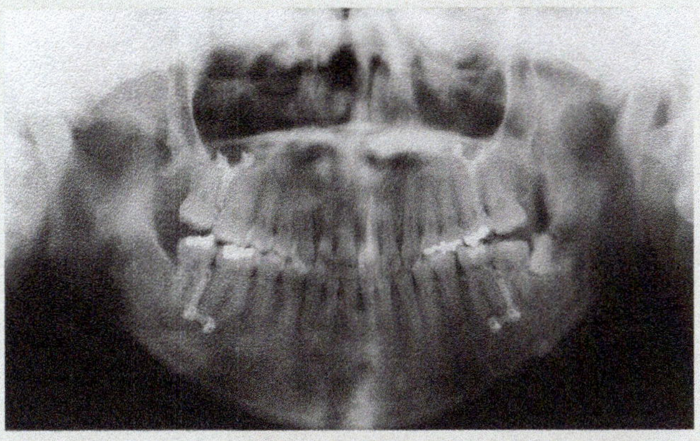

Figure 20-19 Panoramic radiograph immediately after debonding. Four anchor plates were removed and the left lower third molar was extracted after debonding.

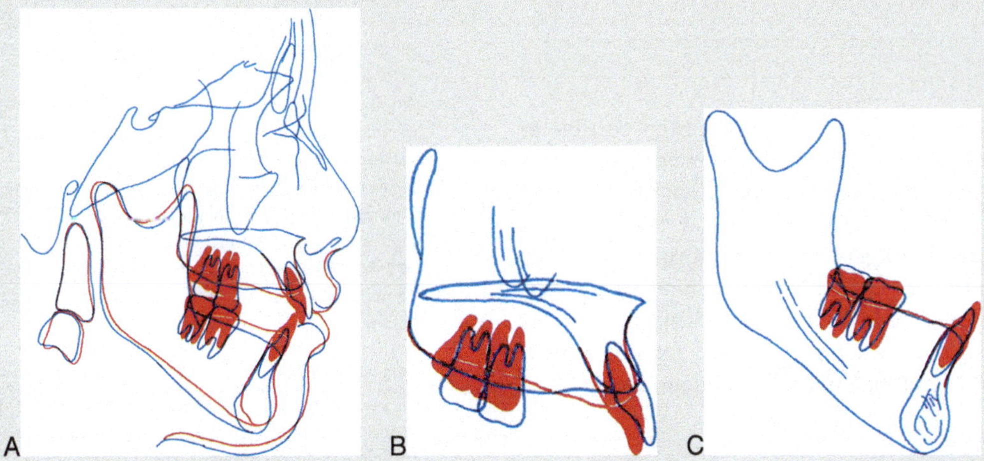

Figure 20-20 Cephalometric superimpositions. **A,** Overall superimposition. **B,** Maxillary superimposition. **C,** Mandibular superimposition.

Continued

CASE REPORT—cont'd

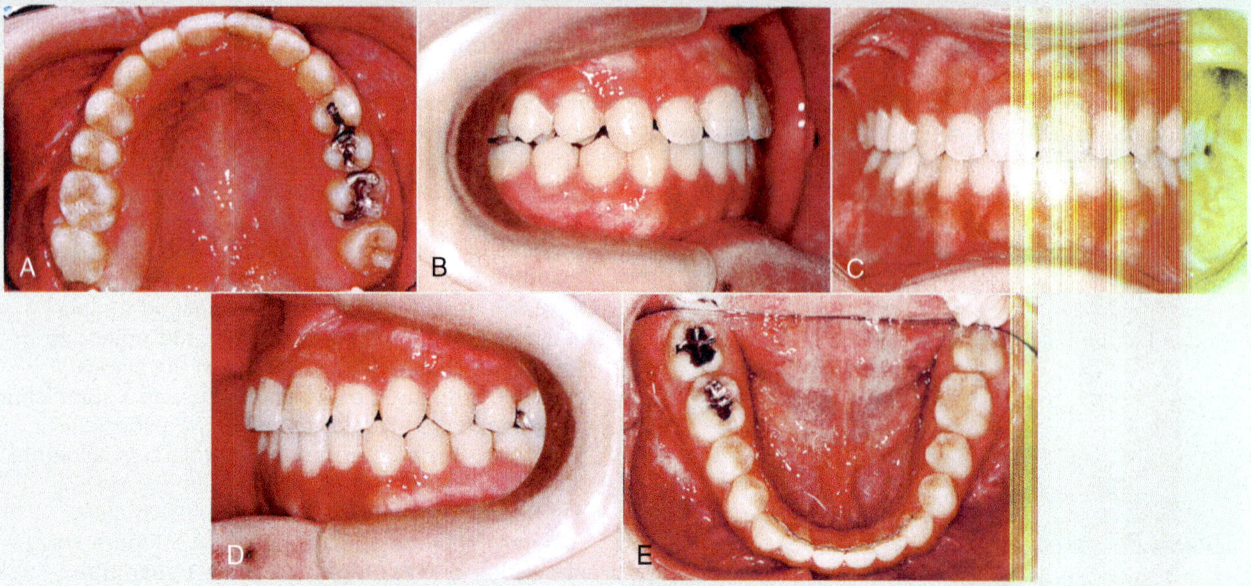

Figure 20-21 **A–E,** Intraoral photographs 1 year after debonding show that the patient is maintaining esthetic and functional occlusion.

SUMMARY

Following the development of SAS, it has been possible to move the molars three-dimensionally. Therefore the extent of camouflage treatment for the correction of crowding without premolar extraction and skeletal malocclusions without orthognathic surgery has drastically increased. Furthermore, SAS provides extremely effective biomechanics for second-phase treatment in developing patients, for patients with complex orthodontic problems, and for retreatment cases. SAS may extend the limits of orthodontic treatment.

REFERENCES

1. Creekmore TD, Eklund MK. The possibility of skeletal anchorage. *J Clin Orthod*. 1983;17:226–269.
2. Jenner JD, Fitzpatrick BN. Skeletal anchorage utilizing bone plates. *Aust Orthod J*. 1985;9:231–233.
3. Sugawara J. JCO interviews: Dr. Junji Sugawara on the skeletal anchorage system. *J Clin Orthod*. 2000;33:689–696.
4. Sugawara J, Nagasaka H, Umemori M, et al. Skeletal anchorage system (SAS). *Dental Outlook*. 2002;99:397–406.
5. Daimaruya T, Nagasaka H, Umemori M, Sugawara J, Mitani H. The influences of molar intrusion on the inferior alveolar neurovascular bundle and root resorption by using anchorage system in dogs. *Angle Orthod*. 2001;71:60–70.
6. Umemori M, Sugawara J, Mitani H, Nagasaka H, Kawamura H. Skeletal anchorage system for open-bite correction. *Am J Orthod Dentofacial Orthop*. 1999;115:166–174.
7. Sugawara J, Baik UB, Umemori M, et al. Treatment and postreatment dentoalveolar changes following intrusion of mandibular molars with application of skeletal anchorage system (SAS) for open bite correction. *Int J Adult Orthod Orthognath Surg*. 2002;17:243–253.
8. Daimaruya T, Takahashi I, Nagasaka H, Umemori M, Sugawara J, Mitani H. Effects of maxillary molar intrusion on the nasal floor and tooth root using skeletal anchorage system in dogs. *Angle Orthod*. 2003;73:158–166.
9. Sugawara J, Umemori M, Mitani H, Nagasaka H, Kawamura H. Orthodontic treatment system for Class III malocclusion using a titanium miniplate as an anchorage. *Orthod Waves*. 1998;57:25–35.
10. Sugawara J, Daimaruya T, Umemori M, et al. Distal movement of mandibular molars in adult patients with the skeletal anchorage system. *Am J Orthod Dentofacial Orthop*. 2004;125:130–138.
11. Sugawara J, Soya T, Kawamura H, Kanamori Y. Analysis of craniofacial morphology using craniofacial drawing standards (CDS): application for orthognathic surgery. *J Jpn Orthod Soc*. 1988;47:394–408.
12. Epker BN, Fish LC. Surgical–orthodontic correction of open bite deformity. *Angle Orthod*. 1977;71:278–299.
13. Kim YH. Anterior openbite and its treatment with multiloop edgewise archwire. *Angle Orthod*. 1987;57:290–321.

CHAPTER 21

Esthetics and New Approaches to Orthognathic Surgery

Carlos Villegas, Flavio Andres Uribe, and Ravindra Nanda

It has long been stated that "beauty is in the eye of the beholder."[1] However, specific facial features are universally associated with attractiveness. Three components in facial esthetics that have been investigated through research in evolutionary psychology and that appear to represent cues for mate selection are *symmetry*, *averageness*, and *secondary sexual characteristics*.[2] Cultural, social, and racial influences may affect one's judgment of attractiveness but they are secondary to these primary three characteristics.[3,4]

As with the other bilateral structures in the human body, symmetry in facial esthetics is evaluated in a right to left relationship. A slight asymmetry between the two facial halves is the norm; however, large asymmetries have been attributed in evolutionary psychology to signal lack of health and poor genetic makeup.[2] Averageness, also referred to as *prototype*, is based on the concept that a computer-generated composite of select features from a group of many individuals will yield better esthetics than any single individual who is part of that group.[5] In treatment planning in orthognathic surgery and orthodontics, the averageness concept is applied when any patient with a dentofacial deformity or malocclusion is compared to a norm. Through the use of cephalometrics, which examines the deviation in magnitude of specific dentofacial angles, lengths, and proportions, the patient is compared to individuals of the same age, gender, and ethnic group. Finally, secondary sexual characteristics are those that distinguish or define both sexes. A specific example is chin prominence in males and high cheekbones and short lower facial height in females.[4,6]

Symmetry, proportionality, and averageness are achievable goals in orthognathic surgery and serve as fundamental concepts that guide the treatment planning process in patients with dentofacial deformities. The esthetic outcomes obtained by following these goals likely result in an improvement in facial esthetics and appearance. Although facial esthetics is significantly affected with orthognathic surgery, other important functional aspects are also improved. Murphy et al.[7] evaluated the quality of life of patients who had undergone orthognathic surgery and found moderate to high improvement in facial appearance (93%), masticatory function (64%), comfort (60%), and speech (32%).

TREATMENT PLANNING FOR ORTHOGNATHIC SURGERY

The treatment plan for patients with dentofacial anomalies must include specific goals, which can be divided into *objective goals* and *subjective goals*. Objective goals are those that can be measured exactly and, in general, are related to symmetry. It is clear that symmetry is measurable and has been regarded as one of the most important parameters in assessing facial esthetics.[2–4] In orthognathic surgery planning, symmetry is mostly related to the transverse dimension; however, it can also be assessed in the vertical dimension (e.g., maxillary cant and ramus height differences). Objectives in the anteroposterior are more subjective, as they relate to averageness. The objectives in the vertical dimension are based on proportions and averageness and goals in this dimension are also prone to subjectivity (Fig. 21-1). Although the transverse dimension is mostly dictated by symmetry, averageness provided by normative values of different dental and skeletal dimensions could affect the surgical plan and therefore should also be included as a subjective goal.

Both objective and subjective goals guide the planning of orthognathic surgery. However, significant subjectivity influences the surgical plan. Although most surgeons and clinicians use cephalometrics as the basis for treatment planning for orthognathic surgery, disagreement can be common due to different clinicians' preferences as to what will constitute an ideal outcome. This is especially the case when patients and surgeons who have different ethnic backgrounds are considered. Lee et al.[8] showed that there were discrepancies between American-trained and Asian-trained oral and maxillofacial surgeons regarding the type of treatment recommended for a group of Asian women with skeletal Class III profiles. While all of the Asian-trained surgeons preferred mandibular setback, approximately 40% of the American-trained surgeons preferred maxillary advancement.

During an orthognathic surgery case planning session it is not uncommon to encounter long discussions on the surgical movements that should be performed. Many complex questions can arise: How much should the maxilla be advanced (i.e., 3- or 5-mm)? Should the procedure include one or both jaws (especially in Class III malocclusions)? Is a genioplasty necessary? These questions arise because clinicians' preferences and biases affect these treatment decisions. Some clinicians prefer that the maxilla or mandible be projected more, or in some instances less, or that the incisor display at rest be a few millimeters more or less compared to other clinicians. This problem of disagreement is more relevant to the anteroposterior and vertical dimensions. However, such discrepancies are not present when symmetry is considered. This is why most clinicians and surgeons would consider a surgical plan with the maxillary midline off by 2-mm or more, a significant maxillary cant, or significant chin point deviation to be completely unacceptable.

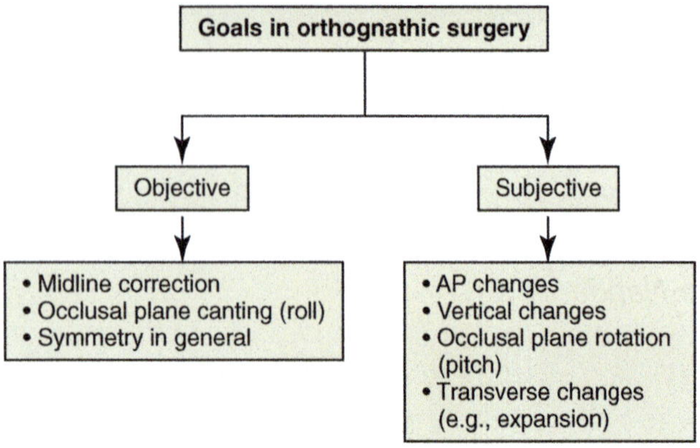

Figure 21-1 Objective and subjective goals in orthognathic surgery. *AP,* Anteroposterior.

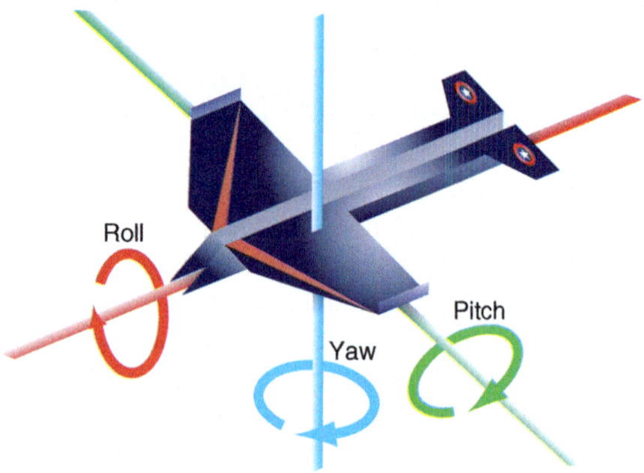

Figure 21-2 Concepts of roll, yaw, and pitch used in aviation and extrapolated to the planning of surgical movements in the three dimensions of space in orthognathic surgery.

To meet the objective goals, new technology consisting of very precise three-dimensional (3D) planning software allows the virtual visualization of the craniofacial anatomy and aids in the surgical planning of patients with dentofacial deformities.[9-11] This 3D planning software is very important in the clinician's ability to quantify with high precision the degree of asymmetry and plan with great detail the surgical movements. When planning occurs in three dimensions, aviation concepts become handy in describing the orientation and planning the surgical movement of a craniofacial structure within an orthogonal coordinate system. Rotational movements (pitch, yaw, and roll) along the three axes (x, y, and z) supplement the traditional two-dimensional movements along the different planes (sagittal, coronal, and axial) (Fig. 21-2).[12] In essence, this 3D planning software allows visualization of the deformity and planning of the surgical movements in a virtual environment with six degrees of freedom.

Pitch refers to rotational movements around a transverse or x axis; in aviation it refers to a situation in which an airplane makes a sudden maneuver to ascend or descend. In orthognathic surgery pitch refers to rotation of both jaws viewed from the sagittal plane, also known as clockwise or counterclockwise rotation (Fig. 21-3). *Yaw* refers to

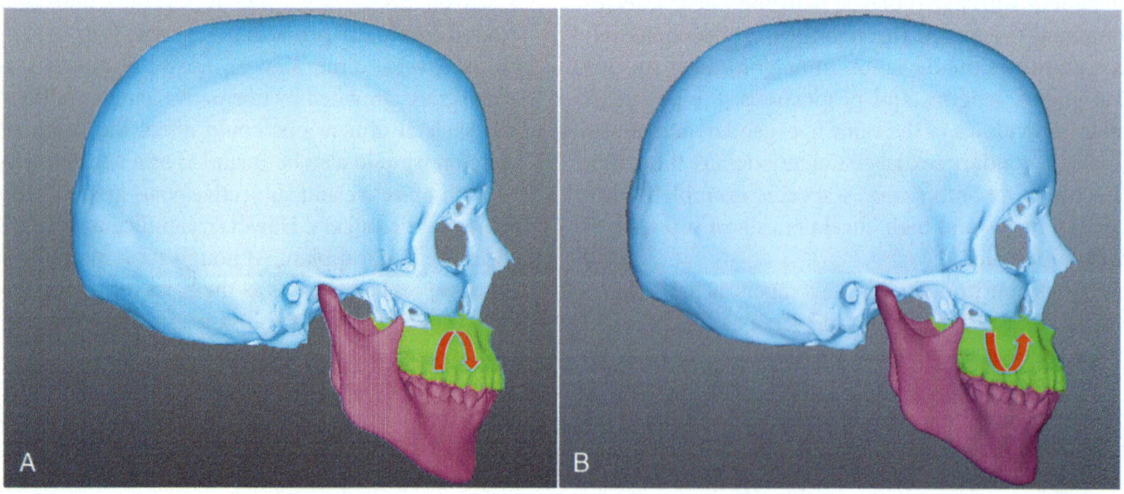

Figure 21-3 Pitch, or inclination movements of the maxilla and mandible in the sagittal plane. **A,** Clockwise rotation. **B,** Counterclockwise rotation.

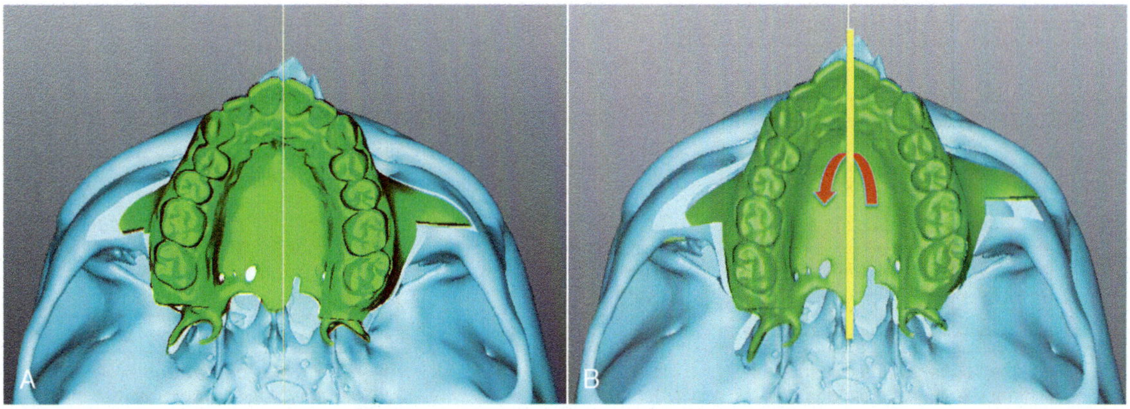

Figure 21-4 Yaw, or rotational movement of the maxilla around a vertical or y axis in order to correct the maxillary skeletal and dental midline. **A,** Maxillary skeletal deviation evaluated in the axial plane. **B,** Correction of the maxillary deviation by counterclockwise rotation in the axial plane.

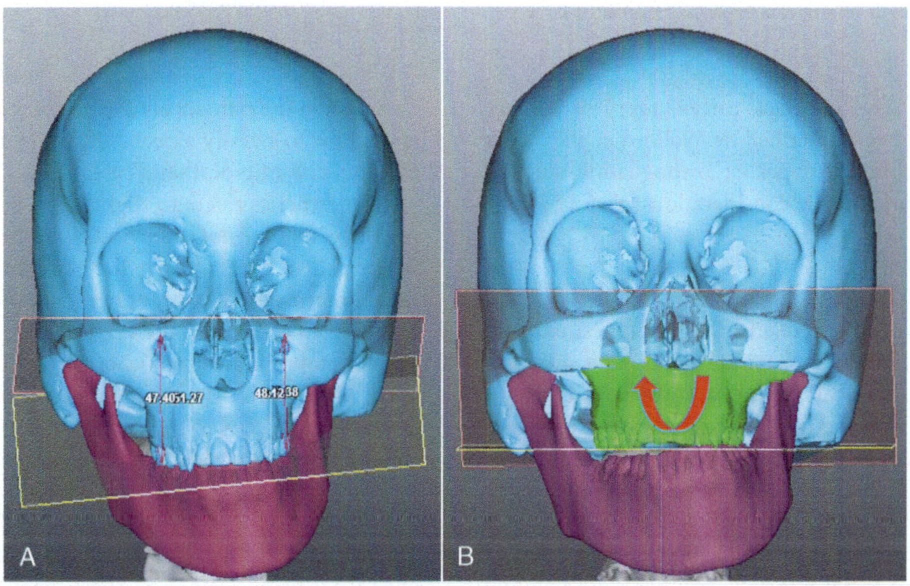

Figure 21-5 Roll, or rotational movements of the maxilla or the mandible around an anteroposterior axis or z axis to correct asymmetries in a vertical direction **A,** Significant occlusal cant evaluated in the coronal plane. **B,** Virtual osteotomy correcting the deformity by addressing the roll deviation.

rotational movements around a vertical or y axis; in aviation it refers to sudden turns to the right or left. In orthognathic surgery yaw refers to the rotation of the maxilla in a lateral direction in order to surgically correct the midline (Fig. 21-4). It could further be described as the rotation of the axial plane around the y axis. *Roll* refers to rotational movements around an anteroposterior or z axis; in aviation it refers to the movement of an airplane when one wing swings upward and the other swings downward. In orthognathic surgery roll refers to the vertical movements made to correct canted occlusal planes evaluated from a frontal view by either descending or impacting one side (Fig. 21-5). In other words, roll is rotation of the coronal plane around the z axis.

Time: The Fourth Dimension in Orthognathic Surgery

Time is another important aspect to consider in orthognathic surgery from two key perspectives. The first relates to the total treatment duration of the combined orthodontic and surgical interventions and the second relates to the appropriate time to execute the surgery. Total treatment time has been reduced with the "surgery first approach."[13,14] With this approach presurgical orthodontics is eliminated, thus reducing the total treatment time compared to the traditional three-phase approach: presurgical orthodontics, orthognathic surgery, and postsurgical orthodontics. In addition, there is immediate resolution of the dentofacial deformity and esthetics are not negatively affected by the dentoalveolar decompensation that accompanies the presurgical orthodontic phase (Fig. 21-6).

The other aspect related to time is the age at which orthognathic surgery is performed, or *surgical timing*. Traditionally, orthognathic surgery was performed once maxillary and mandibular growth was complete. However, we can positively affect patients who have significant dentoalveolar deformities by performing early surgery (during adolescence). This allows for favorable facial change during a key stage of life in which the psychosocial aspect has great

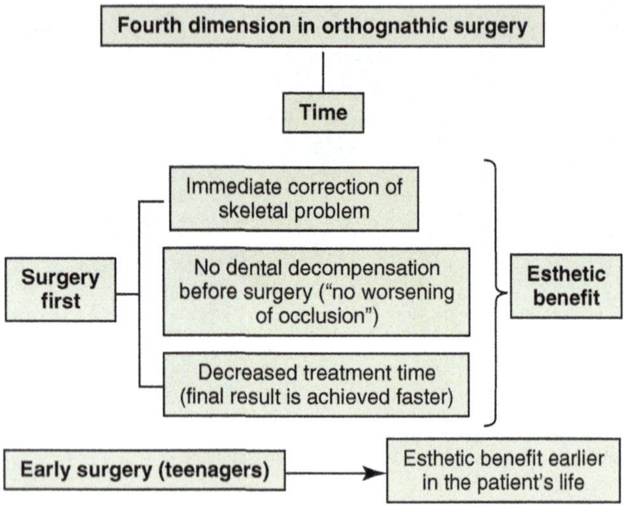

Figure 21-6 Time as the fourth dimension in orthognathic surgery.

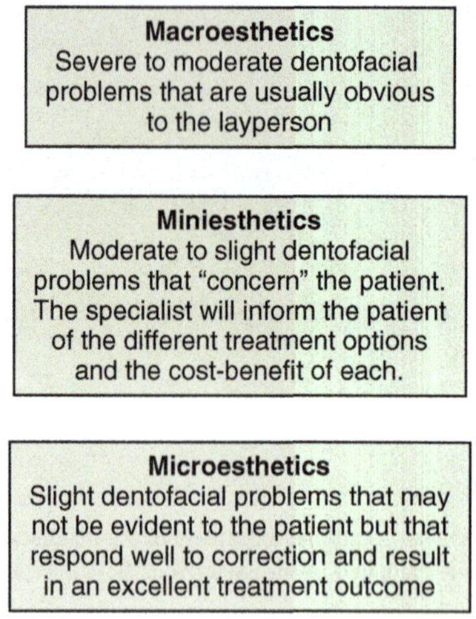

Figure 21-7 Definitions of macroesthetics, miniesthetics, and microesthetics.

influence (see Fig. 21-6). In fact, early surgery or surgery during growth has been described by Wolford et al.[15,16] as a viable option in different types of orthognathic surgical approaches if certain surgical considerations are followed.

Macroesthetics, Miniesthetics, and Microesthetics

There are three major components that define esthetics in surgical cases: macroesthetics, miniesthetics, and microesthetics. These subgroups are based on the size and magnitude of deviation from the norm and should be considered carefully. Macroesthetics refers to the face, miniesthetics refers to the smile, and microesthetics refers to the esthetic characteristics of the teeth and gingival complex.[17]

Although this concept lays a good foundation for a classification system for facial esthetics, macroesthetics should include not only deviations from the norm of the face but also problems that affect the smile. In this line of thinking, macroesthetics is defined as the dentofacial problems that are usually identifiable by a layperson, orthodontist, or surgeon (Fig. 21-7). These problems include moderate to severe Class II or Class III skeletal anomalies, marked asymmetries, and vertical problems. The facial soft tissues would logically include labial or facial fissures and other visibly apparent anomalies that compromise facial esthetics. Intraorally, macroesthetics includes crowding, tooth malposition, missing teeth or teeth in poor condition (teeth with fractures, excessive wear, or discoloration), or severe gingival recession in the esthetic zone. The chief complaint also influences how to classify a problem in the macroesthetic, miniesthetic, and microesthetic categories.

Miniesthetics refers to slight to moderate facial or dental problems that are not so obvious that they can be pinpointed by the patient but that drive the patient to consult a clinician for an improvement in his or her smile. For example, patients consult for problems in the vertical dimension, such as slight or moderate gingival smile or slight to moderate skeletal Class II or Class III with dental compensations. Dentally, miniesthetics refers to tooth malposition, discoloration, diastemas or gingival recession, and other features that are not overtly evident.

Microesthetics refers to slight deviations from the norm that the patient has not identified but, if corrected, will enhance the smile esthetics. These details are what define the difference between a good result and an excellent one. Microesthetics would correspond to the correction of slight tooth malposition in the anterior esthetic zone, gingival recession or uneven gingival margins of more than 1-mm, and excessive tooth discoloration.

CASE REPORTS

The following four cases illustrate the concepts of treatment planning; time as the fourth dimension; and macroesthetics, miniesthetics, and microesthetics in orthognathic surgery.

Text continued on p. 440

CASE REPORT 1

Figure 21-8 depicts the change in the facial profile and occlusion in a 17-year-old patient with a severe skeletal Class III malocclusion from pre-treatment (see Fig. 21-8, A) to 6 weeks after appliance insertion (see Fig. 21-8, B) to post-treatment after 8 months (see Fig. 21-8, C), when the orthodontic-surgical treatment was finished. The facial profile as well as the occlusion and dental appearance were clearly compromised in the initial photographs, which affected the macroesthetics. The patient had a

CASE REPORT 1—cont'd

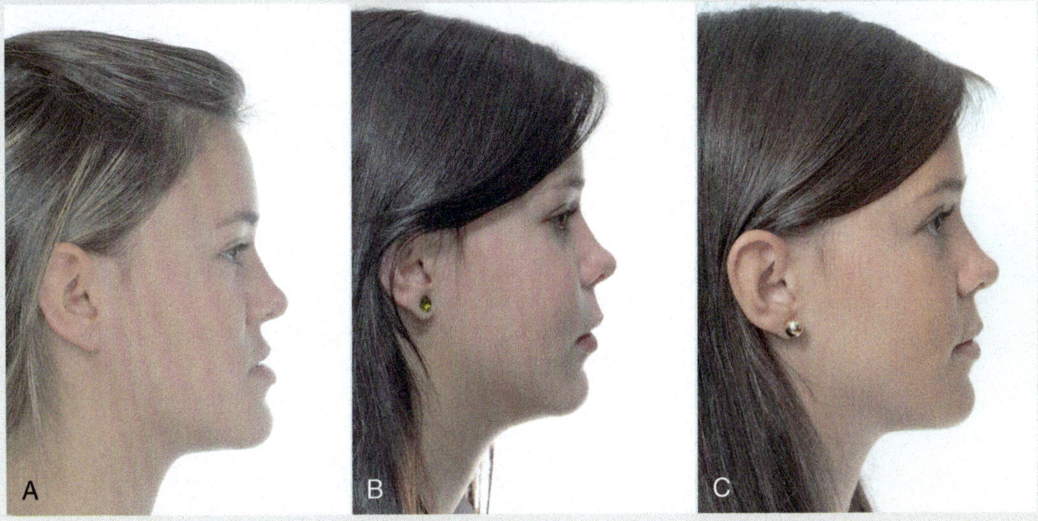

Figure 21-8 **A,** Profile maxillomandibular relationship revealing a severe Class III skeletal dentofacial deformity at pre-treatment. **B,** Correction of the skeletal and dental aspects with a "surgery first approach" (6 weeks after surgery). **C,** Final profile and occlusal outcome after 8 months of treatment.

maxillary advancement and mandibular setback with the benefits of the "surgery first approach," namely (1) no dental decompensations prior to surgery, thereby preventing facial profile deterioration; (2) an immediate facial change after the patient decided to undergo surgery; and (3) completion of orthodontic-surgical treatment 8 months after surgery. Again, this illustrates a very short period of treatment compared to a conventional three-stage approach with presurgical orthodontics, orthognathic surgery, and postsurgical orthodontics treatment.

The anteroposterior and vertical position of the maxillary incisors at rest is one of the most important clinical aspects to evaluate in surgical treatment planning. The determination of the maxillary incisor position in space is the cornerstone used to sequentially position the other structures of the dentofacial complex. It could be regarded as the reference landmark used to plan the key dental and osseous movements. An adequate incisor position at rest in the vertical dimension, approximately 2- to 3-mm of incisor display, will most likely result in a good esthetic outcome in the middle facial third and the smile line.

An important consideration in the determination of the vertical position of the incisors, based on the amount of display on smile, is the evaluation of lip mobility. Patients who have labial hypermobility will most likely have increased gingival display on smiling, regardless of an adequate exposure of the upper incisors at rest. If the maxilla is impacted in such patients, the smile vertical display may be corrected but this will occur at the expense of no display of the incisors during speech, which gives an inadequate appearance of edentulism, a significant negative impact in facial esthetics. Therefore it is very important to evaluate the patient both at rest and on smiling and it is recommended that the final vertical position of the incisors should err in the direction of slightly excessive gingival display on smiling rather than an outcome with no incisor display at rest.

After considering the maxillary incisor position in a vertical dimension, the vertical position of the maxillary buccal segments should follow. Any deviation of the yaw of the maxilla should be appraised and corrected if indicated. The proper positioning of these buccal segments in combination with the adequate display of the maxillary anterior segment will yield optimal smile esthetics from a frontal view (Fig. 21-9). Figure 21-10 shows the inclination or cant of the upper occlusal plane with respect to the bipupilar line. The occlusal plane was more caudal on the right side and more coronal on the left side. Three options were available to level the occlusal cant: (1) impaction of the right buccal segment, (2) inferior repositioning of the left segment, or (3) a combination of both by means of a slight ascent of the right side and a slight descent of the left side. Since the amount of incisor display was reduced on both rest and smile, an inferior repositioning of the left side by 2-mm combined with rotation around the crowns of the right buccal segment was performed (see Figs. 21-10, B and C).

It is very important to keep in mind the effect of sagittal maxillary movements on incisor display.

Continued

CASE REPORT 1—cont'd

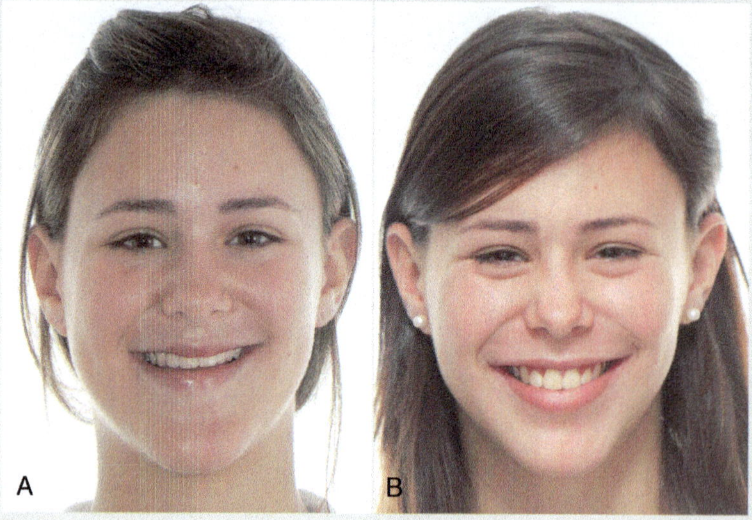

Figure 21-9 **A,** Frontal presurgical and **(B)** postsurgical result showing the macroesthetics and miniesthetics outcomes after an adequate treatment plan and surgical intervention.

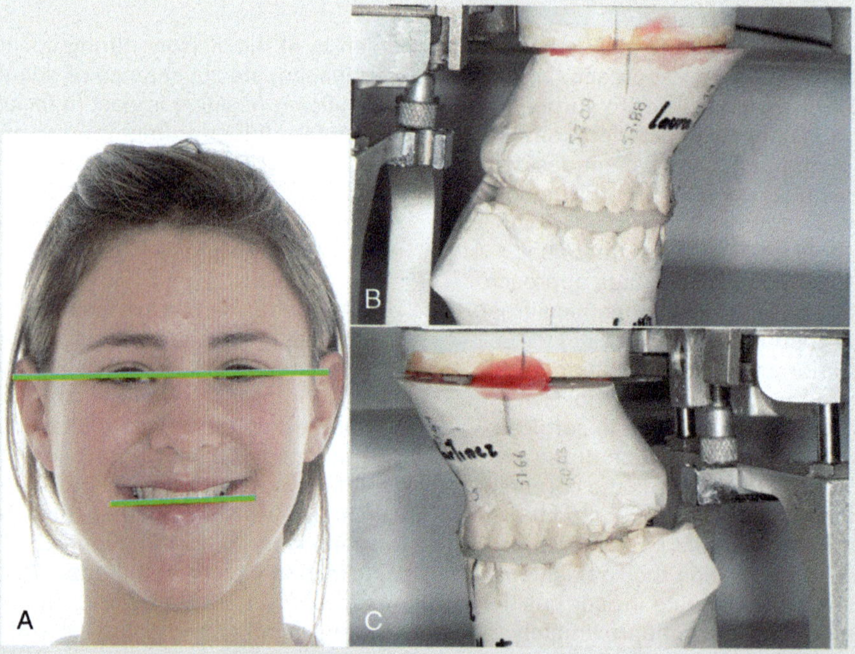

Figure 21-10 **A,** Occlusal cant in relation to the bipupilar line. **B,** No vertical repositioning of the maxilla on the right side for the cant correction. **C,** Inferior repositioning of the left side of the maxilla to improve the tooth display on that side and correct the occlusal cant (roll).

Although the 2-mm of maxillary descent on the left side adequately leveled the occlusal plane, it did not provide sufficient incisor display at rest. However, an important consideration was that the maxilla was to be advanced in order to project the middle third forward. The result of this anterior repositioning of the maxilla is an increase in incisor display, both at rest and on smiling. This effect of the anteroposterior surgical movement of the maxilla on the vertical display of the incisors is important to consider in the planning of the maxillary position in space.

Concurrent with the maxillary positioning of the buccal segments, it is important to evaluate the pitch from a sagittal perspective. Although not very commonly appraised, this inclination has important consequences on the consonance of the smile line with the lower lip. That is, the flatter the plane in

CASE REPORT 1—cont'd

reference to the anterior cranial base plane, the more difficult it is to achieve a consonant smile and the increased chance of a flat or reverse smile arc. Finally, once the maxilla has been positioned correctly in space, the mandible is guided to its correct position based on the maxillary midline and the buccal occlusal relationship. Refinement of the esthetics in all three dimensions can be obtained by means of a genioplasty when indicated.

Once the surgical procedure is completed, treatment continues with the postsurgical orthodontics phase. At the end of orthodontic treatment, minor surgical procedures in gingival contouring further refine the esthetic result. Figure 21-9 shows the changes in microesthetics in the smile after completion of the orthodontic treatment.

The patient showed a low smile line without exposure of the upper incisors, which was corrected with surgery, thereby improving her miniesthetics. Although the postsurgical improvements to her smile line were very adequate, the fact that the upper right lateral incisor was shorter than the left made the asymmetry of the gingival margins more noticeable, thereby compromising the microesthetics (Fig. 21-11). Figure 21-12 depicts a minimally invasive periodontal surgery performed in order to displace the gingival margin apically by 1.5-mm in the upper right lateral incisor. In addition, the patient had tooth whitening, which complemented the microesthetics. Figure 21-13 shows the impact of these procedures, which addressed the microesthetics in the final esthetic outcome.

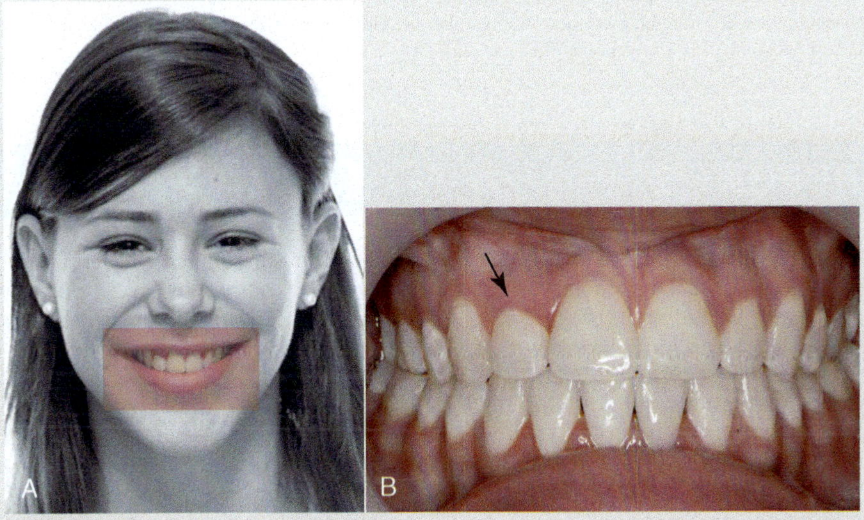

Figure 21-11 **A,** Microesthetics problem noticeable in the smile. **B,** Intraoral photograph showing the asymmetrical maxillary gingival margin of the right lateral incisor with reduced crown length.

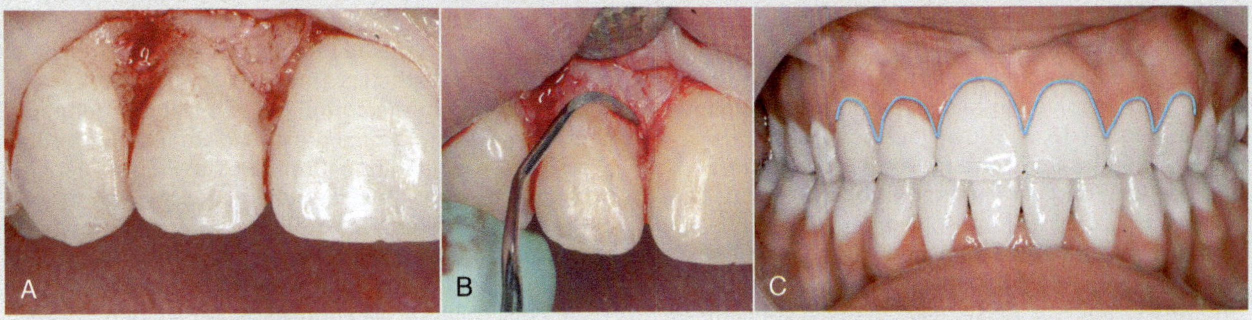

Figure 21-12 Crown lengthening procedure on the right maxillary lateral incisor to match the gingival margin of the maxillary left lateral incisor. **A,** Flap showing the crestal bone level. **B,** Removal of the crestal bone to establish adequate biological width. **C,** Final result showing the improvement in the symmetry and proportion of the anterior teeth in the esthetic zone.

Continued

CASE REPORT 1—cont'd

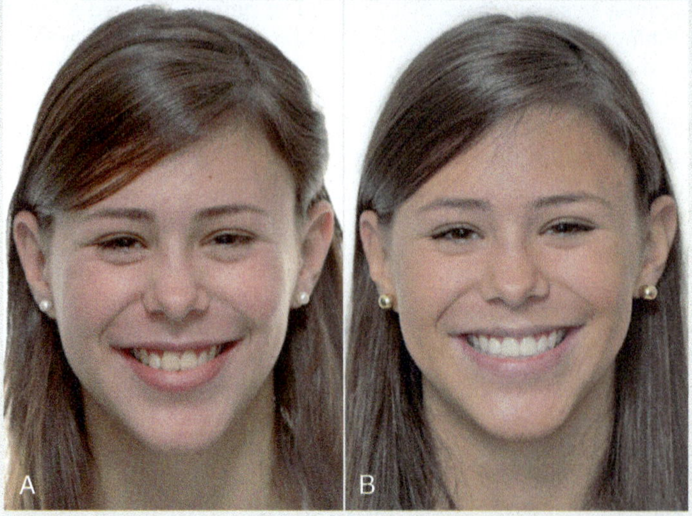

Figure 21-13 Difference in the smile esthetics of the patient **(A)** before and **(B)** after two procedures related to microesthetics (crown lengthening and tooth whitening). These two microesthetic details mark the difference between a good result and an excellent one. (Case from Uribe F, Villegas C, Nanda R. Surgically enhancing the speed of tooth movement: Can we alter the biology? In: McNamara JA Jr, Kapila SD, eds. *Surgical Enhancement of Orthodontic Treatment.* Ann Arbor, MI: The University of Michigan, 2010:323–344.)

CASE REPORT 2

Figure 21-14 shows a 12-year-old female patient who presented with a significant dentofacial deformity involving severe crowding in the maxillary arch, lip incompetence, and excessive and asymmetrical gingival display due to vertical excess of the maxilla. Additionally, mandibular retrognathism due to posterior mandibular rotation was present, compromising her dental and facial macroesthetics.

A surgical plan involving conventional orthognathic surgery was established. In the maxillary arch, presurgical orthodontics without extractions was completed through distalization of the molars using a bone-supported dual-force distalizer (DFD) (Fig. 21-15).[18] Some of the dental macroesthetic problems, such as excessive crowding in the anterior segment and an incisal cant, were resolved in this presurgical orthodontic phase (Fig. 21-16, A). However, the facial macroesthetics involving the excessive gingival display and long vertical proportions with poor chin projection remained unresolved (Fig. 21-16, B).

Early bimaxillary orthognathic surgery and mentoplasty were performed at age 13 years, 6 months to address these macroesthetic concerns, which were having a psychosocial impact on the patient at that stage. A Le Fort I osteotomy was performed to impact the maxilla by 7-mm. Bilateral sagittal split osteotomy (BSSO) of the mandible was also performed to align the occlusion, obtaining a Class I molar relationship. In addition, an 8-mm advancing genioplasty was performed to project the chin point anteriorly and superiorly (Fig. 21-17).

The surgery corrected the facial macroesthetic problems of excessive gingival display at rest and smile, excessive interlabial gap, a convex profile, and poor chin projection. This patient was treated with the traditional sequence of presurgical orthodontics, orthognathic surgery, and postsurgical orthodontics. Total treatment time was 30 months; therefore there was no real benefit regarding treatment time. We did observe that by doing the surgery early (13 years, 6 months), the patient benefited by having her dentofacial esthetic problem corrected without having to wait until age 16 or 18 years to obtain this favorable change.

The macroesthetics and miniesthetics were addressed with the combined surgical-orthodontic plan. However, the microesthetic component of the smile needed additional refinement. Figure 21-18 shows the right maxillary lateral incisor with a shorter clinical crown compared to the contralateral side and not matching the normal maxillary anterior gingival height architecture of the adjacent teeth. This discrepancy was noticeable on smiling; however, the patient had not noticed this issue. Figure 21-19 shows the significant improvement in the smile and overall esthetics that was obtained once gingivectomy was performed to elongate the crown of the right lateral incisor.

CASE REPORT 2—cont'd

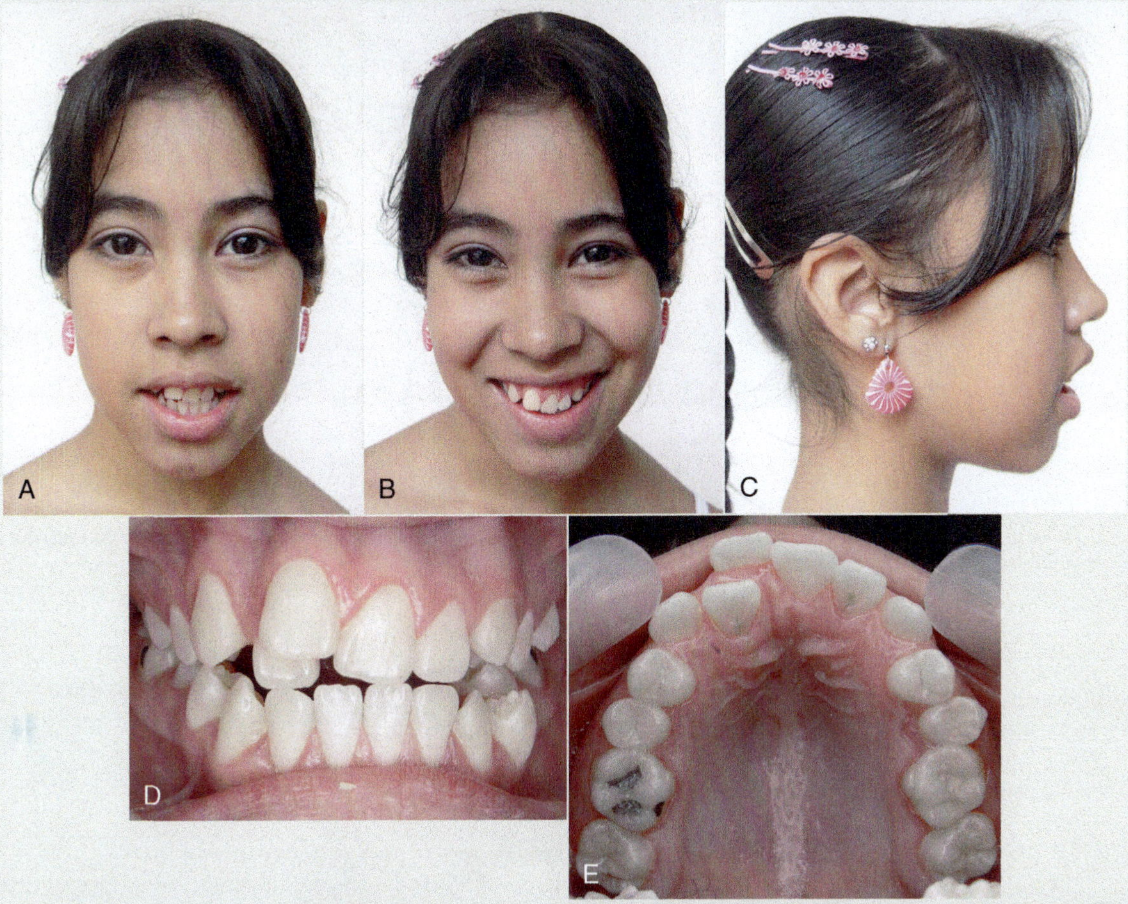

Figure 21-14 Patient with significant dentofacial deformity. **A,** Frontal view depicting the long lower facial height and increased interlabial gap. **B,** Excessive asymmetrical gingival display with incisal cant and maxillary lateral incisor not visible due to excessive crowding (macroesthetic problems). **C,** Profile view displaying an acute nasolabial angle, long lower facial height, increased interlabial gap, and retrognathic mandible. **D,** Frontal intraoral view illustrating excessive crowding, anterior open bite, canted incisal plane, and significant midline discrepancy. **E,** Occlusal view showing the maxillary crowding and blocked-out right lateral incisor.

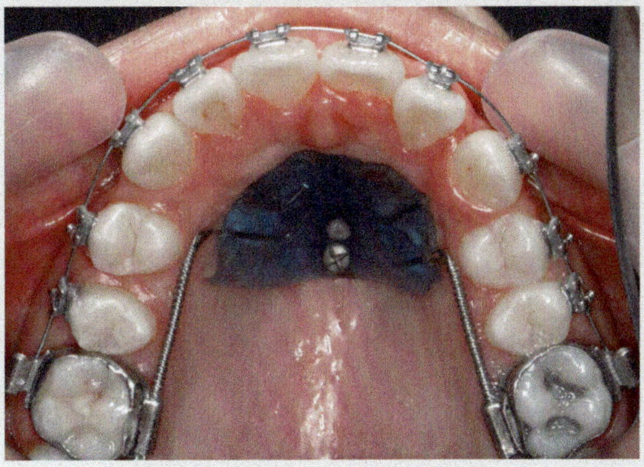

Figure 21-15 Distalization by means of the dual-force distalizer (DFD) to address the crowding.

Continued

CASE REPORT 2—cont'd

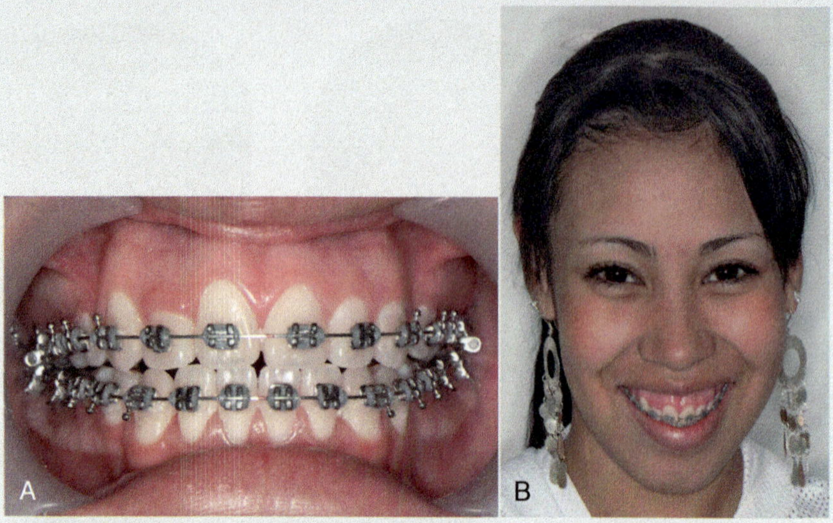

Figure 21-16 **A,** Good arch alignment with incisal cant resolved and maxillary right lateral incisor incorporated in the arch. **B,** Excessive gingival display compromising macroesthetics.

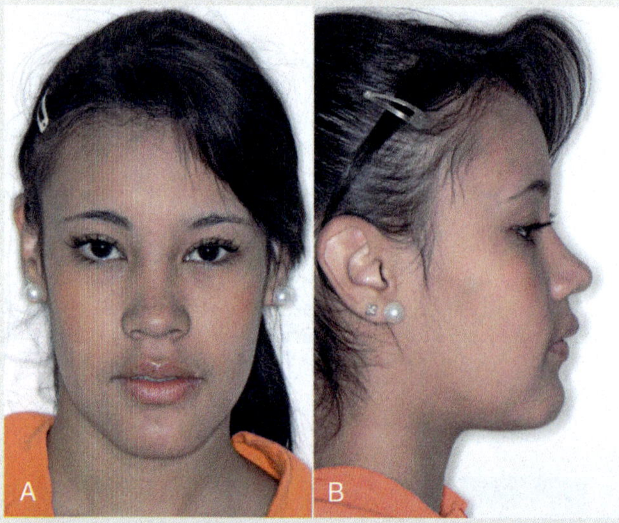

Figure 21-17 Postsurgical result with significant reduction in the interlabial gap and nasolabial angle and improvement in facial proportions and chin projection. **A,** Frontal view. **B,** Profile view.

CASE REPORT 2—cont'd

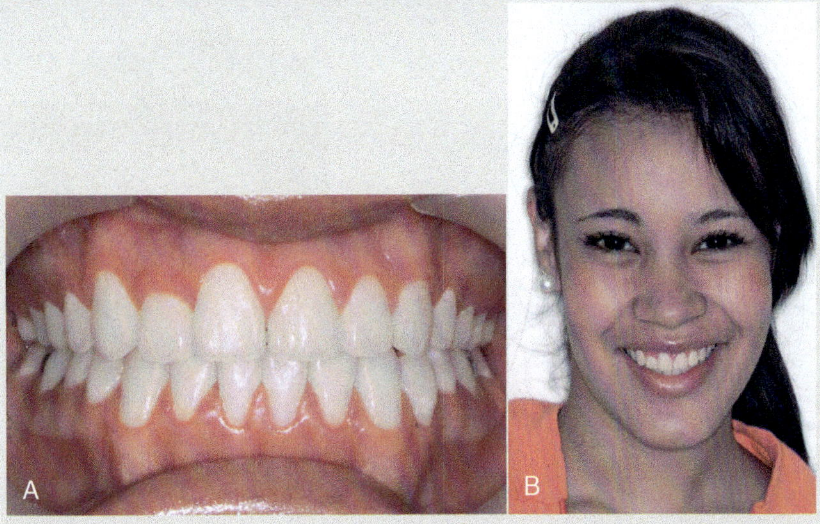

Figure 21-18 Postsurgical result from the frontal view. **A,** Adequate occlusal outcome; however, the microesthetics are still not perfect, with a gingival discrepancy between lateral incisors. **B,** Smile highlighting the microesthetics problem observed in the difference in symmetry and proportions of the maxillary right lateral incisor and the adjacent teeth.

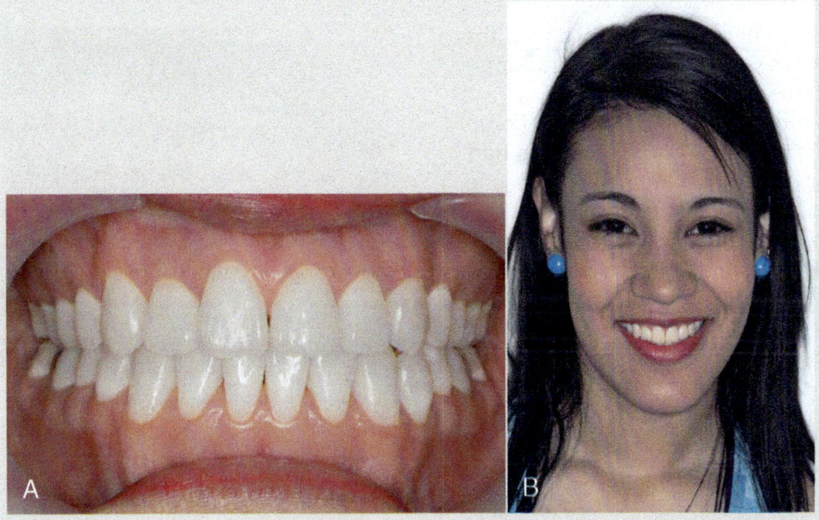

Figure 21-19 **A,** Microesthetics addressed with a gingivectomy of the maxillary right lateral incisor. **B,** Microesthetic detail affecting the overall esthetic outcome.

CASE REPORT 3

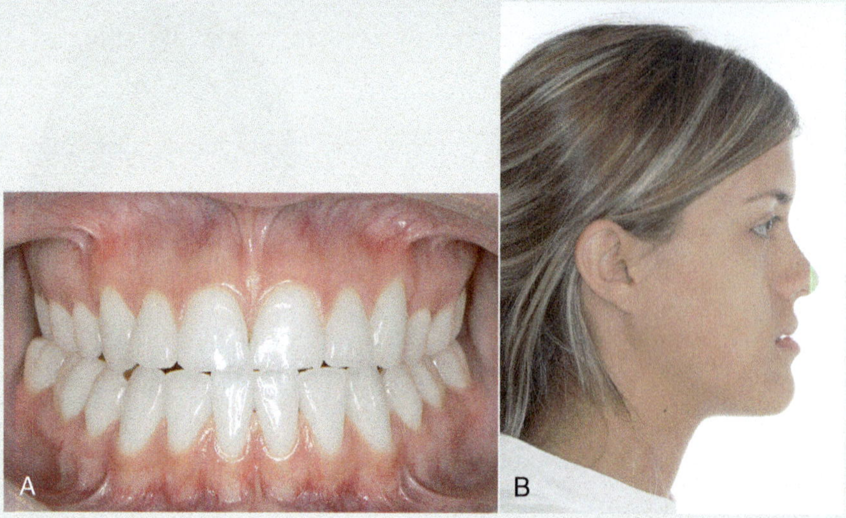

Figure 21-20 **A,** Patient with a Class III malocclusion treated with orthodontics 2 years prior to her consultation. Wear of the incisors was evident, with an edge-to-edge incisor relationship that was not favorable for the integrity of the dentition in the long-term. **B,** Moderate Class III skeletal relationship with obvious midface deficiency.

Figure 21-20 shows an 18-year-old patient with the chief complaint of excessive wear of the anterior teeth. The patient related having completed orthodontic treatment with extractions of all first premolars 2 years prior but over time the bite had reached an anterior edge-to-edge relationship (see Fig. 21-20, A). Facially, the patient presented with a slightly concave profile (see Fig. 21-20, B), with a desire to improve her facial esthetics only if the treatment was not "long and traumatic." The patient had consulted several other orthodontists, who had said that the correction of the dental problem was very risky because of the magnitude of root resorption from the previous orthodontic treatment, mainly in the upper lateral incisors and the upper left second premolar (Fig. 21-21).

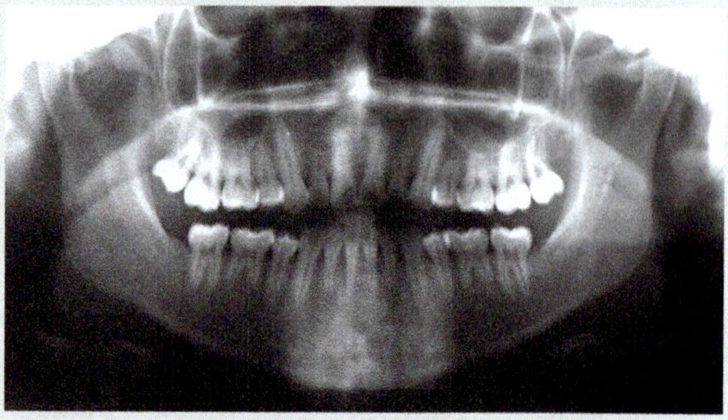

Figure 21-21 Panoramic radiograph depicting the significant root resorption noticed in the maxillary left second premolar and lateral incisors.

A surgical orthodontic treatment with a "surgery first approach" was presented to the patient in order to address the occlusal and esthetics issues, minimizing the time with orthodontic appliances and thus reducing the chances of further root resorption. This treatment plan included a clockwise rotation of the maxillomandibular complex. To accomplish this, a high Le Fort I osteotomy was planned to impact the maxilla 3-mm posteriorly and advance it by 3-mm to project the paranasal region and the upper lip forward (Fig. 21-22, A and B). In addition, a bilateral sagittal osteotomy of the mandible to set back the chin point by 3-mm was planned. This resulted in an orthognathic profile with slightly less chin projection (Fig. 21-22, C).

These procedures evidently produced an orthognathic profile (Fig. 21-23, A) where the middle third was projected forward and the mandible was displaced slightly down and back with a slightly increased postsurgical overjet (Fig. 21-23, B) that was corrected during the postsurgical orthodontic treatment. Figure 21-24 shows the final result after the orthodontic postsurgical phase, which lasted 2 months and 28 days. Once again it can be observed that the "surgery first approach" sequence helps to streamline a treatment that traditionally would have been longer and possibly had a higher biological cost for the teeth that presented root resorption.

Figure 21-25 shows the change in the smile with the combined surgical-orthodontic treatment. The clockwise rotation of the maxilla around the upper central incisors edge had a significant effect on the smile esthetics by steepening the flat presurgical

CASE REPORT 3—cont'd

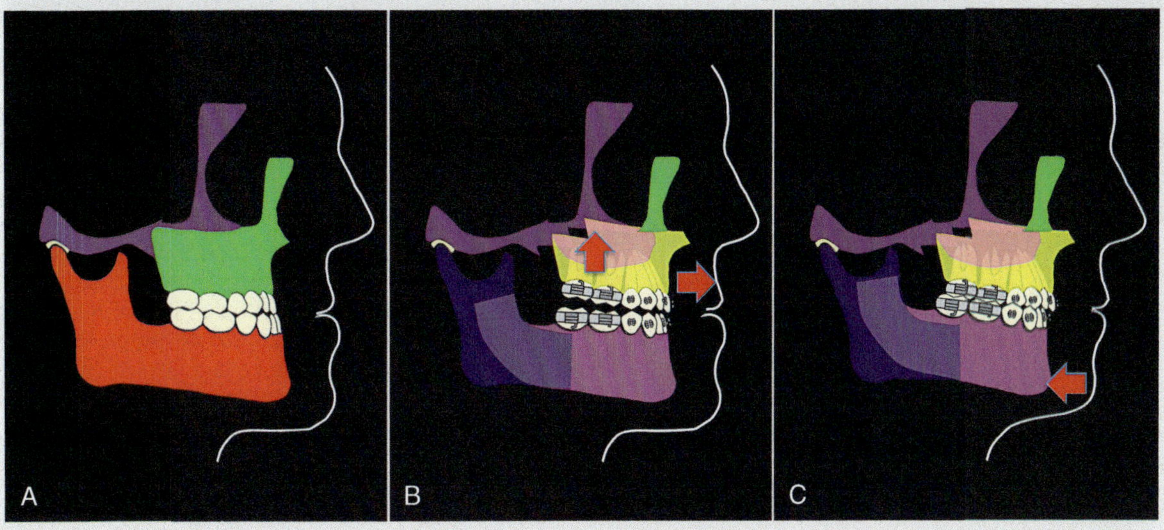

Figure 21-22 Cartoons depicting the surgical movements. **A,** Presurgery. **B,** Maxillary advancement and posterior impaction resulting in clockwise occlusal plane rotation. **C,** Mandibular setback and occlusal plane rotation to match the maxilla.

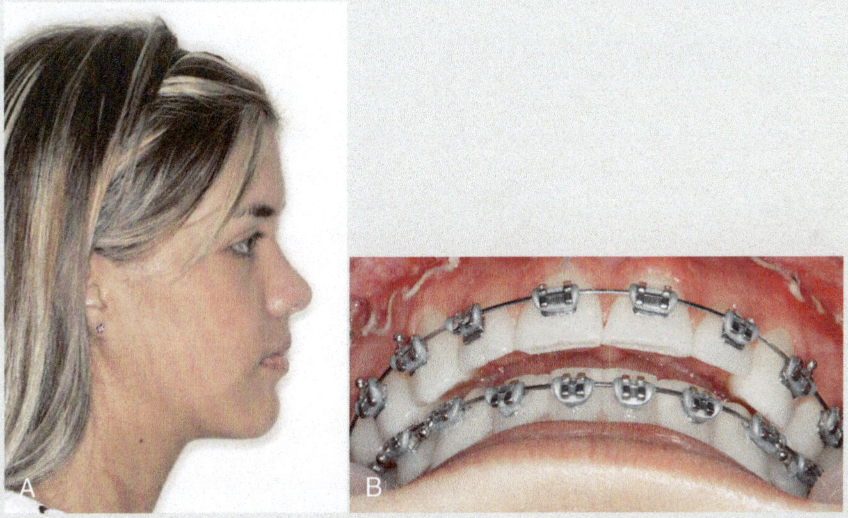

Figure 21-23 **A,** Postsurgical orthognathic profile. **B,** Slightly increased overjet left to decompensate the lower incisors. This is a common practice in the "surgery first approach."

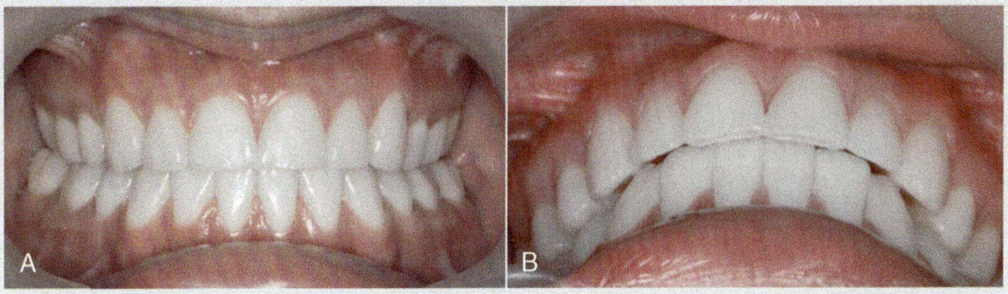

Figure 21-24 Postsurgical occlusion 2 months and 28 days after surgery at debonding. **A,** Adequate overbite, midline relationship, and occlusion. **B,** Note the final overjet.

Continued

CASE REPORT 3—cont'd

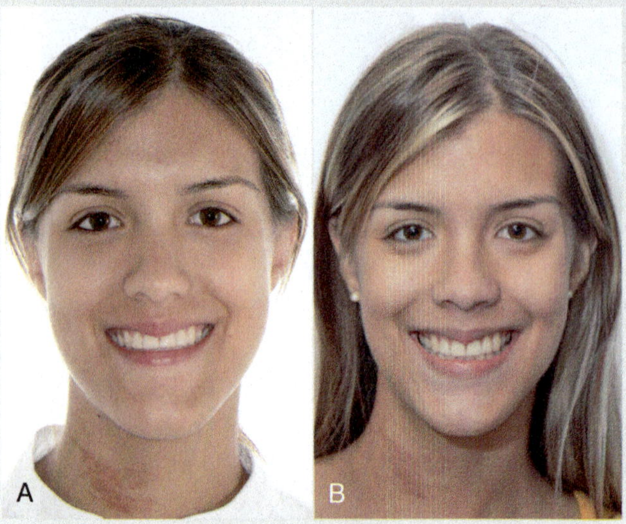

Figure 21-25 **A,** Pre-treatment and **(B)** post-treatment esthetics. Note the difference in macroesthetics and miniesthetics. Positive results are observed in the face and the smile. Notably, the occlusal plane clockwise rotation facilitated the possibility of obtaining a consonant smile and reducing the posterior gingival display.

occlusal plane. This steepening aided in developing a consonant smile arc from the presurgical flat smile arc without affecting vertically the incisor display. Also, by impacting the maxilla posteriorly, the gingival display in the buccal segments was reduced. However, when the microesthetics of the maxillary lip was evaluated at rest and on smiling (Fig. 21-26, A and B), a lip eversion with redundant tissue noticeably compromised the esthetics of the smile. To correct this microesthetic issue, an elliptical excision of a portion of the labial mucosa was performed (Fig. 21-26, C). Although the patient was unaware that the mucosa everted when she smiled, she was pleased that it could be corrected through a simple procedure and had a dramatic improvement in the smile microesthetics (Fig. 21-26, D). This example clearly illustrates that, as clinicians, we are responsible for detecting small microesthetic deviations and advising patients on the viability and complexity of their correction.

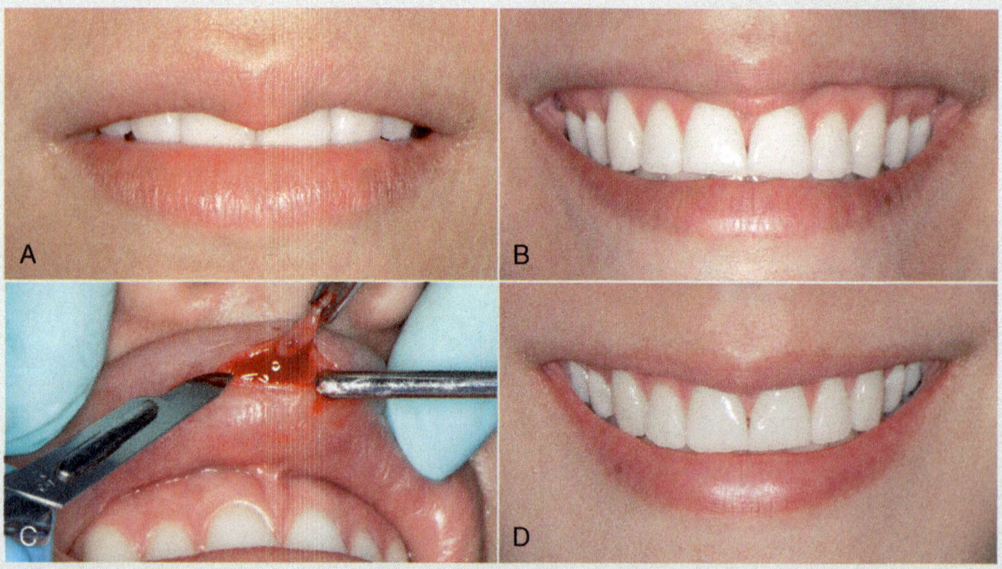

Figure 21-26 Microesthetics in the lip soft tissue are addressed. **A,** Small redundant tissue in the lip philtrum at rest. **B,** Redundant tissue more evident on smile. **C,** Minor excision of the redundant lip tissue. **D,** Improvement in the microesthetics after minimally invasive lip procedure. (Case from Villegas C, Janakiraman N, Uribe F, Nanda R. Rotation of the maxillo-mandibular complex to enhance esthetics using the Surgery First Approach. *J Clin Orthod.* 2012;46[2]:85–91.)

CASE REPORT 4

An 11.2-year-old female patient consulted for a facial asymmetry that had progressed during the last year. The physical exam revealed deviation of the chin toward the left side. An occlusal plane cant was observed as a result of increased vertical growth of the right side (Fig. 21-27, A and B). Deviation of the lower dental midline was not notable since the lower incisors had compensated with their axial inclination for the present mandibular asymmetry (Fig. 21-27, C). A comparative scintigraphy of the mandibular condyles revealed the presence of 60.3% of the contrast media on the right condyle and 39.7% on the left condyle; this confirmed the diagnosis of active hyperplasia of the right condyle (Fig. 21-27, D).[19]

Based on this diagnosis, a high intracapsular condylectomy of the right condyle was performed and an infrazygomatic mini-plate was placed on the right side. In addition, mini-screws were placed in the palate to serve as skeletal anchorage in conjunction with the mini-plate in order to level the occlusal plane without tipping by intruding the teeth on the right side. Figure 21-28 shows the posterior open bite obtained in the right side after the intrusion and the deviation of the lower midline toward the right side after the condylectomy.

Orthodontic treatment with extraction of the first lower premolars was then performed. The patient had extractions of the maxillary first premolars during a prior orthodontic treatment. The infrazygomatic mini-plate was used as anchorage to extrude the mandibular right buccal segment, close the posterior open bite, and level the lower occlusal plane (Fig. 21-29).

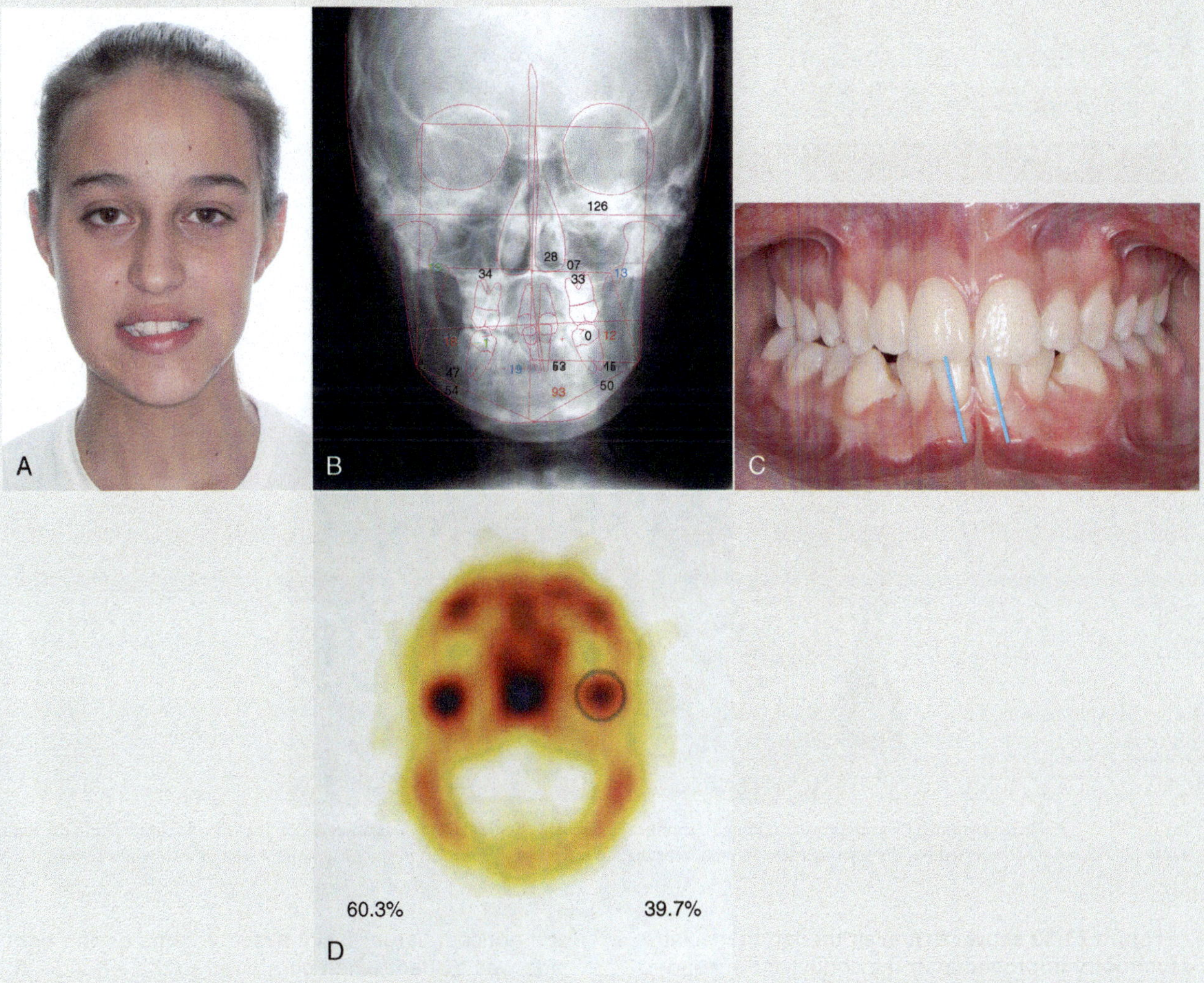

Figure 21-27 **A,** Patient with gross asymmetry noticed during growth. **B,** Posteroanterior cephalogram showing the significant maxillary and mandibular asymmetry. **C,** Lower incisor inclination trying to compensate for the facial asymmetry showing no midline deviation in relation to the maxilla at the incisal edge. **D,** Bone scan reflecting abnormal uptake of the radioactive marker on the right condyle.

Continued

CASE REPORT 4—cont'd

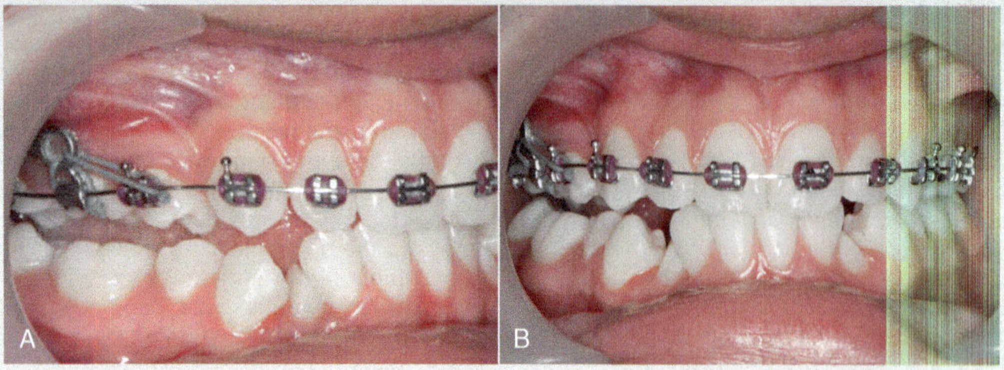

Figure 21-28 **A,** Force from right buccal mini-plate to intrude the buccal segment and correct the occlusal cant. **B,** Intentional lateral open bite created by the intrusion of the right maxillary buccal segment.

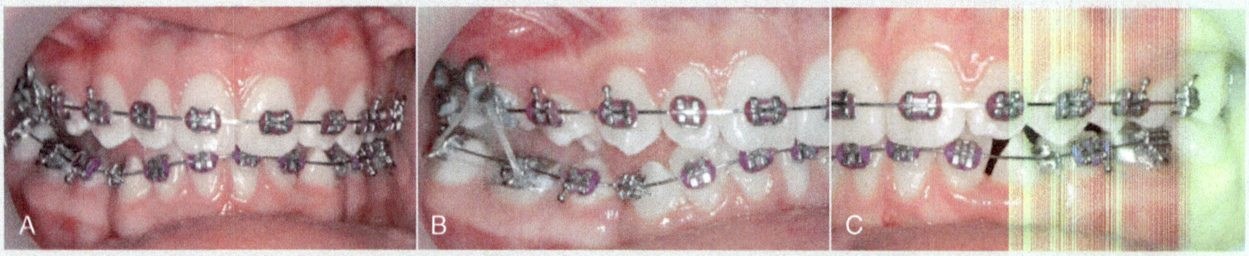

Figure 21-29 **A and B,** Force delivered by an intermaxillary elastic to erupt the lower right buccal segment to match the intruded maxillary right buccal segment. **C,** No intrusive or extrusive mechanics were attempted on the left side.

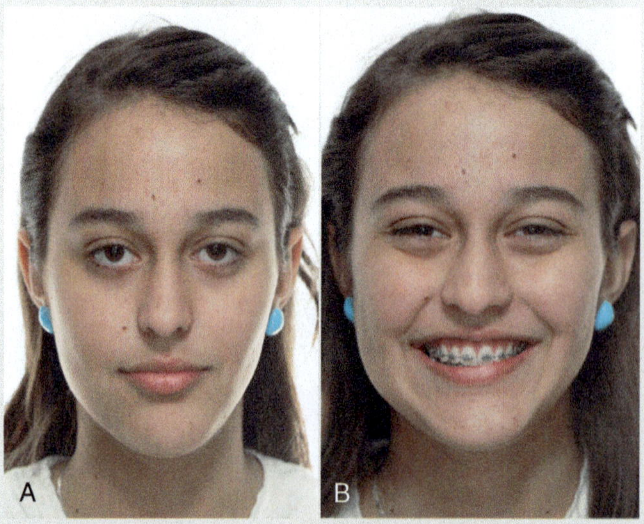

Figure 21-30 **A,** Facial asymmetry was improved, although a significant deficiency in tissue mass was observed on the left side compared to the right. **B,** Maxillary cant was corrected but the asymmetrical animation of the lower lip and general left to right asymmetry was more obvious on smile.

Figure 21-30 shows that even though the facial asymmetry improved after the condylectomy and the leveling of the occlusal plane, a deviation of the chin toward the left side and a difference in volume in the area of the mandibular corpus and ramus was still noticed. Larger facial tissue volume on the right side was evident when compared to the left side. A medical computed tomography (CT) was ordered to quantify the degree of asymmetry and define the amount of volume that was missing (Fig. 21-31, A).

CASE REPORT 4—cont'd

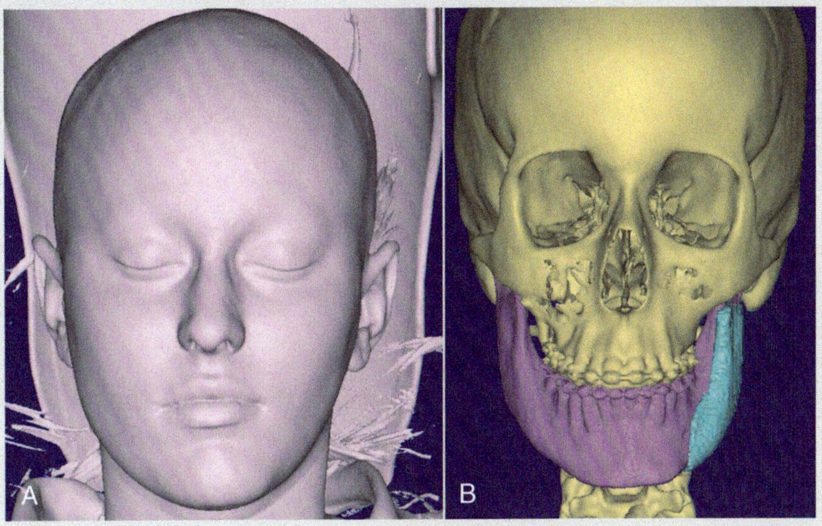

Figure 21-31 Medical computed tomography was used to evaluate the (A) soft tissue and (B) hard tissue asymmetry. Using a mirroring technique, a custom-made implant was designed to fill the missing hard and soft tissue volume on the left lower face.

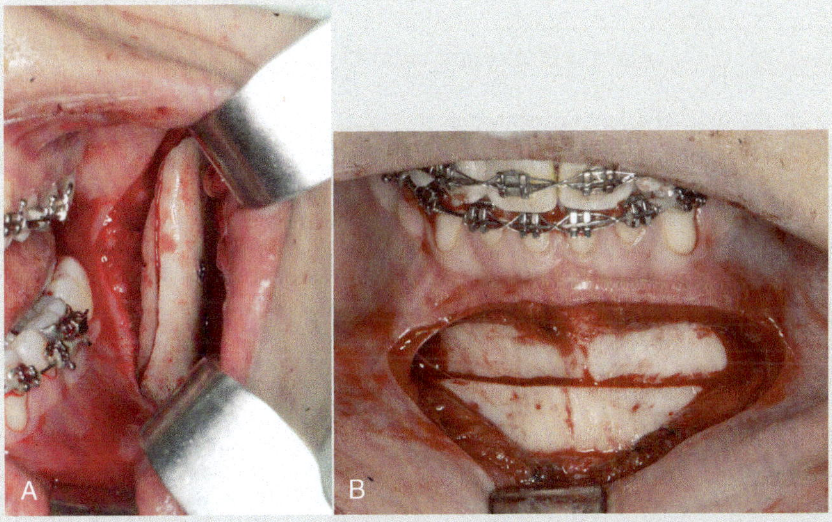

Figure 21-32 **A,** Insertion of the custom-made implant secured with two screws laterally to the left ramus. **B,** Lateral sliding genioplasty complemented the surgical procedure to significantly improve facial asymmetry.

A mirror image of both sides was virtually analyzed and a polymethylmethacrylate (PMMA) implant was designed (Fig. 21-31, B), inserted, and fixed with two 2-mm × 13-mm titanium screws (Fig. 21-32, A) (Lomas, PSM Medical Solutions, Tuttlingen, Germany) on the left side to restitute the missing tissue volume. A lateral sliding genioplasty toward the right side refined the correction of the asymmetry (Fig. 21-32, B).

Figure 21-33 shows the improvement in overall symmetry. The facial contour definition was refined and made symmetrical with secondary effects on the smile. An important aspect to highlight is that the left animation of the lower lip commissure, which was significantly asymmetrical, was improved with the tissue volume augmentation via the facial implant and the lateral displacement of the chin achieved with the genioplasty.

Continued

CASE REPORT 4—cont'd

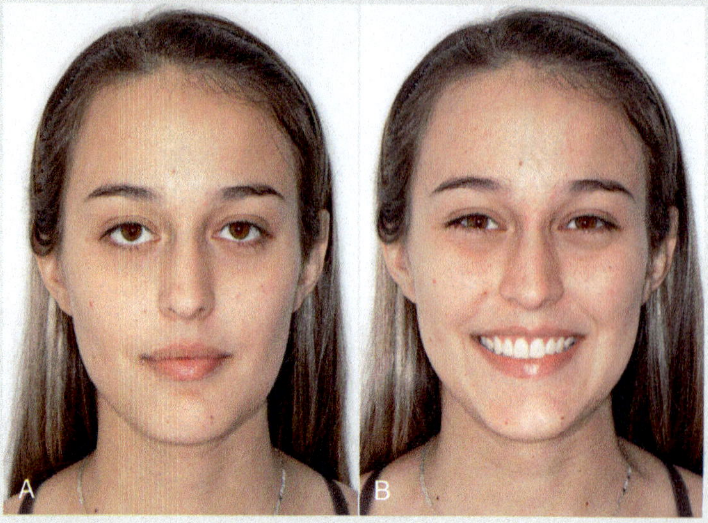

Figure 21-33 Improvement in overall asymmetry evaluated **(A)** at rest and **(B)** on smile. Note the more symmetrical soft tissue volume and animation of the lower lip. (Case from Villegas C, Janakiraman N, Nanda R, Uribe F. Management of unilateral condylar hyperplasia with a high condylectomy, skeletal anchorage, and a CAD/CAM alloplast. *J Clin Orthod.* 2013;47[6]:365–374.)

SUMMARY

It is important to keep in mind several key factors when analyzing patients and deciding how they will benefit from a surgical-orthodontic treatment:

- Treatment plans must be individualized and should not only consider the significant esthetic changes that can be obtained with the proper rearrangement of the facial bones, but also pay close attention to the small details that differentiate a good outcome from an excellent outcome.
- Subjective and objective goals guide the treatment planning process in orthognathic surgery.
- Macroesthetics, miniesthetics, and microesthetics are components of a classification system that can be used as a framework to methodically approach esthetics from a global perspective to a more detailed focus. Symmetry, averageness, and proportion are important pillars in the achievement of optimal facial esthetics.
- The fourth dimension, time, can be addressed with the "surgery first approach," which significantly shortens the duration of treatment. In addition, early surgery during adolescence should be considered in psychosocially compromised patients.
- Technology allows us to evaluate dentofacial deformities in three dimensions with great accuracy. Treatment plans and their execution should address those deviations to the full extent in order to justify the use of these technologies. Small refinements in symmetry may be one of the greatest advantages, where left to right asymmetries can be assessed in detail and corrected by subtraction or addition using these technologies. However, it is important to consider the cost-benefit of using these technologies on a case-by-case basis.

REFERENCES

1. Hungerford MW. *Molly Bawn.* London, England: Smith, Elder, & Co; 1878.
2. Thornhill R, Gangestad SW. Facial attractiveness. *Trends Cogn Sci.* 1999;3:452–460.
3. Bashour M. History and current concepts in the analysis of facial attractiveness. *Plast Reconstr Surg.* 2006;118:741–756.
4. Grammer K, Fink B, Moller AP, Thornhill R. Darwinian aesthetics: sexual selection and the biology of beauty. *Biol Rev Camb Philos Soc.* 2003;78:385–407.
5. Langlois JH, Roggman LA. Attractive faces are only average. *Psychol Sci.* 1991;1:115–121.
6. Grammer K, Thornhill R. Human (*Homo sapiens*) facial attractiveness and sexual selection: the role of symmetry and averageness. *J Comp Psychol.* 1994;108:233–242.
7. Murphy C, Kearns G, Sleeman D, Cronin M, Allen PF. The clinical relevance of orthognathic surgery on quality of life. *Int J Oral Maxillofac Surg.* 2011;40:926–930.
8. Lee LH, Jun JH, Danganan M, Pogrel MA, Kushner H, Lee JS. Orthognathic surgery for the Asian patient and the influence of the surgeon's background on treatment. *Int J Oral Maxillofac Surg.* 2011;40:458–463.
9. Gateno J, Xia JJ, Teichgraeber JF, et al. Clinical feasibility of computer-aided surgical simulation (CASS) in the treatment of complex cranio-maxillofacial deformities. *J Oral Maxillofac Surg.* 2007;65:728–734.
10. Quevedo LA, Ruiz JV, Quevedo CA. Using a clinical protocol for orthognathic surgery and assessing a 3-dimensional virtual approach: current therapy. *J Oral Maxillofac Surg.* 2011;69:623–637.
11. Swennen GR, Mollemans W, De Clercq C, et al. A cone-beam computed tomography triple scan procedure to obtain a three-dimensional augmented virtual skull model appropriate for orthognathic surgery planning. *J Craniofac Surg.* 2009;20:297–307.
12. Ackerman JL, Proffit WR, Sarver DM, Ackerman MB, Kean MR. Pitch, roll, and yaw: describing the spatial orientation of dentofacial traits. *Am J Orthod Dentofacial Orthop.* 2007;131:305–310.

13. Nagasaka H, Sugawara J, Kawamura H, Nanda R. "Surgery first" skeletal Class III correction using the skeletal anchorage system. *J Clin Orthod.* 2009;43:97–105.
14. Villegas C, Uribe F, Sugawara J, Nanda R. Expedited correction of significant dentofacial asymmetry using a "surgery first" approach. *J Clin Orthod.* 2010;44:97–103, quiz 105.
15. Wolford LM, Karras SC, Mehra P. Considerations for orthognathic surgery during growth, part 1: mandibular deformities. *Am J Orthod Dentofacial Orthop.* 2001;119:95–101.
16. Wolford LM, Karras SC, Mehra P. Considerations for orthognathic surgery during growth, part 2: maxillary deformities. *Am J Orthod Dentofacial Orthop.* 2001;119:102–105.
17. Sarver DM. Augmenting and improving esthetics through surgical intervention. In: McNamara JA, Kapila SD, eds. *Surgical Enhancement of Orthodontic Treatment.* Ann Arbor, MI: The University of Michigan; 2010:1–31.
18. Oberti G, Villegas C, Ealo M, Palacio JC, Baccetti T. Maxillary molar distalization with the dual-force distalizer supported by mini-implants: a clinical study. *Am J Orthod Dentofacial Orthop.* 2009;135:282.e1–5, discussion 282–283.
19. Hodder SC, Rees JI, Oliver TB, Facey PE, Sugar AW. SPECT bone scintigraphy in the diagnosis and management of mandibular condylar hyperplasia. *Br J Oral Maxillofac Surg.* 2000;38:87–93.

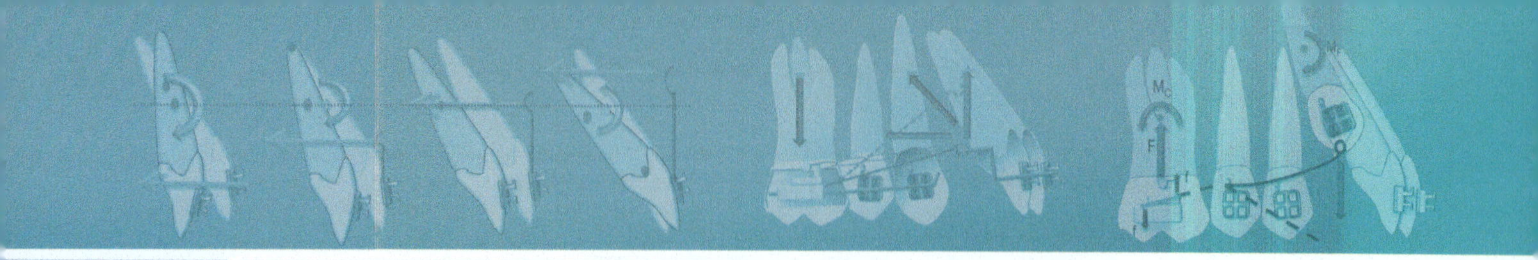

CHAPTER 22

Surgery First: The Protocol of Innovative Surgical Orthodontics

Junji Sugawara, Zaher Aymach, Satoshi Yamada, Hiroshi Nagasaka, Hiroshi Kawamura, and Ravindra Nanda

In recent years, a trend toward implementing treatment plans that achieve rapid facial change has arisen.[1-5] In the surgery first (SF) treatment plan, the presurgical orthodontic treatment phase is completely eliminated, the jaws are surgically repositioned to the desired locations, and orthodontic tooth movement follows. Caution is important when embarking on SF treatment. Even a highly experienced orthodontist/surgeon will not necessarily find it easy to identify the occlusal relationship that will accompany an ideal facial and functional result. This explains why numerous orthodontists prefer to conduct an orthodontic preparation before surgery. Having a stable postoperative occlusion is thought to be important for maintaining the bony stability.[5]

The advent of temporary anchorage devices (TADs), including skeletal anchorage, was a breakthrough in achieving teeth movement beyond traditional orthodontics. The skeletal anchorage system (SAS), which uses titanium mini-plates to control moving teeth in nongrowing patients, has shown that it is possible to achieve predictable three-dimensional movement of teeth and entire dentition with fewer bicuspid extractions.[6,7]

Contemplating SF treatment with the SAS began in 2003 at Tohoku University in Sendai, Japan. The distinguishing feature of this approach is an orthodontics-driven method referred to as Sendai SF. The surgery aims to first correct the skeletal deformity and then the SAS mini-plates, which are placed at the time of orthognathic surgery, manage the dentoalveolar problems and establish the functional and esthetic occlusion postsurgically. The fundamental concept of Sendai SF is to maintain the quality results seen in traditional surgical orthodontics by making a precise prediction of the final outcomes of both orthodontic and surgical correction prior to treatment.

This chapter describes and illustrates the step-by-step protocol used in Sendai SF through four case examples.

SENDAI SURGERY FIRST PROTOCOL

The Sendai SF protocol has 15 steps (Box 22-1). Among these are four major steps, each of which is discussed below and illustrated with a detailed patient case example.

Step 1: Diagnosis (Establishment of Treatment Goals)

Individualized treatment goals in Sendai SF are established at the initial time of treatment.[1-3] This process is led by examining and analyzing the problem list developed for each patient. In our case example, a 37-year-old female presented with a prognathic profile and long face with facial asymmetry, an anterior open bite, and significant retroclination of the lower incisors (Fig. 22-1). According to the posteroanterior (PA) cephalometric radiograph, she had clear mandibular asymmetry. Cephalometric analysis to evaluate skeletal discrepancies was conducted based on five parameters: cephalometric template analysis (CDS analysis),[8] McNamara analysis for points A and B, the A point nasion B point (ANB) angle, Wits appraisal,[9] and Harvold analysis (Fig. 22-2). Results of the cephalometric analysis revealed her mandibular excess and excessive lower facial height due to vertical maxillary excess. These findings indicated her need for surgical correction with mandibular setback and reduction of lower facial height.

Based on the results of the cephalometric analysis, the patient's treatment goals were established (Fig. 22-3). The amount of mandibular setback and the extent of decompensation of the incisors were evaluated as well. The amount of mandibular setback was predicted to be 10-mm on average and her denture relationship changed from Class III to Class II with open bite. In postsurgical orthodontics, 3-mm intrusion of upper molars and 5-mm protraction of lower dentition were needed to achieve the successful decompensation of her lower incisors and good Class I occlusion.

BOX 22-1 The Protocol of Sendai SF

1. Examination
2. Analysis (problem list)
3. Diagnosis (treatment goal)
4. Bonding brackets
5. Passive surgical wires
6. Face bow transfer
7. Mounting models
8. Model prediction
9. Surgical splint
10. Orthognathic surgery
11. Rehabilitation
12. Orthodontic treatment
13. Debonding
14. Retention
15. 5-year follow-up

If using conventional surgical orthodontics, the patient would have been a candidate for two-jaw surgery since she had vertical problems in conjunction with anteroposterior and transverse problems. By using the SAS to intrude the maxillary posterior teeth, the need for two-jaw surgery was eliminated; the less invasive one-jaw surgical approach was all that was required.

At least 1 week before surgery, brackets were bonded indirectly and passive rectangular wires for stabilizing dentition and bone segments were prepared by a dental technician in a laboratory. The brackets and archwires were 0.022-inch and 0.016-inch × 0.022-inch stainless steel, respectively. Surgical hooks were soldered on the archwire (Fig. 22-4).

Step 2: Model Surgery

Model surgery is an essential step in Sendai SF and leads to the fabrication of the surgical splint that will maintain the transit occlusion postsurgically.

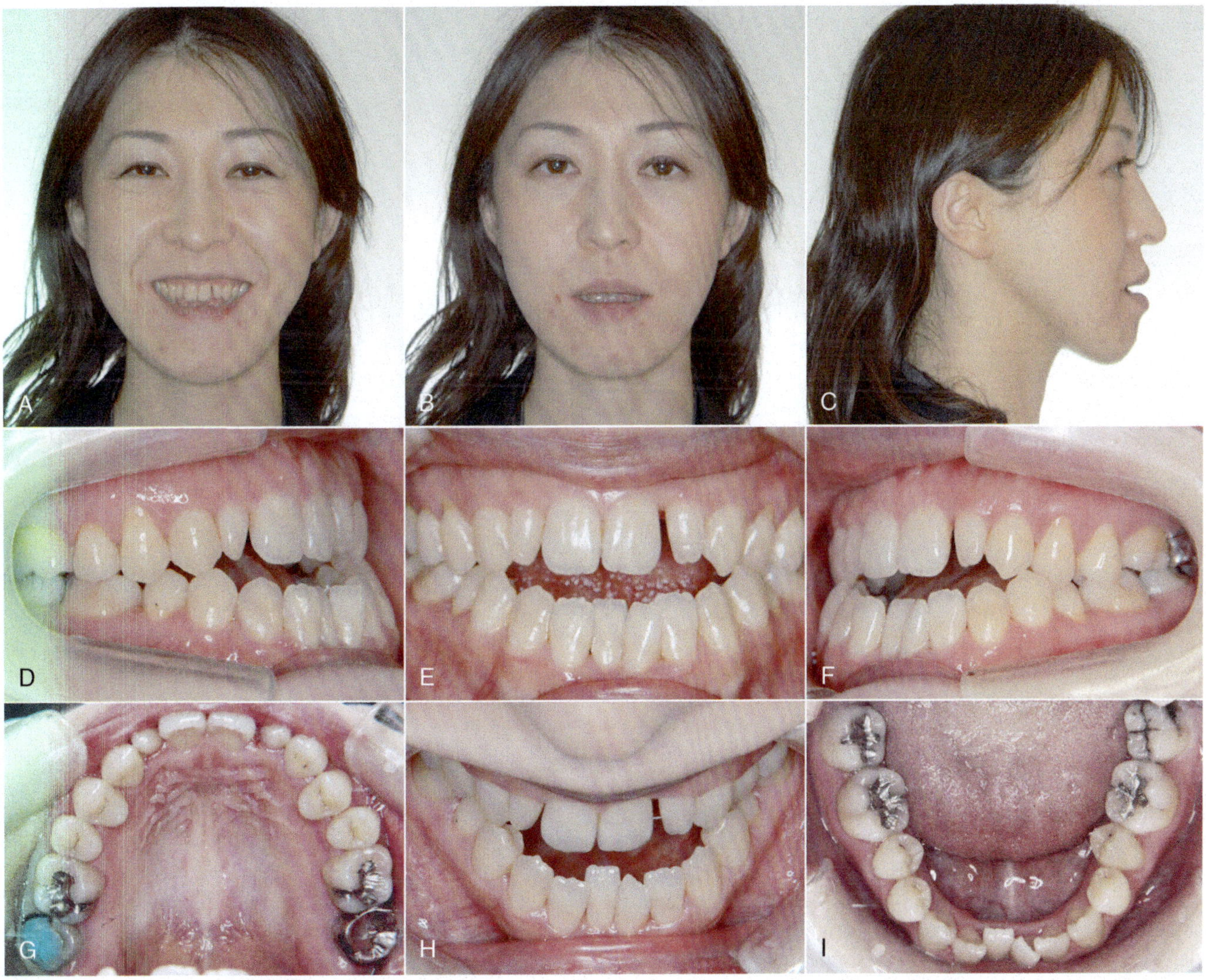

Figure 22-1 Initial (A–C) facial and (D–I) intraoral photos of a 37-year-old female patient show a prognathic profile, long face, Class I dental relationship, anterior crossbite, open bite, and retroclination of the lower incisors.

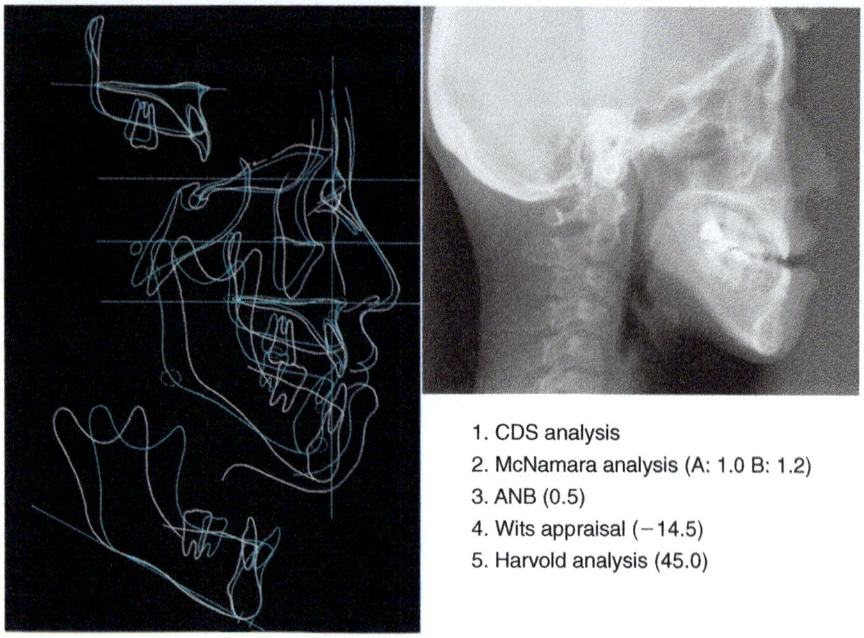

1. CDS analysis
2. McNamara analysis (A: 1.0 B: 1.2)
3. ANB (0.5)
4. Wits appraisal (−14.5)
5. Harvold analysis (45.0)

Figure 22-2 Cephalometric analysis. The line drawing indicates patient (*white*) and norm (*blue*). Clearly, the patient's mandibular protrusion and excessive lower facial height could best be corrected surgically. *A*, A point; *ANB*, A point nasion B point; *B*, B point; *CDS*, cephalometric template analysis.

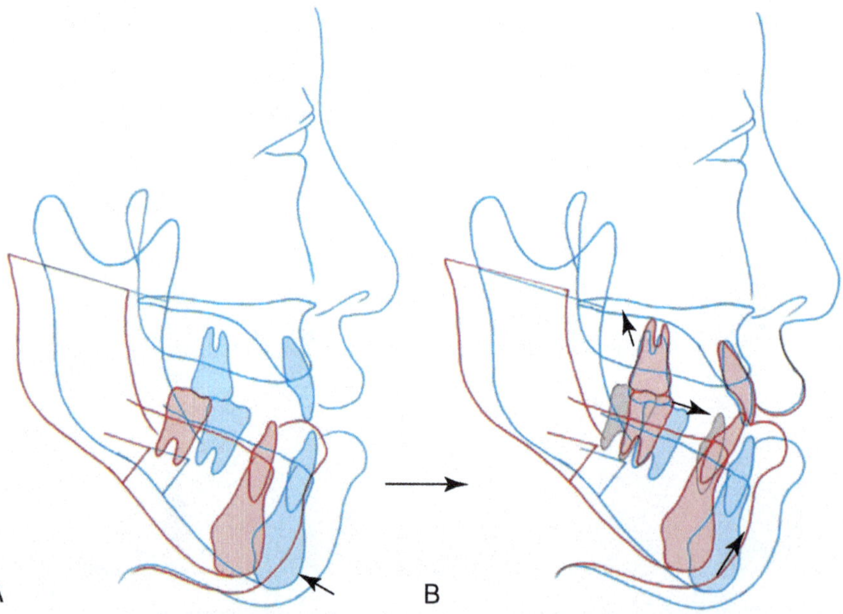

Figure 22-3 Treatment goals. Cephalometric prediction **(A)** immediately after surgery and **(B)** at debonding. The amount of mandibular setback and the extent of decompensation of the incisors were predicted. In postsurgical orthodontics, 3-mm intrusion of upper molars and 5-mm protraction of lower dentition were needed to achieve the successful decompensation of the patient's lower incisors and good Class I occlusion. By using the skeletal anchorage system (SAS) to intrude the maxillary posteriors, the need for two-jaw surgery was eliminated.

The facebow transfer process is used to transfer the maxillary model followed by the mandibular model onto a semi-adjustable articulator. Based on the cephalometric prediction, the surgical movement is simulated. The patient needed mandibular setback of 13-mm on the right and 7-mm on the left (Fig. 22-5, A–C). The surgical simulation of mandibular movement should be parallel to the functional occlusal plane so that the posterior facial height is maintained (Fig. 22-5, D). As a result, many Class III cases will show Class II open bite immediately after surgery due to the occlusal interferences at the molar regions.

Other groups that promote SF treatment recommend establishing three-point contacts in model surgery to acquire stable occlusion and Class I molar relationships immediately after orthognathic surgery.[5,10,11] This is not necessarily required in Sendai SF. The surgical movement is aimed to

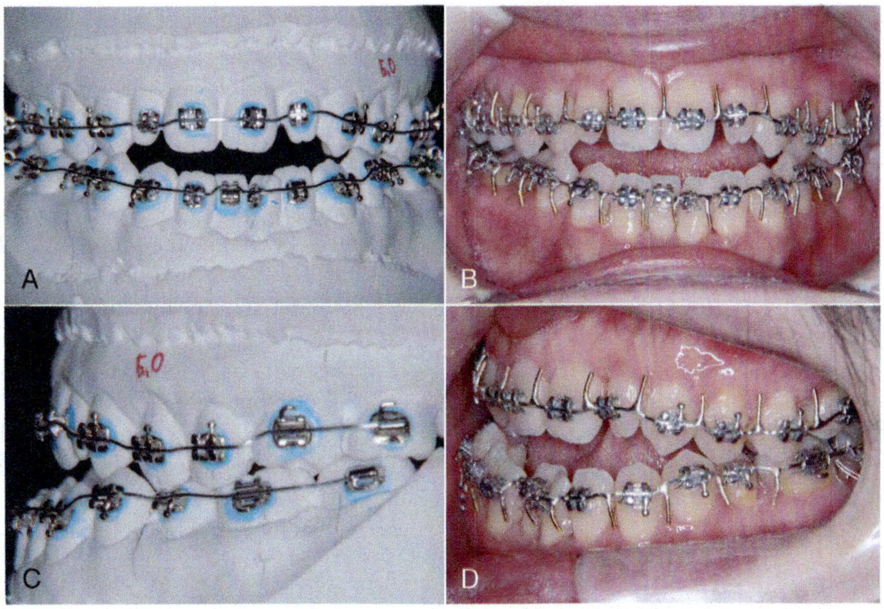

Figure 22-4 Indirect bonding and surgical wires. The passive rectangular surgical wires (0.016-inch × 0.022-inch stainless steel) for stabilizing dentition and bone segments were prepared by a dental technician in a laboratory. **A,** The passive wire bent on a model after the brackets indirectly bonded; frontal view. **B,** The passive wire with the surgical hooks soldered; intraoral frontal view. **C,** Lateral model view. **D,** Lateral intraoral view.

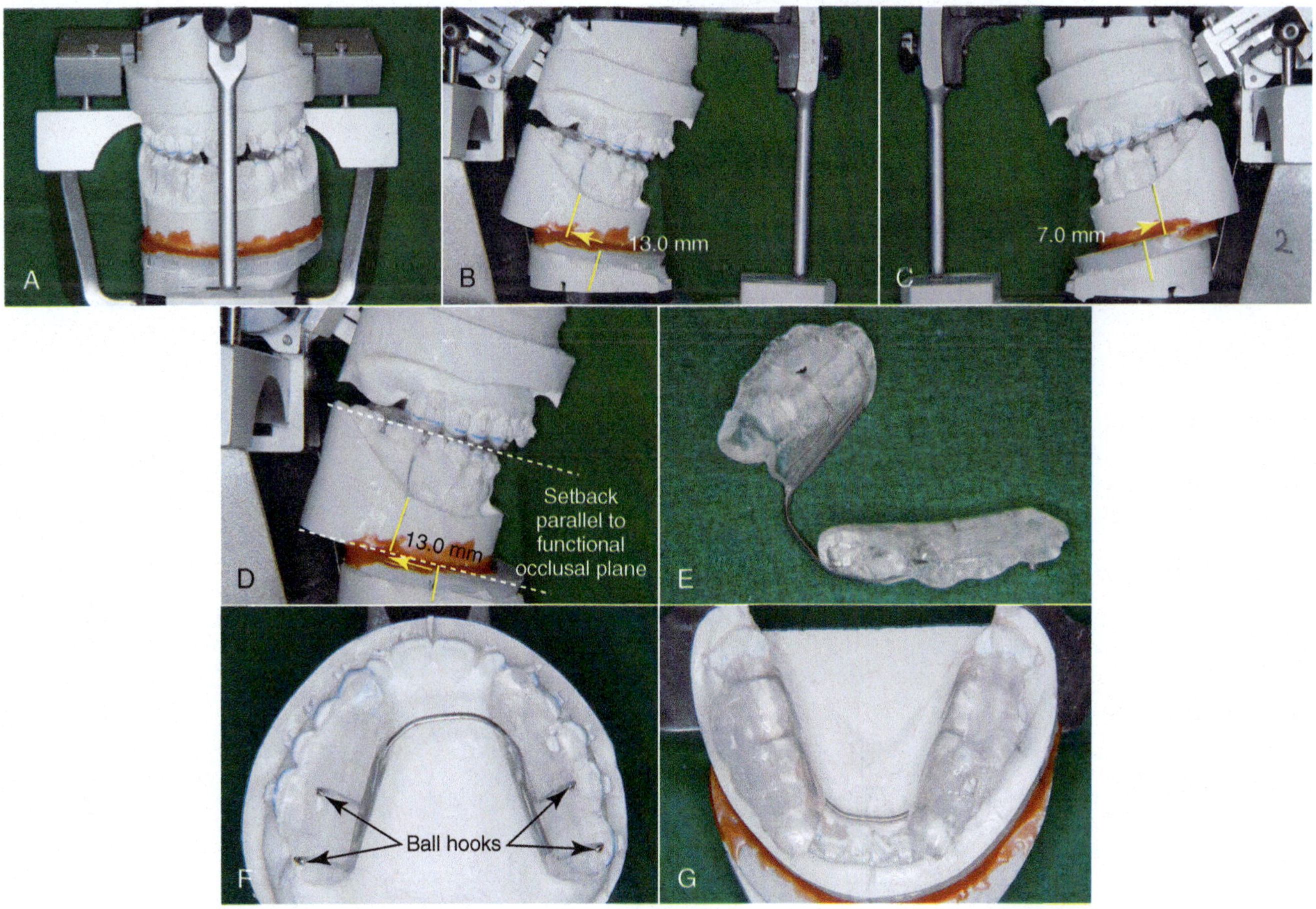

Figure 22-5 **A–C,** Model prediction with semiadjustable articulator. Based on the cephalometric prediction, the patient's mandibular model was setback 13-mm on the right side and 7-mm on the left side. **D,** Mandibular setback should be parallel to the functional occlusal plane to not increase the posterior facial height. Many Class III cases show Class II open bite at that point in the treatment, because of the occlusal interferences at the molar regions. **E–G,** A surgical splint with four ball hooks is essential to maximize the occlusal contact and to stabilize posterior support immediately after surgery. The splint is usually placed at the mandibular dentition in Class III cases.

correct the skeletal disharmony. It is the role of the SAS to achieve the proper occlusion postsurgically. Aymach and Kawamura described the attempt to achieve a three-point contact occlusion and close the open bite by counterclockwise rotation of the mandible will extend the pterygomasseteric sling due to the increase of posterior facial height. Such extension of the sling is closely associated with the postsurgical relapse seen with open bite.[12,13] Therefore other SF groups must apply more invasive two-jaw surgery in order to avoid the increase in posterior facial height.

With the surgical movement simulated, a surgical splint with four ball hooks and a lingual bar is fabricated (Fig. 22-5, E–G). Using a splint is essential to maximize the occlusal contact and to stabilize posterior support. Even though the molars cause occlusal interferences at this point in the treatment process, no cusp grinding of the molars is performed.

Since distalization of the maxillary molars and constriction of the maxillary dentition are needed at the early stage of postsurgical orthodontics, the surgical splint is usually placed at the mandibular dentition in Class III cases.

Step 3: Orthognathic Surgery

Accurate surgical technique has a major role in the success of Sendai SF. Achieving an appropriate osteotomy design, splitting, fixation technique, and proper condyle seating are key in conferring stable results.

The surgeons on the Sendai SF team use a modified design of a bilateral sagittal split osteotomy (BSSO) combined with a T-shaped bone mini-plate fixation.[14-16] The design has a buccal step laid adjacent to the mandibular second molar area. This design prevents condylar dislocation and therefore minimizes relapse (Fig. 22-6). Aymach and Kawamura have shown that for mandibular setback or advancement surgery,

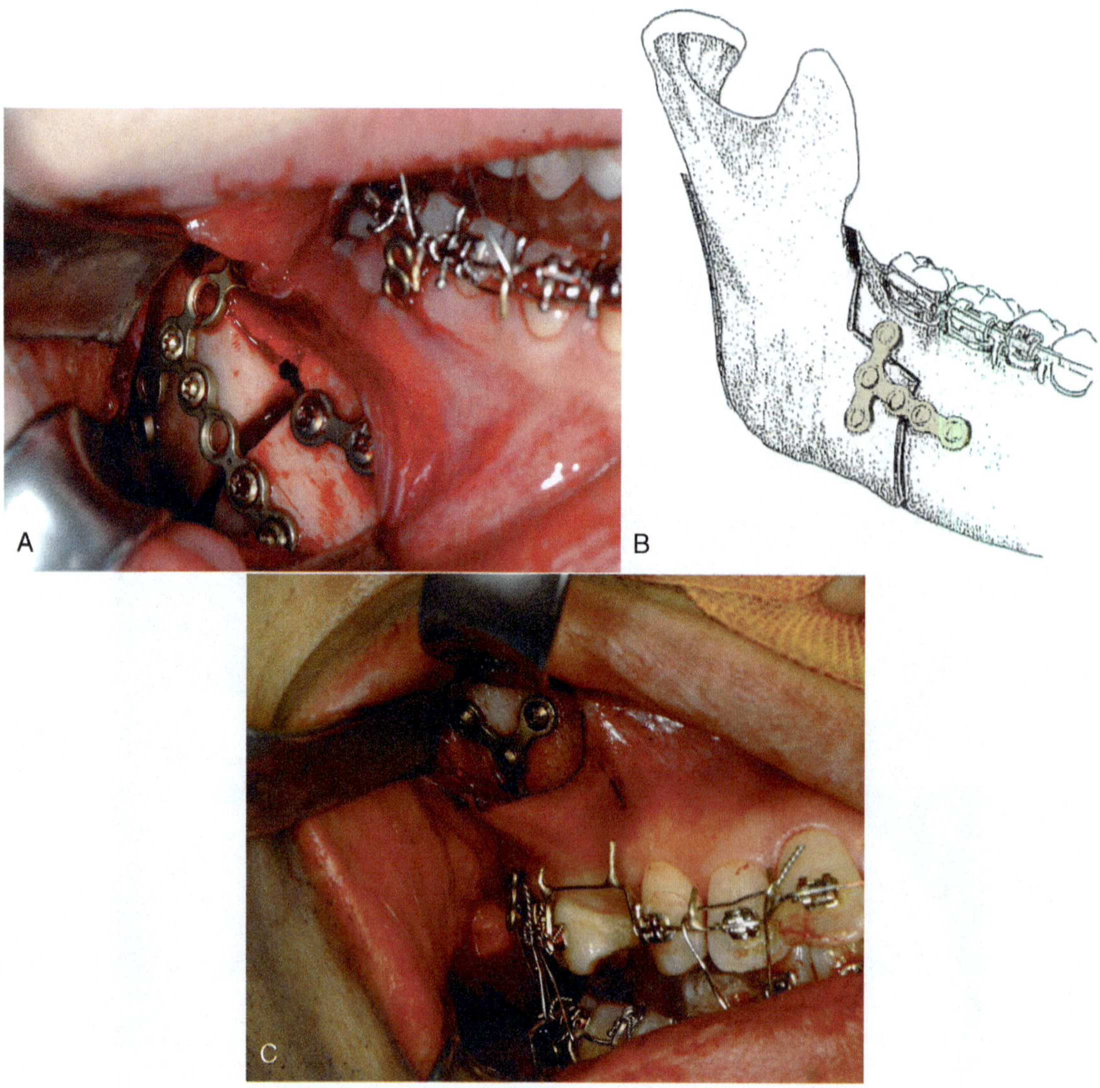

Figure 22-6 **A,** A modified sagittal split ramus osteotomy with buccal step and T-shaped mini-plate fixation; view of the surgical site. Aymach[14] and Kawamura[15] found this technique optimizes the resistance and stability of the fixation when compared with a standard bilateral sagittal split osteotomy (BSSO) fixed with a standard mini-plate. (Note that the orthodontic mini-plates for the skeletal anchorage system [SAS] are placed at the time of surgery). **B,** Schematic view of the T mini-plate fitting and fixating at the site of the buccal step of the osteotomy. **C,** The SAS placed at the maxillary buttress area during surgery. (Note that the hook of the mini-plate extends through the attached gingiva to be used later for orthodontic movement.)

a modified BSSO and buccal step, combined with a T-shaped bone mini-plate fixation, optimizes the resistance and stability of the fixation when compared to a standard BSSO fixed with a single straight bone mini-plate.

The authors suggest avoiding the use of positional screws for osteotomy fixation, as they confer a high potential for torquing the condyle and consequentially shifting the occlusion. Using bone mini-plates provides a sufficient semirigid fixation that allows functional stability under minimal bone movement.[14,17,18]

The patient underwent modified BSSO for mandibular setback. Her maxillary right second molar was extracted because of root fracture. This problem was caused by her general dentist prior to treatment. During the operation, Y-type and L-type orthodontic mini-plates were implanted at the zygomatic buttress and the mandibular body, respectively (Fig. 22-7). Immediately after surgery, the patient showed Class II profile and Class II denture with open bite. Although her profile appeared Class II, her skeletal relationship changed to skeletal Class I. Her mandible was maintained in the proper position using a surgical splint and training elastics at the canine regions (Fig. 22-8). No extraoral appliance, such as a chin cap, was required for maintenance.

Cephalometric superimposition of images at initial presentation and 9 days after surgery showed a 10-mm setback on average, in line with the treatment goal (Fig. 22-9).

Step 4: Orthodontic Treatment

Orthodontic treatment commonly starts 17 days after surgery. Usually 3 to 4 weeks are allowed for recovery and to enhance nutrition. However, in most Sendai SF cases postsurgical treatment begins 2 to 3 weeks after orthognathic surgery.

In the patient, leveling of upper and lower dentition started using 0.016-inch nickel-titanium (Ni-Ti) archwires (Fig. 22-10). The surgical splint was placed at the mandibular posteriors and modified to an occlusal splint by flattening the occlusal surface. It was used in order to not disturb the tooth movement of the upper dentition and to help with eating. Two months after surgery, rectangular Ni-Ti archwires were engaged and intrusion and distalization of maxillary molars and protraction of mandibular dentition were carried out (Fig. 22-11). The occlusal splint was discontinued at that time. In combination with intrusion and distalization of the maxillary posterior teeth and protraction of the mandibular dentition using SAS biomechanics, correction of her Class II denture was started. In addition to correction of the anteroposterior and vertical problems, transverse correction was needed. Constriction of the maxillary arch with buccolingual archwires was performed to allow for transverse decompensation.

Copper-nickel-titanium (Cu-Ni-Ti) archwires (0.019-inch × 0.025-inch) for mandibular use were engaged buccally and a 0.032-inch × 0.032-inch TMA lingual arch was placed (Fig. 22-12). In the lower arch, a 0.019-inch × 0.025-inch Cu-Ni-Ti archwire for maxillary use was engaged for expansion of the mandibular arch, as the mandibular posteriors showed excessive Wilson curve. In most Class III cases, occlusal interferences between the functional cusps of the upper and lower molars occur immediately after mandibular setback osteotomy because of transverse dental compensation. To remedy this problem, transverse decompensation by constriction of the upper arch and expansion of the lower arch is required (Fig. 22-13, A). With SAS biomechanics, the cusp to fossa relationship at the posterior teeth is corrected significantly and counterclockwise rotation of the mandible is then induced (Fig. 22-13, B). Anterior open bite is improved and rigid intercuspation is established (Fig. 22-13, C).

It is important to note that transverse decompensation is a key element in achieving good occlusion quickly and successfully in Sendai SF. To facilitate transverse decompensation the authors frequently apply a variety of different mechanics, including cross elastics in combination with a maxillary constriction lingual arch, an auxiliary expansion arch in the lower dentition, and SAS for unilateral and/or bilateral expansion of the lower arch (Fig. 22-14).

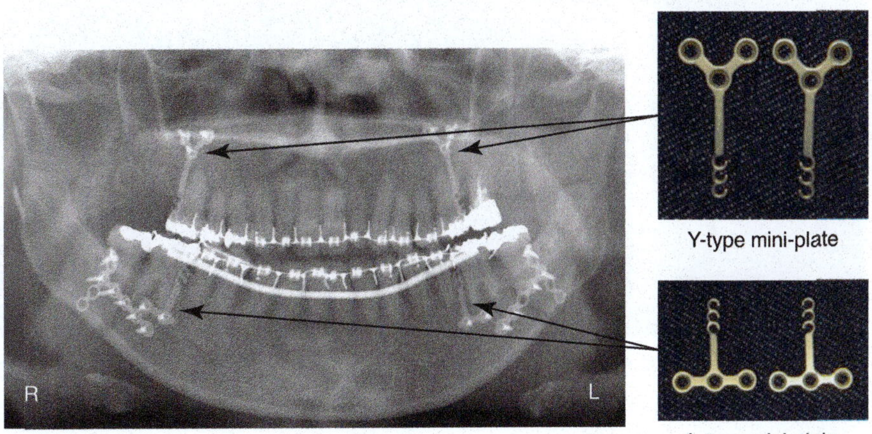

Figure 22-7 Panoramic radiograph obtained immediately after surgery. Orthodontic mini-plates were implanted at the zygomatic buttress and the mandibular body during surgery.

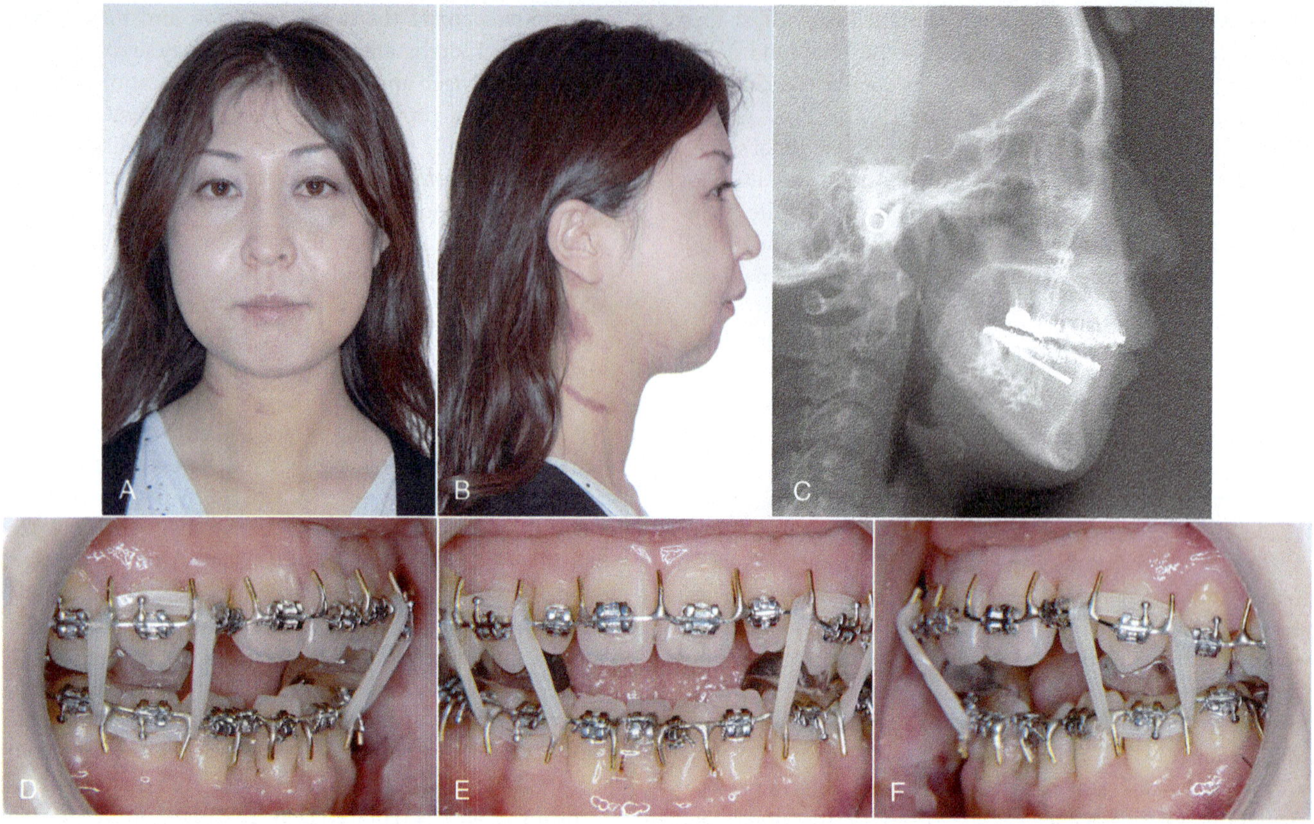

Figure 22-8 **A and B,** Facial photos and **(C)** cephalometric radiograph obtained 9 days after jaw surgery. Patient showed a Class II profile and Class II denture with open bite. **D–F,** Her mandible was maintained in the proper position using a surgical split and up-and-down elastics at the canine regions. Facial swelling takes a little bit longer to resolve.

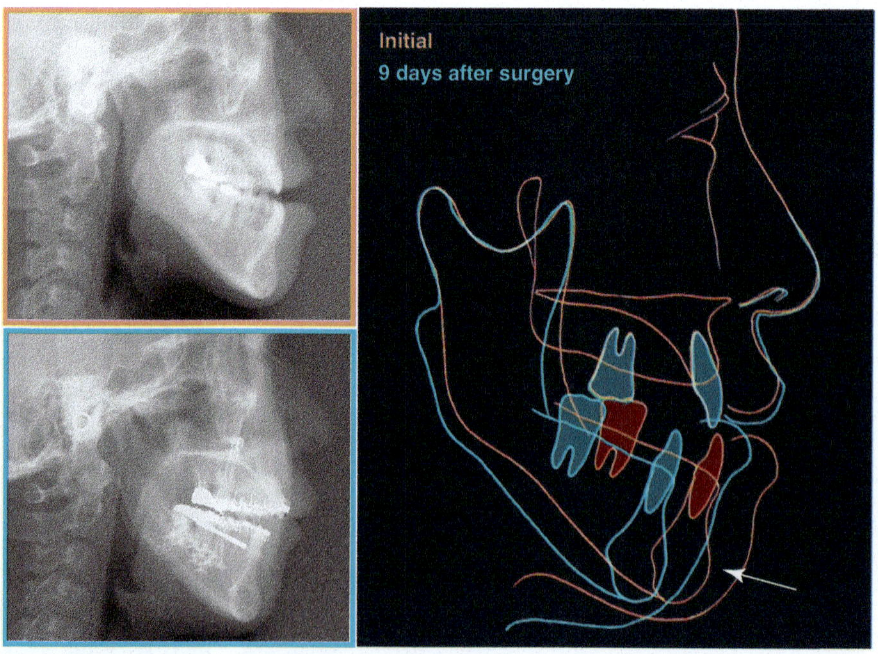

Figure 22-9 Cephalometric superimposition of initial radiograph and radiograph obtained 9 days after surgery. The patient's mandible showed a 10-mm setback on average, in line with the treatment goal.

Four months after surgery, the patient's upper and lower archwires were changed to 0.016-inch × 0.022-inch stainless steel archwires and coordinated (Fig. 22-15). Distalization and intrusion of the upper posteriors were carried out for correction of Class II molar relationship and decompensation of lower incisors, using Y-type mini-plates. At the same time, the protraction of the lower dentition was still in progress using L-type mini-plates. In addition, since tooth #12 and tooth #22 were small and needed to be crowned, Ni-Ti open coil springs were used to make enough space.

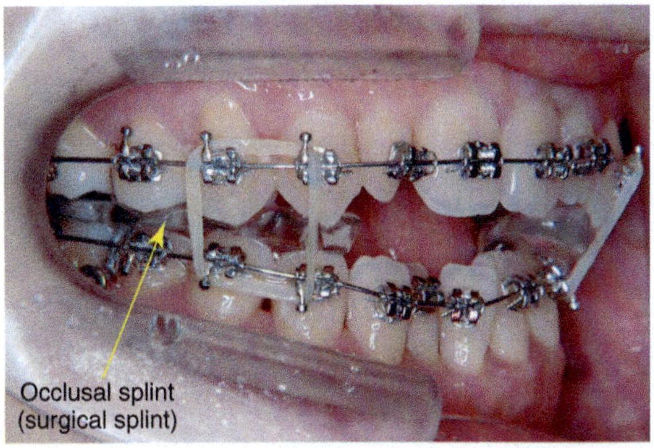

Figure 22-10 Seventeen days after surgery, when orthodontic treatment started. Leveling of upper and lower dentition began using 0.016-inch nickel-titanium (Ni-Ti) archwires. The surgical splint was placed at the mandibular posteriors and modified to an occlusal splint by flattening the occlusal surface.

Distalization of the upper posteriors and protraction of the lower dentition were completed and a Class I canine and molar relationship was established 5.4 months after surgery (Fig. 22-16, A). The bimaxillary arches were stabilized using ligature wires and mini-plates (Fig. 22-16, B).

The cephalometric superimposition of scans obtained immediately after surgery and 6.7 months later showed that the patient's open bite was corrected by counterclockwise rotation of the mandible, following intrusion of the upper molars and transverse decompensation (Fig. 22-17).

Temporary crowns were put on tooth #12 and tooth #22 at 6.7 months after surgery (and after making space). Bull loops were bent in the upper archwire to close minor spaces at the incisors (Fig. 22-18). Detailing and finishing commenced with maxillary and mandibular 0.017-inch × 0.025-inch stainless steel archwires at 7.6 months after surgery (Fig. 22-19). Occlusal equilibrium was carried out 9.2 months after surgery (Fig. 22-20) and debonding occurred at 10.7 months after surgery.

TREATMENT RESULTS AND EVALUATION

Intraoral views of the treatment progress showed that the patient's severe anterior open bite and deviation of lower

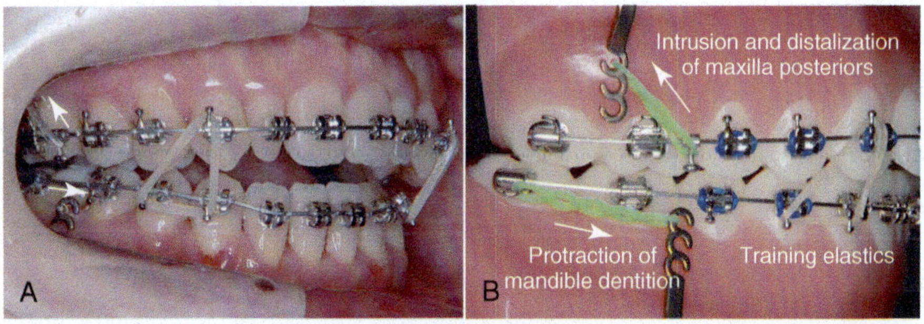

Figure 22-11 Two months after surgery (lateral view). **A,** Rectangular nickel-titanium (Ni-Ti) archwires were engaged and intrusion and distalization of maxillary molars and protraction of mandibular dentition were carried out. The occlusal splint was discontinued at that time. **B,** Skeletal anchorage system (SAS) biomechanics are also applied at this stage. The photo shows SAS biomechanics that were applied to the patient. In combination with intrusion and distalization of maxillary dentition and protraction of mandibular dentition, the patient's Class II denture will be improved quickly.

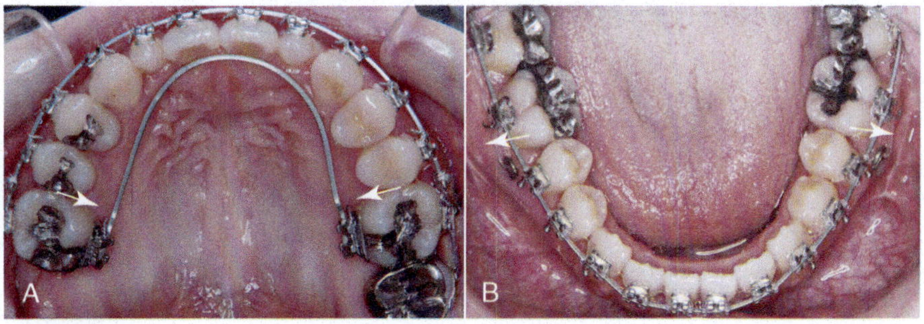

Figure 22-12 Two months after surgery: **(A)** maxillary occlusal view and **(B)** mandibular occlusal view. The transverse correction on the maxillary dentition is shown. Constriction of the maxillary arch with buccolingual archwires was performed to allow for transverse decompensation. Copper-nickel-titanium (Cu-Ni-Ti) wires (0.019-inch × 0.025-inch) 40°C for mandibular use were engaged buccally and a 0.032-inch × 0.032-inch TMA lingual archwire was placed. A Cu-Ni-Ti wire (0.019-inch × 0.025-inch) for maxillary use was engaged for expansion of the mandibular arch since the mandibular posteriors showed excessive Wilson curve.

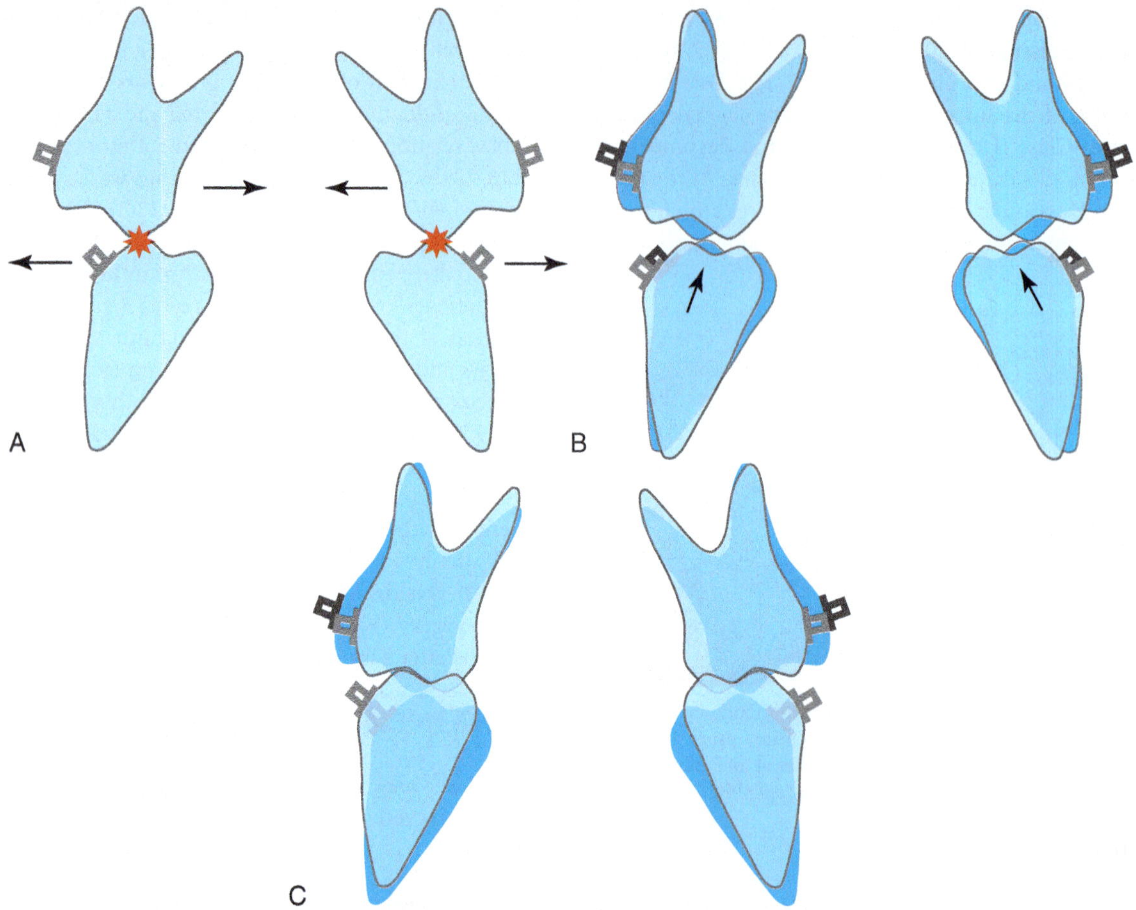

Figure 22-13 **A,** The mechanism of transverse decompensation in Sendai SF (immediately after surgery). In most Class III cases, occlusal interferences between functional cusps of the upper and lower molars occur immediately after mandibular setback osteotomy because of transverse dental compensation. To remedy this problem, transverse decompensation by constriction of the upper arch and expansion of the lower arch is required. **B,** After constriction of the upper arch and expansion of the lower arch. The correction of the cusp to fossa relationship at the posterior teeth is responsible on the counterclockwise rotation seen during the orthodontic phase. **C,** After counterclockwise rotation of the mandible. The anterior open bite is improved and rigid intercuspation is established. Transverse decompensation is key to achieving good occlusion quickly and successfully in Sendai SF.

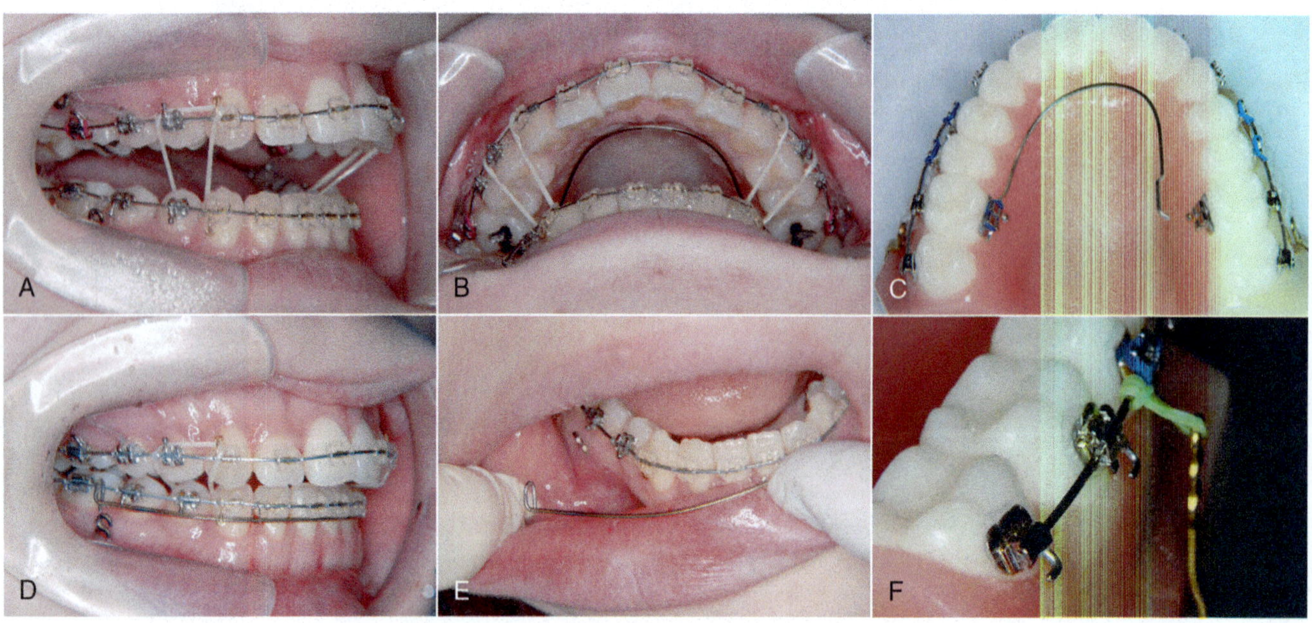

Figure 22-14 Various mechanics for transverse decompensation. **A,** Intermaxillary cross elastics. **B,** Constriction lingual arch for maxillary constriction. **C,** Auxiliary expansion arch for mandibular expansion. **D–F,** Skeletal anchorage system (SAS) for unilateral mandibular expansion.

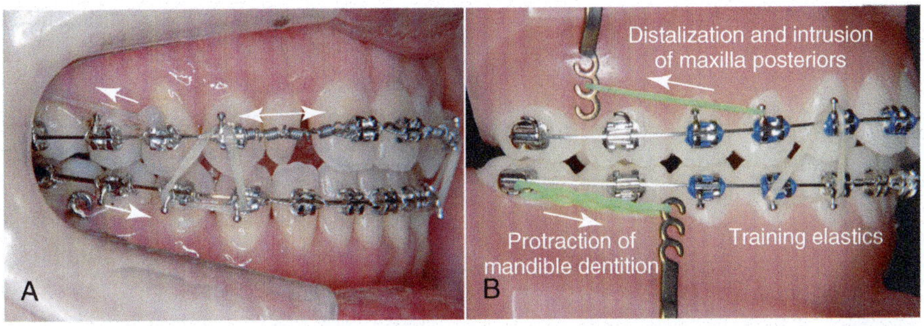

Figure 22-15 Four months after surgery. **A,** Upper and lower 0.016-inch × 0.022-inch stainless steel wires were used. Distalization and intrusion of the upper posteriors were carried out for correction of Class II molar relationship and decompensation of lower incisors using Y-type mini-plates. In addition, since teeth #12 and #22 were small and needed to be crowned, nickel-titanium (Ni-Ti) open coil springs were used to make enough space. **B,** Skeletal anchorage system (SAS) biomechanics for the distalization and intrusion of the upper posterior teeth and the protraction of the entire lower dentition.

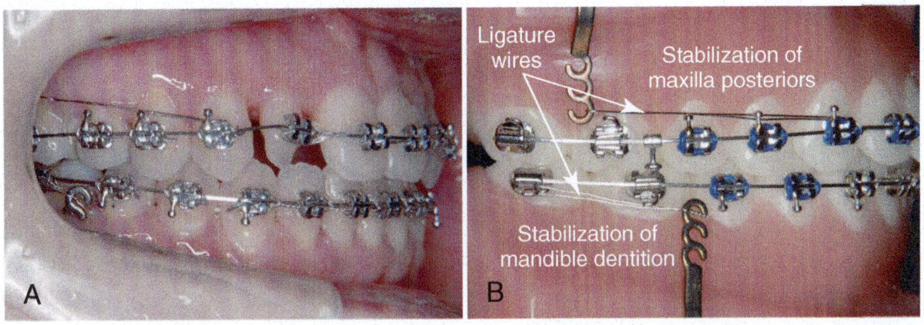

Figure 22-16 At 5.4 months after surgery. **A,** The distalization of the upper posteriors and the protraction of the lower dentition were completed and Class I canine and molar relationship was established. **B,** Skeletal anchorage system (SAS) biomechanics for stabilization of bimaxillary arches using ligature wires and mini-plates.

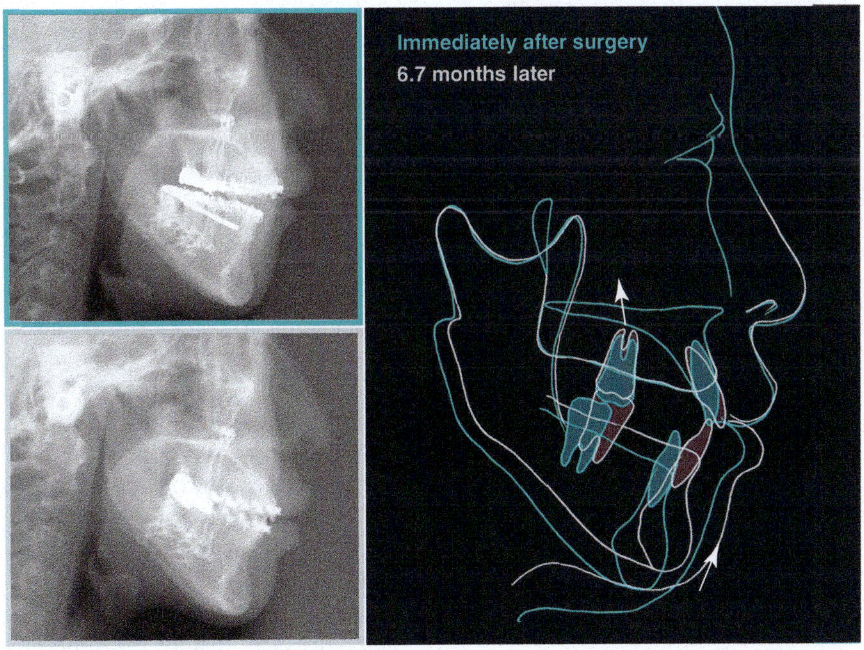

Figure 22-17 Cephalometric superimposition of scans obtained immediately after surgery (*top*) and 6.7 months later (*bottom*). The patient's open bite was corrected by counterclockwise rotation of the mandible following intrusion of the upper molars and transverse decompensation.

dental midline were corrected within 9.7 months of orthodontic work, after surgery (Fig. 22-21, A). Occlusal views of her upper dentition showed that her upper inter-molar width had not changed because of the constriction of the upper arch, which may have been canceled out by the buccal flaring of the molars following intrusion (Fig. 22-21, B). Occlusal views of the mandibular dentition showed that the inter-molar distance at the second molars increased significantly (Fig. 22-21, C). It is clear that, in this case, transverse decompensation was mainly carried out in the mandibular

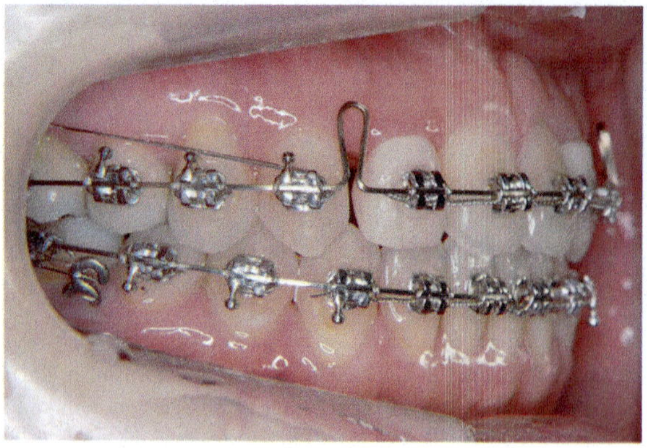

Figure 22-18 At 6.7 months after surgery. After making space, temporary crowns were put on teeth #12 and #22. Bull loops were bent in the upper archwire to close minor spaces at the incisors.

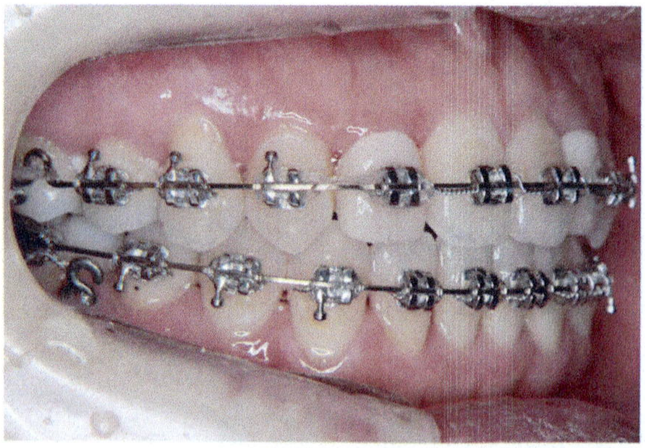

Figure 22-19 At 7.6 months after surgery, detailing and finishing were started.

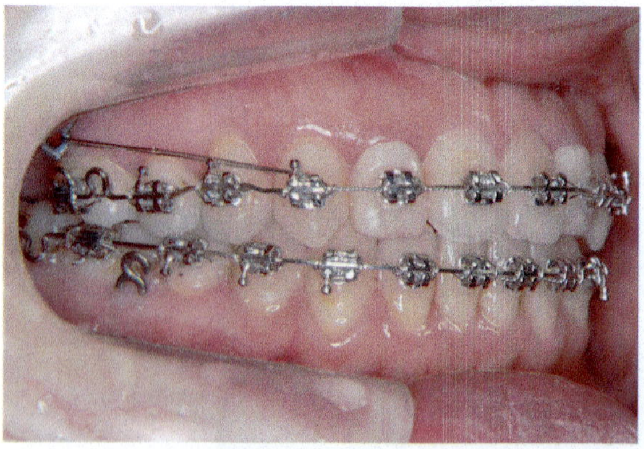

Figure 22-20 At 9.2 months after surgery. Occlusal equilibrium was carried out before debonding.

dentition. Favorable occlusal relationships and proper anterior teeth overlapping were observed at the end of treatment.

According to the cephalometric superimposition of scans obtained 6 months after surgery and at debonding, there was no skeletal change and only minor dental changes were observed. That means that major dentofacial changes occurred in the first 6 months after surgery in Sendai SF (Fig. 22-22).

Figure 22-23 shows the patient's facial and intraoral photos at debonding. Most of her orthodontic problems were solved and she presented a balanced profile, improved smile, and esthetic and functional occlusion. Judging from her cephalometric analysis, her skeletal profile was corrected to skeletal Class I, balanced long face (Fig. 22-24).

The cephalometric superimposition of scans obtained before and after treatment clearly show that her skeletal Class III profile and long face were corrected by modified BSSO. Her dental problems were successfully corrected by intrusion and distalization of the maxillary molars and mesialization of the entire mandibular dentition (Fig. 22-25). The cephalometric comparison of treatment goal and end result indicates that the treatment goal was predictably achieved with the application of Sendai SF (Fig. 22-26).

After postsurgical orthodontic treatment that lasted 9.7 months, all brackets were debonded and the titanium miniplates and screws were removed under local anesthesia. A vacuum-formed retainer was placed in the maxillary arch and a lingual retainer was bonded to the mandibular anterior teeth. The total treatment time from bonding to debonding was 11.7 months. By using SAS to intrude the maxillary posteriors, the need for two-jaw surgery was eliminated and only the less invasive one-jaw surgical approach was required. The patient's 1-year follow-up visit revealed stable outcomes, both dentally and facially (Fig. 22-27).

ADVANTAGES OF SENDAI SF

Combining the SF approach and SAS has a number of advantages. Undoubtedly, one of the most important advantages is shortened treatment time. Dowling et al.[19] reported that conventional surgical-orthodontic treatment usually requires 16 months for preoperative orthodontics and 6 months for postoperative orthodontics. A recent multicenter study by O'Brien et al.[20] on the effectiveness of orthodontic/orthognathic surgery care in the United Kingdom mentioned that treatment duration was longer than commonly expected, with a mean length of 32.8 months.

The authors' research group compared Sendai SF to conventional orthodontics first (COF). Two groups worked in parallel, under almost the same conditions, with a similar number of patients, a similar female/male ratio, similar age of patients at the time of surgery, similar surgical methods, treatment at the same hospital by the same surgeons, and the same period of orthognathic surgery (Fig. 22-28, A). The difference was mainly the procedures performed on the patients. One group used the SF approach with SAS and the other used COF without any TADs. The Sendai SF group got results in 12.7 months on average (Fig. 22-28, B). Many Sendai SF cases intensively distributed between 9 to 15 months. In contrast, the COF group got results in 33.7 months on average. In the patient described, the treatment length of 12.7 months with Sendai SF appears to be significantly shorter than treatment time with COF.

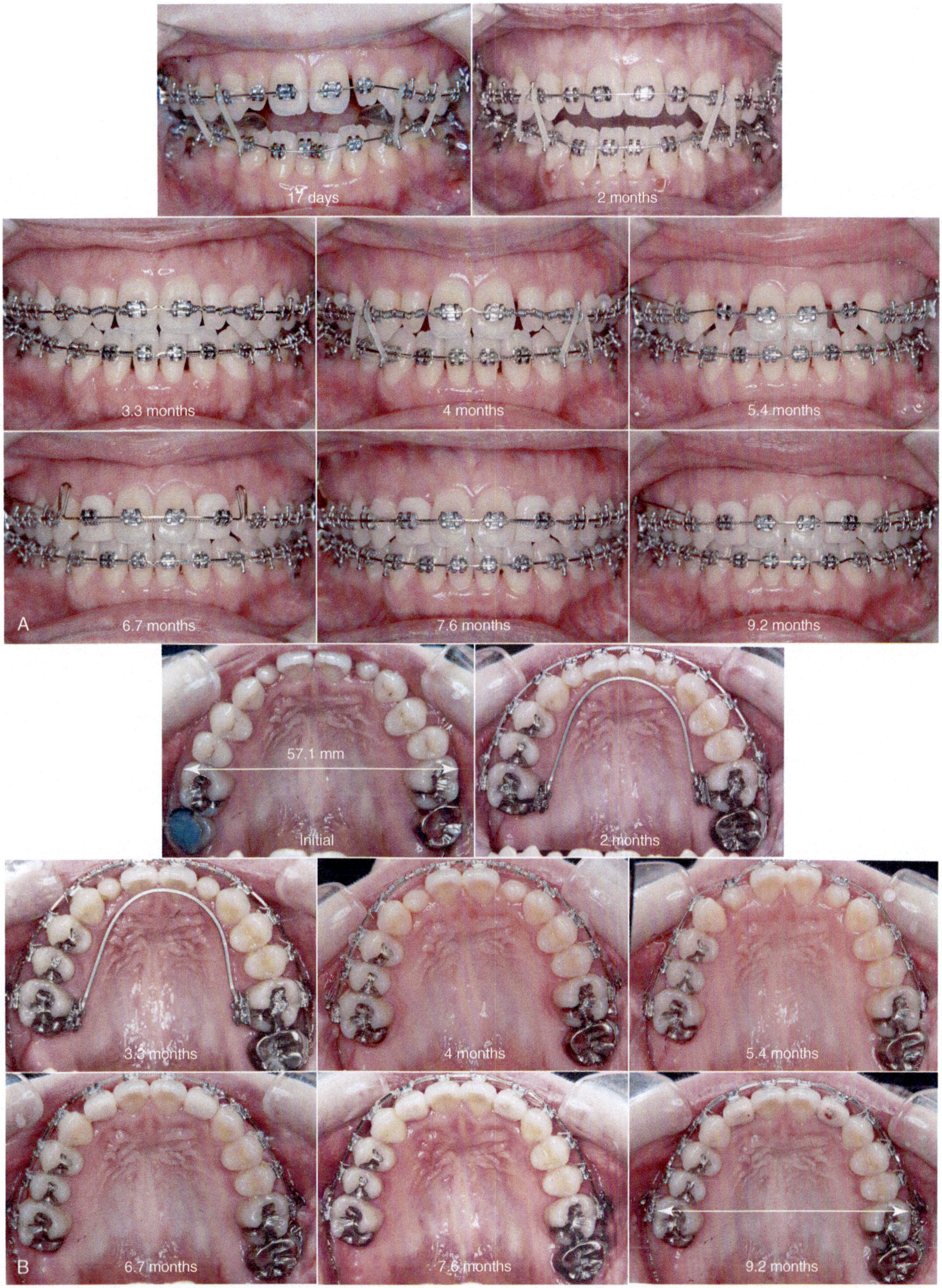

Figure 22-21 **A,** Frontal views of the treatment progress. The severe anterior open bite and the deviation of lower dental midline were corrected within a short period of time. **B,** Occlusal views of upper dentition. Notice that inter–first molar width did not change because constriction mechanics on the upper arch might have been canceled out by the buccal flaring of molar intrusion. *Continued*

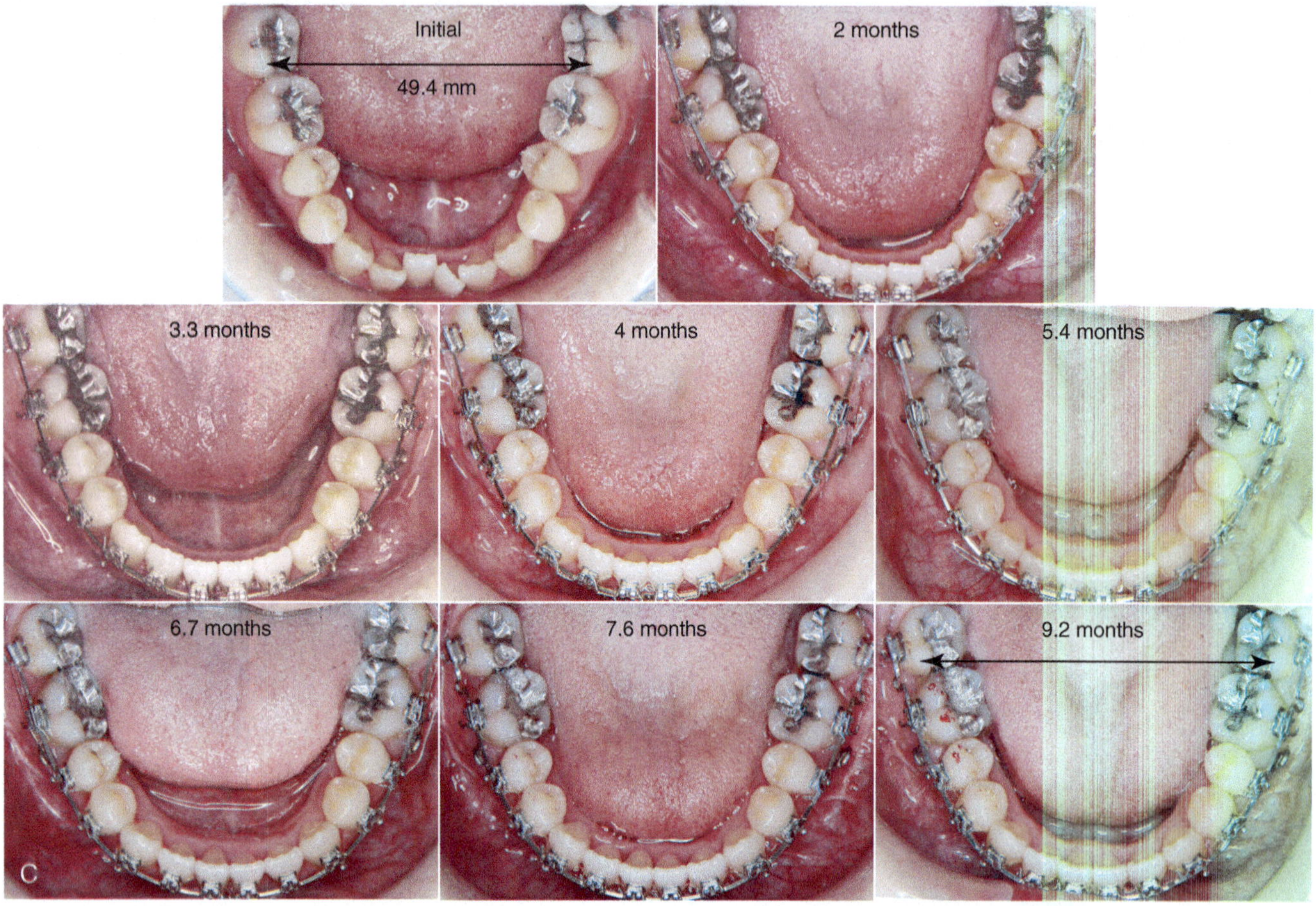

Figure 22-21, cont'd C, Occlusal views of mandibular dentition. Notice that inter–second molar distance increased significantly. It is clear that transverse decompensation was mainly carried out in the mandibular dentition.

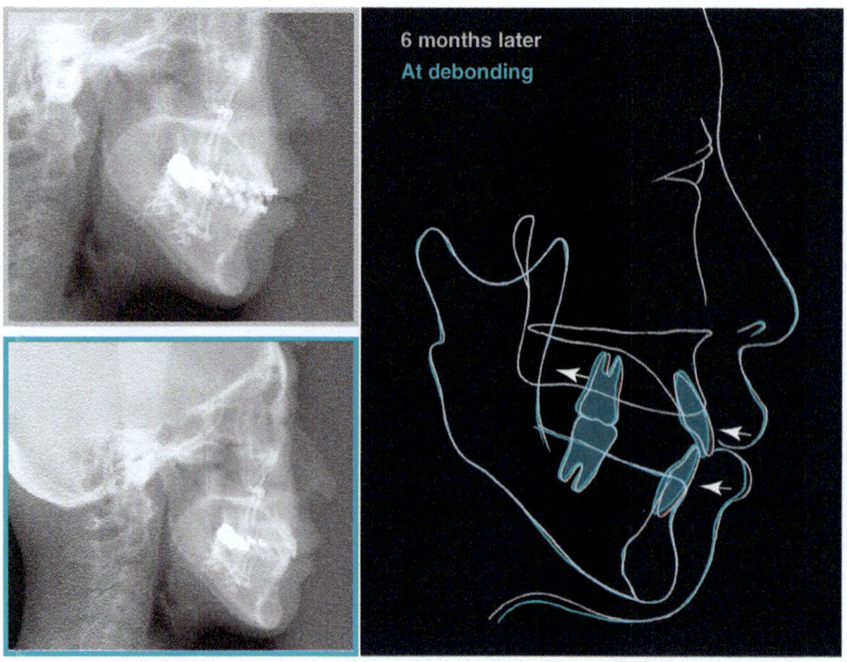

Figure 22-22 Cephalometric superimposition comparing scans obtained 6 months after surgery and at debonding. There was no skeletal change and only minor dental changes were observed.

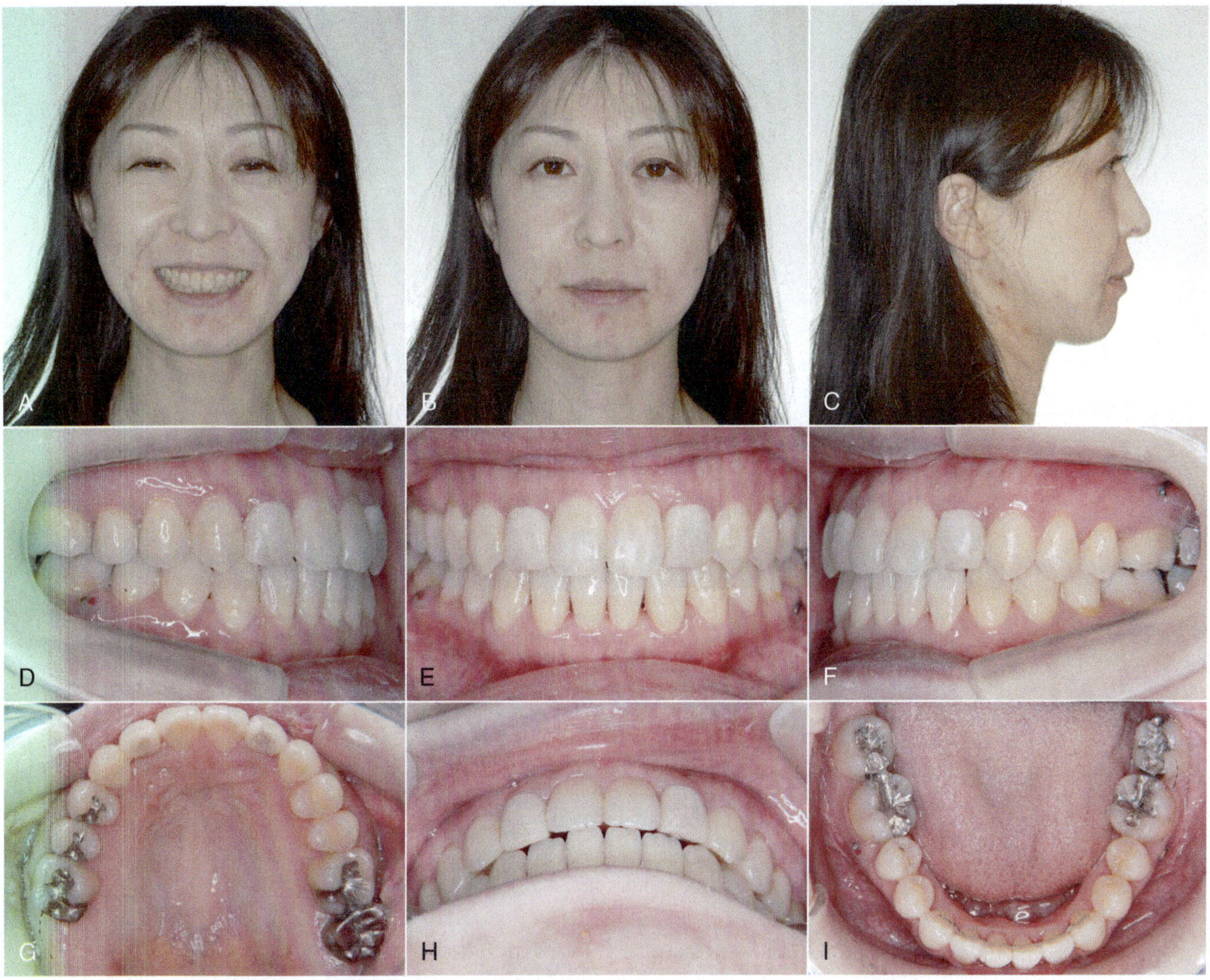

Figure 22-23 **A–C,** Facial and **(D–I)** intraoral photos at debonding. Most of the patient's orthodontic problems were resolved and she showed a balanced profile, improved smile, and good functional occlusion.

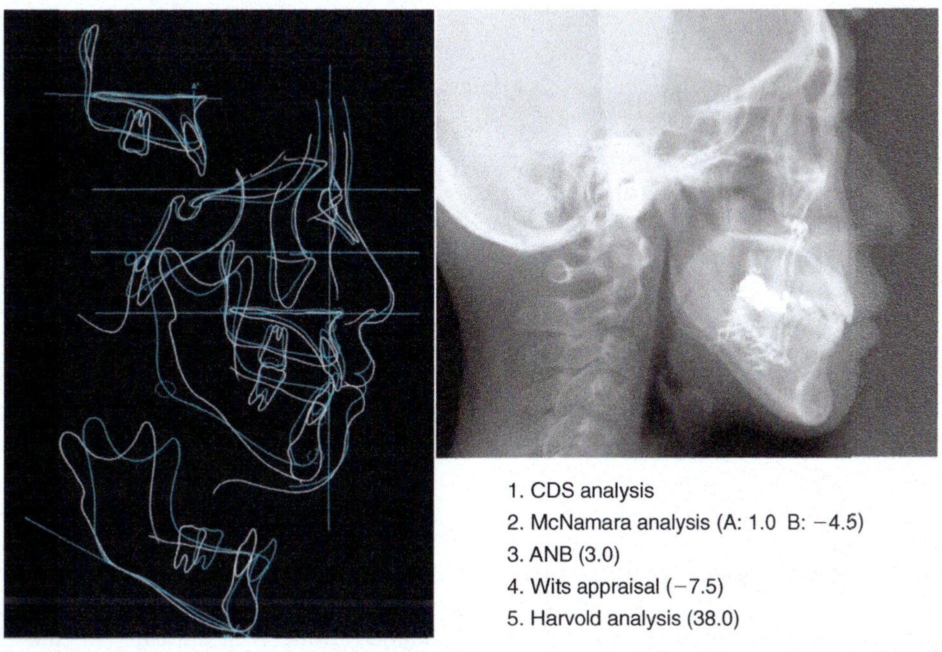

Figure 22-24 Cephalometric analysis at debonding. The patient's mandibular asymmetry was significantly improved. Judging from the cephalometric template analysis, her skeletal profile was corrected to Class I, balanced long face. *A,* A point; *ANB,* A point nasion B point; *B,* B point; *CDS,* cephalometric template analysis.

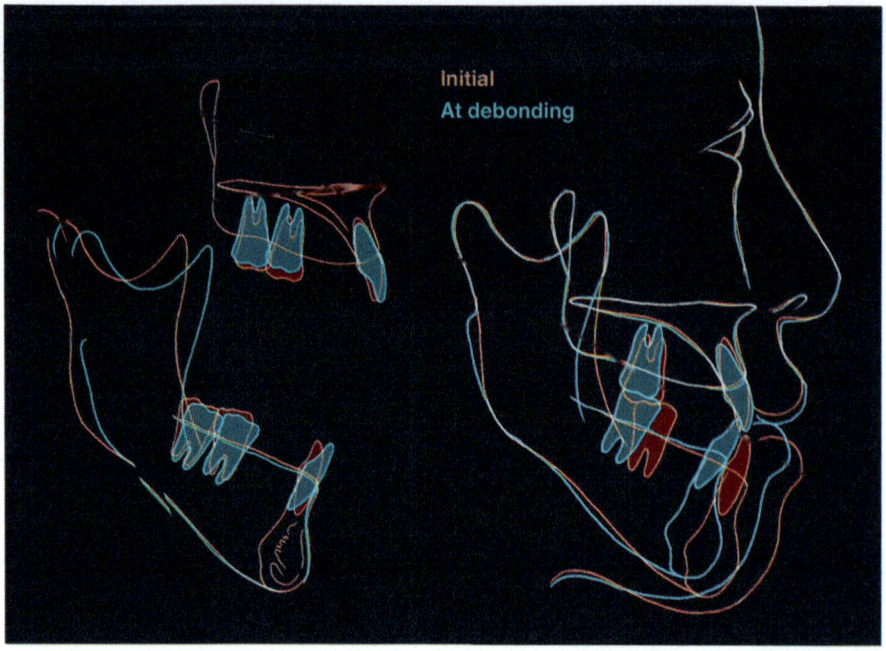

Figure 22-25 Cephalometric superimposition of tracings before and after treatment. Clearly the patient's skeletal Class III profile and long face was corrected by modified BSSO. Her dental problems were successfully corrected by intrusion and distalization of the upper molars and protraction of the entire lower dentition.

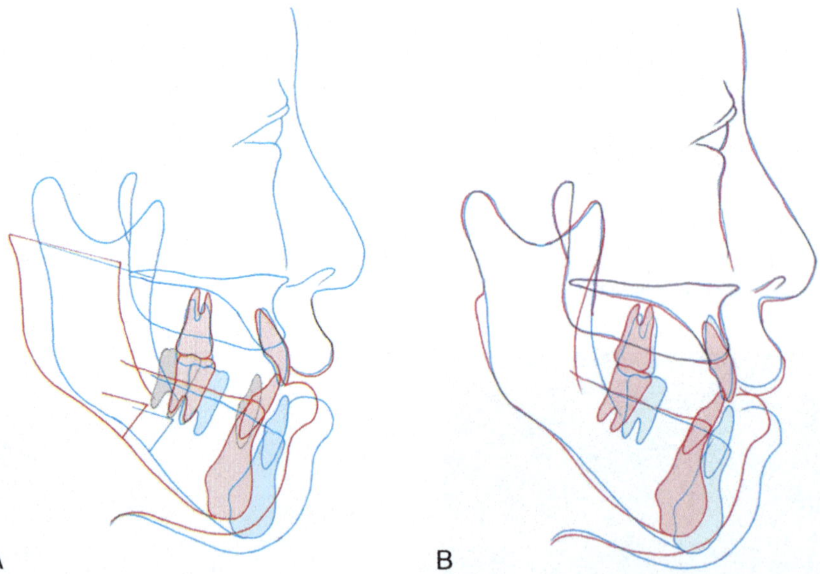

Figure 22-26 Cephalometric comparison of treatment goal (**A**) and the end result (**B**). Notice that the treatment goal was predictably achieved with the application of Sendai SF.

Interestingly, Luther et al.[21] insisted that there was no relationship between the durations of preoperative and postoperative orthodontic treatments. Bone turnover after orthognathic surgery can significantly accelerate orthodontic tooth movement. Teeth respond to the rapid bone turnover rate from the regional acceleratory phenomenon (RAP) in the first 3 to 4 months, resulting in rapid teeth movement, similar to that seen in the accelerated osteogenic orthodontics.[22-23] Difficult orthodontic movements, such as intrusion and distalization, should be efficiently progressed during the postsurgical phase.

Another advantage of Sendai SF is the restored relationship between the jaws and facial soft tissue, as the lips and tongue are considered to be an effective force to move teeth. Consequently, efficient and expedited postsurgical orthodontic work is achieved.[24] In the described patient,

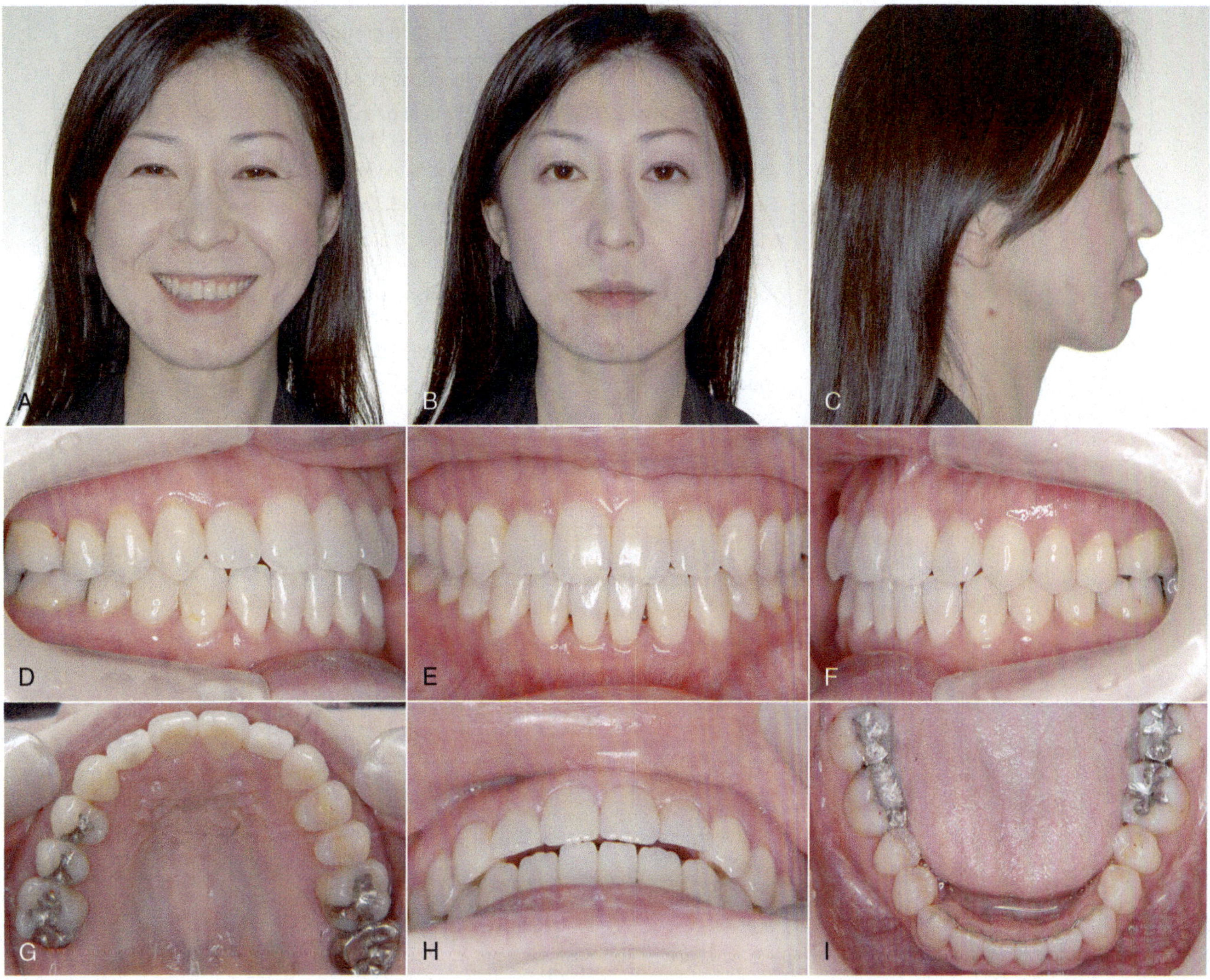

Figure 22-27 **A–C,** Facial and **(D–I)** intraoral views at 1-year follow-up.

following setback of the mandible her tongue was more in touch with the lower incisors, which was expected to help with their decompensation.

In addition, the number of bicuspid nonextraction cases is significantly increased with Sendai SF because SAS enables distalization of the posterior teeth, taking advantage of the third molar spaces created following their extraction prior to orthognathic surgery (Fig. 22-29).

Sendai SF is a less invasive surgery. In many cases, a one-jaw surgical approach is all that is required to correct facial deformities. SAS can play a major role in achieving advanced tooth movement and decompensation, beyond what is possible with conventional orthodontics. In fact, SAS has been shown to be a successful treatment option for patients who need but refuse surgery.[25-27] Other SF teams rely on performing an extensive surgery to use the maximum potential of the regional acceleratory phenomenon, enhance facial aesthetics, and reduce the complexity of the malocclusion.[5,10,28] Two-jaw surgeries are always preferred. As well, severe transverse discrepancies sometimes lead to two-piece or three-piece Le Fort I osteotomies. The increase in the number and complexity of osteotomy procedures poses a greater risk to the patient, higher cost, and higher risk of surgical error or relapse.

DISADVANTAGES OF SENDAI SF

There are some complications and difficulties associated with Sendai SF. The treating orthodontist and orthognathic surgeon must be experienced enough to know the limitations and possible complications of the treatment.

Occlusion cannot be used as a guide to establish treatment goals. Predicting the final occlusion is the hardest part of the Sendai SF approach. In many cases the upper and lower models cannot be placed in an ideal occlusion due to multiple occlusal interferences. If the predicted final occlusion is not achievable or is not planned accurately, the result will be far from ideal.

A surgical splint is essential to guide the repositioning of the mandible. For the first month after surgery, the modified

A

	Sendai SF group	COF group
Clinic	A Orthodontic Clinic	B Orthodontic Clinic
Number of patients	53 Class III patients (Female: 35, Male: 18)	47 Class III patients (Female: 32, Male: 15)
Age	25.6 years old (15.9–41.3)	24.5 years old (17.5–50.2)
OGS	Two-Jaw: 12, One-Jaw: 41	Two-Jaw: 15, One-Jaw: 32
TADs	Mini-plate: 53 cases Mini-screw: 0 case	Mini-plate: 0 case Mini-screw: 0 case
Hospital	Tohoku University Hospital Miyagi Children's Hospital	Tohoku University Hospital Miyagi Children's Hospital
Surgeons	Dr. HK, Dr. SG, Dr. HN	Dr. HK, Dr. SG, Dr. HN
Period of surgery	2004–2009	2004–2009

B

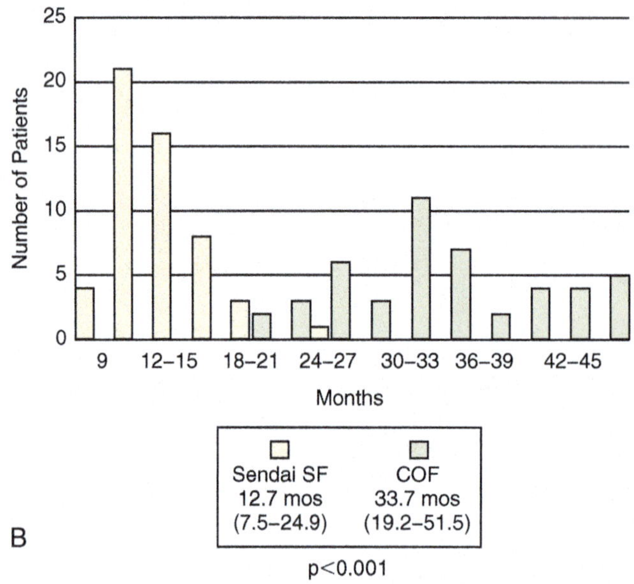

Figure 22-28 **A,** Comparison of the total treatment time between the Sendai SF group and the conventional orthodontics first (COF) group. Total treatment time was defined as the duration from bonding to debonding. The two groups worked in parallel under almost the same conditions. **B,** Results show that the average treatment time in the Sendai SF group was 12.7 months, with many cases distributed around 9 to 15 months. In contrast, treatment time in the COF group was 33.7 months on average. There was a significant difference in treatment time between the two groups. *OGS,* Orthognathic surgery; *SF,* surgery first; *TAD,* temporary anchorage device.

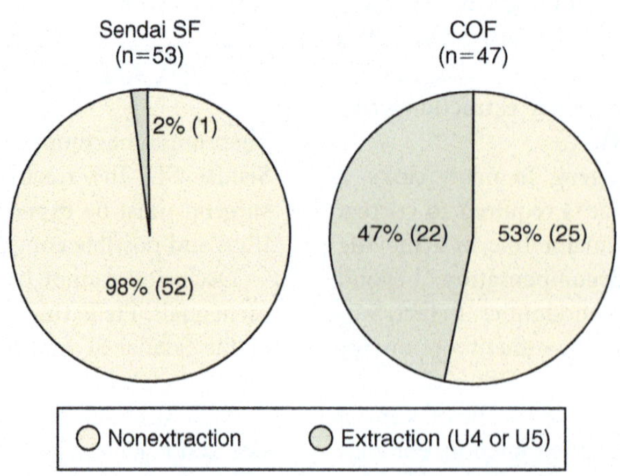

Figure 22-29 Comparison of maxillary bicuspid extraction between Sendai SF and conventional orthodontics first (COF) groups. Only one Sendai SF patient had any upper bicuspids extracted in this survey while almost half of the COF patients had to have their bicuspids extracted. *SF,* Surgery first; *U4,* upper first bicuspid; *U5,* upper second bicuspid.

removable splint (which must be worn while eating) helps to stabilize the jaw position and bring the teeth into proper occlusion, with the aid of seating elastics. When passive stainless steel wires are placed prior to surgery, each wire must be bent to rest passively on the surface of each tooth. This is a challenging and time-consuming procedure for the orthodontist, especially when teeth are severely rotated and misaligned. The indirect bonding technique can be used to allow for accurate bracket positioning and the passive archwires can be bent beforehand by a technician.

The application of SAS for postsurgical orthodontic treatment is the distinguishing feature of the Sendai SF approach. The orthodontist must be experienced and skilled in SAS technique, which is essential to achieving predictable, three-dimensional molar movement and ensuring that individualized treatment goals are predictably achieved.

ADDITIONAL SENDAI SF CASE EXAMPLES

The following case reports all involve a Class III relationship, with varying degrees of complexity. In all of these cases significant improvement is seen in the post-treatment results.

Text continued on p. 472

CASE REPORT 1

The patient presented with a Class III, long face profile with facial asymmetry. This case was addressed with orthognathic surgery (modified BSSO and genioplasty) and SAS for postsurgical orthodontics (Figs. 22-30 to 22-36).

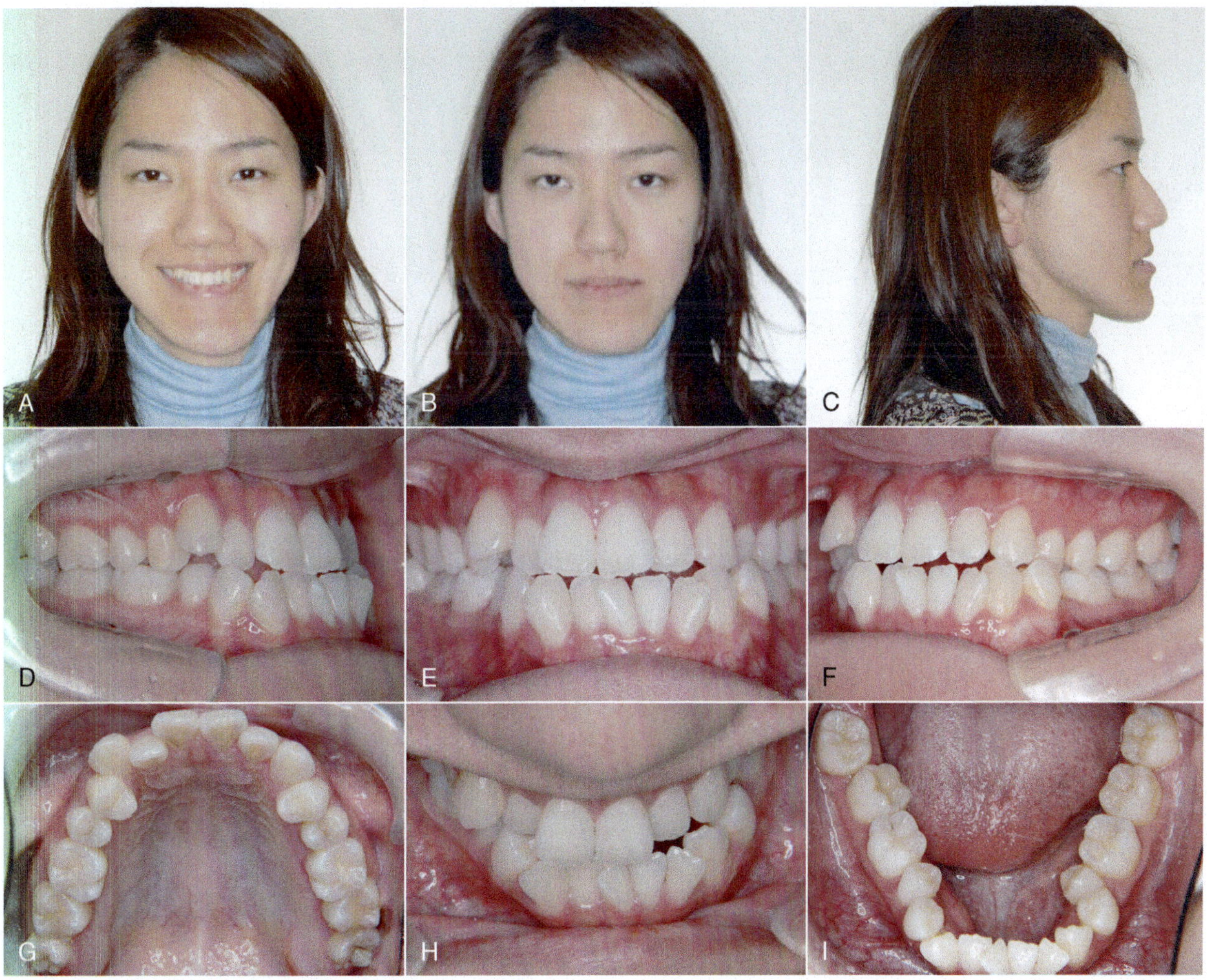

Figure 22-30 Initial (**A–C**) facial and (**D–I**) intraoral photos. A 21-year-old female patient presented with a Class III, long face profile with facial asymmetry. She showed Class III denture, deviation of lower dental midline, retroclination of lower incisors, and anterior crowding.

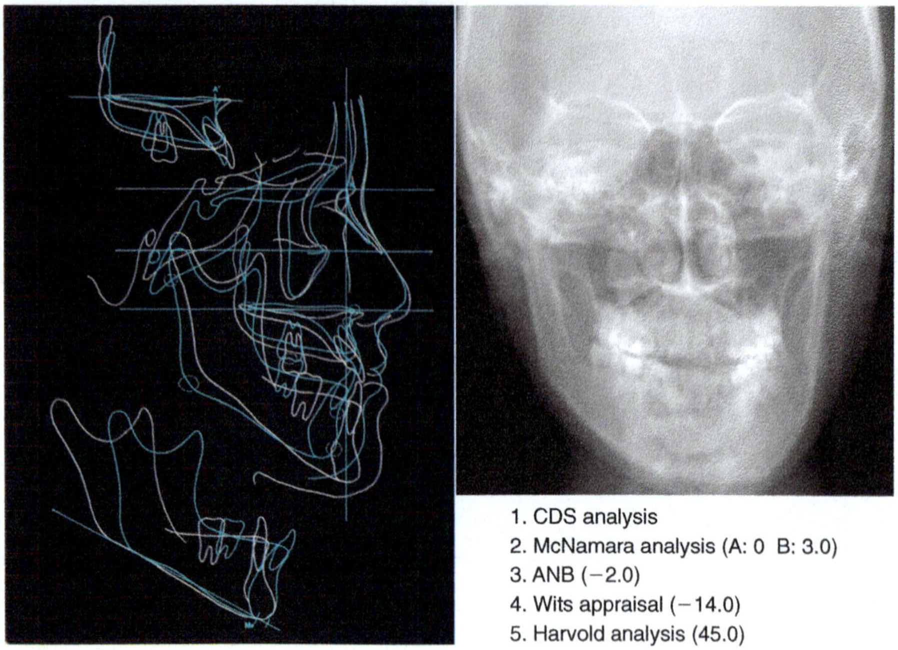

Figure 22-31 Cephalometric template analysis (CDS analysis) revealed that her mandible is extremely large, with retroclination of lower incisors. She was a good candidate for surgery. *A,* A point; *ANB,* A point nasion B point; *B,* B point.

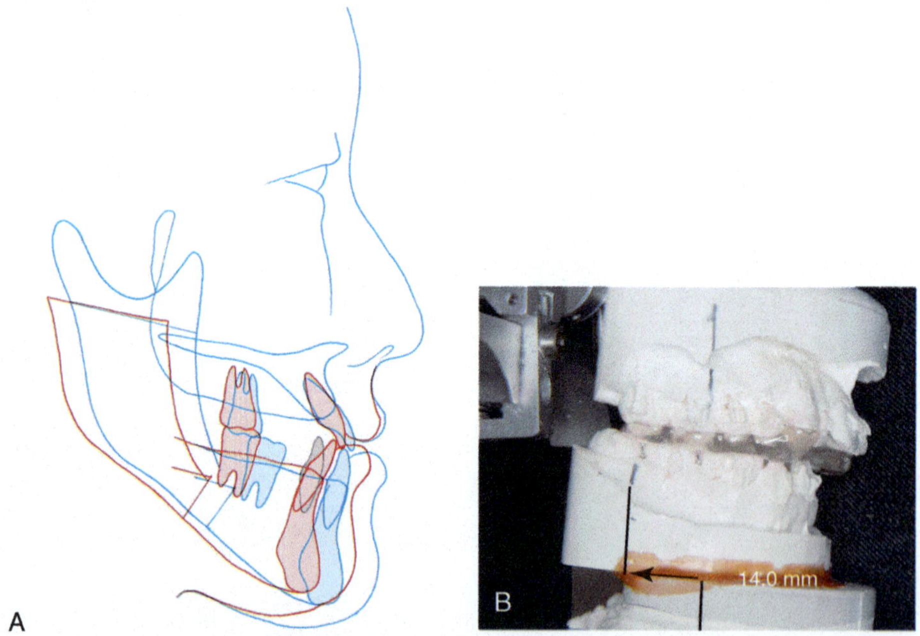

Figure 22-32 **A,** The treatment goal was established and **(B)** the amount of mandibular setback and tooth movement were predicted. Since the patient had a chin deformity, genioplasty was recommended in addition to modified bilateral sagittal split osteotomy (BSSO).

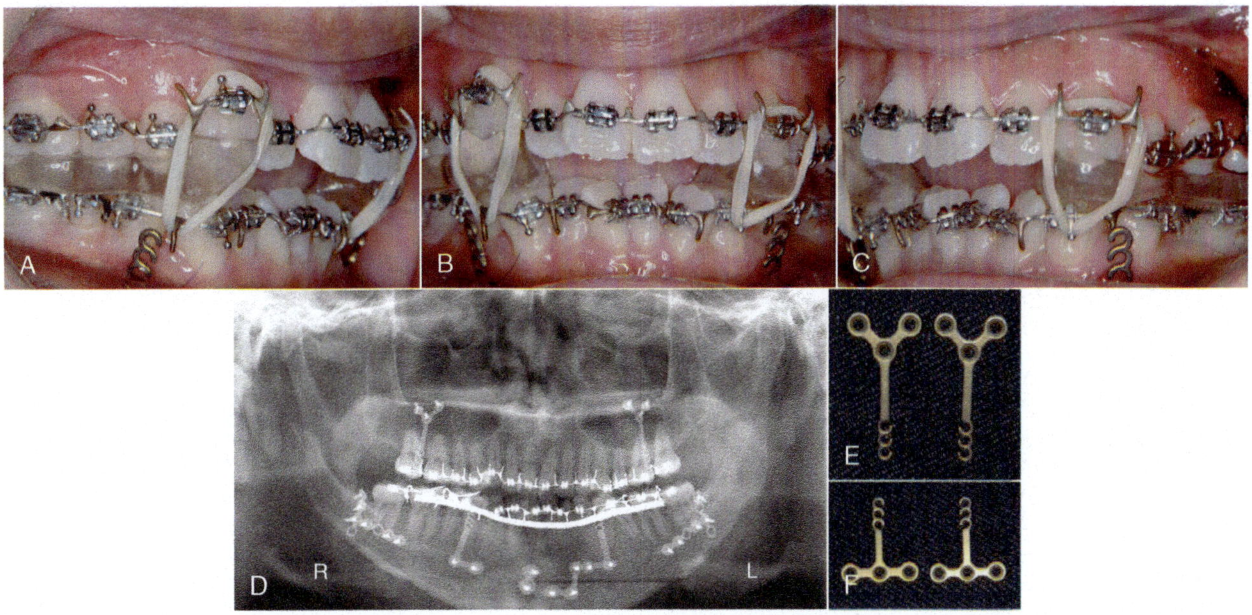

Figure 22-33 Orthognathic surgery. **A–C,** After extracting all of the patient's third molars, brackets and passive surgical hooks were bonded. **D,** The patient then underwent modified bilateral sagittal split osteotomy (BSSO) and genioplasty. Immediately after surgery she showed a Class II open bite with the surgical splint in place. **E,** Two Y-type mini-plates were placed at the zygomatic buttress. **F,** Two L-type mini-plates were fixed at the canine regions of the mandibular body.

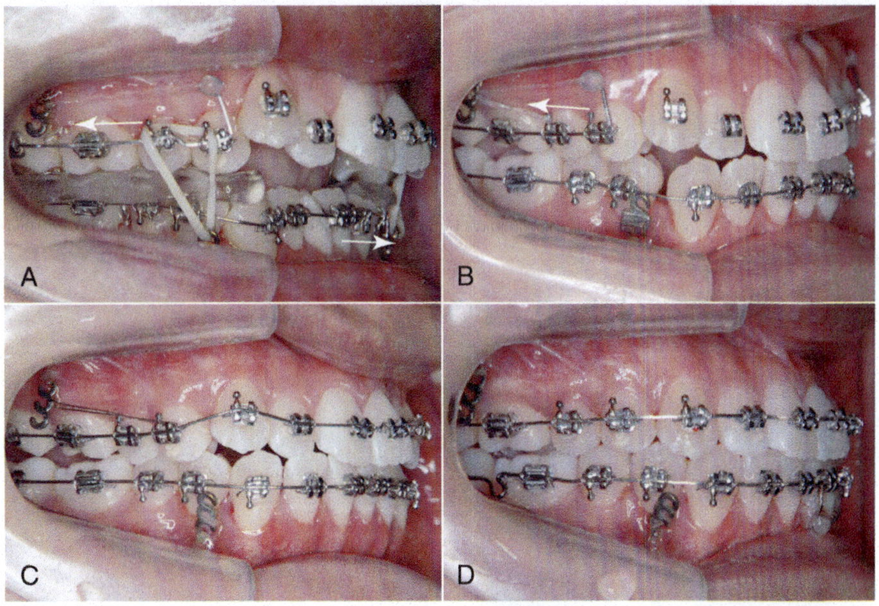

Figure 22-34 Postsurgical orthodontics. Class II open bite and anterior crowding were gradually but radically improved and eventually corrected to a Class I acceptable occlusion. Wires consequence as follows. **A,** Seventeen days: Maxilla (Mx) 0.016-inch × 0.022-inch CNA, mandible (Mn) 0.016-inch nickel-titanium (Ni-Ti), distalization Mx posteriors, occlusal splint. **B,** Three months: discontinued use of occlusal splint; 3.6 months: Mx 0.016-inch × 0.022-inch stainless steel, distalization Mx posteriors 0.016-inch Ni-Ti (decompensation of Mn incisors). **C,** At 5.7 months: Mx 0.018-inch Ni-Ti, leveling, distalization completed, Mn continued leveling. **D,** At 9.8 months: Mx and Mn 0.016-inch × 0.022-inch stainless steel, occlusal equilibrium.

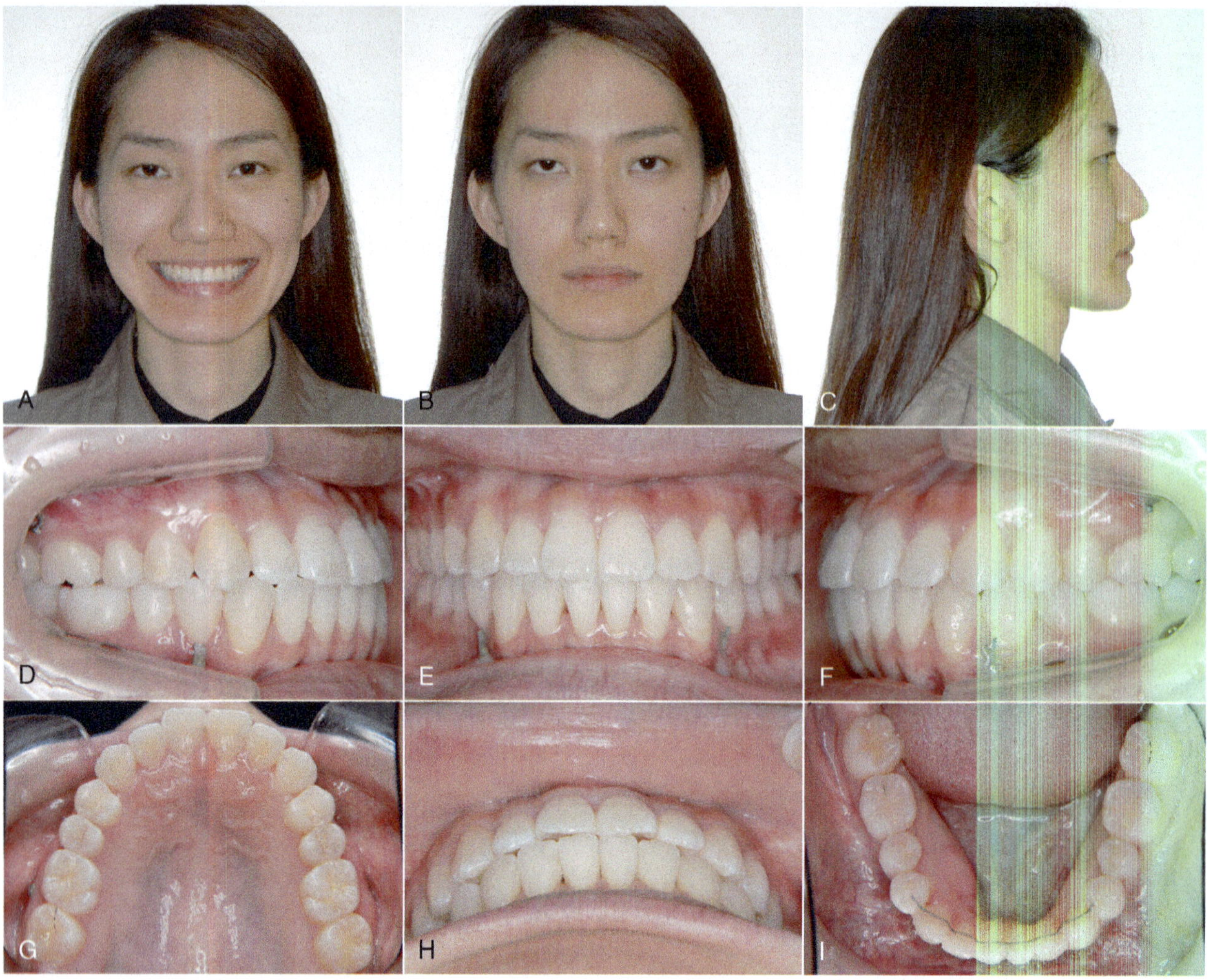

Figure 22-35 **A–C,** Facial and **(D–I)** intraoral photos at debonding. The patient's orthodontic problems were corrected significantly without bicuspid extraction.

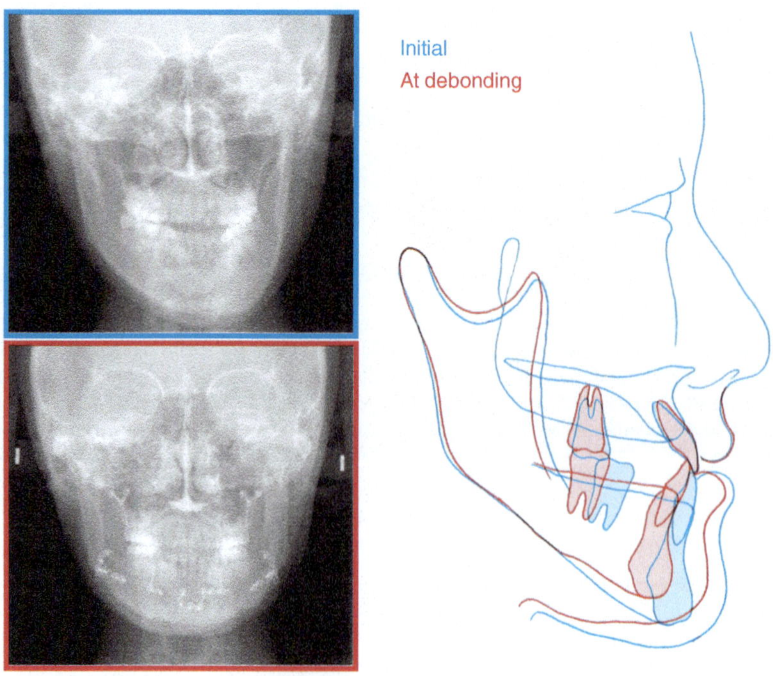

Figure 22-36 Cephalometric superimposition of scans obtained initially and at debonding. With the application of orthognathic surgery with modified bilateral sagittal split osteotomy (BSSO) and genioplasty and skeletal anchorage system (SAS) for postsurgical orthodontics, the patient's complex three-dimensional dentofacial deformities were significantly improved by the course of treatment.

CASE REPORT 2

The patient presented with a long face, Class III relationship with open bite. This case was addressed with Le Fort I osteotomy, modified BSSO, and genioplasty. Postsurgical orthodontics involved SAS, without bicuspid extraction (Figs. 22-37 to 22-43).

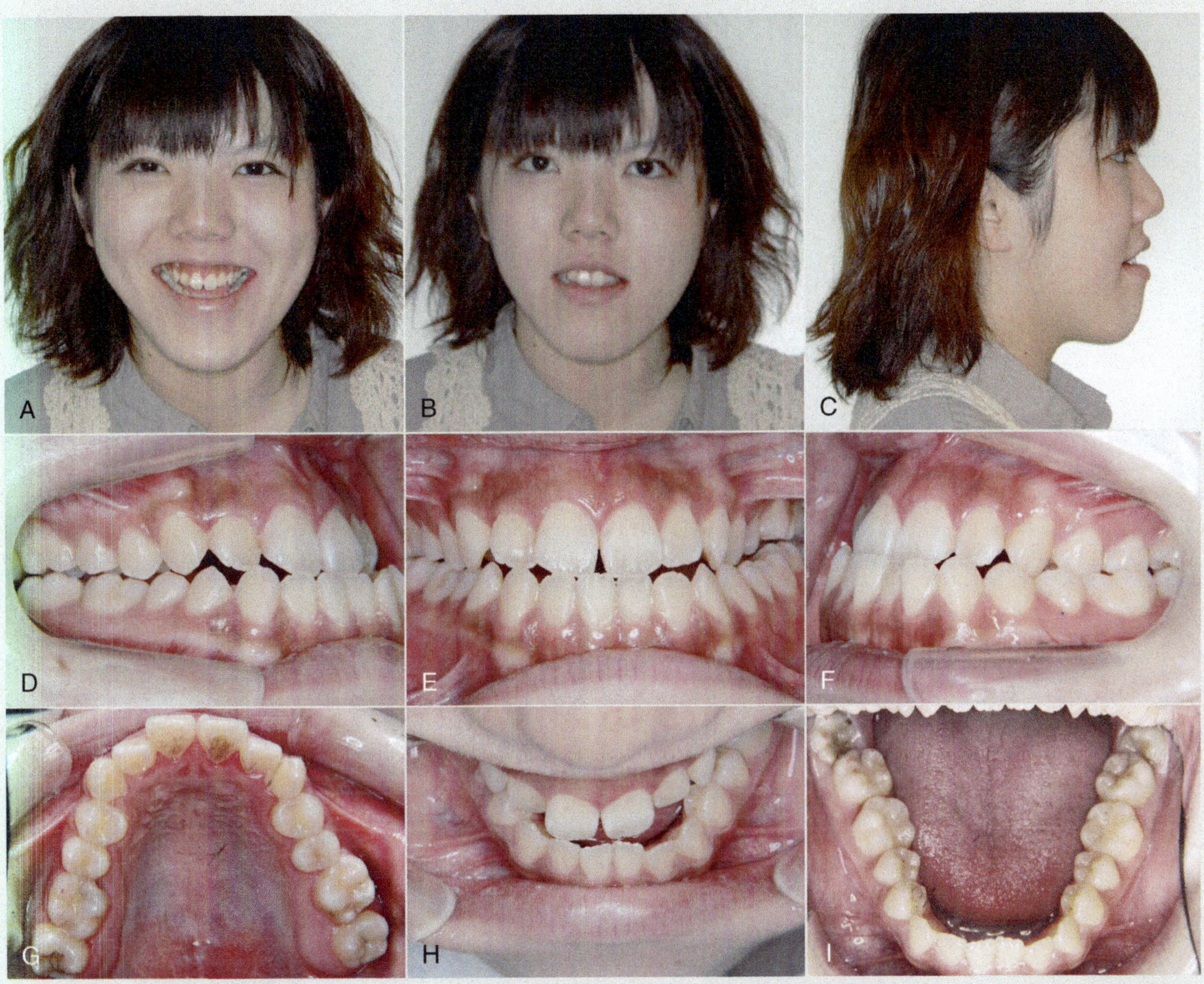

Figure 22-37 Initial **(A–C)** facial and **(D–I)** intraoral photos. An 18-year-old female patient presented with a long face, Class III relationship and open bite. Patient complaints included skewed teeth, mandibular protrusion, facial asymmetry, and a gummy smile.

Continued

CASE REPORT 2—cont'd

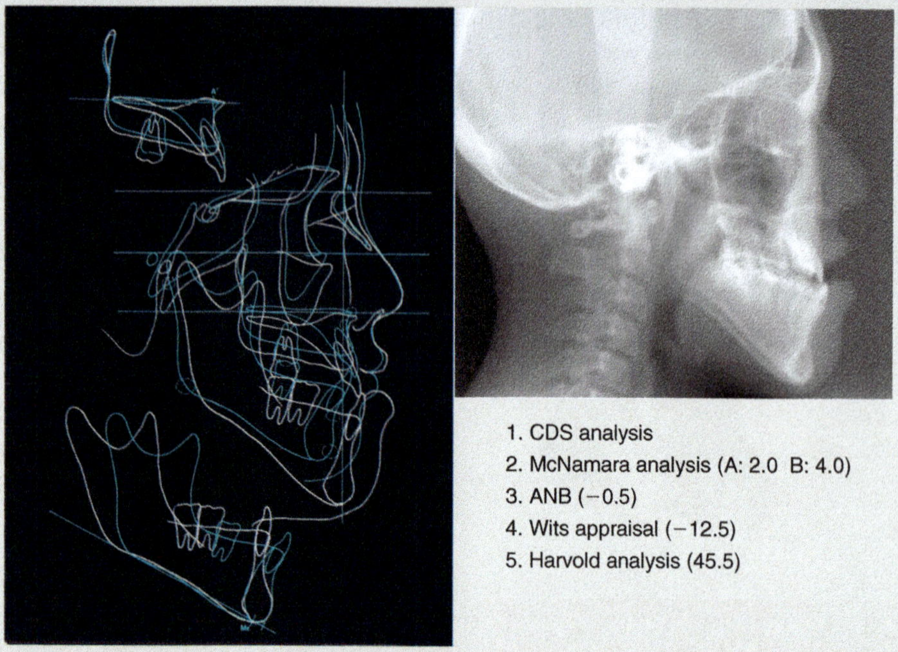

Figure 22-38 Cephalometric template analysis (CDS analysis) exhibited long face syndrome. Mandibular excess was also obvious when plotted against the standard. As shown in the patient example that runs throughout the chapter, generally mild to moderate vertical maxillary excess is successfully treated with one-jaw surgery and skeletal anchorage system (SAS) mechanics. This patient's long face and severe gummy smile indicated that two-jaw surgery was necessary. *A,* A point; *ANB,* A point nasion B point; *B,* B point.

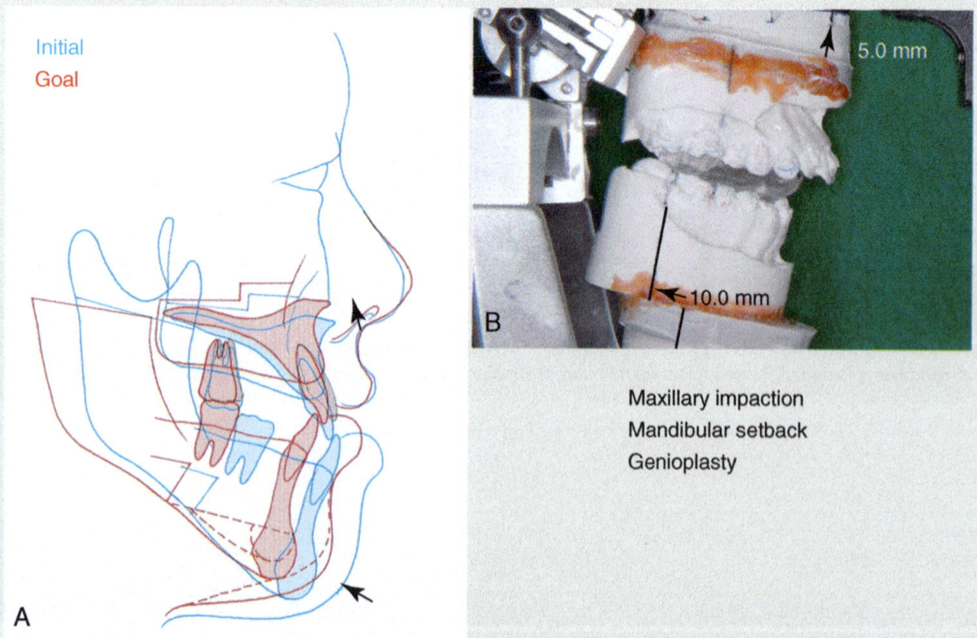

Figure 22-39 Treatment goals. Patient needed 10 mm of average mandibular setback, 5 mm maxillary impaction, and reduction of chin height with genioplasty. Her occlusion relationship changed from Class III to Class II with open bite. **A,** Prediction of treatment goal including the dental and surgical movements. The patient needed a two-jaw surgery of maxillary impaction, mandibular setback, and a genioplasty to enhance the vertical dimension and eliminate the gummy smile appearance. **B,** Model surgery simulation of the planned surgical movement. Based on the final jaw position, an acrylic splint is fabricated to maintain the transitional occlusion.

CASE REPORT 2—cont'd

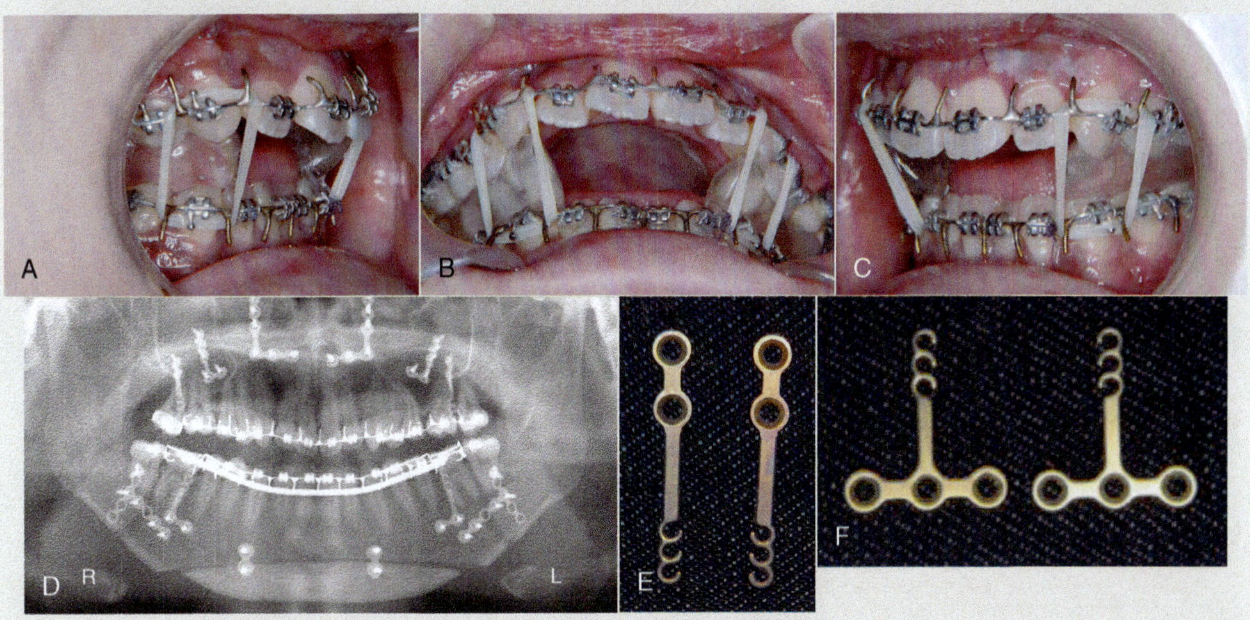

Figure 22-40 Orthognathic surgery. Patient underwent two-jaw surgery: Le Fort I osteotomy, modified bilateral sagittal split osteotomy (BSSO), and genioplasty. Occlusion right after surgery with the splint and training elastics in place: **A,** Right lateral view; **B,** Occlusal view; **C,** Left lateral view; **D,** Panoramic radiograph showing the surgical procedures and rigid fixation used and the skeletal anchorage mini-plates implanted. During surgery **(E)** two I-type mini-plates were placed in the zygomatic buttress and **(F)** L-type mini-plates were placed in the mandible.

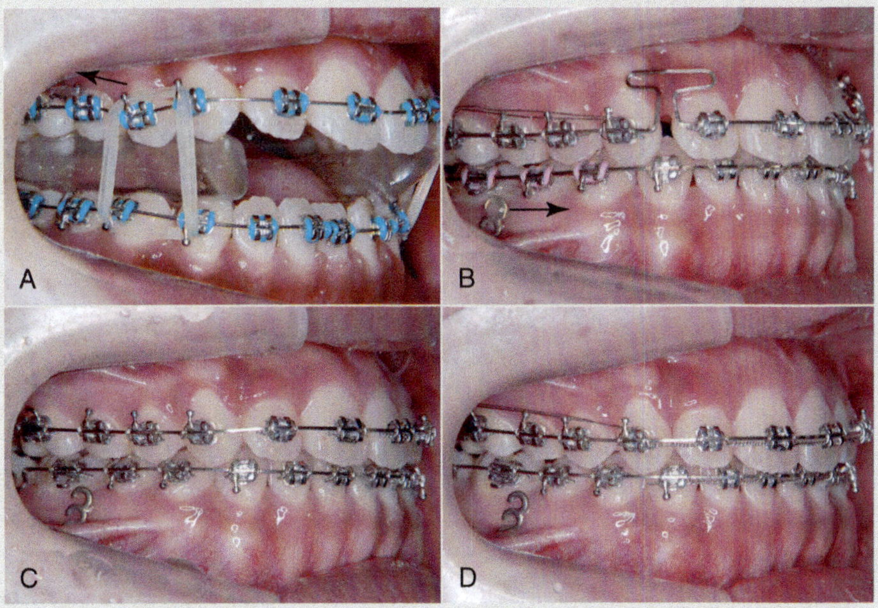

Figure 22-41 Postsurgical orthodontics. The principal skeletal anchorage system (SAS) mechanics used in this case were intrusion and distalization of the upper posteriors and mesialization of the lower dentition. The sequence was as follows. **A,** Eight days: 0.016-inch nickel-titanium (Ni-Ti), surgical splint, intrusion and distalization of maxillary (Mx) posteriors. **B,** At 3.3 months: 0.016-inch × 0.022-inch stainless steel, Mx contraction, protraction of mandibular (Mn) dentition. **C,** At 5.6 months: 0.017-inch × 0.025-inch stainless steel ideal arches. **D,** At 9.2 months: occlusal equilibrium.

Continued

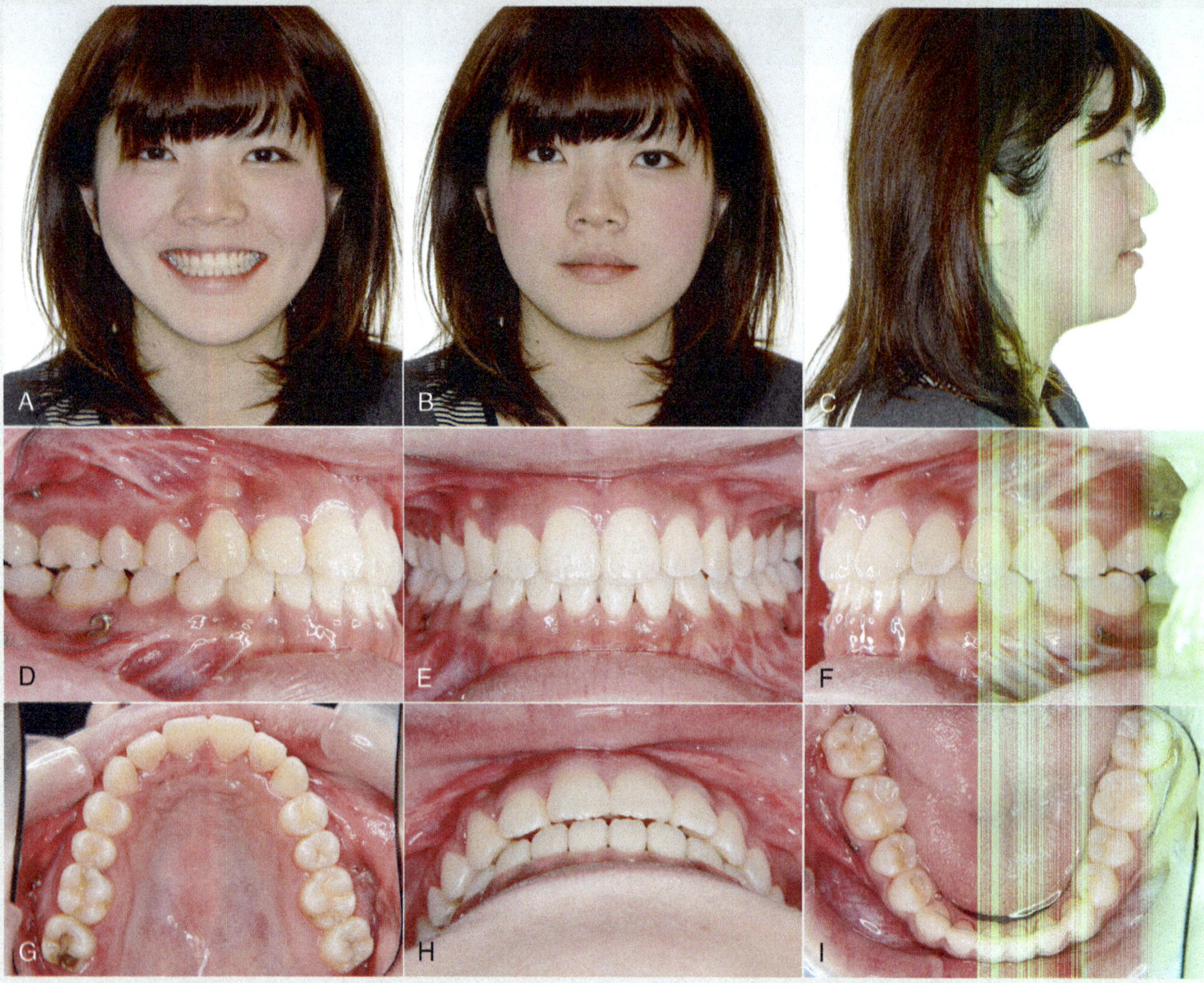

Figure 22-42 **A–C,** Facial and **(D–I)** intraoral photos at debonding. The patient's skeletal and orthodontic problems were corrected significantly by two-jaw surgery and skeletal anchorage system (SAS), without bicuspid extraction.

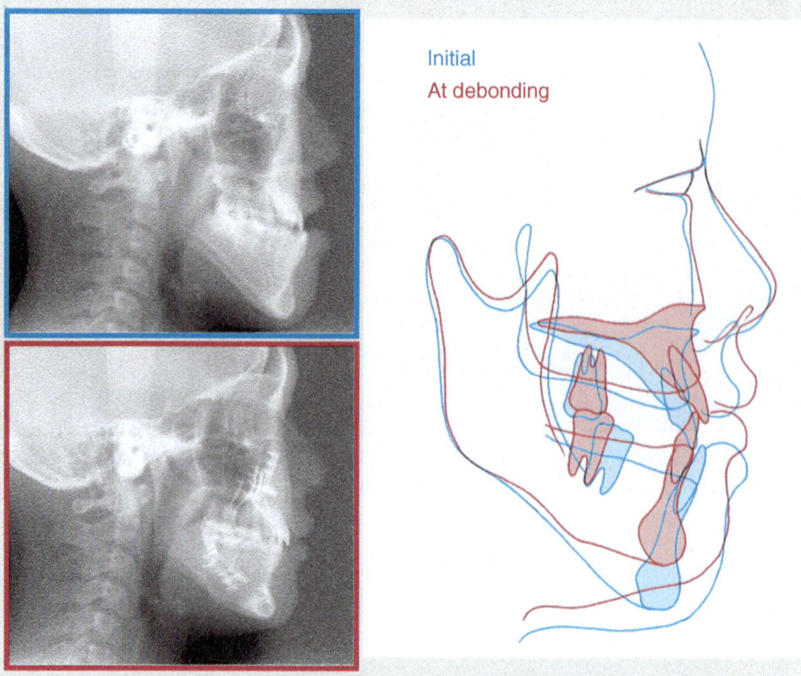

Figure 22-43 Cephalometric superimposition of scans obtained initially and at debonding reveals the improvements realized by the course of treatment, especially in facial height and the normalization of the patient's extremely large interlabial gap.

CASE REPORT 3

The patient presented with a severe Class III profile with maxillary deficiency, severe total crossbite, narrow maxilla, severe crowding in the bimaxillary dentition, and excessive retroclination of the lower incisors. This case was addressed with Le Fort I osteotomy and modified BSSO and postsurgical orthodontic treatment (Figs. 22-44 to 22-51).

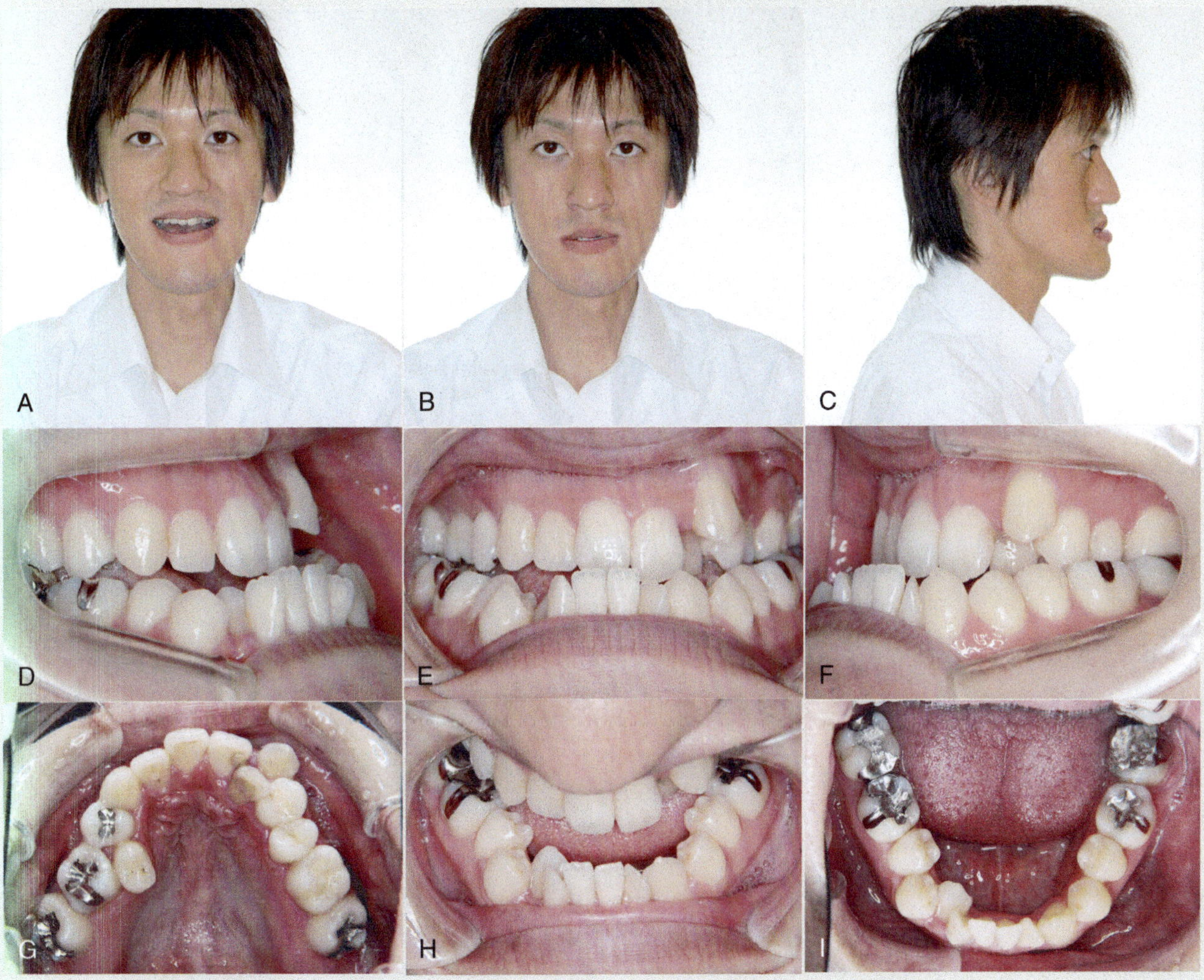

Figure 22-44 Initial **(A–C)** facial and **(D–I)** intraoral photos. A 26-year-old male patient presented with a very severe Class III profile, with maxillary deficiency, severe total crossbite, narrow maxilla, severe crowding in bimaxillary dentition, and excessive retroclination of lower incisors.

Continued

CASE REPORT 3—cont'd

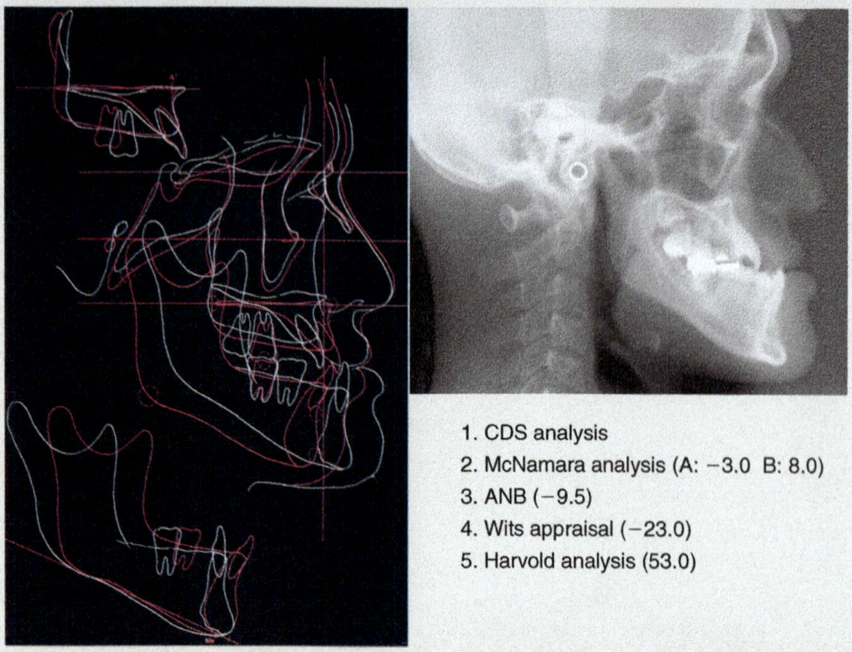

1. CDS analysis
2. McNamara analysis (A: −3.0 B: 8.0)
3. ANB (−9.5)
4. Wits appraisal (−23.0)
5. Harvold analysis (53.0)

Figure 22-45 Cephalometric template analysis (CDS analysis) showed that the patient had a very severe skeletal Class III relationship due to mandibular excess and maxillary deficiency. He was an obvious candidate for two-jaw surgery. *A*, A point; *ANB*, A point nasion B point; *B*, B point.

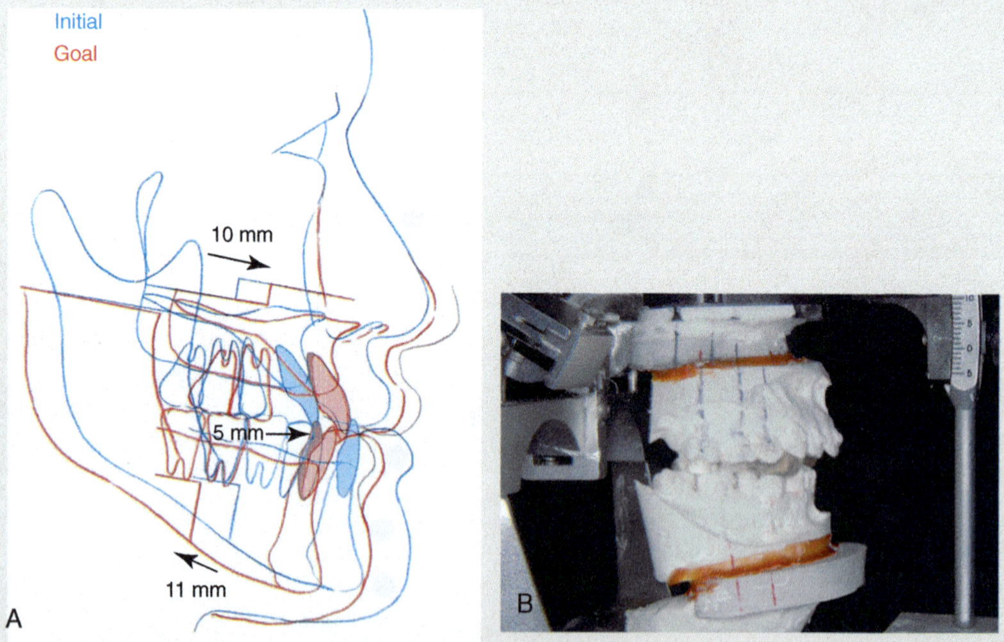

Figure 22-46 **A and B,** Based on the cephalometric template analysis, the patient needed 10-mm of maxillary advancement and 11-mm of mandibular setback. His occlusion relationship changed from Class III to Class II. Significant proclination of the lower incisors was also needed during postsurgical orthodontics.

CASE REPORT 3—cont'd

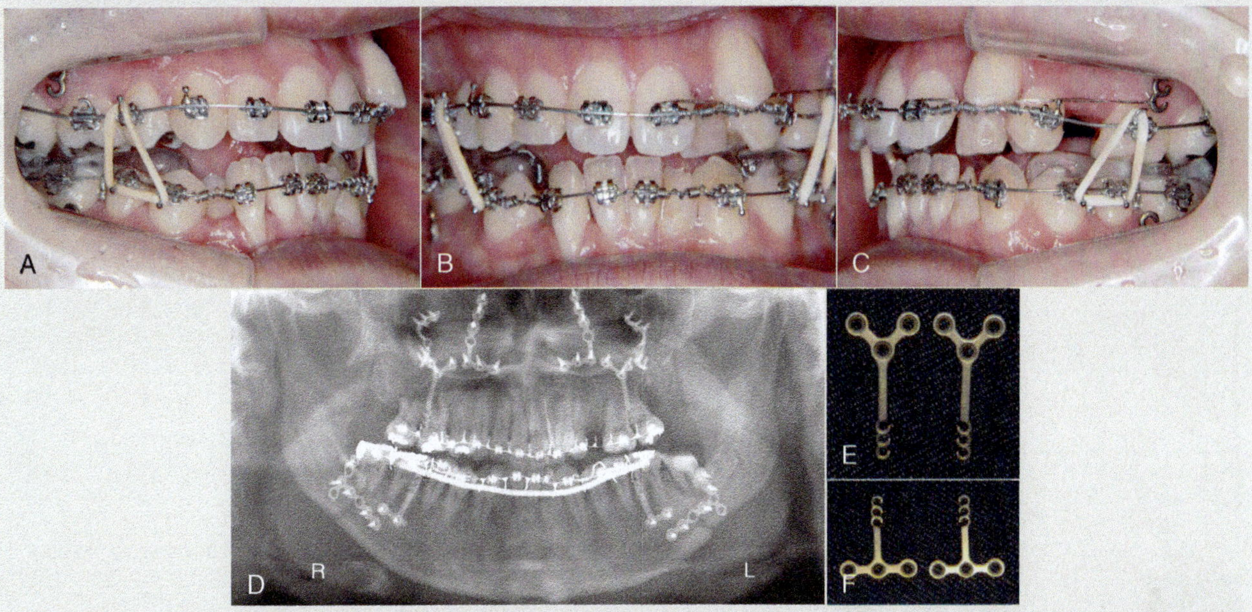

Figure 22-47 Orthognathic surgery. Patient underwent two-jaw surgery: Le Fort I osteotomy and modified bilateral sagittal split osteotomy (BSSO). Occlusion right after surgery with the splint and training elastics in place: **A,** Right lateral view; **B,** Frontal view; **C,** Left lateral view; **D,** Panoramic radiograph showing the surgical procedures and rigid fixation used and the skeletal anchorage mini-plates implanted. **E,** Y-type orthodontic mini-plates were used at the zygomatic buttress during surgery. **F,** L-type mini-plates were placed in the mandible during surgery. His occlusion showed a Class II open bite as predicted.

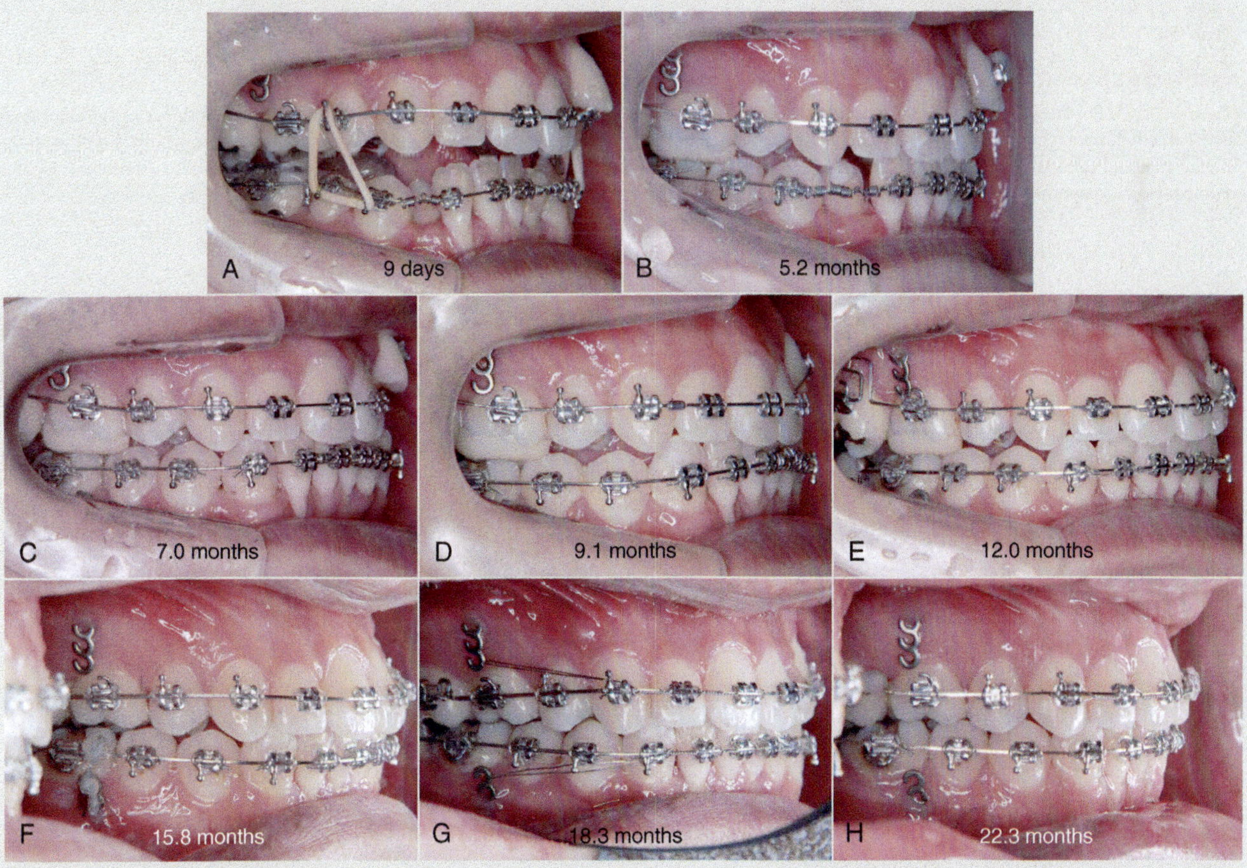

Figure 22-48 Postsurgical orthodontics (lateral intraoral views). After removal of the surgical splint, a resin cap was bonded at the upper left first molar to stabilize posterior support. **A,** At 9 days after surgery. **B,** 5.2 months. **C,** 7.0 months. **D,** 9.1 months. **E,** 12.0 months. **F,** 15.8 months. **G,** 18.3 months. **H,** 22.3 months after surgery.

Continued

CASE REPORT 3—cont'd

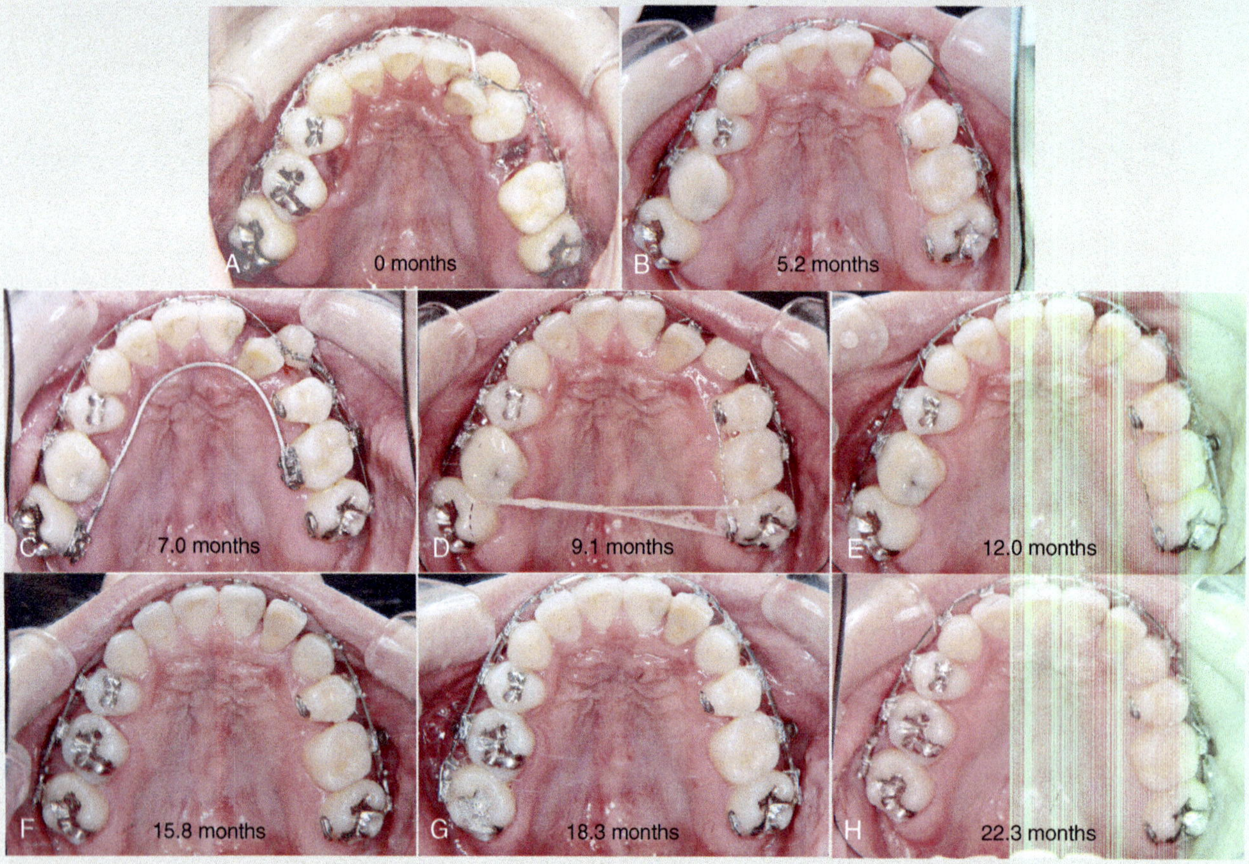

Figure 22-49 Postsurgical orthodontics (maxillary occlusal views). Because of the severe maxillary crowding, the patient's upper second bicuspids were extracted. Interestingly, he showed a total crossbite at initial presentation but after surgery he needed constriction of the maxillary arch with the lingual arch and transpalatal elastics. **A,** At 9 days after surgery. **B,** 5.2 months. **C,** 7.0 months. **D,** 9.1 months. **E,** 12.0 months. **F,** 15.8 months. **G,** 18.3 months. **H,** 22.3 months after surgery.

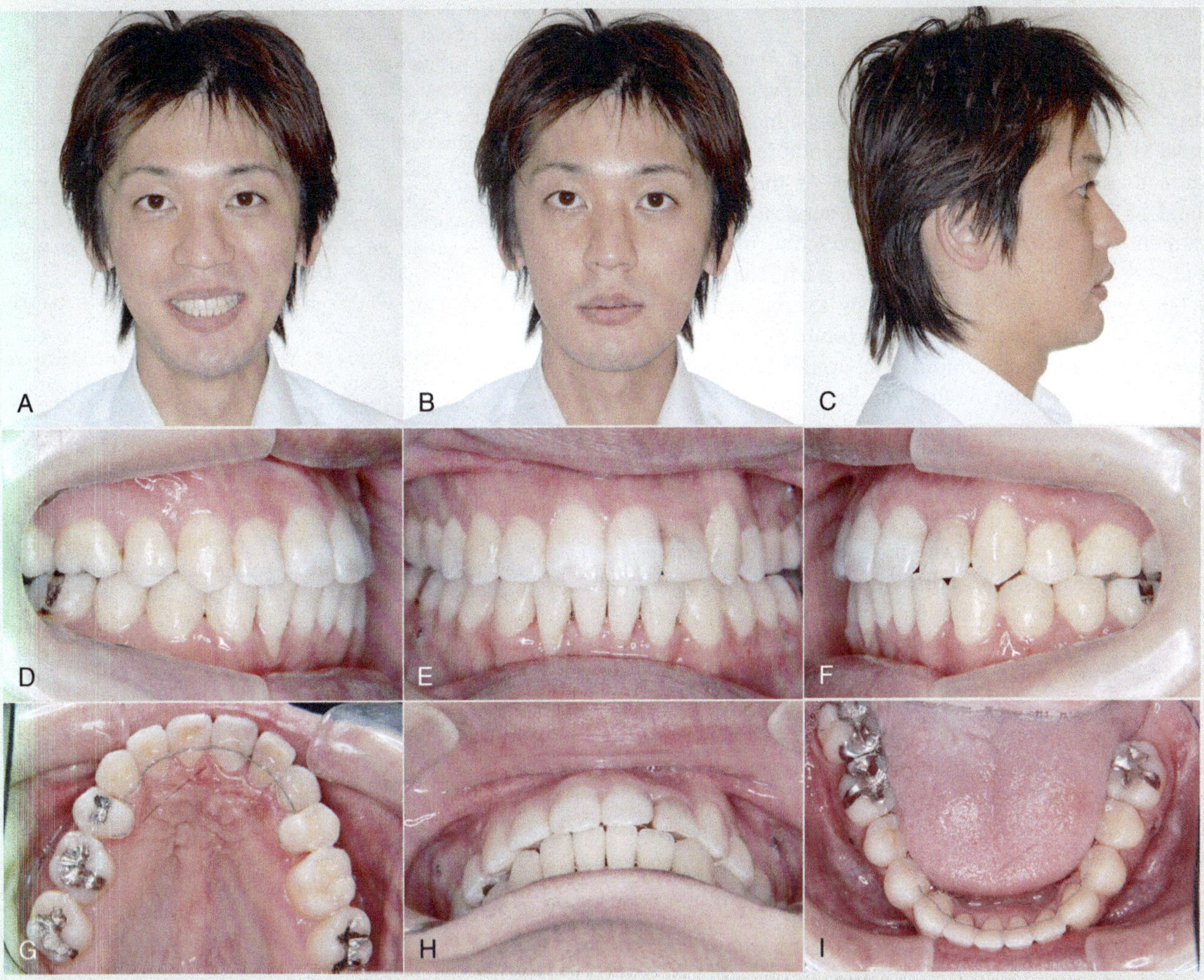

Figure 22-50 **A–C,** Facial and **(D–I)** intraoral photos at debonding. The patient's severe skeletal and dental problems were dramatically corrected.

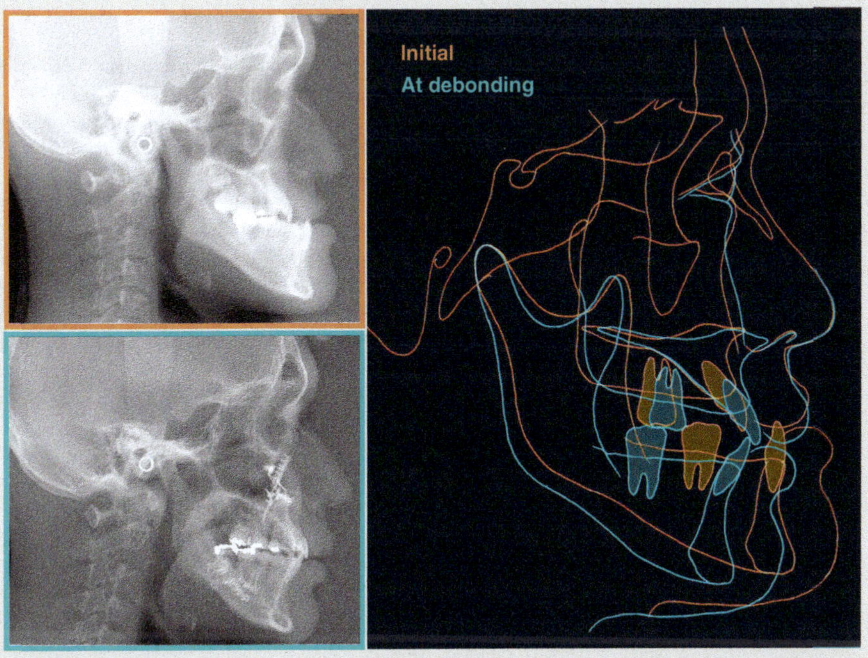

Figure 22-51 Cephalometric superimposition of scans obtained initially and at debonding showed a dramatic improvement, especially in mandibular protrusion and midface deficiency.

FUTURE OF SENDAI SF

With recent developments in cone beam computed tomography (CBCT), virtual model surgery, model visual scan and setup, and wafer fabrication for orthognathic surgery,[29,30] Sendai SF can become a more accurate and predictable procedure than the current state of care. At the same time, Sendai SF remains a new concept in surgical-orthodontic treatment. Further studies on the prediction of treatment goals and long-term stability are necessary. The increased level of cooperation between clinicians is very promising for implementing this technique, as the future of orthognathic surgery is geared toward minimizing overall treatment time without compromising the final results.

SUMMARY

Recently, more attention has been given to the SF approach.[1–5,7,28,31,32] One of the most challenging considerations in the SF technique is that it is a complicated approach that requires close cooperation between a highly experienced orthodontist and a surgeon. Prediction of the desired final occlusion is not easy. This chapter explained the Sendai SF technique step-by-step, including the planning process and application. It should be noted that the severity of a malocclusion is an important factor in determining the length of treatment time. Patients with mildly crowded teeth will have a shorter treatment time compared to patients with severely crowded teeth. In the patient described throughout the chapter, the orthodontic work took nearly 10 months and the total treatment time was 11 months. She was classified as having a moderately crowded occlusion. The authors have experienced longer treatment times in patients with severely crowded occlusions (see Case Reports 1 to 3). Regardless, the treatment time remains significantly shorter than what might be experienced with conventional orthodontic/orthognathic surgery.[20]

Among the benefits of the Sendai SF approach are a greatly reduced treatment time, the rapid improvement of the patient's profile, and the quick improvement of the patient's quality of life. It is the authors' belief that these benefits significantly outweigh the potential problems associated with Sendai SF and that this innovative treatment approach may soon become a standard clinical option.

REFERENCES

1. Sugawara J, Aymach Z, Nagasaka DH, Kawamura H, Nanda R. "Surgery first" orthognathics to correct a skeletal class II malocclusion with an impinging bite. *J Clin Orthod.* 2010;44:429–438.
2. Aymach Z, Sugawara J, Goto S, Nagasaka H, Nanda R. Nonextraction "Surgery First" treatment of a skeletal Class III patient with severe maxillary crowding. *J Clin Orthod.* 2013;47(5):297–304.
3. Nagasaka H, Sugawara J, Kawamura H, Nanda R. "Surgery first" skeletal Class III correction using the skeletal anchorage system. *J Clin Orthod.* 2009;43:97–105.
4. Hernández-Alfaro F, Guijarro-Martínez R, Molina-Coral A, Badía-Escriche C. "Surgery-first" in bimaxillary orthognathic surgery. *J Oral Maxillofac Surg.* 2011;69(6):e201–e207.
5. Liou EJ, Chen PH, Wang YC, Yu CC, Huang CS, Chen YR. Surgery-first accelerated orthognathic surgery: orthodontic guidelines and setup for model surgery. *J Oral Maxillofac Surg.* 2011;69:771–780.
6. White LW, Sugawara J. JCO interviews: Dr. Junji Sugawara on the skeletal anchorage system. *J Clin Orthod.* 1999;33:689–696.
7. Sugawara J. A bioefficient skeletal anchorage system. In: Nanda R, ed. *Biomechanics and Esthetic Strategies in Clinical Orthodontics*. St. Louis, MO: WB Saunders; 2005:295–309.
8. Sugawara J, Soya T, Kawamura H, Kanamori Y. Analysis of craniofacial morphology using craniofacial drawing standards (CDS): application for orthognathic surgery [in Japanese]. *Nippon Kyosei Shika Gakkai Zasshi.* 1988;47:394–408.
9. Jacobson A. The "Wits" appraisal of jaw disharmony, 1975. *Am J Orthod.* 2003;124:470–479.
10. Liou EJ, Chen PH, Wang YC, Yu CC, Huang CS, Chen YR. Surgery-first accelerated orthognathic surgery: postoperative rapid orthodontic tooth movement. *J Oral Maxillofac Surg.* 2011;69:781–785.
11. Villegas C, Uribe F, Sugawara J, Nanda R. Expedited correction of significant dentofacial asymmetry using a "surgery first" approach. *J Clin Orthod.* 2010;44(2):97–103, quiz 105.
12. Aymach Z, Nei H, Kawamura H, Van Sickels J. Evaluation of skeletal stability after surgical-orthodontic correction of skeletal open bite with mandibular counterclockwise rotation using modified inverted L osteotomy. *J Oral Maxillofac Surg.* 2011;69(3):853–860.
13. Aymach Z, Kawamura H. Facilitating ramus lengthening following mandibular-dependent surgical closing of a skeletal open bite with short ramus: a new modified technique. *J Craniomaxillofac Surg.* 2012; 40(2):169–172.
14. Aymach Z, Nei H, Kawamura H, Bell W. Biomechanical evaluation of a T-shaped mini-plate fixation of a modified sagittal split ramus osteotomy with buccal step: a new technique for mandibular orthognathic surgery. *Oral Surg Oral Med Oral Pathol Oral Radiol Endod.* 2011; 111(1):58–63.
15. Kawamura H, Nagasaka H, Sato S, Motegi K, Sugawara J, Mitani H. Sagittal split ramus osteotomy combined with titanium mini-plate internal fixation [in Japanese]. *Jpn J Jaw Deform.* 1991;1:105–112.
16. Ito J, Takahashi I, Umemori M, et al. Postsurgical stability of mandible after sagittal split advancement osteotomy using titanium mini-plate fixation in skeletal class II patients [in Japanese]. *Jpn J Jaw Deform.* 1997; 7:110–119.
17. Ellis E. Rigid versus nonrigid fixation. In: Miloro M, ed. Peterson's Principles of Oral and Maxillofacial Surgery. Vol. 1. Hamilton, Ontario: BC Decker; 2004:371–377.
18. Ochs MW. Bicortical screw stabilization of sagittal split osteotomies. *J Oral Maxillofac Surg.* 2003;61:1477–1484.
19. Dowling PA, Espeland L, Krogstad O, et al. Duration of orthodontic treatment involving orthognathic surgery. *Int J Adult Orthodon Orthognath Surg.* 1999;14:146–152.
20. O'Brien K, Wright J, Conboy F, et al. Prospective, multi-center study of the effectiveness of orthodontic/orthognathic surgery care in the United Kingdom. *Am J Orthod Dentofacial Orthop.* 2009;135:709–714.
21. Luther F, Morris DO, Karnezi K. Orthodontic treatment following orthognathic surgery: how long does it take and why? A retrospective study. *J Oral Maxillofac Surg.* 2007;65:1969–1976.
22. Hajji SS. *The Influence of Accelerated Osteogenic Response on Mandibular Crowding.* St. Louis, MO: St. Louis University, Center for Advanced Dental Education; 2000:1–49.
23. Bailey LTJ, Proffit WR. Combined surgical and orthodontic treatment. In: Fields HW, ed. *Contemporary Orthodontics.* 3rd ed. Philadelphia, PA: Mosby; 1999:674–709.
24. Liou EJ, Chen PH, Wang YC, Yu CC, Huang CS, Chen YR. Surgery-first accelerated orthognathic surgery: postoperative rapid orthodontic tooth movement. *J Oral Maxillofac Surg.* 2011;69:781–785.
25. Sugawara J, Aymach Z, Nagasaka H, Kawamura H, Nanda R. Non-surgical correction of skeletal open bite: a goal-oriented approach evaluated by CBCT. *J Clin Orthod.* 2011;45(3):145–155.

26. Sugawara J, Kanzaki R, Takahashi I, Nagasaka H, Nanda R. Distal movement of the maxillary molars in nongrowing patients with the skeletal anchorage system. *Am J Orthod.* 2006;129:723–733.
27. Umemori M, Sugawara J, Mitani H, Nagasaka H, Kawamura H. Skeletal anchorage system for openbite correction. *Am J Orthod.* 1999;115:166–174.
28. Villegas C, Janakiraman N, Uribe F, Nanda R. Rotation of the maxillomandibular complex to enhance esthetics using a "surgery first" approach. *J Clin Orthod.* 2012;46(2):85–91, quiz 123.
29. Swennen GR, Mollemans W, De Clercq C, et al. A cone-beam computed tomography triple scan procedure to obtain a three-dimensional augmented virtual skull model appropriate for orthognathic surgery planning. *J Craniofac Surg.* 2009;20:297–307.
30. Choi JY, Song KG, Baek SH. Virtual model surgery and wafer fabrication for orthognathic surgery. *Int J Oral Maxillofac Surg.* 2009;38:1306–1310.
31. Park KR, Kim SY, Park HS, Jung YS. Surgery-first approach on patients with temporomandibular joint disease by intraoral vertical ramus osteotomy. *Oral Surg Oral Med Oral Pathol Oral Radiol.* 2013;116:e429–e436.
32. Baek SH, Ahn HW, Kwon YH, Choi JY. Surgery-first approach in skeletal class III malocclusion treated with 2-jaw surgery: evaluation of surgical movement and postoperative orthodontic treatment. *J Craniofac Surg.* 2010;21:332–338.

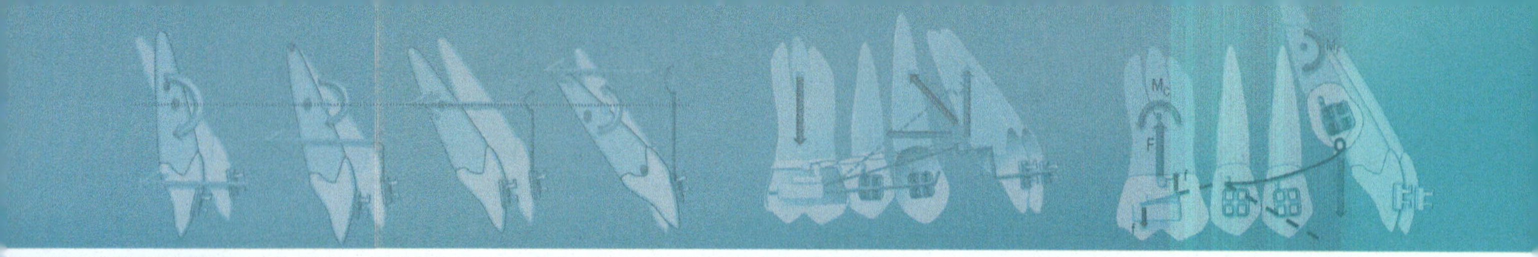

CHAPTER 23

Biomechanical Factors in Surgical Orthodontics

R. Scott Conley and Harry L. Legan

When using orthognathic surgery, application of appropriate diagnosis, treatment planning, biomechanical principles, surgical technique, and timing are all necessary to optimize individual patient treatment outcomes. From the discipline's inception in the mid-nineteenth century through its peak in the 1980s and its continued evolution in the early 2000s, advances have been made in both diagnostic and treatment-related areas. Initial updates made orthognathic surgery a safer and more practical treatment alternative with the development of antibiotics, enhanced surgical techniques, and later rigid fixation. The improved surgical techniques enabled orthodontists to rethink the timing and type of surgical preparation and ultimately enabled orthognathic surgery to become increasingly predictable, with dramatic facial and occlusal improvement the normal outcome.

More recently, diagnostic advances such as cone beam computed tomography (CBCT) and computer aided surgical simulation (CASS) offer tremendous value and new planning opportunities to the orthodontist, the oral and maxillofacial surgeon, and their patients. Both techniques now enable the care team to truly understand the three-dimensional (3D) nature of patient jaw deformities to better simulate and plan treatment before undertaking care. While planning is essential, the greater benefit is the "failure analysis" from the 3D images, which enhances future patient care by preventing adverse outcomes.

Advances have not been restricted to the planning phase but have also included the development of new treatments such as distraction osteogenesis, surgery for the obstructive sleep apnea (OSA) patient, mandibular constriction, earlier surgical intervention, and skeletal anchorage with temporary anchorage devices (TADs) used before, during, and following surgery, each of which potentially alter the biomechanical approach and surgical intervention planned for the patient. While distraction osteogenesis is unlikely to replace traditional orthognathic surgery because, for example, it cannot be used in cases of excessive jaw growth, it offers a treatment alternative for correction of skeletal jaw deficiencies. Unfortunately, few papers describe the detailed biomechanical approach necessary to achieve the correct vectors and movements for optimal treatment results. Orthodontic appliance and TAD placement, localizing the center of resistance of the osteotomized segments, and location of force application are vitally important to minimize treatment complications and enhance treatment outcomes. The same efficient, effective, operator-determined biomechanical principles necessary to produce excellent orthodontic outcomes must be applied to both distraction osteogenesis and TADs. The biomechanical principles are the same whether focusing on tooth-to-tooth movement or bony segment–to-bony segment movement yet few recognize the merging of these disciplines.

Logical, sequential, and appropriate application of these and other related updates and their impact on diagnosis, treatment planning, surgical considerations, methods of efficient leveling, arch coordination, space closure, and other aspects of orthodontic mechanotherapy are discussed in this chapter.

THREE-DIMENSIONAL IMAGING: CEPHALOMETRICS

Cephalometric analysis is one critical step in proper diagnosis and treatment planning for patients with severe skeletal malocclusion. A myriad of analyses are available[1] and preferences vary among orthodontists and surgeons. The most frequently used orthodontic analyses use angular measures,[2,3] which are sufficient for assessing tooth position but are far less precise in accurately assessing jaw position and impossible to translate to the surgical setting. These analyses also use intracranial reference systems (such as porion and orbitale) that are difficult to locate, which has the potential to introduce more error than using an operator-assisted natural head position.[4] To overcome these deficiencies, a cephalometric analysis was developed[5,6] that uses predominantly linear measures that are directly transferable to the surgical setting, uses a natural head position, and can be altered surgically, orthodontically, or with a combined approach. Unfortunately, the improved lateral cephalometric analysis still neglected the transverse (or third dimension), which is highlighted by two significant publications on posterior-anterior (PA) cephalometry.[7,8] While the PA view adds beneficial information, it is fraught with both exposure errors, such as minute patient rotations,[9] and landmark identification and superimposition issues that make the PA cephalogram difficult to read and interpret.[10]

With CBCT, the deficiencies of both lateral and PA cephalometric analyses can be overcome. Several papers[11-14] have shown that two-dimensional (2D) radiographs can be accurately created from the CBCT scan. Creating 2D projections of a 3D structure represents a diagnostic enhancement but developing a true 3D structural analysis that complements the 3D clinical exam and an improved asymmetry analysis would be a much more significant advancement. New 3D techniques such as "mirroring," where the normal side is projected onto the abnormal side, enable the orthodontist and surgeon to precisely recreate what will be performed in the operating room (Fig. 23-1). While these methods are in their infancy and further validation is required,[15-18] time will likely lead to substantial improvement in these areas.

Improved Three-Dimensional Surgical Planning

CBCT not only provides additional information during diagnosis, but also can be used to improve the operative treatment plan. Historically, virtual treatment objectives were created using lateral cephalometric radiographs, photos, dental models, and model surgery. However, this technique is subject to several different sources of error, including facebow registration, model mounting, landmark identification, and poor splint construction. To avoid these complications some surgeons took medical computed tomography (CT) scans, created 3D models, and performed surgery on a plastic model. Now, the presurgical CBCT can be merged with a scanned copy of the patient's models and the surgery can be performed virtually on the computer.[19-21] The surgeon is free to simulate several different surgical plans, including single-piece Le Fort I osteotomy, multisegment Le Fort I osteotomy, mandibular ramus osteotomies, and genioplasties. A 3D summary of the surgical movements is developed and the interim and final surgical splints can be fabricated. The surgical splints can also incorporate stents that will accommodate the precise positioning of the rigid fixation (Fig. 23-2).

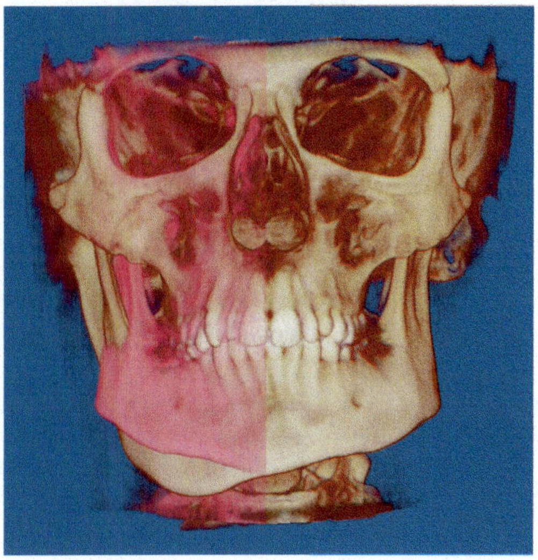

Figure 23-1 The patient's left side is the "normal" side and the patient's right side demonstrates a significant hemimandibular hypertrophy. For treatment planning purposes, the "mirror" function within Dolphin was used to overlay (*in pink*) the "normal" on the affected side to illustrate the amount of bone that will need to be removed for symmetry to be achieved. While this technique is extremely illustrative, it is typically not possible to remove this amount of bone surgically due to the location of the inferior alveolar nerve on the affected side.

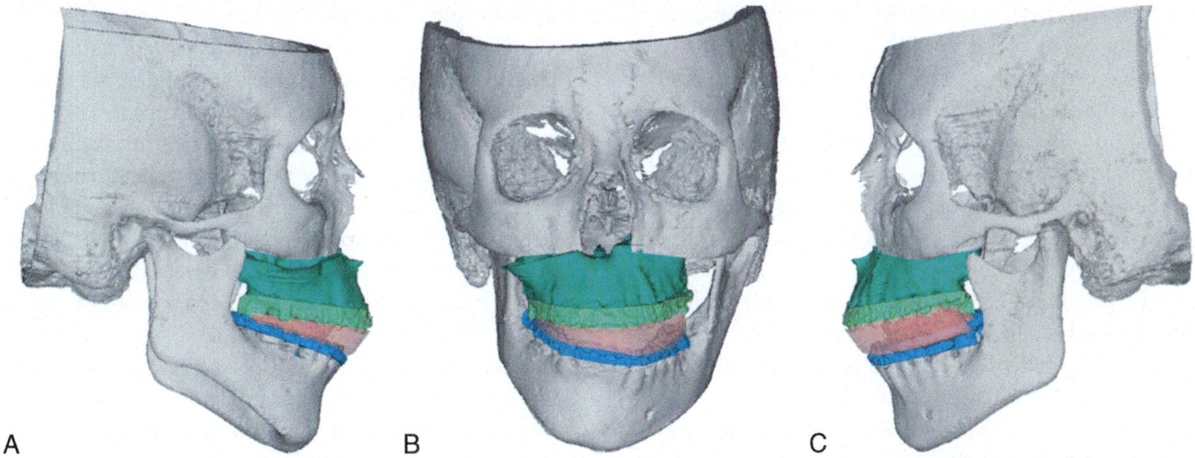

Figure 23-2 **A–C,** This patient with juvenile idiopathic arthritis presented at the presurgical visit with extreme facial asymmetry. Using the computer aided surgical simulation (CASS) technique, the surgeon was able to accurately determine the final position of the maxilla and fabricate the large interocclusal splint required to set the maxilla in the proper position. The next step was to remove the interim splint, complete the mandibular osteotomy, and finally reposition the genial segment (if necessary). (Courtesy Dr. Sean P. Edwards, Ann Arbor, MI.)

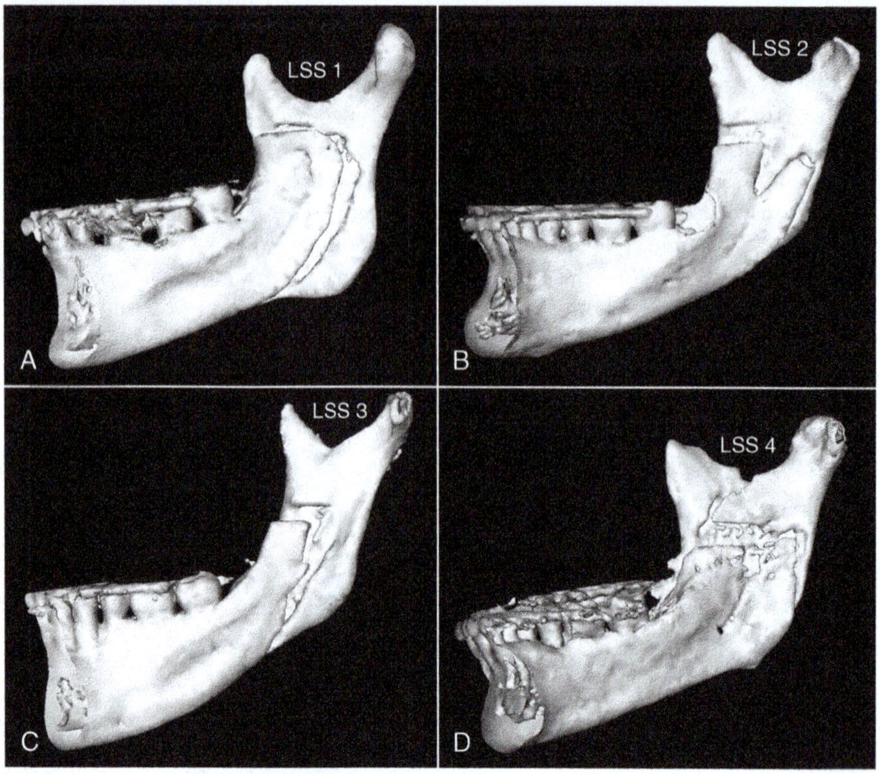

Figure 23-3 The lingual fracture pattern created during the sagittal split ramus osteotomy (SSRO) is considered to be one factor associated with relapse. It was impossible to observe the fracture pattern with conventional two-dimensional imaging techniques but this can be visualized clearly with cone beam computed tomography (CBCT). Additional information such as this can now be used to better understand the possible mechanisms behind unstable or poor treatment results. The goal will be to use this new information prospectively to minimize future negative outcomes. LSS1-4 indicates "lingual sagittal split" for patients 1 to 4. (Reprinted with permission from Plooij JM, Naphausen MT, Maal TJ, et al. 3D evaluation of the lingual fracture line after a bilateral sagittal split osteotomy of the mandible. *Int J Oral Maxillofac Surg.* 2009;38[12]:1244–1249.)

Using immediate postoperative CBCT scans, the shape and form of the fracture that is propagated during the sagittal split ramus osteotomy (SSRO) can be evaluated (Fig. 23-3).[22] This is important, as the muscular influence on the proximal and distal segments varies considerably based on where the fracture pattern occurs and directly influences the surgical stability and success. The authors report only about half of the fracture lines propagated along the line originally described by Hunsuck,[23] even though the surgeon and surgical technique were consistent. They ultimately concluded that the enhanced imaging technique was suitable for analyzing surgical outcome and "has the potential to provide substantial data on the position of the proximal segments as a result of the lingual fracture line."[22]

Another factor in surgical planning is maintaining condylar position during surgery, which is particularly difficult since it is affected by many factors, such as rotational movement of the proximal segment, tensional balance of the surrounding muscles, fixation method, and the surgeon's experience.[24] The ability to detect and assess for these changes following surgery is nearly impossible with 2D imaging but easy with CBCT. Proposed methods for avoiding condylar displacement include intraoperative monitoring by sonography, guiding splints, and intraoperative awakening.[25–29] Because there is substantial evidence of the effect of condylar position on postoperative stability following SSRO,[30–33] presurgical planning and accurate positional assessment of the condyle during and immediately following orthognathic surgery are vital to maximize surgical stability and achieve predictable and favorable treatment outcomes.

Three-Dimensional Surgical Outcome Evaluation: Managing Complications

Surgeons and orthodontists plan each case meticulously to optimize outcomes and minimize complications; however, complications are an unavoidable part of care. CBCT can enhance the clinician's understanding of the root cause, enabling the team to select the most appropriate correction. Options range from adjusting the postsurgical orthodontic course, which is preferred when complications result from a less ideal presurgical orthodontic setup, to additional surgery when complications result from an unexpected skeletal change. Recently a small case series[34] suggested that CBCT may be useful in the management of unfavorable fractures during mandibular surgery. Following unfavorable surgical outcomes, the authors reviewed both presurgical and immediate postsurgical CBCT to examine whether anatomic, surgical, or combined influences could explain the unfavorable splits. The case illustrated in Figure 23-4 involves a patient who was planned for a combined four first premolar extraction pattern and a surgical mandibular advancement. The initial surgical change was quite

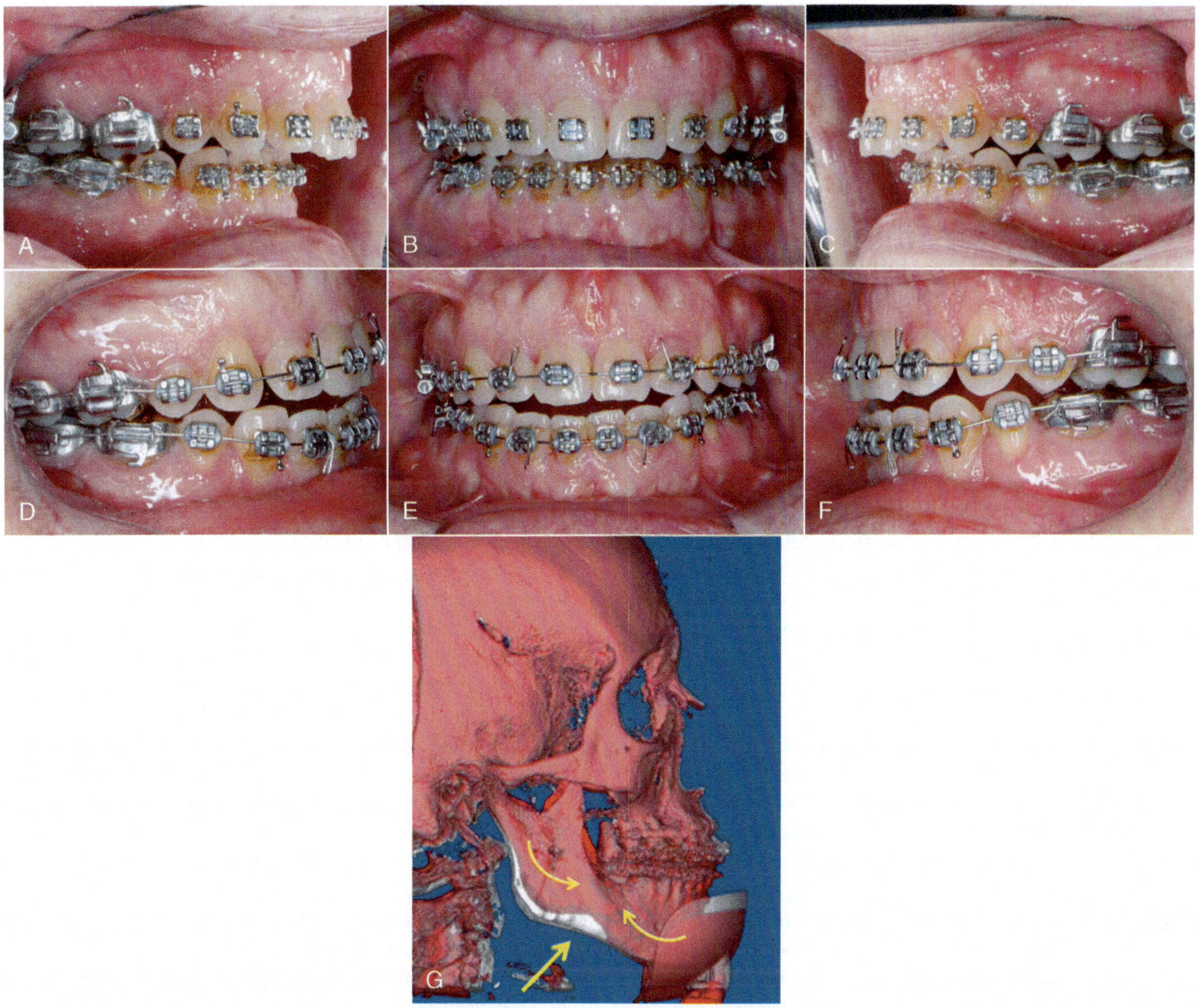

Figure 23-4 **A–C,** Preoperative intraoral views of a patient prior to sagittal split ramus osteotomy (SSRO) to advance the mandible. Note the overbite present. **D–F,** Twelve-week postoperative intraoral views showing the anterior open bite that developed between the 8- and 12-week postoperative evaluations. **G,** Superimposed *(pink)* view of the presurgical *(white)* and 12-week postoperative *(red)* cone beam computed tomography (CBCT) scans. The superimposition depicts the amount of mandibular advancement but also clearly indicates *(arrows)* the rotation of the proximal and distal segments creating both a "V" notch deformity and the anterior open bite.

favorable; however, at the 12-week postoperative follow-up the patient had developed an open bite. To determine the cause, the presurgical, 6-week, and 12-week postoperative CBCT scans were superimposed, showing a dramatic and unfavorable proximal/distal segment rotation. Whether this resulted solely from the muscular influences, fixation difficulties, or poor segment positioning is unclear; however, it is clear that the change resulted at the surgical site rather than from the orthodontic treatment. The patient was given the option to undergo surgical revision to remove the existing fixation, reorient the segments, and replace the fixation or to undergo a potentially unstable orthodontic correction with elastics. Ultimately the patient opted for the "conservative" orthodontic approach but the CBCT enabled everyone to see the root cause and select the most ideal treatment plan.

MAXILLARY ORTHOGNATHIC SURGERY

Several reasons exist for surgical manipulation of the maxilla in all three planes of space. Surgical procedures include maxillary impaction, maxillary advancement, segmentalization of the maxilla, and, more infrequently, maxillary inferior repositioning to lengthen the face. In addition to the direction of movement, the level of the osteotomy must be considered, with options ranging from Le Fort I to Le Fort III with several variations. With each type of surgical intervention, the presurgical and postsurgical orthodontic mechanics must be appropriate for the type of surgery planned, since inappropriate mechanics can reduce the facial improvement and in some cases prevent the proper surgery from occurring. Complete diagnostic records (CBCT or lateral and PA

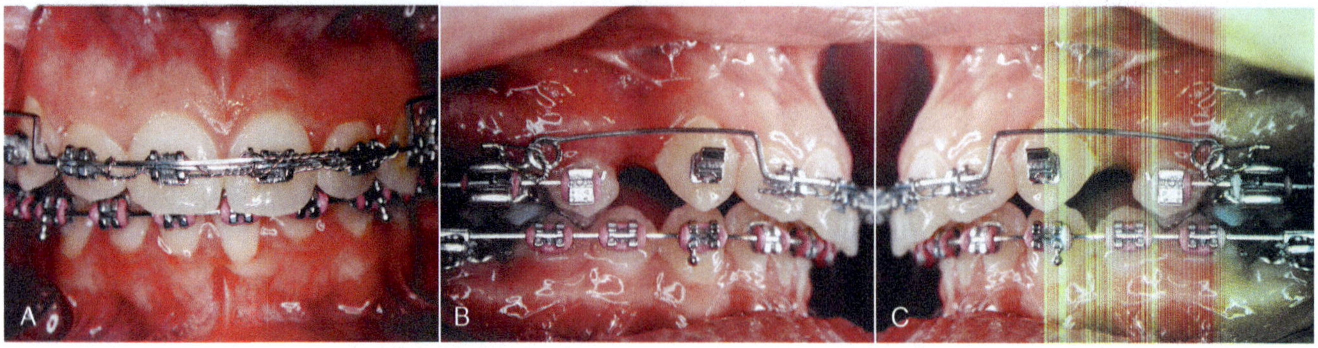

Figure 23-5 **A–C,** A 0.017-inch × 0.025-inch stainless steel intrusive base arch has two and a half helices immediately adjacent to the maxillary first molar. To minimize the side effect of incisal proclination resulting from the application of the intrusive force labial to the center of resistance of the tooth, the base arch is tied back with a stainless steel ligature to the molar band. A Dontrix gauge is used to accurately measure the force magnitude.

cephalogram, models, photographs, hand-wrist x-ray, temporomandibular joint examination) must be obtained and examined in conjunction with a detailed clinical examination to accurately develop the surgical orthodontic database and determine the appropriate mechanics plan for each case. The orthodontic biomechanical considerations for several of the more common surgical procedures are presented below.

Impaction

A common indication for maxillary surgery is vertical maxillary excess. Some of the cephalometric indicators within the cephalometric analysis for orthognathic surgery (COGS)[5,6] are increased upper and lower facial height (N-ANS and ANS-Gn), increased mandibular plane angle (MP-HP), increased posterior facial height (N-PNS), increased gonial angle (Ar-Go-Gn), increased facial height ratio (N-ANS/ANS-Gn), and divergent occlusal planes. A typical clinical presentation includes an increased tooth-to-lip relationship, increased gingival display, an increased interlabial gap, and a *relative* mandibular deficiency. The patient will often have an anterior open bite but this is not always present due to dentoalveolar compensations and hypereruption of the teeth.

Just as the surgical plan must include all three planes of space, the orthodontic biomechanics must evaluate the patient's needs and plan the mode of correction in three dimensions. Of special consideration with vertical maxillary excess is minimizing the orthodontic extrusion that can occur quite rapidly with mechanics, such as the placement of low modulus continuous archwires. Segmented arch mechanics provide an excellent way to predictably control the point of force application and magnitude of force applied and to produce an operator-determined, not appliance-determined, force system. The segmented arch technique has the additional advantage of being able to level each arch without requiring additional arch length.[35]

When divergent occlusal planes exist, a treatment occlusal plane must be selected first and then the appropriate force system designed. Typically a functional occlusal plane (perpendicular to the maxillary posterior teeth) is drawn. Once selected, the anterior teeth may be on, significantly above, or significantly below the treatment occlusal plane. Multiple options regarding arch leveling procedures exist. Should the arches be leveled before, during, or after surgery? Should the leveling be accomplished orthodontically, surgically, or using a combination of the two? The surgical approach to arch leveling is discussed below in the section on maxillary arch segmentalization.

If the maxillary anterior teeth have erupted significantly beyond the treatment occlusal plane, an extremely efficient orthodontic mechanism for leveling the arch is the intrusive base arch. Two stainless steel posterior segments containing the second molar to the first premolar and an anterior stainless steel segment from the lateral incisor to the lateral incisor are fabricated. Either a 0.017-inch × 0.025-inch beta-titanium or a 0.017-inch × 0.025-inch stainless steel base arch with helices is activated to deliver approximately 20 to 25 g of intrusive force per maxillary incisor (Fig. 23-5). The extrusive forces in the posterior segment and the moment of the force created by the base arch are balanced by using a high-pull headgear oriented through a point above and in front of the center of resistance of the maxilla. Without the high-pull headgear setup to balance the adverse effects of the intrusive base arch, a significant steepening of the maxillary posterior occlusal plane can be observed, which can exacerbate the initial clinical presentation of a patient with vertical maxillary excess. In addition, no true anterior intrusion at the level of the center of resistance may occur. Once the anterior and posterior segments are oriented along the same plane (the treatment occlusal plane), a continuous archwire is placed to maintain the arch leveling.

In other vertical maxillary excess patients, the maxillary anterior segment may be more superiorly positioned than the posterior occlusal plane. In this situation the exact opposite orthodontic force system is designed. The segments of teeth are set up in the exact same orientation. The difference is that instead of an intrusive force being applied to the maxillary anterior teeth, an extrusive force of approximately 50 g per tooth is applied to extrude the anterior teeth to the level of the posterior occlusal plane. Once again, when all the teeth are oriented along the treatment occlusal plane, the extrusive base arch is removed, and a continuous stainless steel archwire is placed (Fig. 23-6).

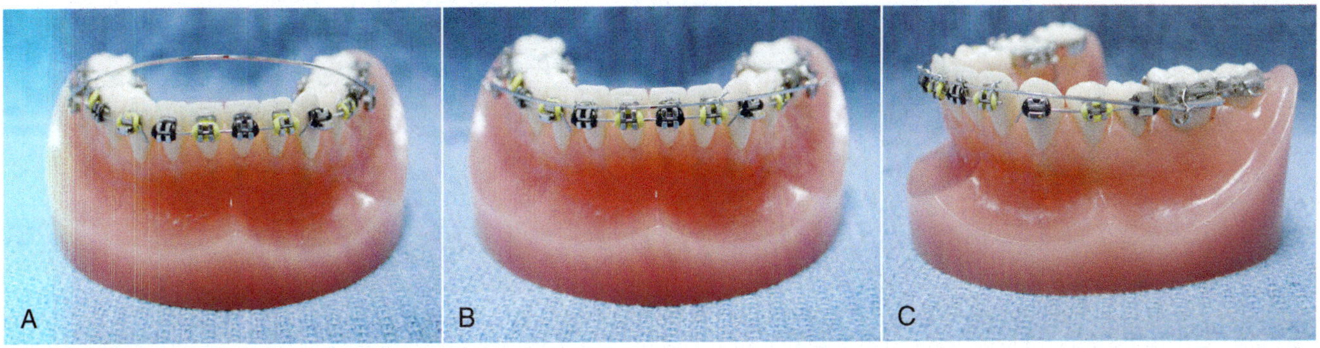

Figure 23-6 Extrusive base arch is essentially the same as intrusive base arch, merely turned upside down. **A,** Extrusive base arch activated but not ligated to the anterior segment. **B,** Ligated to the anterior segment. **C,** Helices in a lateral view. The helix is made so that when the arch is activated, the loop is wound rather than unwound, which results in better load deflection and more constant force delivery.

Many surgeons will perform intermaxillary fixation, orienting the maxilla to the mandible and autorotating the entire maxillomandibular complex to the desired vertical position, and then use rigid fixation. This will typically cause a slight maxillary advancement in addition to the impaction. With vertical maxillary excess, a mandibular osteotomy may or may not be required but attention must still be directed to the setup of the mandibular dental arch to ensure appropriate arch coordination, arch form, and leveling. Within the mandible, attention is directed to the depth of the curve of Spee, lower incisor–menton measurement, and the relative amount of prominence desired at both the soft and the hard tissue pogonion. For specific information on leveling of the mandibular arch, see the section "Mandibular Surgery" later in the chapter.

Advancement

The correction of any severe jaw deformity involved a mandibular osteotomy until the mid-1970s when Bell et al.[36] performed a series of microangiographic studies. Those studies demonstrated the biological basis for surgical manipulation of the maxilla and since then the maxilla has been diagnosed much more frequently as part of the etiology of the Class III malocclusion.[37] Some of the COGS indicators of a maxillary sagittal deficiency with a normal mandibular position include glabella-subnasale (G-Sn), nasion–A point (N-A), nasion–B point (N-B), nasion-pogonion (N-Pg), and glabella–soft tissue pogonion (G-Pg′). Other clinical indications for performing a maxillary advancement in lieu of a mandibular setback include decreased pharyngeal airway, excessive submental adipose tissue, decreased malar convexity, and increased nasolabial grooves on smiling. A helpful clinical diagnostic aid involves using an object, such as a hand, fingers, or cardboard, to "block out" the midface while examining the projection of the lower face. If the chin position is acceptable, it is most likely that the patient has a maxillary sagittal deficiency.

Patients with maxillary sagittal deficiency also frequently exhibit varying degrees of transverse deficiency and may present with a posterior crossbite as part of their Class III malocclusion. The crossbite must be evaluated critically to determine the magnitude and etiology using PA cephalogram (or CBCT) in addition to the clinical examination and models analysis. During the analysis, the transverse dimension must be evaluated in not only the current but also the final sagittal position because the crossbite may not need to be addressed once the maxilla is brought forward. If the patient exhibits an absolute crossbite[38] or has a crossbite in both the presenting and the final position, the magnitude and classification (skeletal versus dental) of the transverse deficiency must be determined. Skeletal crossbites are best corrected skeletally (rapid palatal expansion [RPE], transverse maxillary distraction osteogenesis, or segmented maxillary surgery), while dental crossbites may be corrected skeletally or dentally (RPE, palatal arch, cross-arch elastics, or expansion of the maxillary archwire).

Occlusogram analysis,[39,40] in addition to model analysis, can assist in the differential diagnosis of the transverse dimension. The occlusal aspect of the teeth is traced on a piece of acetate and articulated in the current anteroposterior occlusion. To simulate the surgery, the maxillary member is brought forward the same amount as the anticipated surgical maxillary advancement. Then, using the mandible as the template arch, the appropriate arch form, arch width, and arch length analysis is performed, with the difference between the current and predicted arch width representing the required amount of maxillary expansion or mandibular constriction.

If the etiology of the crossbite is dental or small in magnitude, a transpalatal arch (TPA) provides an efficient method of dental arch expansion and does not require patient compliance. The clinician needs to fabricate a 0.036-inch stainless steel heat-treated TPA (Fig. 23-7). First, the appliance should be fitted passively to ensure that no unintended forces, moments, or vertical couples are present. To activate the TPA, the appliance should not only be expanded but also have buccal root torque placed to reduce the tipping tendency. It is essential to apply an equal amount of buccal root torque bilaterally to prevent a significant vertical couple being produced, which if left in place long enough can result in an iatrogenic occlusal plane cant that can be resolved only by differential vertical positioning of the maxilla as it is

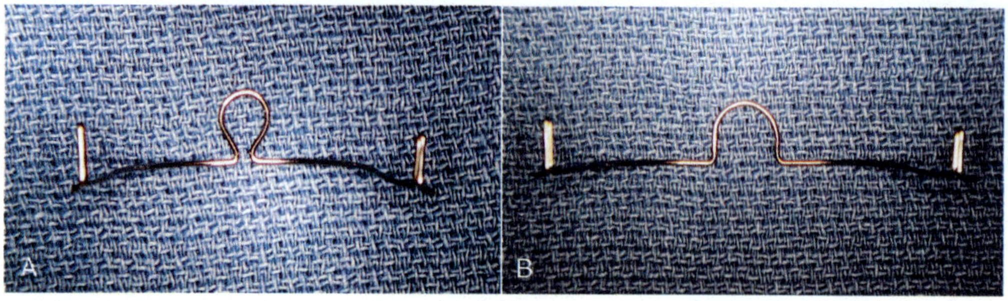

Figure 23-7 **A,** For expansion, a transpalatal arch (TPA) with an omega adjustment loop can be used. The loop introduces more flexibility to the TPA but the advantage is that the wire can be maintained at the same depth within the palate after each activation. Without an adjustment loop the TPA will be brought more occlusally after each activation and increase the potential for tongue irritation and alteration in speech. **B,** Activated TPA.

brought forward. Iatrogenic cants transform a straightforward maxillary advancement to a more technically precise surgery and, worse, can result in an unfavorable outcome and a dissatisfied patient.

For the patient with excess transverse dimension, using a TPA with constriction is an efficient way to reduce arch width. Archwires are far less efficient in these cases because of their smaller cross-sectional dimension and because much arch activation is lost in the act of inserting the wire into the buccal tubes. To be most effective, the TPA must be "overconstricted" and heat treated to prevent a similar loss of activation upon insertion. Palatal root torque must also be placed to minimize tipping of the posterior teeth or posterior segments palatally.

Skeletal maxillary transverse deficiency is typically larger in magnitude and can be measured from the PA cephalogram or CBCT by evaluating both the jugal process (J point) width and the axial inclination of the posterior teeth. In a skeletally mature patient the most stable method[41,42] of correcting the maxillary transverse deficiency is maxillary transverse distraction osteogenesis (also referred to as surgically assisted RPE) or segmentalization of the maxilla (see discussion below).

Patients with maxillary sagittal hypoplasia may also have significant arch length deficiency, which can be assessed using the previously discussed occlusogram analysis, which further allows the clinician to determine the anchorage requirements should extractions be necessary. Occlusogram analysis will provide different anchorage requirements based on where the upper member is placed. If the upper member is left in the pre-treatment position, simulating an "orthodontics-only treatment approach," the anchorage requirements will be the opposite of what is required when the maxilla is advanced surgically. Extractions are performed in surgical orthodontic cases primarily for two reasons: to ideally position the teeth within the basal bone and to resolve significant arch length deficiency. The extraction mechanics should not be directed toward orthodontic correction of the malocclusion; instead, the extraction mechanics should be directed toward making the occlusion reflect the magnitude of the skeletal discrepancy.

The type of extraction mechanics selected should be tailored to meet the specific needs of each case. Cases with significant maxillary anterior crowding are best managed with early extraction of the first bicuspids and alignment of the posterior segments and canines only, bypassing the incisors using a 0.017-inch × 0.025-inch stainless steel track. Once aligned, a segmental precalibrated 0.017-inch × 0.025-inch beta-titanium "A" anchorage T-loop is placed from the first molar to the canine to perform initial canine retraction. "A" anchorage is achieved by placing four 30- to 40-degree moment activations in the posterior leg of the T-loop and three moment activation bends in the anterior leg. The differential moments produce a moment/force ratio of 10:1 (translation) at the canine versus a moment/force ratio of 13:1 (root movement) at the posterior segment. In critical anchorage cases, a high-pull headgear, TPA, or both will be placed to assist in maintaining the position of the posterior teeth and to prevent anchorage loss. If all of the extraction space is required for arch length resolution once the canine is brought back, the maxillary incisors are aligned and there is minimal to no space remaining. If the anchorage requirements are less stringent, the canines may be brought back only enough to allow adequate space for alignment of the maxillary anterior teeth with any residual space closed with a new segmental T-loop activated for "B" or "C" anchorage (Fig. 23-8).[43,44]

Inferior Repositioning (Down Graft)

Vertical maxillary deficiency is much less common than its counterpart, vertical maxillary excess. Some of the cephalometric indicators within COGS are decreased lower facial height (ANS-Gn), decreased mandibular plane angle (MP-HP), decreased gonial angle (Ar-Go-Gn), increased facial height ratio (N-ANS/ANS-Gn), and deep overbite. A typical clinical presentation includes a decreased tooth-to-lip relationship, decreased gingival display, no interlabial gap, and a relative mandibular prognathism and/or prominent chin button.

Much as with vertical maxillary excess, most attention is directed to the vertical relationship of the jaws, with posterior extrusion the primary goal of the presurgical orthodontic mechanics. Continuous low modulus archwires may be used to facilitate orthodontic eruption; however, in many of these short face, low angle, or convergent patients presurgical or nonsurgical orthodontic extrusion is extremely

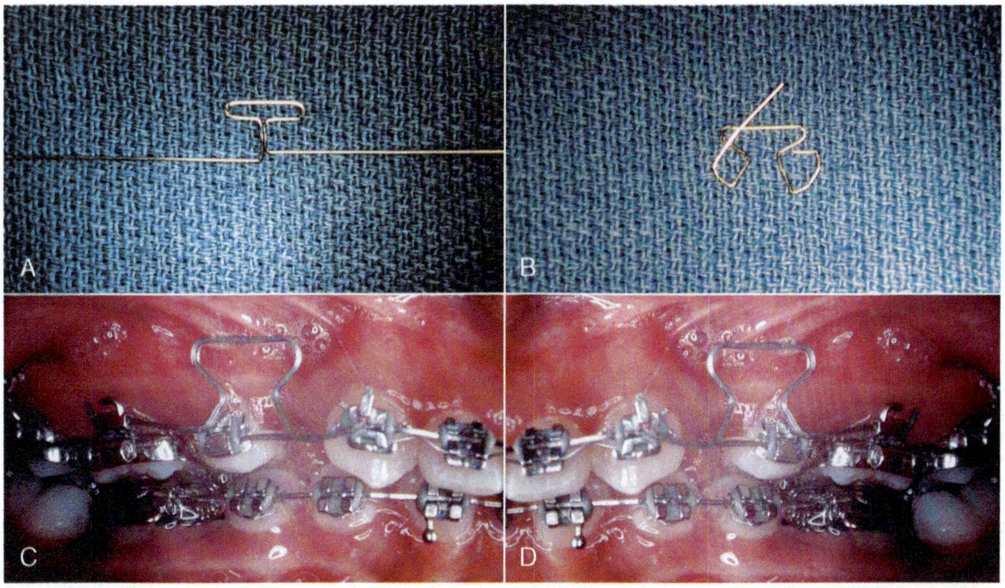

Figure 23-8 **A,** Preactivated 0.017-inch × 0.025-inch beta-titanium T-loop. The anterior leg is more gingival due to the placement of a gingival horizontal tube on the canine. The loop is contoured to the arch and checked for passivity both anteriorly and posteriorly. **B,** Then, depending on the anchorage requirements, the moments are placed within the anterior and posterior legs. **C and D,** Clinical use of an active segmental T-loop.

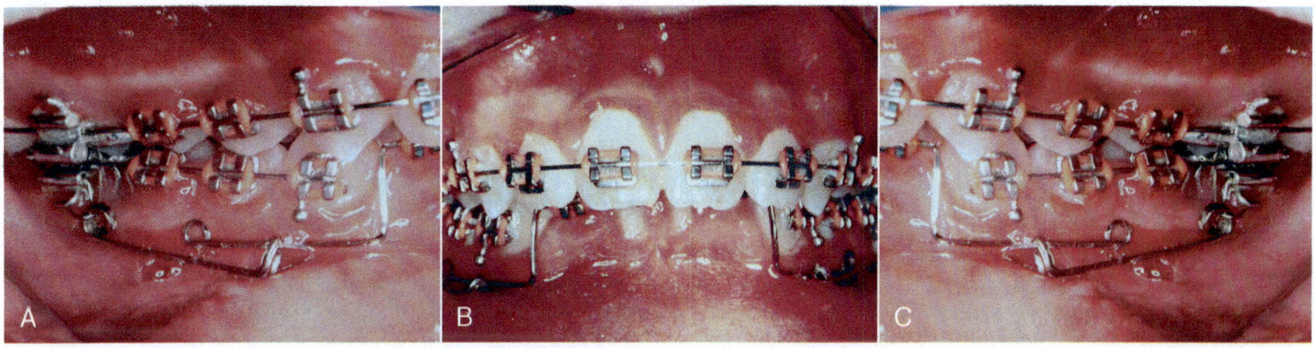

Figure 23-9 **A–C,** Split intrusive base arch allows for precise activation when intruding segments of teeth. The distal extension from the anterior segment allows the operator to place the intrusive force anterior to, at, or posterior to the center of resistance for the segment. This allows for simultaneous intrusion with proclination, intrusion with no axial change, or intrusion with simultaneous uprighting of the anterior segment for increased efficiency, respectively.

difficult to achieve. Extrusive force systems may be placed with continuous low modulus archwires but often the heavy occlusal bite force of the patient will exceed the eruptive force capabilities of the archwire. Instead, extrusive base arches (see Fig. 23-6) can be fabricated to produce an extremely efficient eruptive force (often 200 g or more) to the posterior maxillary and/or posterior mandibular segments while hyalinization of the anterior teeth occurs, producing minimal to no anterior intrusion. Additional benefits derived from the extrusive base arch force system include possible arch length increase resulting from the crown distal or counterclockwise moment and, if not tied back, space will develop between the segments (Fig. 23-9). Once leveling has occurred, this space can be used to retract the maxillary incisors using an "A" anchorage segmented arch T-loop. While the anterior crossbite will worsen presurgically, the maxillary anterior teeth will be appropriately positioned and uprighted within the maxillary basal bone. If simultaneous uprighting of the maxillary incisors during leveling is desired, the extrusive base arch can also be fabricated as a "split" base arch where the force can be applied behind the center of resistance of the maxillary anterior segment.

An alternative method is performing the orthodontic leveling postsurgically, especially when a significant mandibular curve of Spee is present. Immediate postsurgical leveling is extremely effective in part because of the surgically induced change in muscle fiber orientation, which results in a decreased mechanical advantage and decreased bite force (Fig. 23-10). In addition, Frost described a regional accelerative phenomenon due to healing and increased vascularization.[45,46] To assist eruption of the teeth, a continuous light stainless steel archwire with vertical box elastics in the midarch, segmented arch mechanics with an extrusive base arch, or an overlay extrusive base arch can be placed with a light continuous main archwire. Once complete arch leveling is obtained, a rigid continuous stainless steel archwire can be placed to maintain the arch leveling.

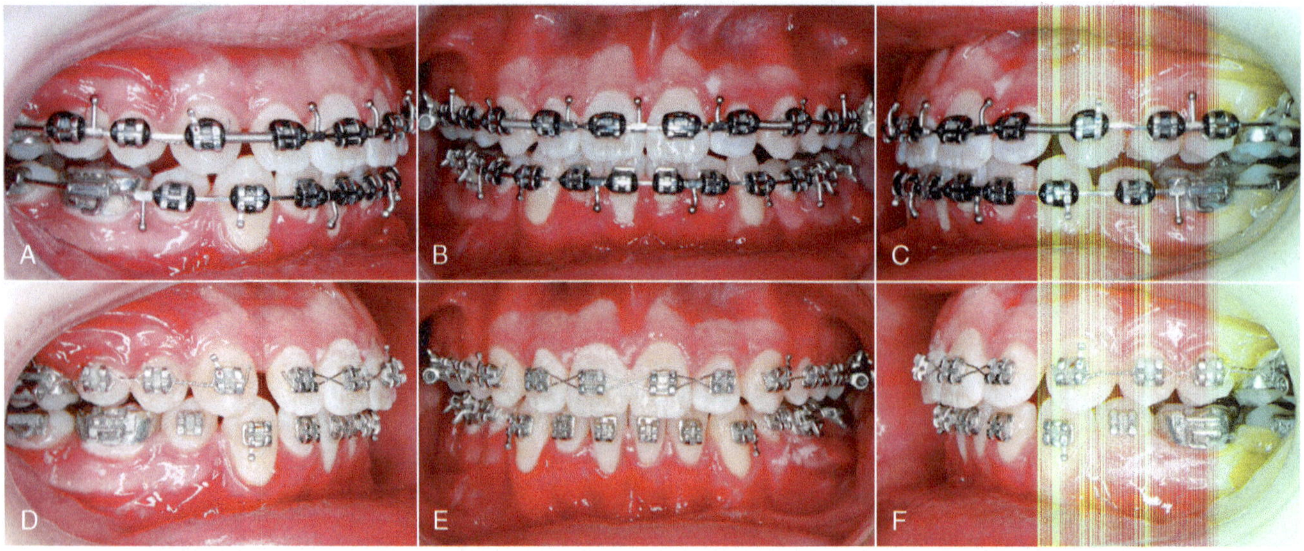

Figure 23-10 **A–C,** This patient is 6 weeks post–mandibular advancement with tripoding. The posterior occlusion remains open because the interocclusal splint was just removed. **D–F,** Six weeks later, following inter-arch vertical elastics with a heavy 0.019-inch × 0.025-inch stainless steel maxillary wire and a "light" 0.016-inch × 0.022-inch stainless steel wire, the patient has nearly completely interdigitated posterior teeth and can begin final finishing orthodontic care.

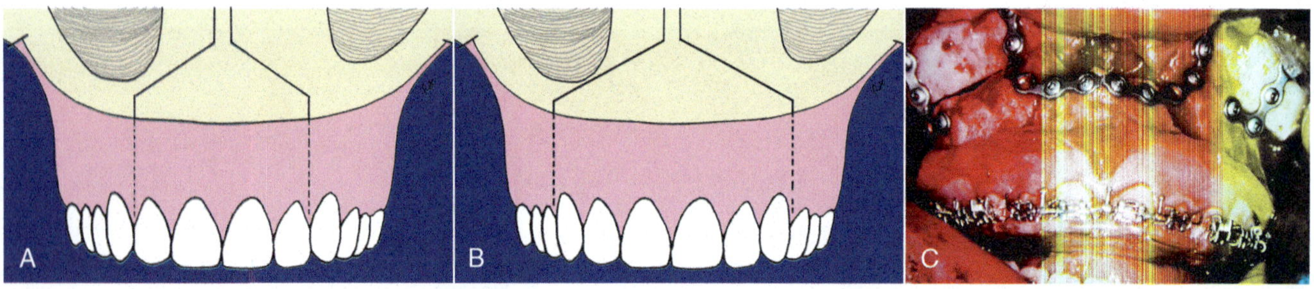

Figure 23-11 Segmental maxillary procedures can be performed in many ways and at many sites. The most common is the three-piece segmental Le Fort I osteotomy either **(A)** between the lateral incisor and canine or **(B)** between the canine and first premolar. The figure demonstrates the approximate area of interdental osteotomy from the frontal view, looking from above the previously down fractured maxilla. It is important to note that the palatal mucosa must be carefully preserved to maintain adequate perfusion of the maxilla and dentition. **C,** Clinical presentation after segmenting between the lateral incisor and canine and placing rigid internal fixation.

Segmentalization

Two main reasons exist for segmental maxillary osteotomies, one being multiple maxillary occlusal planes. The discrepant occlusal planes can be managed orthodontically or surgically and the decision regarding which method is better is largely philosophical and based on the stability of the surgical intervention versus the stability of the vertical orthodontic movement.[47,48] Segmentalization allows for differing amounts of superior or inferior repositioning of the segments surgically. When surgical closure of an anterior open bite is planned, orthodontic eruption of the maxillary anterior teeth is undesirable because this will introduce potential instability to the case and reduce the amount of vertical surgical repositioning. To facilitate segmentalization of the maxilla, segmental or continuous wires with vertical steps that maintain the discrepant occlusal planes are preferred over traditional continuous archwire mechanics because light continuous archwires (nickel-titanium [Ni-Ti]) will generally lead to unwanted extrusion of the maxillary anterior teeth, posterior teeth, or both. Typically, the maxillary arch is segmented either between the lateral incisor and the canine or between the canine and the first premolar depending on the point at which the occlusal planes diverge (Fig. 23-11). One advantage that a four-tooth incisor segment has over a six-tooth anterior segment is that the former can be set deeper surgically without the presence of the maxillary canine and there is a natural root divergence between the maxillary canine and the lateral incisor. To augment this root divergence, a segmental root spring can be placed from the molar to the canine to obtain the necessary root divergence for the osteotomy (Fig. 23-12). For segmental surgery, it is much less important to have space between the crowns than between the roots.[49] A continuous arch technique to obtain root divergence involves placing a centered V-bend with the apex of the "V" pointing apically, creating equal and opposite moments. One common mistake with continuous arch mechanotherapy is placing an open coil spring to create an osteotomy space. The open coil spring is effective in opening space at the level of the crown but will bring the roots of the adjacent teeth into closer proximity and increase rather than

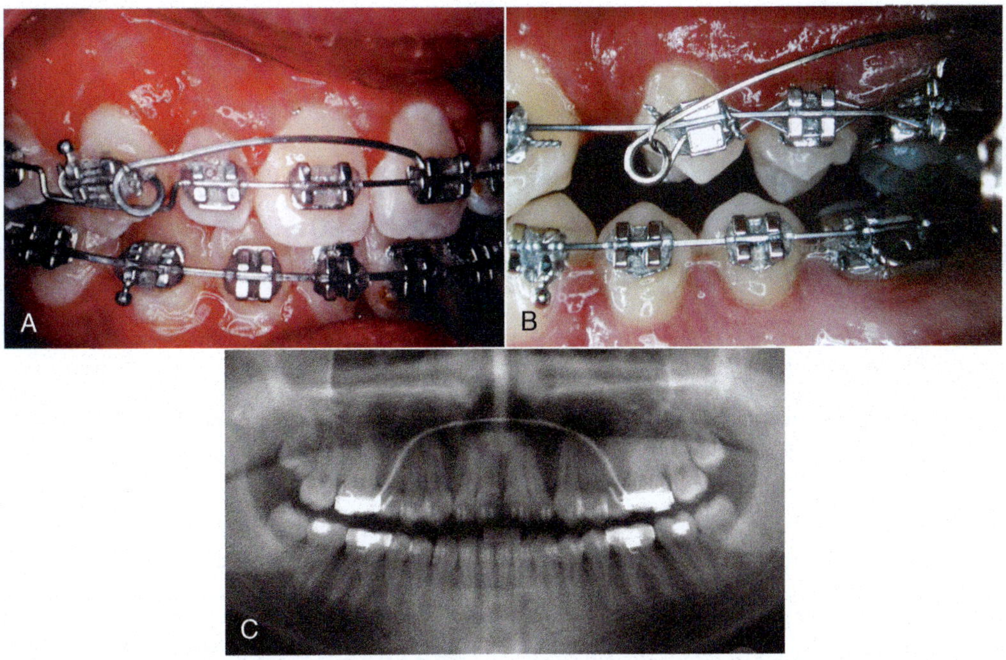

Figure 23-12 Activated root spring is an efficient way to assist in developing an interdental osteotomy site. **A,** Stainless steel main archwire can be stepped occlusally to minimize the extrusive effects of the spring or **(B)** a light nickel-titanium (Ni-Ti) archwire can be placed in the archwire slot. With the archwire in the slot, care must be taken to ensure that the archwire does not negate the effects of the root spring. **C,** Panoramic radiograph must be viewed prior to performing the osteotomy to ensure that the clinical crown angulation is not demonstrating misleading root position. In this patient the osteotomy was planned between the maxillary lateral incisor and canine and adequate divergence of the teeth was obtained. After surgery, the root position must be corrected to place the forces over the long axis of the teeth and to have parallel roots.

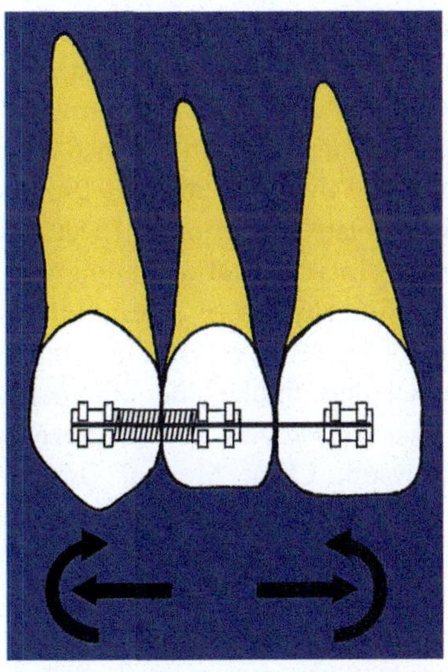

Figure 23-13 The force system created by placing an open coil spring between the crowns of the teeth is exactly the opposite of the desired force system. With an open coil spring the roots are brought closer together rather than farther apart. An appropriate interdental osteotomy site may still be developed but a greater than necessary amount of space may be created, causing inefficient postsurgical orthodontic finishing. The most important area in the interdental osteotomy is the divergence of the roots, not the crowns.

decrease the risk of damage during the interdental osteotomy, as seen in Figure 23-13.

Postsurgically, it is essential to place a continuous archwire along with a TPA to maintain not only the leveling, but also the transverse inter-arch relationship and to prevent postoperative constriction during healing. A panoramic radiograph must be taken to evaluate the root position of the teeth adjacent to the osteotomy site; if increased root divergence remains, this must be corrected during the postsurgical orthodontic finishing.

The second reason for segmenting the maxilla relates to the maxillary transverse dimension. Skeletal crossbites that are mild to moderate in magnitude (less than 5- to 6-mm) can be adequately addressed with segmental Le Fort I osteotomy. The location of the segmental osteotomy depends on the location of the desired arch expansion (see Fig. 23-11). If canine expansion is required, the canine must be in the posterior segment; if only molar and premolar expansion is desired, the canine may be included in the anterior segment. When differing amounts of canine and molar expansion are planned, a four-piece maxilla can be created with an osteotomy in the maxillary midline to increase the canine width and bilateral osteotomies between the maxillary canine and first premolar. When primarily posterior-only expansion is desired, a two-piece maxillary osteotomy with a midsagittal cut may be used. Presurgically, it is important not to make any attempts to orthodontically increase the arch width with the TPA, archwires, or cross-arch elastics because this will introduce the possibility of orthodontic relapse to the surgical procedure or the surgeon may underestimate the necessary amount of expansion (Fig. 23-14).

Postsurgically, intermaxillary fixation remains for 10 to 14 days but patients are typically left in a "horseshoe"-type splint with a palatal strut that is wired to the maxillary arch

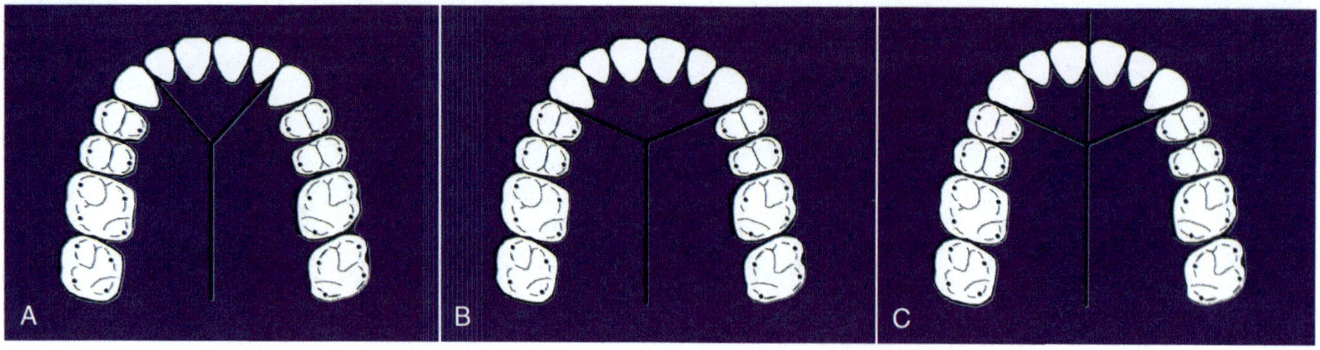

Figure 23-14 Segmental maxillary procedures can be performed in many ways and at many sites. The most common is the three-piece segmental Le Fort I osteotomy either (**A**) between the lateral incisor and canine or (**B**) between the canine and first premolar. **C**, A less common option is the four-piece segmental Le Fort I osteotomy, with segments in the midline and between the maxillary canine and first premolar. The segmentalization is shown here from the occlusal view to depict the ability to expand differentially within the arch.

for approximately 6 to 8 weeks. As close to the day of splint removal as possible (and ideally on the day the splint is removed), a continuous stainless steel maxillary archwire and either a heat-treated TPA or a labial overlay wire with a midline Coffin loop should be placed to retain the surgical expansion during bony healing. Segmental expansion of the maxilla is among the less stable surgical moves and every effort should be made orthodontically to assist in maintaining the increased arch dimension throughout the remainder of treatment. In addition, these patients should be advised of the need for indefinite retention for best long-term results. Transverse discrepancies >6- to 7-mm in the skeletally mature patient are best managed with transverse maxillary distraction osteogenesis (see the section titled "Maxillary Distraction Osteogenesis" below).

Level of Osteotomy

The level of osteotomy is classified based on Le Fort's trauma studies from the nineteenth century.[50]

1. Le Fort I level osteotomies involve movement of only the dentoalveolar portion of the maxilla. Occasionally patients will require anteroposterior augmentation of the malar area in addition to the maxilla. An intermediate surgical procedure is the "high" Le Fort I osteotomy, which goes slightly superior to the typical Le Fort I and includes a portion of the zygomatic process of the maxilla and a small portion of the inferior aspect of the zygoma.
2. Le Fort II osteotomies include the maxilla and nasal bones. One approach for the Le Fort II surgery is a subconjunctival approach. Another more extensive surgical approach involves use of a bicoronal flap.
3. Le Fort III osteotomies include the maxilla, zygoma, and nasal bones, extending superiorly to the zygomaticofrontal suture as well as the frontomaxillary suture. The typical surgical approach for the Le Fort III surgery involves a bicoronal flap.

Most nonsyndromic patients requiring maxillary surgery typically undergo a Le Fort I or high Le Fort I osteotomy when additional malar augmentation is desired. Many syndromic patients with Crouzon, Apert, Binders, Pfeiffer, or other midfacial deficiencies will undergo surgery at a Le Fort II or III level, with others having concomitant frontal bone advancement (Monobloc procedure).

MAXILLARY DISTRACTION OSTEOGENESIS

Craniofacial distraction osteogenesis is still in its relative infancy when compared to orthognathic surgery considering that the first maxillary surgery was performed in the 1860s by Cheever to access a nasopharyngeal carcinoma[51] and the first "distraction" was performed in the 1920s when Wassmund reported on a total Le Fort I osteotomy with orthopedic traction applied later to obtain the desired movement.[52] The most commonly cited person and "father of modern-day distraction osteogenesis" is Gavril Ilizarov, a Russian orthopedic surgeon who developed and refined the contemporary distraction protocol in the 1950s and 1960s.[53] The current protocol requires a latency period of 1 week, to obtain a soft callus, followed by incremental activation with a specific rate (1-mm per day) and rhythm (0.25-mm four times per day). Ilizarov's focus of attention was the long bones, particularly the femur, tibia, and fibula, and craniofacial distraction osteogenesis has developed much more recently, with McCarthy, Grayson, Chin, Molina, Guerrero, and their colleagues[54–58] among the major contributors throughout the 1990s. Maxillary and mandibular distraction have theoretical advantages over orthognathic surgery in that there is both a bony augmentation and expansion (osteogenesis) and a concurrent soft tissue expansion (histogenesis) that may produce enhanced stability. A disadvantage of distraction osteogenesis is that it cannot be used to correct growth excesses, only deficiencies, and as a result distraction is unlikely to completely replace orthognathic surgery as a means of correcting dentofacial deformities.

Maxillary Anterior Distraction

The orthodontic biomechanics for maxillary anteroposterior distraction osteogenesis are very similar to those already described for maxillary advancement surgery. The maxilla and mandible must be evaluated in all three planes of space to obtain the correct transverse, sagittal, and vertical relationship of the teeth to one another and with respect to the opposing arch. The first aspect that must be considered is the transverse relationship to ensure that when the maxilla is distracted forward, it will be wide enough to accommodate the mandible. The second aspect is the vertical relationship of the maxillary anterior and posterior teeth, since it is difficult to fit the maxilla to the mandible until both arches are level. The same intrusive and extrusive mechanisms that are used in standard orthognathic surgery are applied to the distraction.

A major difference in distraction versus surgical advancement of the maxilla is vector control. In orthognathic surgery the maxilla undergoes a single acute movement from its current to its final position, while in distraction the process is incremental. Precise and controlled movement of the maxilla during its transit is required to maximize occlusal contact and facial esthetics. To accomplish these precise movements, determining the location of the center of resistance of the maxilla is essential; then the correct movement can be planned using sound biomechanical diagnosis and treatment planning principles.

Maxillary distraction osteogenesis vector selection is very similar to procedures used for maxillary protraction headgear in growing patients. The primary difference is that the center of resistance in distraction will vary depending on the level of the osteotomy. The higher the osteotomy, the higher the center of resistance will be located. The result is that vector analysis must be unique for each patient. Previous research has localized the center of resistance of the maxilla in patients who have not had a surgical disjunction of the inferior portion of the maxilla from the cranium (Fig. 23-15).[59] Typically, in the lateral cephalogram the center of resistance is located halfway between the inferior aspect of the zygoma and the buccal cusp tip of the maxillary molar. In the PA cephalogram or coronal CBCT view, the center of resistance is approximately 2 cm lateral to the malar base on the infraorbital portion of the zygoma.

After the center of resistance of the dentomaxillary portion of the mobilized maxilla is located, the direction of force application can be determined.[60] A patient with sagittal maxillary hypoplasia with an anterior open bite will be distracted using a vector through a point anterior to and above the center of resistance to produce both advancement and a clockwise moment to bring the anterior maxilla downward and forward, increasing the amount of overbite and anteroposterior projection of the maxilla. The patient with sagittal maxillary deficiency but increased overbite will be distracted using a vector below the center of resistance of the maxilla to produce maxillary advancement and posterior inferior positioning to decrease the amount of overbite. It is essential to closely monitor the distraction weekly as it is proceeding to ensure that the desired vector of distraction is the actual vector of distraction that is obtained. Some patients will distort the distraction appliance and require modification of the original vector, or the center of resistance may be located slightly differently from originally calculated due to factors such as soft tissue attachments and tonicity.

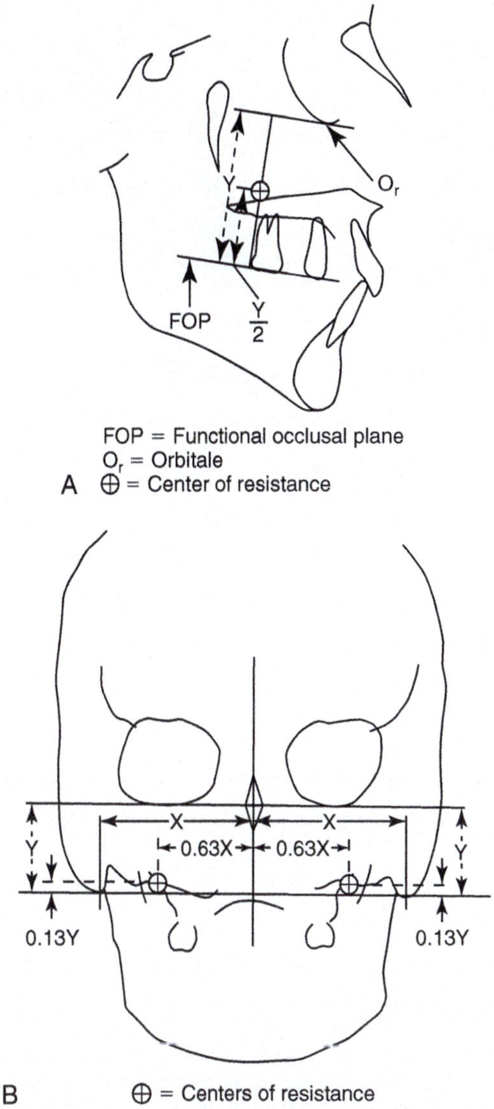

Figure 23-15 Process for localizing the center of resistance of the maxilla. Remember, however, that the level of distraction will dictate the relative position of the center of resistance. The higher the level of osteotomy (high Le Fort I, Le Fort II, or Le Fort III), the higher the center of resistance. The vector of distraction must be adjusted accordingly. (From Braun S, Bottrel JA, Lee KG, Lunazzi JJ, Legan HL. The biomechanics of rapid maxillary sutural expansion. *Am J Orthod Dentofacial Orthop.* 2000;118:257–261.)

Multiple maxillary distraction appliances are currently available. The rigid external distractor (RED) appliance uses an orthopedic halo–type of appliance that is anchored to the outer table of the cranium (Fig. 23-16). The halo serves multiple purposes. First, it is a rigid anchorage device from which to advance the maxilla. Second, and of equal importance, the halo serves as a constant reminder to the patient that the appliance must be worn to achieve the desired movement prior to consolidation of the osteotomy. Typically, a large labiolingual custom framework is fabricated and attached to the maxillary dentition. An extension is fabricated that is brought extraorally and superiorly to give the appropriate choice of vector. A connection from the

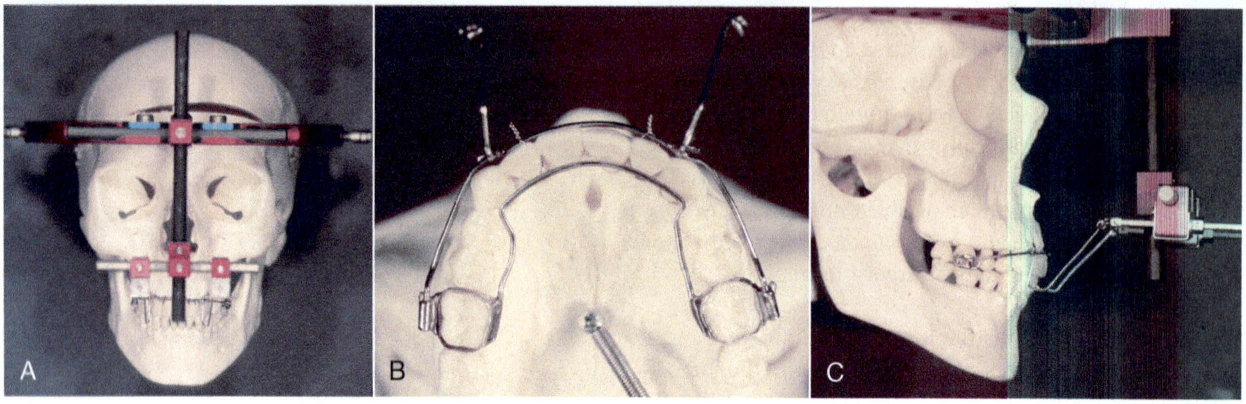

Figure 23-16 The rigid external distractor (RED) appliance is extremely versatile. **A,** From the frontal view, the halo is placed into the outer table of the cranium and serves as an extremely stable anchorage unit. **B,** From the occlusal view, one can see the rigid framework connecting all of the maxillary teeth to minimize the dental effects during distraction. **C,** The vertical pin and the associated wire extension from the rigid dental framework allow for precise force vector application relative to the center of resistance of the mobilized maxilla.

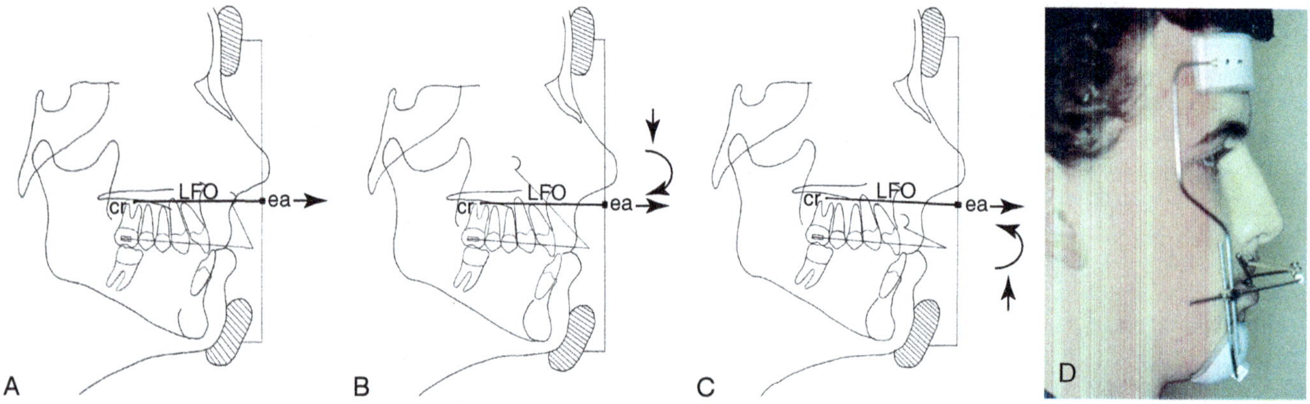

Figure 23-17 Standard protraction headgear can be used when distracting the maxilla downward and forward. For best force application a headgear bow is placed along the dentition, with the outer bow adjusted to deliver the intended vector of force. **A,** The force may be applied through the center of resistance to provide a pure translation of the maxilla. Alternatively, the outer bow may be adjusted (**B**) above or (**C**) below the center of resistance to provide either a clockwise or a counterclockwise moment to assist in bite closing or opening. **D,** A clinical example of protraction headgear using the intraoral facebow approach. *CR,* Center of resistance; *ea,* elastic attachment point; *LFO,* line of force with zero moment. (From Staggers JA, Germane N, Legan HL. Clinical considerations in the use of protraction headgear. *J Clin Orthod.* 1992;26[2]:87–91.)

extraoral wire to the vertical bar extending from the halo on the RED appliance is made with a stainless steel ligature wire. The vertical bar of the RED appliance can easily be moved superiorly, inferiorly, forward, or backward during the distraction phase to alter the vector of distraction. Some surgeons have used a transcutaneous wire from the maxillary bone plates to the vertical rod in cases where the dentition is not a good option for a maxillary handle. A possible negative side effect of the transcutaneous approach is extraoral scarring.

Another appliance is the typical maxillary protraction facemask assembly (Fig. 23-17). Orthodontically, the facemask can be used with or without a facebow but without a headgear bow the direction of distraction is severely limited because the point of force application must pass through the commissure of the lips, which is often too low. With a headgear bow, the outer bow can be adjusted into countless positions to produce the desired direction of distraction. One disadvantage of the orthodontic facemask as a distractor is possible decreased patient compliance since the facemask is not fixated to the cranium, which allows the patient to remove it.

Maxillary Transverse Distraction Osteogenesis

In the mid-1970s Kennedy[60] developed a technique for maxillary expansion of the skeletally mature patient. A subtotal Le Fort I osteotomy was performed using the same cuts as a standard Le Fort I (lateral maxillary wall, lateral nasal wall, septal release, midline osteotomy and pterygoid plate disjunction), except that the dentoalveolar portion of the maxilla was not down fractured. Once the cuts were completed, the appliance was activated approximately 2-mm to ensure complete mobilization of the maxilla and the patient was instructed to activate the appliance two turns in the morning and two turns in the evening until the desired expansion was achieved. This protocol is very similar to that of Ilizarov,[53] with one important distinction: there was no latency period. Because a soft callus was not allowed to form before activating the appliance, this protocol could not truly be called distraction osteogenesis.

The current protocol for maxillary transverse distraction osteogenesis uses Kennedy's osteotomy design and adds a latency period of approximately 1 week to promote formation of a fibrocartilaginous callus to which, once formed, traction is applied to gradually separate the bony segments (Fig. 23-18). Once the maxillary transverse distraction osteogenesis is completed, it is important to stabilize the teeth with a passive open coil spring, placement of two wire segments, or lacing the teeth until there is radiographic evidence of bone formation. Premature movement of the teeth into the distraction gap can lead to a periodontal defect and possible loss of attachment. Once adequate consolidation has occurred, maxillary midline diastema closure can proceed along a stainless steel archwire track to minimize second-order tipping.

After anterior space closure the mechanics required for the rest of the case can be initiated, such as intrusion/extrusion mechanics, space closure mechanics, and torquing arches. It is especially important to evaluate the torque of the maxillary anterior segment after significant transverse expansion, as there is a tendency for the incisors to become much more upright during retraction, which can cause difficulty in obtaining ideal overbite and overjet. An efficient way to apply torque to the four incisors uses a high alpha torquing spring (Fig. 23-19). A full-dimension, rectangular stainless steel archwire is placed, filling the incisor bracket slots. The wire is then stepped gingivally and two helices are placed to deliver a crown labial/root palatal torque. The torquing spring must be tied back to prevent incisor proclination and ensure root movement. Care must be taken to keep the force level low (~100 g) by extending the moment arms posteriorly to approximately the first molar region (~25 mm), which generates a significant proclining moment (~2000 to 2500 g/mm). An incisal step should be made in the main archwire so that it can act as a stop when placed on the incisal wings of the brackets to further minimize the possible extrusive effect.

Maxillary transverse distraction osteogenesis can be performed as an isolated procedure, as a first surgical phase to obtain the necessary space for aligning the dentition and adequate arch width prior to a second surgical phase to correct the sagittal and vertical jaw deformity, or in conjunction with mandibular symphyseal distraction osteogenesis.

Asymmetrical Advancement and Inferior Distraction

Patients with both skeletal and soft tissue deficiencies (such as hemifacial microsomia) are ideal candidates for distraction osteogenesis. The results obtained from distraction can in some cases reduce the need for additional esthetic surgery (e.g., buccal fat and alloplastic grafts) to address the associated soft tissue deficiencies. Diagnostically, the most important aspect is determining the amount of asymmetry from the clinical examination, CBCT, and computer modeling.

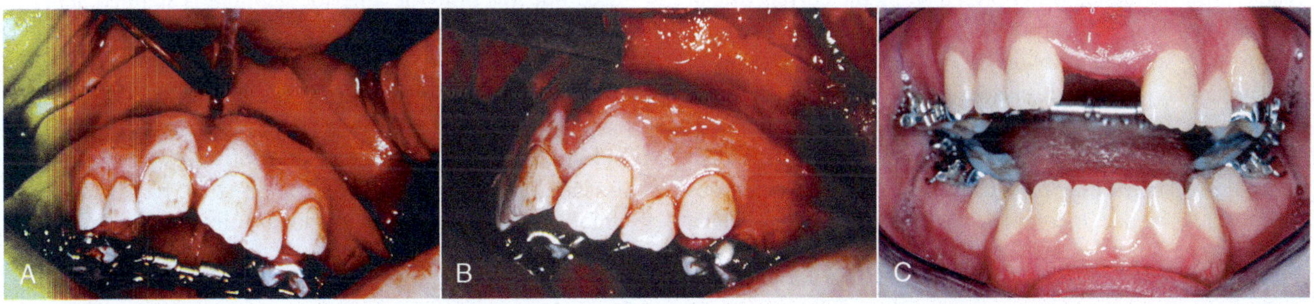

Figure 23-18 Location of the osteotomy from the **(A)** frontal and **(B)** lateral views. The osteotomy is placed at the same time that the appliance is loaded to assist in propagating the midpalatal osteotomy. **C,** Patient after completed maxillary transverse distraction osteogenesis. The total time since completion of the osteotomy is 3 weeks (1 week latency and 2 weeks of activation with two turns twice daily).

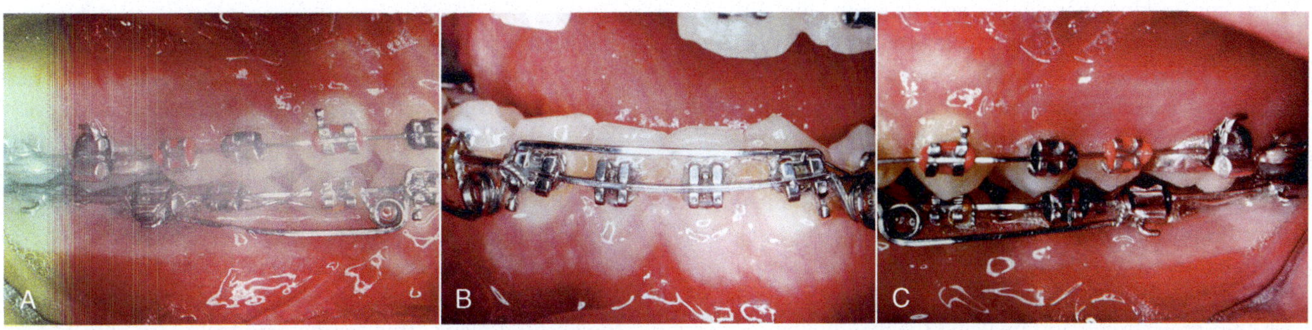

Figure 23-19 **A–C,** High alpha root spring uses a segmental approach to deliver a large moment without requiring a large vertical force. The root spring is placed into the slot of each of the anterior teeth and stepped gingivally and then two and a half helices are wound with the extensions directed posteriorly and inferiorly. A hook is then fabricated so that the spring can be placed over the main archwire in the posterior region. The longer the spring, the lower the force required and the less chance that undesirable vertical forces will be produced.

Particular attention should focus on the presence, location, and magnitude of any occlusal plane cant. The cant may be a frontal occlusal plane cant, posterior cant, or both. With only an isolated frontal occlusal plane cant, intrusive or extrusive base arches are excellent appliances to obtain the necessary correction. A rigid anterior segment can be placed, with the base arch tied only to the tooth or teeth that require intrusion. Once again, a high-pull headgear is placed with a short and elevated outer bow to prevent any posterior extrusion or posterior cant from developing. Once level, a continuous archwire can be placed to obtain coordinated maxillary and mandibular arches. Then, with level and coordinated arches, maxillary distraction can be initiated. When the same amount of cant is present posteriorly and anteriorly, it is best addressed during the distraction phase.

When distracting, extraoral appliances have a distinct advantage in that they are more easily activated, there are almost limitless choices of distraction vectors, and space is plentiful. Unfortunately, patients are more self-conscious with an extraoral appliance and the risk of significant extraoral scarring is much greater. The scars, if objectionable, can be revised by a plastic surgeon but this requires additional surgery. Intraoral appliances have the significant advantage of minimal risk of scarring; however, obtaining the correct distraction vector is more challenging. Intraorally, there is limited space for appliance placement, fewer directional change options, and more difficult visualization. In addition, activation of the appliance is somewhat more complicated, with a finite number of adjustments that can be made. If the appliance is not placed along the correct line of action, very little substantive change can be made without performing surgical revision to change the orientation of the appliance. Inter-arch elastic traction[61] can be a useful adjunct for distraction vector refinement. Unfortunately, any time elastics are placed on the teeth, dental rather than skeletal movement may be occurring, resulting in a reasonable occlusion but incomplete correction of the skeletal asymmetry.

MANDIBULAR SURGERY

Mandibular Advancement

High Angle

When considering mandibular advancement, the clinician must determine if there is a true sagittal skeletal deficiency or if the deficiency is caused by a vertical maxillary excess and an adverse downward and backward mandibular rotation. Some helpful cephalometric measurements to assist the diagnosis include mandibular length (Go-Gn), facial height (N-ANS and ANS-Gn), gonial angle (Ar-Go-Gn), mandibular projection (N-B), chin projection (N-Pg), and angle of skeletal convexity (N-A-Pg). In the high angle (steep mandibular plane, backward rotator, etc.) patient, often the effective chin projection is minimal and the mandibular incisors are extruded (lower incisor to mandibular plane distance measured perpendicular to the mandibular plane). A true mandibular deficient patient with a normal face height but steep mandibular plane can often be treated with isolated mandibular surgery. On the other hand, the patient with increased facial height as well as a steep mandibular plane will often require two-jaw surgery with a maxillary impaction and mandibular advancement.

When leveling the arches, posterior extrusion should be minimized, as it further reduces chin projection; however, if any extrusion is anticipated, it is important that it occurs prior to surgery since postsurgical extrusion could reopen the bite. A better approach focuses on intrusion of the mandibular anterior teeth and true intrusion requires segmentalization of the mandibular arch and use of an intrusive base arch or TADs. If the arch length deficiency is minimal and the position of the mandibular incisors is reasonable (lower incisor to mandibular plane angle) then a rigid anterior segment and two rigid posterior segments are fabricated. A 0.017-inch × 0.025-inch stainless steel intrusive base arch is inserted into the auxiliary tube of the molar and tied either gingival to or just labial to the mandibular incisor brackets. It is important not to insert the wire directly into the incisor brackets as torque might be present, which would produce an indeterminate force system. The torque could be additive, creating a larger intrusive effect, or negative, producing a smaller and clinically ineffective intrusive effect. Once the arch is level, a rigid stainless steel continuous archwire should be placed to maintain the overbite correction.

If the arch length deficiency is more significant or the lower incisors are proclined, a split intrusive base can be fabricated (see Fig. 23-9). The same posterior segments are used but this time the anterior segment is stepped approximately 5-mm gingivally as the wire exits the mandibular lateral incisor. The wire is then contoured to the arch and extended distally with a stop at the distal extent of the segment. Then a cantilever spring can be made (one on each side to deliver approximately 15 g of force per tooth to be intruded) and placed behind the center of resistance of the anterior segment of teeth, producing simultaneous intrusion and uprighting of the anterior teeth. By intruding the anterior teeth, the mandible can be not only advanced but also rotated counterclockwise to increase the chin projection, possibly reducing the need for a genioplasty in borderline patients.

Low Angle

The low angle (low mandibular plane, forward rotator, etc.) patient typically possesses a deep curve of Spee and decreased facial height and often presents with both Class II, Division 2 and a large bony chin button. The facial musculature (masseter, lateral, and medial pterygoids) is typically stronger and posterior dental extrusion can be difficult to achieve and maintain due to high posterior bite force.[62] One goal of treatment focuses on increasing the facial height by both extruding the teeth and advancing the mandible "downhill" along the occlusal plane. This can be extremely easy with a steep maxillary occlusal plane, as the occlusal plane will dictate the relative amount of vertical and horizontal mandibular change in isolated mandibular advancement surgery. Unfortunately, most low angle patients have a normal to flat occlusal plane, so additional techniques must be employed.

Timing of the leveling can dramatically increase the orthodontic efficiency. An extremely efficient way to obtain leveling is to perform the mandibular advancement surgery early in treatment prior to leveling the curve of Spee. Prior to rigid fixation, the mandible is advanced to an edge-to-edge incisor relationship and occlusion on the second molars and the patient is fixated with an anterior and/or superior border wire and an interocclusal splint. After adequate healing time, the splint is removed and intermaxillary elastics in the mid arch are used. The maxilla will have a rigid archwire and the mandible will have a relatively nonrigid wire, such as a 0.018-inch stainless steel wire. Once the elastics have leveled the mandibular arch, a more rigid mandibular wire is placed (see Fig. 23-10). Two processes may be occurring simultaneously to account for the efficiency in leveling. First, it is certainly easier to erupt teeth into air than into heavy bite forces. Second, a regional accelerative phenomenon takes place in the period shortly after surgery. It is speculated that this is due to the increased vascularization that occurs as part of normal wound healing.[47] With rigid fixation, less immediate postsurgical relapse occurs and the mandible does not need to be placed in an edge-to-edge "tripod" occlusion but merely into Class I with a mid arch open bite. The fixation allows for use of elastics almost immediately after surgery, unlike with wire fixation where heavy elastic traction applied too quickly to the mid arch results in "bending" of the bone (similar to that in Fig. 23-4), producing an inferior border notch. If the patient has too much chin projection and some facial lengthening is still desired, a vertical lengthening genioplasty with minimal advancement can also be performed to increase the lower face height.

Mandibular Setback

Isolated mandibular setback procedures are less common today than in the past. More frequently, maxillary advancement with or without mandibular setback is employed.[37] In addition, some advocate that there are few indications for isolated mandibular setback due to the fear that it will cause OSA. Cephalometric measurements that assist in the diagnosis of mandibular hyperplasia include increased mandibular projection (N-B), chin projection (N-Pg), and a normal maxillary projection (N-A, and G′-Sn). Care must be taken during diagnosis to evaluate the soft tissue drape of the lower face and neck, especially the lower face throat angle and lower face throat height/depth ratio to prevent inappropriate setback of the mandibular arch and avoid creating both airway and soft tissue esthetic problems.

One of the most common findings in mandibular hyperplastic patients are dentally compensated, retroclined mandibular incisors. The lower incisor to mandibular plane angle can often be in the mid 70-degree range and the labial mucosa is often thin, making adequate decompensation of the lower incisors quite challenging. An efficient mechanism for lower incisor torque correction is the high alpha root spring (see Fig. 23-19). The root spring is an auxiliary full-size archwire that is placed directly into the lower incisor brackets. The wire exits the brackets and is stepped gingivally, helices are placed bilaterally, and the activated distal archwire extension is then clipped over the main archwire as far posteriorly as possible. The longer the wire, the greater the moment generated and the more efficient the root spring will be. With shorter root springs, significantly higher forces are required to generate the same moment, which has the tendency to cause unwanted mandibular incisor extrusion. To minimize the extrusive component, the main archwire is placed in the posterior brackets and then stepped incisally to rest on top of the incisal tie wings of the mandibular incisor brackets. If incisor proclination is desired, the root spring does not need to be tied back as tightly but the force level should be reduced to prevent overproclination of the incisors.

Many Class III mandibular hyperplastic patients will present with minimal mandibular arch length deficiency and minimal curve of Spee. A crossbite may exist as well but often it is relatively minor when the patient is placed in a Class I molar and canine position. Refer to the section on maxillary advancement for discussion regarding the transverse dimension.

The orthodontic treatment to remove the dental compensations should be the same whether a SSRO or IVRO is performed. Technically, the IVRO is a much simpler, faster, and less morbid procedure compared to the SSRO. When performing the setback, care must be directed toward proximal segment positioning. A critical error that occasionally occurs involves improper positioning of the proximal segment with the condyle pushed too far posteriorly in the fossa. When the intermaxillary fixation is removed, the proximal segment assumes its physiologic position, causing the mandible to rotate forward and reproducing the Class III malocclusion. If the proximal segment is instead positioned anteriorly, the patient will exhibit a Class II open-bite malocclusion upon release from the intermaxillary fixation. To avoid these complications some surgeons elect to perform the IVRO for mandibular setback because without rigid fixation, the condyle assumes a "physiologic" position during intermaxillary fixation while the rigid fixation utilized during SSRO does not.

MANDIBULAR DISTRACTION OSTEOGENESIS

Mandibular Symphyseal Widening

Prior to distraction osteogenesis, attempts were made to widen the mandibular arch by other means[63,64] but most clinical research has suggested that nonsurgical attempts to widen the mandibular arch will not be successful in the long-term.[65] Distraction osteogenesis offers new possibilities for expansion and is the only mandibular expansion alternative with the potential to increase the mandibular basal and alveolar bone in a stable manner.

Many articles have described the diagnostic and treatment planning criteria regarding mandibular symphyseal distraction osteogenesis.[66,67] The classic patient presents with a buccal crossbite that completely encompasses the narrow mandible. In patients with both a narrow maxilla and a narrow mandible, expansion in the maxilla was previously limited by the inability to expand the mandible; now both can be expanded simultaneously.

Presurgically, root divergence of the mandibular anterior teeth is required. Much like the interdental osteotomy in the maxilla, the midsagittal mandibular osteotomy requires adequate interradicular space.[68] A compressed open coil spring will produce crown divergence but can actually produce root convergence since the moment/force ratio is sufficient to produce only simple tipping with the center of rotation between the center of resistance and the root apex. One way to obtain the necessary root divergence preoperatively is by exaggerating the second-order bracket position. If this is done for all mandibular incisors, care must be taken to avoid extrusion of the mandibular central incisors due to the excessive tip placed in the lateral brackets. In addition, a superelastic wire should not be used because it cannot be stepped to minimize the incisor extrusion. Confirmation of the root divergence should be done with periapical or panoramic radiographs. A second method to obtain the root divergence requires a vertical tube/slot in the incisor brackets and fabricating a modified root spring (see Fig. 23-12). The spring should exit the vertical slot, have a helix, and then extend posteriorly and clip over the archwire. This root spring will produce extrusion but also lateral root movement of the incisors. The force should be kept as low as possible to minimize the extrusive effects yet due to the long moment arm the root spring will still be extremely efficient. Once agreement between the surgeon and the orthodontist is reached, the osteotomy can be performed.

Postsurgically, a short latency period (approximately 1 week) is observed to allow for soft callus formation. Then the appliance is activated no more than 1-mm each day until the desired expansion has been obtained. The teeth are prevented from drifting toward the midline for approximately 30 to 60 days. After approximately 3 months or when radiographic evidence of new symphyseal bone is observed, the appliance can be removed and a passive 0.036-inch stainless steel lower lingual arch can be placed to maintain the expansion. At this point continuous stainless steel wires should be used as well. After appliance removal, the space is closed as it would be in any other arch length redundancy case.

An important consideration during distraction osteogenesis relates to the magnitude and direction of movement that occurs at the mandibular condyle.[69] A recent clinical study has shown that there appears to be translation at the condyle with no clinically significant effects or development of any joint symptoms.[70] As the procedure is performed more frequently, larger study groups will provide further information.

Mandibular Advancement

Some patients who have historically been treated with SSRO advancements are now being treated with distraction osteogenesis. While distraction osteogenesis itself is not new, adapting it to the craniofacial skeleton is a more recent application of the procedure. Codivilla first used distraction in 1924 but the process did not become popular until the early 1990s. Grayson and McCormick, Molina, and others have described distraction as an excellent mechanism for craniofacial anomalies such as hemifacial microsomia, Goldenhar syndrome, and Pierre Robin sequence.[55–58]

When considering distraction osteogenesis, the principles of preparing the dentition are the same as those for standard orthognathic surgery. The main difference is that the mandibular skeletal change will be accomplished using small incremental movements rather than a significant and acute positional change in orthognathic surgery. The precise planning of the distraction vector presurgically is critical to obtain and control the correct shape and form of distraction callus.

Prior to orthognathic surgery, either CASS or traditional model surgery is performed, a custom splint is fabricated, and the amount and direction of the jaw movement is determined. The interocclusal splint is then used intraoperatively to determine the final position of the mandible. With distraction, the direction of movement to obtain the desired occlusion is extremely important. Presurgical models must be taken to ensure that the occlusion will fit when the final distraction position is obtained. Once accomplished, the vector of distraction needs to be determined, requiring localization of the center of resistance of the proximal and distal segments, which will depend on the age of the patient, geometry of the osteotomy, size and shape of the bony segments, bone density, and muscle strength and pull. Due to tremendous anatomic and surgical variation, no single common center of resistance for mandibular distraction patients exists.

The correct appliance to deliver the appropriate vertical and horizontal distraction must be selected. The simplest distraction procedure is the uniplaner mandibular distraction where only sagittal distraction is needed. The appliance most often should be oriented to distract the proximal and distal segments parallel to the occlusal plane. Any distraction force applied in a direction other than parallel to the occlusal plane will produce rotation of the segments, creating an iatrogenic malocclusion. Occasionally the newly formed regenerate tissue must be "molded" with extraoral or intraoral forces[61] to obtain the desired result due to anatomic restrictions that limit appliance placement. With a deep bite patient it may be possible to orient the distractor above the level of the center of resistance in the distal segment. A moment will be generated that should produce a clockwise or bite-opening rotation. Too steep an angulation, however, could result in creating an open bite. Open-bite patients may be able to have the same distractor placed but below the level of the center of resistance of the distal segment. That way a counterclockwise or bite-closing rotation can be created. Any time the distractor is placed to produce rotation in addition to sagittal displacement, greater care and observation should be performed. An inadequately supervised distraction can quickly progress in an unanticipated direction with the rotation produced, creating a need for mid-distraction correction.

Biplanar distraction is much more difficult to assess and obtain (Fig. 23-20). Fabrication of a plastic skull constructed from a three-dimensional CT scan can be a useful aid prior to surgery to determine the location of the appliance (Fig. 23-21). Then the relative amount of vertical and horizontal distraction can be calculated with a predetermined activation schedule and sequence. Most importantly, the patient must be observed frequently to evaluate the distraction process to ensure that the protocol is delivering the desired result.

Just as a protraction headgear using a headgear bow can deliver forces in many different directions relative to the center of resistance, the force from a transcutaneous distraction appliance can deliver similar adjustability. The mechanical advantage of the transmucosal appliances comes at a cost, namely the possibility of scar track formation. The scar

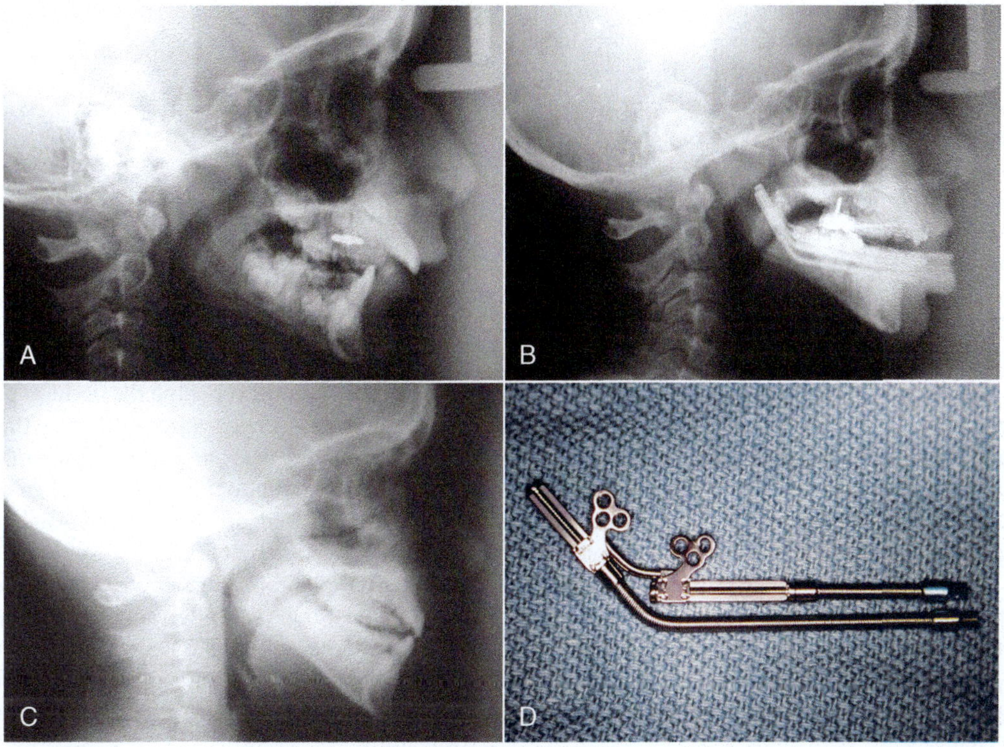

Figure 23-20 Accurate and precise biplanar mandibular distraction is difficult to achieve due to limitations of the intraoral appliances as well as anatomic space limitations. The vector of distraction is just as important here as with maxillary distraction to achieve the optimal result. Here, the appliance is located to attempt to distract the mandible forward with a slight counterclockwise rotation to simultaneously correct the mandibular deficiency and reduce the open bite. No studies are available to determine the center of resistance of the proximal and distal segment, so clinical judgment, relative size of the segments, and anatomic variation must be considered to estimate the proper appliance placement. **A,** Pre-treatment cephalograph. **B,** Cephalograph immediately following distraction. **C,** Post-treatment cephalograph. **D,** Appliance used.

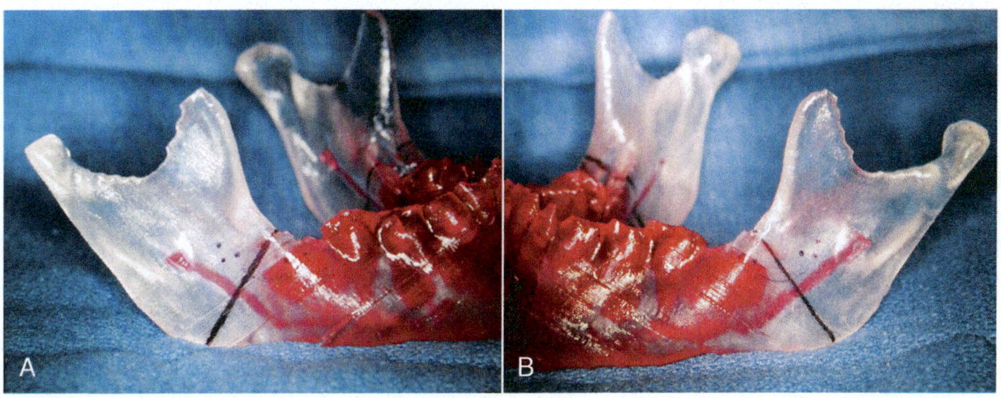

Figure 23-21 **A and B,** To assist in localizing the center of resistance of the proximal and distal segments, a plastic reconstruction of the patient's jaw can be fabricated. The patient is sent for a three-dimensional computed tomography (CT) scan and the model is precisely milled. The planned appliance placement can be attempted on the model to assess feasibility before proceeding to surgery.

tracks, if created, can be revised with plastic surgery procedures but most patients elect to receive the less invasive, less morbid, intraoral appliances.

Occlusal Plane Change

Limited changes in the pitch of the treatment occlusal plane can be performed with isolated maxillary or isolated mandibular surgery. Of course, the occlusal plane alteration is limited by the jaw that is not being surgically manipulated. To obtain an occlusal plane change with isolated mandibular or isolated maxillary surgery, attention is directed to the position of the teeth in each arch relative to the current occlusal plane. High mandibular plane angle patients benefit facially from flattening of the occlusal plane. To accomplish this change the mandible needs to be leveled with anterior intrusion rather than extrusion of the posterior teeth, allowing the mandible to be rotated counterclockwise, closing the gonial angle, and flattening the mandibular occlusal plane. With maxillary advancement patients, the occlusal plane can be flattened or steepened but extreme caution should be exercised as to how the occlusal plane flattening occurs, due to stability concerns. The maxillary occlusal plane may be flattened if the anterior aspect of the maxilla is elevated but it is unwise to inferiorly position the posterior maxilla. Such lengthening produces pterygomasseteric muscle stretch, which is inherently unstable. The maxillary occlusal plane change is limited because it must still articulate with the unchanged mandible. Typically, when the maxillary occlusal plane is changed and no mandibular surgery is performed, a complete Le Fort I osteotomy (with or without segmentalization) is performed, the maxilla is placed in intermaxillary fixation, and the entire complex is rotated to the desired position. In a Class I vertical maxillary excess patient, this requires a slight maxillary advancement along with the occlusal plane change.

For maximal occlusal plane change, two-jaw surgery is required. Then the maxilla, mandible, and occlusal plane can be moved in all three planes of space, depending on the diagnostic and treatment planning goals for ideal stability, function, and esthetics.[49] As a general geometric rule, steepening the occlusal plane will take a patient who is dentally Class II and make him or her closer to Class I (Fig. 23-22). This is not unlike using a cervical headgear, Class II elastics, or some other type of functional appliance in the growing patient. However, steepening the occlusal plane will tend to make the facial profile more convex (i.e., closer to Class II).

Flattening the pitch of the occlusal plane will have a tendency to take a Class III malocclusion and make the apical base discrepancy closer to Class I. However, flattening the occlusal plane with two-jaw surgery will make the facial profile less convex (i.e., flatter and closer to Class III). A common example of manipulating the pitch of the occlusal plane to the patient's benefit occurs in the patient who has a very convex profile yet displays a Class I malocclusion. Since the Class I bite limits the possible advancement of the mandible relative to the maxilla, a desirable change in the profile can be achieved only by surgically flattening the occlusal plane.

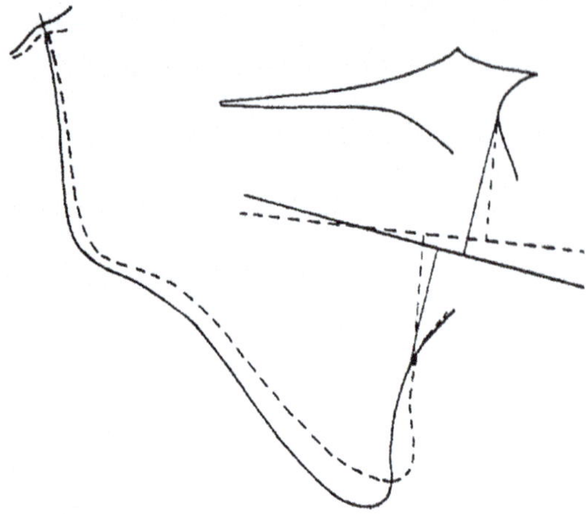

Fig. 23-22 Steepening the occlusal plane can assist in improving the apical base relationship, allowing the Class II dental relationship to be corrected. The clockwise mandibular rotation results in a more convex profile that can negatively affect facial esthetics.

The most common two-jaw surgical patient displays vertical maxillary excess (Fig. 23-23). The goal of treatment typically focuses on steepening the occlusal plane by impacting the maxilla (usually more posteriorly than anteriorly as in an open-bite patient) and allowing the mandible to autorotate. Then either a mandibular advancement or a setback is performed based on the occlusal result after maxillary impaction. Several practitioners have focused on flattening the occlusal plane in the same type of patient to produce greater gonial angle definition and chin augmentation. While the facial results appear excellent, the counterclockwise rotation of the dentomaxillary complex is inherently unstable and few, if any, practitioners routinely perform this type of osteotomy.

Other patients that benefit from occlusal plane changes include some of the Class III maxillary hypoplastic syndromic patients. Typical patients present with Apert syndrome or Crouzon syndrome, achondroplasia, or cleft lip and palate. All of these patients to some degree would benefit from a clockwise rotation of the maxilla and mandible and in some cases of the frontal bone. The occlusion may be near Class I dentally but skeletally presents as Class III. By rotating the entire complex clockwise, the relative mandibular projection is minimized, allowing greater projection of the frontal bone and maxilla. The initial dental malocclusion can be corrected orthodontically and the occlusal change then maintained throughout.

USE OF TADs FOR THE ORTHOGNATHIC SURGERY PATIENT

The use of TADs has increased significantly in routine clinical practice and has made it possible to make orthodontic movements that previously were inefficient, difficult, or impossible. Like any tool, their use must be planned proactively to maximize the potential benefit. TADs can be used

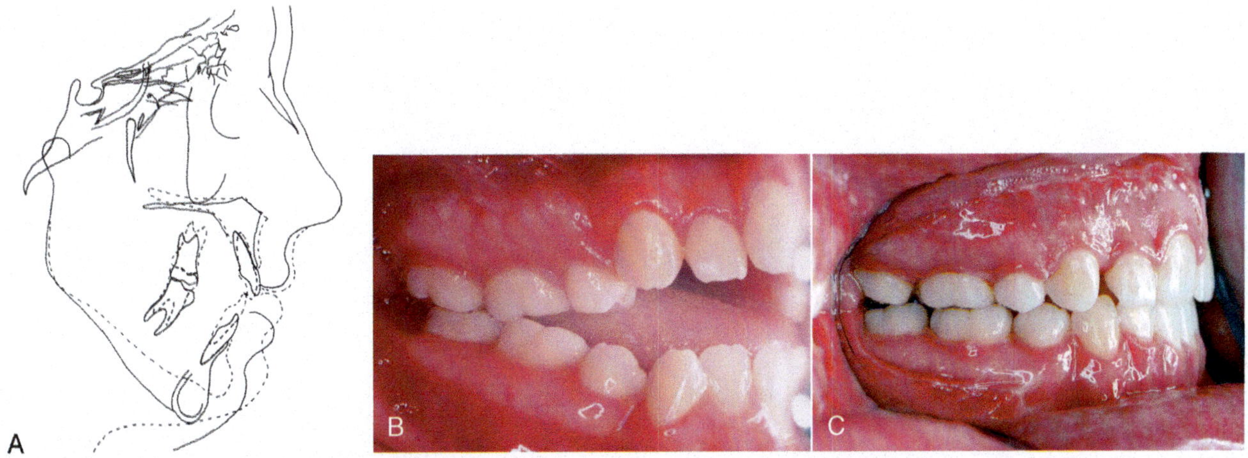

Figure 23-23 **A,** Superimposition depicts the entire surgical manipulation resulting from steepening the occlusal plane in an anterior open-bite patient. **B,** Pre-treatment, a 9-mm anterior open bite was observed. The entire maxilla was impacted, with more impaction posteriorly than anteriorly. **C,** Significant mandibular counterclockwise rotation was observed, which assisted in closing the open bite.

presurgically to assist with orthodontic decompensation, challenging leveling situations, or during space closure to facilitate the ideal anchorage. In some situations TADs are being used as an adjunct intraoperatively during intermaxillary fixation should multiple brackets debond during surgery. Finally, they can be used postoperatively to facilitate the postsurgical finishing that is increasingly more common with the "surgery first" approach to treatment.[71,72] TADs should be used judiciously and should not be used in place of orthodontic mechanics planning; rather, they should be used to facilitate more precise tooth movements when anchorage is critical or traditional orthodontics is unable to deliver the optimal force system. Some have advocated their use in borderline orthognathic cases to intrude posterior teeth[73] but as of yet stability studies have not been performed and the results that appear in the literature may not be sustained post-treatment.

In one case, the patient presented to the office following a failed orthodontics-only treatment approach. Mandibular premolars had been extracted during the first stage of orthodontics, interdental space was created in the maxillary arch, and the previous orthodontist was unable to obtain positive overbite and overjet or an acceptable result. The maxillary incisors were overly proclined and the mandibular incisors were upright. Even though the patient had large spaces remaining, she did not want dental implants. The patient had a Class III skeletal relationship with maxillary hypoplasia and mandibular hyperplasia and a significant facial asymmetry requiring orthodontics and two-jaw surgery. For an optimal facial change, significant retraction and uprighting of the maxillary incisors and protraction of the mandibular posterior teeth were needed. The teeth were aligned, the space was consolidated between segments, and the patient underwent segmental anterior maxillary setback and mandibular anterior subapical surgery to close the majority of the space. Following surgery, TADs were placed in each quadrant for indirect anchorage along with continuous arch beta-titanium T-loops because anchorage was critical so that the Class I canine relationship would not be lost during the postsurgical finishing and final space closure. The patient is now nearing completion with "routine" orthodontics (Fig. 23-24). TADs may be applied to many other presurgical and postsurgical orthodontic movements to further enhance the combined surgical-orthodontics result and treatment efficiency.

ORTHOGNATHIC SURGERY FOR OBSTRUCTIVE SLEEP APNEA

Chronic OSA can be a severely debilitating disorder. People of all ages can be affected but middle-aged adult males who are moderately to severely overweight have the highest prevalence of the disease.[74] Women can be affected by OSA but to a lesser degree.[75] Due to expertise in craniofacial and dentofacial anomalies, orthodontic professionals should be equipped to provide treatment for OSA patients. Several treatment modalities exist to improve a patient's sleep pattern,[76–80] with some of the most successful treatment modalities involving maxillomandibular advancement (MMA) surgery to advance both jaws.[81–84]

Presurgical orthodontic therapy for MMA should focus on all three planes of space just as with any other surgical orthodontic patient and the resulting treatment plan must include where the teeth will be positioned within each jaw and where each jaw will be positioned relative to the cranial base. However, with the significant sagittal movements performed in sleep apnea surgery (10- to 12-mm routine advancement with occasional advancement of 20-plus mm), routine orthognathic surgery planning, timing, and orthodontic preparation may need to be modified.

One modification affects the transverse dimension. Surgeons who may not hesitate to segment the maxilla in routine cases are often quite concerned about this technique when combined with the large MMA advancements, due to concern that the palatal pedicle that provides the vascular support for the maxilla is being stretched significantly with

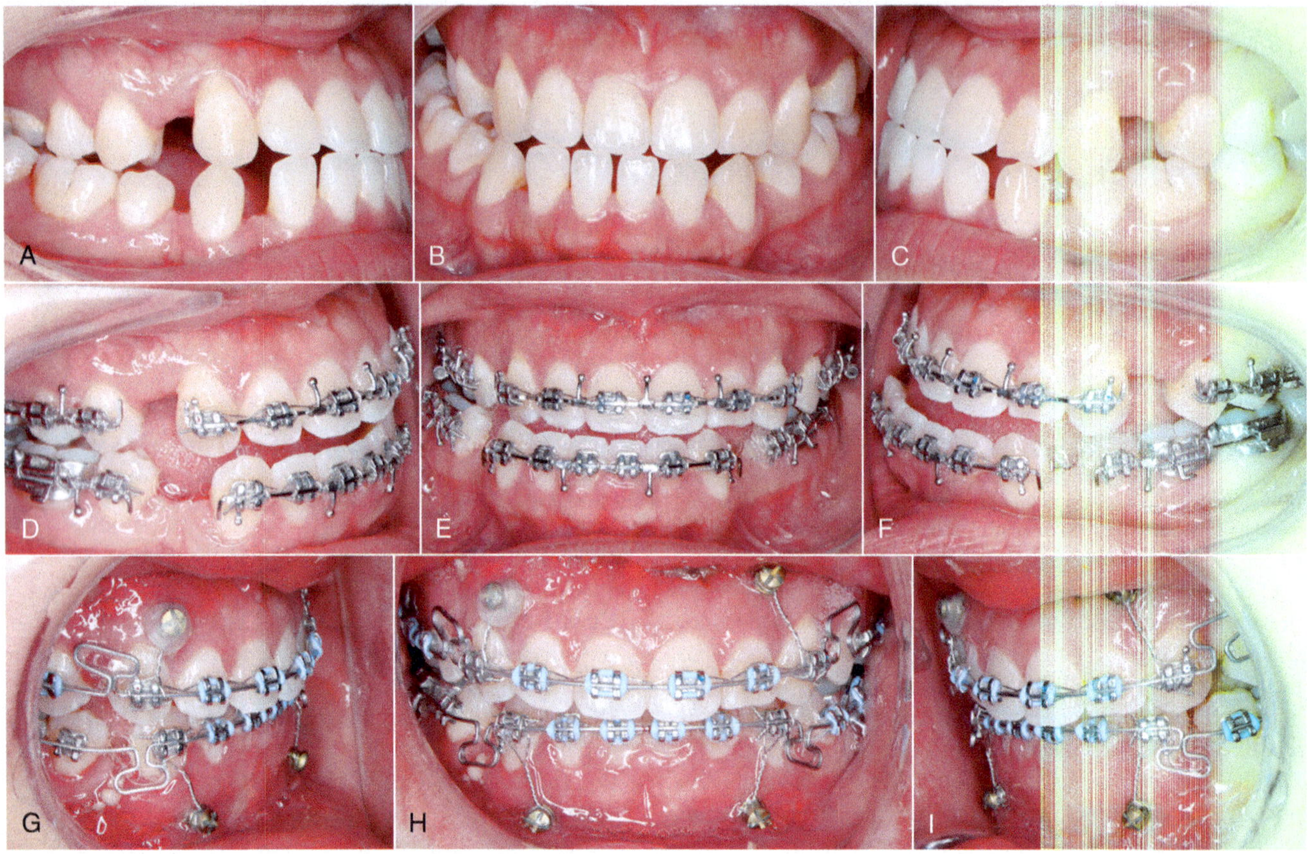

Figure 23-24 The patient underwent previous orthodontic treatment with attempts at camouflage that were unsuccessful, leading to debonding. The patient was not satisfied with care and sought a combined orthodontic and surgical treatment plan. **A–C,** Pre-treatment frontal and lateral intraoral views showing significant spacing created in the maxillary arch and incomplete space closure in the lower arch following lower first premolar extraction. **D–F,** Presurgical frontal and lateral intraoral photographs showing consolidation of the spacing into segments in preparation for segmental osteotomies in both arches. **G–I,** Six-week postsurgical frontal and lateral intraoral views taken on the day the splint was removed. TADs were placed due to the critical anchorage requirements necessary to close the space while maintaining overjet and overbite.

the maxillary advancement alone. Additional stretch of the pedicle by segmentation raises the risk of kinking the pedicle, possibly resulting in a decrease of the vascular supply and an increased risk of segment necrosis.

A second modification affects the orientation of the occlusal plane. Even with the positive effect that significant MMA advancements have on airway, steepening of the occlusal plane (clockwise rotation of the maxillary occlusal plane) should be avoided whenever possible, as it tends to make the face more convex and can reduce the favorable effect on airway dimension. As a result, many patients will have the occlusal plane maintained or more likely flattened (counterclockwise rotation) during the MMA for maximum chin projection and airway opening. Should the chin projection be too extreme, a genial recontouring that maintains the position of the genial tubercles rather than a reduction genioplasty is more likely to be performed than a sagittal reduction genioplasty because the goal is to put tension on the soft tissue for airway opening rather than decrease tissue tension.

A third modification is the timing of the surgery. Patients with OSA have often struggled with the condition for years and undergone multiple forms of treatment, including previous soft tissue surgery that proved ineffective. To maximally benefit these patients, earlier surgery (ideally within 6 months or less of starting orthodontics) is extremely advantageous, as it can free them from their dependence on continuous positive air pressure machines and allow them to resume normal lives. Earlier surgery may require accepting a presurgical setup that is "close" but may not be ideal as long as appropriate postsurgical orthodontic care will still provide a functional occlusion. Patients must also be informed that the decreased presurgical orthodontic time may result in a longer postsurgical orthodontic finishing phase. While the goal of MMA is a favorable effect on airway, postoperative malocclusion, though a published risk, should be avoided at all costs so that one function limitation is not traded for another (Fig. 23-25).

SUMMARY

Appropriate orthodontic planning and treatment strategies can be the difference between simply treating a patient and treating a patient successfully. When jaw surgery is combined with orthodontic tooth movement, greater care must be taken with the diagnosis and treatment plan as well as with the treatment mechanics. Proper mechanics contribute

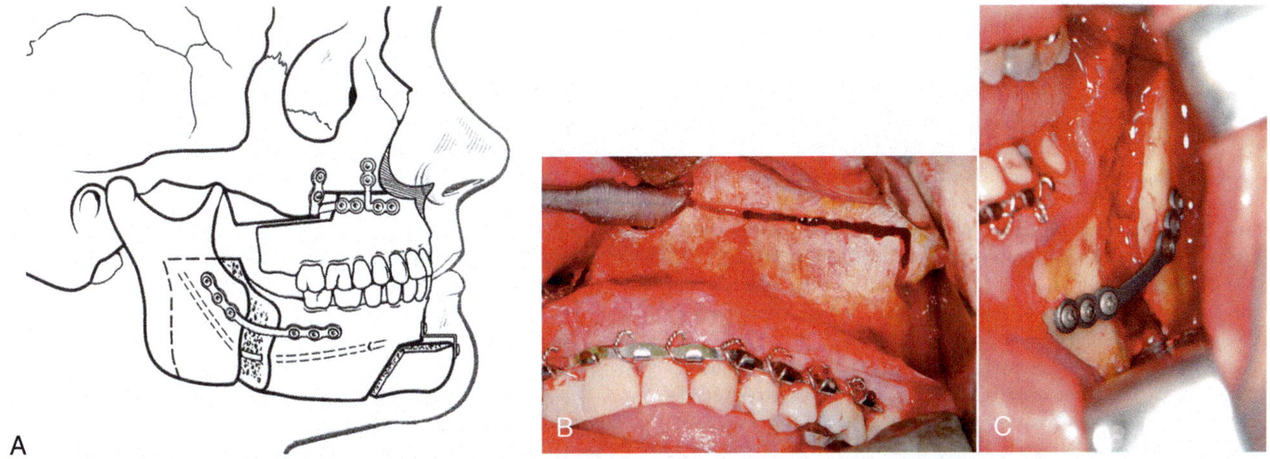

Figure 23-25 **A,** The diagram represents the maxillomandibular advancement (MMA) surgery that is performed to successfully treat the obstructive sleep apnea (OSA) patient. Clinical photos demonstrate the osteotomy design and fixation for **(B)** the maxilla and **(C)** the mandible. (**A** courtesy Vanderbilt University Medical Arts Group, with consultation from Scott B. Boyd, DDS, PhD.)

efficiency, stability, enhanced esthetics, and better function to the surgical-orthodontic patient's result. The approach to orthodontic planning and mechanical strategies presented here is an attempt to provide an accurate, precise, planned, and predictable operator-determined treatment delivery system. In this manner, harmony among the dental, skeletal, and soft tissue components may be achieved in all three planes of space.

REFERENCES

1. Wylie GA, Fish LC, Epker BN. Cephalometrics: a comparison of five analyses currently used in the diagnosis of dentofacial deformities. *Int J Adult Orthodon Orthognath Surg.* 1987;2(1):15–36.
2. Ricketts RM. Perspectives in the clinical application of cephalometrics: the first fifty years. *Angle Orthod.* 1981;51(2):115–150.
3. Steiner C. Cephalometrics for you and me. *Am J Orthod.* 1953;39(10): 729–755.
4. Broca M. Sur les projections de la tete et sur un noveau procede de cephalometrie. *Bull Soc Antropol.* 1862;3:514–544.
5. Burstone CJ, James RB, Legan H, Murphy GA, Norton LA. Cephalometrics for orthognathic surgery. *J Oral Surg.* 1978;36(4):269–277.
6. Legan HL, Burstone CJ. Soft tissue cephalometric analysis for orthognathic surgery. *J Oral Surg.* 1980;38(10):744–751.
7. Betts NJ, Vanarsdall RL, Barber HD, Higgins-Barber K, Fonseca RJ. Diagnosis and treatment of transverse maxillary deficiency. *Int J Adult Orthodon Orthognath Surg.* 1995;10(2):75–96.
8. Grummons DC, Kappeyne van de Coppello MA. A frontal asymmetry analysis. *J Clin Orthod.* 1987;21(7):448–465.
9. Major PW, Johnson DE, Hesse KL, Glover KE. Effect of head orientation on posterior anterior cephalometric landmark identification. *Angle Orthod.* 1996;66(1):51–60.
10. Major PW, Johnson DE, Hesse KL, Glover KE. Landmark identification error in posterior anterior cephalometrics. *Angle Orthod.* 1994;64(6): 447–454.
11. Bholsithi W, Tharanon W, Chintakanon K, Komolpis R, Sinthanayothin C. 3D vs 2D cephalometric analysis comparisons with repeated measurements from 20 Thai males and 20 Thai females. *Biomed Imaging Interv J.* 2009;5(4):e21.
12. Papé R, Pizelle C, Foucart JM. Measurement errors in 3D cephalometrics: about the buccal cranio-facial analysis [in French]. *Orthod Fr.* 2012;83(1):37–44.
13. van Vlijmen OJ, Maal T, Bergé SJ, Bronkhorst EM, Katsaros C, Kuijpers-Jagtman AM. A comparison between 2D and 3D cephalometry on CBCT scans of human skulls. *Int J Oral Maxillofac Surg.* 2010; 39(2):156–160.
14. Zamora N, Llamas JM, Cibrián R, Gandia J, Paredes V. A study on the reproducibility of cephalometric landmarks when undertaking a three-dimensional (3D) cephalometric analysis. *Med Oral Patol Oral Cir Bucal.* 2012;17(4):e678–e688.
15. Chenin DL. 3D cephalometrics: the new norm. *Alpha Omegan.* 2010;103(2):51–56.
16. Fuhrmann R, Feifel H, Schnappauf A, Diedrich P. Integration of three-dimensional cephalometry and 3D-skull models in combined orthodontic/surgical treatment planning. *J Orofac Orthop.* 1996;57(1): 32–45.
17. Noguchi N, Tsuji M, Shigematsu M, Goto M. An orthognathic simulation system integrating teeth, jaw and face data using 3D cephalometry. *Int J Oral Maxillofac Surg.* 2007;36(7):640–645.
18. Olszewski R, Cosnard G, Macq B, Mahy P, Reychler H. 3D CT-based cephalometric analysis: 3D cephalometric theoretical concept and software. *Neuroradiology.* 2006;48(11):853–862.
19. Gateno J, Xia JJ, Teichgraeber JF, et al. Clinical feasibility of computer-aided surgical simulation (CASS) in the treatment of complex cranio-maxillofacial deformities. *J Oral Maxillofac Surg.* 2007;65(4):728–734.
20. Xia JJ, Gateno J, Teichgraeber JF. Three-dimensional computer-aided surgical simulation for maxillofacial surgery. *Atlas Oral Maxillofac Surg Clin North Am.* 2005;13(1):25–39.
21. Xia JJ, Shevchenko L, Gateno J, et al. Outcome study of computer-aided surgical simulation in the treatment of patients with craniomaxillofacial deformities. *J Oral Maxillofac Surg.* 2011;69(7):2014–2024.
22. Plooij JM, Naphausen MT, Maal TJ, et al. 3D evaluation of the lingual fracture line after a bilateral sagittal split osteotomy of the mandible. *Int J Oral Maxillofac Surg.* 2009;38(12):1244–1249.
23. Hunsuck EE. A modified intraoral sagittal splitting technic for correction of mandibular prognathism. *J Oral Surg.* 1968;26(4):250–253.
24. Lee W, Park JU. Three-dimensional evaluation of positional change of the condyle after mandibular setback by means of bilateral sagittal split ramus osteotomy. *Oral Surg Oral Med Oral Pathol Oral Radiol Endod.* 2002;94(3):305–309.
25. Helm G, Stepke MT. Maintenance of the preoperative condyle position in orthognathic surgery. *J Craniomaxillofac Surg.* 1997;25(1): 34–38.
26. Landes CA. Proximal segment positioning in bilateral sagittal split osteotomy: intraoperative dynamic positioning and monitoring by sonography. *J Oral Maxillofac Surg.* 2004;62(1):22–28.
27. Landes CA, Sterz M. Proximal segment positioning in bilateral sagittal split osteotomy: intraoperative controlled positioning by a positioning splint. *J Oral Maxillofac Surg.* 2003;61(12):1423–1431.

28. Politi M, Toro C, Costa F, Polini F, Robiony M. Intraoperative awakening of the patient during orthognathic surgery: a method to prevent the condylar sag. *J Oral Maxillofac Surg*. 2007;65(1):109–114.
29. Renzi G, Becelli R, Di Paolo C, Iannetti G. Indications to the use of condylar repositioning devices in the surgical treatment of dental-skeletal class III. *J Oral Maxillofac Surg*. 2003;61(3):304–309.
30. Baek SH, Kim K, Choi JY. Evaluation of treatment modality for skeletal Class III malocclusion with labioversed upper incisors and/or protrusive maxilla: surgical movement and stability of rotational maxillary setback procedure. *J Craniofac Surg*. 2009;20(6):2049–2054.
31. Gu G, Nagata J, Suto M, et al. Hyoid position, pharyngeal airway and head posture in relation to relapse after the mandibular setback in skeletal Class III. *Clin Orthod Res*. 2000;3(3):67–77.
32. Jakobsone G, Stenvik A, Sandvik L, Espeland L. Three-year follow-up of bimaxillary surgery to correct skeletal Class III malocclusion: stability and risk factors for relapse. *Am J Orthod Dentofacial Orthop*. 2011; 139(1):80–89.
33. Mucedero M, Coviello A, Baccetti T, Franchi L, Cozza P. Stability factors after double-jaw surgery in Class III malocclusion: a systematic review. *Angle Orthod*. 2008;78(6):1141–1152.
34. Lloyd T, Drage N, Cronin A. The role of cone beam computed tomography in the management of unfavorourable fractures following sagittal split mandibular osteotomy. *J Orthod*. 2011;38(1):48–54.
35. Braun S, Hnat WP, Johnson BE. The curve of Spee revisited. *Am J Orthod Dentofacial Orthop*. 1996;110(2):206–210.
36. Bell WH, Fonseca RJ, Kenneky JW, Levy BM. Bone healing and revascularization after total maxillary osteotomy. *J Oral Surg*. 1975;33(4): 253–260.
37. Bailey LT, Proffit WR, White RP Jr. Trends in surgical treatment of Class III skeletal relationships. *Int J Adult Orthodon Orthognath Surg*. 1995;10(2):108–118.
38. Jacobs JD, Bell WH, Williams CE, Kennedy JW 3rd. Control of the transverse dimension with surgery and orthodontics. *Am J Orthod*. 1980;77(3):284–306.
39. Faber RD. Occlusograms in orthodontic treatment planning. *J Clin Orthod*. 1992;26(7):396–401.
40. Marcotte MR. The use of the occlusogram in planning orthodontic treatment. *Am J Orthod*. 1976;69(6):655–667.
41. Bays RA, Greco JM. Surgically assisted rapid palatal expansion: an outpatient technique with long-term stability. *J Oral Maxillofac Surg*. 1992;50(2):110–115.
42. Phillips C, Medland WH, Fields HW Jr, Proffit WR, White RP Jr. Stability of surgical maxillary expansion. *Int J Adult Orthodon Orthognath Surg*. 1992;7(3):139–146.
43. Kuhlberg AJ, Burstone CJ. T-loop position and anchorage control. *Am J Orthod Dentofacial Orthop*. 1997;112(1):12–18.
44. Kuhlberg AJ, Priebe D. Testing force systems and biomechanics: measured tooth movements from differential moment closing loops. *Angle Orthod*. 2003;73(3):270–280.
45. Frost HM. The biology of fracture healing; an overview for clinicians, part II. *Clin Orthop Relat Res*. 1989;(248):294–309.
46. Frost HM. The biology of fracture healing: an overview for clinicians, part I. *Clin Orthop Relat Res*. 1989;(248):283–293.
47. Nemeth RB, Isaacson RJ. Vertical anterior relapse. *Am J Orthod*. 1974;65(6):565–585.
48. Proffit WR, Turvey TA, Phillips C. Orthognathic surgery: a hierarchy of stability. *Int J Adult Orthodon Orthognath Surg*. 1996;11(3): 191–204.
49. Legan HL. *Orthodontic Considerations*. Philadelphia, PA: Lippincott; 1992.
50. Gerlock AJJ, Sinn DP, McBride KL. *Clinical and Radiographic Interpretaion of Facial Fractures*. Boston, MA: Little Brown, & Co; 1981.
51. Moloney F, Worthington P. The origin of the Le Fort I maxillary osteotomy: Cheever's operation. *J Oral Surg*. 1981;39(10):731–734.
52. Wassmund M. *Lehrbuch der Praktischen Chirurgie des Mundes und der Kiefer*. Leipzig, Germany: Meuser; 1935.
53. Ilizarov GA. Clinical application of the tension-stress effect for limb lengthening. *Clin Orthop Relat Res*. 1990;(250):8–26.
54. Guerrero CA, Bell WH, Meza LS. Intraoral distraction osteogenesis: maxillary and mandibular lengthening. *Atlas Oral Maxillofac Surg Clin North Am*. 1999;7(1):111–151.
55. McCarthy JG, Stelnicki EJ, Grayson BH. Distraction osteogenesis of the mandible: a ten-year experience. *Semin Orthod*. 1999;5(1):3–8.
56. McCarthy JG, Stelnicki EJ, Mehrara BJ, Longaker MT. Distraction osteogenesis of the craniofacial skeleton. *Plast Reconstr Surg*. 2001; 107(7):1812–1827.
57. Molina F, Ortiz Monasterio F. Mandibular elongation and remodeling by distraction: a farewell to major osteotomies. *Plast Reconstr Surg*. 1995;96(4):825–842.
58. Toth BA, Kim JW, Chin M, Cedars M. Distraction osteogenesis and its application to the midface and bony orbit in craniosynostosis syndromes. *J Craniofac Surg*. 1998;9(2):100–122.
59. Lee KG, Ryu YK, Park YC, Rudolph DJ. A study of holographic interferometry on the initial reaction of maxillofacial complex during protraction. *Am J Orthod Dentofacial Orthop*. 1997;111(6):623–632.
60. Kennedy JW III, Bell WH, Kimbrough OL, James WB. Osteotomy as an adjunct to rapid maxillary expansion. *Am J Orthod*. 1976;70(2): 123–137.
61. Hanson PR, Melugin MB. Orthodontic management of the patient undergoing mandibular distraction osteogenesis. *Semin Orthod*. 1999;5(1):25–34.
62. Braun S, Bantleon HP, Hnat WP, Freudenthaler JW, Marcotte MR, Johnson BE. A study of bite force, part II: relationship to various cephalometric measurements. *Angle Orthod*. 1995;65(5):373–377.
63. McDougall PD, McNamara JA Jr, Dierkes JM. Arch width development in Class II patients treated with the Frankel appliance. *Am J Orthod*. 1982;82(1):10–22.
64. Weinberg M, Sadowsky C. Resolution of mandibular arch crowding in growing patients with Class I malocclusions treated nonextraction. *Am J Orthod Dentofacial Orthop*. 1996;110(4):359–364.
65. Little RM, Riedel RA, Stein A. Mandibular arch length increase during the mixed dentition: postretention evaluation of stability and relapse. *Am J Orthod Dentofacial Orthop*. 1990;97(5):393–404.
66. Conley R, Legan H. Mandibular symphyseal distraction osteogenesis: diagnosis and treatment planning considerations. *Angle Orthod*. 2003;73(1):3–11.
67. Contasti G, Guerrero C, Rodriguez AM, Legan HL. Mandibular widening by distraction osteogenesis. *J Clin Orthod*. 2001;35(3): 165–173.
68. Legan HL. Orthodontic treatment planning and biomechanics for transverse distraction osteogenesis. *Semin Orthod*. 2001;7:160–168.
69. Samchukov ML, Cope JB, Harper RP, Ross JD. Biomechanical considerations of mandibular lengthening and widening by gradual distraction using a computer model. *J Oral Maxillofac Surg*. 1998;56(1): 51–59.
70. Braun S, Bottrel JA, Legan HL. Condylar displacement related to mandibular symphyseal distraction. *Am J Orthod Dentofacial Orthop*. 2002;121(2):162–165.
71. Sugawara J, Aymach Z, Nagasaka DH, Kawamura H, Nanda R. "Surgery first" orthognathics to correct a skeletal class II malocclusion with an impinging bite. *J Clin Orthod*. 2010;44(7):429–438.
72. Villegas C, Uribe F, Sugawara J, Nanda R. Expedited correction of significant dentofacial asymmetry using a "surgery first" approach. *J Clin Orthod*. 2010;44(2):97–103.
73. Shu R, Huang L, Bai D. Adult Class II Division 1 patient with severe gummy smile treated with temporary anchorage devices. *Am J Orthod Dentofacial Orthop*. 2011;140(1):97–105.
74. Young T, Palta M, Dempsey J, Skatrud J, Weber S, Badr S. The occurrence of sleep-disordered breathing among middle-aged adults. *N Engl J Med*. 1993;328:1230–1235.
75. Strollo PJ, Rogers RM. Obstructive sleep apnea. *N Engl J Med*. 1996; 11;33:99–104.

76. Smith PL, Gold AR, Meyers DA, Handnick EF, Bleecker ER. Weight loss in mildly to moderately obese patients with obstructive sleep apnea. *Ann Intern Med.* 1985;103:850–855.
77. Scrima L, Broody M, Nay KN, Cohn MA. Increased severity of obstructive sleep apnea after bedtime alcohol ingestion: diagnosis and potential and proposed mechanisms of action. *Sleep.* 1982;5:318–328.
78. Sanders MH, Moore SE, Eveslace J. CPAP via nasal mask: a treatment for obstructive sleep apnea. *Chest.* 1983;83:144–145.
79. Coleman JA Jr. Laser-assisted uvulopalatoplasty: long-term results with a treatment for snoring. *Ear Nose Throat J.* 1998;77:22–34.
80. Prinsell JR. Maxillomandibular advancement surgery for obstructive sleep apnea syndrome. *J Am Dent Assoc.* 2002;133:1489–1497.
81. Campos-Rodriguez F, Pena-Grinan N, Reyes-Nunez N, et al. Mortality in obstructive sleep apnea hypopnea patients treated with positive airway pressure. *Chest.* 2005;128(2):624–633.
82. Lavie P, Lavie L, Herer P. All-cause mortality in males with sleep apnea syndrome: declining mortality rates with age. *Eur Respir J.* 2005;25: 514–520.
83. Milleron O, Pillière R, Foucher A, et al. Benefits of obstructive sleep apnea treatment in coronary artery disease: a long-term follow-up study. *Eur Heart J.* 2004;25:728–734.
84. Marti S, Sampol G, Muñoz X, et al. Mortality in severe sleep apnoea/hypopnoeas syndrome patients: impact of treatment. *Eur Respir J.* 2002; 20:1511–1518.

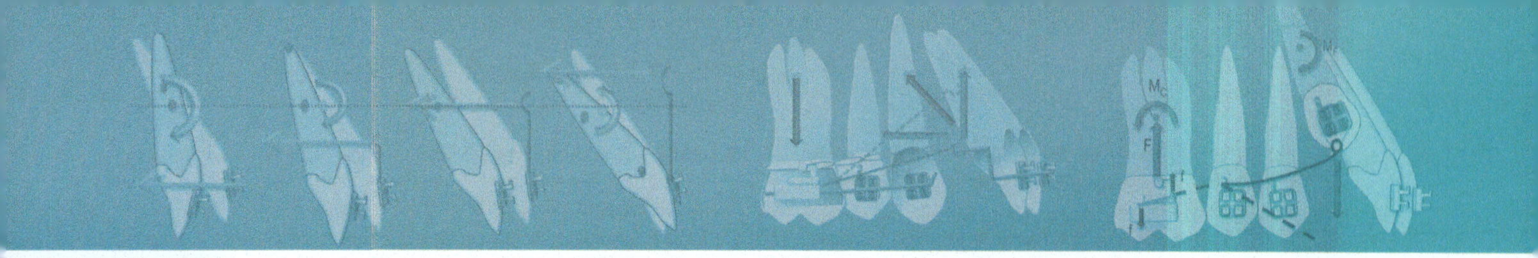

CHAPTER 24

Interdisciplinary Strategies for Treating Adult Patients

Mithran S. Goonewardene and Bradley G. Shepherd

The contemporary clinician is generally presented with a patient or parent who is well informed because of the significant opportunities to research treatment options on electronic media. Patients often present with certain expectations resulting from these search activities and are generally aware of possibilities to modify tooth form and color using contemporary methods. Moreover adult patients now represent a significant proportion of individuals seeking orthodontic treatment for esthetic improvement because of changing opportunities or the need for comprehensive rehabilitation.[1,2]

Adult patients present significant challenges across many spheres of concern.[3-5] Often adults have been affected by periodontal disease, attrition, abrasion, and erosion. The most significant challenge to successful treatment may be the effects of long-term and sometimes unsatisfactory restorative dentistry, which may be contributing to the progression of multifaceted deterioration. Moreover adult patients are generally more fastidious but have a degree of psychological tolerance to treatment that must be considered carefully. Adults also measure the compromise of treatment very carefully and must make difficult decisions for themselves, factors that are not as significant for adolescent patients. Finally, from the orthodontist's perspective, biomechanical side effects usually compensated by growth changes demand more precise execution of tooth movement strategies.

Adult patients often engage in the treatment process and play an active role in decision-making. It is important to realize that there is often a lack of concordance between the clinician's and the patient's perception of treatment success. Therefore contemporary clinicians attempt to achieve realistic treatment goals that aim to marry the objectives of both clinician and patient.

CONCEPTS OF INTERDISCIPLINARY TREATMENT PLANNING

Approximately two-thirds of the population exhibit malocclusion, with some individuals able to progress to later adulthood with minimal intervention from a restorative dentist.[6] However, a combination of caries-related restorative dentistry procedures, tooth loss, periodontal problems, and tooth surface loss may contribute to challenges for the restorative dentist.[7] These issues may result in significant migration of teeth into positions that make routine dentistry problematic. Moreover a significant number of individuals may have had a preexisting malocclusion with some degree of skeletal discrepancy and associated dental compensations, which place unrealistic demands on the restorative dentist and their materials as they attempt to manage patients' concerns (Fig. 24-1).

The majority of orthodontic patients present following referral from a restorative dentist but some may present spontaneously without referral. In well-established offices with an excellent history of communication between many practitioners, the patients are usually well informed about the problems prior to orthodontic referral. However, a number of patients may be referred for assessment without any preliminary knowledge related to their problems and the issues associated with management (Fig. 24-2). The management of these patients is critical and sometimes challenging. The orthodontist often takes on the role of facilitator among a new group of clinicians to ensure that the patient and all associated clinicians have similar appreciation of the diagnosis, treatment goals, and possible solutions for the patient's circumstances. In patients with more complex treatment needs that may require periodontal and restorative intervention, treatment requires a consistently coordinated approach for successful management.[8,9]

UNIDISCIPLINARY TREATMENT

Unidisciplinary treatment occurs when a clinician attempts to treat a complex problem in isolation.[9] It is often disappointing to see a patient who has been treated with a succession of restorative procedures alone, in an attempt to manage a complex dental problem that may be the result of an interaction of tooth loss and periodontal disease on an aberrant

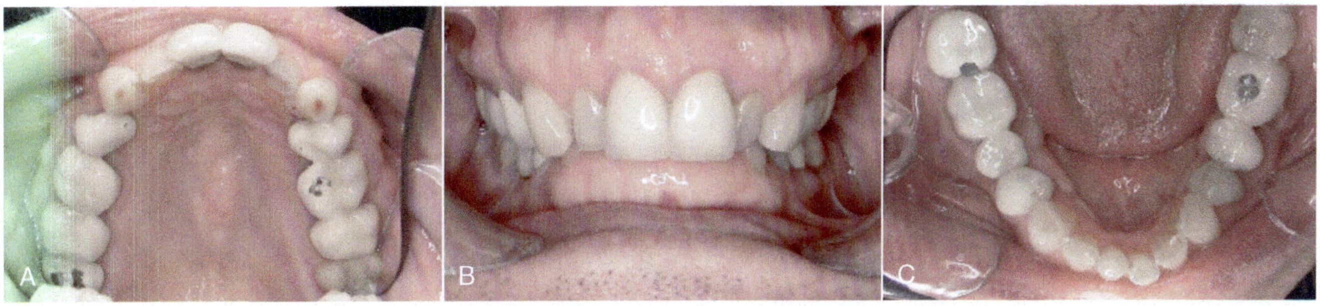

Figure 24-1 **A–C,** A 57-year-old male patient has been partially restored in an attempt to address cosmetic issues related to tooth surface loss and a generally heavily restored dentition. The impact of the significant Class II relationship, deep overbite, and nocturnal bruxism were not considered in the treatment planning process and significant acceleration of lower anterior wear occurred.

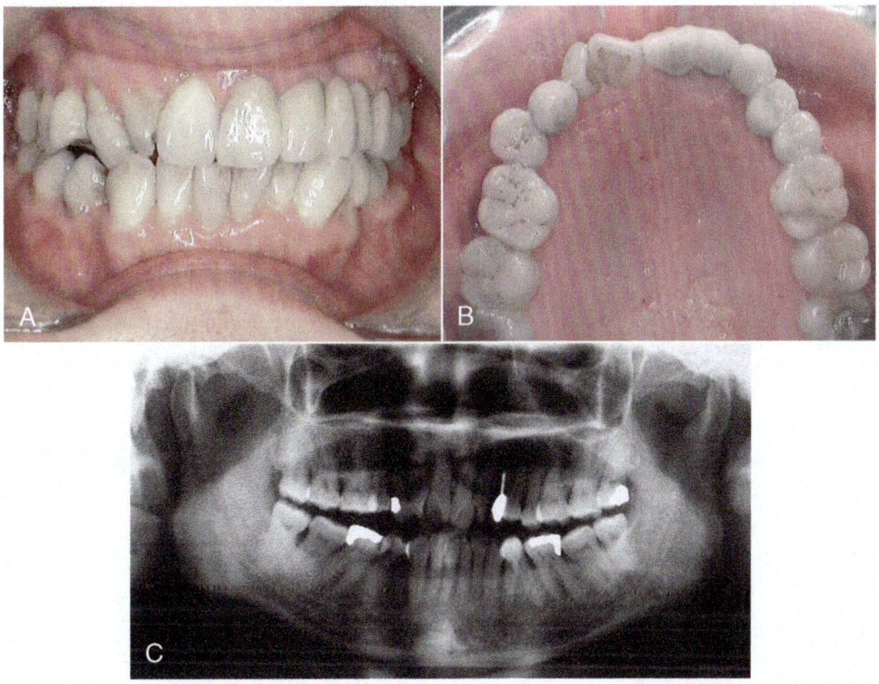

Figure 24-2 A 50-year-old female patient presented soon after placement of a fixed prosthesis by her general dentist. **A and B,** Intraoral photographs reveal an attempt to replace five dental units after removal of the upper left canine due to failure of post and core crown. There has been no regard for the preexisting malocclusion and the resultant aberrant contours in the compromised final prosthesis. **C,** The pre-treatment radiograph clearly reveals significant periodontal problems and irregularity that were not addressed as part of the overall treatment plan.

skeletal jaw base (Fig. 24-3). Some clinicians even attempt to deliver care in periodontics, endodontics, and orthodontics without the skills and knowledge needed to consider all of the risks and benefits of various therapies. Moreover, these clinicians might not have the skills required to deliver the appropriate therapy to the expected standard of care.

MULTIDISCIPLINARY TREATMENT

Multidisciplinary treatment progresses beyond unidisciplinary treatment in that clinicians from multiple disciplines are integrated into the treatment in a haphazard way. Often the course of multidisciplinary treatment is dependent on which clinician is seen first.

There are many examples of orthodontic or restorative dentistry initiated in patients with undiagnosed periodontal disease. Orthodontists often complete treatment in partially edentulous patients without consulting the restorative dentist. This may result in inadequate spatial arrangements, with too much space or too little space for an optimal prosthetic outcome.

The characteristic shortcoming of multidisciplinary treatment is poor communication between clinicians who independently might be excellent clinicians but who do not understand the considerations of all specialty areas and their prospective influence on the overall management of the patient (Fig. 24-4).[9]

INTERDISCIPLINARY TREATMENT

Interdisciplinary treatment is characterized by a group of clinicians from numerous backgrounds all contributing to

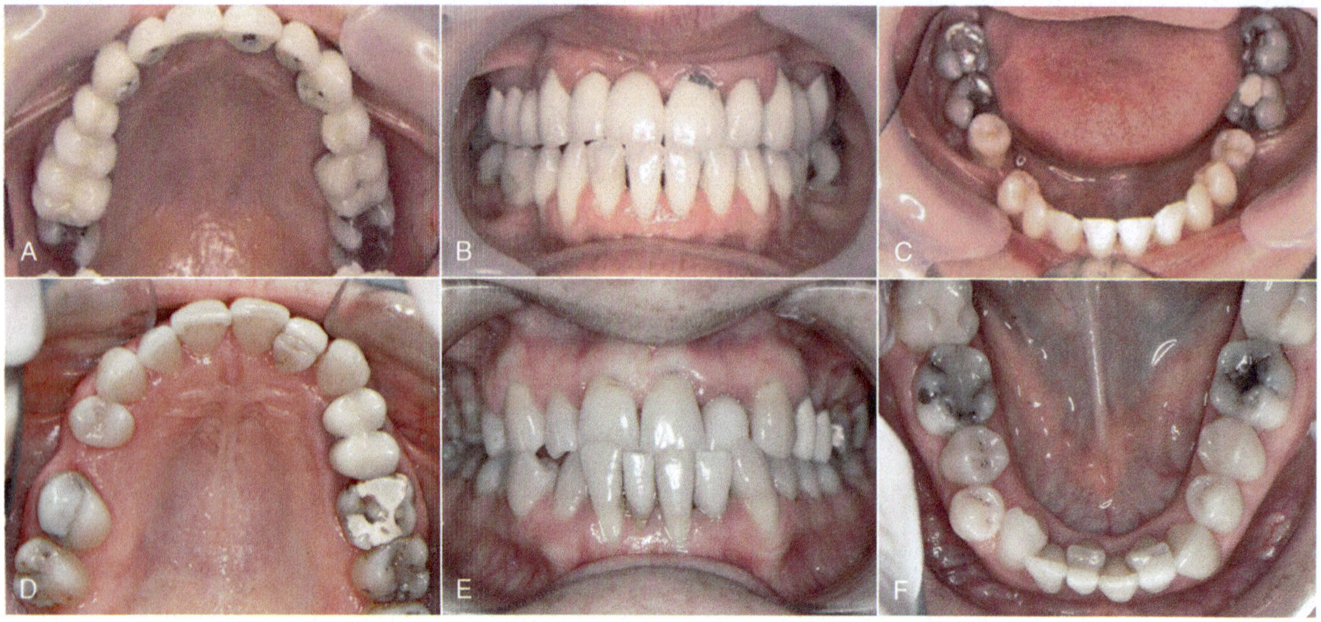

Figure 24-3 **A–C,** A 53-year-old female patient with a significant Class III malocclusion has been restored with a near complete prosthetic maxillary rehabilitation with no regard to the skeletal relationship. An attempt was made to compensate the prosthetic tooth position for the aberrant jaw relationship, which resulted in excessive loads concentrated on the prosthesis and resultant porcelain fractures. **D–F,** A 40-year-old female patient presented 7 years after consulting her general dentist for improvement in her esthetics. She has experienced periodontal problems resulting from a combination of labial positioning of the lower incisors, plaque-induced periodontal inflammation, and aggressive tooth brushing. The "overcontoured" veneers have also directly contributed to her periodontal problems. Unfortunately the general dentist did not appreciate the impact of the underlying malocclusion on future stability and simply offered her a veneer option. Orthodontics was never presented to the patient as a potential solution.

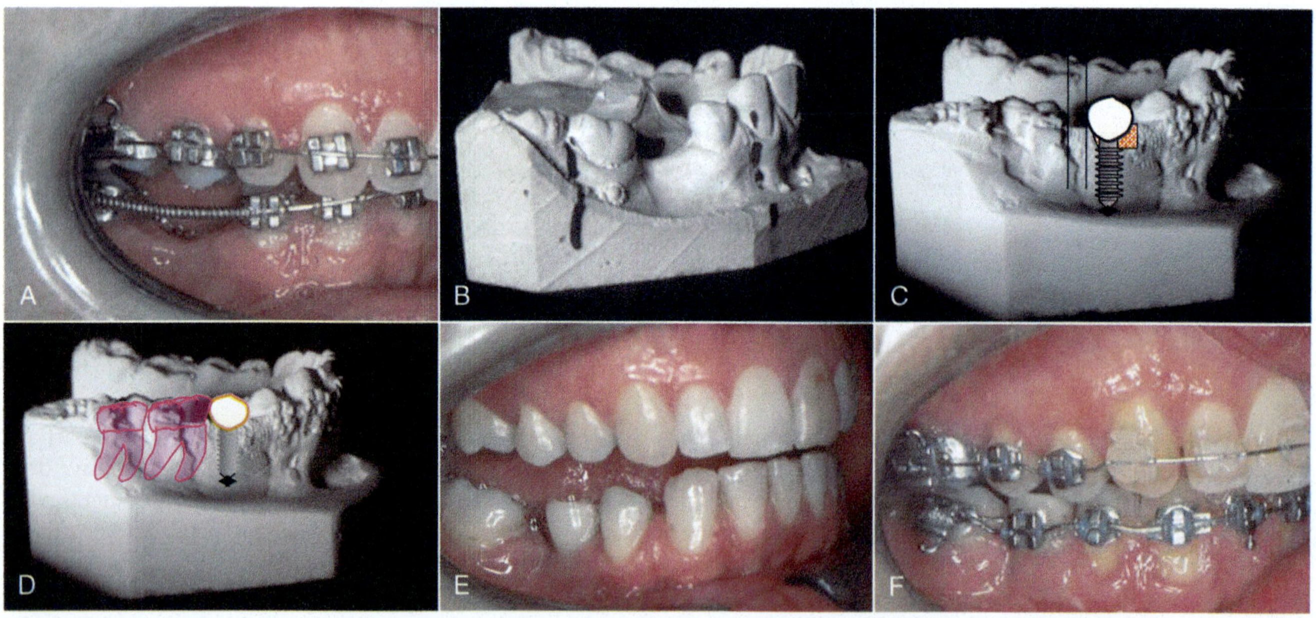

Figure 24-4 **A,** Adult patient presented to the office in appliances for completion of her orthodontic treatment, which included mandibular advancement surgery and preparation for prosthetic teeth. The transferring orthodontist indicated that the patient was ready for the mandibular surgery and implant placement. **B,** The pre-treatment model demonstrates a tipped molar. The treatment plan aimed to move the molar distally and open up the space. **C,** A progress model clearly demonstrates inadequate consideration by the orthodontist for the prosthetic replacement. The decision was made without the input of a prosthodontist. **D–F,** The appliances were removed and a new plan was formulated. This plan included placement of a premolar-sized implant in the lower right second premolar region, which would be used to protract the molars and close the excess space. The mandible was advanced and the occlusion was detailed into this position. This case demonstrates the need for a coordinated approach with several clinicians involved in the decision-making process.

the management of a patient for which their expertise is needed. It is important to establish a working team of specialists who can communicate effectively and meet regularly.[8,9]

Once a patient has been recognized as needing interdisciplinary management, a specific series of procedures must be considered and adhered to. This ensures that the patient's interest is foremost.

Preliminary Discussion: Establish Interest

Not all patients are suitable candidates for complex interdisciplinary treatment. After careful consideration of the patient's primary complaint, it is important to clearly determine the patient's needs. A common mistake in advising patients with complex needs is to immediately assume that the patient will progress through complex and costly diagnostic processes and interdisciplinary consultations. One clinician should take responsibility for briefly outlining the nature of the problem, the time commitment, and the possible financial cost by establishing a well-defined roadmap for treatment. Often the orthodontist assumes the role of facilitator and he or she must recognize that there are occupational biases between practitioners in various disciplines that may influence the balance of information transfer.[10]

A simple patient-specific set of records may be considered at this stage to satisfy the requirements of the initial evaluation and information exchange between clinicians (Fig. 24-5).

In patients with moderate to extreme deterioration of the dentition it is important to reflect on how the patient arrived at this juncture. Often the situation has resulted from an unfortunate combination of opportunity and finances; occasionally it has resulted from neglect by the patient, the dental care provider, or both. It is important for the clinician to exercise good judgment and consider whether the patient is a candidate for complex treatment and its associated demands on the patient.

Patients with Significant Periodontal Problems

In patients with significant long-standing pathology such as periodontal disease, caries, and/or periapical pathology, a period of periodontal and caries control therapy may be necessary to establish optimal health prior to initiating orthodontic treatment.[11] This period is therefore seen as a provisional or therapeutic diagnostic test. In fact, this may be an ideal method of screening possible interdisciplinary patients. The cost and significant time commitment will identify problematic patients prior to committing to potentially risky tooth movement and placement of complex prostheses in the presence of uncontrolled disease (Fig. 24-6).

There is nothing more disastrous for the interdisciplinary clinician than to encounter a patient who fails to attend regular treatment sessions or fails to adhere to the rudimentary home care regime. It is beneficial for all concerned to

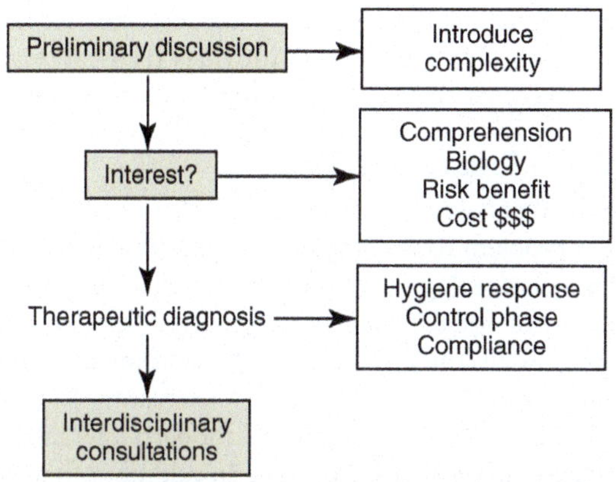

Figure 24-5 The sequence of managing patients from initial consultation to interdisciplinary consultations. It is important that this is performed in a progressive manner to ensure that the patient understands the complexity and general goals of treatment. This may include a period of preliminary treatment that may be considered a therapeutic diagnostic process and may determine the suitability of patients for more extensive treatment.

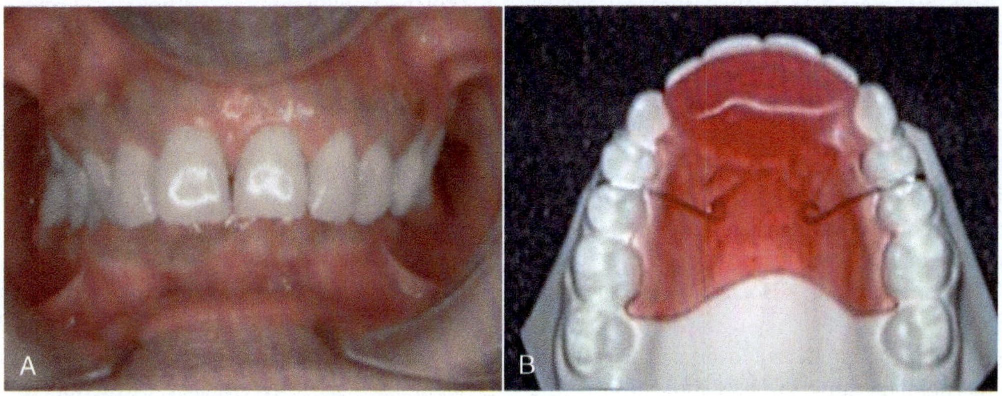

Figure 24-6 **A,** A 42-year-old patient presented with significant restorative dentistry, periodontal problems, and a deep overbite that required comprehensive interdisciplinary treatment. The patient was sent for stabilization of the periodontal problems and provisional restorations prior to definitive interdisciplinary treatment. **B,** A removable biteplate serves a dual purpose of relieving the direct gingival impingement on the palatal tissue margins and helping in a preliminary assessment of the patient's capacity to conform to the demands of treatment. In such patients it is often important to assess whether they will comply with the challenges of multiple appointments over the treatment time, particularly if their history has included periods of neglect and irregular dental attendance.

identify these issues at the outset. In some circumstances patients are placed in a removable biteplate or occlusal splint in addition to the periodontal treatment. This enables the orthodontist to evaluate patient compliance with an appliance as well as the patient's attention to appointments for orthodontic review.

Patient Review and Definitive Record Taking

Once the patient has been stabilized and is considered a favorable candidate for treatment, he or she may progress to a more complex stage of acquiring complete diagnostic records and referral for interdisciplinary consultations with appropriate clinicians. These may include an orthodontist, restorative dentist or prosthodontist, periodontist, oral surgeon, endodontist, physician, and oral radiologist and computer scientist.[8]

Numerous developments in information technology enable clinicians to share material in electronic format and, with patient consent, even to share the treatment records of multiple clinicians. This is a time- and cost-effective method for clinicians and patients that provides ready access to all available records and treatment progress by team members.

Establish Treatment Goals

Once the database has been established, a detailed and prioritized problem list is developed.[12] The problem list forms the basis for developing a list of "ideal treatment goals." One clinician will usually take the responsibility of developing this list and circulating the findings to all members of the treatment team.

Communication is facilitated by modern interactive software that enables sharing of data. In addition, many clinicians will meet regularly using a roundtable discussion format to discuss complicated cases. This is valuable time for clinicians even if a case does not involve consideration of a specific specialist's skills,[8,9] as the discussion will enable all clinicians to remain current with developments in other specialty areas. In formal training or treatment institutions, patients are often consulted in comprehensive multidisciplinary clinics and this interaction facilitates interdisciplinary management with all clinicians present.

Considerations in Goal Setting

There are many factors to consider when establishing the goals for a patient's treatment, including:

- Cost-benefit analysis
- Patient values and quality-of-life issues
- Growth and maturation issues
- Treatment outcomes and associated maintenance requirements

The patient's primary complaint and dental history are significant at this point because the best indication of the need for intervention is the observation of any deteriorating status in the dentition. It is often more difficult to make a decision to treat a younger adult with a malocclusion than to treat an older individual. Older patients may reveal signs of breakdown such as tooth wear, soft tissue impingement, and/or tooth migration related to their occlusal relationships or they may show no adverse effects from their malocclusions. This is perhaps the most significant aspect in decision-making after the patient's primary complaint.

In young children it is usually a simpler decision to treat malocclusion to an ideal Class I occlusion. The biological and psychological cost is usually reduced in the presence of optimal oral health. However, in adults careful consideration must be given to achieving realistic goals, which may not be the same as the ideal goals.[8] For example, it is not always necessary to treat a posterior crossbite with a shift as part of interdisciplinary treatment nor to achieve an ideal Class I posterior occlusion in every circumstance, particularly if this relationship is not considered to be problematic to the patient's primary complaint and treatment stability.

A series of treatment solutions with modified goals may be considered by the interdisciplinary group and often team members will be surprised by a totally satisfactory solution that they had not considered that is introduced by a colleague in another discipline (Fig. 24-7).[9] Clinicians tend to have an occupational bias when considering treatment options and this type of decision-making environment ensures a thorough evaluation of many possible scenarios.

It is important to consider the risks and benefits and the patient's perspective when outlining the best treatment solution for the patient. One clinician will usually be responsible for carefully and systematically finalizing the discussion with the patient to ensure agreement on a solution that encompasses the patient's and clinicians' desires, acknowledged risks and sacrifices, and associated financial considerations. This is particularly important when considering replacement of missing teeth.

Many interdisciplinary treatment plans include replacement of missing teeth and the restorative dentist or prosthodontist must have a comprehensive discussion with the patient on the risks and benefits of the range of replacement options, including removable partial dentures, fixed prostheses, and/or implants. Historically, the success of a restorative option has been simplistically reported as retention of the prosthesis with limited pathology. A more contemporary view of success includes esthetics and periodontal health outcomes as well as factors such as the longevity versus indexed cost, invasiveness and biological cost, and esthetic outcome.[4,10–14] These contemporary studies have included a complex assessment of quality-of-life issues from the patient's perspective in seeking and receiving therapy.

Diagnostic Model Setup

In patients who require routine orthodontic treatment it is fairly easy for the experienced clinician to visualize the final occlusion. However, in patients who require atypical treatment such as lower incisor extraction, canine or incisor substitution, or complex interdisciplinary treatment involving prosthetic replacement of several teeth and even jaw surgery, it may be difficult for clinicians to visualize the final outcome (Fig. 24-8). Technological advances have seen the application of digital study models and the development of

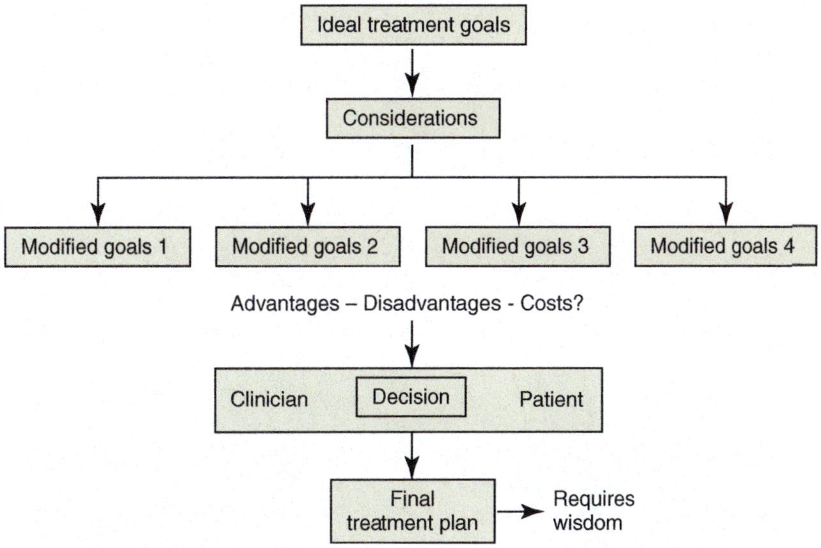

Figure 24-7 Possible complex considerations that influence attainment of ideal treatment goals. A carefully considered treatment plan that represents a joint decision between the patient and clinicians based on their relative value systems will be formulated.

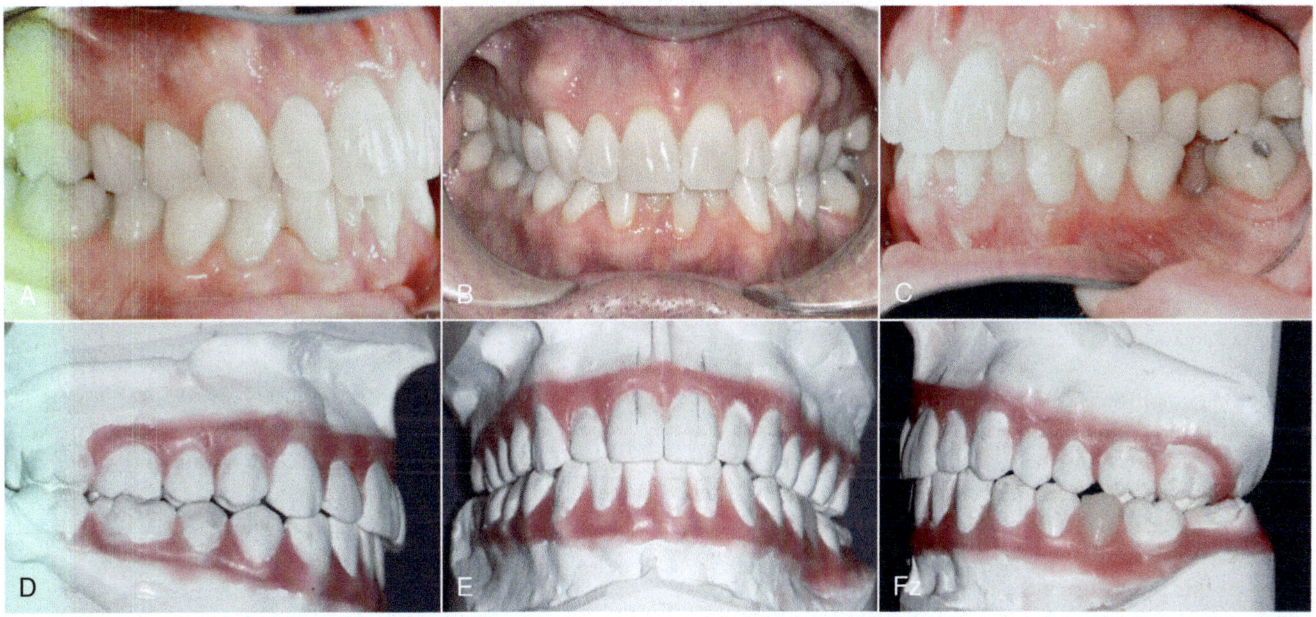

Figure 24-8 **A–C,** Patient presented with missing lower left first molar and Class I malocclusion. **D–F,** Plaster and wax diagnostic setup clearly demonstrates alignment of teeth and uprighting of lower left molars in preparation for a prosthetic replacement. All clinicians involved in treatment are now able to visualize the final outcome.

digitally assisted setups that facilitate assessment of numerous treatment options on a three-dimensional imaging program but many clinicians still prefer plaster and wax setups (Fig. 24-9).

The diagnostic setup is usually prepared after consultation with key clinicians involved in the specific plan. It enables the clinicians to realistically assess:

- Proposed occlusal relationship
- Anticipated space requirements for alignment and/or compensatory tooth movements that may necessitate extractions and/or interproximal reduction
- Anteroposterior and vertical space requirements for restorative dentistry particularly relevant to tooth replacement
- Anchorage requirements for orthodontic tooth movement

The diagnostic setup is the key communication tool used by all clinicians and the patient.[13] Various simulations may be presented with their relative merits and risks, which will assist in developing the final treatment plan. Moreover once the plan has been accepted by all concerned, it is a key reference point to which all parties, clinicians, and the patient may refer through the course of treatment.

Facilitating Communication: Treatment Sequencing

The final treatment plan will reflect the combined decision of the group of clinicians and the patient. It is now critical

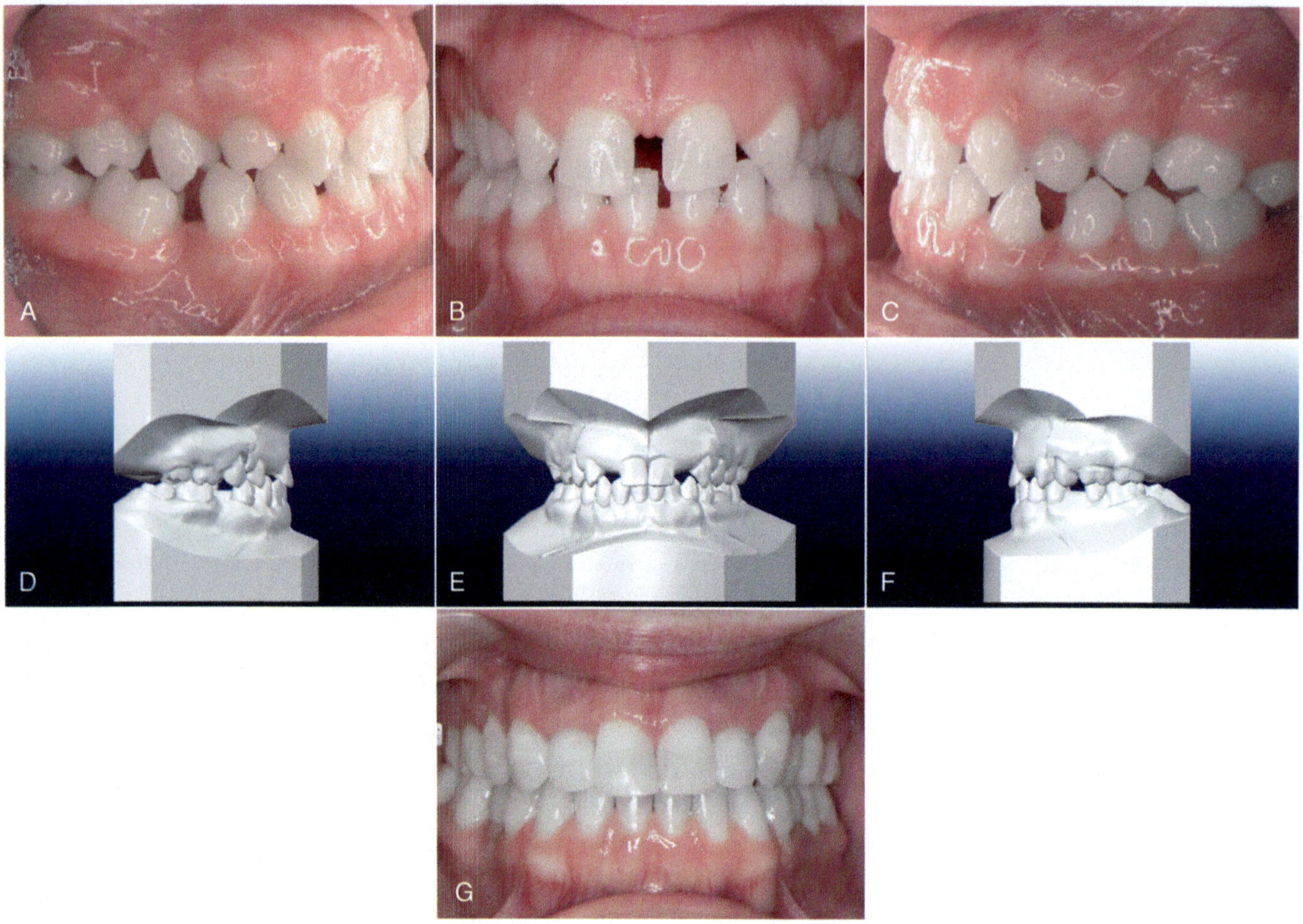

Figure 24-9 **A–C,** Pre-treatment intraoral views of a partially edentulous patient who requires preprosthetic orthodontics. **D–F,** Digitally generated diagnostic setup. **G,** Postorthodontic restorative outcome.

to ensure that all clinicians recognize their specific role and the sequence of treatment.

The absence of a treatment sequencing document often results in poor communication and less than optimal outcomes. Clinicians may be surprised when a patient attends for a specific procedure if the recollection of the goals at this stage is not immediately apparent. Significant effort may have to be expended by the clinicians to reacquaint themselves with the treatment plan. Inherent complications in treatment efficiency and possibly inappropriate treatment procedures can result if a clear outline of the goals is not understood.

An interdisciplinary plan will be formulated, principally by the team leader. The orthodontist frequently facilitates this process, as he or she often spends significantly more time with the patient during the course of treatment (Figs. 24-10 and 24-11). Equally so, other team members may find themselves assuming this role at specific phases of the plan. The team leader must ensure that a comprehensive list of procedures with specific goals and timelines is outlined and circulated to all clinicians and to the patient.[8] This is a key component in ensuring excellent communication between all parties. It ensures that all clinicians are familiar with the stages of treatment and ensures an efficient transition through treatment. Moreover patients may wish to review their progress by referring to the treatment sequencing document.

PERIODONTAL IMPLICATIONS IN INTERDISCIPLINARY TREATMENT

Adults represent a significant number of patients referred for interdisciplinary treatment. The adult patient often has preexisting periodontal problems that need to be evaluated. These may include:

- Malocclusion that has resulted from tooth drift secondary to the periodontal tissue destruction. This is a significant challenge, as these patients often have complex factors (including compliance with dental procedures) that need to be addressed.
- Tooth drift and tipping secondary to loss of teeth that has predisposed the tissues to periodontal problems.
- Recession-like defects and patients with thin gingival biotype, which may influence the clinician's ability to move teeth and maintain tissue integrity.

Referral for assessment and management of periodontal problems is probably the most significant step in interdisciplinary treatment.[14] Many patients find themselves in this

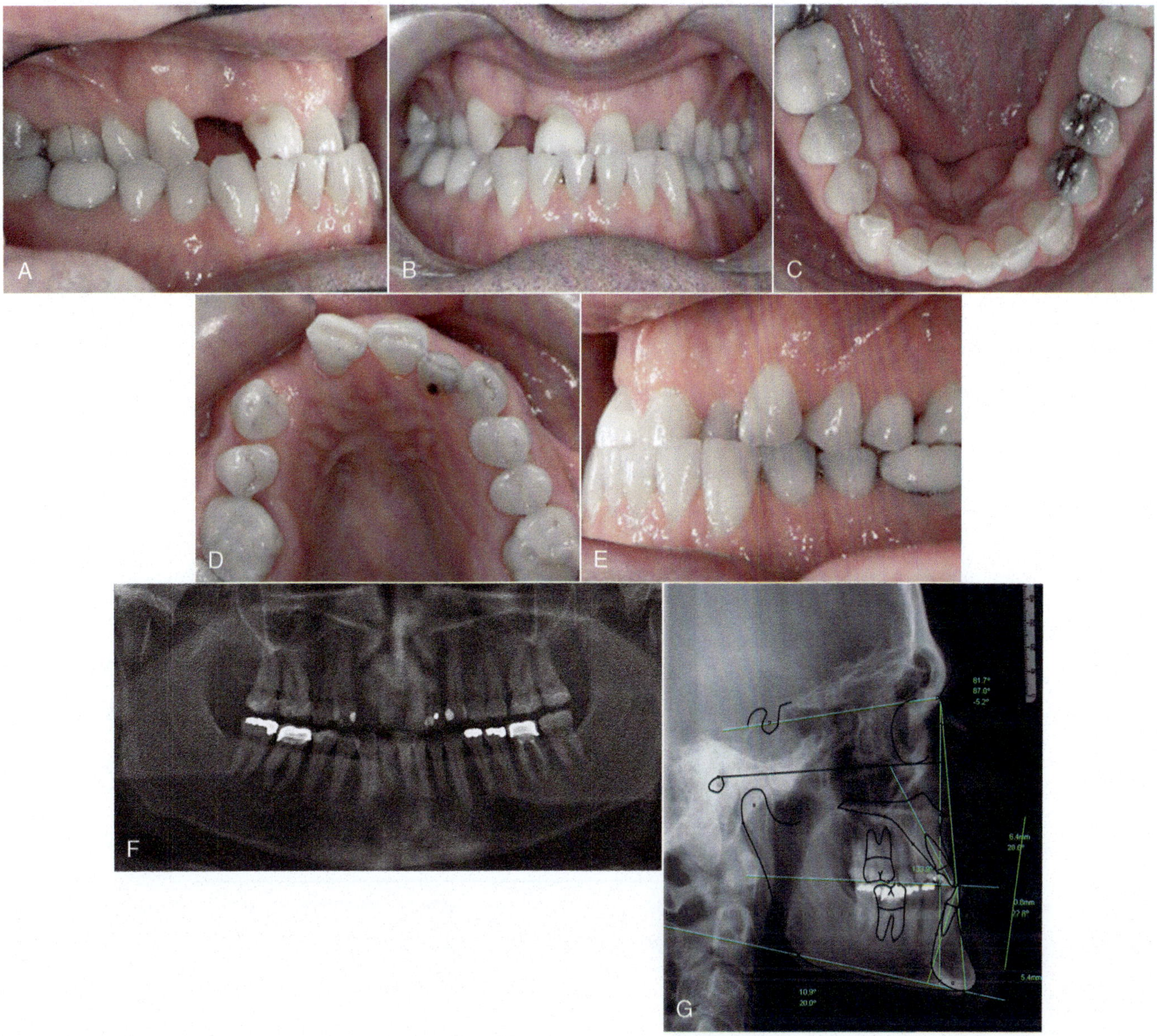

Figure 24-10 **A–E,** Intraoral views of a 42-year-old male patient who presented with a Class III malocclusion, advanced periodontal problems, a missing lateral incisor, and attrition of the upper central incisors. **F,** Panoramic radiograph revealed advanced attachment loss around the upper central incisors. **G,** Cephalometric radiograph revealed a significant Class III skeletal relationship with a retrognathic maxilla that will be managed by maxillary advancement surgery.

circumstance because of a historical lack of home care and regular dental review. It is often difficult to gauge whether adult patients are committed to what will be a challenging treatment regime in terms of both time and cost. The initial periodontal assessment is often considered a preliminary screening process during which adherence to issues of home care,[11] regular appointment attendance, and suitability for a potentially extended course of treatment may be determined.[15]

The periodontal assessment may include a process of therapeutic diagnosis in which tissue response to treatment is assessed. The primary goal of this treatment is to eliminate and stabilize the disease process. It also enables the clinicians to identify the specific location and architecture of bony and soft tissue lesions.[16] These include crater defects; one-, two-, and three-wall defects; furcation defects; and localized horizontal bone loss.[17] Through careful consideration of the relative prognoses of various treatment procedures, the interdisciplinary team will determine whether periodontal treatment alone is indicated or the orthodontist may modify the position of the teeth to effect changes in the bony architecture.[18,19]

Consideration may be given to bone regeneration procedures[16,20,21] but often the orthodontist is called on to level teeth by selective vertical repositioning to establish a balanced and healthy bone level across associated teeth, particularly if they are intimately associated with restorative procedures (Fig. 24-12).[18,19] These specific procedures

Patient: John Doe

Interdisciplinary Treatment Sequence

1. Connective tissue graft to lower incisors a. Thicken tissue prior to labial movement (decompensation)	Periodontist
2. Placement of orthodontic appliances a. Align and coordinate upper teeth b. Add prosthetic tooth to fixed braces c. Bring lower teeth forward (9 months approximately)	Orthodontist
3. Periodontal maintenance every 2–3 months during orthodontics	Periodontist
4. Presurgical assessment	Oral Surgeon
5. Placement of surgical hooks 1–2 days prior to surgery	Orthodontist
6. Jaw surgery—upper jaw advancement	Oral Surgeon
7. Removal of surgical splint 2–3 weeks after surgery	Orthodontist
8. Postsurgical orthodontics—6–8 months duration	Orthodontist
9. Removal of fixed appliances and placement of retainer with teeth	Orthodontist
10. Review for prosthodontic treatment following debanding	Prosthodontist
11. CT scans and assessment for implant replacement	Prosthodontist
12. Removal of both central incisors, placement of implants a. Minor bone augmentation b. At least 6 months after debonding	Oral Surgeon
13. Placement of provisional prostheses supported and retained on implants 1 week after implant surgery	Prosthodontist
14. Final ceramic prostheses 5–6 months after implant surgery	Prosthodontist

A

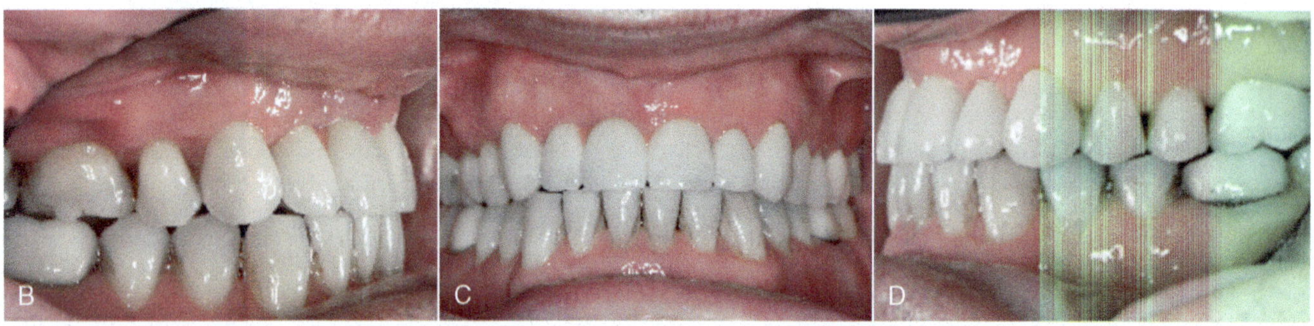

Figure 24-11 **A,** Interdisciplinary treatment sequence for the patient shown in Figure 24-10. It addresses his periodontal problems first, followed by complex orthodontics, restorative dentistry, and oral surgery. The key elements in this treatment plan are to establish the sequence of events and determine whether his upper central incisors need to be replaced, as they were considered to have a questionable prognosis. The decision by the periodontist and prosthodontist was that implant replacement would offer a more predictable outcome than attempting to retain these teeth. The timing of extraction and implant replacement (with or without grafting) must be determined carefully by the team to ensure that treatment flows smoothly. **B–D,** Final intraoral photos of the patient following orthodontic treatment, maxillary surgery, and implant replacement. *CT,* Computed tomography.

may be incorporated into the biomechanical plan (Fig. 24-13).

The periodontist may consider soft tissue augmentation procedures to prevent further breakdown of the gingival tissues either because the tissues are predisposed to recession by the dental history or because the tooth movement proposed by the interdisciplinary team may predispose the patient to further attachment loss (Fig. 24-14).[22–27]

PREPROSTHETIC TOOTH MOVEMENT

The restorative dentist or prosthodontist is routinely challenged by the task of restoring teeth that are not ideally positioned.[8] Often minor modifications to tooth preparation and crown form may compensate for a less than ideal position of teeth and the restorative dentist is able to achieve excellent esthetic and functional results. However, in many

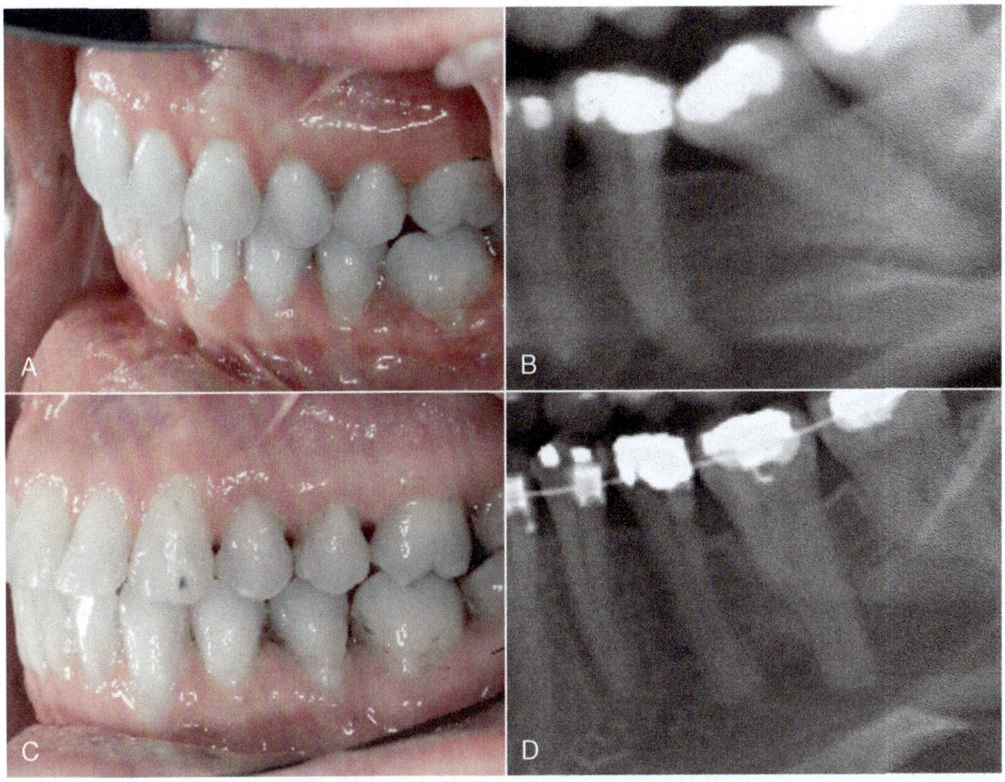

Figure 24-12 The orthodontist may assist in uprighting significantly tipped molars. **A and B,** A lower second molar tipped significantly due to earlier extraction of the lower first molar. A significant angular periodontal defect has developed. **C and D,** Uprighting of the molar improved the bony morphology and eliminated the angular bony defect.

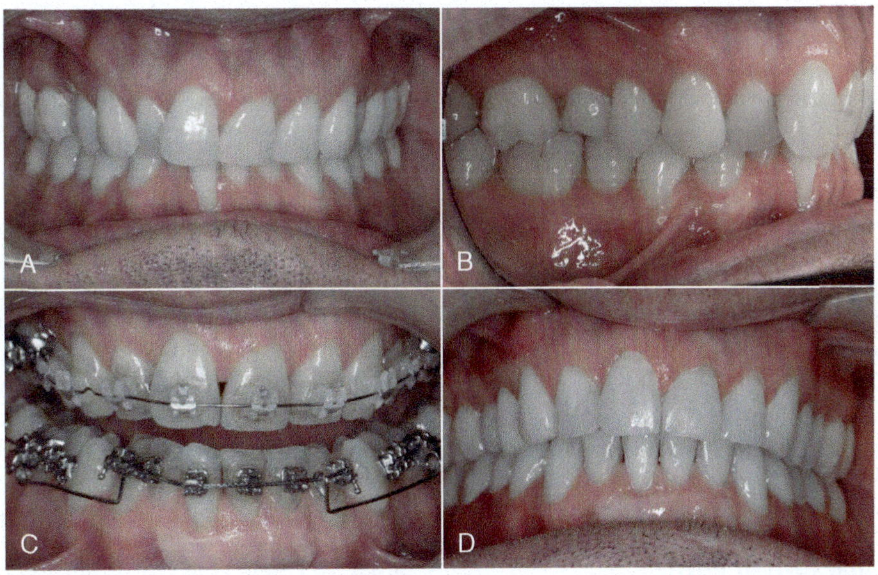

Figure 24-13 An adult patient presented with a deep overbite and significant tooth wear. **A and B,** Pre-treatment intraoral photographs revealed significant loss of attachment on the lower central incisor. **C,** Management of the deep overbite involved lower incisor intrusion and proclination. A gingival graft was performed to cover the defect and thicken the gingiva prior to bonding of appliances and orthodontic treatment. **D,** The gingival graft was successful in covering the defect and contributed to a most satisfactory treatment outcome.

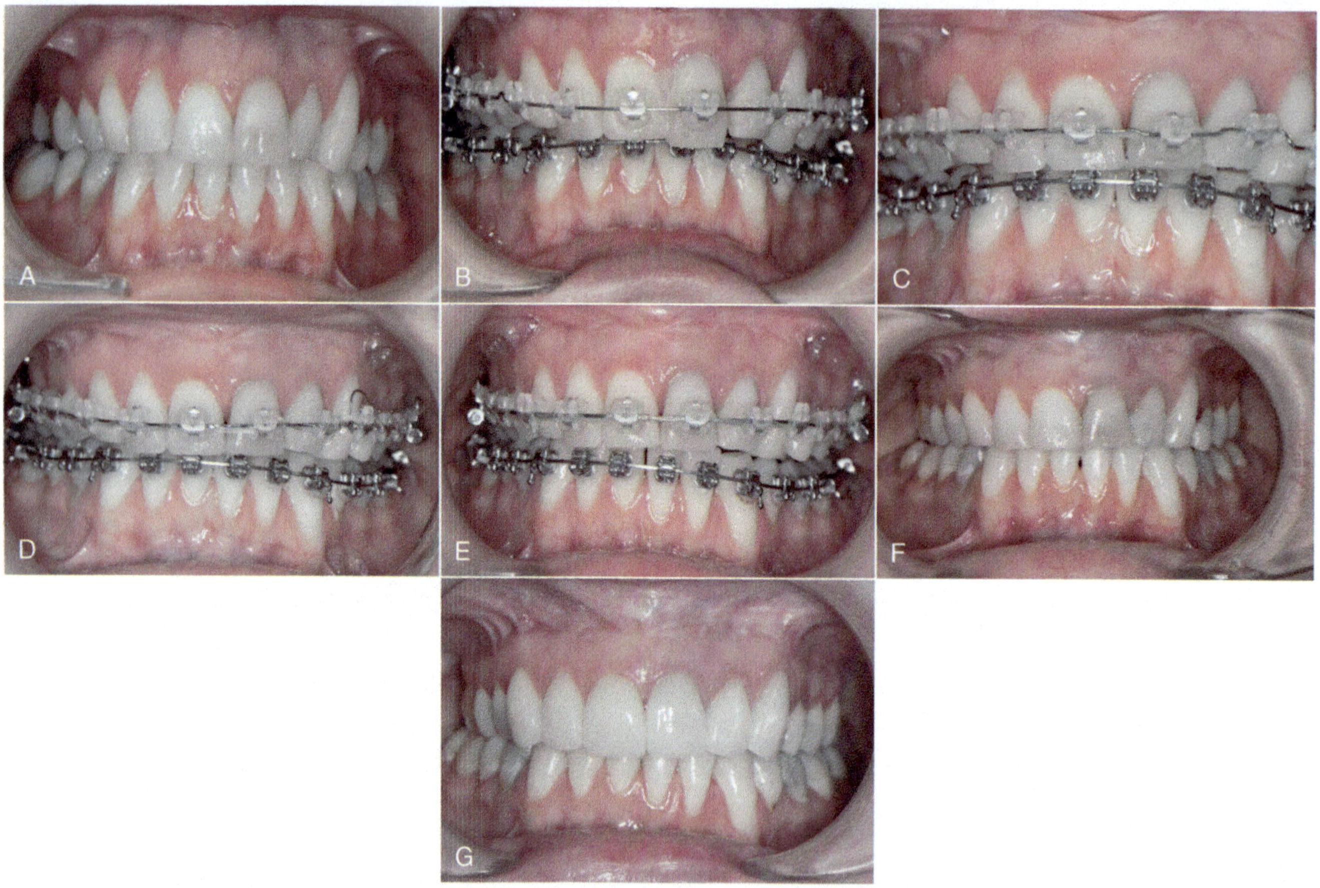

Figure 24-14 **A,** A 30-year-old female patient presented with a complex problem related to previous restorative dental treatment, which was performed to address her significant recession. The overcontoured restorations facilitated plaque retention and, when combined with a skeletal constriction of the maxilla and a thin periodontal biotype, recession progressed quite rapidly. **B,** The narrow maxilla was managed with a surgically assisted expansion procedure. Fixed appliances were placed strategically to facilitate selective extrusion of the periodontal attachment, as seen by the irregular incisor edges. **C,** Further extrusive adjustments of the teeth were performed on the left central incisor and canine. **D,** The upper left canine root was torqued palatally with a torquing auxiliary. **E and F,** The lower arch was leveled and the left lower canine root was moved lingually. It will be considered for grafting. **G,** The final upper veneers were placed on significantly improved soft tissue and bony attachment levels.

circumstances tooth movement is required to ensure that the optimal form and position are achieved in the final outcome. These may include:

- Teeth with atypical crown form
  - Teeth such as peg lateral incisors and other deviations in morphodifferentiation
  - Teeth that have been subjected to wear and/or erosion and subsequent compensatory tooth movements
- Teeth that have drifted and tipped, associated with tooth extraction or congenital absence

Teeth with Atypical Crown Form

Absence of normal tooth structure often results in compensatory tooth movements and may be accompanied by other malocclusion traits. It is important to evaluate the spatial position of the crown and associated gingival anatomy before planning tooth movements in three dimensions.

Ideally the abnormally shaped tooth should be restored with a provisional restoration (usually a composite resin or heat-cured temporary crown) prior to tooth movement to an ideal position.[8,28–30] Often tooth movement is required prior to buildup to create the necessary space to achieve ideal form. Teeth may have to be intruded and ideally positioned mesiodistally in an initial stage of treatment prior to a mid-treatment restoration, in preparation for finishing, and detailing of the occlusion.

This should not be a random act and careful consideration must be given to the final occlusal outcome, whether it be a Class I ideal relationship or, in some specific circumstances, a realistically stable occlusal scheme (Fig. 24-15). This is often best visualized by the diagnostic setup. However, the esthetic balance of the smile, which includes the mesiodistal and incisogingival proportions of the teeth, must always be considered.[3,31] There are many proposed guides, including the mathematically derived golden proportions, as significant deviations in form are recognized to influence the esthetics significantly.[32,33]

Restoration of the tooth prior to or during treatment is often more predictable than following removal of appliances, when the uncertainties of retainer wear may allow minor tooth movement to occur before the patient presents to the restorative dentist (Fig. 24-16).

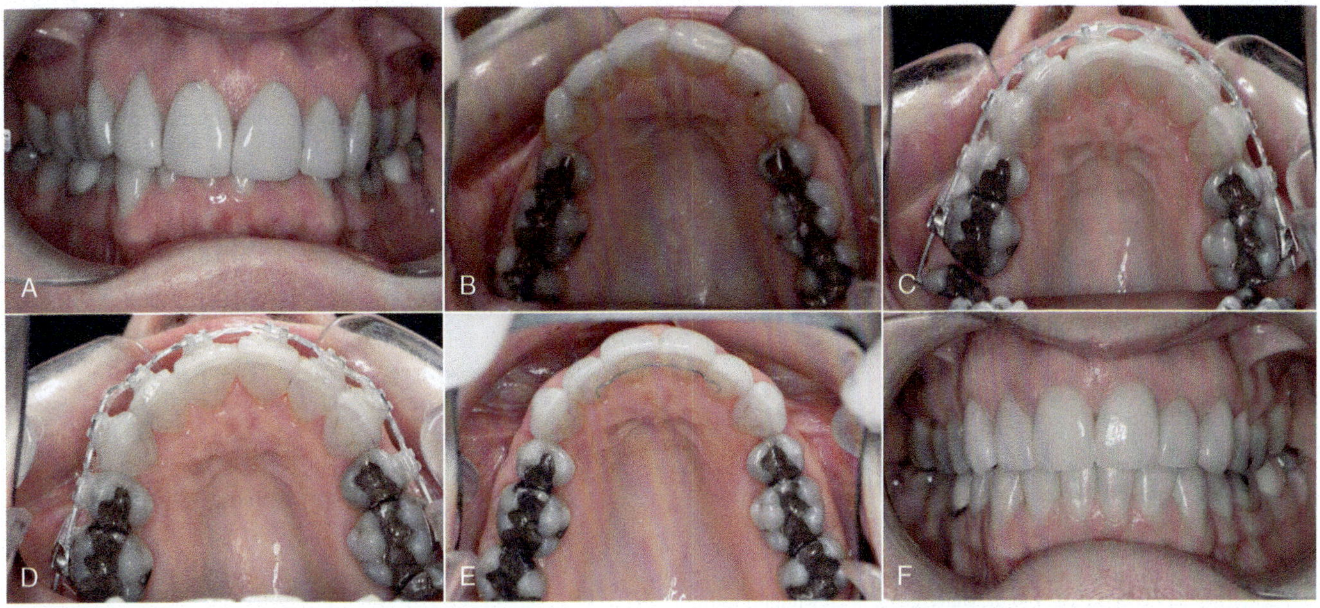

Figure 24-15 **A and B,** A 40-year-old female patient presented with the primary compliant that her teeth appeared too large and she was very aware of her increased overbite. She was sensitive to the issue of her teeth feeling overbuilt, as a dentist had attempted to camouflage the irregularity by overcontouring the teeth with veneers. Intrusion mechanics were used to address the deep overbite and careful attention was given to reducing the mesiodistal dimensions of the existing veneers. **C,** Variations in veneer thickness is seen after initial alignment. **D,** Artistic bends were placed in the archwire to align the palatal surfaces of the teeth in order to idealize positions of the underlying crowns and roots. Note the significant irregularity of the upper incisors. **E and F,** Final veneers were placed, which restored the original mesiodistal and buccolingual dimensions of the teeth. The outcome is most pleasing.

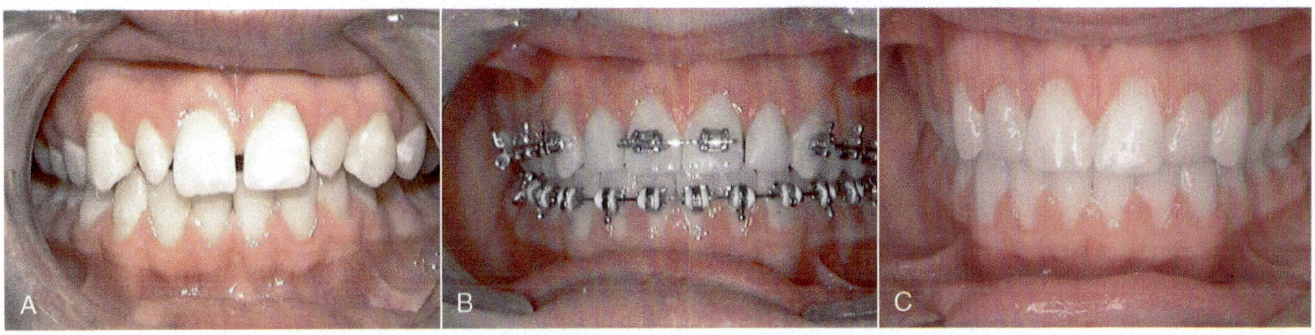

Figure 24-16 **A,** A 13-year-old male patient presented with peg-lateral incisors and a midline diastema. **B and C,** Closure of the diastema and placement of the lateral incisors in the ideal position, as dictated by the prosthodontist, will facilitate composite buildups to their ideal form. If sufficient space is available prior to bonding, these type of teeth may be built up prior to banding.

Attrition of the dentition is a complex problem, with compensatory tooth movements possible in all three dimensions (Fig. 24-17).[34,35] It is not uncommon to experience vertical eruption, anteroposterior uprighting, and mesiodistal dimension reduction because of the convergent crown form. In preparing for restoration of the teeth it is important to establish the nature of the compensatory movements that have occurred. It is often necessary to intrude, procline, and redistribute the teeth mesiodistally to facilitate restoration in all dimensions (Fig. 24-18).[36-39] In circumstances in which a significant skeletal jaw discrepancy has occurred, vertical space may be created by inferiorly repositioning the mandible to create space for restoration (Fig. 24-19).

In periodontally sound dentition, again it is important to use the cementoenamel junction or gingival margins as a vertical guide to establish the normal periodontal architecture, bone levels, and optimal esthetic balance.[40] This can be difficult to determine, particularly when the dimensions of the free gingiva may vary dependent on the labiolingual position of the tooth and the gingival biotype (Fig. 24-20).

The restorative dentist will carefully consider the restorative material of choice in patients with previous attrition to ensure that the wear properties are matched with natural teeth and/or the dentition in the opposing arch.[41] This may require further refinement when considering the need for optimal esthetic outcome and the ubiquitous techniques available for final prosthetic reconstruction (Fig. 24-21).

It is often necessary to consider an occlusal splint as part of the retention regime and the interdisciplinary team must ensure that the delegated clinician takes responsibility for the construction and maintenance of the appliance. Often the

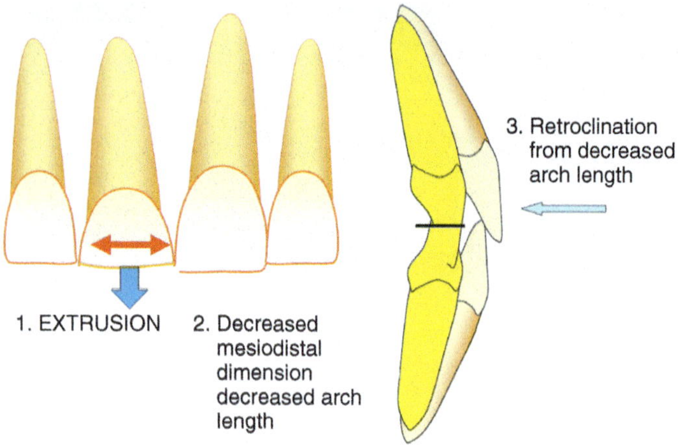

Figure 24-17 Attrition of teeth is a complex problem that results in tooth position compensations. The most significant effect is the loss of crown height and accompanying extrusion of the tooth or teeth, which will affect the level of the gingival margin. Often the extent of the attrition may be determined by the variation in the level of the respective gingival margins. (1) The secondary effects related to the convergence of crown form to the gingival margin is a reduction in mesiodistal dimension of the teeth, (2) which may in turn result in uprighting of the teeth to assume a more vertical relationship. (3) Comprehension of these effects is paramount in effecting movements to remove these compensatory tooth movements. Often teeth must therefore be intruded selectively, spaces regained between the incisal edges and proclined to assume their original positions prior to experiencing tooth wear. This will create space that facilitates the restorative dentistry procedures and reduces the need for significant further tooth reduction required to restore the teeth.

orthodontist will construct a routine orthodontic retainer such as a Hawley or vacuum-formed retainer and, once the full-time period of retention is complete, refer the patient to the restorative dentist for an occlusal splint.

Complex Tooth Movements in Partially Edentulous Patients

A patient may present with permanent tooth loss related to pathology or congenital absence. Frequently these patients require careful consideration of the treatment goals to manage issues related to tooth drift, tipping, and eruption in addition to the tooth replacement.[8] This may involve a course of orthodontic therapy to idealize tooth position prior to prosthetic replacement (Figs. 24-22 and 24-23).

The goals of treatment may include alignment of teeth to:

- Facilitate replacement of a prosthetic tooth of optimal size and form
- Idealize loading of the tooth, which may function in isolation or as part of a fixed prosthesis
- Facilitate improvement of periodontal architecture and plaque control mechanisms
- Reduce the number and complexity of prosthetic tooth replacements with consideration given to eliminating the need for a prosthesis

Historically there have been some biomechanical limitations on the clinician to management of severely tipped or extruded teeth, occasionally requiring consideration of

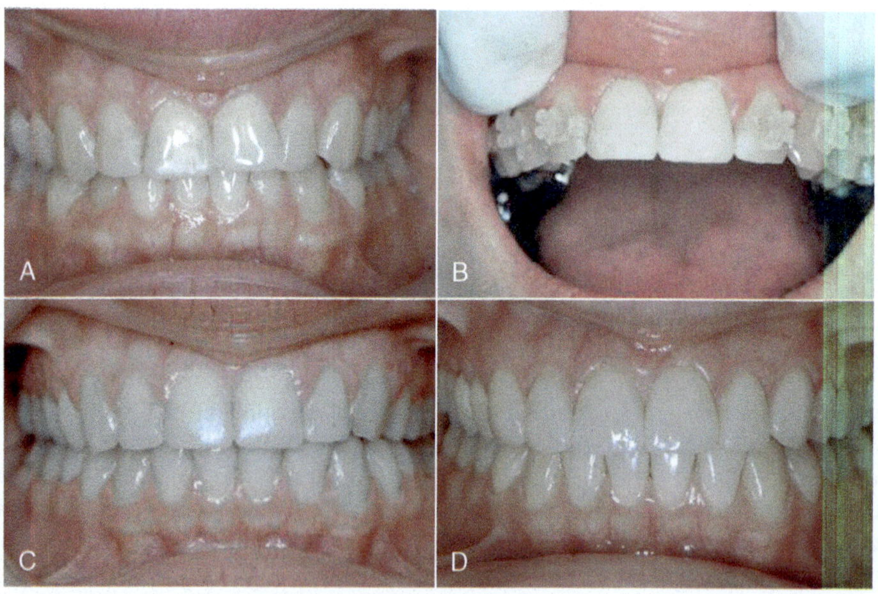

Figure 24-18 **A,** A 29-year-old female patient presented with a history of numerous failed composite restorations on the upper central incisors and a report of nocturnal bruxism. The restorative dentists who treated her in the past continually removed more natural tooth substance to create space for the composite bonding and the patient has become frustrated with their short clinical life. Due to the failure of her composite restorations, she consulted a prosthodontist. **B,** Fixed appliances were placed on upper and lower teeth to procline the upper and lower incisors. In addition, there was significant intrusion of the upper central incisors. Note the gingival margin heights relative to the lateral incisors after the brackets were removed and the composite buildups were performed mid-treatment. **C,** The brackets were debonded, the treatment was completed, and the prosthodontist carefully monitored the patient for any wear facets. The patient was provided with a splint to wear at night as a retainer. **D,** After 9 months and no significant wear facets on the composite restorations, the prosthodontist was confident enough to proceed with ceramic veneers.

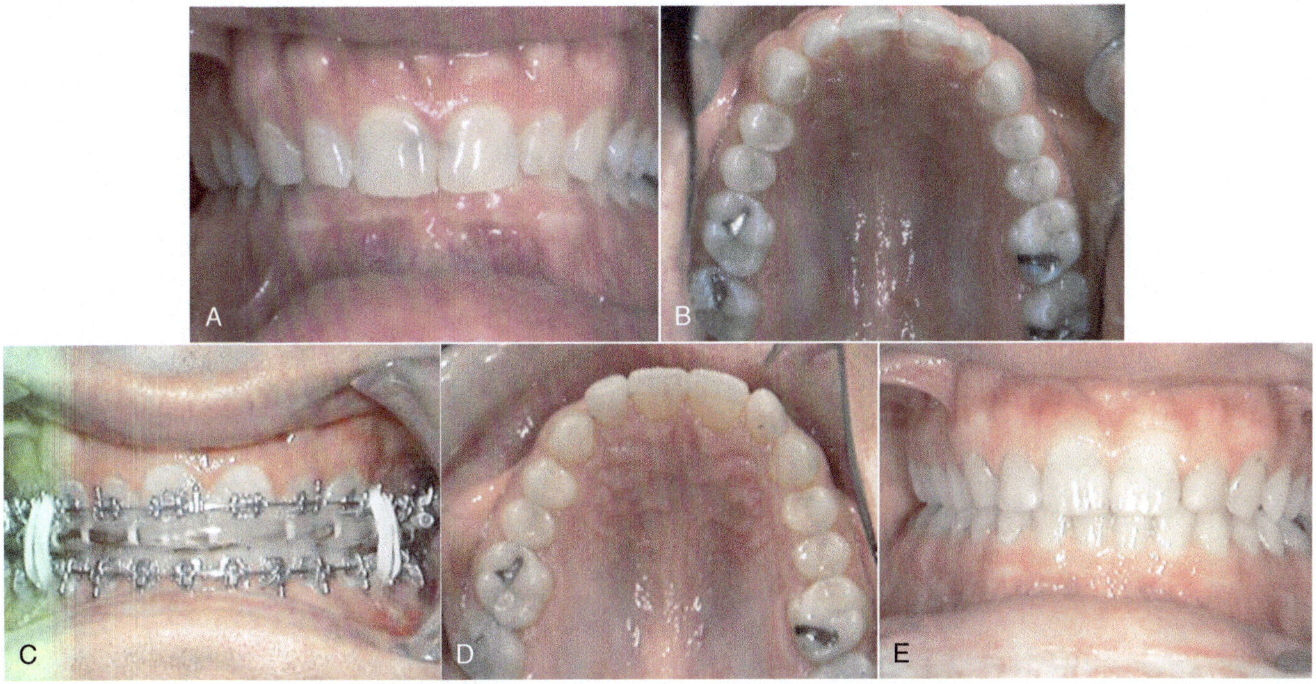

Figure 24-19 **A and B,** Occasionally a combination of a significant skeletal problem and bruxism may predispose the patient to a major attrition problem. In this case, the significant Class II skeletal deep bite contributed to a major wear effect, nearly exposing the pulp. The darkened appearance on the labial surface of the central incisors reflected the near penetration of the attrition lesion through to the labial surface. **C,** Surgical repositioning of the mandible created vertical space, which allowed for buildup and restoration of the teeth by addition of composite-type materials. **D and E,** The combination of addressing the aberrant jaw morphology and restoring the lost tooth substance has contributed to an excellent clinical outcome. The patient will be provided with a splint to wear as a retainer.

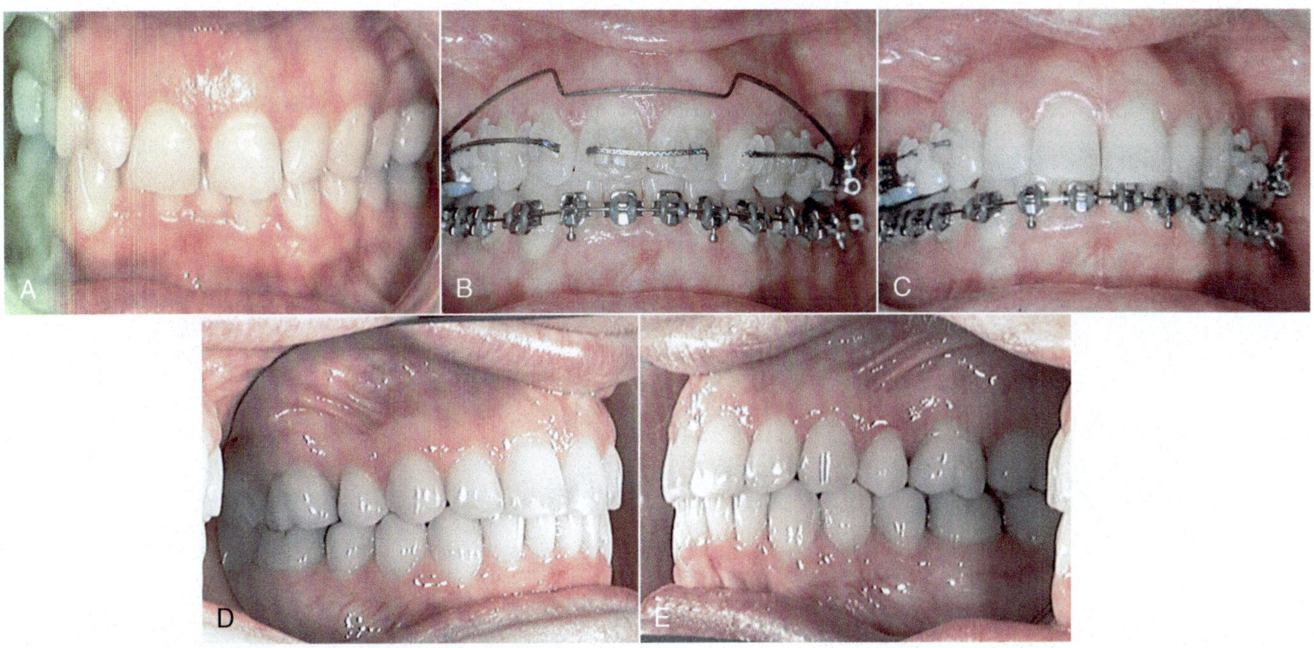

Figure 24-20 **A,** A 38-year-old female patient presented with the primary complaints of her teeth "wearing away" and deteriorating esthetics. She had upper premolar extractions, but no orthodontics, as a child. The upper and lower incisors were retroclined and significant attrition was observed on the upper central incisors, reflected in the level of the gingival margins. **B,** Treatment commenced with a 0.021-inch × 0.025-inch multistranded nickel-titanium (Ni-Ti) segmental maxillary arch and a beta-titanium intrusion arch to intrude and procline the upper centrals. In this view the wire has been untied to reassess activation and change the discolored elastometrics. **C,** When sufficient vertical and mesiodistal space was created, the brackets were removed from the teeth to facilitate restoration. The teeth were then rebonded with brackets and the final detailing was performed. **D and E,** The final outcome showed that normal gingival heights were regained.

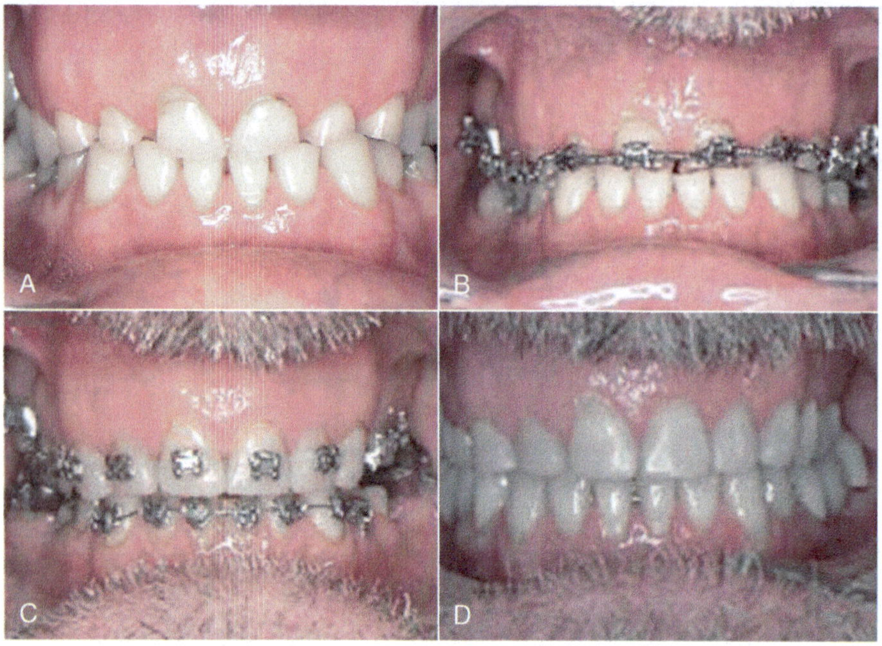

Figure 24-21 **A–D,** Significant attrition may necessitate a sequential approach to treatment, with one arch followed by a progressive addition of the other arch and composite restorations added as the dimensions of the teeth are progressively restored. This patient required an increase in vertical dimension of both upper and lower arches and composite restorations.

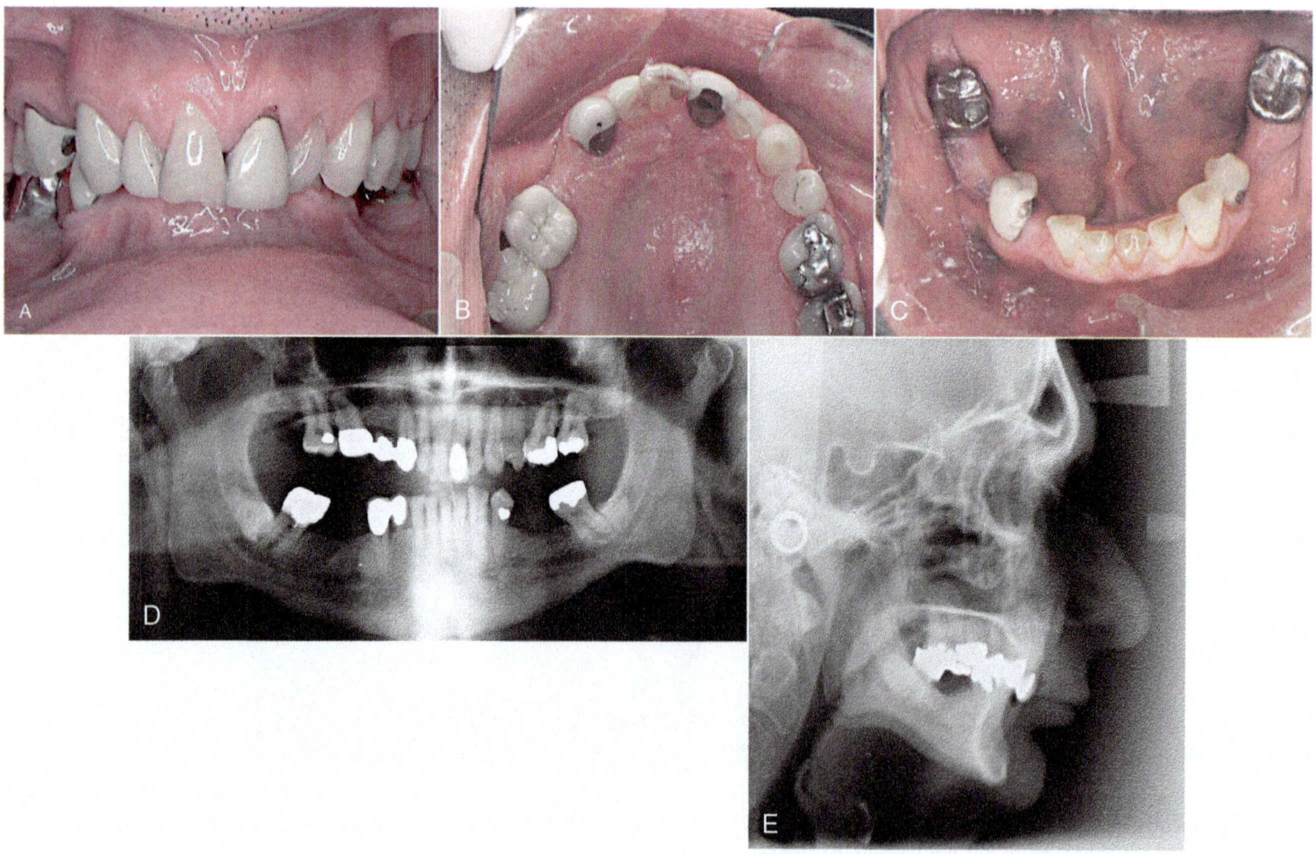

Figure 24-22 **A–C,** A 65-year-old male patient presented with the primary concerns of progressive tooth loss and tooth wear. He recently had a bridge fail, which had been placed to restore the upper right first premolar. The prosthodontist removed the pontic because of the traumatic relationship of the lower arch loading the bridge pontic. The patient showed a typical pattern of heavily restored teeth, placed erratically, as numerous dentists responded to minor dental crises through his life. **D,** The panoramic radiograph revealed heavily restored teeth, partial edentulism, and an unerupted lower right third molar. **E,** The cephalometric headplate revealed a significant Class II skeletal relationship, characterized by a retrognathic mandible and decreased vertical dimension. The upper incisors were significantly retroclined.

localized osteotomies and occasionally extraction of healthy teeth to address significant deviations in tooth position. Severely mutilated dentitions may challenge the clinician in finding a sufficient number of teeth to use as anchorage for efficient tooth movement.

The introduction of osseointegrated dental implants has made a significant contribution to dental rehabilitation with what is now considered to be a relatively predictable prosthetic replacement (Figs. 24-24 and 24-25).[42] Dental implants may now be considered for the majority of replacement options but may be limited by anatomic factors such as sufficient bone volume, space requirements, and issues related to dentofacial growth (Fig. 24-26).

INTERDISCIPLINARY TREATMENT SEQUENCE	
• Control phase	
– Preventive/perio/restorative	VH
– Oral surgery (extract 48)	BA
• Orthodontic decompensation	MG
• Periodontal maintenance (3-4m)	VH
• Mandibular surgery	BA
• Restore lower anteriors	VH
• Postsurgical orthodontics	MG
• Retention appliances	MG
• Reassessment	VH
– (exo 44)	BA
• Implant placement	BA/VH
• Provisional restorations	VH
• Final restorations	VH
• Maintenance	VH/MG

F

Figure 24-22, cont'd **F,** An interdisciplinary treatment plan (sequence outlined) was developed to decompensate the patient and address the missing and worn teeth, the skeletal relationship, and the impacted molar.

Treatment plans may even include placement of osseointegrated implants prior to or during orthodontic treatment to facilitate tooth movement.[43-50] In fact, the use of dental implants has expanded the envelope of possible tooth movements to enable significant mesiodistal tooth position changes, which may include edentulous space closure without the biomechanical side effects encountered during unsupported orthodontic treatment. Moreover, control of vertical tooth movements, including significant intrusive movement, may be achieved using dental implants for anchorage.

More recently a range of temporary anchorage devices (TADs), including micro-screws and bone plates, has been introduced.[51-54] These devices may be placed outside the field of tooth movement and have been shown to be effective in facilitating significant tooth movements by reducing biomechanical side effects.

Missing Lateral Incisors

The patient with congenitally missing lateral incisors presents the clinician with the dilemma of either replacing the lateral incisors with a prosthesis or closing the space and in so doing eliminating the need for a prosthesis.[55,56] Before the introduction of osseointegrated dental implants, patients with a Class II malocclusion with favorable color and form of the canine teeth would be considered for space closure and canine substitution[57]; however, the implant has been promoted as the standard of care in most circumstances.[58-61]

In minimally restored abutment teeth, implant replacement seems to be more reliable and predictable to reestablish function and aesthetics. Although treatment time may be longer than replacement via conventional bridges, a

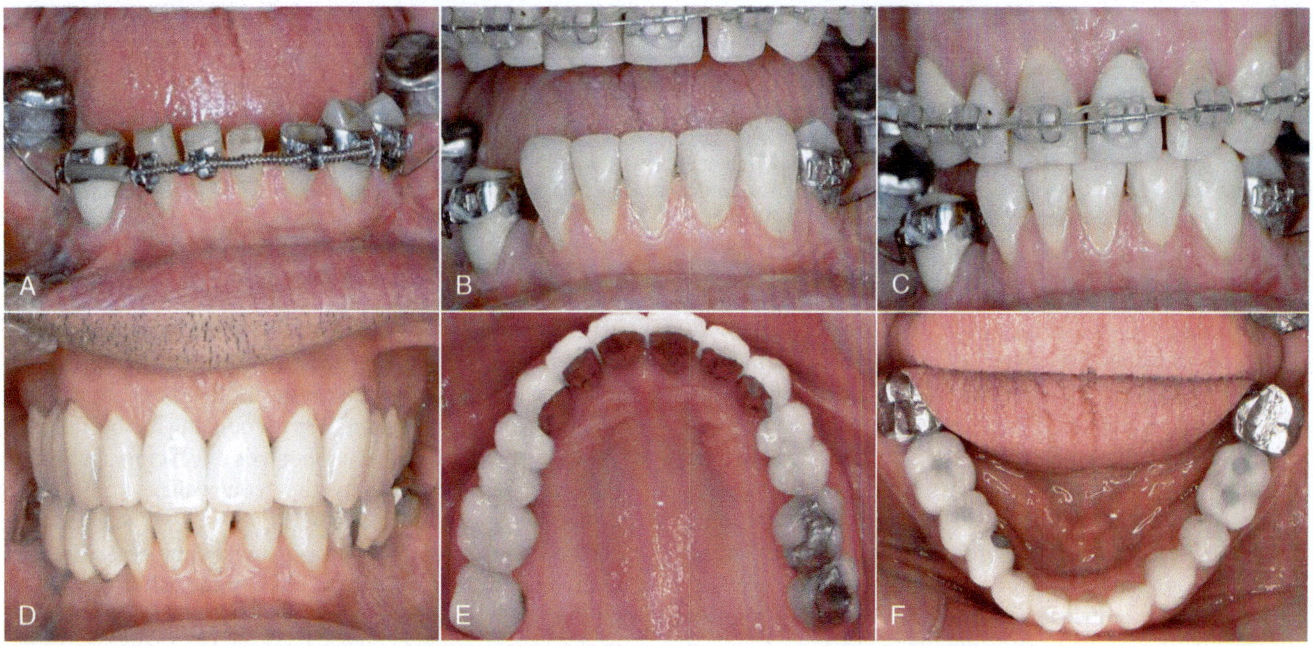

Figure 24-23 **A-C,** Management of attrition typically involves intrusion and space opening and removal of the fixed appliances to facilitate restoration with composite. In this case (the same patient shown in Figure 24-22), the maxillary incisors were decompensated, the mandible was advanced, and the teeth were restored. The lower right first premolar was considered a risk to the implant placed in this region, so it was extracted. **D-F,** The final outcome of fixed appliances, orthognathic surgery, implant placement, composite restoration of the lower incisors, and extensive crown and bridge treatment is most pleasing.

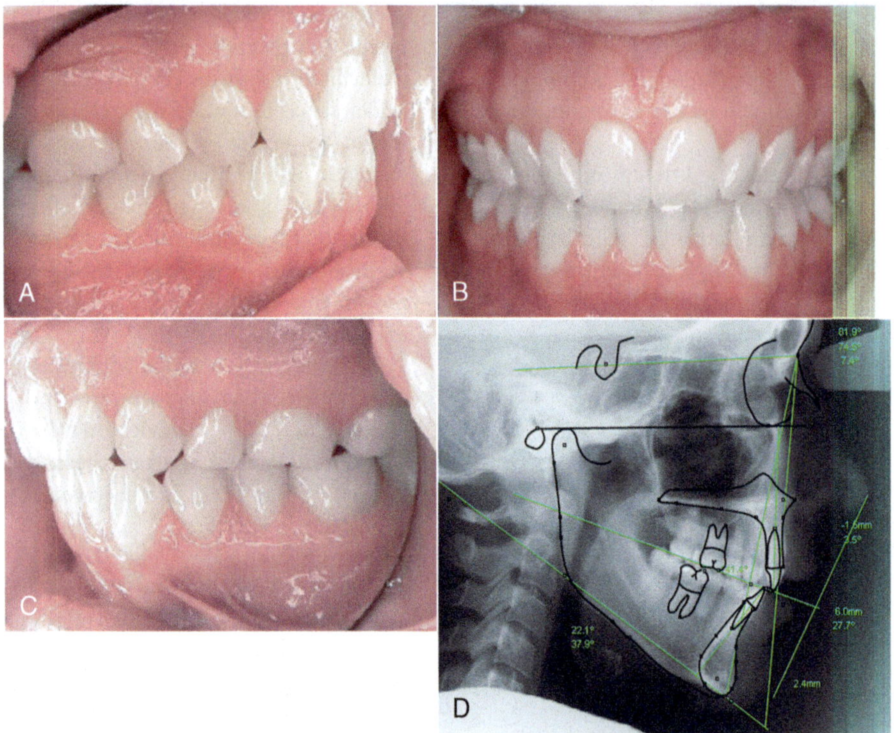

INTERDISCIPLINARY TREATMENT SEQUENCING

• Place maxillary expander	MG
• Surgically assisted expansion	BA/MG
• Orthodontic decompensation	MG
– Open space for upper premolars	
– Place teeth on fixed appliances	
• Mandibular surgery	BA
• Postsurgical orthodontics	MG
• Implant placement	BA
– 6 mos after debanding upper premolars	
• Provisional restorations	BS
• Final restorations	BS
• Maintenance	BS/MG

E

Figure 24-24 **A–C,** A 23-year-old female patient presented with the primary complaints of a narrow dental arch and a flat smile. Her history included treatment of a significant Class II, Division 1 malocclusion as a teenager, with extraction of the first premolars and headgear for anchorage. An acceptable occlusal result was achieved after retraction of the upper incisors. **D,** The cephalometric radiograph revealed a significant skeletal Class II skeletal relationship characterized by mandibular retrognathism. The maxillary incisors were retracted and uprighted within the limits of the alveolar process. **E,** An interdisciplinary treatment plan (sequence outlined) was developed and involved expanding the upper arch and moving the upper incisors back to their protrusive position, opening the spaces for the extracted upper first premolars. The mandible would then be advanced and implants placed in the premolar region.

systematic review has reported an estimated 96.8% 5-year survival rate.

When implants have been chosen to replace missing lateral incisor teeth, often adjacent teeth have erupted into the edentulous region. Fixed orthodontic appliances are required to create sufficient space for the lateral incisor implant and crown.[62] Thorough assessment of the patient's skeletal and dental relationships is required. First, planning for space creation should be preceded by careful evaluation of a diagnostic setup to ensure that an ideal occlusal relationship will enable sufficient space to be prepared for implant placement. The implant will require at least 5.5- to 6-mm of space between the adjacent roots (Fig. 24-27).[63]

Orthodontic tooth movement within the confines of the alveolar ridge has been recommended to develop the mesiodistal dimensions of the bone (Fig. 24-28). Moreover, extrusive alveolar ridge development has been proposed to increase the hard and soft tissue dimensions in circumstances where the prognosis for the tooth is poor and implant replacement is contemplated. Space opening has been shown in a canine model to develop bone of satisfactory trabeculation and density to satisfy the requirements for optimal osseointegration and loading (Fig. 24-29). There is some controversy related to bony ridge developmental changes, with reports suggesting that the canine acts to promote development of the bony ridge volume when it has erupted in the edentulous ridge. Distal movement of the canine has been proposed to leave a significant volume of bone from its point of origin[8,64] but this was not a consistent finding in a recent report.[65]

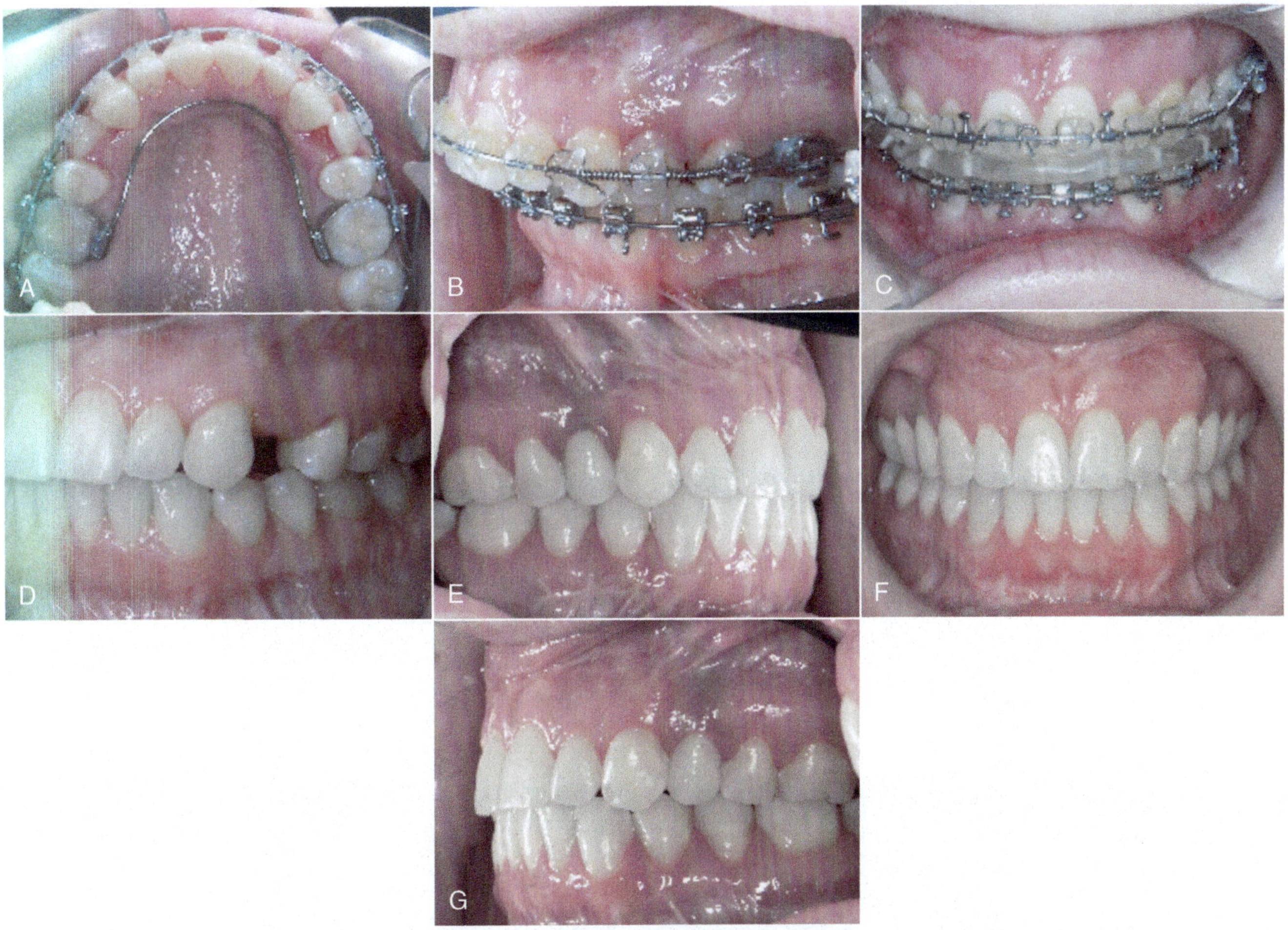

Figure 24-25 **A and B,** Surgical maxillary expansion was performed (same patient shown in Figure 24-24) to broaden the maxillary arch. Fixed appliances were then placed to open space for the extracted upper first premolars and flare the upper incisors to their normal inclinations. Acrylic pontics were added to the extraction spaces. **C,** The mandible was advanced (seen with the surgical splint in place). **D,** Intraoral view of the patient at debanding showed the premolar space. **E–G,** Final intraoral photographs showed excellent occlusal outcomes, improved incisor inclinations and arch width, and premolar implants in place.

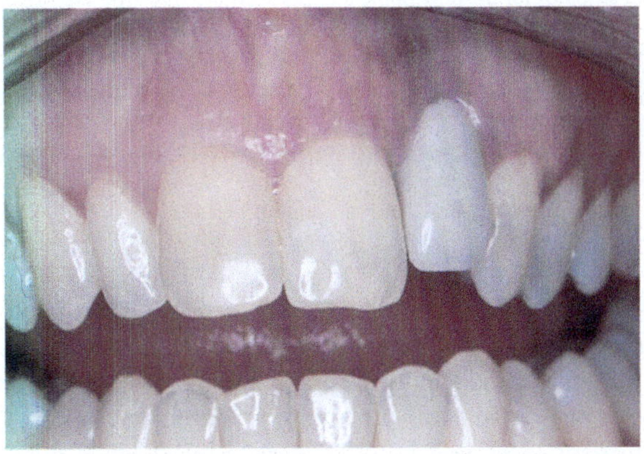

Figure 24-26 Placement of implants in the esthetic zone is extremely difficult, as many patients experience maturational changes in the dentofacial complex even in adulthood. This intraoral view demonstrates a lateral incisor implant supported crown submerged several years after the dentist considered growth to be complete. As the face grows, bone is often resorbed from the anterior surface of the maxilla. The soft tissue fenestration above the gingival margins indicates that very little bone would overlie the implant and that even with grafting procedures it will be difficult to recover from this circumstance.

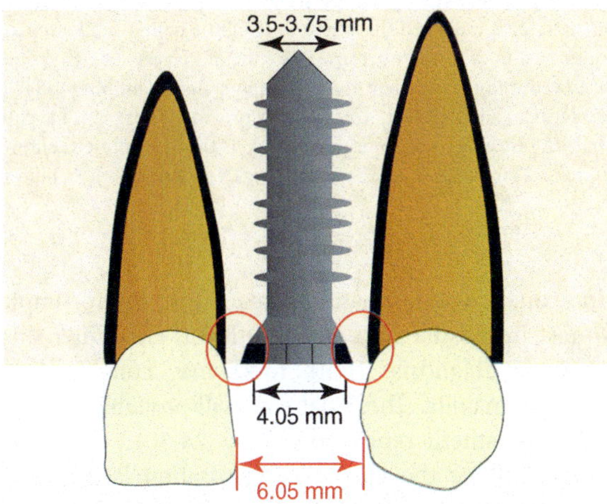

Figure 24-27 At least 6-mm of space is required between adjacent teeth for a satisfactory implant replacement. This dimension may be reduced to 5.5-mm but it should be stressed that at least 1-mm of bone is required between the implant structure and the adjacent tooth to enable the bone to act as a stimulus for adequate soft tissue papilla development and satisfactory emergence form. Less than 6-mm of space may be problematic at the time of implant placement, with possible root damage and an esthetic outcome that may be disappointing for both the clinician and patient, as insufficient soft tissue papilla will be allowed to develop.

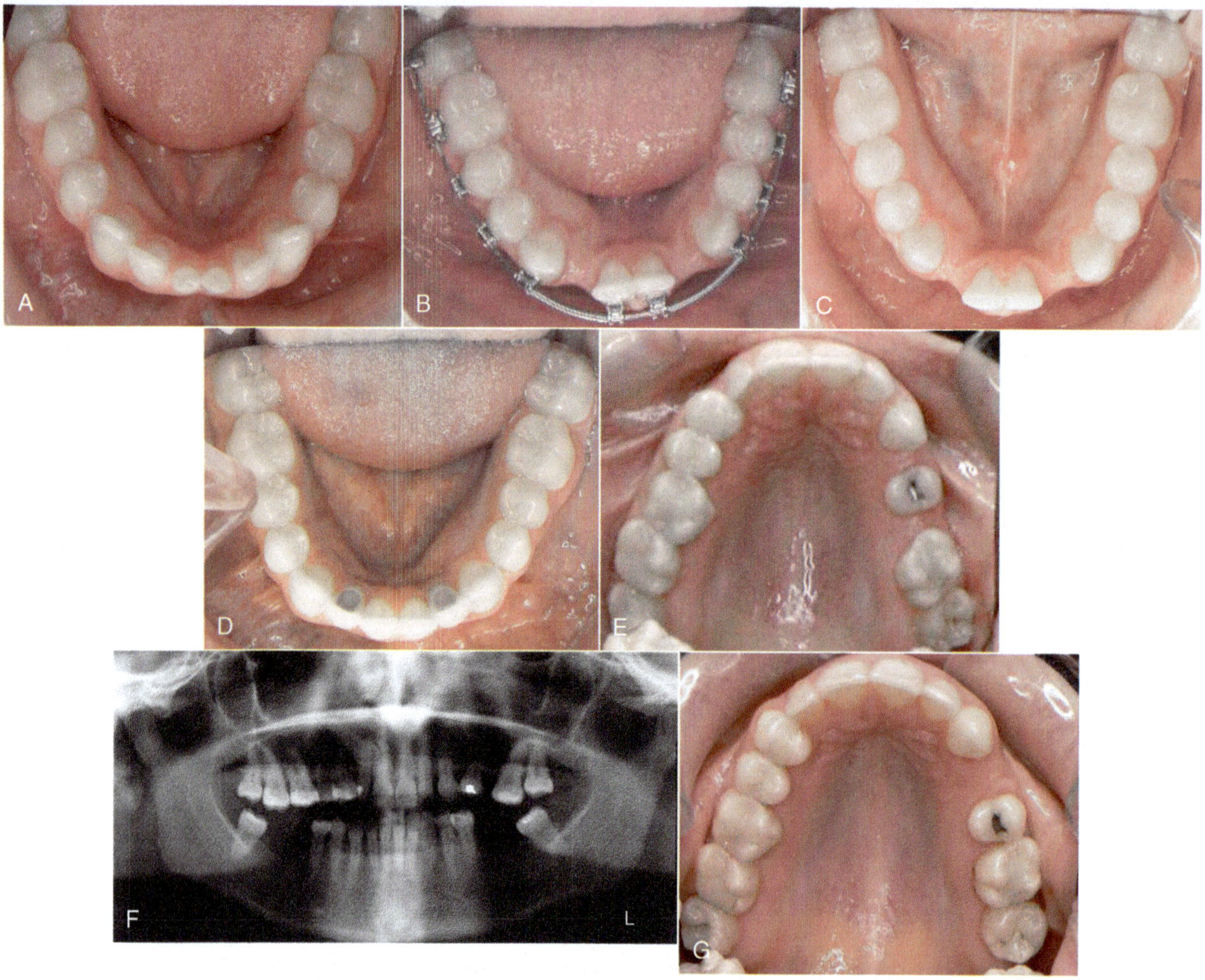

Figure 24-28 **A–D,** Orthodontic tooth movement may be used to develop bone. This young adult patient presented with missing lower central incisors and retained deciduous incisors. The presence of erupting permanent teeth was an excellent stimulus for the development of the bony alveolus. The absence of the permanent teeth indicated that there will be little bone volume to place two incisor implants without bone grafting. Moreover, it is problematic to place two implants next to each other because it is difficult to create enough bone between the implants to generate an adequate papilla. Therefore the two lateral incisors were moved into the deficient ridge, leaving a significant bony ridge behind. Two lateral incisor implants can now be placed. **E–G,** A similar circumstance occurred in an adult patient. This patient's prosthodontist sent the patient for treatment to create space for an implant in the upper left second premolar site. A sinus lift procedure was to be performed, as the sinus projected down vertically. A treatment plan was devised to move the first premolar back through the sinus, taking bone with it and leaving a large volume of bone behind for a more simple implant placement.

In a small group of patients, space opening for implants is almost impossible and often clinicians encounter this by therapeutic diagnosis. Tooth roots may converge into a diminutive maxilla. These patients will probably require an alternate prosthetic replacement (Fig. 24-30).

Regardless of the choice of restoration, some type of interim prosthesis will be required, especially in growing children who require maintenance of tooth positions with a specific retention protocol until the cessation of facial growth. During the period the clinician waits for growth to cease, the ridge volume has been shown to be remarkably stable,[8] unlike extraction sites where the healing response includes significant remodelling.[66] In preparation for implant replacement, up to 11% of patients may require orthodontic retreatment to realign the roots of adjacent teeth due to significant relapse during the retention phase.[67]

Biological and technical complications with implant prostheses are frequent, with peri-implantitis (9.7%), screw/abutment loosening (12.7%), darkening of labial gingival, and resorption of the endosteally derived labial bone being the most commonly reported events even within the first 5-year observation period.[68–72] The prosthetic crown on the implant independently also has failure issues related to color and integrity. Implants are invasive to the bone and soft tissue, leaving little margin for error and potentially a larger penalty to pay esthetically and functionally if there is a less than desirable outcome in the short- to medium-term. Moreover, the inability of implants to adapt to dynamic

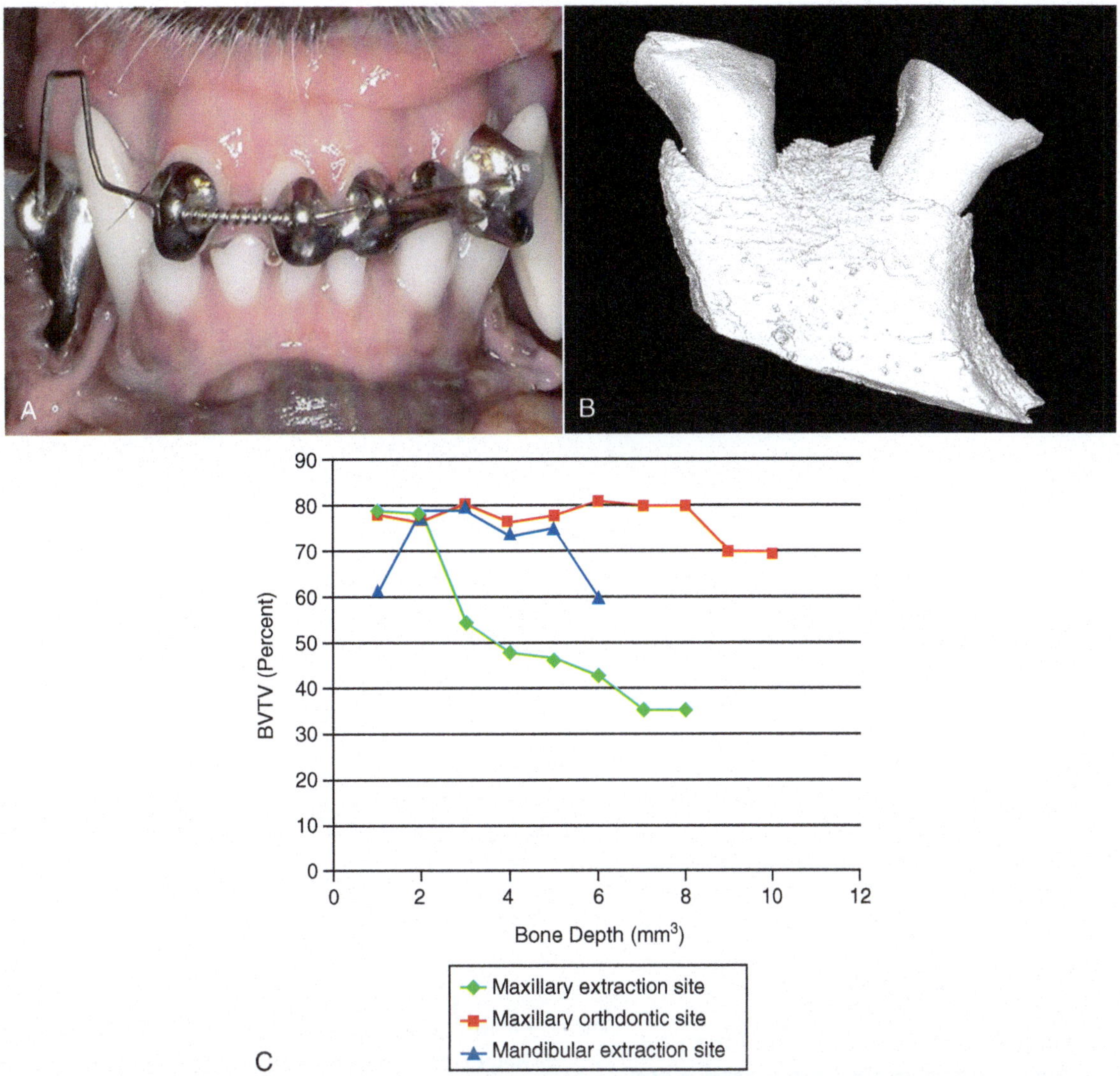

Figure 24-29 A canine study demonstrated that when a ridge is created by opening space between incisors, the quality of the bone is as dense as normal bone and denser than a healing extraction site. **A,** The upper right third incisor and the upper left second incisor were extracted and a cast appliance cemented with an archwire and opening coil to move the right second incisor distally. A ridge will be created between the right central and second incisor. **B,** A 3D reconstruction of a scanning electron microscopic exposure demonstrates the bony ridge created by the distal movement. **C,** The graph reveals the fractional bone volume (BVTV) at different depths through the bony ridge for the created ridge, and an extraction site in both the maxilla and mandible.

maturational changes experienced during adulthood may result in minor vertical and anteroposterior discrepancies even when the optimal time has been established following serial cephalometric review.[73–80]

These long-term findings and the development of TADs, which have extended the biomechanical possibilities, have stimulated orthodontists to consider space closure and canine substitution when it had been ruled out historically.

On the contrary, management of hypodontia may include consideration for space closure.[81] This offers the advantage of completing treatment during adolescence, leaving the growing child with some case-specific retention considerations, such as bonded upper retainers during growth to prevent spaces from reopening. The patient may then be left with a naturally embedded occlusion that grows and adapts to normal craniofacial maturational changes (Fig. 24-31).[82]

Nevertheless, orthodontic space closure is not without controversy. The problems often associated with moving the posterior teeth one unit forward in patients with missing lateral incisors relate to the larger, darker canine crown and the smaller first premolars. Thin porcelain veneers, selective bleaching, and even significant selective vertical repositioning of premolars and canines have been proposed, each of which has biological issues (Figs. 24-32 and 24-33).

This may be dealt with by several strategies either in isolation or combined as the individual circumstances dictate (Table 24-1 and Fig. 24-34). The canine may be recontoured to assume the shape of a lateral incisor and the premolar palatal cusp may have to be reduced, with minimal biological impact. The canine root may also be moved palatally if it is overly bulbous.[83,84]

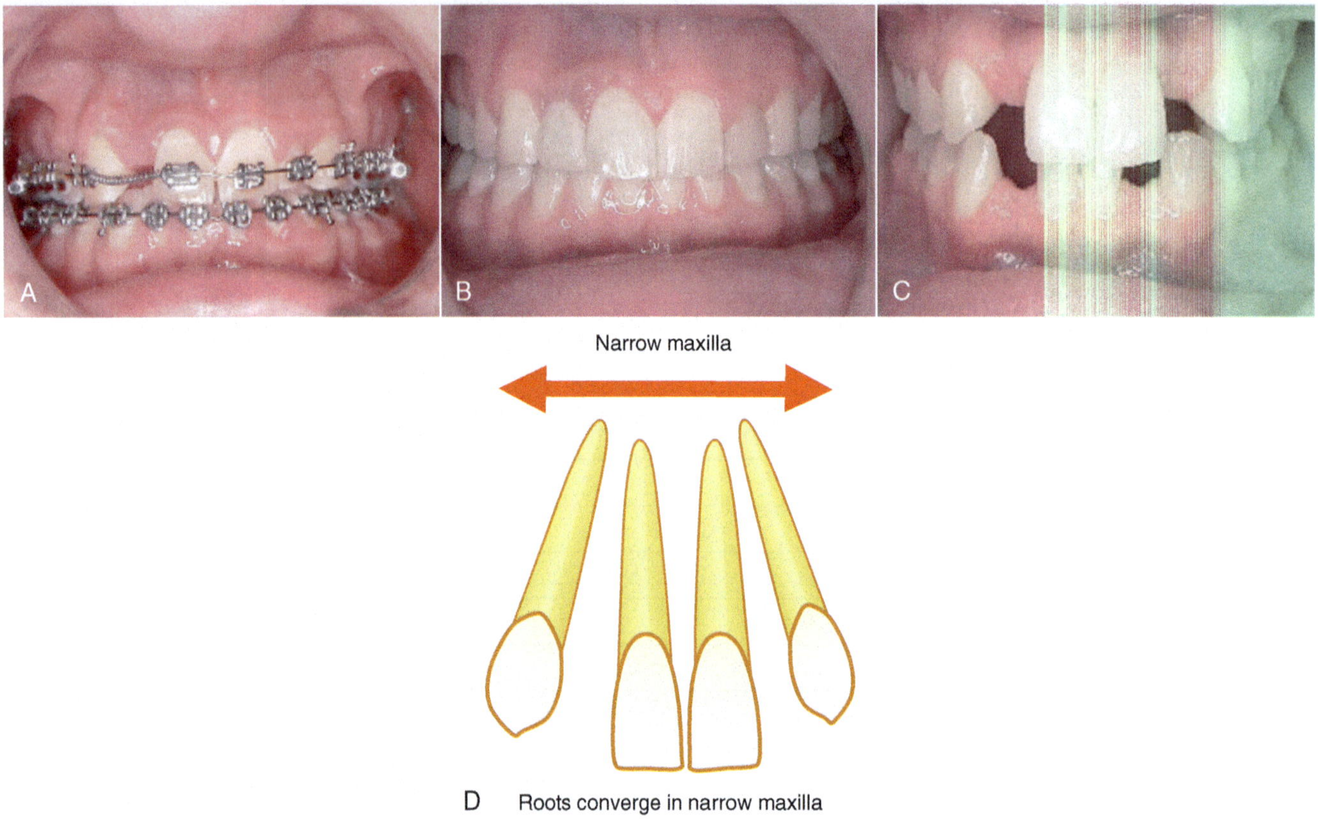

Figure 24-30 **A and B,** Opening space for an implant to replace the lateral incisor was relatively simple in this patient, who had an implant to replace the right lateral incisor and a composite buildup to enlarge the left lateral incisor. **C and D,** Significant difficulty was encountered in this patient, who presented with a compensated Class III relationship in which the roots converge back to the diminutive maxilla, sometimes transversely and often anteroposteriorly. As shown in **D,** it is almost impossible to create space at the apices to place an implant in some people and alternative strategies may have to be considered.

TABLE 24-1 Modifications in Tooth Position and Form That May Be Considered when Canine Substitution for Lateral Incisors Is Performed

Tooth	Modification
Canine	• Recontour • Mesiodistally • Incisal edge • Cingulum • Labial contour • Extrude and level gingival margin • Move root palatally to reduce root bulge • Build up with composite or ceramic
Premolar	• Rotate mesially • Intrude carefully • Recontour palatal cusp • Build up with composite or ceramic
Molar	• Rotate mesially if left as Class II relationship

In patients with a high smile line, the gingival margin height differences between the canine and first premolar may need to be modified by selective vertical tooth positioning.[82,85,86] The premolar tooth may be smaller than the canine for which it substitutes and it may be rotated mesially to occupy more space, if restorative procedures have not been considered to reshape the premolar.[84,85,87] A word of caution is required regarding significant vertical repositioning of canines and premolars, as there is an issue of biological width when teeth are leveled irregularly, introducing angular bony variation between teeth that may introduce some confounders to the periodontal health in addition to any proposed restorative therapy. To date there have been no long-term reports of the outcome on the periodontium from this strategy, although the esthetic outcomes are most impressive.

Something that should never be overlooked is the time factor involved in achieving a satisfactory treatment outcome in space closure, as an extended period in fixed appliances is often required. It is recognized that some patient factors may contraindicate a protracted course of therapy.

It is interesting to note that when the esthetic outcome of space closure or space opening strategies was compared in a group of patients, laypersons, dentists, and orthodontists all rated the esthetic outcome of canine substitution above all prosthetic outcomes (i.e., conventional fixed prostheses or

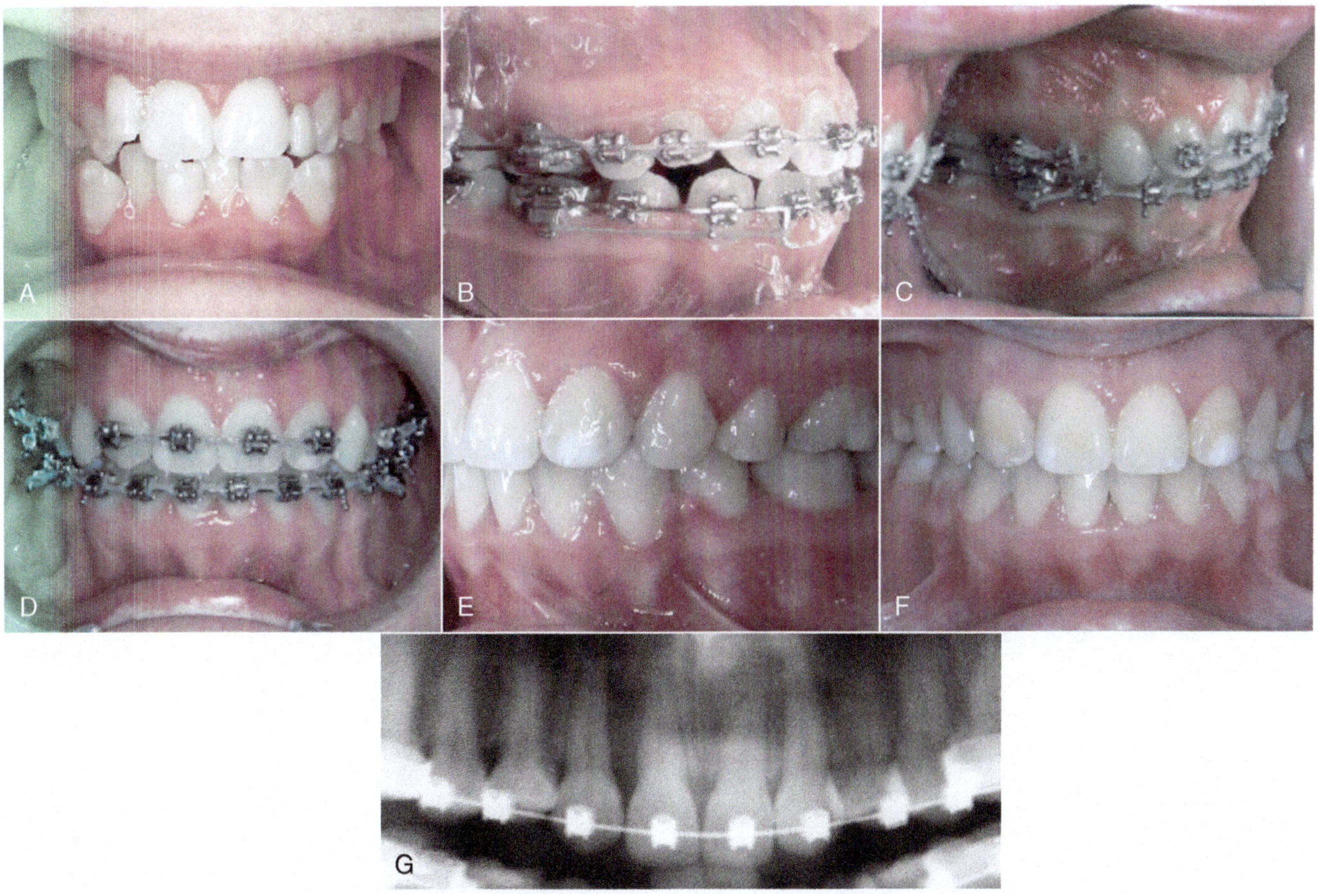

Figure 24-31 **A,** An adult female patient presented with a Class I malocclusion and a missing lateral incisor that was replaced with a Maryland bridge. The remaining lateral incisor was peg-shaped. **B–D,** A treatment plan was devised to extract the peg lateral, remove the bridge, and remove two lower premolars. Fixed appliances were placed and all spaces were closed. The upper first premolars were intruded during treatment to position the gingival margin apically to facilitate composite buildup so that the premolar would assume canine form. The canine root was moved lingually and the canine was reshaped to assume incisor form. **E and F,** The functional and esthetic outcome was excellent. **G,** Although the esthetic outcome is excellent, on reviewing the treatment progress panoramic radiograph it is clear that this strategy does create an angular bony defect and the long-term periodontal outcome is yet to be reported.

implants), although the dentists suggested that they anticipated a better esthetic outcome following implant replacement.[88–92]

Acceptable functional relationship in the periodontium and occlusion can be achieved after space closure, with results that are well accepted by patients and encourage periodontal health without compromising temporomandibular joint (TMJ) function in comparison with prosthetic replacements.

Missing Second Premolars

Similarly, for missing second premolars the two major approaches used are orthodontic space closure by allowing the mesial drifting of the permanent first molars and space maintenance by retaining the deciduous molar and subsequent prosthetic replacement.[87] Esthetic considerations may not be as influential in a posterior tooth prosthesis and therefore the clinician may be more likely to accept a posterior prosthesis or be optimistic about the deciduous molar's prognosis. Occasionally, ideal intercuspation of the posterior teeth may not be achieved without modification to the crown form of the deciduous molar. Despite the absence of its successor, physiological resorption and/or infraclusion of clinically healthy deciduous molars may still occur but approximately 50% of deciduous molars have been reported to remain healthy and functional after 2 to 3 decades.

As with the missing lateral incisor, similar issues have now confronted the contemporary clinician, with serious consideration given to space closure with the assistance of TADs.

SUMMARY

Interdisciplinary treatment plans may be extremely rewarding for both treating clinicians and patients. However, irrespective of the individual clinician's technical skill, significant regret is often encountered when a rigorous systematic approach is not pursued in developing a coordinated, patient-centered, goal-oriented treatment plan (Figs. 24-35 to 24-37).

It is critical to establish the needs of the individual patient within his or her own value system and to establish a realistic plan to address these needs. In the patient who presents with a degree of neglect, it is important to control disease

Text continued on p. 524

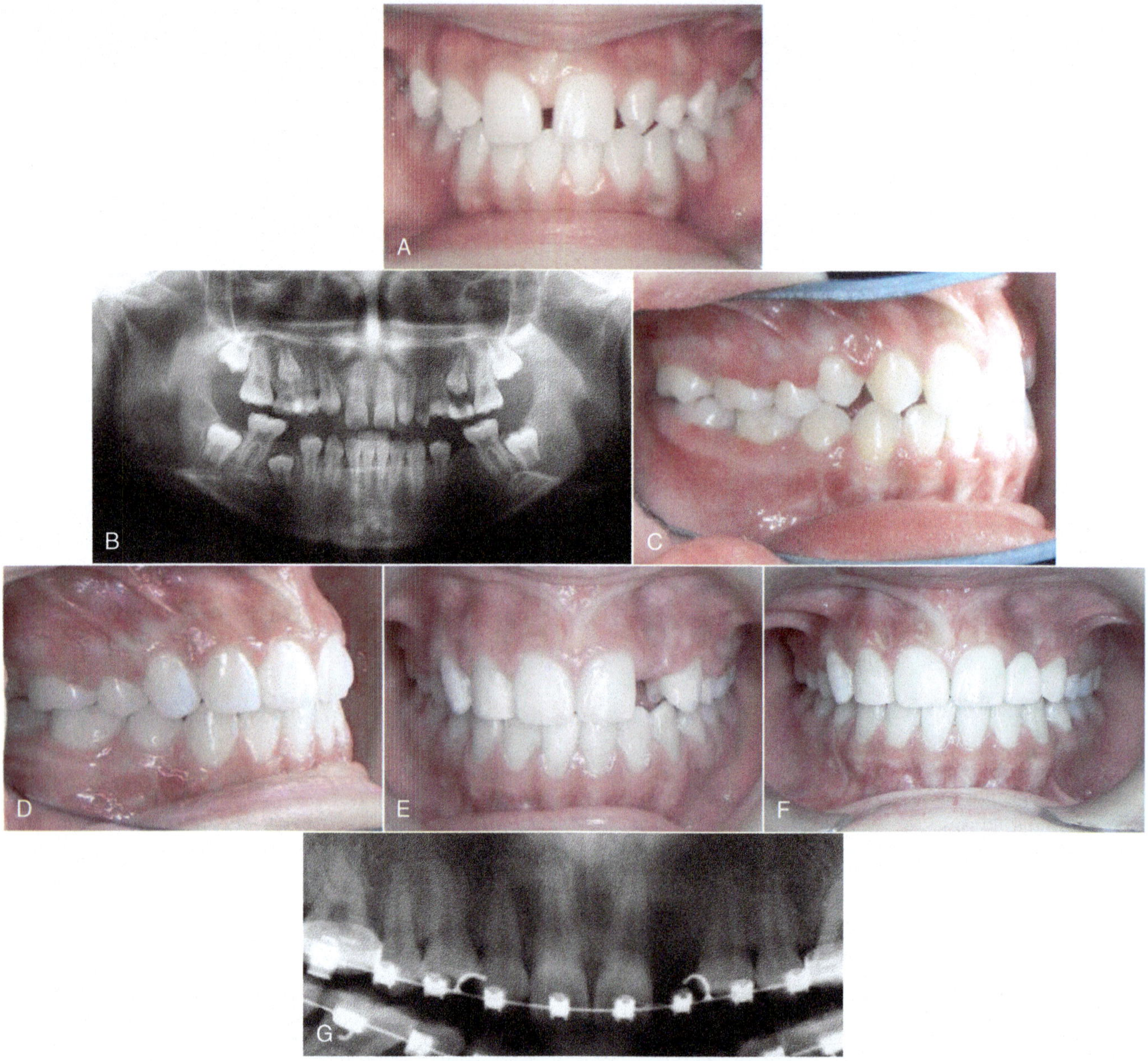

Figure 24-32 **A and B,** A young female patient presented with a missing right lateral incisor, left upper canine, and lower left second premolar. The upper left lateral incisor had a periapical lesion, as it was a dens invaginatus. (This case is similar to the one shown in Figure 24-31.) **C–E,** A treatment plan was developed to extract the upper left lateral incisor (on the endodontist's advice), extract the lower right second premolar, and close all spaces except for that left by the upper left lateral incisor. The upper first premolars were intruded during treatment to position the gingival margin apically in order to facilitate composite buildup so that the premolar would assume canine form. The canine root was moved lingually and the canine was reshaped to assume incisor form on the right. **F and G,** The functional and esthetic outcome was excellent but it is clear that an angular bony defect developed around the premolar and the long-term periodontal outcome is yet to be reported.

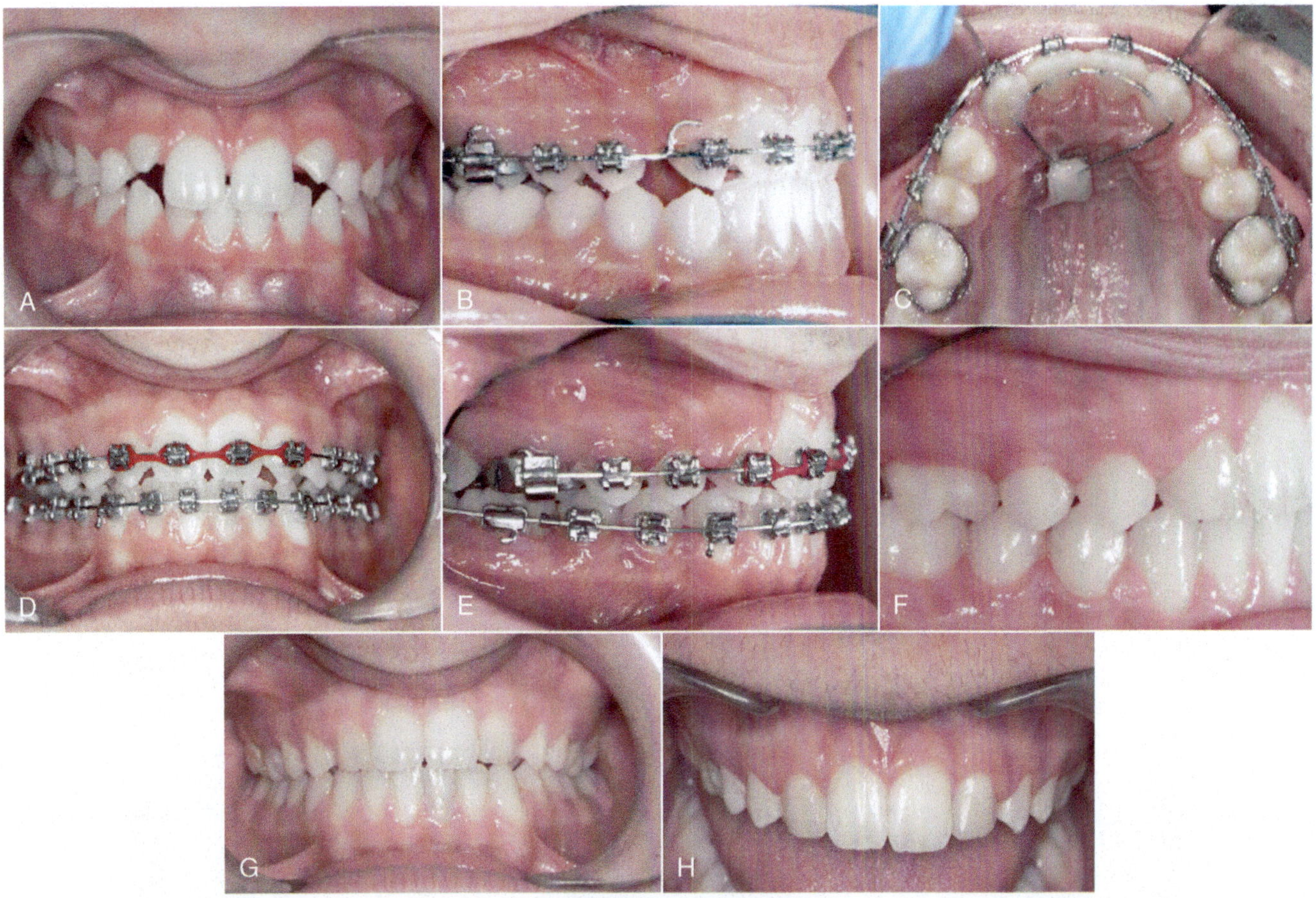

Figure 24-33 **A,** An adolescent male patient presented with a Class I malocclusion and missing lateral incisors and canines. Historically this presentation would have been treated with space creation for implant replacement and all associated issues with adaptive changes in the adult dentition. **B–E,** Temporary anchorage devices (TADs) have provided increased opportunities to close spaces and substitute canines for lateral incisors in most cases. These TADs may be placed in the palate and used indirectly (as in this case) or placed in the alveolus and used directly for force application. This simplifies the mechanics, as simple sliding mechanics may be used. **F–H,** The entire maxillary arch was effectively moved forward by one dental unit and the premolar size was considered to be a suitable substitute for the canine. The canine root was moved lingually and the canine was reshaped to assume lateral incisor form.

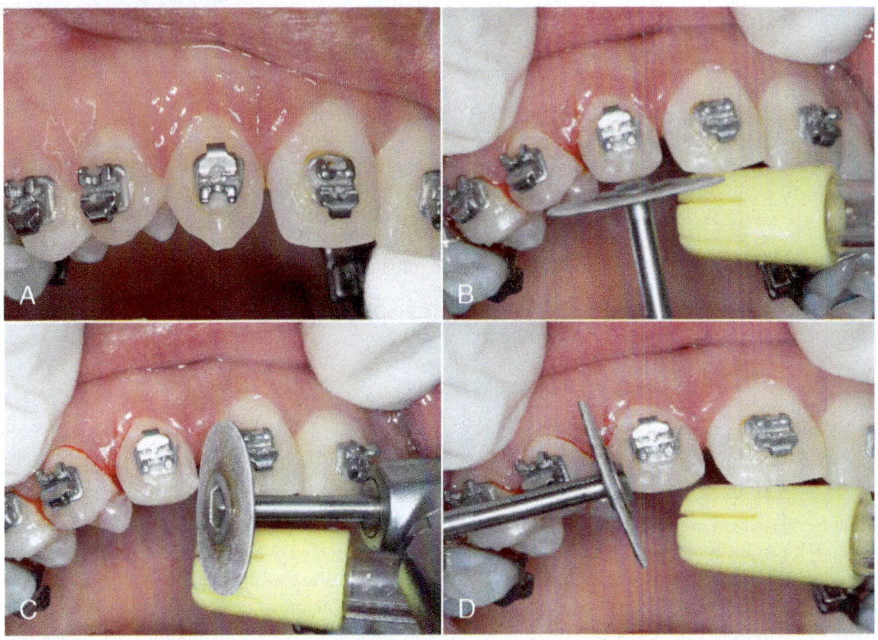

Figure 24-34 **A,** Modification in canine root position may be achieved by placing a lower second premolar bracket upside down on the upper canine. This will move the canine root lingually. **B–D,** Modification to canine form, when replacing a lateral incisor, includes reduction in incisal tip, mesial and distal recontouring, and careful flattening of the labial contour.

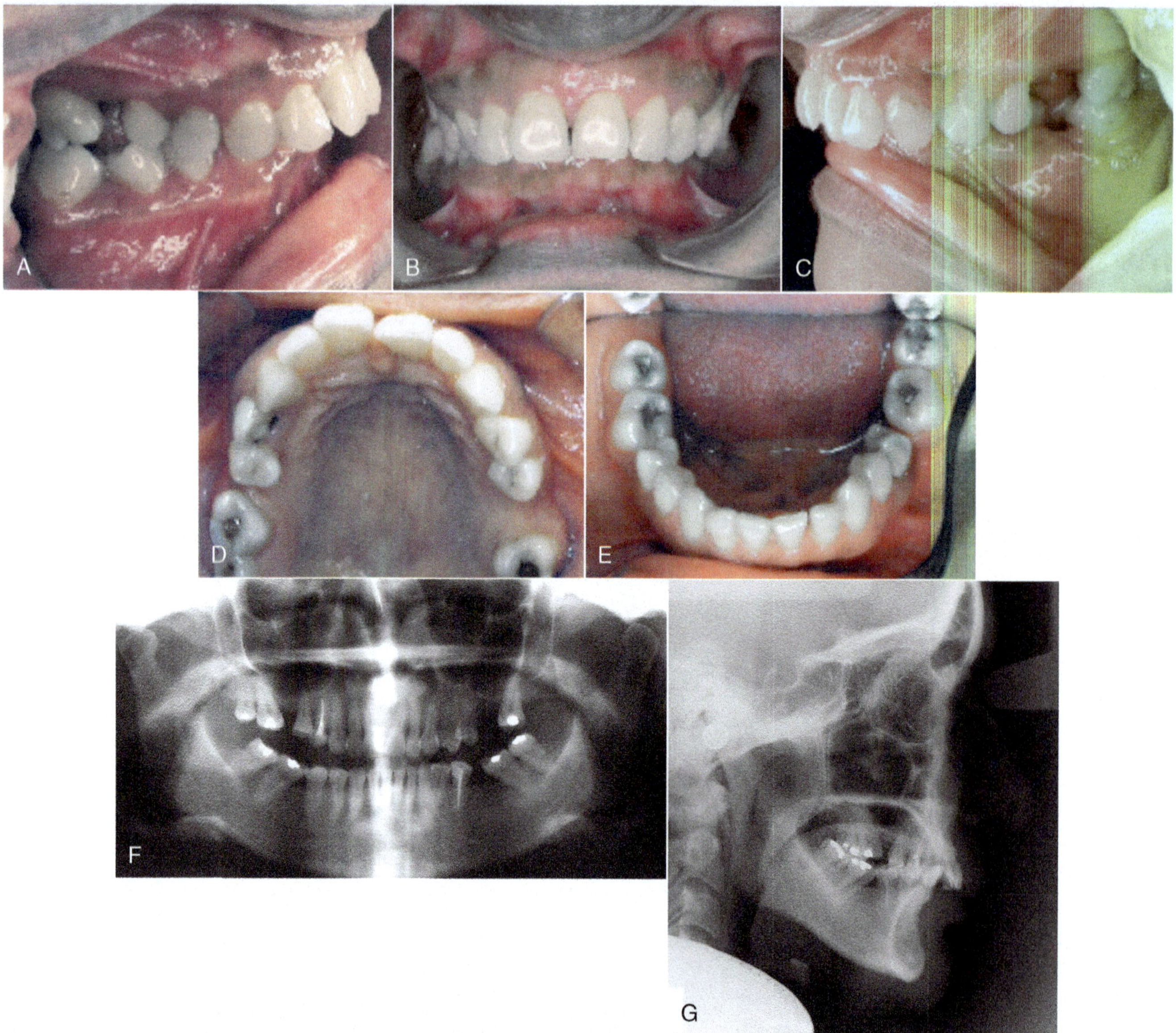

INTERDISCIPLINARY TREATMENT SEQUENCING

• Control phase	
– Preventive/perio/restorative	DC
– Oral surgery (extract 14, 35)	BA
• Implant placement and provision crowns 14, 35	BA/BG
• Orthodontic decompensation	
– Move 24 back open space, close 16, close 36	
– Using implants for anchors	MG
• Periodontal maintenance (3-4 months)	DC
• Mandibular surgery and implant 25	BA
• Provision crown 25	BG
• Postsurgical orthodontics	MG
• Retention appliances	MG
• Final restorations	BG
• Maintenance	DC/BG/MG

H

Figure 24-35 **A–E,** An adult female patient presented with the primary complaints of her teeth sticking out and the lower incisors impinging in the gingiva behind the upper incisors. She felt that her teeth were moving. She had several teeth extracted as a young child, with associated tipping of posterior teeth. **F,** The panoramic radiograph revealed two teeth with unsatisfactory root canal treatment. The treating endodontist determined that these teeth have a questionable prognosis because of the apical extent of the carious lesions. Moreover, the bone volume available to restore the upper left quadrant was minimal. A sinus lift procedure may have to be considered. **G,** The lateral cephalometric radiograph revealed a significant Class II skeletal problem characterized by mandibular retrognathism. A mandibular surgical procedure will have to be considered. **H,** A treatment plan was devised in which the first step was to control the periodontal disease and determine whether the patient was a candidate for such a complex treatment plan. The sequencing plan outlined the following treatment: the upper left second premolar will be moved back through the sinus to create bone between the premolars and simplify the implant placement. The left lower and upper right first premolars will be extracted, replaced by implants and provisional crowns and used as anchors for orthodontic tooth movement.

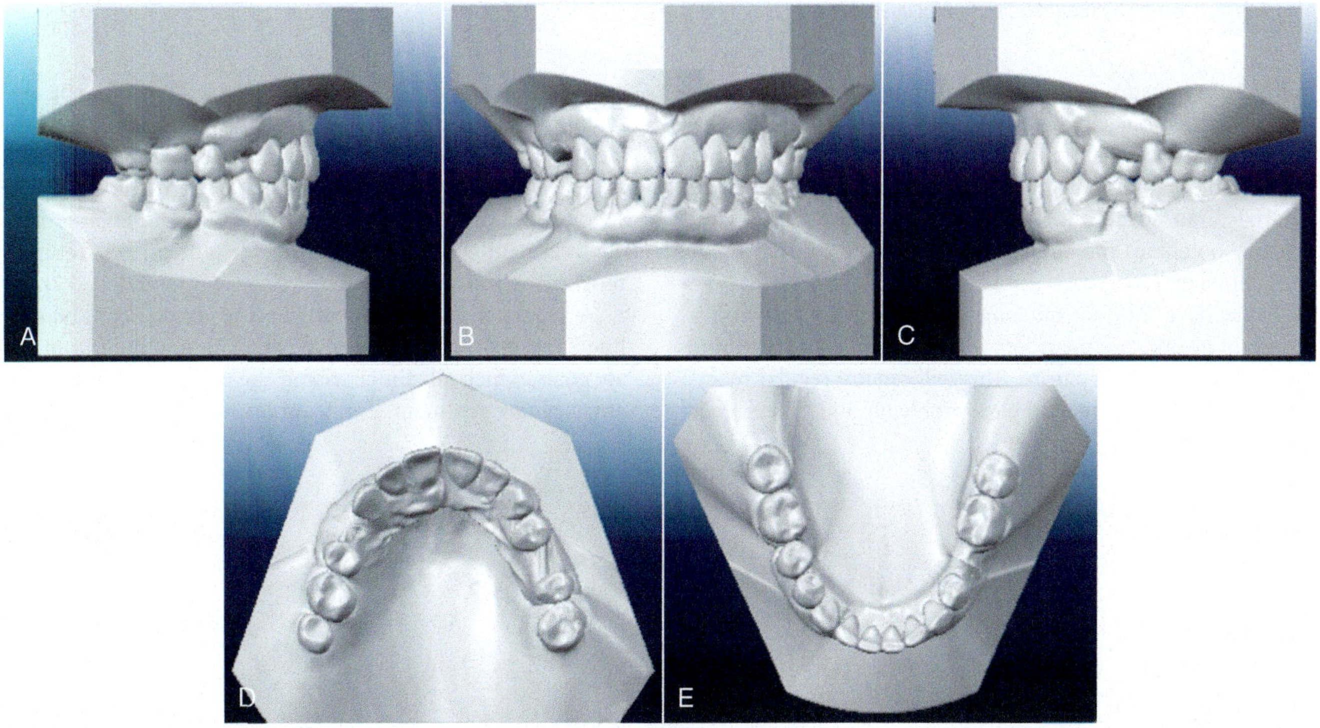

Figure 24-36 **A–E,** The digital diagnostic setup (for the patient shown in Figure 24-35) revealed the anticipated final tooth positions, including locations for final implant-supported prostheses after orthodontics and orthognathic surgery.

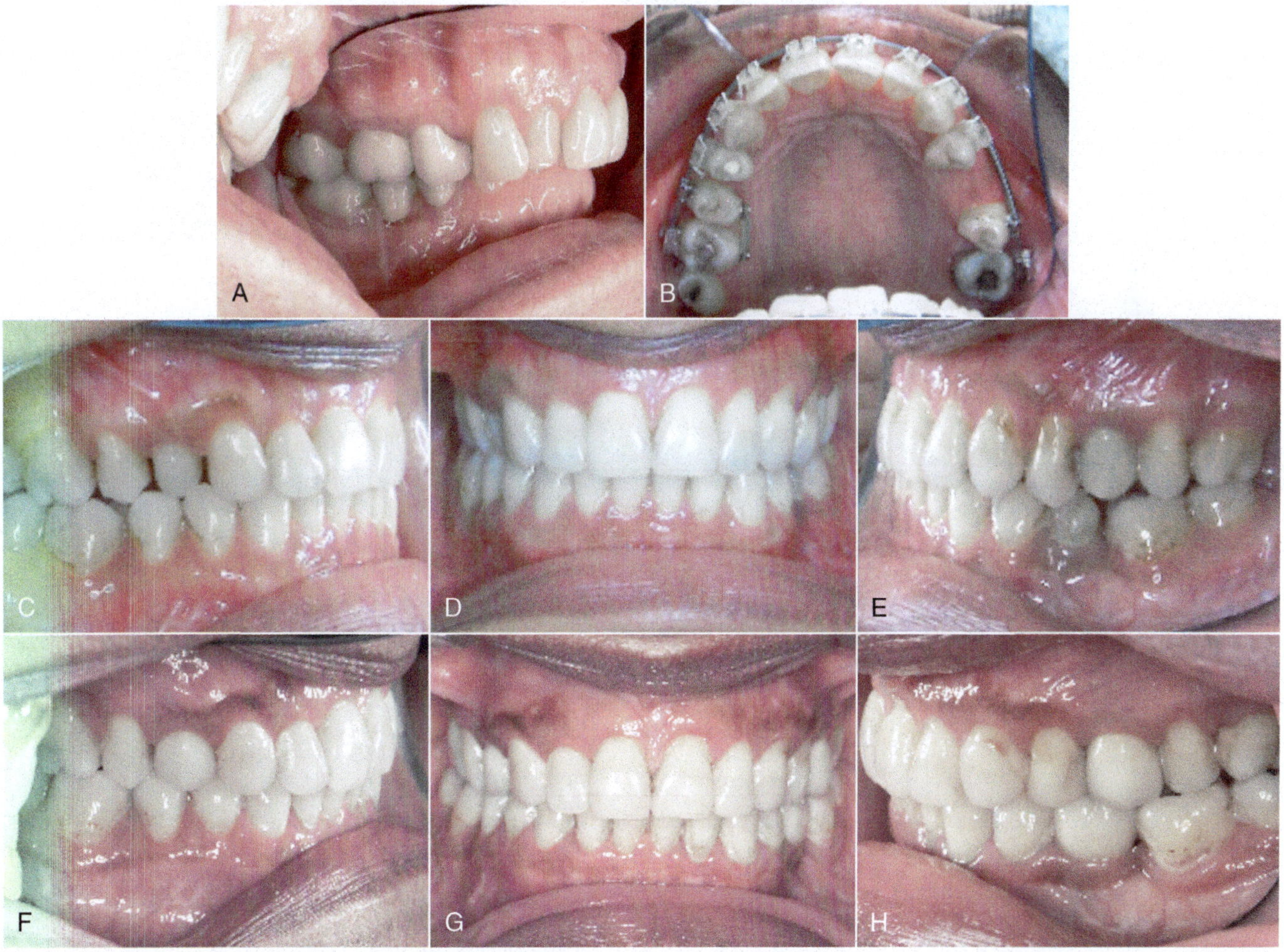

Figure 24-37 Upper arch treatment of the patient shown in Figures 24-35 and 24-36. **A,** Opening coils moved the upper left second premolar back through the sinus and the upper right first premolar was replaced with an implant and provisional crown. This will be used as anchorage to move the upper right posterior teeth forward. **B,** Outcome of the mechanics described in **A,** with space opened between the upper left premolars, creating bone and space closure by posterior movement forward on the right. **C–E,** Intraoral photographs following orthodontics and orthognathic surgery, with provisional crowns in place. **F–H,** Three years post debanding, with final implant-supported crowns in posterior teeth.

initially and ensure that the patient is well informed of the complexities associated with interdisciplinary treatment. This disease control stage is often considered a screening tool for suitable patients. In many circumstances the plan may approach an ideal but, commonly, alternate plans with various outcomes may be equally acceptable to the patient and clinician.

To achieve the best outcome clinicians must establish a group of health care providers who are willing to contribute to an interdisciplinary team. This will require regular meetings to discuss more complex problems and share their respective expertise with other clinicians. They must be able to communicate regularly and effectively through appropriate media. A rigorous, systematic, case-specific database of clinical records must be established; a team leader for the specific treatment plan must be identified; and an appropriate treatment goal, which will include a diagnostic setup in most cases, must be established (Figs. 24-38 and 24-39).

A sequence of activity with specific goals should be outlined, identifying the respective clinicians and their immediate goals, which all clinicians and the patient may refer to at any stage in treatment. The team leader takes responsibility

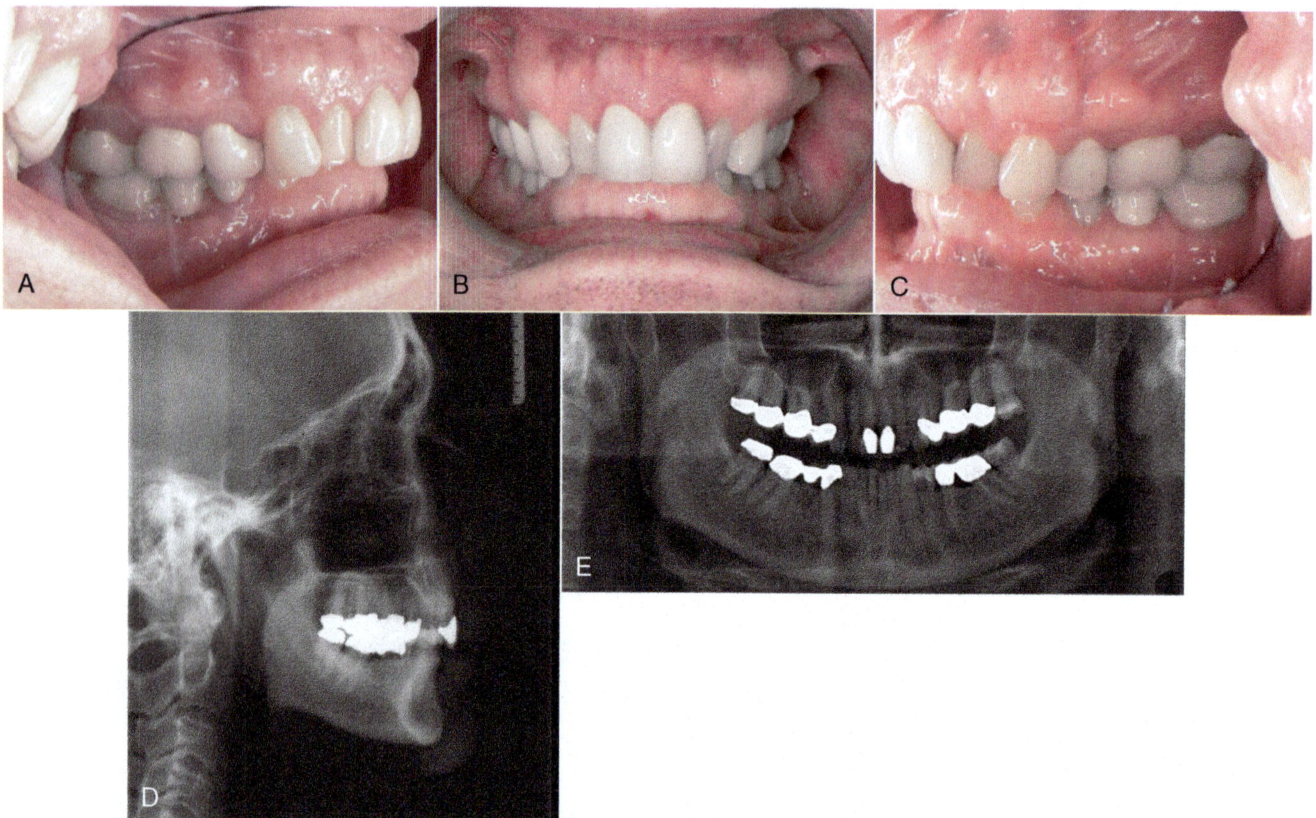

INTERDISCIPLINARY TREATMENT SEQUENCING

• Periodontal assessment and maintenance	JM
– Maintenance every 2-3 months during orthodontics	
• Remove existing posterior teeth and investigate	BS
– Possible extraction of tooth 36	BA
• Provisional restorations	BS
• Presurgical orthodontics	MG
• Mandibular advancement	BA
• Postsurgical orthodontics	MG
• Provisional restorations (bridges and crowns)	BS
• Final restorations	BS

F

Figure 24-38 **A–C,** A 57-year-old male patient presented with a significant Class II malocclusion, pain in the lower left molar region, and heavily restored upper and lower posterior teeth. These teeth were splinted in a rather unconventional manner and it was almost impossible for the patient to maintain. In addition, the crowns on the upper incisors contributed to significant wear on the lower incisors. **D,** The lateral cephalometric radiograph revealed a significant Class II skeletal problem characterized by mandibular retrognathism. A mandibular surgical procedure will have to be considered. **E,** The panoramic radiograph revealed a heavily restored dentition with several missing premolars and a periapical lesion associated with the lower left molar. Further follow-up revealed a poor prognosis for this tooth and it was extracted. **F,** An interdisciplinary treatment plan outlined periodontal therapy, removal of the splinted posterior crowns, and provisional restoration prior to orthodontics to prepare the patient for a mandibular surgical procedure. Final restorations would be placed after 6 to 12 months of retention in provisional crowns.

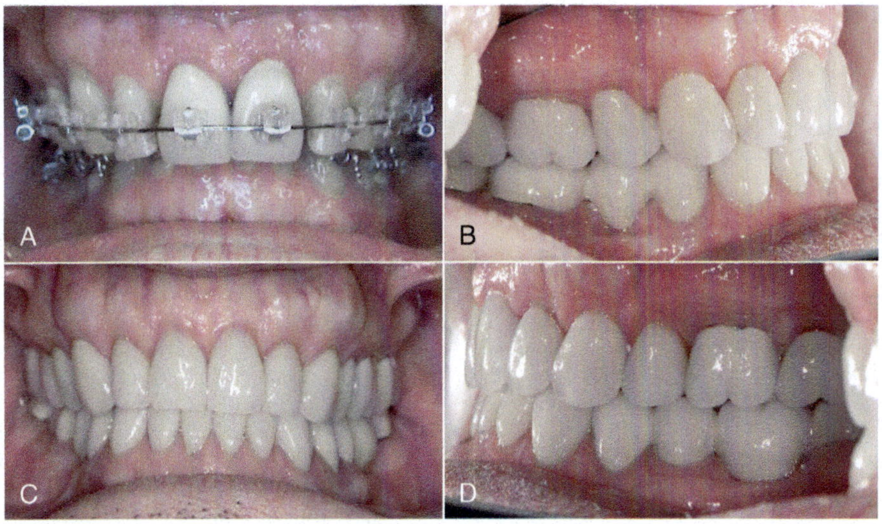

Figure 24-39 **A,** Presurgical intraoral photograph of the patient shown in Figure 24-38. **B–D,** The final outcome of orthodontics and orthognathic surgery and full upper and lower rehabilitation with crowns, bridges, and selective lower incisor veneers.

for ensuring that the patient and clinicians are all cognizant of the stage the patient has reached and what will be performed next, in turn facilitating communication.

If these processes are adhered to, the patient and the team can anticipate a mutually rewarding experience with consistently reproducible outcomes.

REFERENCES

1. Nattrass C, Sandy JR. Adult orthodontics: a review. *Br J Orthod.* 1995;22:331–337.
2. Pabari S, Moles DR, Cunningham SJ. Assessment of motivation and psychological characteristics of adult orthodontic patients. *Am J Orthod Dentofacial Orthop.* 2011;140(6):e263–e272.
3. Spear FM, Kokich VG, Mathews DP. Interdisciplinary management of anterior dental esthetics. *J Am Dent Assoc.* 2006;137(2):160–169.
4. Musich DR, Crossetti HW. Assessment and description of the treatment needs of adult patients for orthodontic therapy: III. Characteristics of the multiple provider group. *Int J Adult Orthodon Orthognath Surg.* 1986;1(4):251–274.
5. Musich DR. Assessment and description of the treatment needs of adult patients evaluated for orthodontic therapy: II. Characteristics of the dual provider group. *Int J Adult Orthodon Orthognath Surg.* 1986;1(2): 101–117.
6. Proffit WR, Fields HW, Moray LJ. Prevalence of malocclusion and orthodontic treatment need in the United States (estimates from the NHANES III survey). *Int J Adult Orthod Orthognath Surg.* 1998;13: 97–106.
7. Abdullah A, Sherfudhin H, Omar R, Johansson A. Prevalence of occlusal tooth wear and its relationship to lateral and protrusive contact schemes in a young adult Indian population. *Acta Odontol Scand.* 1994;52:191–197.
8. Kokich VG, Spear FM. Guidelines for managing the orthodontic-restorative patient. *Semin Orthod.* 1997;3(1):3–20.
9. Roblee RD. Interdisciplinary dentofacial therapy (IDT): a comprehensive team approach. *Ann R Australas Coll Dent Surg.* 1998;14:41–47.
10. Kokich V. Enhancing restorative, esthetic and periodontal results with orthodontic therapy. In: Schluger S, Youdelis R, Page R, et al, eds. *Periodontal Therapy.* Philadelphia, PA: Lea and Febiger; 1990:433–460.
11. Mathews DP, Kokich VG. Managing treatment for the orthodontic patient with periodontal problems. *Semin Orthod.* 1997;3(1):21–38.
12. Proffit WR, Fields HW, Sarver D. *Contemporary Orthodontics.* 5th ed. St. Louis, MO: Mosby; 2013.
13. Kokich VG. Create the vision. *Am J Orthod Dentofacial Orthop.* 2011; 140(6):751.
14. Knocht A, Zohn H, Deasy M, et al. Screening for periodontal disease: radiographs versus PSR. *J Am Dent Assoc.* 1996;127:749–756.
15. Axelsson P, Lindhe J. The significance of maintenance care in the treatment of periodontal disease. *J Clin Periodontol.* 1981;8:281.
16. Becker W, Becker BE. Treatment of mandibular 3-wall intrabony defects by flap debridement and expanded polytetrafluoroethylene barrier membranes: long-term evaluation of 32 treated patients. *J Periodontol.* 1993;64:1138–1144.
17. Schluger S. Osseous resection: a basic principle in periodontal surgery. *Oral Surg.* 1949;2:316.
18. Ingber J. Forced eruption: part I: A method of treating isolated one and two wall infrabony osseous defects: rationale and case report. *J Periodontol.* 1974;45:199–206.
19. Brown IS. The effect of orthodontic therapy on certain types of periodontal defects: I. Clinical findings. *J Periodontol.* 1973;44:742–756.
20. Shallhorn R, McClain P. Combined osseous composite grafting, root conditioning and guided tissue regeneration. *Int J Periodont Rest Dent.* 1988;8:9–31.
21. Kramer GM. Surgical alternatives in regenerative therapy of the periodontium. *Int J Periodont Rest Dent.* 1992;12:11–31.
22. Langer B, Langer L. Subepithelial connective tissue graft technique for root coverage. *J Periodontol.* 1985;56:715–720.
23. Miller PD. Root coverage using a free soft tissue autograft following citric acid application: part I. *Int J Periodont Rest Dent.* 1982;2:65–70.
24. Dorfmann H, Kennedy J, Bird W. Longitudinal evaluation of free autogenous gingival grafts: a four-year report. *J Periodontol.* 1982;53: 349–352.
25. Dorfman HS. Mucogingival changes resulting from mandibular incisor tooth movement. *Am J Orthod.* 1978;74:286.
26. Steiner GG, Pearson JK, Ainamo J. Changes of the marginal periodontium as a result of labial tooth movement in monkeys. *J Periodontol.* 1981;52:314.
27. Gartrell JG, Mathews DP. Gingival recession: the condition, process, and treatment. *Dental Clin North Am.* 1976;1:199–213.
28. Kokich V. Anterior dental esthetics: an orthodontic perspective: II. Vertical relationships. *J Esthet Dent.* 1993;5:174–178.
29. Chiche G, Kokich V, Caudill R. Diagnosis and treatment planning of esthetic problems. In: Pinault A, Chiche G, eds. *Esthetics in Fixed Prosthodontics.* Chicago, IL: Quintessence; 1994:33–52.
30. Kokich V. Esthetics: the ortho-perio-restorative connection. *Semin Orthod.* 1996;2:21–30.

31. Kokich V. Anterior dental esthetics: an orthodontic perspective: III. Mediolateral relationships. *J Esthet Dent.* 1993;5:200–207.
32. Kokich V. Anterior dental esthetics: an orthodontic perspective: I. Crown length. *J Esthet Dent.* 1993;5:19–23.
33. Kokich V, Nappen D, Shapiro P. Gingival contour and clinical crown length: their effects on the esthetic appearance of maxillary anterior teeth. *Am J Orthod.* 1984;86:89–94.
34. Berry DC, Poole DFG. Attrition: possible mechanism of compensation. *J Oral Rehab.* 1976;3:201–206.
35. Silness J, Berge M, Johannessen G. Prevalence, pattern, and severity of incisal wear in dental students. *Acta Odontol Scand.* 1994;52: 178–181.
36. Dahl B, Krogstad O, Karlson K. An alternative treatment in cases with advanced localised attrition. *J Oral Rehab.* 1975;2:209–214.
37. Dyer K, Ibbetson R, Grey N. A question of space: options for the restorative management of worn teeth. *Dent Update.* 2001;28(3):118–123.
38. Evans RD. Orthodontics and the creation of localised inter-occlusal space in cases of anterior tooth wear. *Eur J Prosthodont Rest Dent.* 1997;5(4):169–173.
39. Mizrahi B. The Dahl principle: creating space and improving the biomechanical prognosis of anterior crowns. *Quintessence Int.* 2006;37(4): 245–251.
40. Kokich VG. Managing orthodontic-restorative treatment for the adolescent patient. In: McNamara JA, Brudon WI, eds. *Orthodontics and Dentofacial Orthopedics.* Ann Arbor, MI: Needham Press; 2001: 423–452.
41. Dahl B, Carlsson GE, Ekfeldt A. Occlusal wear of teeth and restorative materials. *ACTA Odont Scand.* 1993;51:299–309.
42. ADA Council of Scientific Affairs. Dental endosseous implants: an update. *J Am Dent Assoc.* 2004;135:92–97.
43. Branemark PI, Breine U, Adell R. Intraosseous anchorage of dental prostheses: I. Experimental studies. *Scand J Plast Reconstr Surg.* 1969;3: 81–100.
44. Buser D, Mericske-Stern R, Bernard JP, et al. Long-term evaluation of non-submerged ITI implants: part 1: 8-year life table analysis of a prospective multi-center study with 2359 implants. *Clin Oral Implants Res.* 1997;8:161–172.
45. Linkow LI. The endosseous blade implant and its use in orthodontics. *Int J Orthod.* 1969;18:149–154.
46. Roberts WE, Smith RK, Zilberman Y, Mozsary PG, Smith RS. Osseous adaptation to continuous loading of rigid endosseous implants. *Am J Orthod.* 1984;86:95–111.
47. Roberts WE, Marshall KJ, Mozsary PG. Rigid endosseous implant utilized as anchorage to protract molars and close an atrophic extraction site. *Angle Orthod.* 1990;60:135–152.
48. Wehrbein H, Merz BR. Aspects of the use of endosseous palatal implants in orthodontic therapy. *J Esthet Dent.* 1998;10:315–324.
49. Odman J, Lekholm U, Jemt T, Thilander B. Osseointegrated implants as orthodontic anchorage in the treatment of partially edentulous adult patients. *Eur J Orthod.* 1994;16:187–201.
50. Umemori M, Sugawara J, Mitani H, Nagasaka H, Kawamura H. Skeletal anchorage system for open-bite correction. *Am J Orthod Dentofacial Orthop.* 1999;115:166–174.
51. Kanomi R. Mini-implant for orthodontic anchorage. *J Clin Orthod.* 1997;31:763–767.
52. Freudenthaler JW, Haas R, Bantleon HP. Bicortical titanium screws for critical orthodontic anchorage in the mandible (a preliminary report on clinical applications). *Clin Oral Implants Res.* 2001;12: 358–363.
53. Daimaruya T, Nagasaka H, Umemori M, Sugawara J, Mitani H. The influences of molar intrusion on the inferior alveolar neurovascular bundle and root using the skeletal anchorage system in dogs. *Angle Orthod.* 2001;71:60–70.
54. Nagasaka H, Sugawara J, Kawamura H, Kasahara T, Umemori M, Mitani H. A clinical evaluation on the efficacy of titanium miniplates as an orthodontic anchorage. *Jpn J Orthod Soc.* 1999;58:136–147.
55. Spear FM, Mathews DM, Kokich VG. Interdisciplinary management of single-tooth implants. *Semin Orthod.* 1997;3(1):45–72.
56. Sabri R. Management of missing maxillary lateral incisors. *J Am Dent Assoc.* 1999;130:80–84.
57. Tuverson DL. Orthodontic treatment using canines in place of missing maxillary lateral incisors. *Am J Orthod.* 1970;58:109–112.
58. Kokich VG. Maxillary lateral incisor implants: planning with the aid of orthodontics. *Int J Oral Maxillofac Surg.* 2004;62:48–56.
59. Noack N, Willer J, Hoffmann J. Long-term results after placement of dental implants: longitudinal study of 1,964 implants over 16 years. *Int J Oral Maxillofac Implants.* 1999;14:748–755.
60. Weng D, Jacobson Z, Tarnow D, et al. A prospective multicenter clinical trial of 3i machined-surface implants: results after 6 years of follow-up. *Int J Oral Maxillofac Implants.* 2003;18:417–423.
61. Mayer TM, Hawley CE, Gunsolley JC, Feldman S. The single-tooth implant: a viable alternative for single-tooth replacement. *J Periodontol.* 2002;73:687–693.
62. Kinzer GA, Kokich VO. Managing congenitally missing lateral incisors: part II: tooth-supported restorations. *J Esthet Restor Dent.* 2005;17: 76–84.
63. Kan JY, Rungcharassaeng K, Umezu K, Kois JC. Dimensions of peri-implant mucosa: an evaluation of maxillary anterior single implants in humans. *J Periodontol.* 2003;74:557–562.
64. Novackova S, Marek I, Kaminek M. Orthodontic tooth movement: bone formation and its stability in time. *Am J Orthod Dentofacial Orthop.* 2011;139:37–43.
65. Uribe F, Chau V, Padala S, Neace WP, Cutrera A, Nanda R. Alveolar ridge width and height changes after orthodontic space opening in patients congenitally missing maxillary lateral incisors. *Eur J Orthod.* 2013;35:87-92.
66. Carlson G. Changes in contour of the maxillary alveolar process under immediate dentures. *Acta Odont Scand.* 1967;25:1–31.
67. Olsen TM, Kokich VG. Postorthodontic root approximation after opening space for maxillary lateral incisor implants. *Am J Orthod Dentofacial Orthop.* 2010;137:158–159.
68. Esposito M, Ekestubbe A, Gröndahl K. Radiological evaluation of marginal bone loss at tooth surfaces facing single Brånemark implants. *Clin Oral Implants Res.* 1993;4:151–157.
69. Belser UC, Grütter L, Vailati F, Bornstein MM, Weber HP, Buser D. Outcome evaluation of early placed maxillary anterior single-tooth implants using objective esthetic criteria: a cross-sectional, retrospective study in 45 patients with a 2- to 4-year follow-up using pink and white esthetic scores. *J Periodontol.* 2009;80:140–151.
70. Fürhauser R, Florescu D, Benesch T, Haas R, Mailath G, Watzek G. Evaluation of soft tissue around single-tooth implant crowns: the pink esthetic score. *Clin Oral Implants Res.* 2005;16:639–644.
71. Chang M, Wennström JL, Ödman P, Andersson B. Implant supported single-tooth replacements compared to contralateral natural teeth: crown and soft tissue dimensions. *Clin Oral Implants Res.* 1999;10: 185–194.
72. Robertsson S, Mohlin B. The congenitally missing upper lateral incisor: a retrospective study of orthodontic space closure versus restorative treatment. *Eur J Orthod.* 2000;22:697–710.
73. Fudalej P, Kokich VG, Leroux B. Determining the cessation of vertical growth of the craniofacial structures to facilitate placement of single-tooth implants. *Am J Orthod Dentofacial Orthop.* 2007;131(suppl): S59–S67.
74. Jemt T, Ahlberg G, Henriksson K, Bondevik O. Changes of anterior clinical crown height in patients provided with single-implant restorations after more than 15 years of follow-up. *Int J Prosthodont.* 2006; 19:455–461.
75. Thilander B, Ödman J, Lekholm U. Orthodontic aspects of the use of oral implants in adolescents: a 10-year follow-up study. *Eur J Orthod.* 2001;23:715–731.
76. Oesterle LJ, Cronin RJ. Adult growth, aging, and the single-tooth implant. *Int J Oral Maxillofac Implants.* 2000;15:252–260.

77. Iseri H, Solow B. Continued eruption of maxillary incisors and first molars in girls from 9 to 25 years, studied by the implant method. *Eur J Orthod.* 1996;18:245–256.
78. Zachrisson BU. Single implant-supported crowns for the anterior maxilla: potential esthetic long-term (>5 years) problems. *World J Orthod.* 2006;7:306–312.
79. Bernard JP, Schatz JP, Christou P, Belser U, Kiliaridis S. Long-term vertical changes of the anterior maxillary teeth adjacent to single implants in young and mature adults: a retrospective study. *J Clin Periodontol.* 2004;31:1024–1028.
80. Nordquist GG, McNeill RW. Orthodontic vs. restorative treatment of the congenitally absent lateral incisor: long-term periodontal and occlusal evaluation. *J Periodontol.* 1975;46:139–143.
81. Kinzer GA, Kokich VO. Managing congenitally missing lateral incisors: part I: canine substitution. *J Esthet Restor Dent.* 2005;17:5–10.
82. Thordarson A, Zachrisson BU, Mjör IA. Remodeling of canines to the shape of lateral incisors by grinding: a long-term clinical and radiographic evaluation. *Am J Orthod.* 1991;100:123–132.
83. Zachrisson BU, Mjör IA. Remodeling of teeth by grinding. *Am J Orthod.* 1975;68:545–553.
84. Rosa M, Zachrisson BU. Integrating esthetic dentistry and space closure in patients with missing maxillary lateral incisors. *J Clin Orthod.* 2001; 35:221–234.
85. Rosa M, Zachrisson BU. Integrating esthetic dentistry and space closure in patients with missing maxillary lateral incisors: further improvements. *J Clin Orthod.* 2007;41:563–573.
86. Rosa M, Zachrisson BU. The space-closure alternative for missing maxillary lateral incisors: an update. *J Clin Orthod.* 2010;44:540–549.
87. Swift EJ, Friedman MJ. Critical appraisal: porcelain veneer outcomes, part II. *J Esthet Restor Dent.* 2006;18:110–112.
88. Dueled E, Gotfredsen K, Damsgaard MT, Hede B. Professional and patient-based evaluation of oral rehabilitation in patients with tooth agenesis. *Clin Oral Implants Res.* 2009;20:729–736.
89. Jørnung J, Fardal Ø. Perceptions of patients' smiles: a comparison of patients' and dentists' opinions. *J Am Dent Assoc.* 2007;138: 1544–1553.
90. Armbruster PC, Gardiner DM, Whitley JB, Flerra J. The congenitally missing maxillary lateral incisor: part 1: esthetic judgment of treatment options. *World J Orthod.* 2005;6:369–375.
91. Armbruster PC, Gardiner DM, Whitley JB, Flerra J. The congenitally missing maxillary lateral incisor: part 2: assessing dentists' preferences for treatment. *World J Orthod.* 2005;6:376–381.
92. Dueled E, Gotfredsen K, Damsgaard MT, Hede B. Professional and patient-based evaluation of oral rehabilitation in patients with tooth agenesis. *Clin Oral Implants Res.* 2009;20:729–736.

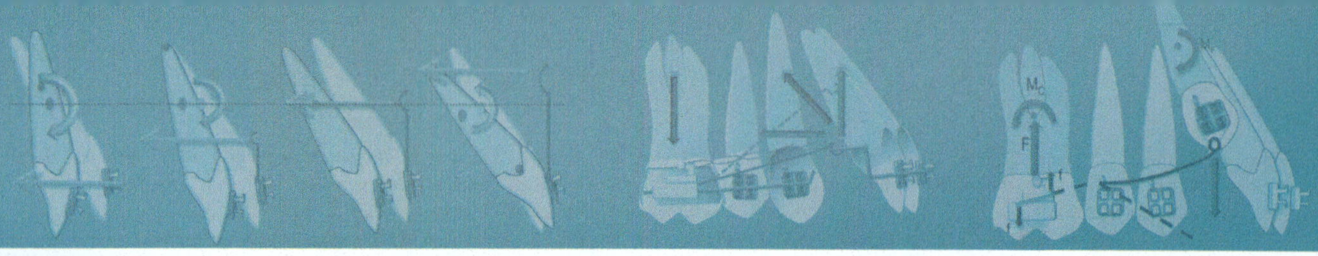

CHAPTER 25

Missing Maxillary Lateral Incisors: New Procedures and Indications for Optimal Space Closure

Marco Rosa and Bjørn U. Zachrisson

The maxillary lateral incisor is the second most common congenitally absent tooth. There are three treatment options to replace missing lateral incisors: canine substitution,[1-8] a single-tooth implant,[9-11] or a tooth-supported restoration.[12]

Available evidence indicates that proper orthodontic space closure is well accepted by patients, does not produce a major risk for temporomandibular joint disorder (TMD) problems, and from a periodontal standpoint is safer than prosthetic replacements.[13-15]

The advent of osseointegrated implants decreased the popularity of the space closure alternative among many orthodontists and referring dentists and the implant substitution became their first option. Although it may appear preferable from an esthetic and functional point of view to create space to replace the missing lateral incisor with a single-tooth implant crown, recent studies have demonstrated that frequent biological complications may occur in the long-term.[16-28] Such problems may include blue coloring of the marginal gingiva following labial bone resorption,[19] peri-implantitis,[18] bone loss around neighboring teeth,[20] abutment exposure due to retraction of the labial gingiva,[28] and progressive infraocclusion.[20] Infraposition of the clinical crown may occur even when the implant has been placed in a mature adult, due to continuous eruption of the adjacent teeth (Fig. 25-1).[21,23-26,29-31] The cessation and degree of vertical growth is unpredictable.[21,23-27,30,31] Even if some evidence exists to help define the "end of growth" period, at present the individual variation is high and it is not possible to predict when unforeseen changes will appear.[29] This could itself contraindicate the single-tooth implant restoration in the esthetic zone of patients who show the gingival margins when smiling.

Another drawback of the space reopening alternative for a teenage patient is that several years must elapse between completion of orthodontic treatment and implant placement. After successful orthodontic opening of the implant space, the central incisor and canine roots may reapproximate during retention and prevent implant placement. Olsen and Kokich[32] have reported that retreatment and orthodontic space reopening was needed in 11% of their patients. At this stage of treatment, related problems and questions arise, such as:

- What is the optimal retention device?
- Will a temporary resin-bonded bridge be esthetically acceptable?
- How long must we wait to place the implants?
- Will the newly regenerated alveolar bone undergo atrophy?
- Will a second orthodontic finishing phase be needed?

In contrast, the canine substitution option has the indisputable advantage that the entire treatment is accomplished in one phase and the result is permanent and independent of residual maxillary growth.[2-8] This point is particularly important since the majority of patients with missing maxillary lateral incisors are diagnosed at an early age.

It has to be stated, however, that even if space closure treatment results are well accepted by the patient and parents and acceptable from a functional standpoint,[13,14] the simple substitution of the missing lateral incisor with the canine is not sufficient for today's high esthetic standards. The reasons for this are several:

- The gingival margins frequently became unnatural. The borders are too high apically on canines moved to replace the lateral incisors and too short on the first premolars moved in the place of the canines (Fig. 25-2).

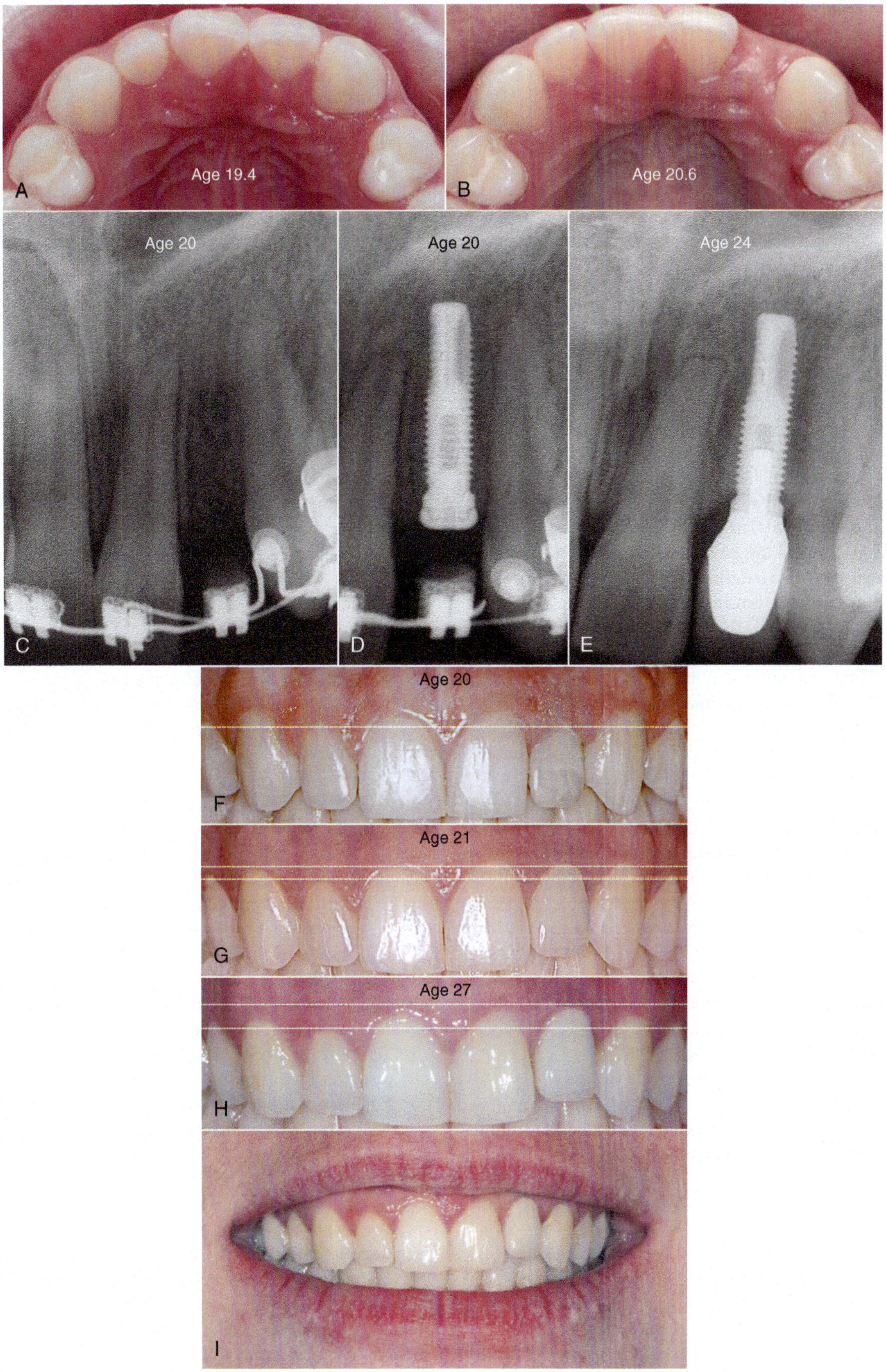

Figure 25-1 Infraocclusion of an implant crown placed at the "end of growth." **A and B,** An adequate implant site was orthodontically opened in a 19-year-old woman. **C and D,** The osseointegrated implant was inserted during orthodontic treatment and a temporary resin restoration was cemented 1 month after the end of orthodontic treatment when the patient was 20 years old. **F,** The periodontal tissues were leveled similarly to the contralateral natural tooth. Due to continued eruption of adjacent teeth, **(G)** the gingival margin of the porcelain crown was already 2- to 3-mm higher than the implant restoration after 1 year and **(E)** uneven bone peaks were evident after 4 years. **H and I,** After 7 years the clinical situation was even worse. There is no reason to believe that this situation will remain stable. *(The treatment was performed by the same team of professionals, in the same years and using similar procedures and implants, as the case shown in Fig. 25-18. It is impossible to explain why in this case an evident amount of infraocclusion occurred while in the case shown in Fig. 25-18 it did not.)* (Periodontist: Dr. Francesca Manfrini; Prosthodontist: Dr. Giovanni Manfrini, Riva del Garda, Italy; Ceramist: Antonio Bertoni, Brescia, Italy.)

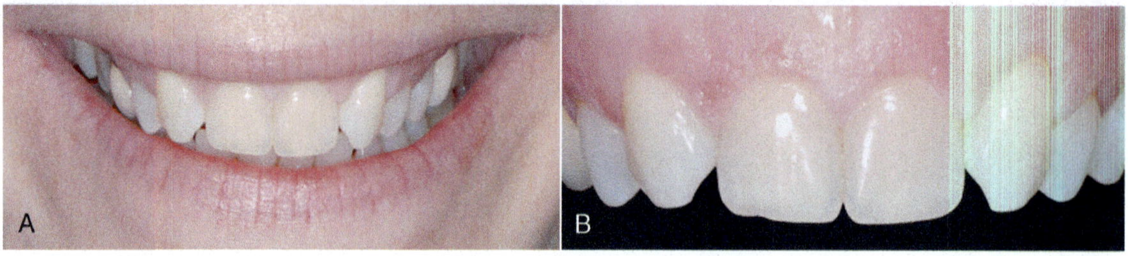

Figure 25-2 Long-term appearance after space closure. **A,** Twenty-five years after orthodontic space closure the result is stable and the periodontal tissues are healthy, although the esthetic result is not ideal and the smile is not natural. **B,** The gingival margins are not natural. They are too high on the canines, which were moved in place of the lateral incisors, and too short on the first premolar, which was moved to replace the canines.

- Canines are generally more yellow than lateral incisors.
- The canine is sometimes too large. This may make it impossible to grind it to the proper size of a lateral incisor and achieve good balance with the adjacent teeth.
- The closed spaces may reopen in some patients.

Over the last decade, new clinical procedures have been proposed to improve the esthetic and occlusal outcome for canine substitution treatment by combining carefully detailed orthodontic finishing with techniques used in esthetic dentistry.[5-8] Together, these procedures are able to provide the improvements needed to approach the appearance of a natural intact dentition, both functionally and esthetically, and provide predictable final results that are stable in the long-term (Figs. 25-3 and 25-4). It is the authors' opinion that this will make orthodontic space closure a more attractive treatment alternative than before.

The goal of this chapter is to:

1. Describe the method for optimal space closure.
2. Define priorities in treatment planning.
3. Suggest new indications and contraindications for the space closure alternative.
4. Recognize and address the most frequent hidden problems.
5. Suggest possible treatment alternatives.
6. Suggest what needs to be improved further in the future.

CLINICAL METHOD FOR OPTIMAL SPACE CLOSURE

When the goal is the appearance of a naturally intact dentition, both functionally and esthetically, the patient needs a long, sometimes difficult two-phase interdisciplinary treatment approach.

Orthodontic Treatment

The overall goal of orthodontic treatment is not only space closure while correcting the malocclusion, but also proper finishing in the esthetic zone to create a well-balanced exposure of the upper front teeth, allowing the restorative dentist to perform minimally invasive, ideal restorations.

The specific goals of the orthodontic finishing phase are:

- On posterior teeth:
  - Stable occlusion with no prematurities and no centric occlusion–centric relation (CO-CR) discrepancy.
  - Class I or Class II molar occlusal relationship (depending on the need for extractions in the lower arch) (see Figs. 25-3 and 25-4; Figs. 25-5 to 25-7).
- On anterior teeth:
  - Alignment of the incisal edges of the central incisors with the cusps of the canines and the buccal cusps of the restored first premolars ("new" canines) (see Fig. 25-7, N; Figs. 25-8 and 25-9).
  - Ideal frontal exposure. Compared to the lateral incisor width, the central incisors should be about 160% and the canines 70%.[33]
  - Leveling with torque control of the upper six front teeth to achieve natural "high-low-high" gingival margins. The new canines (i.e., the first premolars) are at the same level as the central incisors and the new lateral incisors (i.e., the canines) are at a lower level (see Fig. 23-6). Such adjustments can be made using archwire bends or, more easily, by bonding the canine brackets higher than normal and the first premolar brackets in an incisal position.[5-8] The gingival leveling is particularly important in patients who show much gingiva when smiling.

Restorations

The goals of the restoration phase for canines and first premolars (and possibly central incisors) are:

- Temporary hybrid-composite direct restorations made just after the orthodontic treatment.
- Final restorations as porcelain veneers, which should be made after an adequate stabilization period.

Six-Step Clinical Procedure (Box 25-1)

Step 1: Space Closure and Correction of the Malocclusion

The extraction of two premolars in the mandibular arch is sometimes necessary, depending on the extent of lower arch crowding, incisor protrusion, lip posture, and expected growth pattern. Typically, a normal mandibular arch form should not be expanded and should maintain the pretreatment shape. The maxillary archwires should be coordinated with the lower ones.

The space closure in the upper arch may be performed without major problems in crowded cases and in Class II malocclusions. If the diagnosis is made in the early mixed

BOX 25-1 Six-Step Clinical Procedure to Properly Achieve Optimal Space Closure

1. Space closure and correction of the malocclusion.
2. Orthodontic finishing in the maxillary front area.
   a. Alignment and overjet (taking into consideration size and morphology, function, and long-term stability).
   b. Leveling of the gingival margins by extrusion and grinding of the canines and intrusion of the first premolars.
   c. Torque control of the canines and first premolars to prevent periodontal tissue complications and to allow optimal restorations.
3. Local gingivectomies in selected cases.
4. Resin buildups for esthetic, functional, and stability reasons.
5. Vital bleaching of yellowish teeth.
6. Occlusal finishing, final porcelain restorations, and long-term stability.

dentition, a serial extraction strategy may sometimes be effective to shorten the treatment time stage with fixed appliances (see Fig. 25-3).

The problems become more relevant when treatment must be achieved with maximum anterior anchorage. In such cases, conventional biomechanics (Fig. 25-10, A and B) are usually sufficient to close the spaces.[3] However, moving each tooth individually is time consuming and the patient's compliance with intermaxillary elastics is essential to achieve the treatment goal in a reasonable time span. Usually space closure is made with a heat-treated 0.016-inch × 0.022-inch stainless steel archwire, using brackets of different slot sizes: 0.018-inch on the central incisors and canines and 0.022-inch on the premolars and molars.

With recent technical advances, including absolute skeletal anchorage with two connected palatally inserted mini-screws,[34–38] maximum anchorage problems can be overcome and all posterior teeth can be moved simultaneously forward without compliance problems. This system

Text continued on p. 537

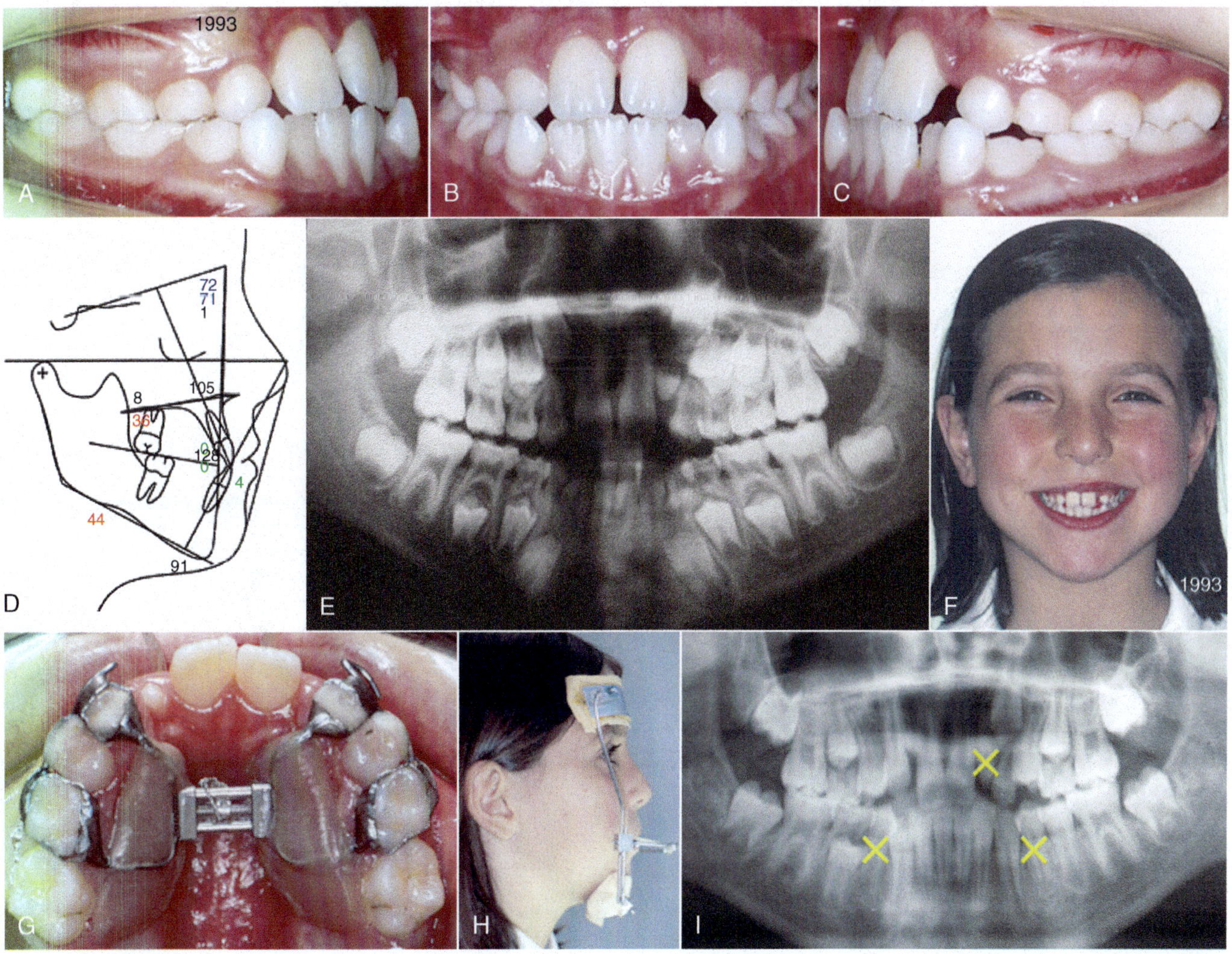

Figure 25-3 Long-term stability of space closure and gingival remodeling. **A–F,** An 8-year-old girl with hyperdivergent Class III malocclusion, narrow maxilla, lower crowding, and unilateral missing upper right lateral incisor in the early mixed dentition. Early orthopedic treatment included **(G)** rapid maxillary expansion (RME) and **(H)** maxillary protraction using deciduous teeth as anchors. *Continued*

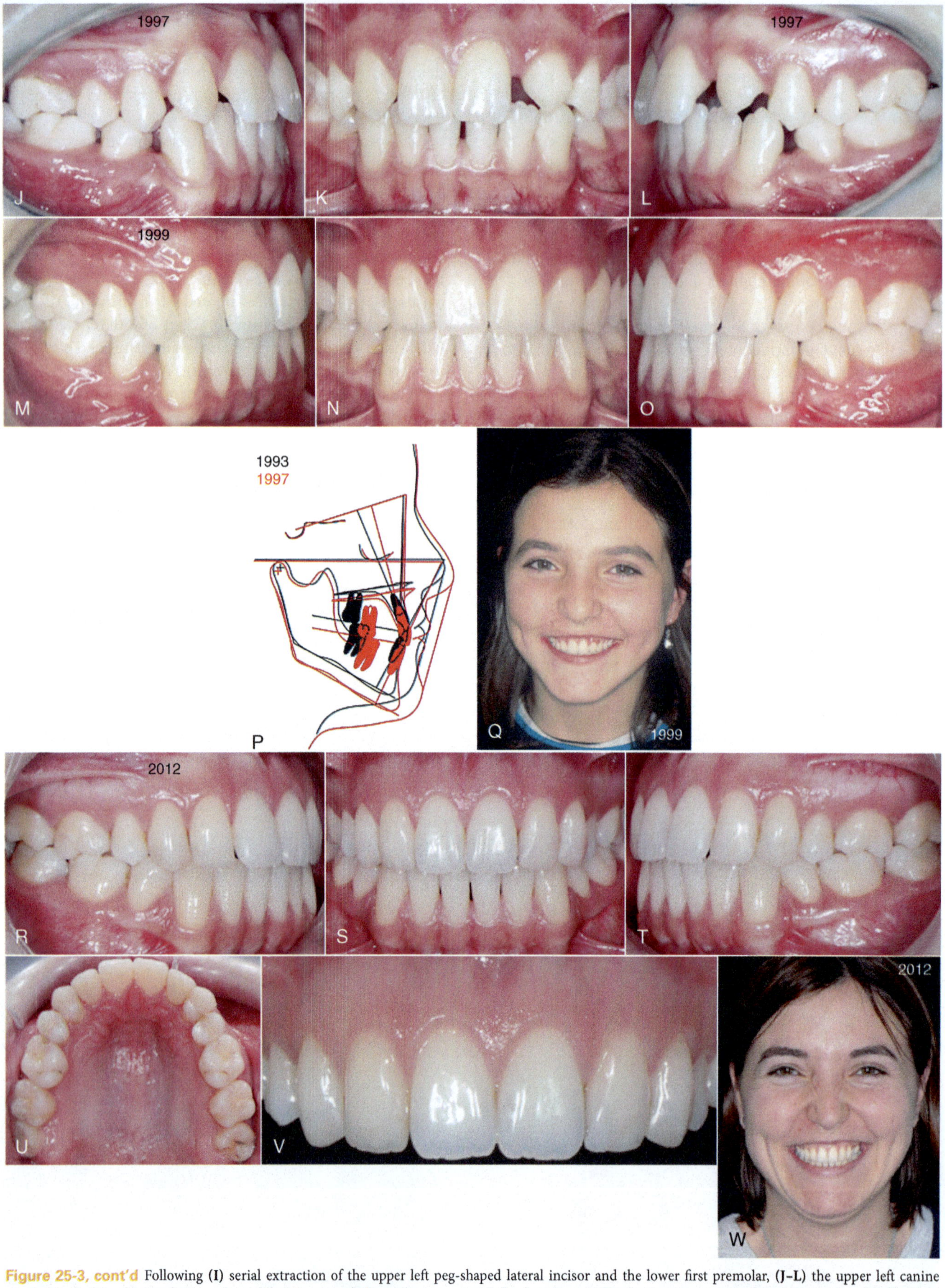

Figure 25-3, cont'd Following **(I)** serial extraction of the upper left peg-shaped lateral incisor and the lower first premolar, **(J–L)** the upper left canine erupted in the lateral incisor's site and simplified the second phase of treatment with fixed appliances. The fixed appliance stage lasted 11 months and effectively closed the spaces with a good occlusion **(M–P)**. On the same day that debonding occurred, the upper canines were ground and restored with composite resin to close the "black triangles" and the first premolars were built up to resemble and function as canines. **Q,** The patient showed gingival margins when smiling and the overall exposure of teeth and periodontal tissues was in good balance. Twelve years after the end of treatment the patient was 27 years old. **R–V,** The occlusion is stable and **(W)** the overall esthetics remains satisfactory. Minimal maintenance of the composite buildups was needed, although substitution with porcelain veneers would increase the esthetic outcome and improve the long-term prognosis. (Composite buildups: Dr. Patrizia Lucchi, Trento, Italy.)

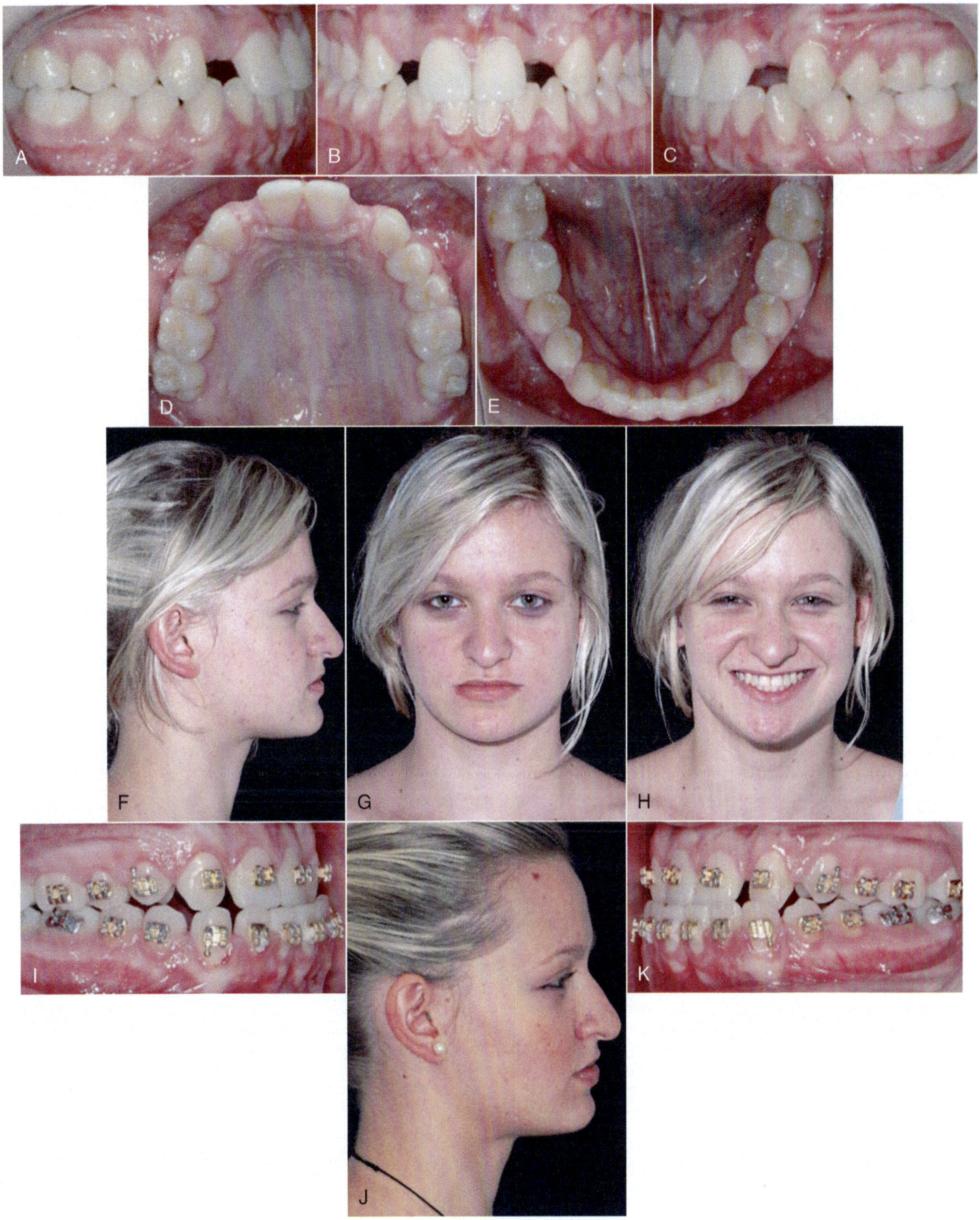

Figure 25-4 Space closure and facial surgery after unsatisfactory space reopening. **A–H,** In a previous treatment performed elsewhere, spaces were reopened for implant substitution in a 17-year-old female. The occlusion appears normal and maxillary lateral incisor spaces were prepared bilaterally for implants. Because of the Class III tendency with retruded maxilla, the upper incisors were protruded in an attempt to correct the overjet and improve the profile. The lateral incisors were temporarily replaced with a removable plate. **I–K,** The revised treatment plan included closure of all spaces in the maxilla. Uprighting of the maxillary incisors produced an anterior crossbite. **J,** Note that the soft tissue profile after the 7 mm incisor retraction didn't change significantly when compared to the initial profile. The overjet was corrected surgically together with the skeletal discrepancy.

Continued

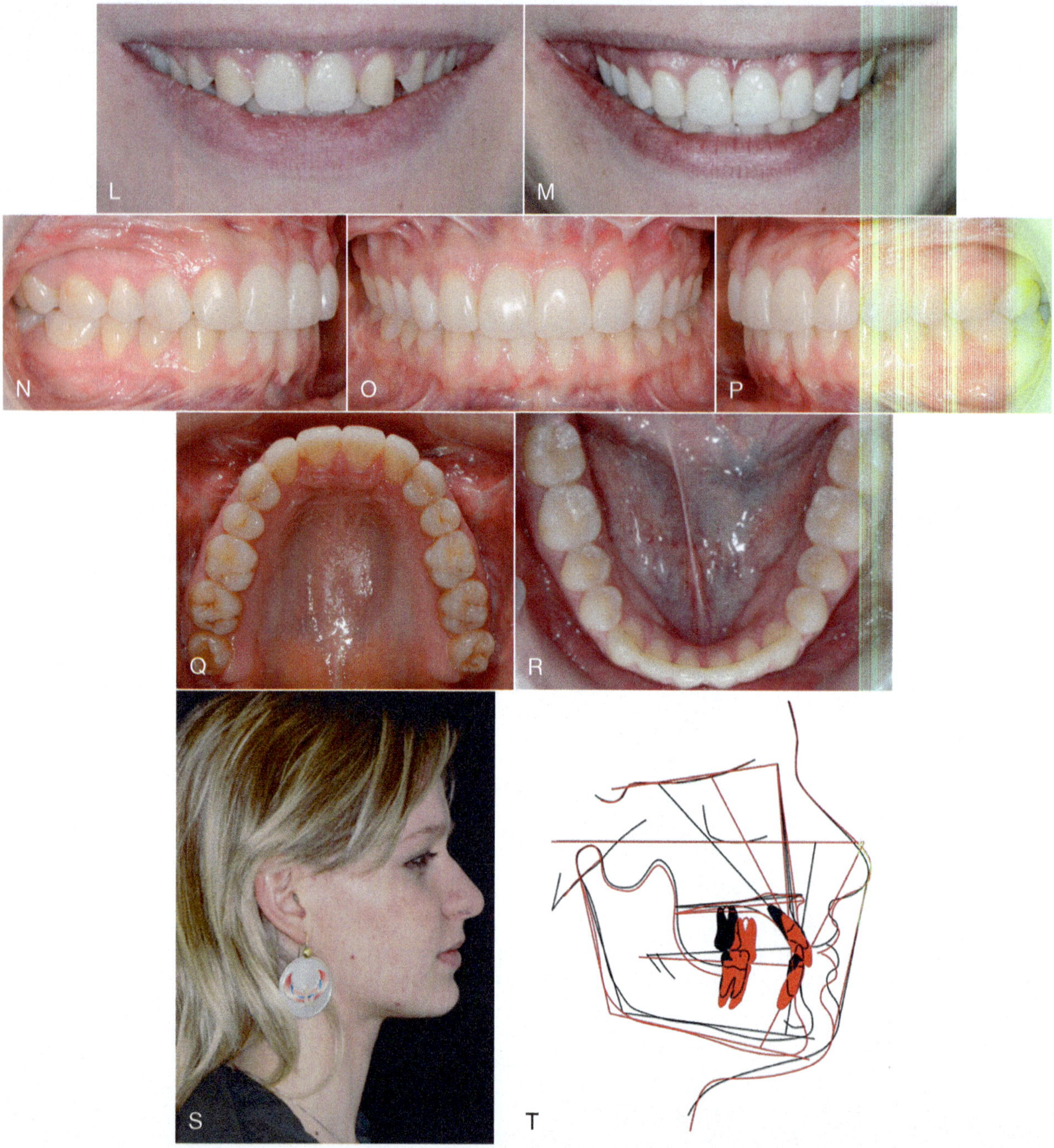

Figure 25-4, cont'd **L,** The first premolars were intruded to achieve ideal levels of the gingival margins. **L and M,** On the day that debonding occurred, temporary composite direct restorations were made on the six front teeth. **M–Q,** Five years postop, the direct composite build-ups were substituted with resin veneers. **M,** The incisor display while smiling is ideal for a young adult woman. **N–P,** Final results show maxillary molars in Class II relationship. **R,** Retention consisted of one bonded six-unit retainer in the lower arch. The profile **(S)** improved significantly due to **(T)** the surgical vertical/sagittal maxillary repositioning and the concomitant mandibular rotation. **T,** Surgery involved just the maxilla, which was moved forward and down to increase the overall vertical dimension. The superimposition in **T** also shows that the upper lip did not move forward. (Surgeon: Dr. Mirco Raffaini, Parma, Italy; Composite restorations and veneers: Dr. Patrizia Lucchi, Trento, Italy.)

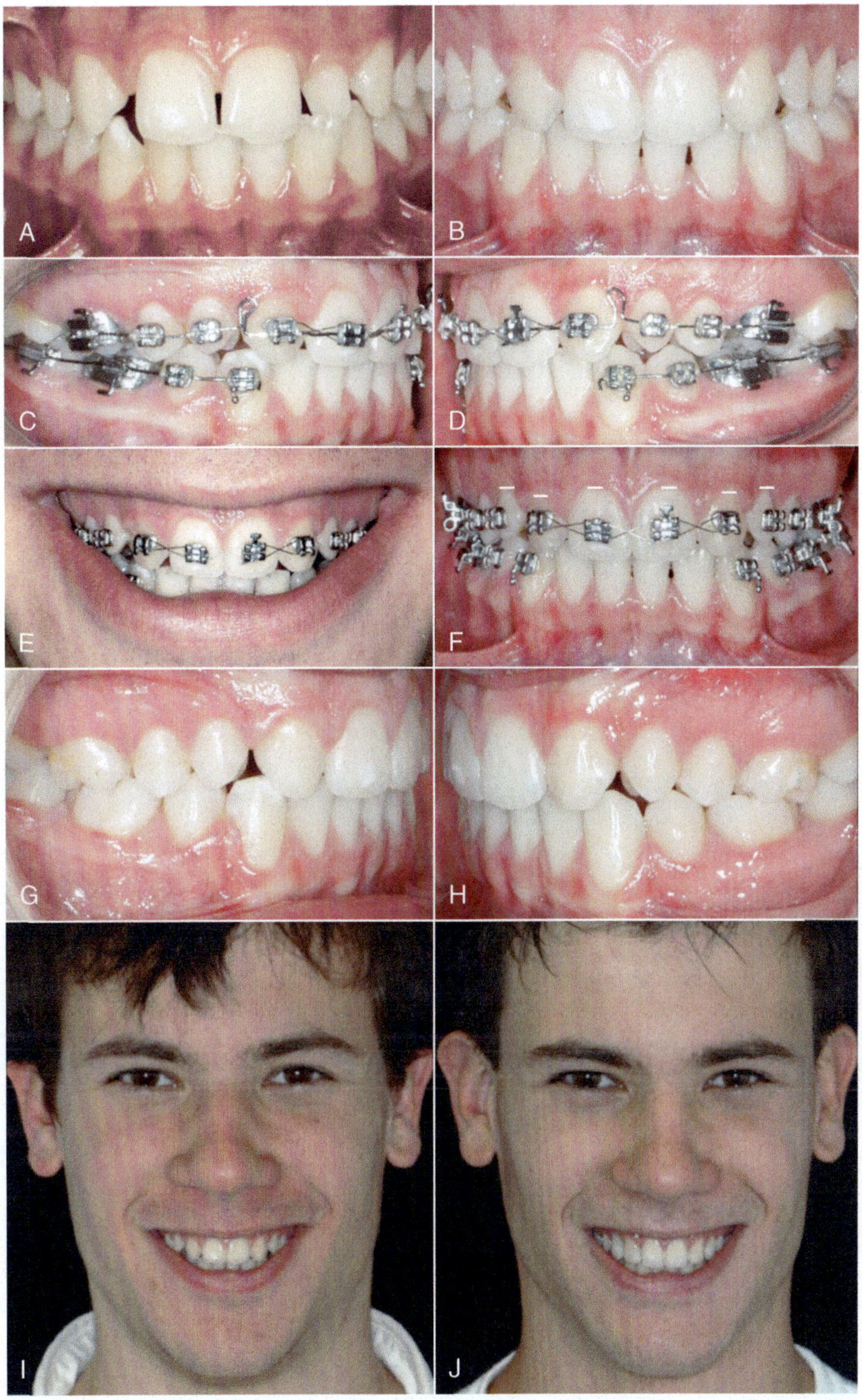

Figure 25-5 Space closure with lower premolar extractions. **A,** A 13-year-old boy with unilateral agenesis. Peg-shaped left lateral incisor and lower first premolars were extracted. **C–F,** Treatment lasted 22 months and **(B and E–I)** included gingival leveling by extrusion of the canines and intrusion of the first premolars. **J,** Composite resin buildups on six teeth included elongation of the central incisors to produce a nice smile arc. (Composite restorations: Dr. Patrizia Lucchi, Trento, Italy.)

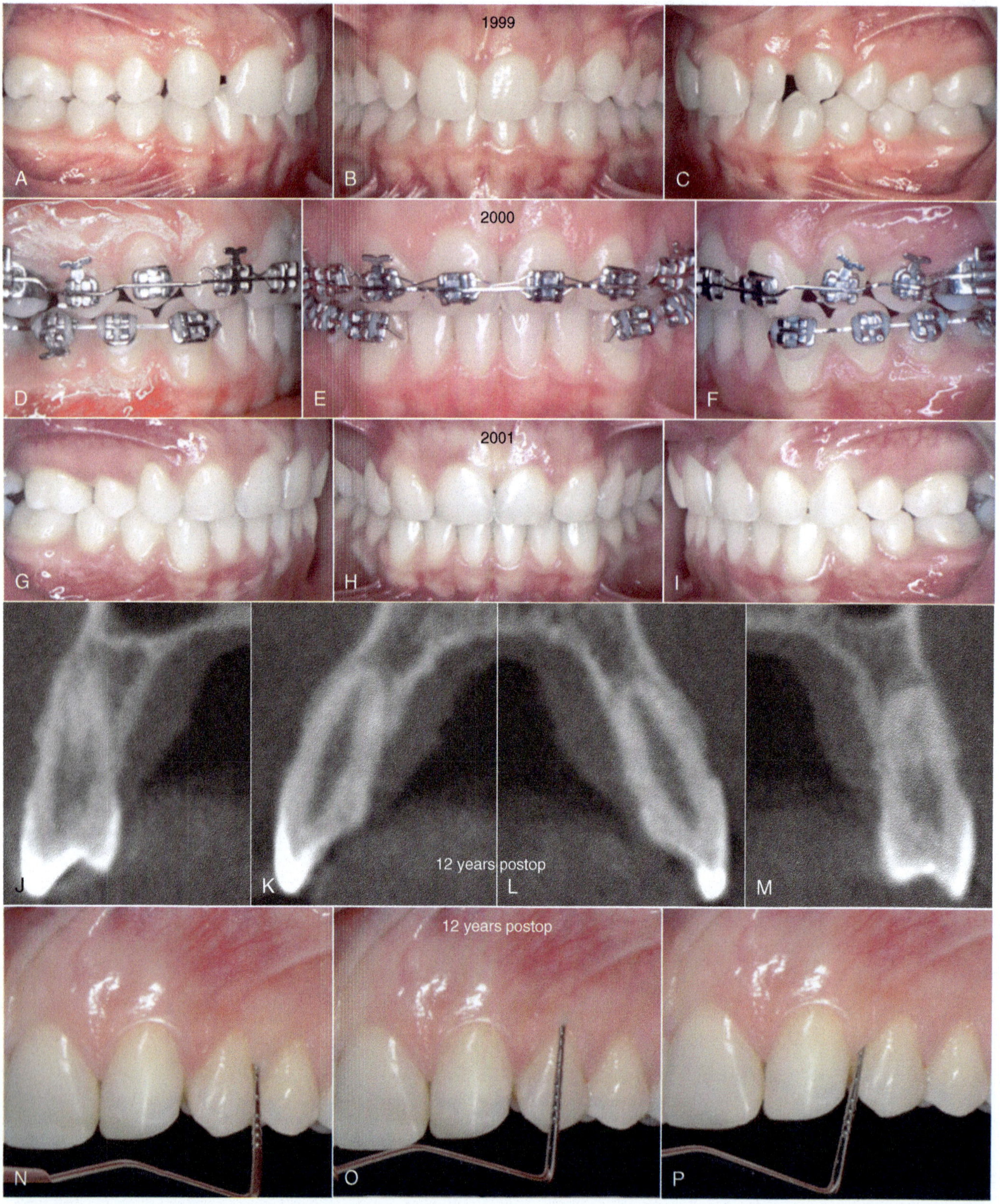

Figure 25-6 Long-term stability of space closure and gingival remodeling. **A–C,** An 11-year-old girl presented with Class II, subdivision and a missing maxillary lateral incisor. The small left lateral incisor was extracted. The lower arch was treated with minor stripping to flatten the curve of Spee and solve the 2-mm crowding. **D–F,** Upper space closure was performed with maximum anchorage on the upper central incisors, extrusion of the canines, and intrusion of the first premolars to create a natural-looking gingival profile. At the end of active treatment (25 months), the patient was 14 years old. **G–I,** The result was satisfactory: good intercuspation with Class II molar relationship and natural-looking front teeth, mainly due to the "big" canines. Resin buildups were made directly on the canines and first premolars. **J–M,** Twelve years after treatment, cone beam computed tomography (CBCT) shows the adequate tissues were achieved by the palatal root torque of the canines during their extrusion and the labial root torque/palatal crown tip of the premolars during their intrusion. The occlusion is stable and the periodontal tissues are healthy. **N–P,** Twelve years after treatment, there is no bleeding on probing and probing depth (PD) is within the normal range.

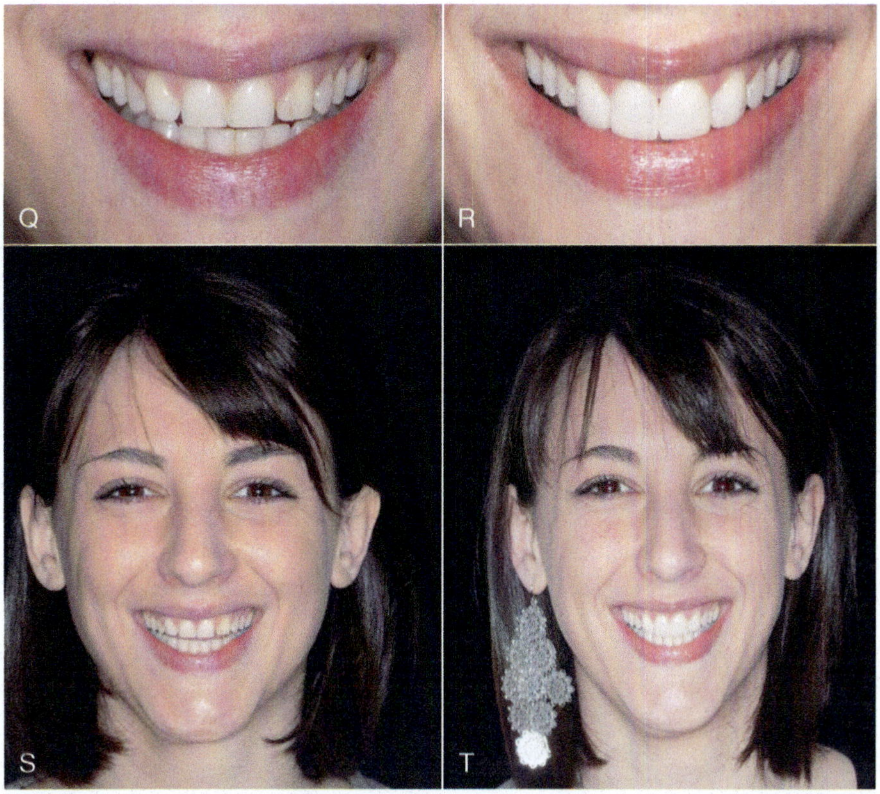

Figure 25-6, cont'd **Q and S,** Ten years postop and despite the satisfactory occlusal result and periodontal stability, the overall esthetics of the smile was not ideal due to the small teeth, especially the central incisors. **R and T,** After buildups on the central incisors and canines, the macroesthetic elements of the smile were improved. (Buildups: Dr. Patrizia Lucchi, Trento, Italy.)

allows mesial movement of molars and premolars with no extra anchorage and/or Class III elastics[39] (Fig. 25-10, C-H).

The mesial movement of the first premolar may be complicated in the presence of two divergent roots. It may be indicated to slightly rotate such premolars to prevent the buccal root from moving into the cortical plate, which would slow down the movement and potentially produce a risk for periodontal tissue breakdown.

Furthermore, the curve of Spee should be flattened to allow proper orthodontic finishing. Fixed appliances are necessary in the mandibular arch, at least in the final stages of treatment. A correct cusp to fossa relationship should be achieved on the upper second premolars, together with a solid stable occlusion with no notable CO-CR discrepancy. Sometimes slight selective grindings are necessary.

Another possible alternative treatment plan for agenesis patients who show much gingiva when smiling is to close the spaces anteriorly and open up space for a third premolar in the posterior areas (see Fig. 25-9; Fig. 25-11).

Step 2: Orthodontic Finishing in the Maxillary Anterior Region

Alignment of the Six Maxillary Front Teeth. To achieve an optimal alignment, some adjustment bends must be made on the maxillary archwires. An offset bend is necessary between the central incisors and the mesially moved canine, while inset bends may be needed mesially and distally to the first premolars (see arrows on Fig. 25-14).

Mesiodistal enamel reduction of the canines may be necessary to make them more similar in width to a lateral incisor. Minor diastemas may be left mesially and/or distally to the first premolars and restored to proper canine shape later. The zenith (most apical point of the gingival tissue) should be distal to the long axis of the central incisors and canines but should coincide with the long axis of the lateral incisors.[33]

The overjet relationship is usually ideal on the "new" lateral incisors (i.e., canines ground on the palatal surface), while it may be 1- to 3-mm on well-aligned central incisors[7] (see Fig. 25-9, M).

Extrusion of the Canines and Intrusion of the First Premolars to Achieve Ideal Levels of the Gingival Margins. Canines that replace lateral incisors must be extruded to move the gingival margins 1- to 2-mm below those of the central incisors (see Fig. 25-5, F). During extrusion the canine needs to be ground not only on the cusp but also on the palatal surface in order to provide a good occlusion. To avoid abrasion of the lower lateral incisors due to contact with the thick palatal surface of the canines, the canine's palatal surface can be reduced or an artificial "canine protection" can be developed through a composite buildup on the first premolar.

The gingival contours also must be considered in cases of canine substitution. First premolars should be intruded until the cementoenamel junction (CEJ) is close to the level of the

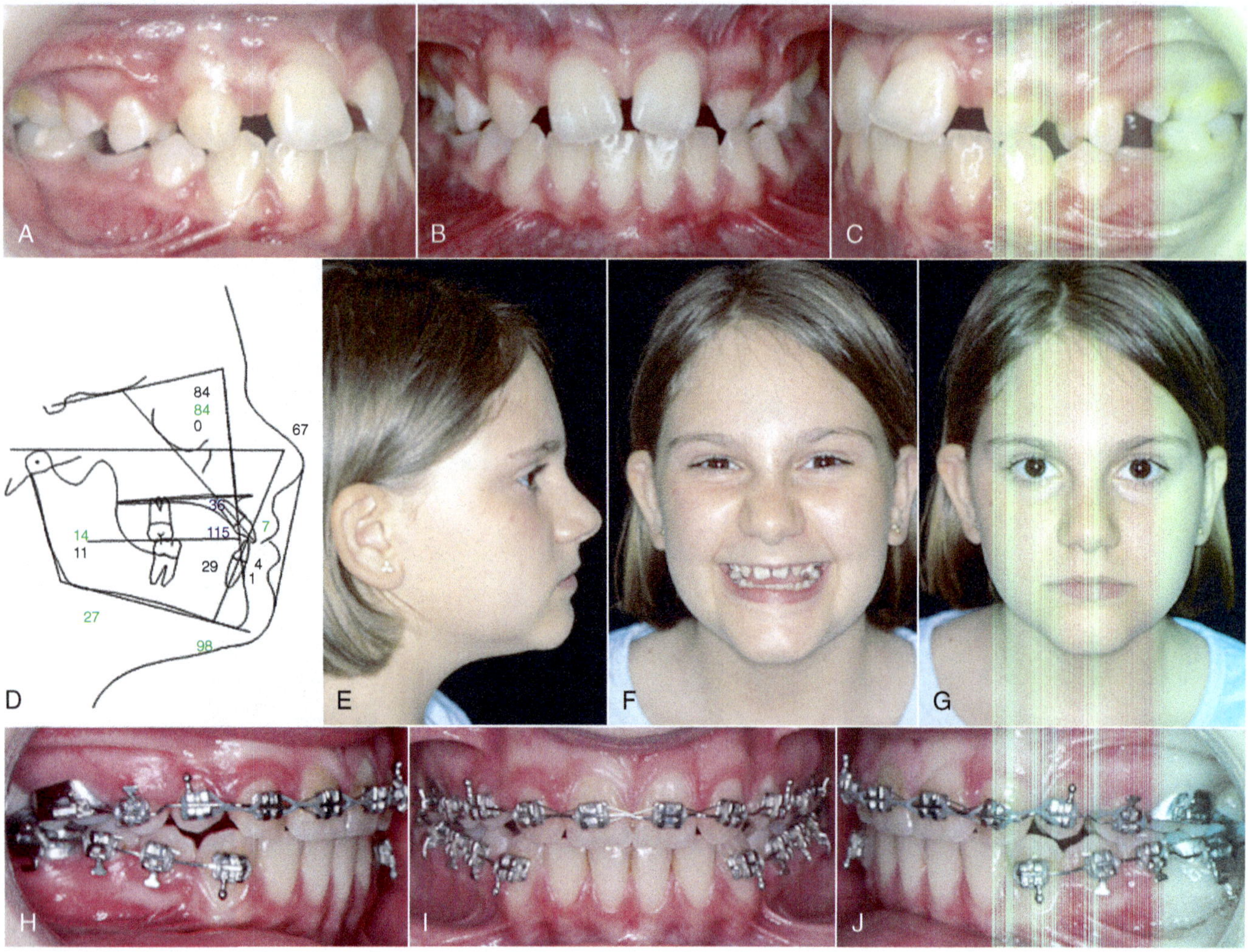

Figure 25-7 Space closure in Class III malocclusion with narrow maxilla and spaced upper arch. **A–G and M,** A 12-year-old girl presented with bilateral maxillary lateral incisor agenesis, Class III malocclusion, narrow maxillary arch, and pronounced spacing. Because of optimal motivation of and cooperation by the patient, the treatment plan was to close all spaces. **H–J,** After rapid maxillary expansion (RME), fixed appliances were used for space closure to obtain good intercuspation of the second premolars with Class II molar occlusion. Canine extrusion and first premolar intrusion, as well as torque control of anterior and posterior teeth, was achieved by archwire bending.

central incisor but at a higher level than the "new" lateral incisors (see Fig. 25-5, F). Extrusion and intrusion will move the periodontal supporting tissues together with the tooth. Intrusion will move the gingival margin about 70% to 80% of the tooth movement and a small pseudopocket may appear.[40] Extrusion may move the gingival margin down 80% of the tooth movement.[41] The vertical movements not only produce changes in the soft tissues but may also produce uneven bone peaks (Figs. 25-12 and 25-13). These are not true vertical defects and the patient can brush and floss effectively. During retention often the alveolar bone and the bone peaks remodel while the gingival margins remain unchanged (see Fig. 25-12).

The starting point in planning the amount of extrusion and intrusion is the position of the maxillary central incisor edge relative to the upper lip at rest and when smiling.[42] The position of the maxillary incisal edge with resting lips correlates with their display and can be acceptable or unacceptable, depending on age (see discussion in Chapter 3).

It is important to prevent central incisor intrusion as a side effect in the leveling stage and to maintain a good vertical exposure. The vertical position of the central incisor brackets is decided on, with the goal of having 4- to 5-mm incisal show with relaxed lips in young patients, and having 2- to 3-mm of gingiva exposed on full smiling at the end of treatment (see Figs. 25-4, L, and 25-5, I). The brackets on the canine and first premolars should be positioned intentionally high and low, respectively, at the beginning of treatment in order to achieve optimal gingival levels in the first months of treatment (see Fig. 25-12, B).

Torque Control of Extruded Canine and Intruded First Premolar to Prevent Periodontal Complications and Enable Correct Restorations. The root of the canine is bigger than the root of the lateral incisor and it is critical to consider the thickness of the alveolar ridge and soft periodontal tissues. The risk for development of labial gingival recession is obvious, particularly in patients with a

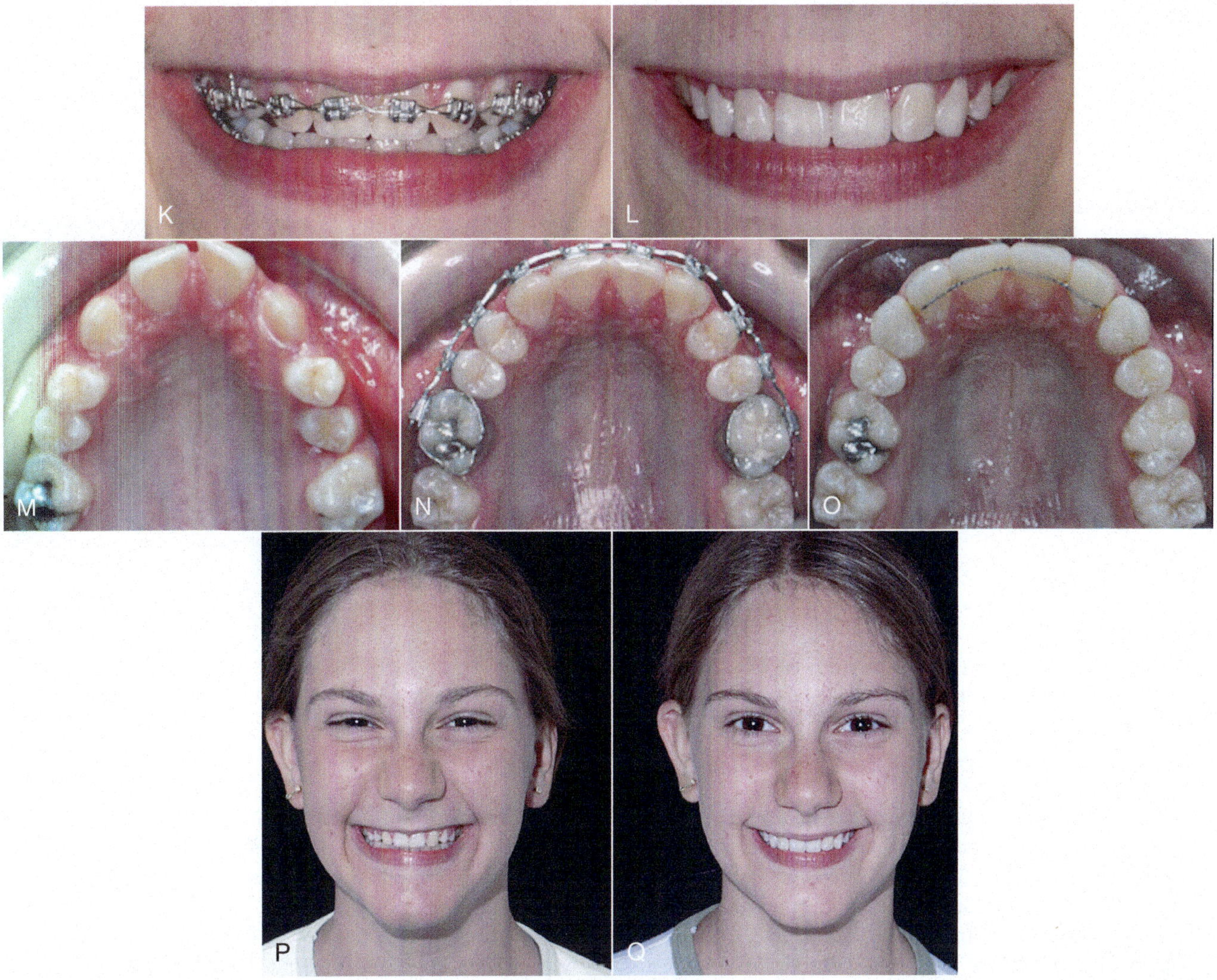

Figure 25-7, cont'd As shown in **K and L,** the maxillary anterior teeth may need further elongation to improve their relationship to the lips. **N,** Note the detailed alignment on rectangular stainless steel archwires, with mesial and distal offset bends for the canines in lateral incisor position and distal offsets for the first premolars in canine position. At the end of treatment **(R–T)** the occlusion was good and **(O)** a fixed retainer was bonded on four teeth. The **(V)** profile and **(W and X)** frontal facial appearance improved significantly due to the mandibular posterior rotation, which increased the vertical dimension. The selective extrusion and intrusion of the canines and first premolars, respectively, leveled the gingival margins to **(R–T)** a natural high-low-high relationship. The composite resin buildups were made on the day of debonding for esthetic reasons and to stabilize the occlusion. The canines in lateral incisor position were not ground and shortened. **P and Q,** The clinical crown length of the central incisors was increased with the buildups to an improved proportion compared to the new lateral incisors and **(Q and X)** to provide a good smile arc.

Continued

thin periodontal biotype. In addition, when the canine is extruded with labial appliances the root tends to move buccally. For this reason, palatal root torque should be applied at the start of the extrusion. Application of lingual root torque results in less enamel grinding near the labial CEJ, where the enamel layer is sometimes thin.[2] This can be accomplished by using a bracket with a higher torque prescription or by placing third-order bends in the archwire prior to extrusion (Fig. 25-14).

During intrusion of the first premolars with labial appliances and preformed nickel-titanium (Ni-Ti) archwires, their crowns tend to tip buccally. This is not a problem for the roots, which will move toward the palate, but the labial crown tip may impair the smile esthetics and produce an excessive overjet, which will create problems for the restorative dentist who is trying to restore the premolar to canine shape (see Fig. 25-14, D). To avoid the buccal tip of the premolar during intrusion, the upper stainless steel (0.016-inch × 0.022-inch) archwire must be shaped straight in this segment and sometimes an inset bend is needed mesial to the second premolar and distal to the canine (see Fig. 25-14, E; Fig. 25-15, B).

To check the proper torque and angulation of the roots a cone beam computed tomography (CBCT) examination is useful after the space closure in the finishing stages of the treatment (see Figs. 25-13 and 25-14).

Step 3: Gingivectomy

In select cases, localized gingivectomies are required to level the gingival margins (see Fig. 25-15).[5] While rare in adult

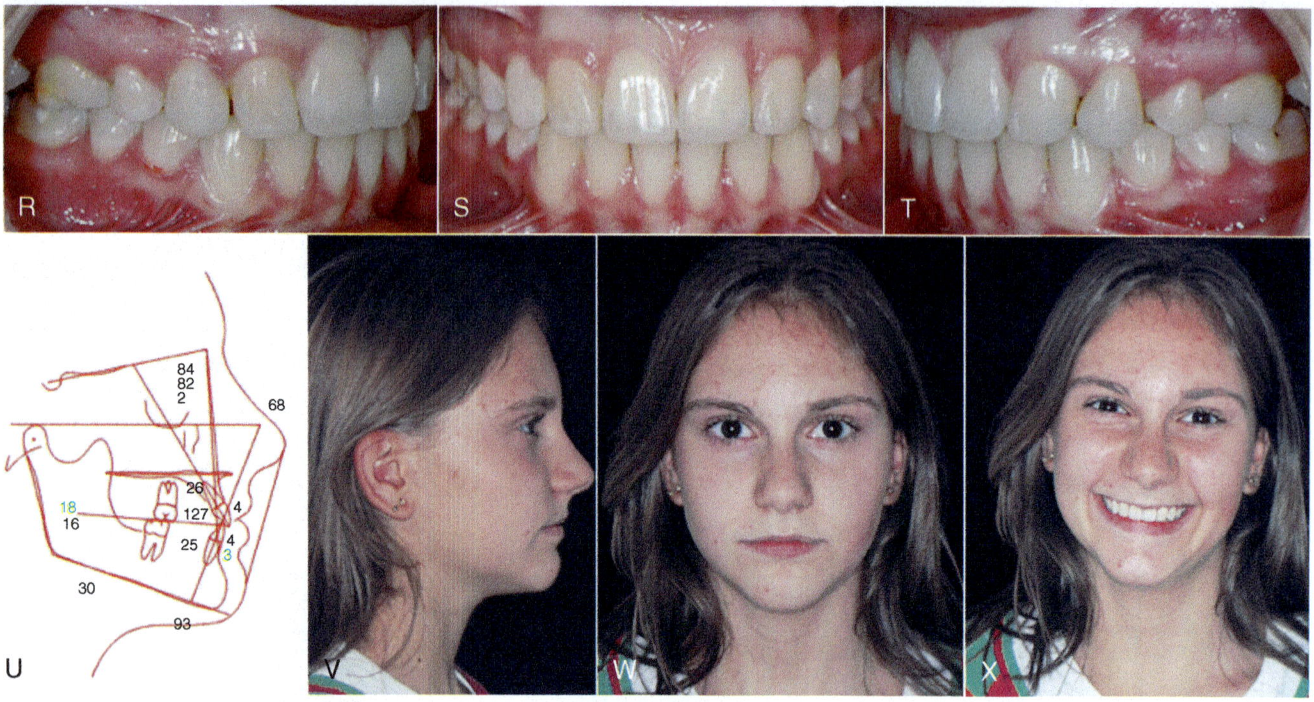

Figure 25-7, cont'd **Q and X,** After the cosmetic phase with composite resin buildups on all six front teeth and whitening (vital bleaching) of the canines, a balanced and naturally looking appearance was achieved. The smile is pleasant not because of the new lateral incisors but because of the restored first premolars in canine position and central incisors. (Composite resin buildups: Dr. Patrizia Lucchi, Trento, Italy.)

patients, surgery is sometimes necessary in growing patients to modify hypertrophic gingivae due to poor oral hygiene or allergies and/or to correct negative aspects of altered passive eruption.[43,44] A gingivectomy involving the marginal gingiva should be done post-treatment and after repeated sessions of professional oral hygiene instruction. The excision must be wide since up to half of the excised tissue will regenerate.[45] Even if the excision is extended into the alveolar mucosa, the coronal part of the regenerated gingiva will still be keratinized.[46]

When the gingiva is swollen or hypertrophic during orthodontic treatment, it may be difficult to probe the CEJ and plan the amount of intrusion and extrusion needed for individual teeth. It may be even more problematic if the teeth are abraded and have lost their anatomic integrity. If there is altered active eruption in growing patients (i.e., persistence of alveolar bone and periodontal attachment coronally to the CEJ), a gingivectomy is not enough. In such instances open flap surgery is needed during the orthodontic treatment to remodel the levels of the alveolar bone and the gingival margins (see Fig. 25-15).

In all cases, it is very important to motivate and educate patients regarding proper oral hygiene measures before, during, and after the orthodontic treatment, to maintain normal healthy tissues.

Step 4: Esthetic Restorations

At the end of the orthodontic treatment, the malocclusion should be corrected, the spaces closed, and the gingival margins optimally leveled due to canine extrusion and first premolar intrusion. At this point, since the final goal is to achieve an optimally esthetic incisor exposure, restorations are necessary on the canines and the first premolars for esthetic and functional reasons.[6–8]

The extruded canine, even if properly ground, often requires restoration to correct a "black triangle" and embrasures[47,48] (see Figs. 25-5 and 25-13, A).

The intruded first premolars must be suitably restored to resemble natural canines. A wide restoration is necessary to build up the cusp, lingual surface, and contact points. The lingual surface of the buildup may provide canine guidance but more often participates in group function. The palatal cusp of the first premolar does not need to be ground and is sometimes covered by the restoration (see Fig. 25-13).

The final goal is to achieve a balanced and attractive exposure of the upper front teeth (see Figs. 25-3 to 25-5, 25-9, and 25-15):

- Transversally: 70% for the canines and 160% for the central incisors[33]
- Vertically: correct periodontal levels and smile arc[47]

For a truly satisfactory result, not only do the restorations need to be intraorally ideal, but the overall result needs to incorporate macroesthetic elements, such as the relationship between teeth, lips, and face.[49] A consonant smile arc is important to consider and the parallelism between the arc formed by the maxillary teeth and the inner contour of the lower lip when the patient is smiling needs to be harmonious.[47] In some cases the central incisors may need to be made longer and wider to achieve an optimal smile arc[6–8] (see Fig. 25-6).

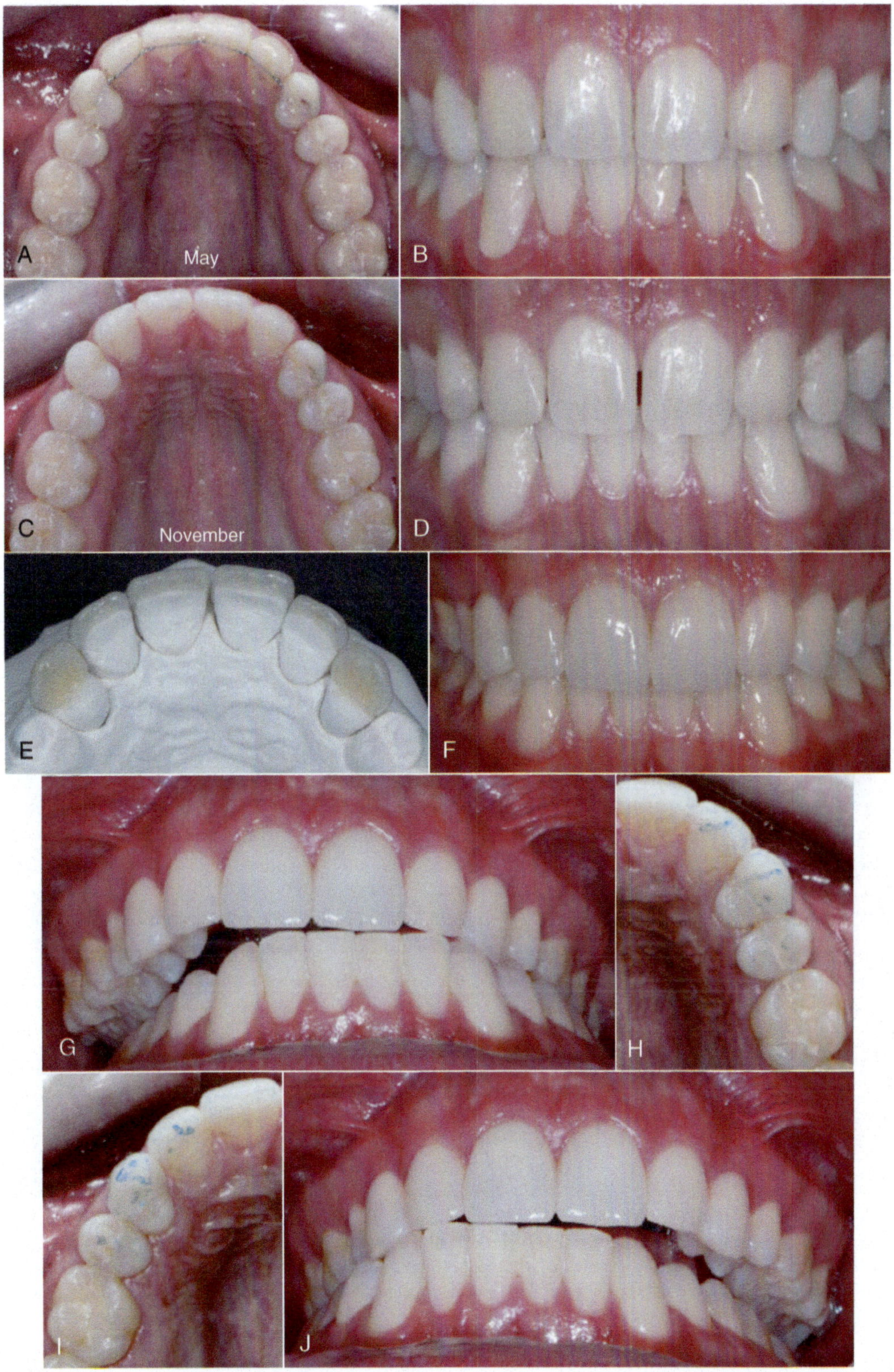

Figure 25-8 Porcelain laminate veneers (PLV) and long-term stability. **A–D,** At least 10 months before the PLV are made, the upper bonded retainer must be removed, which will allow small spaces to reopen. During this time the patient should not use any removable retainer in the upper arch. Selective grinding may become necessary to stabilize the occlusion. **E and F,** When the occlusion and the small spaces are stable, the PLV are made and will close the spaces. **G–J,** Two years after the porcelain restorations, the result was stable and no spaces were noticeable among the upper front teeth. The porcelain veneers will also optimize the functional occlusion. In the absence of a lingually bonded retainer, group function may be better than a cuspid protected occlusion to ensure long-term stability. **G to J** show simultaneous contacts on the second, third, and fourth tooth (blue marks in **H and I**). (Prosthodontist: Dr. G. Manfrini, Riva d G, Italy. Ceramist: A. Berto.)

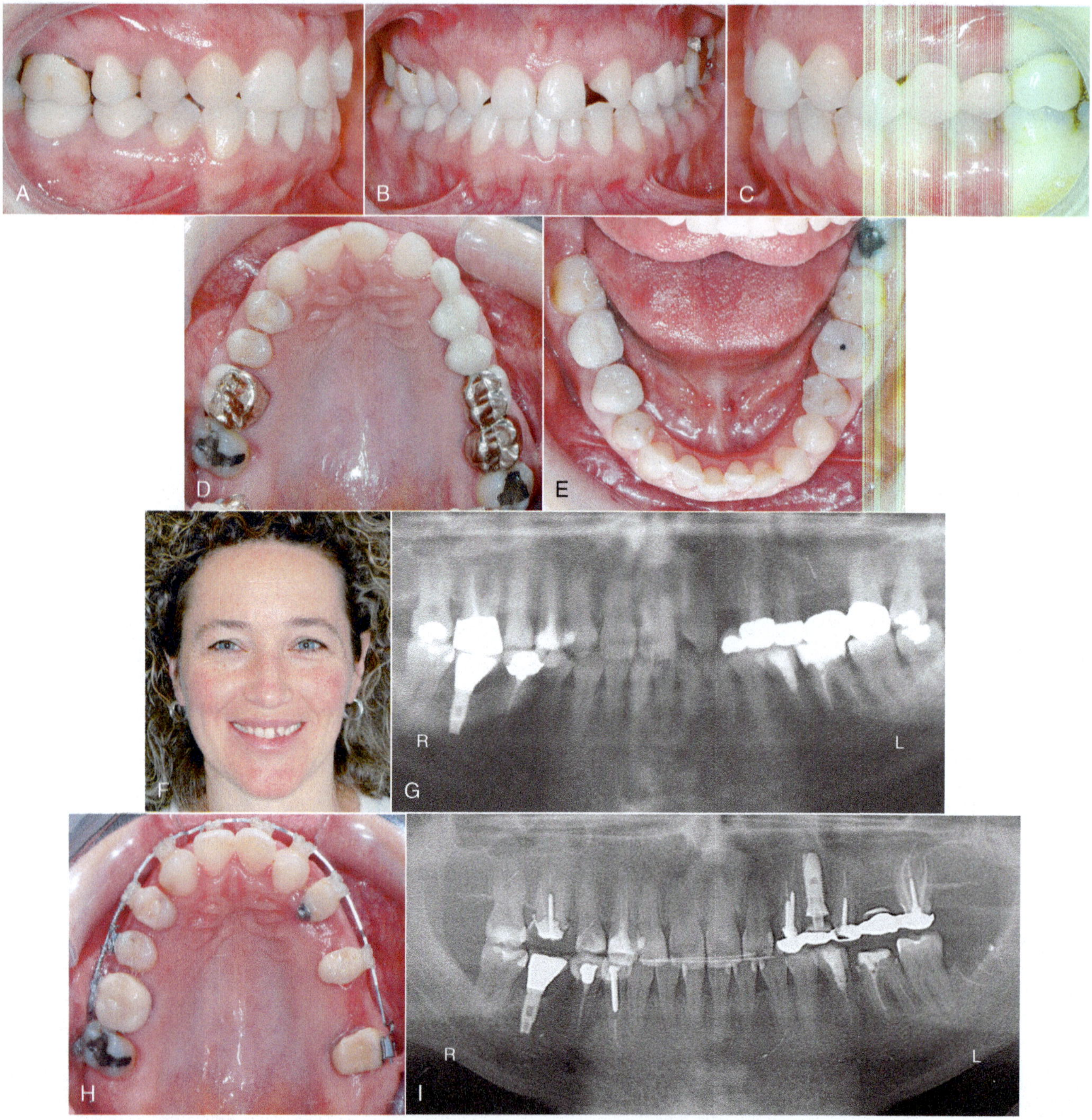

Figure 25-9 **A–G,** A 37-year-old female patient with bilateral agenesis of the maxillary lateral incisors and severe asymmetry of the upper small-sized front teeth. A 5-unit bridge restoration replacing the upper left first molar and a small canine (cantilever) is evident in the upper left arch. The treatment plan was to close the spaces in the smile area and correct the upper midline while reopening a space (implant site) between the upper left premolars. During treatment, adequate diastemas were opened mesially and distally on the central incisors to allow resin buildups on those teeth. **I,** An implant was inserted into the orthodontically regenerated alveolar bone during orthodontic treatment.

Recent studies have demonstrated that subjects with unilateral or bilateral agenesis of maxillary lateral incisors may have smaller teeth than those with normal dentition.[50–52] Therefore if the goal is to obtain a balanced, ideal smile, restorations should also be considered on the central incisors in many patients with agenesis. This is also valid for patients in whom space opening is planned.

Generally, buildup restorations should be made directly with hybrid composite material immediately after the debonding (on the same day, if possible). The hybrid composite allows for easy finishing and adjustments until ideal esthetics are achieved. The restorations should be whiter than the yellowish enamel of the canines and the color should be chosen with consideration given to the subsequent

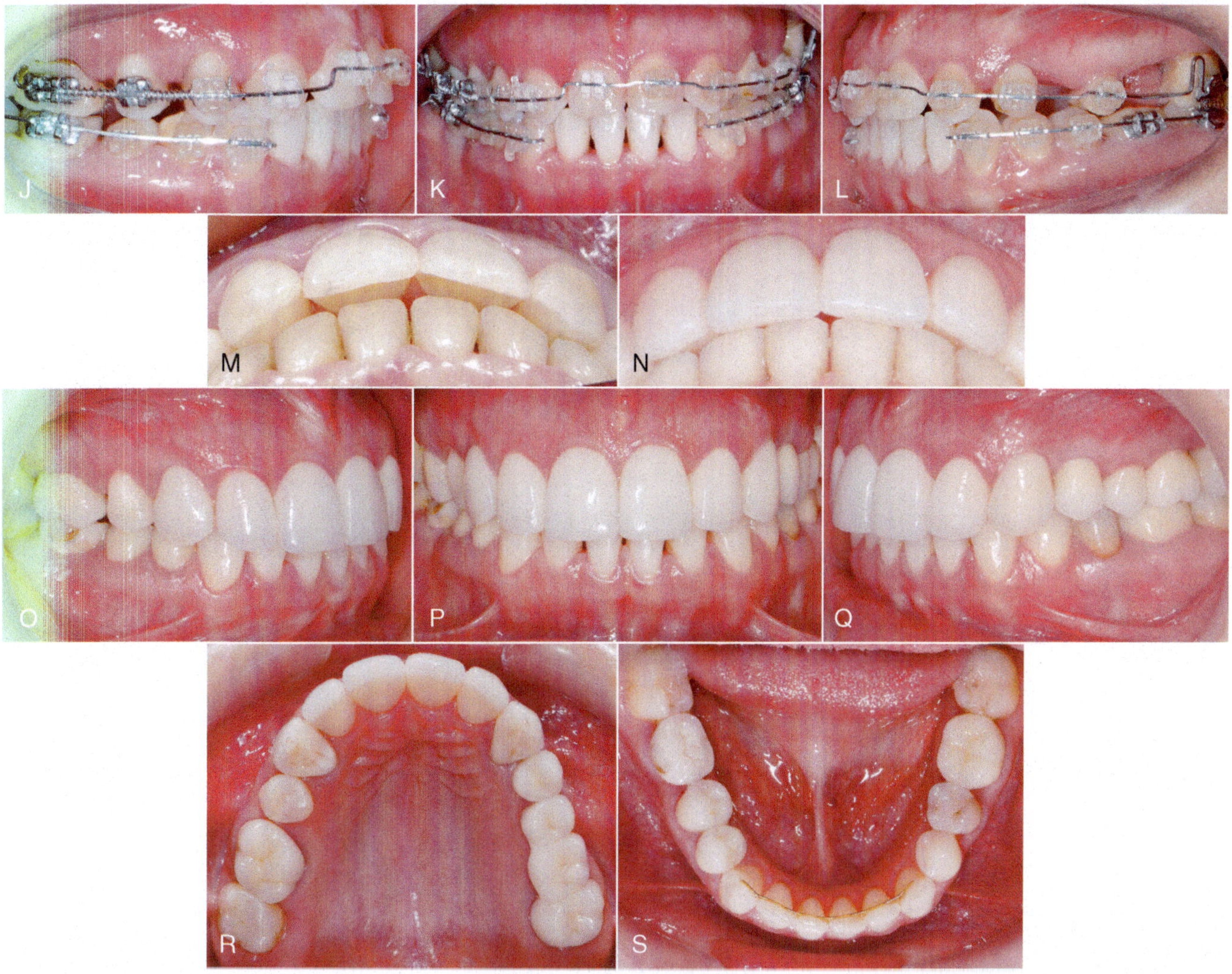

Figure 25-9, cont'd **J–L,** The canines were extruded and the first premolars in canine position were intruded. **D and H,** The maxillary arch form was corrected and the symmetry was reestablished. **M,** A 3-mm overjet was left intentionally after the orthodontic treatment, to be filled by restorations of the small central incisors: **(N)** two different porcelain veneers in the palatal and buccal side. **O–Q,** Four years post-treatment, with porcelain restorations on the implant and on the six upper front teeth, the result was stable. *Continued*

bleaching procedure (see step 5). It is easier and more convenient to adapt the bleaching to the color of the composite resin than vice versa.

Step 5: Vital Bleaching

Relocated canines may be more yellow than intact central and lateral incisors. This problem can be solved relatively easily and predictably with either at-home or in-office vital bleaching procedures.[53,54] Nocturnal use of 10% hydrogen peroxide gel in an Essix-type retainer is a preferred way of bleaching teeth in young patients, when the risk of developing increased sensitivity is significant.

The thermoplastic tray is applied after the composite restorations have been made. The whitening procedure starts on the canines with the bleaching gel injected only in the canine reservoirs (see Fig. 25-15). Once the enamel of the canine is sufficiently whitened, the same procedure can start on the adjacent teeth. In-office bleaching may be preferable for adult patients.

Step 6: Occlusal Finishing, Final Restorations, and Long-Term Stability

Proper occlusal finishing is important for long-term success and stability. It is accomplished in the last months of treatment and during the first year after removal of the orthodontic appliances. Fundamental points are as follows:

- Do not expand the lower arch and keep normal pretreatment arch forms.
- A long-term bonded retainer should be placed on the lower front teeth.
- Lip competence should be achieved at the end of orthodontic treatment (consider lower premolar extractions, maxillofacial surgery to correct skeletal discrepancies, and/or speech therapy).
- There should be secure stable occlusion in the posterior areas with no CO-CR discrepancy.
- Group function occlusion anteriorly without balancing interferences (see Figs. 25-8 and 25-9) may be preferable to pure cuspid protected occlusion.[55]

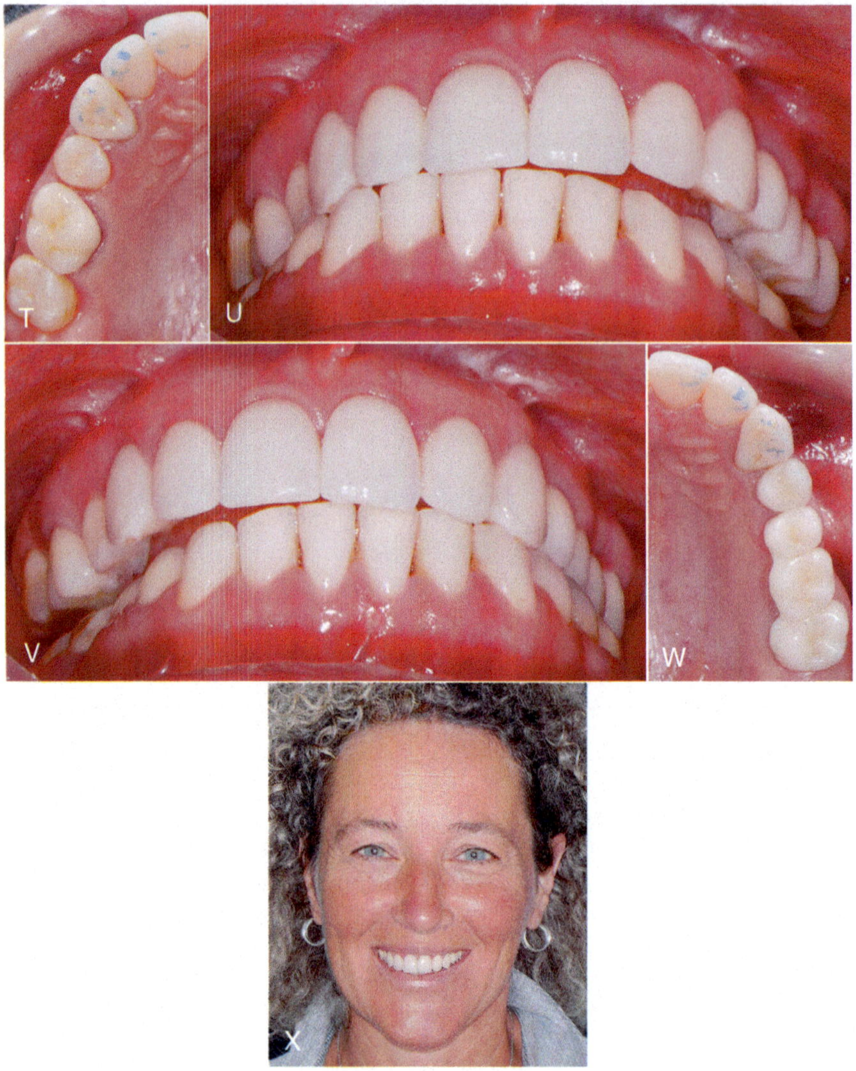

Figure 25-9, cont'd **T–W,** The anterior occlusal guidance is a group function and was ideal after the restoration of upper central incisors. **O–W,** With no retention in the upper arch, the upper space closure remained stable with no reopening of the spaces. **X,** The overall smile is better than what could have been possible with two restorations replacing the missing laterals because of the ideal size of the central incisors, which are in good balance with the face. The long-term prognosis is more predictable because of the presence of natural roots instead of foreign bodies. (Prosthodontist: Giovanni Manfrini, Riva del Garda, Italy; Ceramist: Antonio Bertoni; Brescia, Italy.)

Since it is common that spaces may reopen after debonding, long-term retention is mandatory in the maxillary arch. The thermoplastic retainers used for vital bleaching are not adequate for retention. A fixed bonded retainer on the maxillary six front teeth is presumably the best option, as it needs no patient compliance and allows the first premolars to bear some weight in function.[56] The optimal retention time is still to be documented. The authors' clinical experience indicates that spaces may reopen after retainer removal as much as 5 to 6 years after the end of treatment.

Spaces may reopen especially:

- After excessive upper incisor compensation (i.e., excessive palatal tip) in hyperdivergent skeletal Class II patients
- In lateral agenesis patients with small teeth
- In the presence of parafunctions or dysfunctional habits
- In cases where the occlusal finishing was not sufficiently detailed

The long-term stability of composite resin buildups is inadequate and, because of large individual variation, the restorations must be maintained regularly throughout the patient's life. Smokers and patients with parafunctional habits show small breakages and unesthetic shadowing of the buildups. This is the main reason why definitive porcelain restorations should be proposed to patients before treatment (see Fig. 25-8).

For porcelain veneers the following procedure is advisable:

- Carefully check the occlusion and perform selective grinding when indicated.
- Remove the upper fixed retainer.
- Allow 8 to 12 months for stabilization, during which time small diastemas may reopen between the front teeth in some patients (see Fig. 25-8). During this period the resin buildups can be adjusted further.

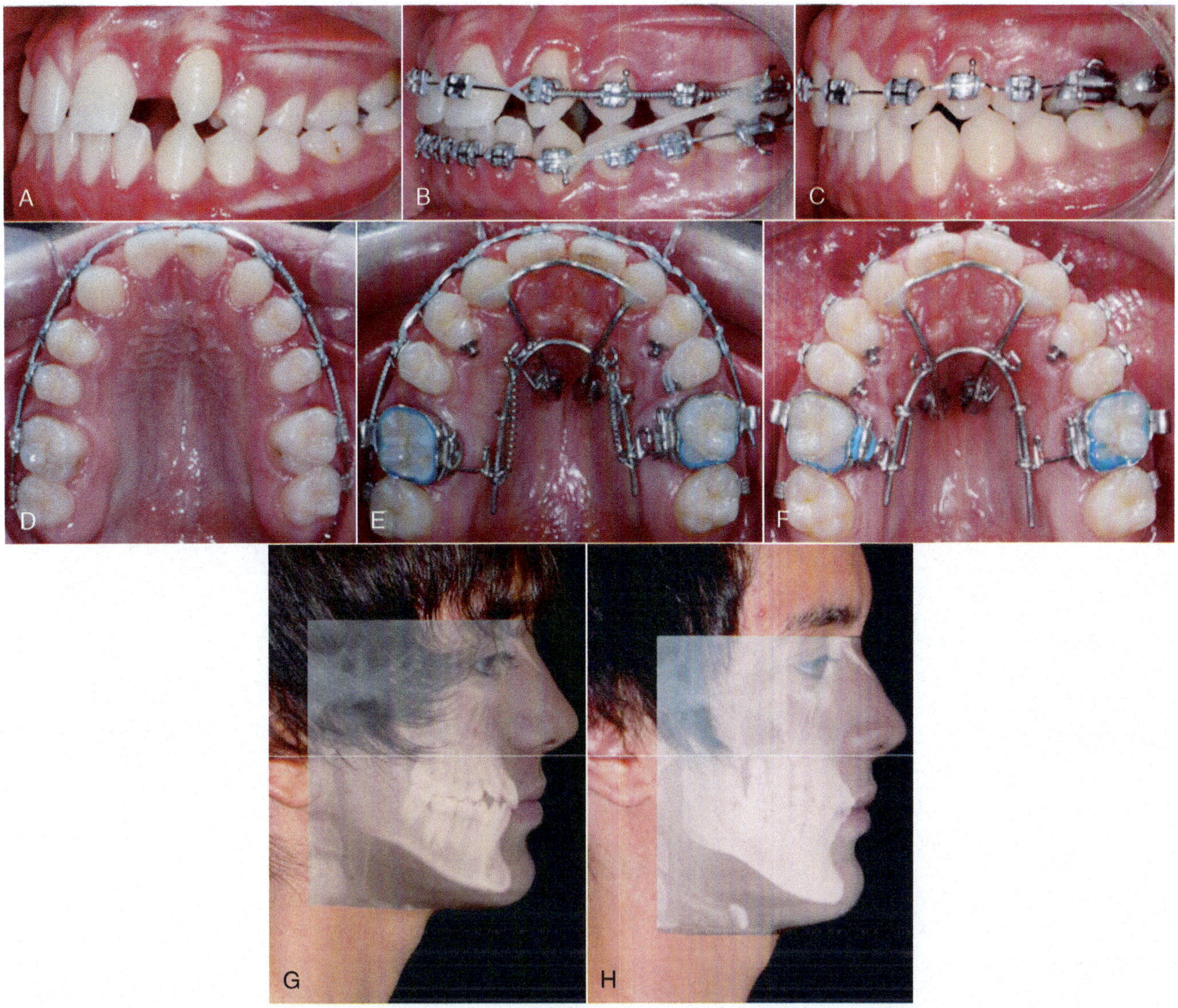

Figure 25-10 Noncompliance space closure. **A,** A 15-year-old boy presented with missing maxillary lateral incisors. The lower arch was not crowded and the lower incisors were well positioned on the A-Pogonion line. **B,** The upper space closure was difficult due to poor cooperation in wearing Class III elastics. Two mini-screws were inserted in the palatal vault at the level of the first premolars. **C,** Appliances were removed in the lower arch and **(D–F)** a sliding structure, which acted as absolute anchorage in supporting the mesial movement of the premolars and molars with pulling springs for 14 months, was tied to the mini-screws. **G and H,** It was possible to move the whole posterior dentition in the upper arch mesially while maintaining a good interincisal angle and lip posture and profile.

The porcelain veneers will match the resin restorations and will optimize function and esthetics. The porcelain restorations should provide group function on the mesially moved upper canines and first and second premolars (see Figs. 25-8 and 25-9, T-W) as well as provide new embrasures and closure of small spaces that have reopened in the months after the retainer removal. Supragingival preparations secure long-term periodontal health (see Fig. 25-8).

Even when porcelain veneers are planned, it may be advisable to use direct hybrid resin restorations to determine the optimal size and morphology of the new lateral incisors and cuspids. They can be reevaluated and adjusted at subsequent visits and the porcelain veneers can be placed when the patient is well out of treatment with a settled occlusion.

At the end of treatment the use of a bonded or removable retainer or a biteplate (to be worn at night) is advisable in patients who are seeking long-term excellence and those who show parafunctions.

PRIORITIES IN TREATMENT PLANNING

Before starting a long, complicated, and expensive interdisciplinary orthodontic and restorative treatment, it is important to define the priorities of the treatment plan. This includes an understanding of what the patient expects from the treatment and an evaluation of his or her motivation and potential cooperation.

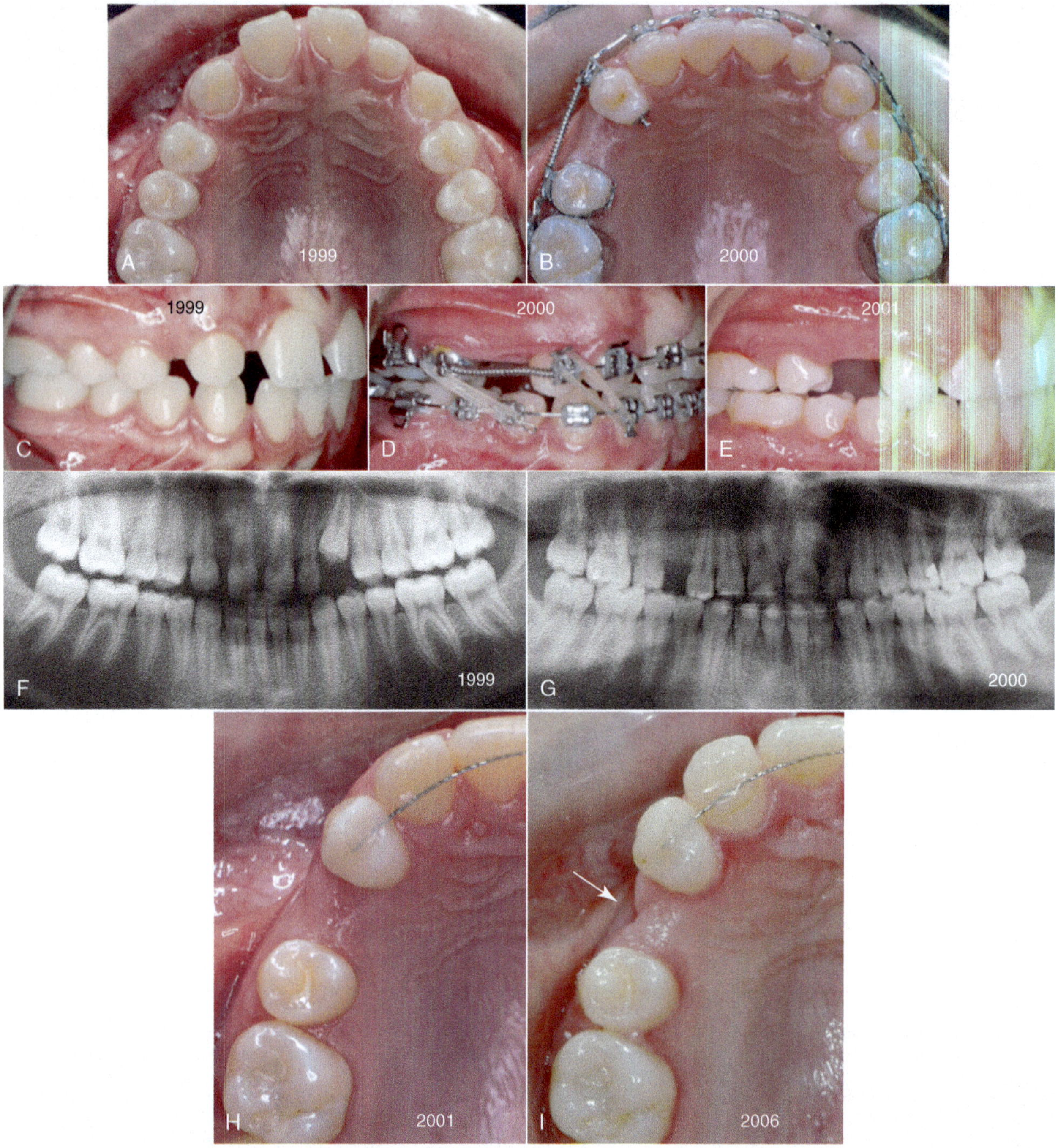

Figure 25-11 Atrophy of the orthodontically regenerated alveolar bone in the interim between orthodontic treatment and the implant, after unilateral space closure and space reopening in the back. **A, C, F, and N,** A 13-year-old girl presented with a gummy smile and unilaterally missing upper right lateral incisor. **B, D, E, and G,** She was treated with space closure while a space was reopened between the premolars. At the end of the orthodontic treatment, the implant site was adequate in **(E)** width, **(G)** height, and **(B and H)** thickness. Since the patient was then 15 years old, the final restoration was delayed until the "end of growth" and a lingual retainer was bonded on the six upper front teeth. Placement of an osseointegrated implant was planned for when the patient was 21 years old. **I,** During the 6-year interim the thickness of the alveolar crest decreased due to bone atrophy *(arrow)*.

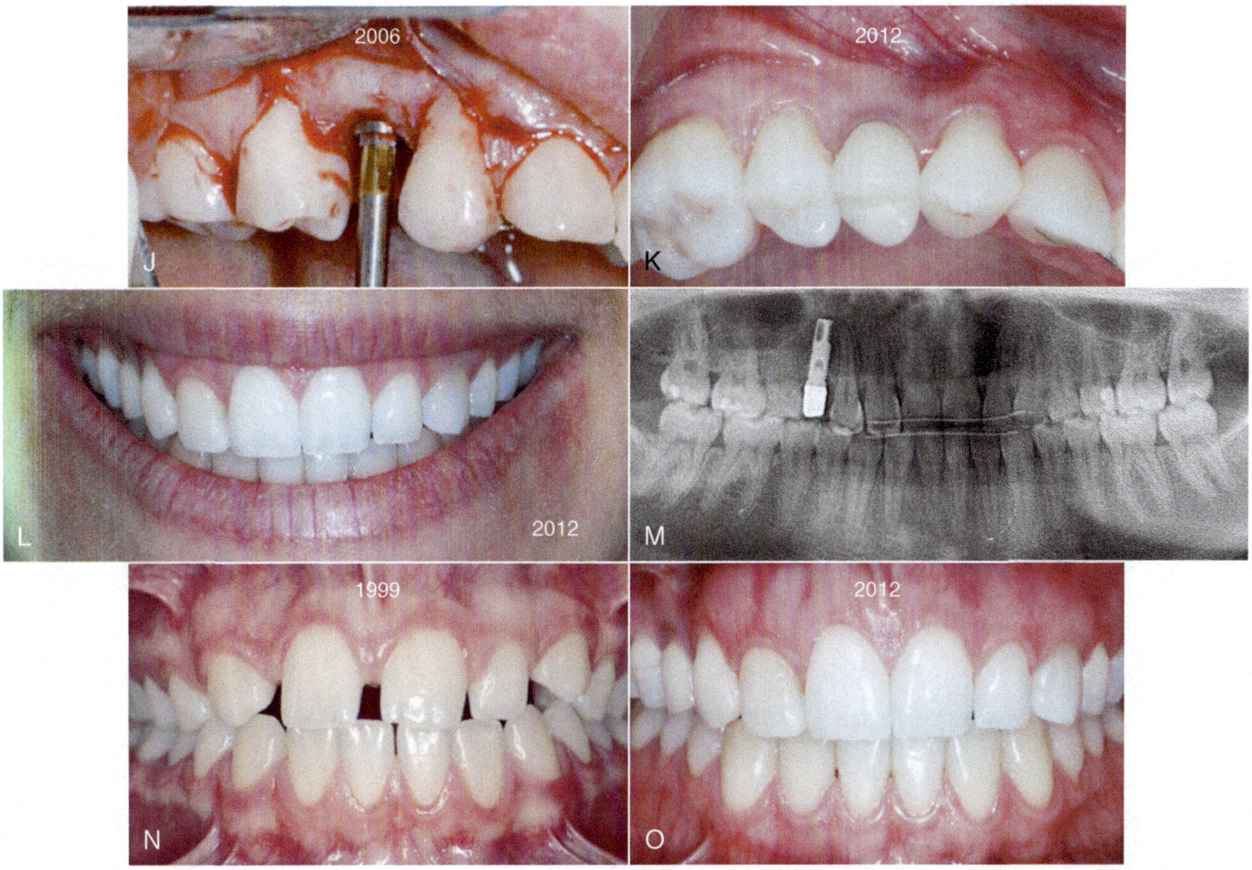

Figure 25-11, cont'd **J,** The implant was placed at age 21 years. **K, L, M, and O,** Six years after the implant restoration, further bone loss and bluish gingival discoloration was evident. The composite buildups on the right premolar and canine were substituted with porcelain restorations. **L and O,** The upper right lateral incisor (the canine) looked healthy, with the gingival margin at the same level as the left lateral incisor. **L,** The loss of periodontal tissue thickness was evident in the buccal side of the implant area and created a severe esthetic impairment in this "gummy smile" woman, who was not satisfied with the final result after a very long and expensive treatment. The long-term prognosis is uncertain and it is not possible to exclude the necessity of maintenance, adjustments, periodontal procedures, or possible remaking of the implant crown. (Periodontist: Dr. Francesca Manfrini, Riva del Garda, Italy; Prosthodontist: Dr. Giovanni Manfrini, Riva del Garda, Italy; Ceramist: Mr. Antonio Bertoni, Brescia, Italy.)

Predictability

The first priority is the predictability in achieving the desired treatment objectives and the long-term stability of the outcome. From a biological and periodontal point of view, clinical experience and scientific evidence have demonstrated that the long-term results with all types of prosthetic replacement of missing laterals are unpredictable in terms of periodontal health and less satisfactory when compared to the natural root substitution.[13,14,16–26]

Overall Esthetics

In cases with missing maxillary lateral incisors, esthetics is naturally the main focus for the patient and expectations of achieving an attractive tooth display and smile have increased in recent years. Therefore the goals cannot simply be replacement of the missing tooth and correction of the malocclusion. The goal, especially in young patients, is *overall esthetics*. Overall esthetics is the ideal alignment of beautiful teeth, surrounded by intact gingiva, displayed attractively in the face during conversation and when smiling.[5–8,57]

In a recent study, tipping of incisors, interdental gingival recessions ("black spaces"), and diastemas in the esthetic zone were the least tolerated aspects of the smiles in patients with agenesis of the maxillary lateral incisors, as judged by different categories of observers (specialists in orthodontics, adult orthodontic patients, general practitioners, and laypersons).[58]

Symmetry is another critical esthetic goal. For this reason, unilateral agenesis of a lateral incisor can often be treated more successfully with extraction of the contralateral lateral incisor, especially when it is peg-shaped (see Figs. 25-3, 25-5, and 25-6).

When examining the possibility of changing facial esthetics and profile by opening or closing the spaces for absent maxillary lateral incisors, some myths and biases need to be discussed.

In hypodivergent Class III cases with a narrow maxilla, concave profile, and congenitally absent lateral incisors, the assumption that orthodontic maxillary sagittal expansion can improve the facial profile is not supported by the literature and is probably not true. As shown in Figure 25-4, protrusion of maxillary incisors will not improve a concave profile and the overall face esthetics. Increasing the vertical dimension by clockwise rotation of the mandibular and

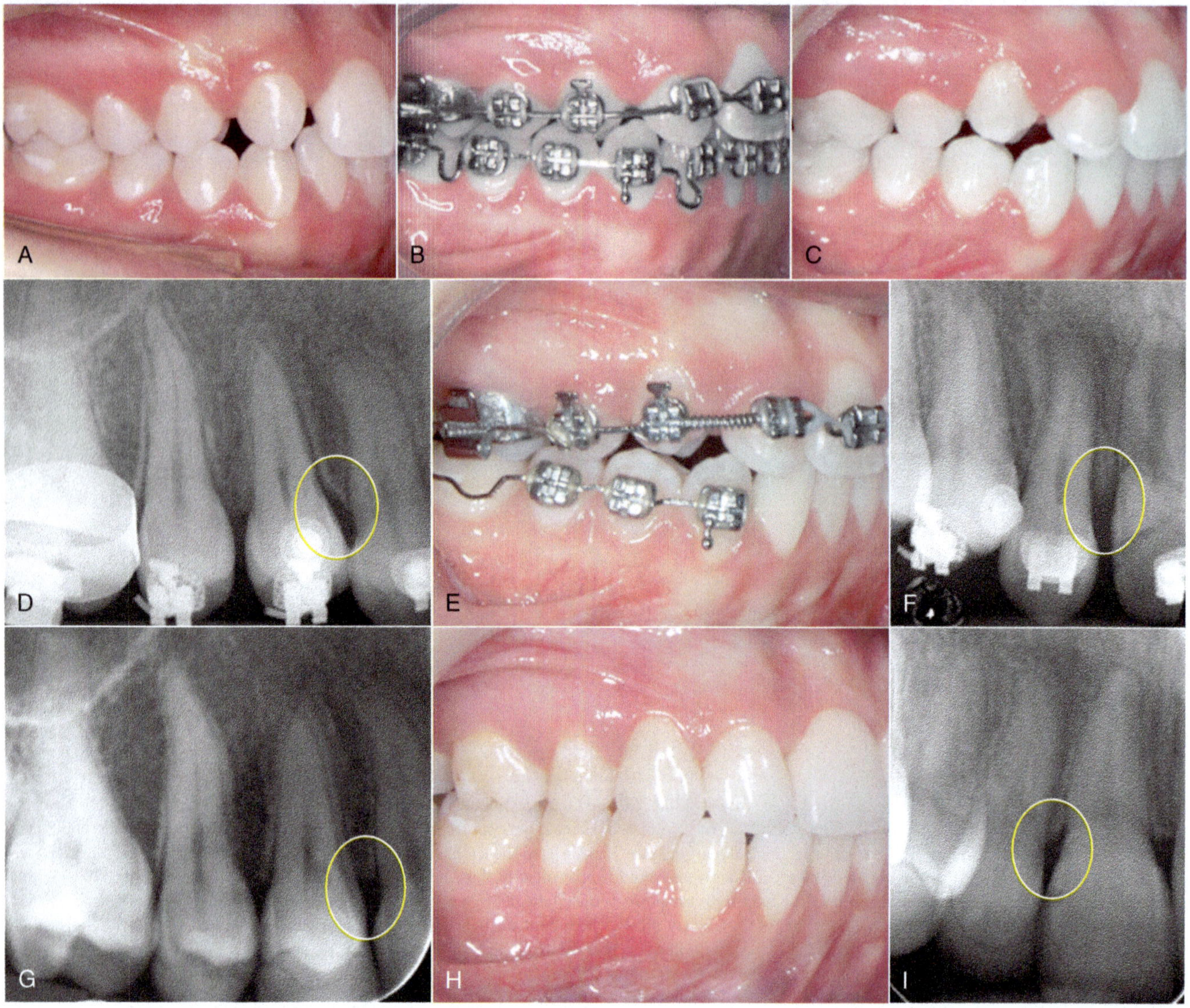

Figure 25-12 Long-term stability of gingival margins and alveolar bone remodeling. **A and B,** A 15-year-old girl with Class I malocclusion and agenesis of the upper right lateral incisor was treated for 23 months to close spaces. **C,** Simultaneous intrusion of the first premolars and extrusion of the canines with torque control remodeled the periodontal tissues to natural leveling of the gingival margins. **D–F,** The intrusions and extrusions moved the entire periodontal apparatus, not only the soft tissues, but also the bone peaks *(yellow circles)*. **D, F, G, and I,** Six years after the orthodontic treatment, the gingival margins are stable **(H)** and the alveolar bone has remodeled *(yellow circles)*. The front teeth were restored with porcelain veneers. (Prosthodontist: Dr. Giovanni Manfrini, Riva del Garda, Italy; Ceramist: Antonio Bertoni, Brescia, Italy.)

occlusal planes is much more effective (see Fig. 25-7). On the other hand, it is possible to close spaces for the missing lateral incisors without collapsing the maxilla and, in doing so, worsen the profile[6] (see Figs. 25-7 and 25-10). In this type of malocclusion, the only way to really improve the profile and smile is to use a surgical approach[7] (see Fig. 25-4).

In contrast, in the case of a hyperdivergent patient, sagittal changes of the upper incisors can affect the position of the lips. As a consequence, space reopening can produce lip incompetence. In Class II, Division 1 malocclusions, correction of the overjet by space closure could worsen the posture of the upper lip, causing a "dished-in" profile, and should be avoided, especially in females. Thus the common opinion that the space closure alternative in Class II, Division 1 malocclusions has no contraindications should be regarded with caution, as we are entering into the era of "overall esthetics." In some patients (as described in Fig. 25-9) it may be preferable to finish the treatment and leave some overjet, which will be filled by restorations. Such inclination of the upper central incisors is also more stable.

Patient's Age

Most patients with congenitally absent maxillary lateral incisors are younger than 20 years. The first obligation when dealing with adolescent patients is to provide them with an attractive tooth display at a young age. These patients not only need a smile, but need it as soon as possible. Adolescent patients are entering the most critical part of their lives, when a balanced smile is fundamental to creating the

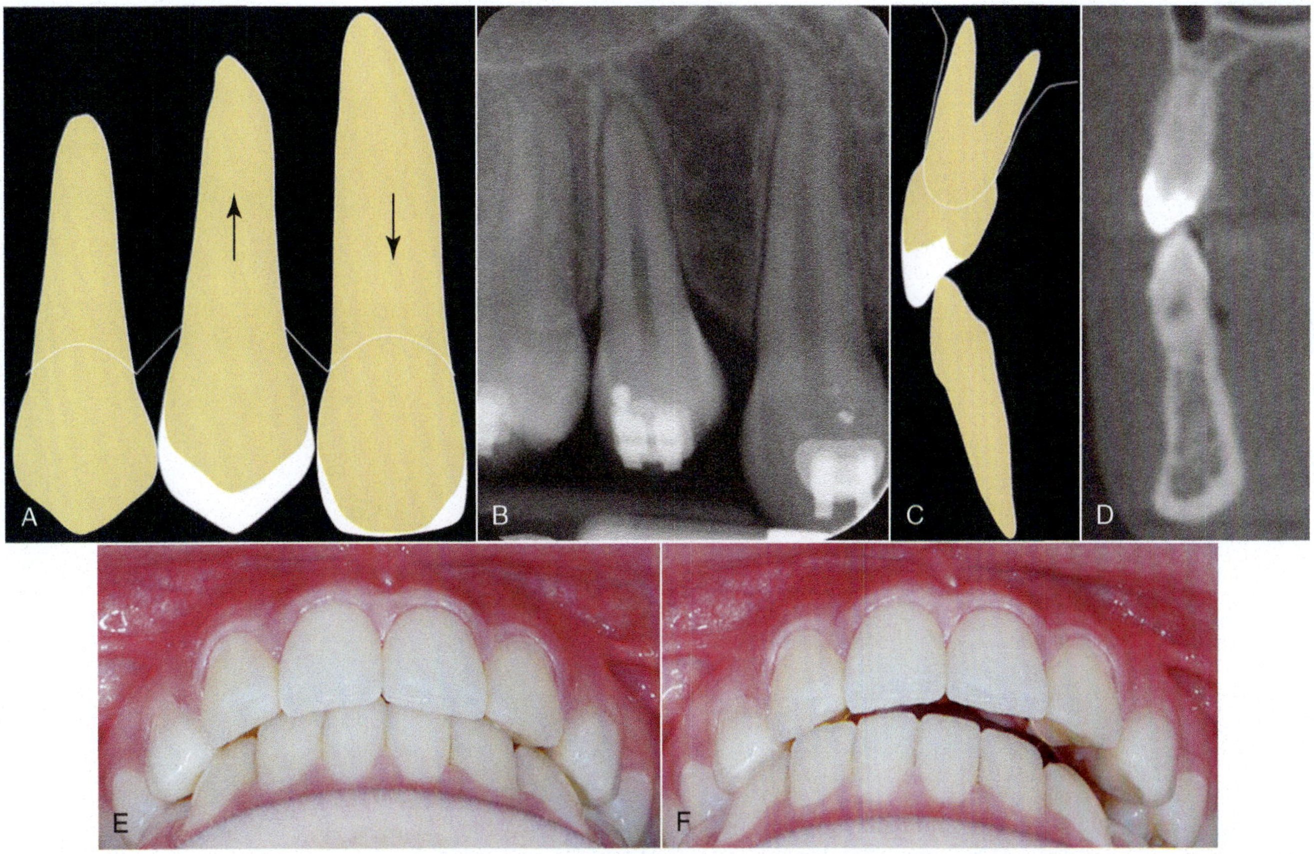

Figure 25-13 Premolar buildup to resemble a canine. After **(A and B)** intrusion, the premolar **(B–D)** needs to be built up for esthetic and functional reasons in order to participate in **(E and F)** proper group protection during lateral movements of the mandible. **C and D,** The palatal cusp of the premolar remains untouched and not ground.

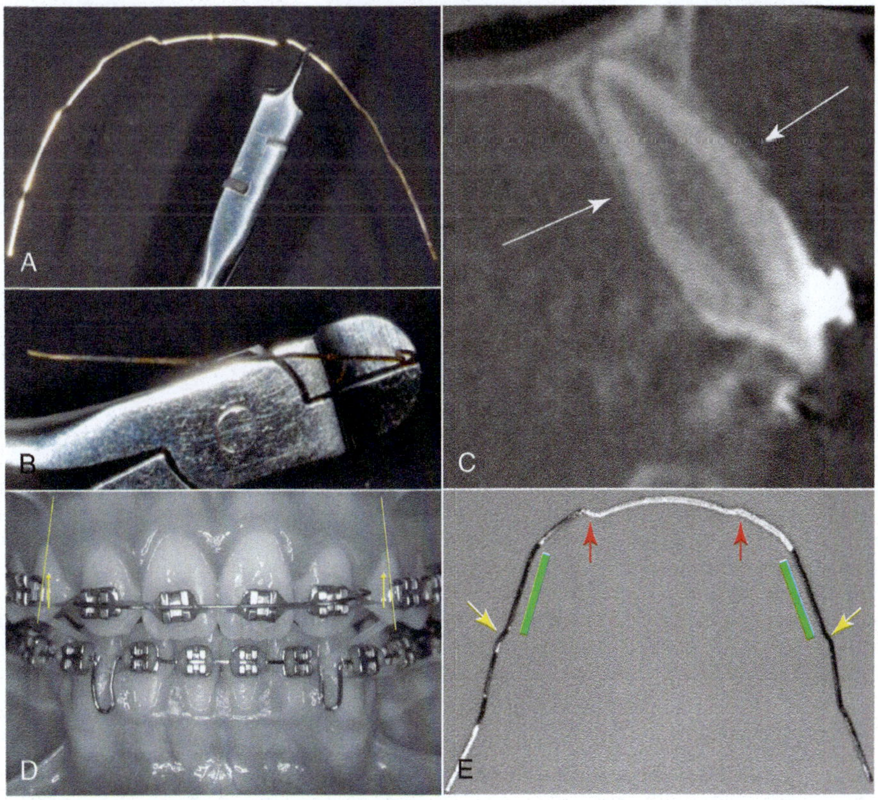

Figure 25-14 During extrusion of canines with labial appliances, the root may tip labially and reduce the thickness of the periodontal tissues. This can lead to a predisposition to gingival recession in the years after treatment. **A–C,** It is important to maintain the root of the canine inside the periodontal envelope, with proper palatal root torque on the finishing archwire. **D,** During their intrusion the premolars tend to tip labially, with resulting excessive overjet, and during premolar intrusion with straight-wire technique, buccal tip of the crown is a common side effect. **E,** To prevent this, the maxillary stainless steel archwire must be shaped straight in this segment *(green lines)*; sometimes an inset bend is necessary mesial to the second premolar *(yellow arrows)*. The *red arrows* in **E** indicate the offset bends for proper alignment of the canines.

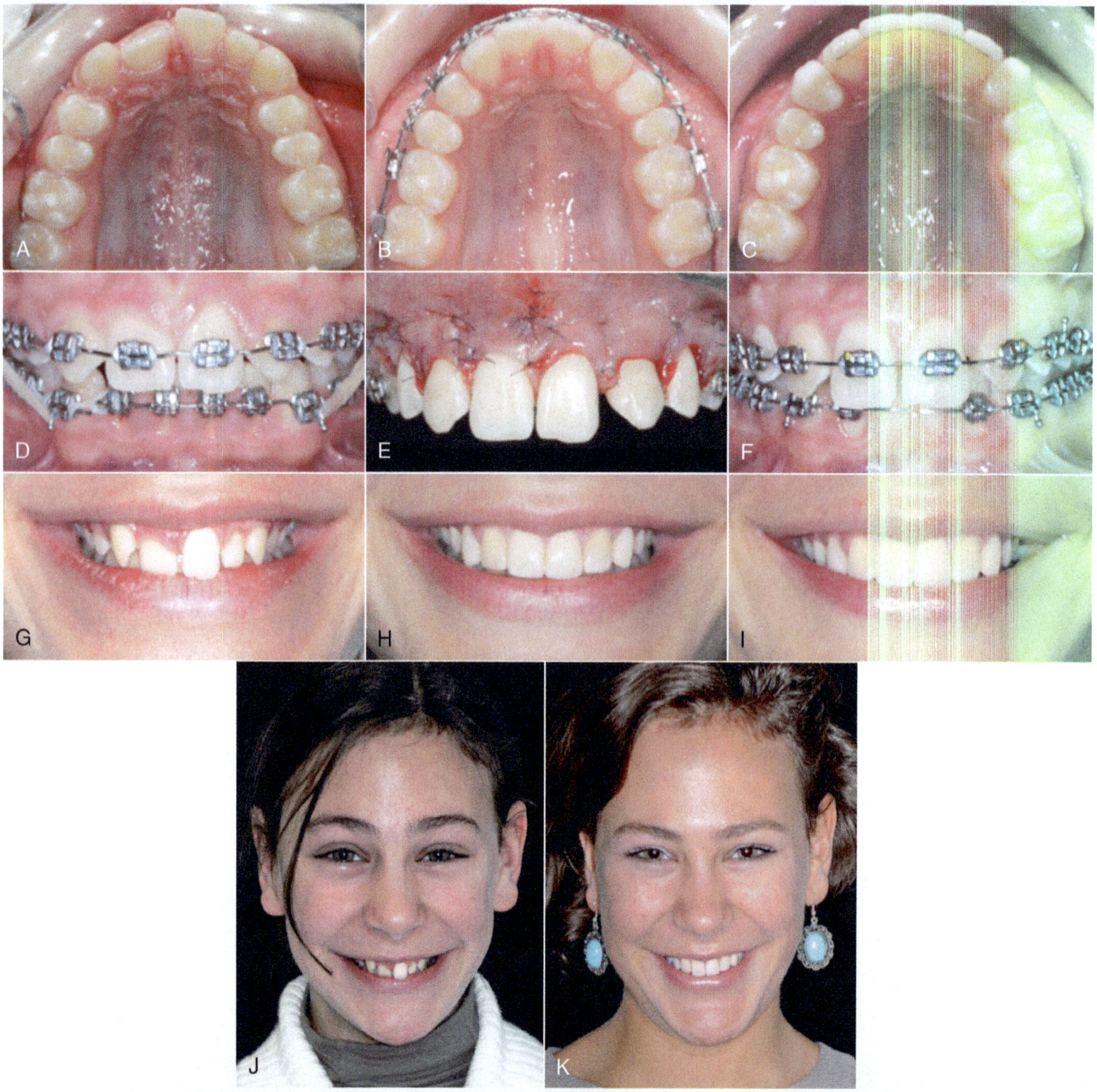

Figure 25-15 Gingivectomy and resective surgery during orthodontic treatment. **A, G, and J,** A 14-year-old girl presented with Class II malocclusion and a unilaterally missing upper right lateral incisor. **B and C,** She was treated with space closure after the extraction of the contralateral lateral incisor. **D,** During the orthodontic finishing phase, it was difficult to identify the cementoenamel junction (CEJ) and plan the amount of intrusion and extrusion because of the swollen marginal soft tissues and the altered active eruption. The removal of the brackets and professional oral hygiene maintenance was not successful. **E,** After a check of the alveolar bone crest (with the patient under local anesthesia), the periodontist diagnosed the presence of alveolar bone coronally to the CEJ and performed surgical remodeling of the bone crest and gingival margins. **F,** Three months after surgery the brackets were rebonded and the orthodontic treatment was finished more effectively. **C,** After treatment, on the same day as debonding occurred, a bonded retainer was made for the upper four front teeth and direct resin buildups were made on the upper left central incisor, which was smaller than the upper right one. **H and I,** Vital bleaching was performed at home with an Essix removable plate. **K,** The smile is well balanced and the result was stable 2 years after the end of treatment. (Periodontist: Dr. Francesca Manfrini, Riva del Garda, Italy; Direct resin buildups: Dr. Patrizia Lucchi, Trento, Italy.)

self-esteem they need to approach many crucial life decisions. Psychosocial pressures are also of concern for parents, who want an early resolution of their children's esthetic problems. These adolescents should not have to wait until the "end of growth" to achieve the finished result. Temporary restorations to replace missing lateral incisors may break, debond, and otherwise need maintenance. Adolescents and young adults often travel for their education and problems with a temporary tooth may create discomfort in several ways and for many years.

INDICATIONS AND CONTRAINDICATIONS

Due to recent improvements in clinical procedures, the traditional indications and contraindications for the space closure alternative in patients with missing maxillary lateral incisors should be reviewed.[5–8,39]

Indications for Space Closure

The optimal canine substitution patient is one who has small canines with crowns that match the shade of the central incisors as well as:

- Crowding, normally inclined anterior teeth, and a well-balanced profile
- Dentoalveolar protrusion
- Canines and premolars of similar size
- Class II dental relationship

In the authors' opinion, space closure interdisciplinary treatment should be proposed as the best treatment option in three categories of patients:

1. Adolescents and young adults
2. Patients who show the gingival margin when smiling
3. Patients who will also undergo maxillofacial surgical procedures

In light of recent clinical research findings, some traditional contraindications for space closure should be reevaluated and can be considered obsolete. This may be valid for cases with pronounced spacing in the maxillary arch, no malocclusion, and normal intercuspation of posterior teeth. In such cases, the space closure is more difficult than reopening and it takes longer but it can be done without the risk of causing "dished-in" profiles. Patient cooperation with Class III elastics is generally sufficient to close the spaces without losing anchorage in the front areas. Even more relevant are the findings that skeletal anchorage, provided by two connected mini-screws inserted in the palatal vault (see Fig. 25-10), will allow for compliance-free space closure in a shorter time than tooth-by-tooth movement.[39]

Large Difference in Size Between Canines and First Premolars

A large canine cannot be ground to resemble a small lateral incisor in good balance with the adjacent teeth. Since patients with unilateral or bilateral agenesis of lateral incisors generally have smaller teeth than patients without any dental anomalies,[50–52] the correct question often is not "How do we make the canine smaller?" but rather "Do the central incisors need widening and/or elongation?" If the goal is to create a well-balanced, attractive smile and optimal incisor display at rest and during speech, restorations may be necessary on the central incisors and the large canines can become excellent lateral incisors (see Figs. 25-4 to 25-7 and 25-9). Widening of the central incisors may result in a tooth-size discrepancy (with maxillary excess) and increased overjet, as the tooth widths are generally reduced in both the maxillary and the mandibular teeth in patients with agenesis of the lateral incisors. Therefore procedures such as enlargement of the mandibular incisors or, better, thickening of maxillary restorations may need to be executed to achieve ideal esthetic and functional results[7] (see Fig. 25-9).

Class III Cases with Retrognathic Profile

In hypodivergent Class III patients, some improvement of the profile can be achieved by increasing the vertical dimension through occlusal plane and mandibular clockwise rotation (see Fig. 25-7), while the inclination of the upper incisors may be irrelevant to obtaining improved changes in lip posture[6,7] (see Fig. 15-4).

Contraindications for Space Closure

The detailed orthodontic and restorative interdisciplinary treatment is contraindicated in:

- Elderly patients who have no gingival exposure when smiling
- Patients who have low esthetic expectations
- Patients who indicate lack of cooperation and motivation

In such instances the alternative is space reopening or patient-oriented, limited treatment (see "Alternatives to Space Closure" below).

MOST FREQUENT PROBLEMS

The interdisciplinary space closure treatment is sometimes difficult due to several problems, which can come as a surprise or be overlooked during treatment. The most frequent problems are discussed here.

Excessive Buccal Tip of the Intruded First Premolar Crowns

Excessive buccal tip of the intruded first premolar crowns may occur and result in excessive overjet in the canine area (see Fig. 25-14, D). This is one of the most common mistakes and will make it difficult for the restorative dentist to achieve correct esthetics and functional occlusion. To diagnose the problem clinically, the patient must be examined while standing in an eye-to-eye position.[42] To correct this problem when it occurs, the stainless steel finishing archwire must be shaped straight in the segment of the intruded premolar (see Fig. 25-14, E). Sometimes an inset bend is needed mesially to the second premolar (see Figs. 25-14 and 25-15).

Uncontrolled Buccal Root Torque of the Canines During Extrusion

Uncontrolled buccal root torque of the canines during extrusion will decrease the width and volume of the periodontal tissues and produce a risk for gingival recession several years after treatment in patients with a thin periodontium. A bracket with a minimum 20-degree palatal torque prescription together with rectangular superelastic archwires during extrusion in the first months of treatment, as well as proper third-order bends on a stainless steel rectangular archwire during the finishing phase, should be used to prevent this problem.

Undefined Marginal Periodontal Tissue in Young Patients

Undefined marginal periodontal tissue in young patients (altered passive or active eruption and poor hygiene) can make it difficult to properly locate the CEJs. A strict hygiene protocol must be applied from the beginning of orthodontic treatment. Careful bracket positioning and regular checks of anatomic details during treatment are necessary to level the front teeth properly.

Unilateral Space Closure

Unilateral space closure can also create problems and is often a dilemma for the orthodontist. In unilaterally missing incisor patients, the upper midline is often asymmetrical and deflected relative to the midline of the face and necessitates extraction of one tooth on the contralateral side. A generally safe decision is to extract the other lateral incisor, particularly if it is narrow or peg-shaped (see Figs. 25-3, 25-5, 25-6, and 25-15). In cases where the lateral incisor and the canines are of similar size, the first premolar can be extracted as an alternative.[5–8,57]

An orthodontist may decide to close the space unilaterally because this treatment appears easier and is more acceptable to the patient and/or the patient's parents. However, bilateral space closure should require similar treatment time compared to the unilateral approximation and the final result may be more symmetrical and easier to finish with the restorations.

The main indication for unilateral space closure is a Class II subdivision case on the agenesis side, with a symmetrical upper midline in a patient who does not show the gingival margins when smiling (Fig. 25-16).

ALTERNATIVES TO SPACE CLOSURE

Limited Treatment

Limited treatment refers to treatment solutions in which the result is not the ideal occlusion but ones that can be achieved in a shorter time and in an easier way with both space closure and space reopening with prosthetic replacement. It is usually an interdisciplinary treatment involving orthodontics and cosmetic restorative dentistry (Fig. 25-17).

The prerequisites for limited treatment include the following:

- It takes a short time.
- It is not invasive for teeth and periodontal tissues.
- It is efficient (optimal cost to benefit ratio).
- It effectively solves the main complaints of the patient.
- It leaves other treatment alternatives to be reconsidered at a later date.

Indications

Limited treatment is indicated in situations where there is no reason to propose a long, difficult, sometimes invasive, and expensive interdisciplinary treatment. Examples of such situations are:

- Adolescents who can be treated better or more efficiently at the "end of growth":
  - Space reopening cases. The interim between the orthodontic treatment and the restoration will be shorter (Fig. 25-18).
  - Surgical discrepancies. The surgical option should be discussed with the patient after growth and psychological maturity (see Figs. 25-4 and 25-17).
  - Adolescents with little motivation who will not cooperate during treatment.
- Patients who cannot afford a long and invasive treatment for financial or biological reasons (e.g., external root resorption, periodontal problems, high caries activity).
- Patients with low expectations and little motivation to achieve an ideal result.
- Patients with Class III deep bites with a "hidden smile" not showing the gingival margins when smiling (usually associated with vertical skeletal maxillary hypoplasia) and who do not want to undergo surgical correction to make the upper dentition more visible.

The primary goal of limited treatment is to correct the essential problems related to esthetics and function. The goals can sometimes be achieved with direct composite restorations but a short orthodontic treatment is usually necessary first to reduce spaces and correct incisor angulations.

A retention strategy is necessary to ensure stability. Fixed bonded retainers and/or a removable biteplate will stabilize the temporomandibular joint (TMJ) and prevent extrusion and abrasion of the mandibular front teeth.

After limited treatment in adolescents, the treatment plan should be reevaluated and discussed with the patient again at the "end of growth." For adult and elderly patients, limited treatment may represent the best option.

Limited treatment is not a compromise. It is a precise treatment option with clear and predictable goals. It is not necessarily easy. When only a few teeth have to be moved, it is sometimes difficult to prevent undesired movements of the anchor teeth and temporary anchorage devices may be needed.

Space Reopening and Autotransplantation

A tooth with a single, partially developed root is suitable for autotransplantation in anterior or posterior regions that have been developed by orthodontic space reopening. Ideally, the root to be transplanted should fit the alveolar ridge and its root development should range from one-half to two-thirds. Teeth that may fit are lower premolars, upper second premolars, and sometimes diminutive upper third molars or a contralateral supernumerary incisor. The predictability and long-term stability of this procedure are supported by scientific evidence to a greater extent than exists for implants.[59,60]

Space Closure in the Front and Space Opening Posteriorly

In selected patients, when the goal is to shorten the treatment time or simplify the biomechanics, while also keeping a natural root in the smile area, the treatment plan can be to

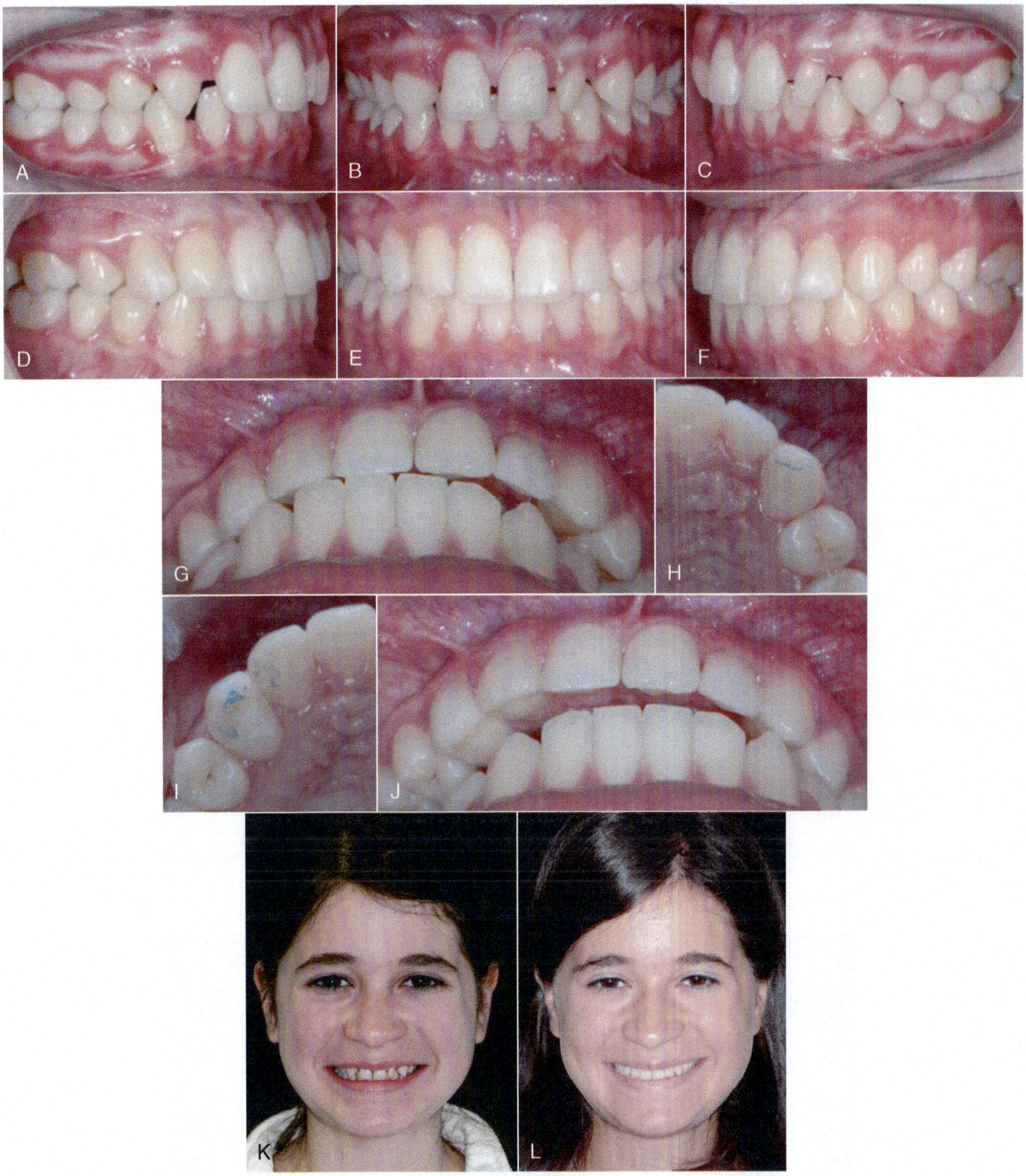

Figure 25-16 Unilateral space closure. **A–C,** A 14-year-old girl presented with ideal conditions for unilateral space closure: hypodivergent Class II subdivision (molar Class II only on the right side) with a solid occlusion in the posterior segments and the upper midline deflected a few millimeters to the right relative to the facial midline. **K,** On smiling, the patient did not show the gingival margins. **D–F,** After orthodontic treatment the occlusion was still Class II subdivision, a subdivision with coincident midlines. The upper right canine was ground during orthodontic treatment. Composite buildups were done on the upper right first premolar, canine, peg-shaped upper left lateral incisor, and small central incisors. **L,** Two years later the smile arc was correct, with incisal margins tangent to the lower lip. **E, K, and L,** The asymmetry of the gingival margins does not impair the overall smile esthetics because of the low smile line. Lateral movements of the mandible are guided by (**H** [*blue mark*] **and J**) a canine protected occlusion in the left side, while (**G and I** [*blue marks on the canine and first premolar*]) group function is evident on the mutilated right side. (Composite buildups: Dr. Patrizia Lucchi, Trento, Italy.)

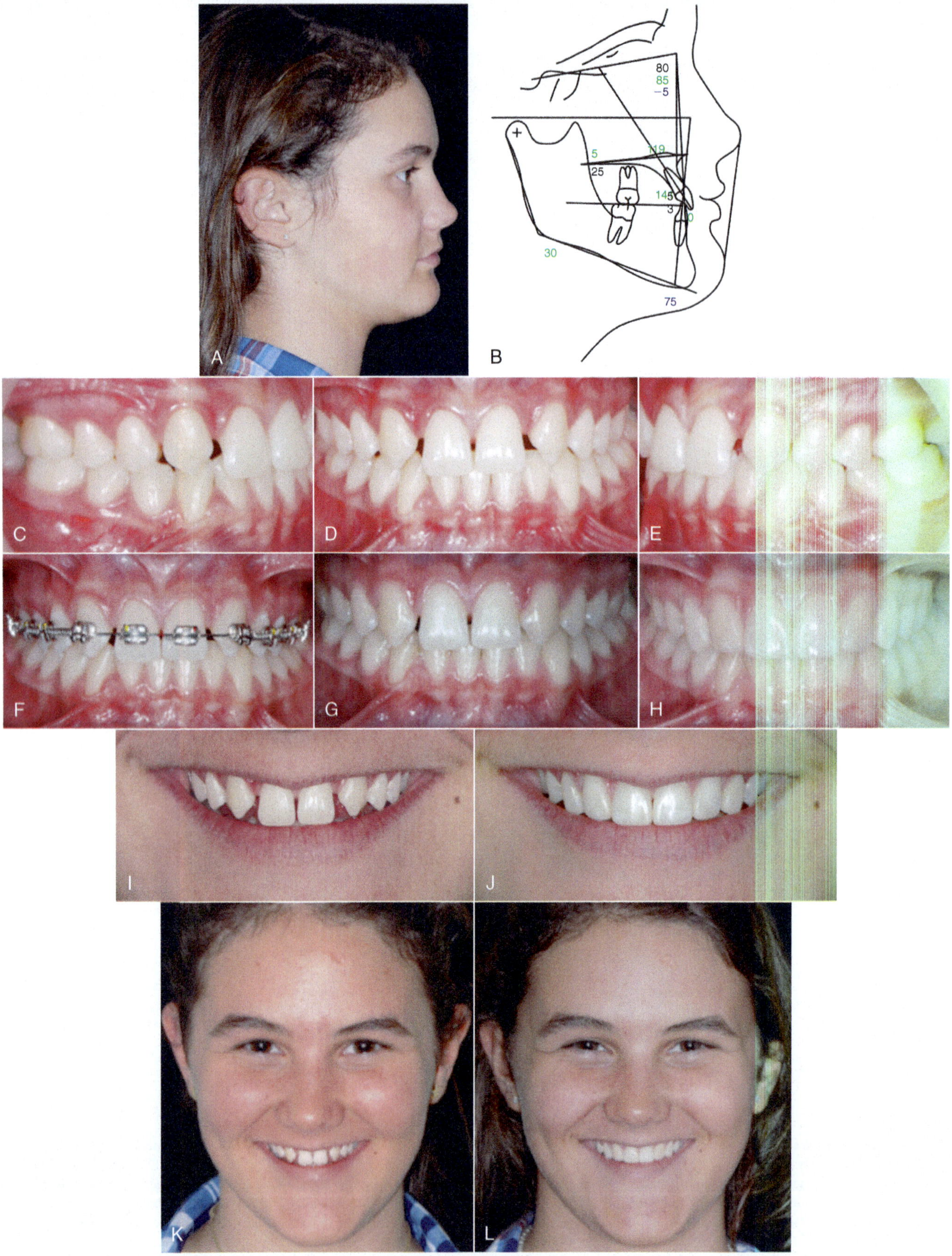

Figure 25-17 Limited treatment. **A and B,** A 12-year-old girl presented with congenitally missing lateral incisors, skeletal Class III, and maxillary sagittal and vertical deficiency. **C–E, I, and K,** The occlusal relationship was a Class II subdivision with the upper midline well positioned when smiling. No centric occlusion–centric relation (CO-CR) discrepancy was noticed and the occlusion was stable with acceptable group function. **D, I, and K,** Since the chief complaint was the presence of black spaces when smiling and the treatment goals to correct the malocclusion (space closure, space opening, surgery) would be better focused at the "end of growth," a phase of noninvasive, inexpensive, limited treatment was chosen to solve the patient's complaints in a short time, while leaving all possible treatment alternatives open later. **F and G,** The spaces between upper anterior teeth were reduced in 3 months with fixed appliances and **(H, J, and L)** the residual black spaces were filled with composite restorations. At the end of the limited treatment, the result was satisfactory from an esthetic and functional point of view. The treatment goals will be reevaluated at the "end of growth." (Composite restorations: Dr. Patrizia Lucchi, Trento, Italy.)

close anterior spaces and reopen space in the premolar area for an implant crown. Usually an implant site is created between the premolars. The orthodontic treatment involves developing an effective implant site, one that is adequate in volume and does not need any further surgical improvement[7] (see Figs. 25-9 and 25-11). In the years after space reopening in the maxillary posterior areas, the regenerated bone seems to undergo atrophy (see Fig. 25-11) to a greater extent than in spaces opened up for implants in the lateral incisor area.[61,62] This can be explained by differences in embryological origin. For this reason, osseointegrated implants should be inserted as soon as possible after posterior space reopening and, when possible, during the orthodontic treatment[7] (see Fig. 15-9).

For the very demanding patient, this alternative could require the highest number of restorations: four or six porcelain veneers on front teeth and implant restoration in the posterior segments. The esthetic effectiveness, biological health, and long-term stability are predictable but the financial cost of such a solution is high.

Space Reopening and Prosthetic Replacement of the Congenitally Missing Lateral Incisor

The available scientific evidence concludes that, in the long-term, any type of restoration is less favorable and less predictable in terms of periodontal health and patient satisfaction when compared to a natural root substitution.[13,14,16] The total treatment time for frontal space opening in children is extended because the final restoration generally can be done only at the "end of growth." When the orthodontic reopening is done during adolescence, the interim may last many years and the temporary restorations could create many problems and discomfort for the patient (as discussed earlier in the chapter). Therefore orthodontic treatment should be delayed with the specific goal of shortening the interim as much as possible. If the appearance at a young age is not acceptable and some treatment is necessary during adolescence, it is preferable to choose a limited treatment to solve only the esthetic problems (black spaces, diastemas, and evident asymmetries). The long, difficult, and expensive procedures, including space opening, can then take place at the "end of growth."

After orthodontic space reopening, the lateral incisor can be replaced with a removable plate, an implant-supported restoration, or a tooth-supported restoration.[63]

Removable Plate

The removable plate can be esthetically satisfactory and is the most conservative solution, although it is the solution least accepted by patients. It is usually the first option in the interim immediately after debonding. It can also be used as a retainer while waiting for a fixed restoration. A removable

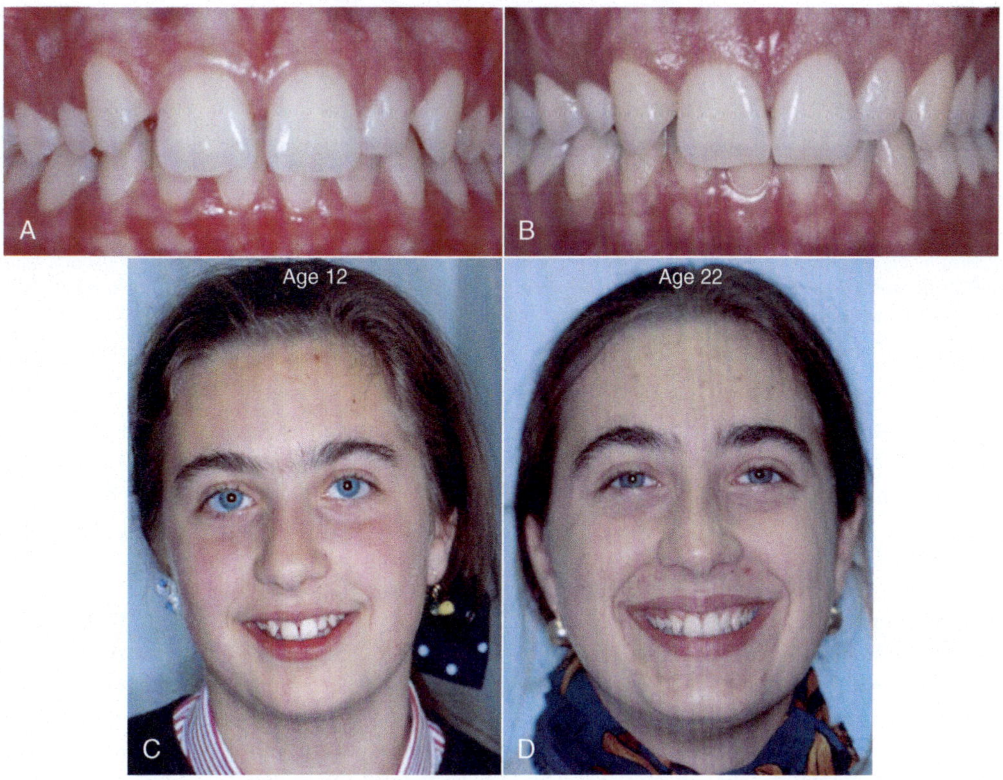

Figure 25-18 Ideal timing for space reopening for an implant-supported porcelain restoration. **A, C,** A 12-year-old girl presented with a unilaterally missing right lateral incisor and persistent primary canine. Since space reopening and implant restoration were planned for later and she did not complain about her esthetic appearance (no noticeable spaces), orthodontic treatment was delayed until toward the "end of growth." **B, D, and E,** Orthodontic treatment began when the patient was 22 years old and lasted 20 months.

Continued

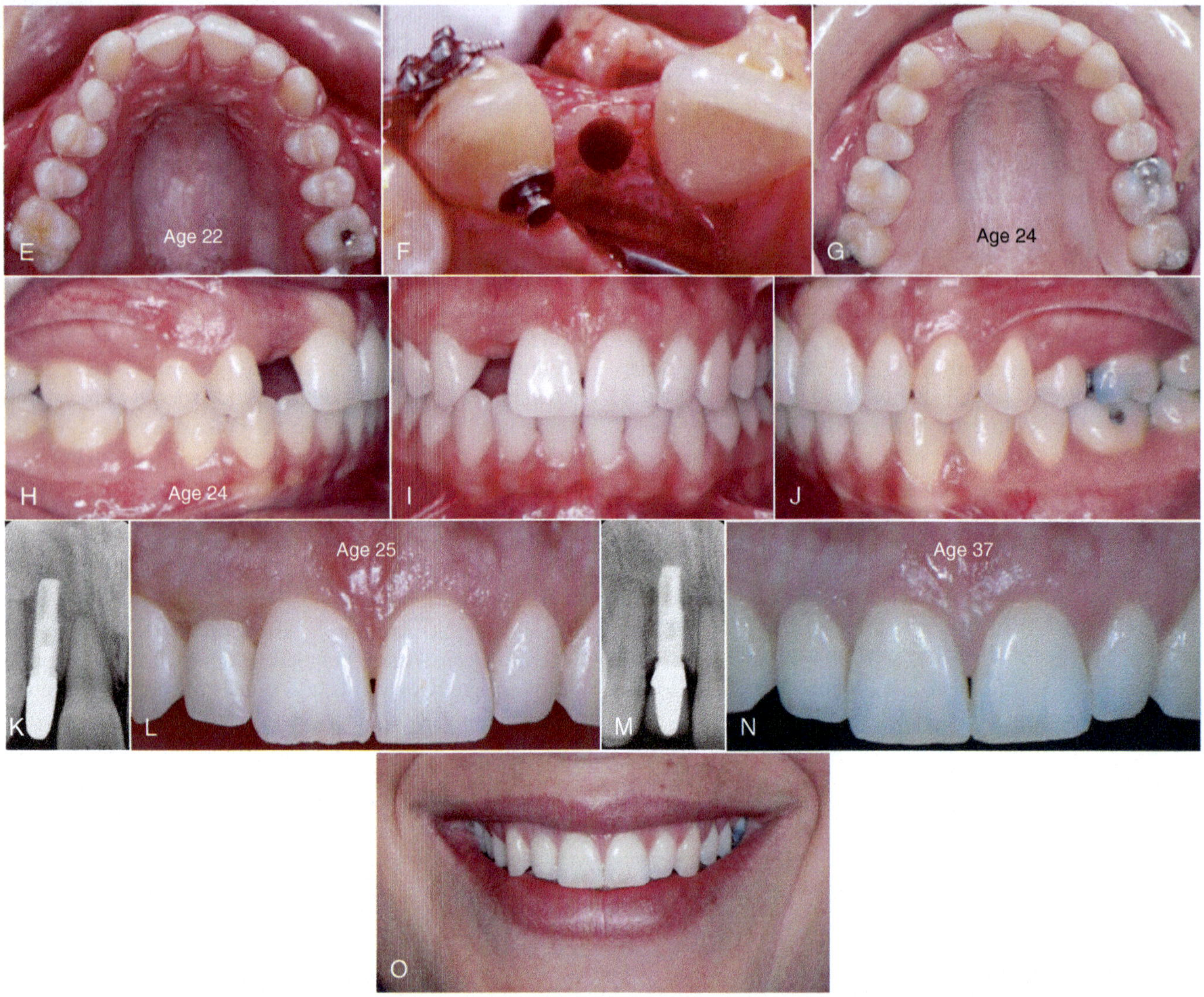

Figure 25-18, cont'd **G, H, and I,** An adequate implant site was developed by orthodontic movement. **F,** The implant was inserted during the orthodontic treatment. **J–L,** A temporary resin crown was cemented on the implant 8 weeks after the end of orthodontic treatment. **M–O,** Twelve years after the implant insertion, the stability was good, the alveolar bone was healthy (although the papilla is shorter on the implant site), and there was no infraocclusion. *(The treatment was performed by the same team of professionals, in the same years and using similar procedures and implants, as the case shown in Fig. 25-1. It is impossible to explain why evident infraocclusion happened in the case shown in Fig. 25-1 but did not occur in this one.)* (Surgeon: Dr. Francesca Manfrini; Prosthodontist: Dr. Giovanni Manfrini, Riva del Garda, Italy; Ceramist: Antonio Bertoni, Brescia, Italy.)

plate cannot provide stability of the root position[32] and therefore should be substituted quickly with a fixed bonded retainer in cases where an implant restoration is planned.

Tooth-Supported Restoration

Resin-Bonded Fixed Partial Denture. The resin-bonded fixed partial denture (FPD) is the most conservative tooth-supported restoration because it is possible to leave the adjacent teeth almost untouched. This type of restoration must fulfill stringent criteria to provide an esthetic and stable result. For this reason the long-term predictability is poor, with debonding the most common cause of failure.[64] The zirconia resin-bonded FPDs provide a better esthetic result than what was possible with the metal-supported resin-bonded FPDs (Fig. 25-19).[65,66]

The cases that can be restored with a resin-bonded FPD are those with a shallow overbite and no mobility of the adjacent teeth. Contraindications for this restoration are the presence of parafunctions, deep overbite, and proclined abutment teeth.

Cantilevered Fixed Partial Denture. The cantilevered FPD is less conservative than the resin-bonded 3-unit bridge because it needs full or partial coverage of the canine. It is more secure in use than a resin-bonded FPD. The key factor for long-term success is careful removal of all eccentric contacts from the pontic.[67]

Conventional Full-Coverage Fixed Partial Denture. The conventional full-coverage FPD is the least conservative

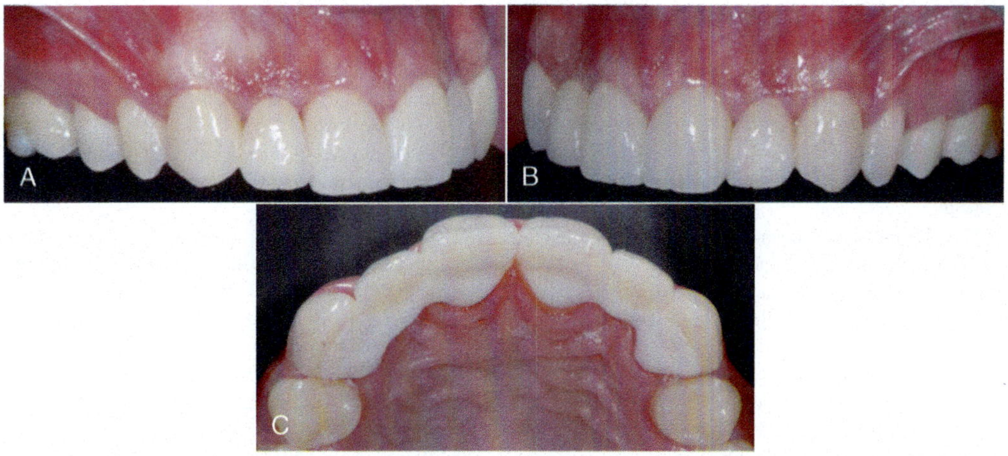

Figure 25-19 Zirconia resin-bonded fixed partial denture (FPDs) can provide a better esthetic result than what was possible with the metal-supported resin-bonded FPDs. (Prosthodontist: Dr. Giovanni Manfrini, Riva del Garda, Italy; Ceramist: Antonio Bertoni, Brescia, Italy).

procedure. Its indication is limited to patients who need full-coverage crown restoration on the central incisors and canines for other reasons than merely lateral incisor prosthesis.

Implant-Supported Restoration

The most commonly used treatment alternative is the single-tooth implant porcelain crown. This solution is the most conservative since the adjacent teeth may remain untouched. The orthodontic treatment should not only provide ideal position of the adjacent crowns and roots, but also develop the implant site (see Fig. 25-9). This is most predictable when the canine is close to the central incisor before the orthodontic treatment (see Fig. 25-18). It has been reported that the bone created through orthodontic tooth movement is largely stable in both horizontal and vertical directions.[62,63] However, other authors have found a significant decrease in alveolar ridge width and height during and immediately after the space opening.[68,69] As discussed earlier in the chapter, the preferred procedure when an implant-supported restoration is planned is to delay the orthodontic space opening treatment so it is as close as possible to the time of implant insertion (see Fig. 25-18), to try to avoid the central incisor and canine converging toward each other during the retention phase, making future implant placement difficult or impossible.[32]

SUMMARY

The main problem in treating patients with missing maxillary lateral incisors and any coexisting malocclusion is not closing or opening spaces, but to achieve overall esthetics. Since a long and difficult interdisciplinary treatment is required, the challenge is to obtain predictably satisfactory results with long-term stability, regardless of the alternative treatment plan. This is an obligation when treating adolescents and young patients.

Until recently, space closure is the treatment alternative that scientific evidence has proven to be the most predictable in the long-term. Such treatment can be completed during adolescence and the result can be considered permanent.

The restorations, which can be done directly at the end of orthodontic treatment, provide ideal esthetics and function in a conservative way. The tooth preparation is minimal, with supragingival restoration margins that do not intrude into the gingival sulcus.

On the other hand, space reopening always requires root and tooth replacement and restorations, which are more invasive and less predictable in the long-term. The total treatment time can be frustrating for young patients who must wait several years until the difficult-to-define "end of growth" period before final restorations can be implemented.

Even though the introduction of osseointegrated implants has decreased the popularity of the space closure alternative among dentists, the natural root is the best solution in the esthetic zone, as discussed in this chapter. In the future, it is expected that the canine substitution, supplemented with proper interdisciplinary restorative treatment, will experience a renaissance among clinicians.

REFERENCES

1. Tuverson DL. Orthodontic treatment using canines in place of missing maxillary lateral incisors. *Am J Orthod.* 1970;58:109–127.
2. Zachrisson BU, Mjör IA. Remodeling of teeth by grinding. *Am J Orthod.* 1975;68:545–553.
3. Zachrisson BU. Improving orthodontic results in cases with maxillary incisors missing. *Am J Orthod.* 1978;73:274–289.
4. Thordarson A, Zachrisson BU, Mjör IA. Remodeling of canines to the shape of lateral incisors by grinding: a long-term clinical and radiographic evaluation. *Am J Orthod.* 1991;100:123–132.
5. Rosa M, Zachrisson BU. Integrating esthetic dentistry and space closure in patients with missing maxillary lateral incisors. *J Clin Orthod.* 2001; 35:221–234.
6. Rosa M, Zachrisson BU. Integrating space closure and esthetic dentistry in patients with missing maxillary lateral incisors: further improvements. *J Clin Orthod.* 2007;41:563–573.
7. Rosa M, Zachrisson BU. The space-closure alternative for missing maxillary lateral incisors: an update. *J Clin Orthod.* 2010;44:540–549.

8. Zachrisson BU, Rosa M, Toreskog S. Congenitally missing maxillary lateral incisors: canine substitution: point. *Am J Orthod Dentofacial Orthop*. 2011;139:434, 436, 438 passim.
9. Kinzer GA, Kokich VO Jr. Managing congenitally missing lateral incisors, III: single-tooth implants. *J Esthet Restor Dent*. 2005;17: 202–210.
10. Spear FM, Mathews DM, Kokich VG. Interdisciplinary management of single-tooth implants. *Semin Orthod*. 1997;3:45–72.
11. Kokich VG. Maxillary lateral incisor implants: planning with the aid of orthodontics. *J Oral Maxillofac Surg*. 2004;62:48–56.
12. Kinzer GA, Kokich VO Jr. Managing congenitally missing lateral incisors, II: tooth-supported restorations. *J Esthet Restor Dent*. 2005;17: 76–84.
13. Nordquist GG, McNeill RW. Orthodontic vs. restorative treatment of the congenitally absent lateral incisor: long-term periodontal and occlusal evaluation. *J Periodontol*. 1975;46:139–143.
14. Robertsson S, Mohlin B. The congenitally missing upper lateral incisor: a retrospective study of orthodontic space closure versus restorative treatment. *Eur J Orthod*. 2000;22:697–710.
15. Armbruster PC, Gardiner DM, Whitley JB Jr, Flerra J. The congenitally missing maxillary lateral incisor, I: esthetic judgment of treatment options; II: assessing dentists' preferences for treatment. *World J Orthod*. 2005;6(4):369–381.
16. Arnoux JP, Weisgold AS, Lu J. Single-tooth anterior implant: a word of caution: part II. *J Esthet Dent*. 1997;9:285–294.
17. Jung RE, Pjetursson BE, Glauser R, Zembic A, Zwahlen M, Lang NP. A systematic review of the 5-year survival and complication rates of implant-supported single crowns. *Clin Oral Implants Res*. 2008;19: 119–130.
18. Fransson C, Wennstrom J, Tomasi C, Berglund T. Extent of peri-implantitis-associated bone loss. *J Clin Periodontol*. 2009;36:357–363.
19. Dueled E, Gotfredsen K, Damsgaard MT, Hede B. Professional and patient-based evaluation of oral rehabilitation in patients with tooth agenesis. *Clin Oral Implants Res*. 2009;20:729–736.
20. Thilander B, Odman J, Lekholm U. Orthodontic aspects of the use of oral implants in adolescents: a 10-year follow-up study. *Eur J Orthod*. 2001;23:715–731.
21. Bernard JP, Schatz JP, Christou P, Belser U, Kiliaridis S. Long-term vertical changes of the anterior maxillary teeth adjacent to single implants in young and mature adults: a retrospective study. *J Clin Periodontol*. 2004;31:1024–1028.
22. Zachrisson BU. Single implant-supported crowns for the anterior maxilla: potential esthetic long-term (>5 years) problems. *World J Orthod*. 2006;7:306–312.
23. Kuijpers MA, de Lange J, van Gool AV. Maxillofacial growth and dental implants in the maxillary anterior region [in Dutch]. *Ned Tijdschr Tandheelkd*. 2006;113:130–133.
24. Jemt T. Measurements of tooth movements in relation to single-implant restorations during 16 years: a case report. *Clin Implant Dent Relat Res*. 2005;7:200–208.
25. Jemt T, Ahlberg G, Henriksson K, Bondevik O. Changes of anterior clinical crown height in patients provided with single-implant restorations after more than 15 years of follow-up. *Int J Prosthod*. 2006;19: 455–461.
26. Jemt T. Single implants in the anterior maxilla after 15 years of follow-up: comparison with central implants in the edentulous maxilla. *Int J Prosthod*. 2008;21:400–408.
27. Björk A, Palling M. Adolescent age changes in sagittal jaw relation, alveolar prognathy, and incisal inclination. *Acta Odont Scand*. 1955; 12:201–232.
28. Chang M, Wennström JL, Odman P, Andersson B. Implant supported single-tooth replacements compared to contralateral natural teeth: crown and soft tissue dimensions. *Clin Oral Implants Res*. 1999;10: 185–194.
29. Fudalej P, Kokich VG, Leroux B. Determining the cessation of vertical growth of the craniofacial structures to facilitate placement of single-tooth implants. *Am J Orthod Dentofacial Orthop*. 2007;131(4 suppl): S59–S67.
30. Iseri H, Solow B. Continued eruption of maxillary incisors and first molars in girls from 9 to 25 years studied by the implant method. *Eur J Orthod*. 1996;18:245–256.
31. Solow B, Iseri H. The continued eruption of teeth in relation to the timing of treatment with osseointegrated implants. *Tandlægebladet (57 Dent J)*. 1996;100:500–506.
32. Olsen T, Kokich VG Sr. Postorthodontic root approximation after opening space for maxillary lateral incisor implants. *Am J Orthod Dentofacial Orthop*. 2010;137:158.e1–158.e8.
33. Sarver DM. Principles of cosmetic dentistry in orthodontics: part I: shape and proportionality of anterior teeth. *Am J Orthod Dentofacial Orthop*. 2004;126(6):749–753.
34. Wilmes B, Drescher D. A miniscrew system with interchangeable abutments. *J Clin Orthod*. 2009:42:574–580.
35. Wilmes B, Drescher D, Nienkemper MA. Miniplate system for improved stability of skeletal anchorage. *J Clin Orthod*. 2009:43:494–501.
36. Ludwig B, Baumgaertel S, Bowman SJ. *Mini-Implants in Orthodontics: Innovative Anchorage Concepts*. Hanover Park, IL: Quintessence Publishing; 2008.
37. Antoszewska J, Papadopoulos MA, Park HS, Ludwig B. Five-year experience with orthodontic miniscrew implants: a retrospective investigation of factors influencing success rates. *Am J Orthod Dentofacial Orthop*. 2009;136:158.e1–158.e10.
38. Ludwig B, Glasl B, Bowman SJ, Wilmes B, Kinzinger GSM, Lisson JA. Anatomical guidelines for miniscrew insertion: palatal sites. *J Clin Orthod*. 2011;45:433–441.
39. Ludwig B, Zachrisson BU, Rosa M. Non-compliance space closure in patients with missing maxillary lateral incisors. *J Clin Orthod*. 2013;47: 180–187.
40. Erkan M, Pikdoken L, Usumez S. Gingival response to mandibular incisor intrusion. *Am J Orthod Dentofacial Orthop*. 2007;132:143.e9–143.e13.
41. Kajiyama K, Murakami T, Yokota S. Gingival reactions after experimentally induced extrusion of the upper incisors in monkeys. *Am J Orthod Dentofacial Orthop*. 1993;104:36–47.
42. Spear FM, Kokich VG, Mathews DP. Interdisciplinary management of anterior dental esthetics. *J Am Dent Assoc*. 2006;137:160–169.
43. Evian CI, Cutler SA, Rosenberg ES, Shah RK. Altered passive eruption: the undiagnosed entity. *J Am Dent Assoc*. 1993;124:107–110.
44. Cairo F, Graziani F, Franchi L, Defraia E, Pini Prato GP. Periodontal plastic surgery to improve esthetics in patients with altered passive eruption/gummy smile: a case series study. *Int J Dent*. 2012;2012:837658. doi:10.1155/2012/837658.
45. Monefeldt I, Zachrisson BU. Adjustment of clinical crown height by gingivectomy following orthodontic space closure. *Angle Orthod*. 1977:47:256–264.
46. Wennström JL. Regeneration of gingiva following surgical excision: a clinical study. *J Clin Periodontol*. 1983;10:287–297.
47. Sarver DM. The importance of incisor positioning in the esthetic smile: the smile arc. *Am J Orthod Dentofacial Orthop*. 2001;120:98–111.
48. Fields HW Jr. Orthodontic-restorative treatment for relative mandibular anterior excess tooth size problems. *Am J Orthod*. 1981; 79:175–183.
49. Morley J, Eubank J. Macroesthetic elements of smile design. *J Am Dent Assoc*. 2001;132:39–45.
50. Olivadoti A, Doldo T, Treccani M. Morpho-dimensional analysis of the maxillary central incisor clinical crown in cases of congenitally missing upper lateral incisors. *Prog Orthod*. 2009;10:12–19.
51. Yaqoob O, DiBiase AT, Garvey T, Fleming PS. Relationship between bilateral congenital absence of maxillary lateral incisors and anterior tooth width. *Am J Orthod Dentofacial Orthop*. 2011;139(3):e229–e233.
52. Mirabella AD, Kokich VG, Rosa M. Analysis of crown widths in subjects with congenitally missing maxillary lateral incisors. *Eur J Orthod*. 2012;34:783–787.

53. da Silva Marques DN, Silveira JM, Marques JR, Amaral JA, Guilherme NM, da Mata AD. Kinetic release of hydrogen peroxide from different whitening products. *Eur J Esthet Dent*. 2012;7:344–352.
54. He LB, Shao MY, Tan K, Xu X, Li JY. The effects of light on bleaching and tooth sensitivity during in-office vital bleaching: a systematic review and meta-analysis. *J Dent*. 2012;40:644–653.
55. Rinchuse DJ, Kandasamy S, Sciote J. A contemporary and evidence-based view of canine protected occlusion. *Am J Orthod Dentofacial Orthop*. 2007;132:90–102.
56. Zachrisson BU. Long-term experience with direct-bonded retainers: update and clinical advice. *J Clin Orthod*. 2007;41:728–737.
57. Zachrisson BU. Master clinician: Björn U. Zachrisson, DDS, MSD, PHD: interviewed by Dr. Peter M. Sinclair. *J Clin Orthod*. 2012;46(9): 531–557.
58. Rosa M, Olimpo A, Fastuca R, Caprioglio A. Perceptions of dental professionals and laypeople to altered dental esthetics in cases with congenitally missing maxillary lateral incisors. *Prog Orthod*. 2013;14: 34-41.
59. Czochrowska EM, Stenvik A, Bjercke B, Zachrisson BU. Outcome of tooth transplantation: survival and success rates 17–41 years posttreatment. *Am J Orthod Dentofacial Orthop*. 2002;121:110–119.
60. Zachrisson BU, Stenvik A, Haanæs HR. Management of missing anterior teeth with emphasis on autotransplantation. *Am J Orthod Dentofacial Orthop*. 2004;126:284–288.
61. Kokich VG. Maxillary lateral incisor implants: planning with the aid of orthodontics. *Int J Oral Maxillofac Surg*. 2004;62(9 suppl 2):48–56.
62. Novackova S, Marek I, Kaminek M. Bone formation by orthodontic tooth movement and its stability in time. *Am J Orthod Dentofacial Orthop*. 2011;139:37–43.
63. Kokich VO Jr, Kinzer GA, Janakievski J. Congenitally missing maxillary lateral incisors: restorative replacement. *Am J Orthod Dentofacial Orthop*. 2011;139:434–445.
64. Williams VD, Thayer KE, Denehy GE, Boyer DB. Cast metal, resin-bonded prostheses: a 10-year retrospective study. *J Prosthet Dent*. 1989; 61:436–441.
65. Pröbster B, Henrich GM. 11-year follow-up study of resin-bonded fixed partial dentures. *Int J Prosthodont*. 1997;10:259–268.
66. Duarte S Jr, Park JH, Tada T, Sadan A. Resin-bonded fixed partial dentures with a new modified zirconia surface: a clinical report. *J Prosthet Dent*. 2009;102:68–73.
67. Kern M. Clinical long-term survival of two-retainer and single-retainer all-ceramic resin-bonded fixed partial dentures. *Quintessence Int*. 2005; 36:141–147.
68. Beyer A, Tausche E, Boening K, Harzer W. Orthodontic space opening in patients with congenitally missing lateral incisors. *Angle Orthod*. 2007;77:404–409.
69. Uribe F, Chau V, Padala S, Neace WP, Cutrera A, Nanda R. Alveolar ridge width and height changes after orthodontic space opening in patients congenitally missing maxillary lateral incisors. *Eur J Orthod*. 2013:35(1):87–92.

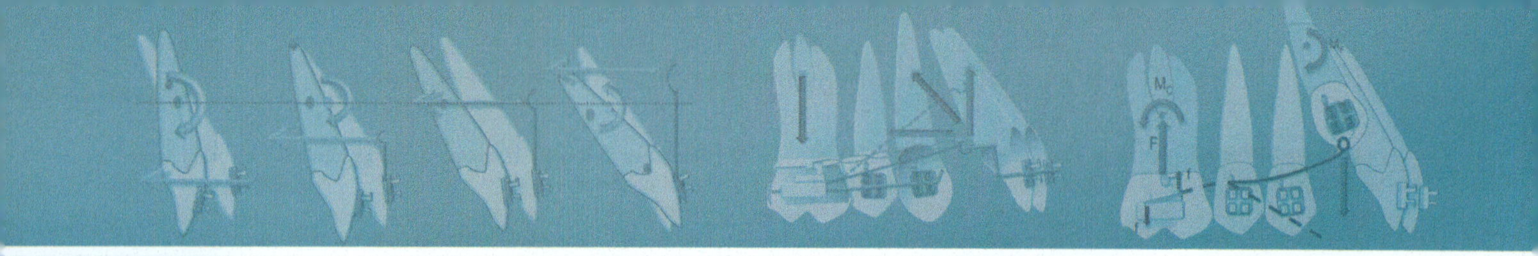

CHAPTER 26

Interrelationship of Orthodontics with Periodontics and Restorative Dentistry

Vincent G. Kokich and Vincent O. Kokich

Today, orthodontics is not just for children and adolescents. For the past two decades, increasing numbers of adults have been referred to orthodontists to correct their malocclusions. Adults are usually wonderful patients because they are cooperative, clean their teeth, show up for appointments, and are appreciative of the clinician's efforts. However, adults may have problems other than malposed teeth and jaws that make their orthodontic treatment more challenging. Whereas children and adolescents have intact dentitions with few restorations and a healthy periodontium, adults may have old failing restorations, edentulous spaces, abraded teeth, periodontal bone defects, gingival level discrepancies, hopeless teeth, and a variety of other restorative and periodontal problems that could compromise the orthodontic result. In the past orthodontists made all decisions about the treatment plan for a child or adolescent. However, in the compromised adult malocclusion, a team consisting of an orthodontist, oral and maxillofacial surgeon, periodontist, endodontist, and restorative dentist must interact to make prudent treatment decisions for the patient.

This chapter elucidates the dilemmas encountered in the orthodontic patient with multidisciplinary problems and describes a series of 10 guidelines to help manage the interrelationship of orthodontics with periodontics and restorative dentistry.

GENERATE REALISTIC TREATMENT OBJECTIVES

The first step in any type of dental therapy is to establish the treatment objectives. It is impossible to achieve the correct end result if the appropriate goals or objectives have not been identified before treatment. In nonrestored, adolescent patients with complete dentitions, orthodontic treatment objectives tend to be idealistic. After all, if patients have intact dentitions without restorations, it is appropriate to expect that ideal esthetic and occlusal treatment should be attainable, if the patient cooperates. Because of this tendency, most orthodontists are trapped into applying these same idealistic treatment objectives to adult patients with missing teeth, abraded teeth, old restorations, or other restorative and periodontal complications. Idealistic treatment objectives may not be appropriate for ortho-perio-restorative patients. For these patients it is important to establish realistic, not idealistic, treatment objectives. Realistic treatment objectives generally should be economically realistic, occlusally realistic, periodontally realistic, and restoratively realistic.[1]

If an adult orthodontic patient is missing several teeth, the edentulous spaces created during orthodontic treatment will require restoration after the removal of the orthodontic appliances. Several restorative alternatives may exist to replace the missing teeth. The cost of these restorative treatment plans may differ widely. Furthermore, each type of restoration may require slightly different tooth positioning. Therefore it is mandatory for the team to establish a treatment plan that is economically realistic for each patient. If the team fails to establish economically realistic objectives, the patient might not complete the restorative treatment following orthodontic therapy.

In young patients it is important to establish ideal occlusal objectives, such as a Class I canine relationship with normal overbite and overjet relationships. When planning occlusal treatment for young patients, the orthodontist is missing two critically important pieces of information: (1) because of their young age, there is no occlusal history and (2) the orthodontist unfortunately cannot predict the future habits or problems that a young patient will encounter during his or her lifetime. Therefore in these situations it is appropriate for the orthodontist to create an ideal occlusion. However, in the adult patient, orthodontists often overlook the most valuable piece of information: the patient's dental history. Has the adult patient demonstrated parafunctional occlusal habits, evidence of temporomandibular disorders, cracked teeth or restorations, wear facets, abraded incisors, or other

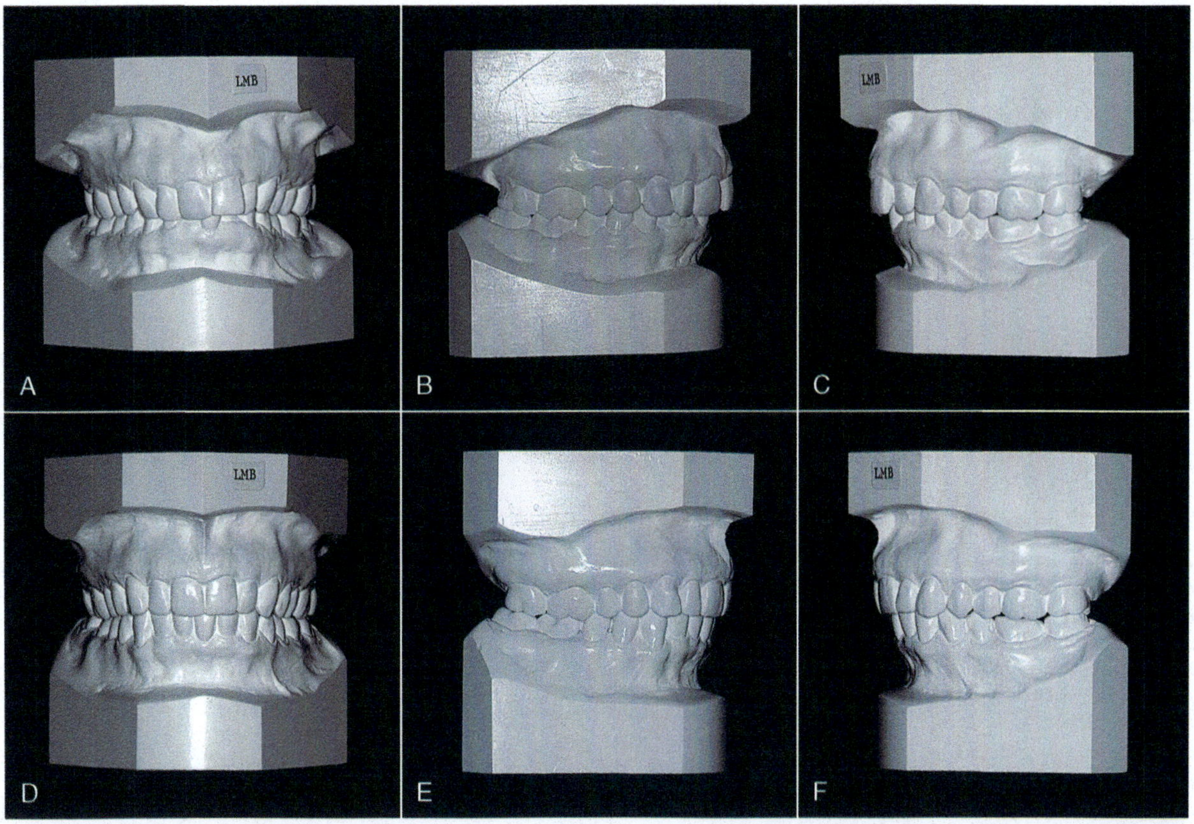

Figure 26-1 A 68-year-old female had **(A)** a deep anterior overbite with **(B)** Class I molar and canine relationships on the right and **(C)** Class II molar and canine relationships on the left. She had no temporomandibular joint symptoms and a healthy periodontium. **D,** Treatment objectives included alignment of teeth in both arches and reduction of the deep overbite. Because of an anterior tooth size discrepancy, proclined mandibular incisors, and upright maxillary incisors, her treatment objectives did not include correction of the Class II molar and canine relationships on the left. **E and F,** At the end of treatment all treatment objectives were achieved, including maintaining the original posterior occlusal relationships.

signs and symptoms that would suggest that the treatment plan should alter the existing occlusion? Not all existing occlusions in adult patients need to be corrected to an adolescent ideal (Fig. 26-1). In all adult patients the dental history, as well as the future restorative requirements, plays a greater role in determining the final occlusion (Fig. 26-2). For example, it may not be necessary to correct posterior crossbites in adults who have no occlusal interferences and no shift of the mandible and who can be restored adequately in a posterior crossbite relationship (Fig. 26-3).

If patients are missing many teeth, it may not be prudent to establish idealistic occlusal objectives. An ideal Class I posterior occlusion is achievable in a patient with a complete nonrestored, nonabraded dentition. However, if the patient is missing several teeth and will require extensive restorative treatment after orthodontics, it may be more prudent to establish treatment objectives that are occlusally realistic for the specific patient. For example, if the patient will require extensive restorations after orthodontic treatment, the restorative dentist may suggest altering a Class I occlusion to facilitate restoration of the teeth (Fig. 26-4). It is critical for the orthodontist to be aware of these alterations before bracket placement to achieve an occlusally realistic relationship for the restorative patient.[1]

A common occlusal treatment objective in children is to align the marginal ridges of the posterior teeth in order to produce a uniform vertical relationship between the maxillary and mandibular posterior teeth.[2] In a nonabraded, periodontally healthy adolescent dentition, aligning the marginal ridges helps to establish even contact of the posterior teeth, when they are brought into occlusion. However, in the adult patient with interproximal bone loss and uneven wear of the posterior teeth, the marginal ridges are poor guides for positioning the posterior teeth.[3] In these patients the periodontal objectives outweigh the occlusal objectives. The role of the orthodontist in the periodontal patient is to level the bone during orthodontic treatment. This could require equilibration and reshaping of the posterior teeth in order to maximize the occlusal contacts. In most of these situations the teeth that have been equilibrated will require restoration anyway after orthodontic treatment.

Certain types of restorations require specific positioning of adjacent or opposing teeth. As a result, orthodontists must not establish idealistic treatment objectives for patients who will require extensive restoration. If teeth are worn or abraded, it may be more important to position the teeth in a restoratively realistic location to facilitate the appropriate restoration.

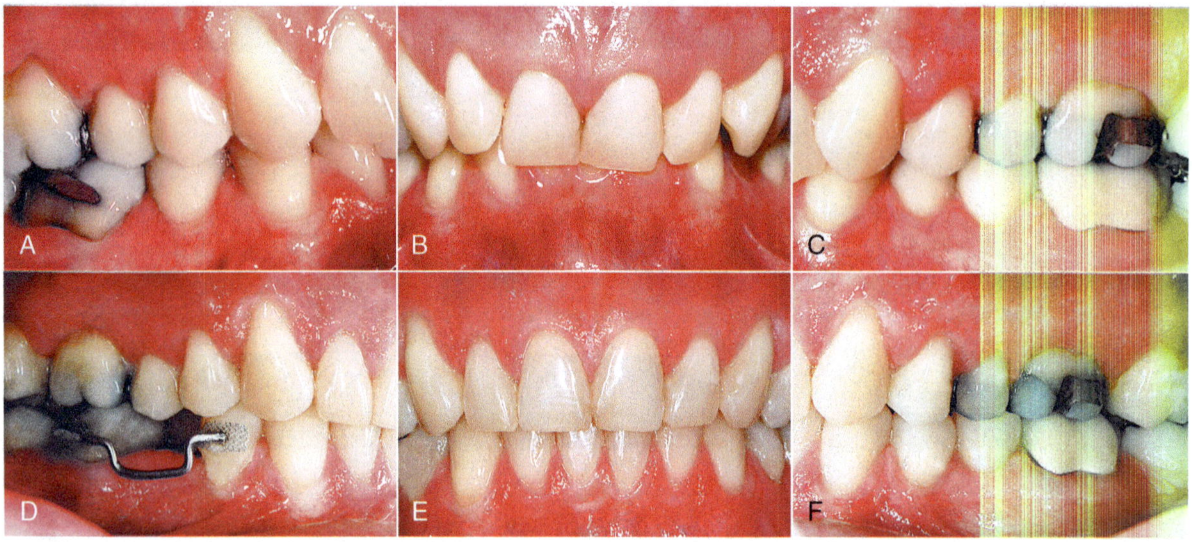

Figure 26-2 A 52-year-old male had (A) a bilateral Class II, Division 2 malocclusion with a deep anterior overbite, (B and C) retroclined maxillary incisors, a missing mandibular second premolar, and a mandibular dental midline that deviated to the right. The patient had no temporomandibular joint symptoms and the periodontium was healthy. Treatment objectives included (D) reduction of the deep overbite, opening space for the missing premolar, correction of the dental midline, and establishing normal overjet. Because of the inclination of the anterior teeth and the anterior tooth size relationships, (E) a Class I canine relationship was established on the right and (F) a Class II relationship was maintained on the left. The objectives were achieved without correcting the Class II canine relationship on the right side.

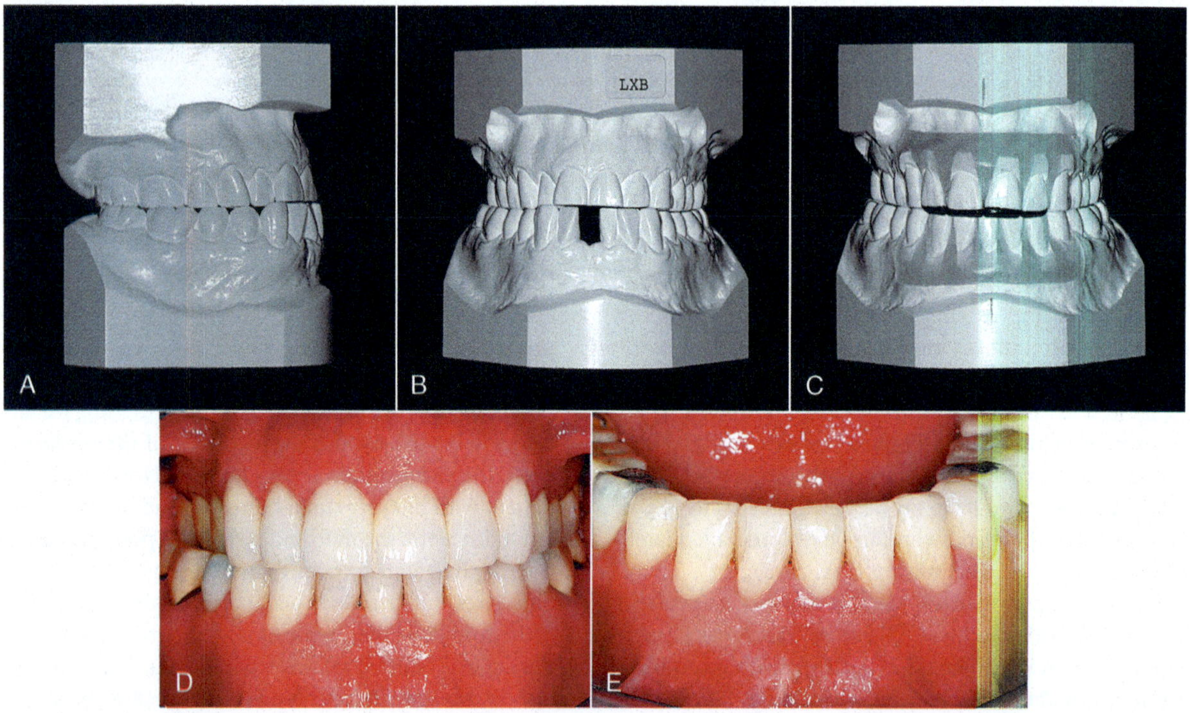

Figure 26-3 A 57-year-old male had (A) a Class III end-to-end posterior occlusion with an anterior dental crossbite, a missing mandibular incisor (failed endodontic therapy), severe wear of the maxillary incisors, and (B) bilateral posterior dental crossbites with no lateral shift of the mandible. He had no temporomandibular joint symptoms and the periodontium was healthy. Treatment objectives included correction of the anterior crossbite to create an overjet to restore the abraded maxillary incisors. Correction of the bilateral dental crossbites was not a treatment objective. C, A diagnostic setup showed that the mandibular space could be closed to create restorative space. The final photographs of the restored (D) maxillary and (E) mandibular incisors show that correction of the posterior crossbites was not necessary to achieve the restorative objectives.

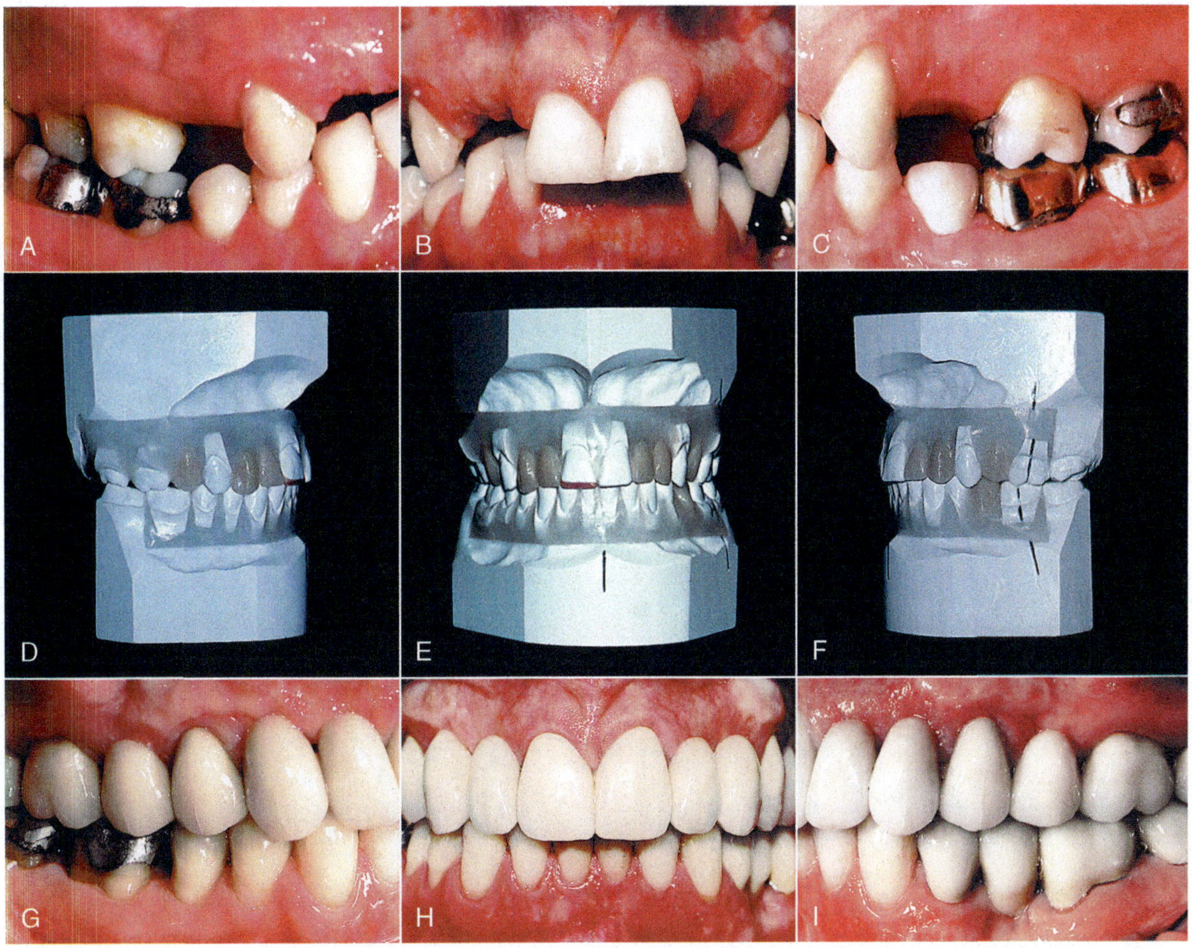

Figure 26-4 **A–C,** A 32-year-old female had a Class II, Division 1 malocclusion with a deep anterior overbite. She was congenitally missing both maxillary lateral incisors and all four maxillary premolars. The restorative dentist wanted the maxillary canines positioned in the first premolar positions in order to restore the maxillary arch with three segments of fixed restorations connected at the canines with a semirigid connector. **D–F,** A diagnostic wax setup provided the guide for the orthodontist to position the canines in their appropriate position. **G–I,** After the final restorations were placed, the widths of the pontics and abutments in the maxillary arch were functionally and esthetically correct because the vision had been created with the diagnostic setup.

CREATE THE VISION

After an orthodontist has treated several hundred adolescent patients with complete dentitions, it is easy for him or her to visualize or foresee the final orthodontic result before beginning treatment. However, some adult orthodontic patients may be missing several permanent teeth. If teeth have been absent for several years, the remaining teeth may have drifted. In other situations it may be necessary to position teeth in unusual situations. These patients may require a combination of orthodontics and restorative dentistry to rehabilitate their occlusion. In these patients it may be difficult for the orthodontist to visualize or foresee the final result, as he or she may not be aware of the restorative requirements or the eventual restorative treatment plan. Similarly, it may be difficult for the restorative dentist to visualize the final result, as he or she may be unaware of the orthodontic possibilities.

However, it is possible to predetermine the final occlusal and restorative outcome by completing a diagnostic wax setup for these types of patients. A diagnostic setup is mandatory for any patient who is missing multiple permanent teeth[4] and will require a combination of orthodontics and restorative dentistry (see Fig. 26-4). In addition, patients who will have implants used first for orthodontic anchorage and later for restorative abutments will require a diagnostic setup[5] to position the implants properly prior to the beginning of orthodontics (Fig. 26-5). The orthodontist should never make the restorative decisions but rather should consult with the restorative dentist when planning treatment for these types of patients. In that way the orthodontist may reposition the teeth to simulate realistic orthodontic objectives that will be in harmony with the patient's restorative requirements. Both practitioner and patient can visualize the result. The diagnostic wax setup is the blueprint for treatment in these types of patients.

A diagnostic wax setup is also necessary for patients who have unusual combinations of missing teeth and in whom the orthodontist is planning to substitute one tooth for another. For example, if a patient were missing maxillary lateral incisors and the orthodontist were planning canine

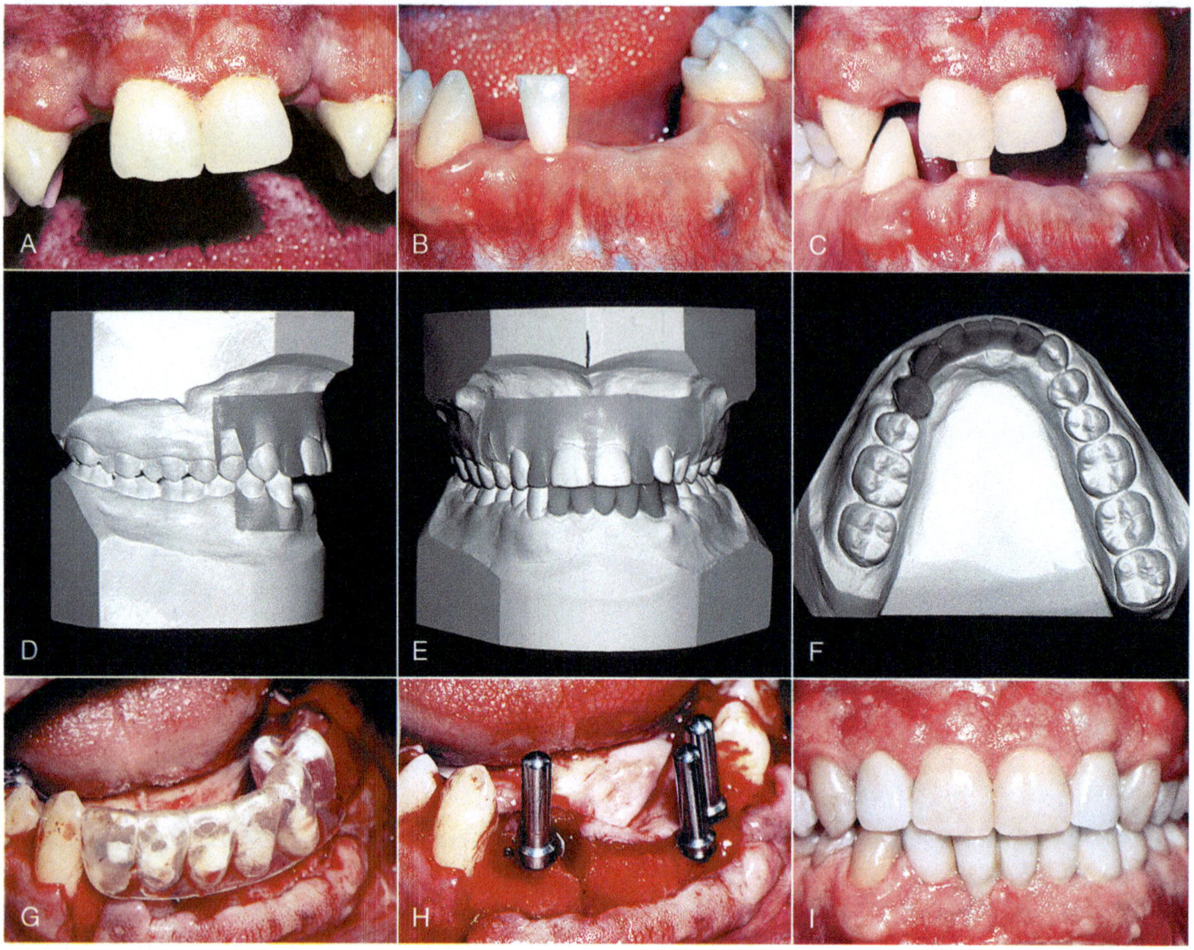

Figure 26-5 A 24-year-old male was the victim of a robbery during which he was shot in the face and lost (**A**) his maxillary lateral incisors and (**B**) most of his mandibular anterior teeth. The restorative plan involved single-tooth implants in the maxilla and an implant-supported bridge in the mandible to replace the missing teeth. The implants were also to be used as anchors to intrude the mandibular right canine and first premolar. **D–F,** A diagnostic setup was constructed to determine the appropriate implant position prior to orthodontics. **G,** A placement guide was constructed from the setup so the surgeon could (**H**) guide the placement of the implants. **I,** After orthodontics, the same implants that were used as orthodontic anchors were used to restore the missing teeth.

substitution, a diagnostic wax setup would be mandatory to determine whether the occlusion will fit properly and if the teeth can be shaped accordingly. Occasionally a patient is missing a central incisor[6] and a treatment option could be to restore the opposite lateral incisor as a central incisor in order to avoid an implant or fixed bridge (Fig. 26-6). A diagnostic wax setup would be necessary to determine whether the tooth arrangement will be both esthetic and functional.

Finally, adult malocclusions with significant mandibular incisor crowding occasionally are treated with extraction of a single mandibular incisor.[7] This type of extraction improves long-term stability, easily eliminates the crowding, simplifies the mechanics, preserves facial esthetics, and improves periodontal health in certain adults. However, before extracting the incisor the orthodontist must know whether the occlusion will fit properly, especially in the canine and incisor region (Fig. 26-7). A diagnostic wax setup will give the clinician the appropriate information to make the correct decision when planning incisor extraction in crowded adult malocclusions.

ESTABLISH THE SEQUENCE OF TREATMENT

Many orthodontic-restorative patients also require adjunctive periodontal therapy and orthognathic surgery. As the number of dentists involved in a patient's treatment increases, the complexity of the treatment also increases. In many of these situations, different specialists must interact at varying intervals during the patient's overall treatment. Therefore the team of specialists not only must establish a realistic plan of treatment, but also should determine the sequence of interaction between the different specialists (Fig. 26-8).

This critical step is often overlooked. It requires that the team members meet to discuss the patient's treatment before the initiation of therapy. After the sequence of intervention has been determined, it should be recorded by one of the clinicians.[1] A copy of the treatment sequence should be given to each of the participating dentists and to the patient. Then, at any time during treatment, any of the team members can

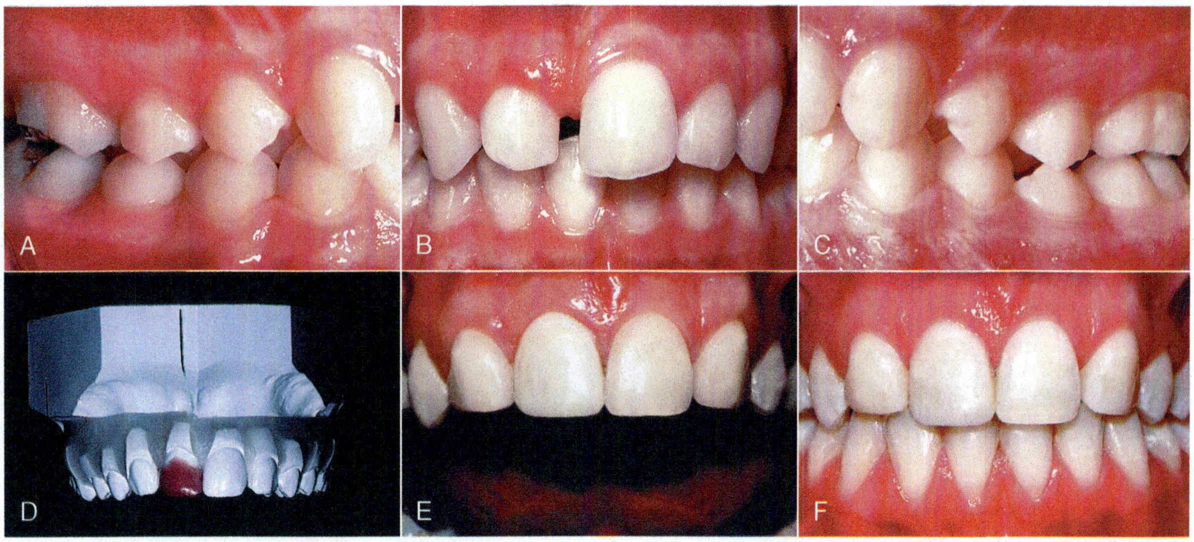

Figure 26-6 **A–C,** A 14-year-old female lost her maxillary right central incisor in a horseback riding accident as a child. No treatment was done at the time and the edentulous space had closed partially. She had a bilateral Class II malocclusion, no crowding in either dental arch, and a good facial profile. Although various treatment options were considered initially, the final plan involved extraction of the left lateral incisor, restoration of the right lateral as a central incisor, and bilateral canine substitution. **D,** A diagnostic wax setup was necessary to confirm that the treatment plan would satisfy the objectives. The setup helped the orthodontist to achieve an excellent **(E)** esthetic and **(F)** occlusal result.

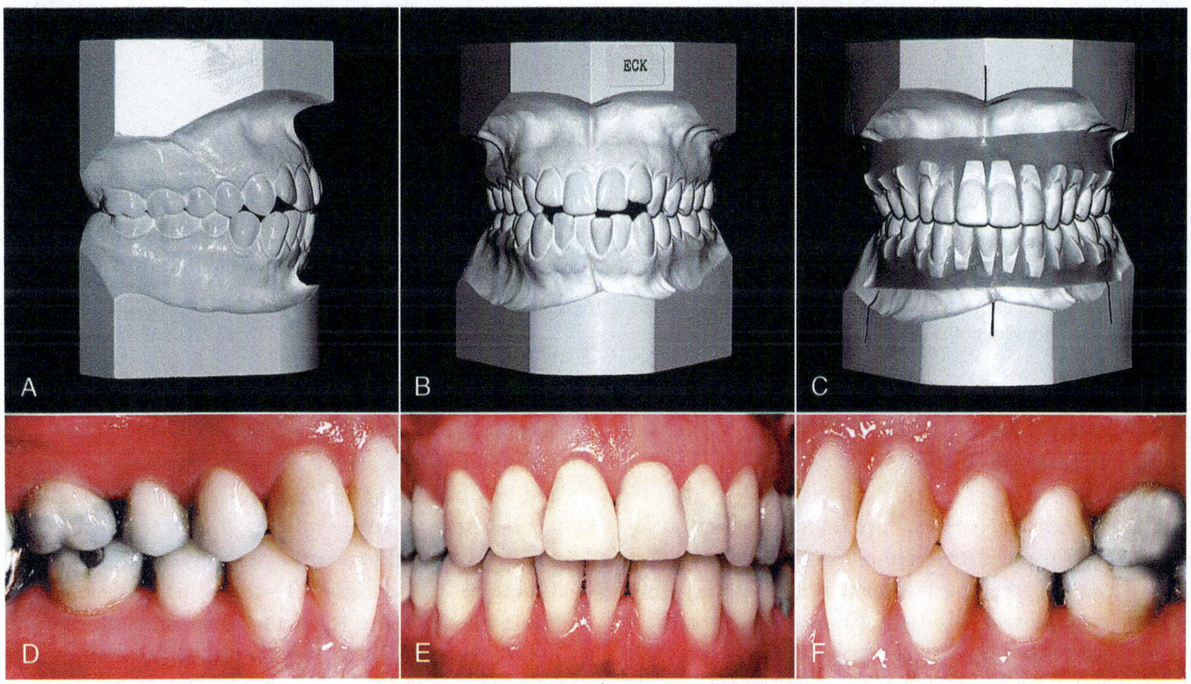

Figure 26-7 A 32-year-old female had **(A)** a bilateral Class I occlusion with **(B)** mild crowding of the maxillary teeth and moderate crowding of the mandibular incisors. **C,** A diagnostic setup was constructed to determine whether extraction of a mandibular incisor would eliminate the crowding and permit satisfactory overbite and overjet. **D–F,** The setup was invaluable in creating the vision and allowing the orthodontist to achieve a well-interdigitated occlusal result.

review the sequence, determine his or her point of interaction, and feel secure that the plan is proceeding properly. In addition, the patient is aware of the pathway toward completing treatment. The importance of this step in interdisciplinary treatment cannot be overemphasized. Success in treating a patient with complex restorative, periodontal, orthognathic, and orthodontic problems is dependent on not only the correct plan of treatment, but also the correct sequence of interaction among different practitioners during the course of treatment.

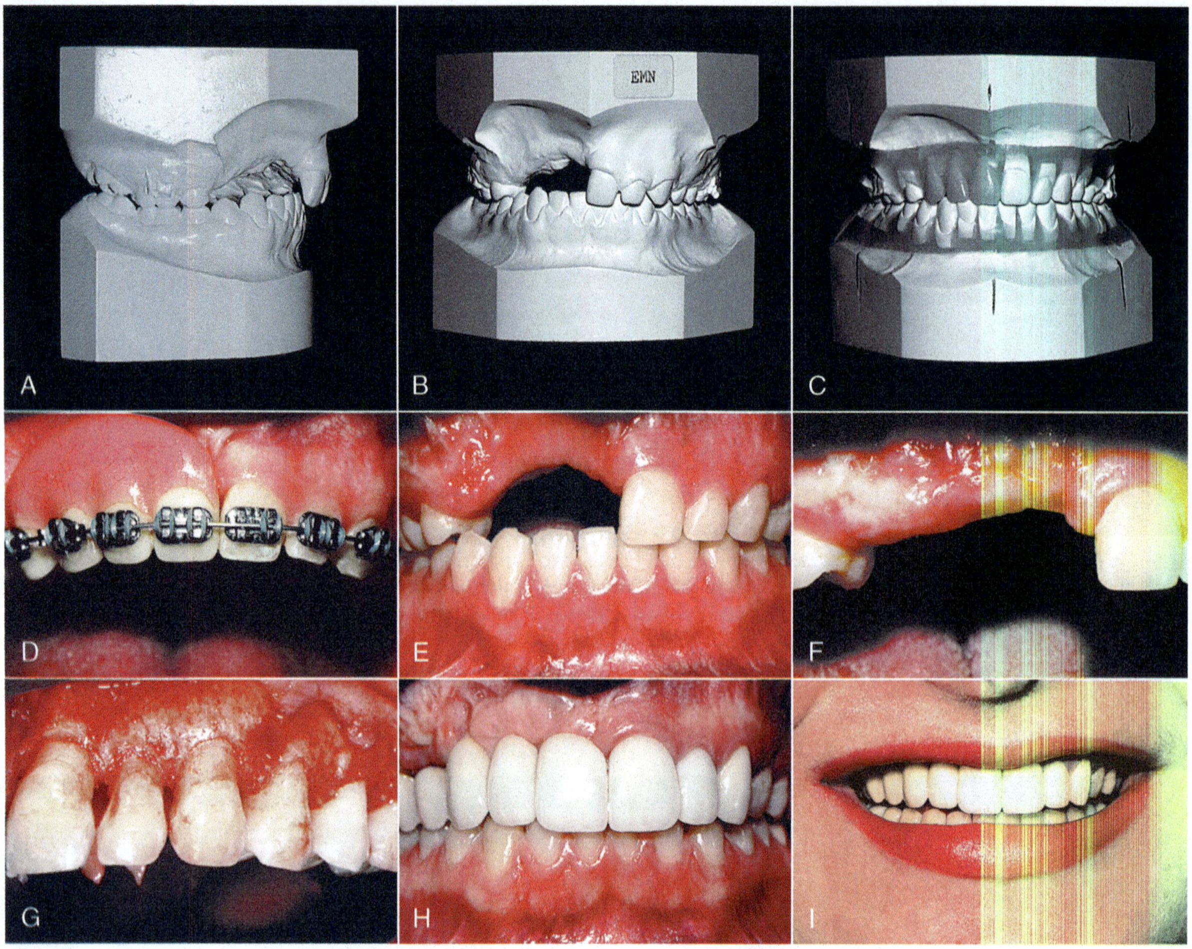

Figure 26-8 **A and B,** A 14-year-old female lost her maxillary anterior teeth in a water skiing accident, which left a huge void in the maxillary alveolus. **C,** A diagnostic setup was constructed to create the vision for the practitioners and patient. Several treatment options were discussed but the final plan involved **(D and E)** orthodontics, segmental maxillary jaw surgery, sagittal split ramus osteotomy, **(F)** autogenous soft tissue ridge grafting, **(G)** crown lengthening, provisionalization, and **(H and I)** final restoration. Because of the complexity of the treatment plan, the four practitioners on the patient's team established the sequence of treatment before beginning therapy. Having the flow chart or treatment sequence facilitated the smooth treatment of this complicated case by keeping all practitioners aware of the timing of each step along the way.

IDENTIFY WHO WILL CORRECT THE PERIODONTAL DEFECTS

Many adult orthodontic patients have underlying periodontal defects that will need to be resolved before, during, or after the orthodontic therapy. It is mandatory that the orthodontist and periodontist discuss the management of these patients to determine who will be responsible for correcting the periodontal problems.[8] These problems are generally divided into two categories: soft tissue or gingival discrepancies and hard tissue or bony defects. Gingival discrepancies include recession, lack of attached gingiva, and open gingival embrasures. Bony alveolar defects include interproximal craters; one-, two-, and three-wall defects; furcation defects; and generalized or localized horizontal bone loss secondary to periodontal disease. Each of these defects must be discussed prior to the initiation of orthodontic bracketing to determine who will be responsible for correcting them.

Gingival recession and inadequate attached gingiva often will require the placement of a connective tissue graft. In some cases it is best to perform the grafting prior to orthodontic treatment. This is especially important when the adult patient has preexisting recession and dental crowding and will be treated without the extraction of teeth.[3] If there is a dehiscence labial to the tooth and recession has already occurred, it could get worse during orthodontic treatment. Therefore the periodontist will probably place a connective tissue graft prior to the orthodontic therapy to ensure that the recession will not progress and to cover the exposed root with gingiva.

Open gingival embrasures often occur during orthodontic therapy. If not corrected, these dark spaces between the teeth create an esthetic compromise after orthodontic therapy. The presence of a space above the central incisor interproximal contact may be caused by one of three factors.[9] The first possible cause is diverging roots of the maxillary central incisors. This is usually the result of improper bracket placement (Fig. 26-9). In patients with overlapping and abraded maxillary central incisors, brackets may be placed inadvertently at an angle that is not perpendicular to the long axis of the central incisor. As the teeth are aligned, the roots

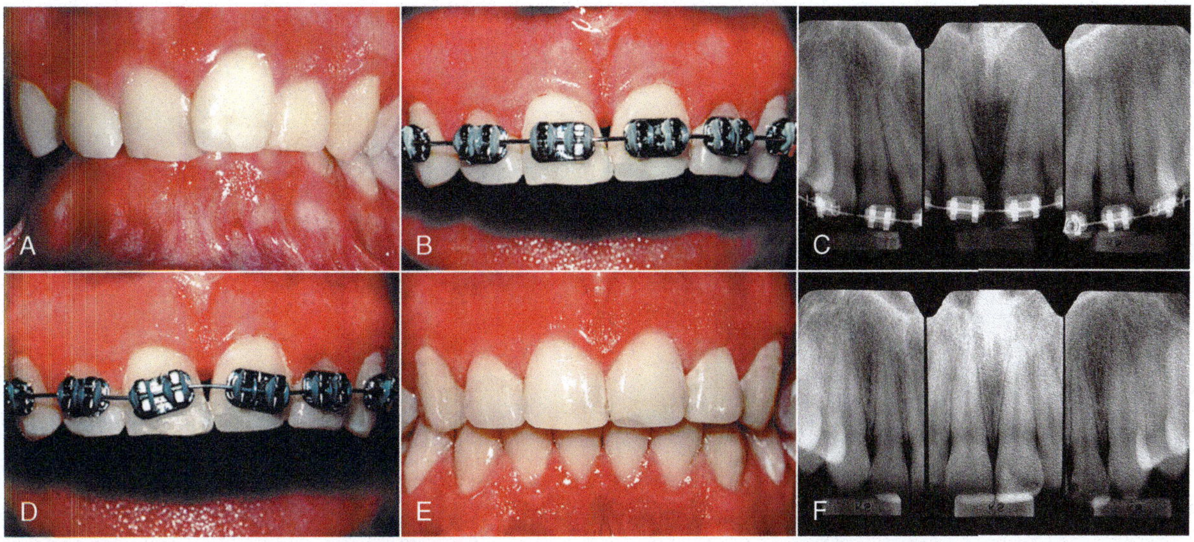

Figure 26-9 **A,** A young adult male had a Class II deep overbite malocclusion with mild crowding in both arches. **B,** During alignment of his overlapped maxillary incisors, an open embrasure developed between the maxillary central incisors. **C,** Progress periapical radiographs showed that the central incisor roots were diverted distally, causing the open embrasure. **D,** Therefore the teeth were rebracketed with the bracket slot perpendicular to the long axis of the roots. **E and F,** This permitted uprighting of the central incisor roots, which moved the contact gingivally and the papilla incisally to close the open embrasure.

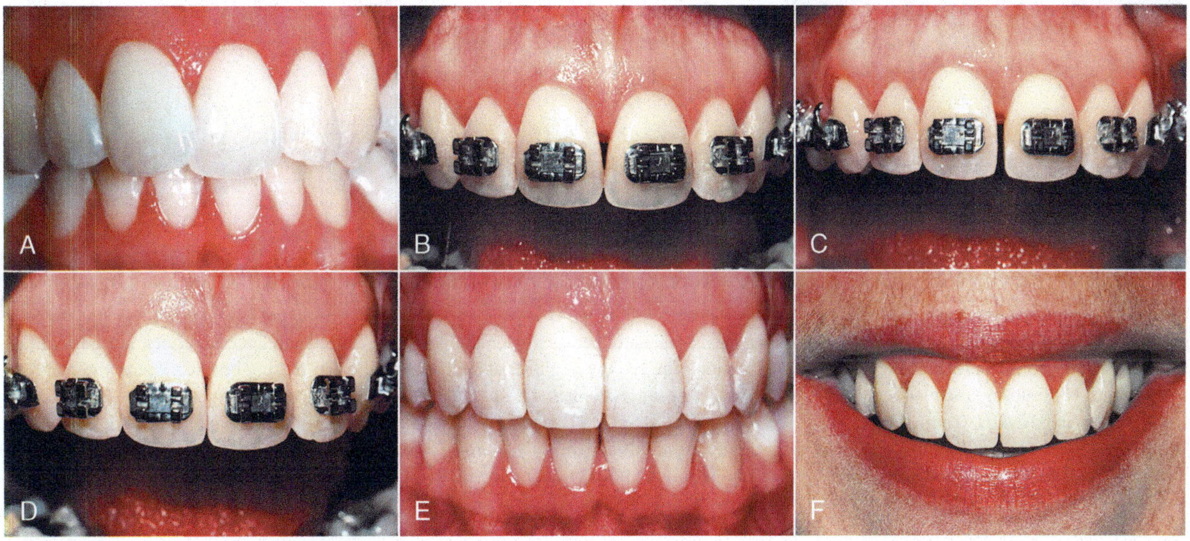

Figure 26-10 **A,** A 28-year-old female had a mildly crowded Class I malocclusion. Four premolars were extracted early in her life but no orthodontic treatment was performed. The objectives were to align the teeth and reduce the overbite. **B,** During alignment an open embrasure developed between the central incisors. The papilla height was normal but the contact between the centrals was too low, due to the triangular shape of the maxillary central incisors. **C,** The mesial surfaces of both centrals were reshaped with a diamond disc and **(D)** the space was closed, moving the contact gingivally toward the normal papilla. **E and F,** After orthodontics, the open embrasure had been eliminated and the occlusion and esthetics were satisfactory.

may diverge distally. To identify this cause the clinician should evaluate a periapical radiograph. If the roots diverge, the brackets should be removed and repositioned with the bracket slots perpendicular to the long axes of the roots. As the roots align, the interproximal contact lengthens and moves apically toward the papilla. Usually the distal-incisal corners of the centrals also move apically. This reflects the amount of incisal wear that may have occurred before orthodontic treatment. These teeth usually require an incisal restoration to restore proper incisal contour.

A second possible cause of space above the interproximal contact of the central incisors is abnormal tooth shape.[9] In some patients the crowns of the central incisors are much wider at the incisal edges than at the cervical region (Fig. 26-10). In these situations the contact between the incisors is located in the incisal 1-mm between the two centrals. This is an unusual contact relationship, as the contact should occupy about half the distance between the gingival margin and the incisal edge. One method of correcting this problem is to recontour the mesial surfaces of the central incisors and

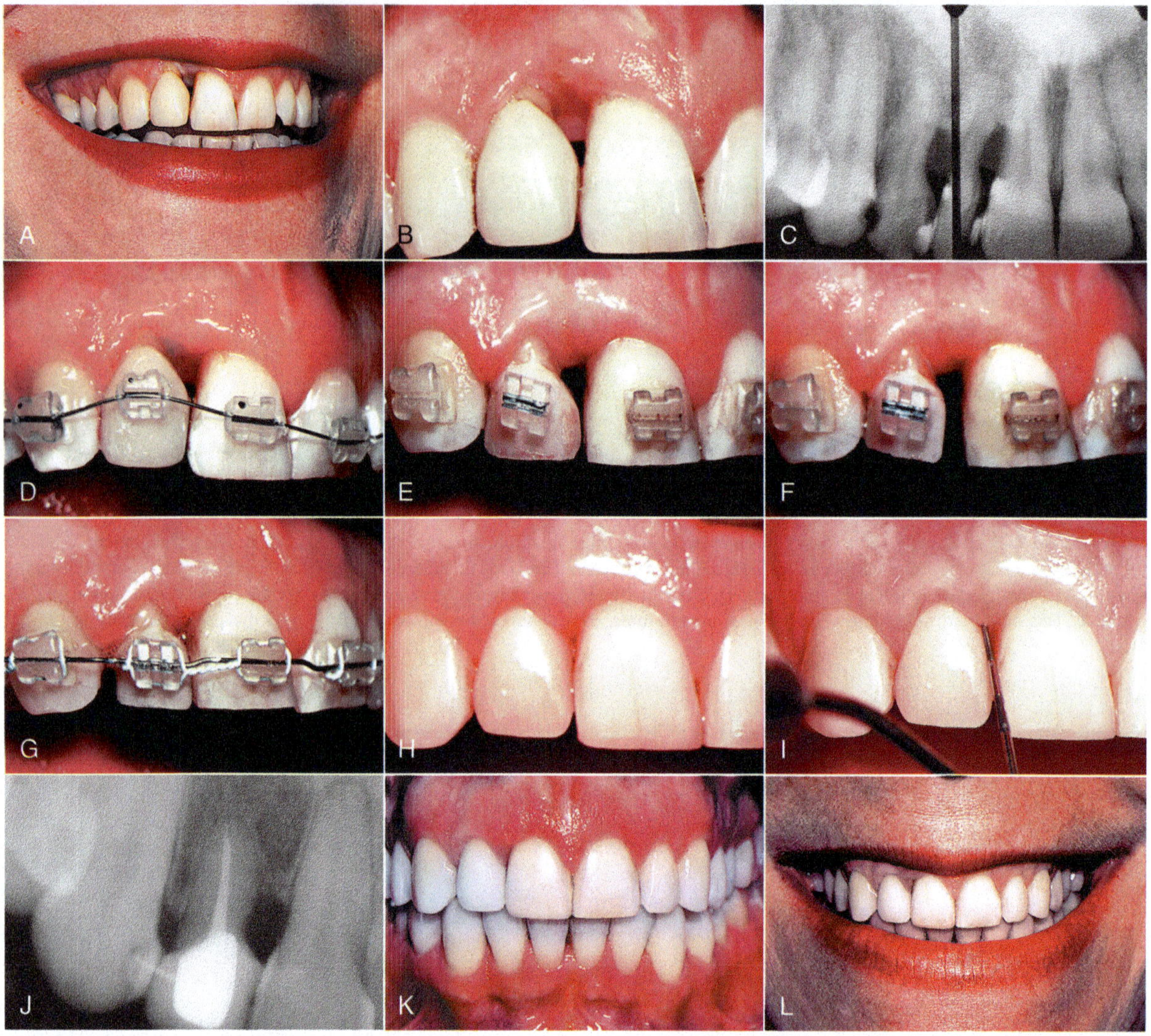

Figure 26-11 An adult female had **(A and B)** a significant open embrasure between the maxillary right central and lateral incisors, caused by a periodontal abscess with resultant **(C)** interproximal bone loss. The correction required moving the papilla coronally by **(D)** placing brackets nearer the gingival margins of the incisors and **(E)** erupting the two teeth. Then, to correct the contact problem, **(F)** the bracket was repositioned, the mesial of the lateral was reshaped, and **(G)** the space was closed. **H,** A provisional crown was placed after orthodontics and **(I)** the sulcular depth was reduced significantly. **J,** The post-treatment radiograph shows the amount of bone that was created by erupting the tooth incisally. **K and L,** The final restoration looked much more esthetic after the open embrasure was closed by orthodontics, periodontics, endodontics, and restorative dentistry.

close the space (see Fig. 26-10). The other method is to restore the contact with either a composite or a porcelain laminate restoration. If recontouring of the tooth will make it too narrow, then restoration is appropriate. In all other cases, recontouring of the teeth and space closure is the easiest way to correct the open embrasure. The amount of enamel that must be removed from each tooth is equal to half the distance between the mesial surfaces of the incisors at the level of the tip of the papilla. Usually this will be about 0.5- to 0.75-mm and does not penetrate into the dentin. After this diastema has been created, the space between the teeth is consolidated. As this occurs, the contact lengthens and moves toward the papilla.

In patients with advanced generalized or localized periodontal disease and destruction of the crestal bone between anterior teeth, the papilla may be absent. This produces an unesthetic large gap after orthodontics. Several methods may be needed to resolve this problem (Fig. 26-11). In some cases reshaping the adjacent teeth, altering the root angulation, eruption of the adjacent teeth, and restoration will be necessary to move the bone coronally and to squeeze the gingival tissue between the adjacent crowns to establish a papilla between adjacent teeth after orthodontic therapy.

Adult orthodontic patients may also have osseous defects that could compromise the patient's ability to clean his or her teeth adequately and that require correction prior to or during orthodontic therapy.[8] These osseous defects include interproximal craters; one-, two-, and three-wall defects; furcation defects; and horizontal defects. Interproximal craters can be the most volatile intrabony defects in the orthodontic patient. These are two-wall defects, where the remaining walls are the buccal and lingual walls. Attachment loss occurs on the mesial and distal surfaces of the adjacent roots. Orthodontic movement cannot improve interproximal craters.[8] If the crater is mild to moderate but the patient cannot maintain the area adequately, it may require resective bone removal and recontouring prior to orthodontic bracketing.

One-wall defects are treated most efficiently by the orthodontist.[10] In these situations, periodontal pathogenic bacteria have destroyed the attachment on three of the four interproximal walls, leaving one wall remaining. These defects are difficult for a periodontist to manage because resective surgery could be too destructive and regenerative therapy is inappropriate. However, orthodontic eruption of the tooth will eliminate the defect (Fig. 26-12). In these situations, the orthodontist must place the bracket more apically on the facial surface of the crown and perpendicular to the long axis of the root of the tooth. As the tooth erupts, the orthodontist must equilibrate the crown to avoid premature contact with teeth in the opposing arch and increased mobility of the erupting tooth. The orthodontist should evaluate a progress periapical radiograph to determine when the tooth has erupted sufficiently. When the interproximal bone is flat between adjacent teeth and the one-wall defect has been eliminated, the extrusion of the tooth is complete. Most of these erupted and equilibrated teeth will require a crown to cover the dentin that may have been exposed during the eruption process.

Two-wall defects are best treated with orthodontics and periodontal surgery.[8] When two walls remain in an interproximal region and the patient cannot maintain the area, it is difficult for a periodontist to completely resolve the defect with resective or regenerative treatment. These defects often require orthodontic eruption of the affected tooth, followed by crown lengthening to improve the restorability of the tooth. Three-wall defects are not resolvable with orthodontics. If the patient cannot maintain a three-wall defect during orthodontic therapy, it must be resolved prior to bracket placement. These defects are generally treated with regenerative therapy, using either autogenous or alloplastic bone grafts in the affected area.[8] Generally, orthodontic tooth movement can begin a short time after placement of the bone graft in order to enhance the fibroblastic and osteoblastic turnover that is necessary to heal the defect and move the adjacent teeth.

Furcation defects are typically divided into three classifications: class 1, 2, or 3. Class 1 furcation defects are typically very shallow and do not enter the molar furcation deeply and usually are observed or monitored during orthodontic therapy. Class 2 furcation defects extend into the furcation

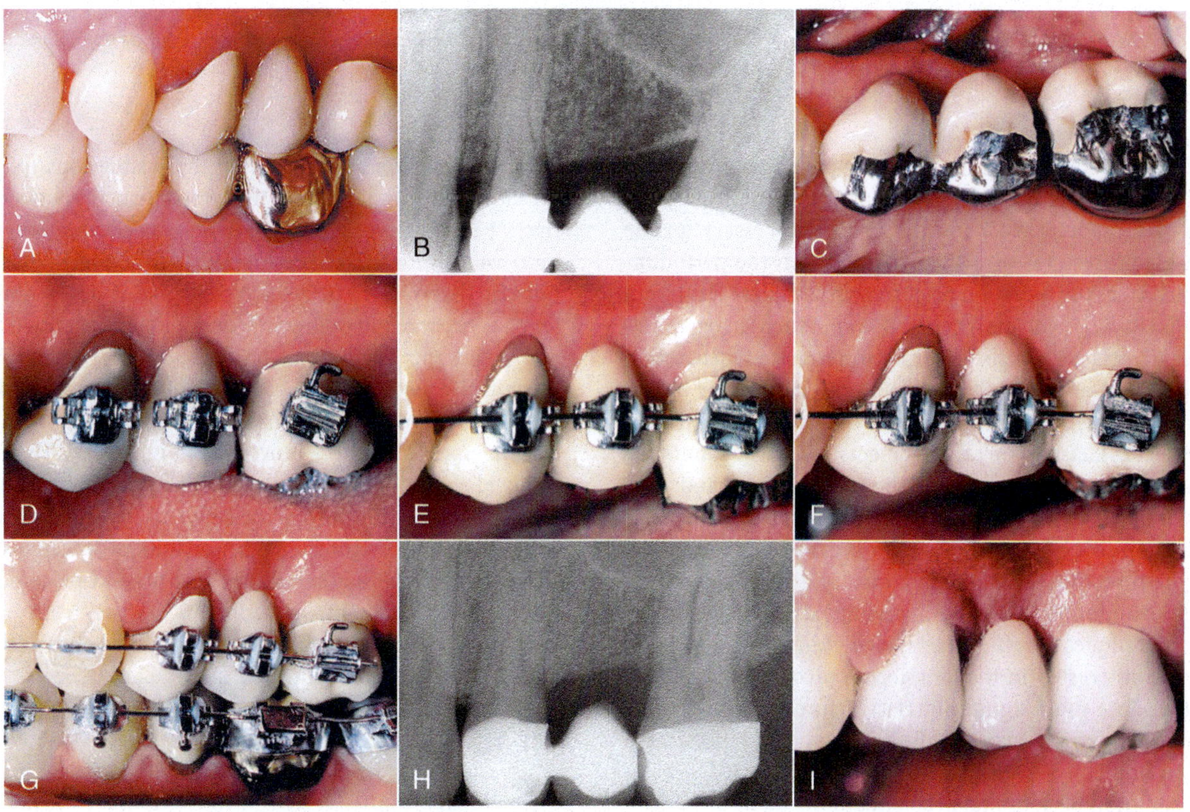

Figure 26-12 **A,** A 43-year-old veterinarian had a 6-mm bleeding pocket on the mesial surface of the maxillary left first molar. This tooth was an abutment for an existing three-unit bridge. **B,** The periapical radiograph shows the one-wall defect that was present mesial to the tipped first molar. The treatment plan involved **(C)** sectioning of the bridge, **(D)** placing the molar bracket perpendicular to the long axis of the root, and **(E)** inserting an archwire to upright and erupt the tooth. Because the crown had been overcontoured, **(F)** the occlusal surface was equilibrated to establish **(G)** satisfactory occlusal contact. The post-treatment radiograph showed **(H)** the amount of molar extrusion that was accomplished in order to eliminate the one-wall defect, so that **(I)** the final bridge could be placed on a periodontally healthy tooth.

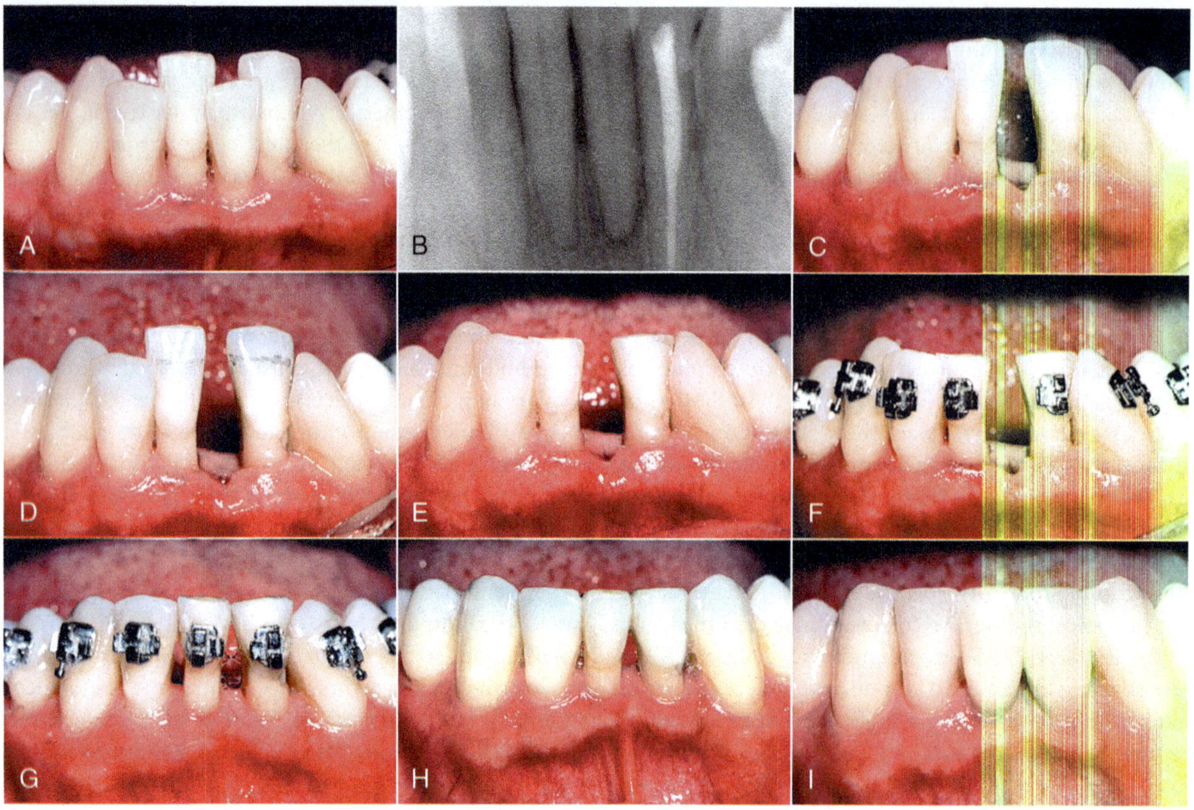

Figure 26-13 A 61-year-old female had **(A)** severe crowding of her mandibular incisors and **(B)** significant horizontal bone loss around her mandibular incisors. **C,** A diagnostic wax setup showed that the mandibular left lateral incisor could be extracted to eliminate the crowding. Since the bone levels were flat, **(D and E)** the incisal edges were equilibrated prior to bracket placement in order to maintain **(F–H)** a flat bony architecture during orthodontics. **I,** After bracket removal, the restorative dentist placed porcelain veneers on the teeth to close the open embrasures.

but do not communicate with the opposite side or interproximal region of the tooth. If the patient cannot maintain a class 2 furcation defect and the tooth is necessary for the occlusal and restorative treatment plan, then the periodontist must treat the furcation prior to orthodontics. Treatment most likely will involve a regenerative approach[8] using membranes to isolate the defect in order to promote regeneration of the periodontal membrane, while the membrane blocks the ingrowth of the epithelium that would recreate the furcation defect. Class 3 furcation defects typically cannot be maintained by patients during orthodontic therapy and decisions about their outcome must be made during the treatment planning process before beginning orthodontics. In the past, hemisection, root amputation, and root separation using orthodontics have been attempted.[3] In some cases these techniques worked nicely. However, clinicians today are more interested in the long-term outcome of treatment and therefore most significant class 3 furcation defects are treated with extraction of the affected tooth and replacement with an implant.[8]

A common periodontal problem among adult orthodontic patients is generalized horizontal bone loss in the anterior region of the mouth. In these situations, if significant bone loss has occurred on all anterior teeth, then often the teeth have disproportionate crown/root ratios. The orthodontist must recognize this problem prior to bracket placement (Fig. 26-13). It may be appropriate in these situations to reduce the clinical crown lengths of these teeth to achieve two objectives.[3,8] First, if the crown length is reduced, the crown/root ratio will improve and the mobility of the tooth after orthodontic therapy will be reduced. Second, if horizontal bone loss has occurred in only one area, reduction of crown length will avoid the creation of bony defects between adjacent teeth as the teeth are aligned. The orthodontist should draw on the tooth with a pencil or pen to identify how much crown length must be removed (see Fig. 26-13). Then tooth removal should be accomplished slowly with water spray to avoid damaging the pulp of the tooth.[11] Once the new incisal edge has been established, the orthodontist can use this surface of the tooth as a reference for bracket placement. At the end of treatment, the mobility of the teeth will be improved and the periodontal defect will be eliminated.

NEGOTIATE THE EXTRACTION OF HOPELESS TEETH

Occasionally, adults present for orthodontic treatment with teeth that are either periodontally or restoratively hopeless and that require extraction at some point during interdisciplinary treatment (Fig. 26-14). In these situations it is important for all members of the team (restorative dentist, periodontist, orthodontist, and oral and maxillofacial

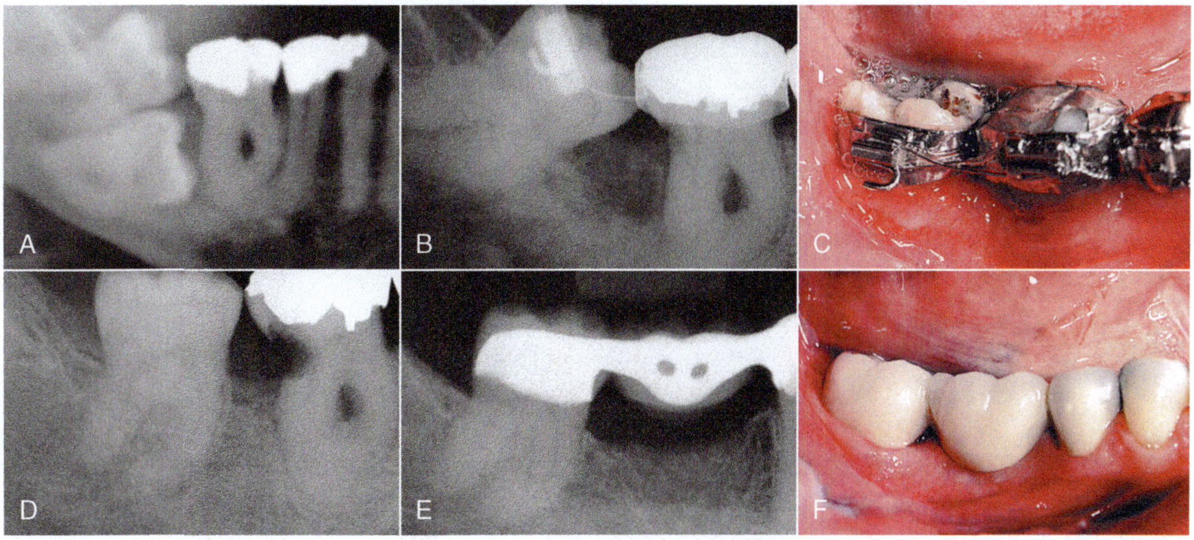

Figure 26-14 **A,** A 55-year-old female had an impacted mandibular right second molar and the third molar had erupted over the occlusal surface. The first molar had severe bone loss on the distal root and a class 3 furcation defect and was considered hopeless. **B,** The second molar was extracted and **(C and D)** the first molar was used as an anchor to upright the third molar. Although the first molar would eventually be extracted, the timing of the extraction was delayed until after the orthodontics and **(E and F)** a bridge was chosen to restore the edentulous space. Timing the extraction of hopeless teeth until after orthodontics can help to facilitate difficult tooth movement.

surgeon) to participate in the decision regarding timing of the extraction.[1] If the tooth has a periodontal or pulpal infection that cannot be maintained by the patient, dentist, or periodontist during treatment, then the tooth may require extraction before orthodontic bracketing. However, orthodontic treatment becomes more complicated with each edentulous space that is created prior to orthodontics, especially if that space must be maintained during and after orthodontic therapy. In addition, the mechanics could be more complicated if several teeth must be removed prior to orthodontic treatment. The fewer teeth the patient has, the more difficult it is to anchor the remaining tooth movement. If possible, it is advantageous for the orthodontist to maintain hopeless teeth in the dental arch during orthodontic treatment (see Fig. 26-14). They provide anchorage and space maintenance for the orthodontist and occlusal function and intraoral comfort for the patient. Therefore it is desirable to extract hopeless teeth after orthodontic treatment as long as the periodontal health of adjacent teeth can be maintained.

RESHAPE AND REBUILD TEETH WITH UNUSUAL CROWN FORM

Some orthodontic-restorative patients have small, malformed teeth that will require restoration after the completion of orthodontic treatment. In some of these situations, the orthodontist must create additional space to restore these teeth. In other situations, the malformed teeth are too large and must be reduced in width. Ideally, restoration of these small or malformed teeth should be performed before the initiation of orthodontic therapy. However, often there is not enough space to restore the tooth before bracket placement. The team must decide how much space to create for these restorations and the timing of restoring these small or malformed teeth. Two situations are common: retained primary teeth and peg-shaped lateral incisors.

When patients are congenitally missing their mandibular second premolars, the primary second molar may be unrestored, caries free, not submerged, and not ankylosed. If the patient will not have an implant placed for several years after orthodontics because of the potential for further jaw growth, it may be advantageous to reduce and retain the primary molar during orthodontics.[12] After all, it will maintain the width of the alveolar bone, prevent supereruption of opposing teeth, and help to maintain mesiodistal width after orthodontics. However, these teeth are too wide and must be reduced to the size of a premolar (Fig. 26-15). After reduction, these teeth have exposed cementum on the mesial and distal surfaces, so it is often advantageous to build up these teeth with composite. These temporary, inexpensive restorations will help to prevent interproximal caries and provide a better-shaped buccal surface for bonding of an orthodontic bracket.[12] If the primary molar roots do not resorb excessively during orthodontics, these primary teeth may remain for several years until the patient is old enough to have an implant placed.

Another common orthodontic-restorative problem is peg-shaped or malformed maxillary lateral incisors. In some patients the best choice for treating a peg-shaped lateral incisor is to restore the malformed tooth to its correct dimension. If sufficient space exists, a composite restoration may be placed before orthodontic treatment (Fig. 26-16). However, in most situations there is insufficient space to restore the malformed lateral incisors. Therefore orthodontics is often necessary to create space to build up peg-shaped lateral incisors. The space is usually acquired by placing open coil springs on either side of the tooth.[1] This will create space

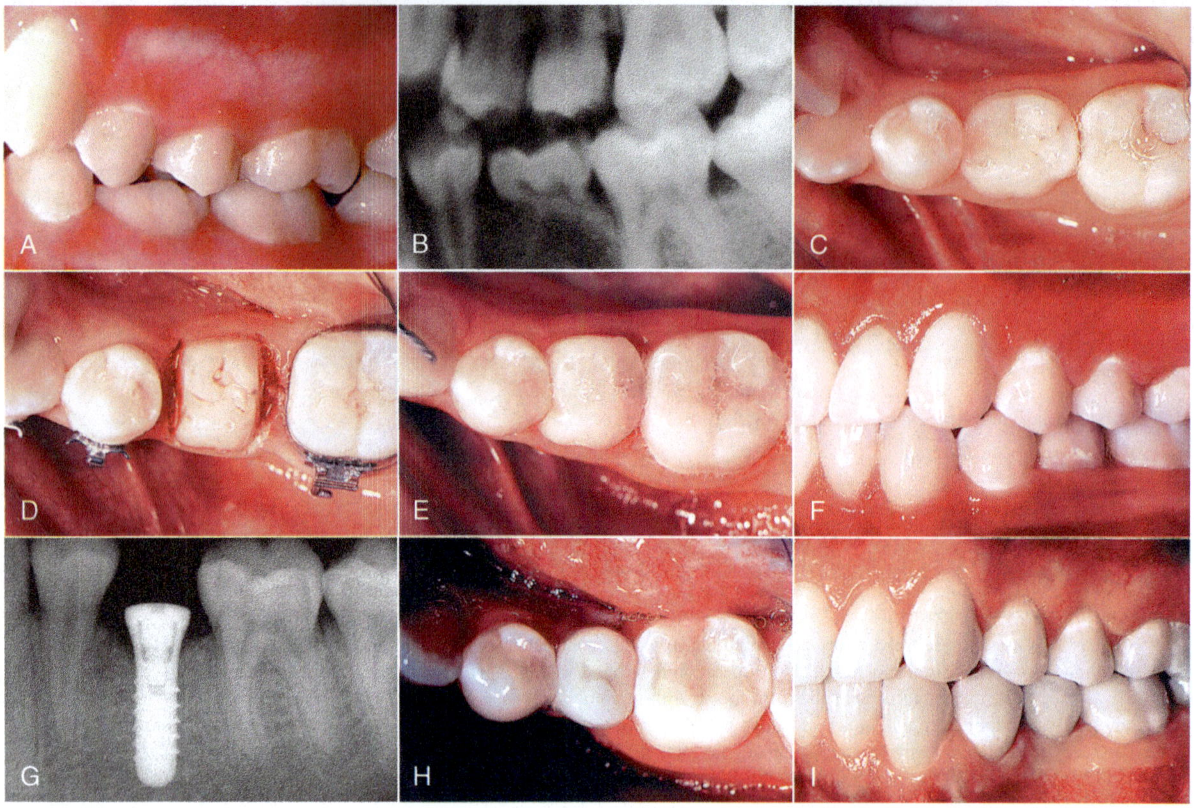

Figure 26-15 A 15-year-old female was congenitally missing **(A and B)** her mandibular left second premolar and **(C)** the primary second molar was retained. The restorative plan was to replace the missing tooth with an implant. To maintain the alveolar ridge width for the implant but to create the appropriate space for the implant crown, **(D)** the width of the primary tooth was reduced significantly and the exposed dentin was restored with composite. Two years later, at the end of orthodontics, the primary molar was still present and **(E)** helped to maintain the intra-arch space and **(F)** provide an occlusal stop for the opposing premolar. One year later, the primary molar was extracted, **(G)** an implant was placed, and then 6 months later **(H and I)** it was restored with a porcelain crown.

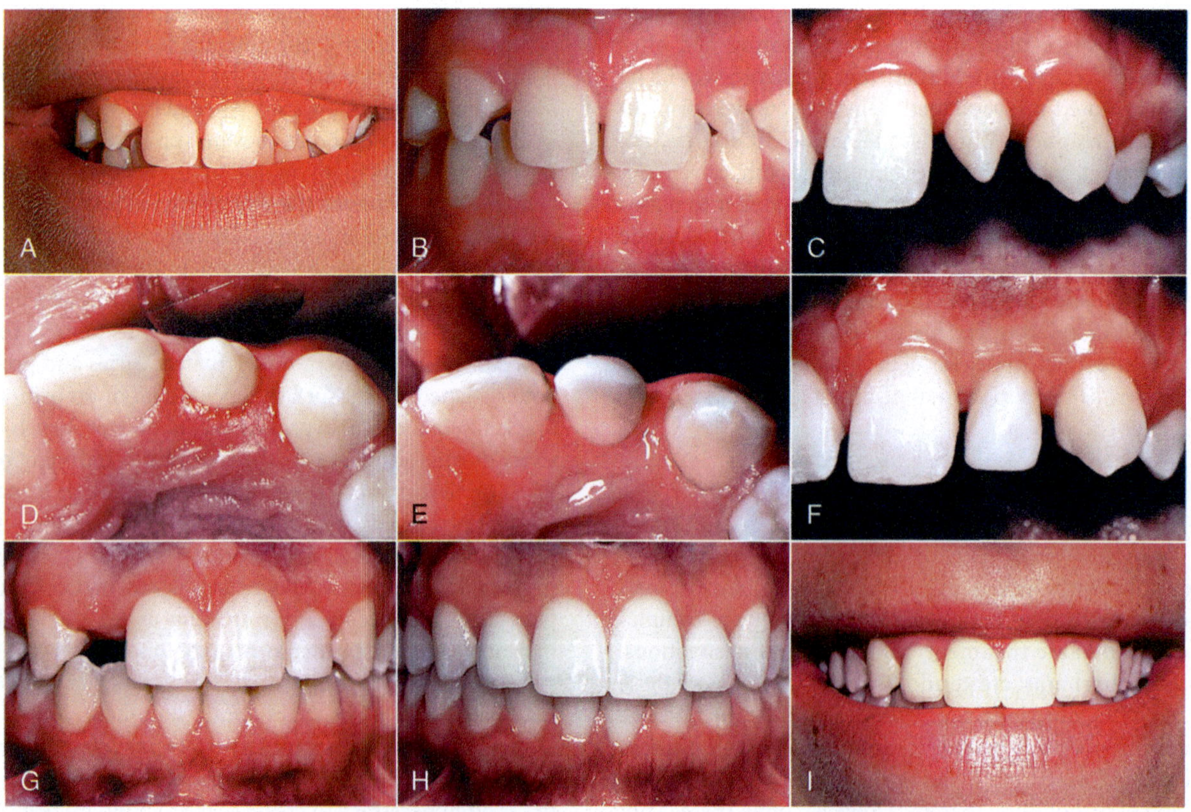

Figure 26-16 A 12-year-old female was congenitally missing **(A and B)** her maxillary right lateral incisor and **(C and D)** the left lateral incisor was cone shaped. The restorative plan involved replacing the missing tooth with an implant and restoring the malformed lateral incisor with a porcelain crown. A diagnostic wax setup was constructed **(E and F)** to determine the appropriate size of the temporary restoration of the malformed lateral incisor and **(G)** facilitated the orthodontic correction of the malocclusion. When the patient completed facial growth 3 years later, an implant was placed and **(H and I)** porcelain crowns were placed on the implant and malformed lateral incisors.

on the mesial and distal surfaces for future restoration. It is generally advantageous to position the tooth closer to the central incisor than the canine, so the emergence profile of the restoration on the mesial surface is rather flat and matches the adjacent incisors. In this way, most of the overcontouring is on the distal surface, which is less obvious esthetically. In addition, the gingival margin of the peg-shaped tooth should be aligned with the contralateral lateral incisor in order to create symmetrical gingival levels and crown lengths after restoration. If these principles are followed, the restored peg-shaped lateral incisor will match the contralateral lateral incisor in size and shape.

POSITION TEETH TO FACILITATE RESTORATIVE DENTISTRY

In the nonrestored adolescent patient, orthodontic positioning of teeth is determined by the size and shape of the teeth. Ideally, if the sizes of all teeth are compatible, a Class I occlusion with complete interdigitation is possible. However, in the orthodontic-restorative patient it may not be prudent to position teeth ideally. If restorations are planned for the patient, it may be advantageous to position teeth to facilitate this restorative treatment. Specific restorations require different types of tooth positioning.

A common orthodontic-restorative situation involves the patient who is congenitally missing one or two maxillary lateral incisors and will have implants to replace the missing tooth or teeth after orthodontic therapy. If the patient were missing one maxillary lateral incisor, the contralateral lateral incisor would determine the amount of space for the implant and crown. However, in some patients the existing lateral incisor may be peg-shaped (see Fig. 26-16). In other situations, both lateral incisors are congenitally absent (Fig. 26-17) and the amount of space is determined by two factors[12]: esthetics and occlusion (see Fig. 26-17). An esthetic relationship exists between the size of the maxillary central and lateral incisors. The size relationship has been called the "golden proportion."[13] Ideally, the maxillary lateral incisor should be about two-thirds the width of the central incisor.[14] Since most central incisors are about 9-mm wide, the width of the lateral incisor space should be no less than 6-mm. Today the narrowest implants are about 3.2-mm in diameter. If the edentulous space were 6-mm wide, then about 1.4-mm would exist between the implant and the adjacent roots (see Fig. 26-17). Studies have documented that narrower distances between the implant and adjacent root are more likely to show a reduction in bone height over time.[15,16] So at least 1-mm between the implant and adjacent root is desirable.

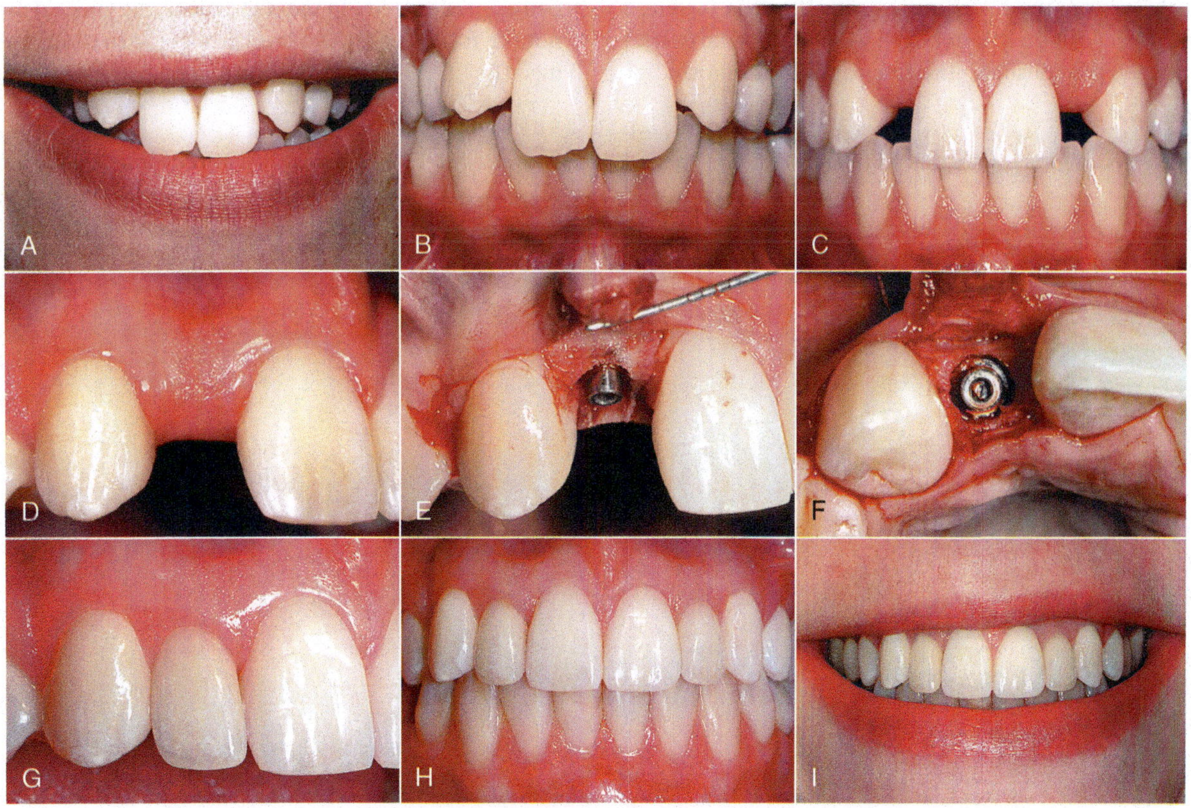

Figure 26-17 **A and B,** A 14-year-old female was congenitally missing both maxillary lateral incisors. **C,** The treatment plan involved opening space for two implants and two crowns. **D,** The labial sulcus depths of the central incisor and canine were 1-mm, there was no incisal wear of either tooth, and the width-to-length proportions of these teeth were normal. **E and F,** Therefore the position of the head of the implant was determined by the future gingival margin of the lateral incisor implant crown. When **(G)** the implant crown was placed, **(H and I)** the gingival margin level was positioned correctly relative to the adjacent teeth as well as the contralateral incisor.

However, in some situations the orthodontist may create less than the ideal width for a lateral incisor implant and crown because of the patient's occlusal relationships. The orthodontist should assess the posterior intercuspation as well as the appropriate amount of overbite and overjet. If the correct occlusion has been achieved and the space for the implant crown is too narrow, the orthodontist should remove interproximal enamel from the central incisors and canines to provide additional width for the lateral incisor implant. In some cases, if the interproximal surfaces of the canines and central incisors are already flat, the orthodontist must remove enamel interproximally from the premolars.[17] The maxillary premolars generally have tapered crowns with sufficient thickness of enamel, so they can be reduced without penetrating the dentin interproximally. By reducing the widths of adjacent anterior or posterior teeth, the orthodontist can create sufficient space for lateral incisor implants.

Another method for temporarily replacing congenitally missing maxillary lateral incisors is a resin-bonded bridge. Although this type of restoration has a high incidence of failure caused by debonding, it is a conservative means of replacing a missing maxillary lateral incisor, until an implant can be placed at a later time. If the teeth are in the proper position, the life of a resin-bonded bridge can be increased and the tendency for debonding may be decreased. Since a resin-bonded bridge depends on surface coverage for retention,[18,19] the greater the area of coverage on the lingual of the teeth, the greater the retention (Fig. 26-18). It is therefore important to position anterior teeth with appropriate overjet and overbite relationships. The anterior overbite should not be excessive but should be enough to provide disocclusion of the posterior teeth when the mandible is protruded forward. The anterior overjet should produce contact of the maxillary and mandibular incisors in centric occlusion. The angulation of the maxillary anterior teeth should be upright and oriented more vertically after orthodontic treatment. This will produce a shear force on the major connector of the resin-bonded bridge, which will enhance retention and stability of the bridge.[20] If incisors are proclined, the force on the bonded metal connector will be a tensile force, which could cause debonding of the bridge.

Another common problem in the adult orthodontic patient is wear or abrasion of the maxillary incisors causing uneven gingival levels and unequal crown length of adjacent central incisors (Fig. 26-19). Treatment for this problem could consist of periodontal crown lengthening to level the gingival margins, orthodontic extrusion of the longer central incisor, or intrusion and restoration of the short tooth or teeth. To diagnose this problem adequately, the clinician must first evaluate the labial sulcular depth of the maxillary incisors.[21] If the sulcular depth is uniformly 1-mm, the discrepancy in gingival margins may be due to uneven wear or trauma of the incisal edges of the anterior teeth. In these situations, the clinician must decide if the amount of gingival discrepancy will be noticeable (see Fig. 26-19). If it will be, bracketing and alignment of these teeth must be accomplished in a way that improves the esthetics and restorability of the abraded teeth. In these situations, the gingival margins, not the incisal edges, are used as a guide in tooth positioning.[22] As the gingival margins are aligned, the discrepancy in

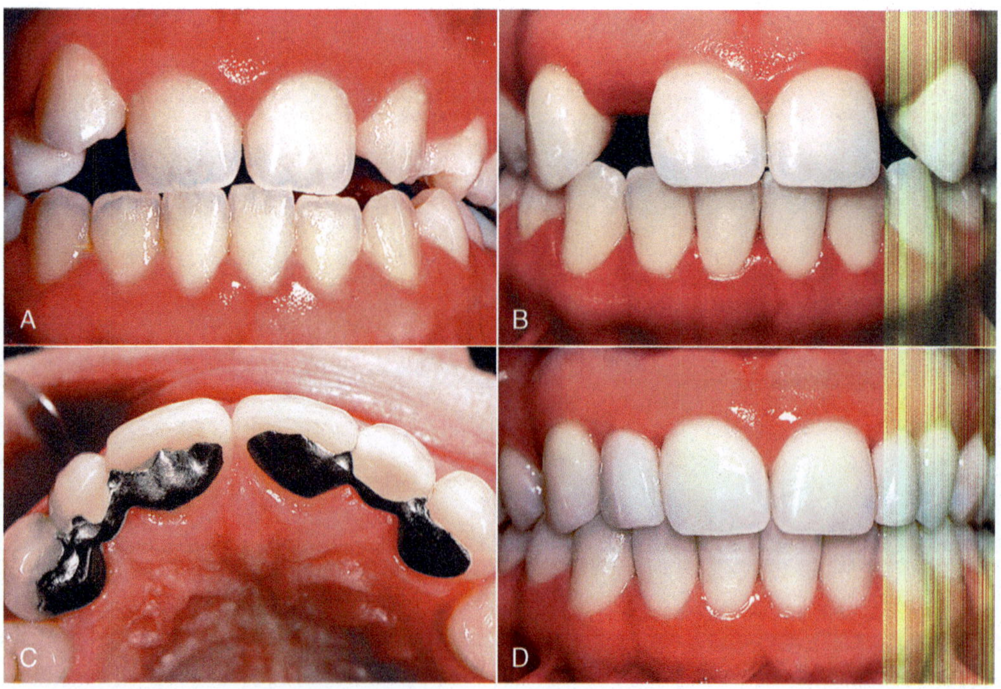

Figure 26-18 **A,** A 22-year-old female was congenitally missing both maxillary lateral incisors. The orthodontic-restorative plan involved **(B)** opening space for **(C)** bilateral resin-bonded bridges. **B,** To enhance retention and provide sufficient space for bonding of the metal connectors, the overbite should be minimal and only sufficient to permit posterior disocclusion in protrusive function. **D,** Seven years later, the original bridge was still in place and the esthetic appearance was satisfactory.

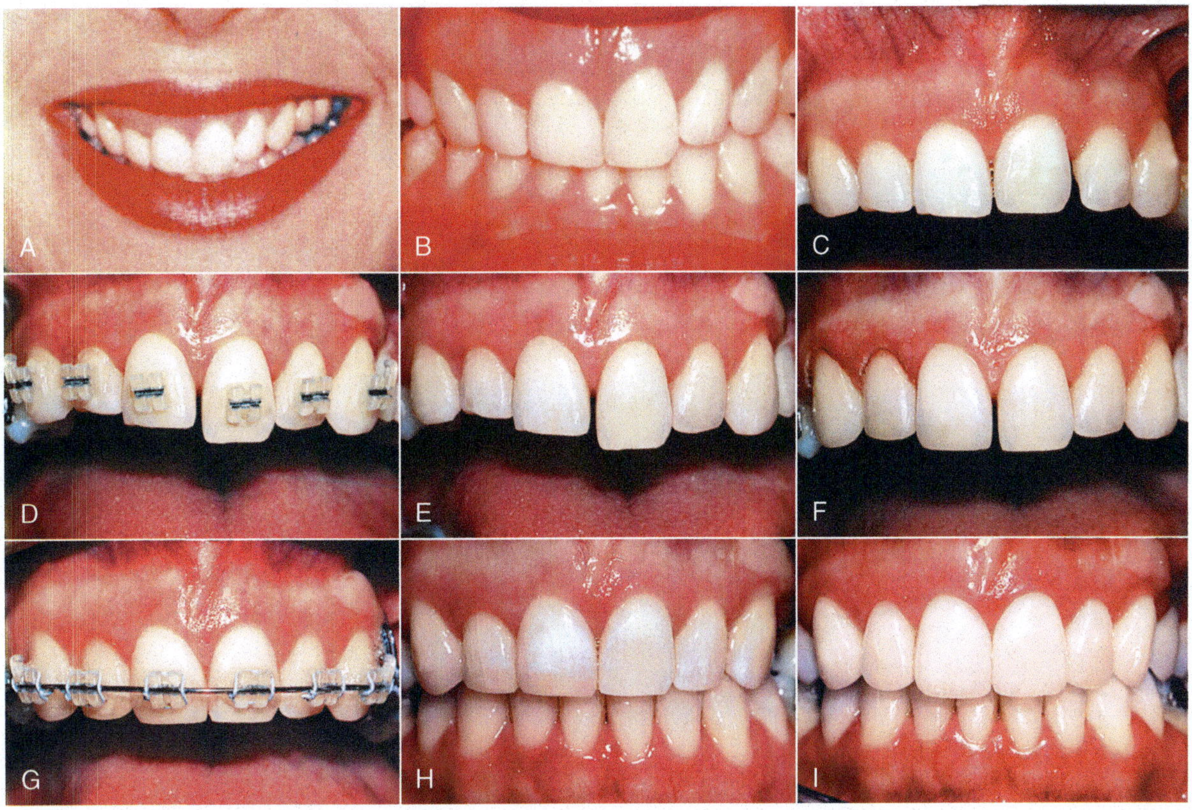

Figure 26-19 **A–C,** A 29-year-old female had crown length discrepancies between the maxillary right and left central and lateral incisors and canines. The labial sulcular depths of all anterior teeth were 1-mm and the cementoenamel junctions were at the bottom of the sulcus. The anterior teeth on the right had been abraded and the teeth had continued to erupt. Therefore the correct treatment plan involved **(D)** intrusion of the right central and lateral incisors and canine, **(E and F)** temporary restoration of these teeth with composite, and **(G)** replacement of the orthodontic brackets for 6 months to stabilize the intruded teeth. **H,** At the end of orthodontics the lengths of the right and left anterior teeth were equivalent. **I,** Two years later, after final restoration with porcelain veneers, the intruded position of the anterior teeth was stable.

the incisal edges becomes more apparent (see Fig. 26-19). These incisal discrepancies are restored temporarily with composite restorations and then restored permanently with porcelain veneer restorations after the teeth have stabilized. If the gingival margin discrepancies are corrected by leveling the gingival margins orthodontically, these tooth positions should be maintained for at least 6 months to avoid relapse. As teeth are intruded, the orientation of the periodontal fibers changes and becomes more oblique.[23] It typically takes at least 6 months for these fibers to reorient themselves in the horizontal position and to stabilize the tooth position.

Mandibular incisal edge abrasion is also a common problem in the adult orthodontic-restorative patient (Fig. 26-20). When this occurs, the mandibular incisors typically erupt in order to maintain contact. This presents a restorative dilemma for the general dentist, because it leaves no space to place the incisal restoration. Without orthodontics to intrude the lower incisors and create restorative space, the patient would require periodontal crown lengthening with bone removal and apical positioning of the gingival margin. If severe wear has occurred, this could also require root canal therapy and a post and coping on the short and abraded mandibular incisors. However, orthodontics is of tremendous benefit to restorative patients with significant wear of their mandibular incisors. By intruding the lower incisors (see Fig. 26-20), the orthodontist can create space for the restoration, avoid gingival surgery, eliminate the need for endodontic treatment, and thereby simplify the restoration of the abraded teeth.

When patients are congenitally missing their mandibular permanent second premolars, the clinician must monitor the vertical position of the primary second molar. Occasionally, the mandibular primary second molar will become ankylosed and fused to the alveolus (Fig. 26-21). In these situations, leaving the primary molar may result in a significant vertical bone defect in the edentulous ridge. If an implant is planned in the edentulous site, the vertical defect may be difficult to implant. If an ankylosed primary molar is not extracted early enough and a vertical ridge defect is produced, one option is to place a bone graft in the area either at the same time or prior to implant placement. Another option is to move the mandibular first premolar into the second premolar position[20] and to place the implant in the first premolar position (see Fig. 26-21). Studies have shown that it is possible, within limits, to move a tooth into a narrower edentulous ridge[24,25] in order to create an implant site. The bone that is created behind the moving tooth typically will be as wide as the root of the tooth that was moved. This

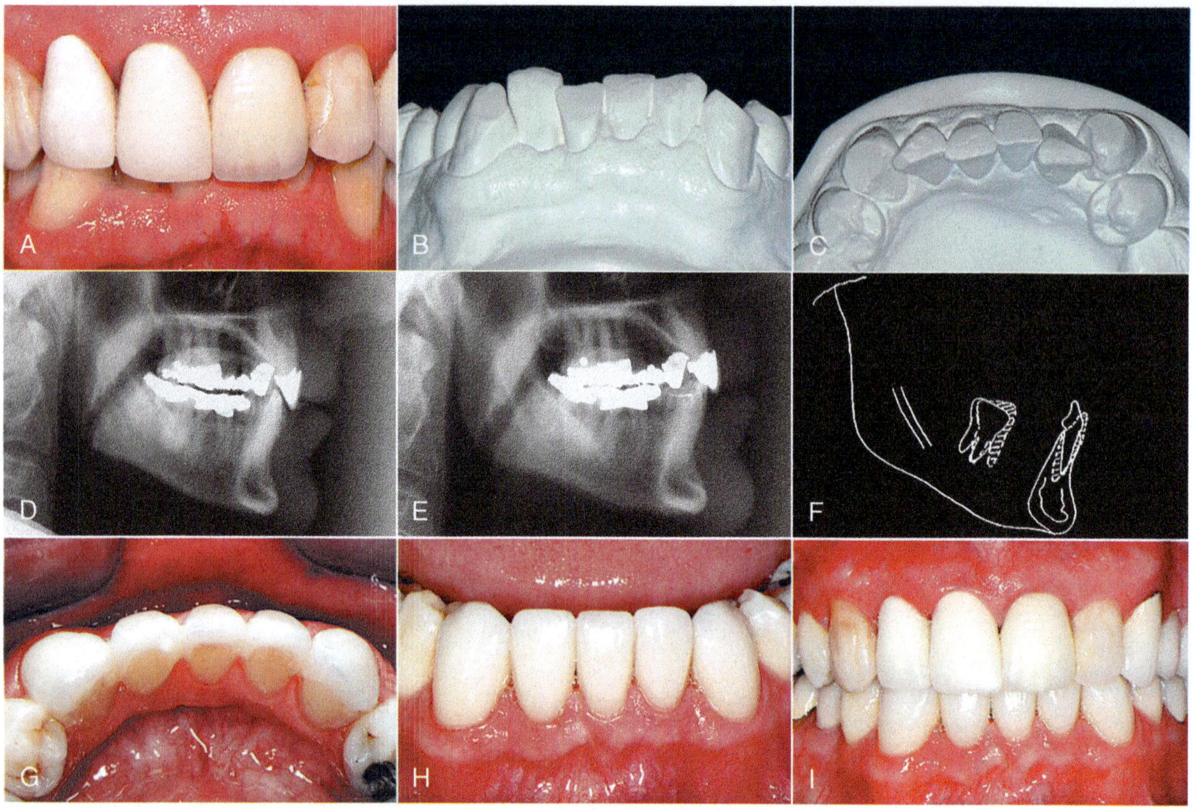

Figure 26-20 A 52-year-old male had **(A)** a deep anterior overbite and **(B and C)** a protrusive bruxing habit that produced significant wear of the mandibular incisors. **D,** There was no space for the restorative dentist to restore these teeth. Orthodontic treatment was initiated **(E and F)** to intrude the mandibular incisors so they could be restored with **(G and H)** porcelain veneers. **I,** Not only was the deep overbite corrected, but the orthodontic intrusion had permitted the restoration of esthetics and function to this debilitated dentition.

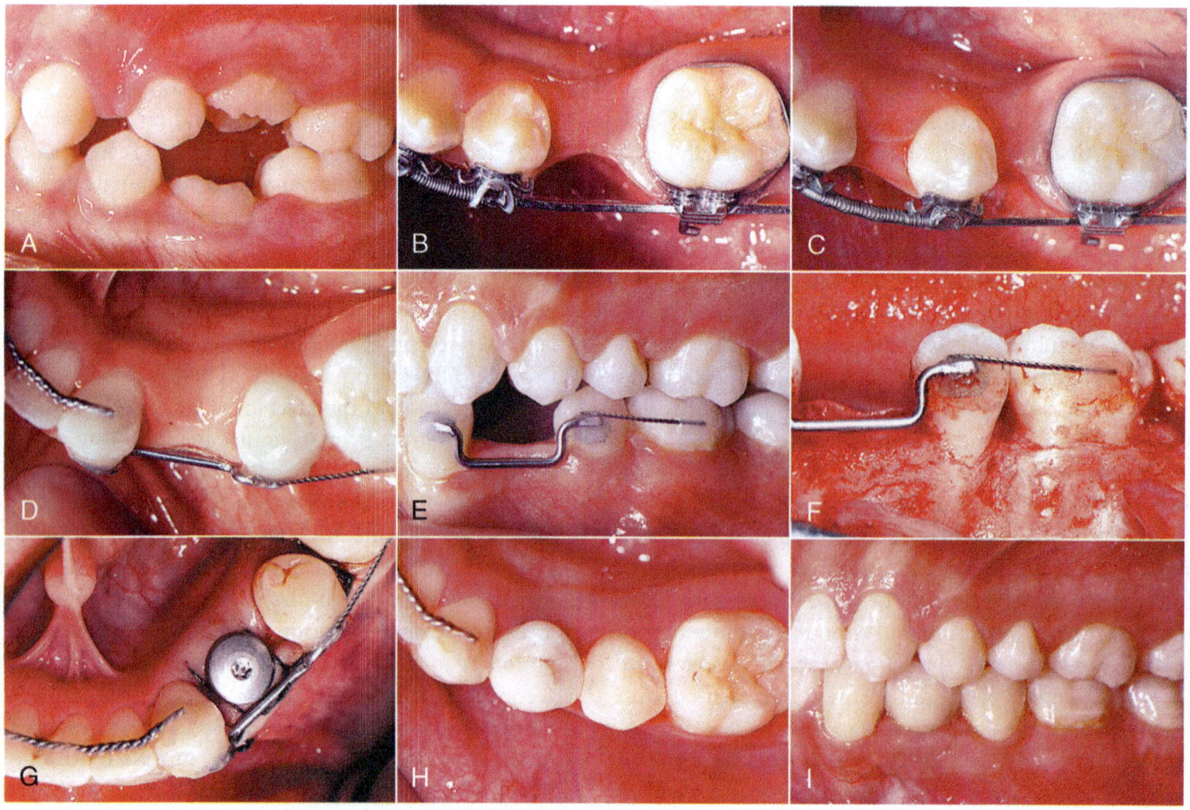

Figure 26-21 **A,** A 16-year-old female was congenitally missing the mandibular left second premolar and the primary molar had ankylosed and was submerged. **B,** After extraction of the primary molar, the alveolar ridge width decreased significantly. To create adequate ridge width for placement of an implant, **(C–E)** the first premolar was moved distally into the second premolar position and **(F and G)** the implant was placed in the first premolar position. **H and I,** The process of "orthodontic implant site development" is an excellent method to facilitate implant placement in sites with deficient bone.

type of orthodontic movement (called orthodontic implant site development) may eliminate the need for a bone graft in the edentulous site.

CONSIDER IMPLANTS TO FACILITATE DIFFICULT TOOTH MOVEMENT

In recent years dental implants have become an accepted method of replacing missing teeth.[26] Today millions of implants are placed annually to rehabilitate and reestablish patients' occlusions. In many of these individuals the teeth may be in a less than ideal position to accept the integration of a single implant or groups of implants with the remaining teeth. These patients could benefit from orthodontics to reposition malposed teeth and enhance the overall occlusal scheme.[27] However, if significant numbers of teeth are missing, the orthodontist is at a disadvantage because of the lack of anchorage to effect the desired tooth movement.

Several types of implant systems are available to provide anchors for tooth movement. These include subperiosteal implants,[28-30] interproximal transitional implants,[31] palatal implants,[32-34] mini-implants,[35-37] and titanium plates.[38-40] These auxiliaries are typically placed between the roots of teeth, apical to the roots of teeth, or in the retromolar regions of the maxilla and mandible. Although they are efficient anchors for tooth movement and are very versatile, they are also expendable. Usually they are removed after orthodontic treatment and discarded. Although this may be an extra expense for the patient, in a completely dentulous patient this technology may be appropriate. However, in a partially edentulous patient, where implants will be used as anchors to restore the occlusion, these restorative implants could be used initially for orthodontic anchorage and later as restorative abutments after orthodontics has been completed.[27]

The indications[27] for using a restorative implant as an orthodontic anchor include intra-arch intrusion of teeth that have overerupted, intra-arch retraction of teeth that are proclined, and intra-arch protraction of teeth that are positioned distally (Fig. 26-22). In each of these situations the implant must be placed prior to orthodontic bracketing. However, the implant must be positioned appropriately so it will not only satisfy the orthodontic requirements, but also be in a suitable position for the final restoration. The orthodontist must construct a diagnostic wax setup, after consultation with the restorative dentist and surgeon. The diagnostic wax setup must be constructed in a series of specific steps to ensure accuracy. These steps have been documented elsewhere.[27,41,42] The diagnostic wax setup permits construction of a placement guide for the surgeon to provide accurate positioning of implants.

After placement the implants must integrate with the bone prior to orthodontic loading. The timing of implant

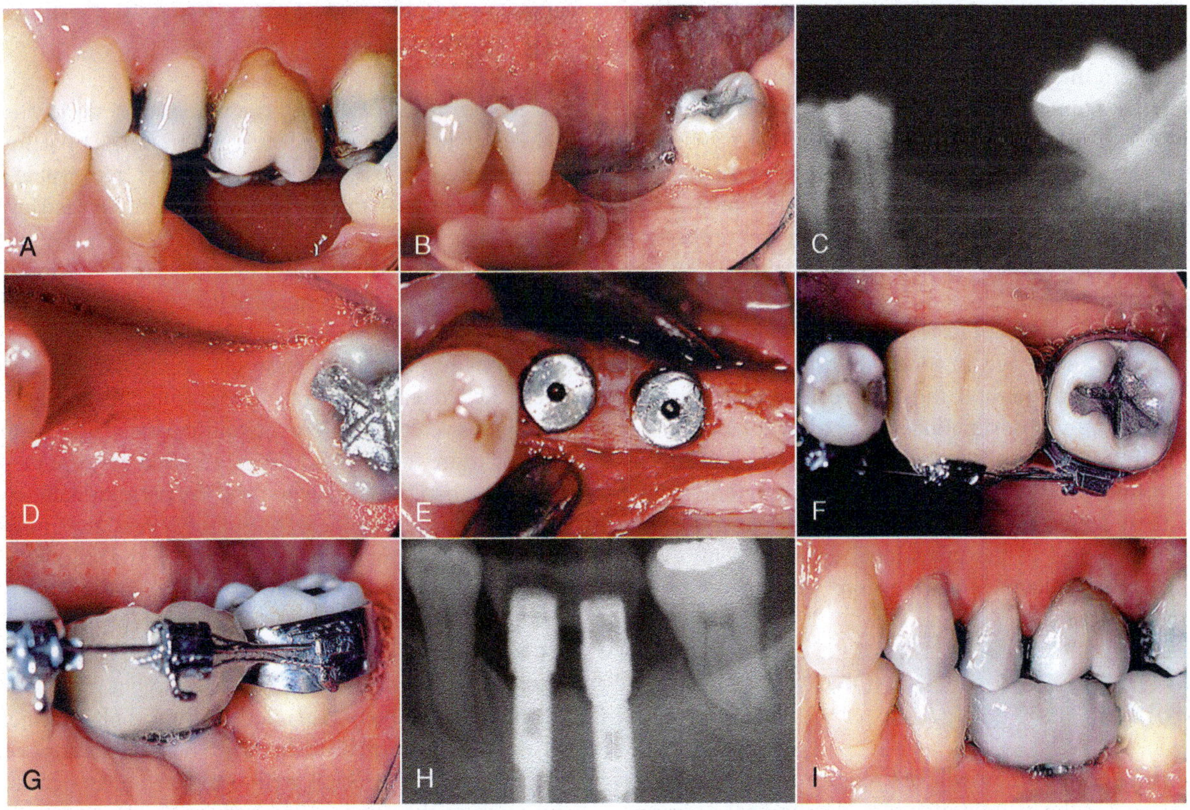

Figure 26-22 **A,** An adult female had lost her mandibular left first and second molars due to dental caries and the maxillary first molar had supererupted. **B–D,** In addition, the mandibular third molar had tipped mesially. **E,** The restorative plan was to place two premolar implants to replace the missing teeth. The implants would be used as anchorage to upright the third molar and move the **(F and G)** tooth and **(H)** roots mesially. **I,** By using the implants as anchorage, the posterior occlusion was maintained and the implants were restored to provide occlusion for the maxillary left first molar.

loading for single implants is determined by the amount of time required by the bone adjacent to the implant to undergo secondary osteon (remodeling) formation around the implant.[43] If multiple implants are placed at the same time, they are often loaded immediately after placement, using a provisional prosthesis. Even though the bone around the implant has not completely remodeled, the rigidity supplied by cross-arch splinting allows for integration to occur around the functioning implants.[44] Recent research has shown that when implants are loaded with static or continuous load in the same direction, the bone on the implant surface develops more rapidly.[45,46] However, when a dynamic load is applied to the implant (not continuous and in different directions), much less bone develops on the implant surface.[46] When the implant is loaded continuously, the same biomechanical message is delivered to the bony surface, which is to stimulate bone formation on the compressed surface in order to form more supporting bone. When the force on the implant is dynamic or intermittent, the biomechanical message is not clear and less bone is formed. Therefore if implants are to be used for orthodontic anchorage, they could be loaded immediately since an orthodontic load is continuous and in the same direction.

Animal studies have shown that when implants are loaded, more bone develops on the pressure or compressive side of the implant.[47] This is the opposite of what happens around teeth. When the periodontal ligament of a tooth is loaded with a compressive force, bone resorbs on the pressure side and deposits on the tension side. However, implants do not have a periodontal ligament and therefore the bone that forms on the pressure side of the implant is referred to as buttressing bone, which develops in response to implant loading.

After the implant has been uncovered, a provisional restoration must be placed so that the orthodontic force can be attached to the implant. The type of provisional restoration varies, depending on the type of orthodontic mechanics.[27] In some situations a tooth-shaped plastic restoration is required. However, in other situations a metal abutment is sufficient to provide the anchorage. In general, if orthodontic brackets are not to be used, a simple metal cap can be placed on top of the implant. In most situations, if the teeth adjacent to the implant are to be moved toward the implant, a provisional plastic restoration is necessary to permit accurate positioning of these teeth during the orthodontic process. In these situations the size of the provisional crown can be ascertained from the diagnostic wax setup used to create the placement guide.

EVALUATE TOOTH POSITION PRIOR TO BRACKET REMOVAL

If an orthodontic patient will not require restorations, it is appropriate for the orthodontist to make the final decisions regarding tooth position and appliance removal. However, if the patient will require restorations after orthodontics, the restorative dentist should play a part in the finishing process. It is advantageous to request input from the restorative dentist during final tooth positioning and the patient should be referred back to the restorative dentist during the final 6 months of treatment. A note or letter should be sent asking for input from the restorative dentist or periodontist about final tooth positioning, especially in areas where restorations are planned. Not only does the patient benefit from having several individuals evaluate the final result, but the orthodontist will learn from this interaction about the individual requirements of certain types of restorative patients.

In most orthodontic patients, aligning the crowns of the teeth will produce proper root angulation. Ideally, the roots of the teeth should not be in close interproximal contact. In that way, sufficient bone will be present between the roots of each tooth. Proper root angulation may be even more important for the orthodontic-restorative patient. When implants are planned for missing maxillary lateral incisors, it is important to create adequate space for the implant between adjacent roots.[12] As the central incisor and canine are pushed apart, the apices of the roots move toward one another (Fig. 26-23). During orthodontic finishing, radiographs must be taken to assess whether proper root angulation has been achieved. If it has not been achieved, the archwire must be removed and either the teeth should be rebracketed or bends should be placed in the archwire to achieve proper root angulation. If the roots are too close together, an implant cannot be placed.

DETERMINE THE APPROPRIATE TYPE OF RETENTION

Fixed and/or removable retainers are used routinely to maintain tooth position immediately after removal of orthodontic appliances. In most orthodontic patients, removable retainers include either maxillary and mandibular Hawley appliances or custom-fit Essix retainers. Fixed retainers typically consist of braided or solid stainless steel or gold wires that are bonded to the lingual surfaces of the maxillary or mandibular anterior teeth. In some patients it is beneficial to place combinations of fixed and removable retainer types. If patients wear their retainers for a sufficient time, the teeth will stabilize. However, the adult orthodontic patient may be missing one or more teeth. In addition, an adult restorative patient may have had prior bone loss and the periodontally involved teeth could be significantly mobile. If so, the purpose of retention is not only to stabilize the teeth and reduce mobility, but also to maintain posterior and anterior edentulous spaces until they are restored with either bridges or implants.

If a patient is missing three or more adjacent anterior or posterior teeth after orthodontic treatment, fixed retention is probably unlikely. Therefore a removable retainer with prosthetic teeth will be necessary to help stabilize the remaining teeth in that arch, as well as to provide an occlusal stop for teeth in the opposing arch (Fig. 26-24). However, when constructing the removable retainer, occlusal stops are necessary in order to prevent occlusal loads from damaging the edentulous ridge. These stops are constructed from wire and/

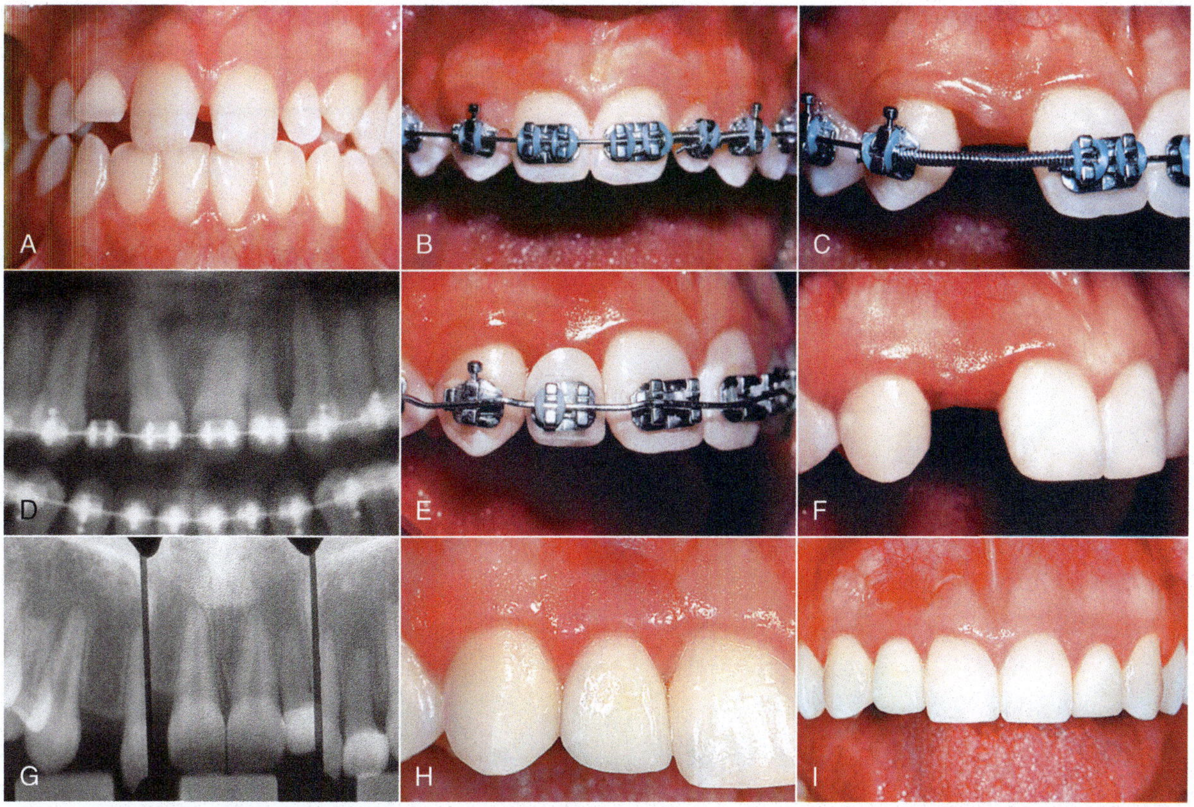

Figure 26-23 **A,** A 16-year-old female was congenitally missing her maxillary right lateral incisor and the left lateral incisor was malformed. The restorative plan involved restoration of the malformed left lateral incisor and placement of an implant and crown to replace the missing right lateral incisor. After **(B)** aligning the teeth and **(C)** opening space for the implant, **(D)** a progress radiograph was indispensable in determining **(E)** the appropriate tooth and root movement necessary to create the correct final **(F)** crown and **(G)** root position prior to **(H and I)** implant placement and restoration.

or acrylic and can cover the cingula of the anterior teeth or insert onto the occlusal surfaces of posterior teeth.

If one tooth is missing and an implant or bridge is planned to restore the edentulous space, a fixed bonded wire is more desirable for several reasons (see Fig. 26-24). First, the fixed retainer does not require patient compliance. Second, it can stop the opposing occlusion from overerupting. Third, teeth can be attached to the bonded wire to provide an esthetic temporary replacement for the patient. Whatever the choice of retainer, the important step is to make a decision about the responsibility for retention in perio-restorative patients prior to orthodontic treatment. It is much easier to coordinate the appointments and appliances if the team members make the decisions collectively, so that the patient will be provided with the optimum method of retention for his or her specific ortho-perio-restorative situation after appliance removal.

SUMMARY

This chapter discussed and illustrated a series of 10 guidelines for managing the orthodontic patient with periodontal or restorative complications. One of the most important steps is to generate realistic treatment objectives that will address the needs, desires, and financial capabilities of the patient and the goals of the team members. Then a visual representation of the final result must be created in the form of a diagnostic wax setup. This provides the blueprint or endpoint of treatment for the entire team. Next, the sequence of treatment must be established for patients who will require several steps performed by multiple team members at varying points during the treatment. This structured list of steps and responsibilities becomes the road map for treating the patient. Then the periodontal problems must be identified and the person responsible for the treatment of these soft tissue or osseous defects must be determined. If certain teeth are hopeless, the timing of extraction must be sequenced to facilitate the needs of all practitioners on the team. Prior to appliance placement, any malformed, abraded, or broken-down teeth should be built up to facilitate bracketing. The future position of teeth should be determined by the specific restorative or periodontal needs of the patient. If insufficient anchorage exists for tooth movement, implants could be considered for orthodontic as well as restorative anchorage during and after tooth movement. Prior to appliance removal, the orthodontist should ask the restorative dentist and/or periodontist to evaluate the patient's tooth position in order to achieve appropriate crown and root position for restorative treatment and to determine the type of retention necessary, especially for missing teeth prior to appliance removal. If the team of periodontist, surgeon, orthodontist, and restorative dentist follows these 10 guidelines, the management of ortho-perio-restorative patients will be simplified, predictable, and pleasurable.

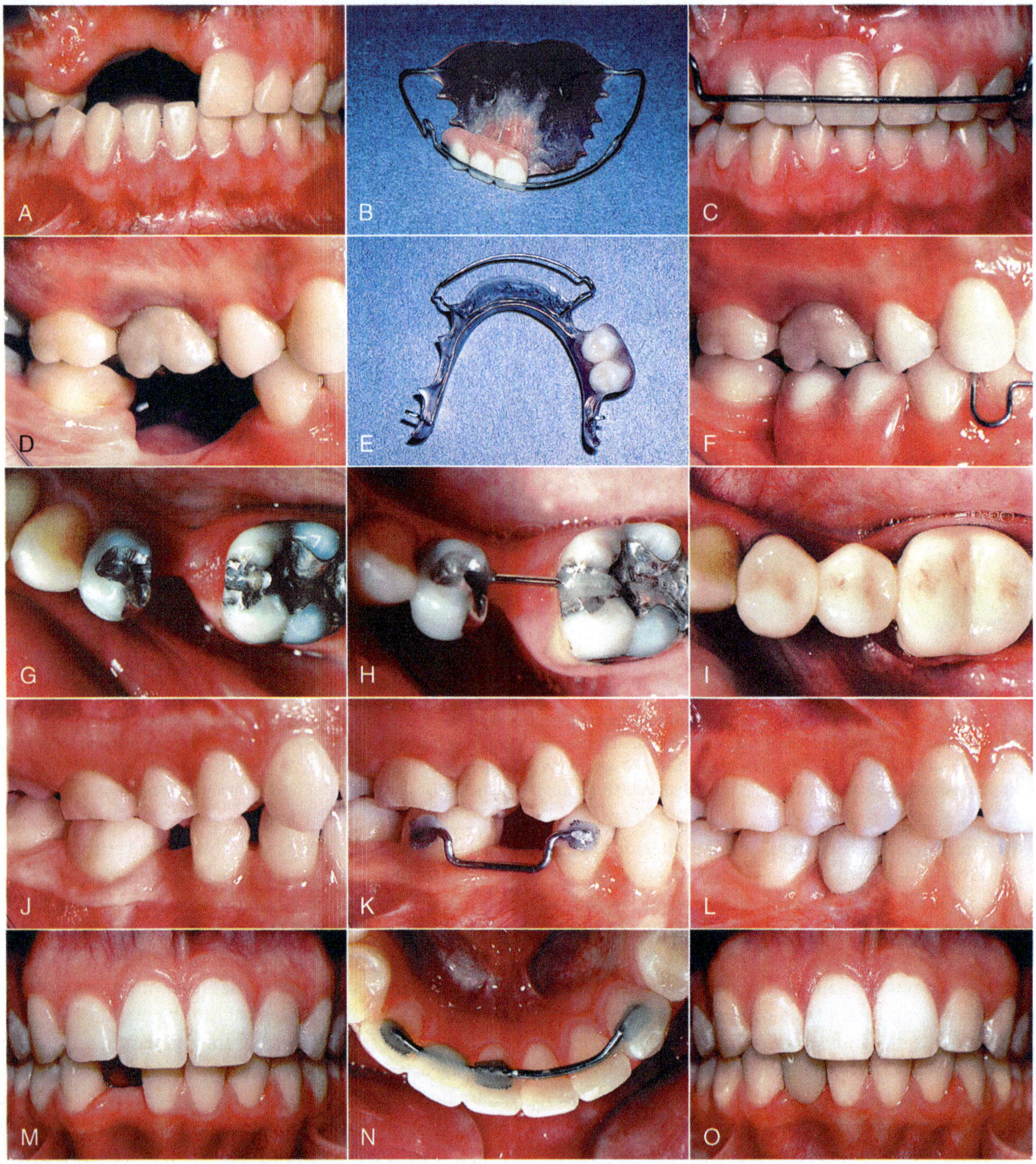

Figure 26-24 An important step in any interdisciplinary treatment plan is to select the appropriate method of retaining the orthodontic tooth movement prior to restoration. In patients who are missing several **(A–C)** maxillary or **(D–F)** mandibular teeth after orthodontic treatment, it may be prudent to maintain tooth position with a removable retainer with prosthetic teeth to establish satisfactory esthetics and function. If the patient will have a posterior fixed bridge placed after orthodontic treatment, **(G–I)** an intracoronal wire and acrylic splint is an excellent method to prevent supereruption of teeth in the opposing arch and to rigidly maintain tooth position prior to bridge construction. If an implant will be used to replace a missing mandibular second premolar after orthodontic treatment, it is advantageous to place **(J–L)** an extracoronal wire and acrylic splint to maintain the space rigidly during implant placement, osseointegration, and final restoration. If a mandibular incisor is missing and the space will be maintained after orthodontics, **(M–O)** a fixed mandibular lingual retainer with an attached tooth is a convenient method of retaining the space until the bridge or implant is placed.

REFERENCES

1. Kokich V, Spear F. Guidelines for managing the orthodontic–restorative patient. *Semin Orthod.* 1997;3:3–20.
2. Casko J, Vaden J, Kokich V, et al. American Board of Orthodontics grading system for dental casts and panoramic radiographs. *Am J Orthod Dentofacial Orthop.* 1999;114:18–23.
3. Mathews D, Kokich V. Managing treatment for the orthodontic patient with periodontal problems. *Semin Orthod.* 1997;3:21–38.
4. Kokich V. Anterior dental esthetics: an orthodontic perspective: III. Mediolateral relationships. *J Esthet Dent.* 1993;5:18–22.
5. Kokich V. Managing complex orthodontic problems: the use of implants for anchorage. *Semin Orthod.* 1996;2:153–160.
6. Kokich V, Nappen D, Shapiro P. Gingival contour and clinical crown length: their effects on the esthetic appearance of maxillary anterior teeth. *Am J Orthod.* 1984;86:89–94.
7. Kokich VG, Shapiro PA. Extraction of a mandibular incisor to facilitate orthodontic treatment. *Angle Orthod.* 1984;54:139–153.
8. Kokich V. The role of orthodontics as an adjunct to periodontal therapy. In: Newman MG, Takei HH, Carranza FA, eds. *Clinical Periodontology.* 9th ed. Philadelphia, PA: WB Saunders; 2002:704–718.
9. Kokich V. Esthetics: the orthodontic–periodontic–restorative connection. *Semin Orthod.* 1996;2:21–30.
10. Ingber J. Forced eruption: part I: a method of treating isolated one and two wall infrabony osseous defects—rationale and case report. *J Periodontol.* 1974;45:199–206.
11. Zachrisson B, Mjor I. Remodeling of teeth by grinding. *Am J Orthod.* 1975;68:543–553.
12. Spear F, Mathews D, Kokich V. Interdisciplinary management of single-tooth implants. *Semin Orthod.* 1997;3:35–74.
13. Lombardi R. The principles of visual perception and their application to dental esthetics. *J Prosthet Dent.* 1973;29:359–382.
14. Rufenacht C. Structural esthetic rules. In: Rufenacht C, ed. *Fundamentals of Esthetics.* Chicago, IL: Quintessence Publishing; 1992:67–134.
15. Esposito M, Ekkestube A, Grondahl K. Radiological evaluation of marginal bone loss at tooth surfaces facing single-tooth implants. *Clin Oral Implant Res.* 1993;4:151–157.
16. Thilander B, Odman J, Grondahl K, Friberg B. Osseointegrated implants in adolescents: an alternative in replacing missing teeth? *Eur J Orthod.* 1994;16:84–95.
17. Kokich V. Single-tooth implants: planning with the aid of orthodontics. *J Oral Maxillofac Surg.* 2004;62:48–56.
18. Creugers N, Kayser A, Van't Hof M. A seven-and-a-half year survival study of resin-bonded bridges. *J Dent Res.* 1992;71:1822–1825.
19. Boyer D, Williams V, Thayer K, Dennehy G. Analysis of debond rates of resin-bonded bridges. *J Dent Res.* 1993;72:1244–1248.
20. Kokich V. Orthodontic–restorative management of the adolescent patient. In: McNamara JA Jr, ed. *Orthodontics and Dentofacial Orthopedics.* Ann Arbor, MI: Needham Press; 2001:425–452.
21. Kokich V. Anterior dental esthetics: an orthodontic perspective: I. Crown length. *J Esthet Dent.* 1993;5:19–23.
22. Kokich VG, Kokich VO, Spear F. Maximizing anterior esthetics: an interdisciplinary approach. In: McNamara JA Jr, Kelly K Jr, eds. *Frontiers in Dental and Facial Esthetics.* Ann Arbor, MI: Needham Press; 2001:1–18.
23. Reitan K. Clinical and histologic observations of tooth movement during and after orthodontic treatment. *Am J Orthod.* 1967;53:721–745.
24. Stepovich M. A clinical study of edentulous closing spaces in the mandible. *Angle Orthod.* 1979;49:277–283.
25. Hom B, Turley P. The effects of space closure on the mandibular first molar area in adults. *Am J Orthod.* 1984;85:475–489.
26. ADA Council on Scientific Affairs. Dental endosseous implants: an update. *J Am Dent Assoc.* 2004;135:92–97.
27. Kokich V. Comprehensive management of implant anchorage in the multidisciplinary patient. In: Hiiguchi K, ed. *Orthodontic Application of Osseointegrated Implants.* Chicago, IL: Quintessence Publishing; 2000:21–32.
28. Block M, Hoffman D. A new device for absolute anchorage for orthodontics. *Am J Orthod Dentofacial Orthop.* 1995;107:251–258.
29. Kluemper GT, Spalding PM. Realities of craniofacial growth modification. *Atlas Oral Maxillofac Surg Clin North Am.* 2001;9:23–51.
30. Armbruster PC, Block MS. Onplant-supported orthodontic anchorage. *Atlas Oral Maxillofac Surg Clin North Am.* 2001;9:53–74.
31. Gray JB, Smith R. Transitional implants for orthodontic anchorage. *J Clin Orthod.* 2000;34:659–666.
32. Keles A, Erverdi N, Sezen S. Bodily distalization of molars with absolute anchorage. *Angle Orthod.* 2003;73:471–482.
33. Giancotti A, Greco M, Docimo R, Arcuri C. Extraction treatment using a palatal implant for anchorage. *Aust Orthod J.* 2003;19:87–90.
34. Celenza F. Implant-enhanced tooth movement: indirect absolute anchorage. *Int J Periodontics Restor Dent.* 2003;23:533–541.
35. Ohmae M, Saito S, Morohashi T, et al. A clinical and histological evaluation of titanium mini-implants as anchors for orthodontic intrusion in the beagle dog. *Am J Orthod Dentofacial Orthop.* 2001;119:489–497.
36. Kyung SH, Choi JH, Park YC. Mini-screw anchorage used to protract lower second molars into first molar extraction sites. *J Clin Orthod.* 2003;37:575–579.
37. Cheng SJ, Tseng IY, Lee JJ, Kok SH. A prospective study of the risk factors associated with failure of mini-implants used for orthodontic anchorage. *Int J Oral Maxillofac Implants.* 2004;19:100–106.
38. Chung KR, Kim YS, Linton JL, Lee YJ. The miniplate with tube for skeletal anchorage. *J Clin Orthod.* 2002;36:407–412.
39. Sherwood KH, Burch J, Thompson W. Intrusion of supererupted molars with titanium miniplate anchorage. *Angle Orthod.* 2003;73:597–601.
40. Sugawara J, Daimaruya T, Umemori M, et al. Distal movement of mandibular molars in adult patients with the skeletal anchorage system. *Am J Orthod Dentofacial Orthop.* 2004;125:130–138.
41. Smalley W. Implants for orthodontic tooth movement: determining implant location and orientation. *J Esthet Dent.* 1995;7:62–72.
42. Smalley WM, Blanco A. Implants for tooth movement: a fabrication and placement technique for provisional restorations. *J Esthet Dent.* 1995;7:150–154.
43. Roberts WE, Smith R, Zilberman Y, et al. Osseous adaptation to continuous loading of rigid endosseous implants. *Am J Orthod.* 1984;86:95–111.
44. Tarnow DP, Emtiaz S, Classi A. Immediate loading of threaded implants at stage 1 surgery in edentulous arches: ten consecutive case reports with 1 to 5-year data. *Int J Oral Maxillofac Implants.* 1997;12:319–324.
45. Piatelli A, Corigliano M, Scarano A, Costigliola G, Paolantonio M. Immediate loading of titanium plasma-sprayed implants: an histologic analysis in monkeys. *J Periodontol.* 1998;69:321–327.
46. Duyck J, Ronold HJ, Van Oosterwyck H, Naert I, Vander Sloten J, Ellingsen JE. The influence of static and dynamic loading on marginal bone reactions around osseointegrated implants: an animal experimental study. *Clin Oral Implants Res.* 2001;12:207–218.
47. Turley P, Shapiro P, Moffett B. The loading of bioglass coated aluminum oxide implants to produce sutural expansion of the maxillary complex in the pigtail monkey. *Arch Oral Biol.* 1980;25:459–464.

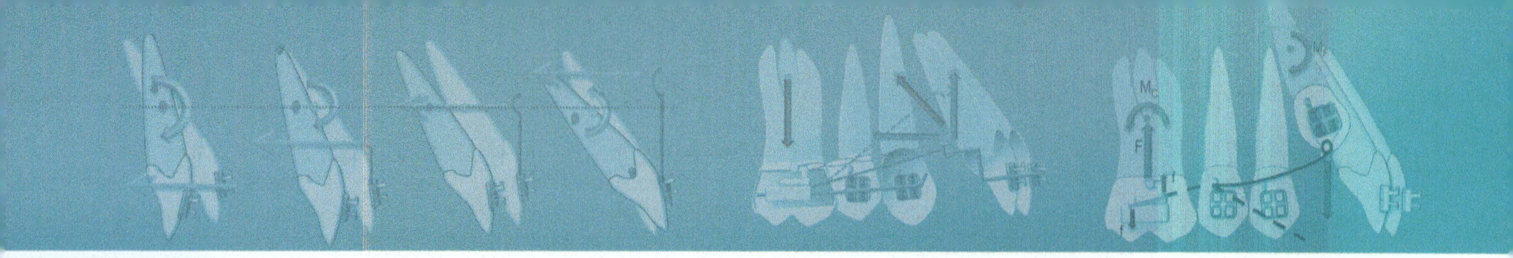

CHAPTER 27

Biomechanical Strategies for Optimal Finishing

Flavio Andres Uribe, Padma Mukherjee, and Ravindra Nanda

Orthodontic finishing is described as an "art" composed of individual perceptions and small detailing. Finishing distinguishes a true master of the profession from an average orthodontist. It is a critical step that involves fine-tuning individual tooth positions and intra-arch and inter-arch relationships and optimizes the treatment results.[1] This step can be especially challenging to the clinician since the minor changes performed generally are not appreciated by patients.

Finishing is the last phase of "active" treatment and thus is heavily dependent on the previous stages of treatment. It is extremely difficult, if not impossible, to achieve an acceptable end result when the treatment objectives have not been met and the mechanics have not been delivered properly. Major tooth movement should have been executed properly so that the minute tooth movements can be achieved with precision in the final finishing phase of treatment. When the treatment mechanics are less than optimal, the finishing stage often includes indiscriminate use of intermaxillary elastics and quick-fix therapies such as interproximal reduction. Although there are definite indications for these procedures, they should not be used routinely to compensate for deficiencies in treatment planning and/or application of mechanics. Overall, the finishing stage of treatment should be evaluated according to four major categories: intraoral, extraoral, radiographic, and functional objectives. In each category specific objectives must be met to obtain a desirable finish (Fig. 27-1).

INTRAORAL OBJECTIVES

Intraoral objectives are arguably the most important of the four major categories.[2] The intraoral objectives are classified into two subcategories: intra-arch and inter-arch objectives. The primary objective in both is to achieve ideal occlusion with well-aligned arches. Most of these intraoral objectives are described in the American Board of Orthodontics (ABO) grading criteria.[2]

Intra-Arch Analysis

Each tooth must be evaluated with reference to its first-, second-, and third-order position. When evaluating the first order, teeth should have no rotations and have tight interproximal contacts.[1] In addition, tooth morphology must be taken into consideration and the cusp tips and fossae should follow the perfect arch form. An occlusal mirror can be very useful to identify minor rotations and buccolingual displacement of teeth outside of the perfect arch form (Fig. 27-2). The upper first molar has special considerations regarding its first-order position. A mesial-out rotation of the mesiobuccal cusp[3] is considered to be ideal. It has also been advocated that the buccal surface of the upper first molar should be parallel to the palatal suture (Fig. 27-3).[4]

In the second order, the root parallelism and marginal ridges are evaluated. The marginal ridges should be at the same level, particularly in the buccal segments. Often when marginal ridges between adjacent teeth coincide, root parallelism also will. A panoramic x-ray is an adjunct to evaluate second-order discrepancies. In extraction cases, a small degree of crown tipping most likely will occur and root parallelism will be required. Small adjustments in the second-order angulation of the anterior teeth (i.e., accentuating the distal tip) can help to decrease any excess space in the anterior region (Fig. 27-4).[1] The third order is most relevant to the inter-arch objectives (i.e., the occlusal relationship) and to the esthetics of the smile (an extraoral category, discussed below). Regarding the intraoral objectives, a small curve of Monson between the buccal segments allows for proper occlusal function (i.e., adequate intercuspation without balancing interferences). An accentuated curve of Monson usually results in balancing interferences, especially in the second molar area.[5] This clinical situation is commonly encountered in adults after the dental correction of buccal crossbites without expansion of the basal bone and palatal suture (Fig. 27-5). Proper third-order angulation of anterior teeth is also important for good occlusion (Fig. 27-6). Furthermore, regarding the extraoral category, third-order

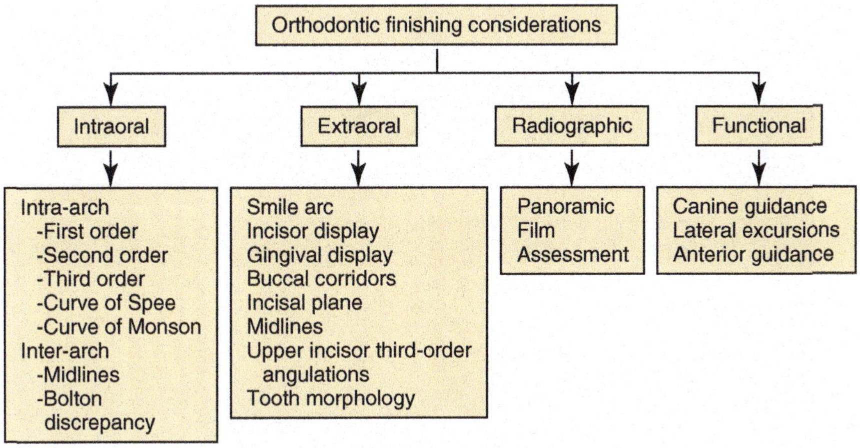

Figure 27-1 Systematic approach to finishing.

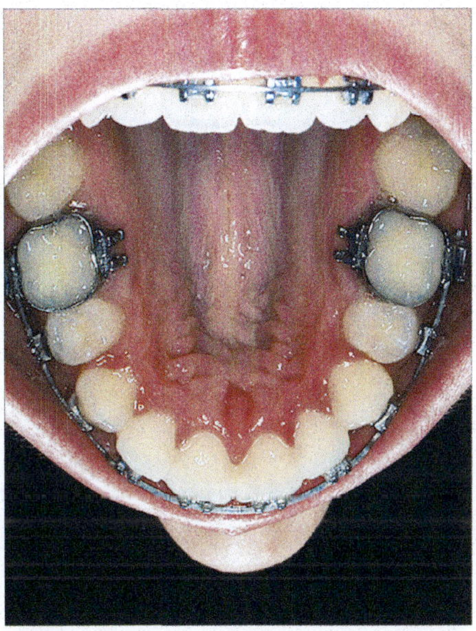

Figure 27-2 Occlusal mirror used as an aid to evaluate intra-arch discrepancies during finishing. This view is used to identify first-order rotations, spacing, and any arch form problems.

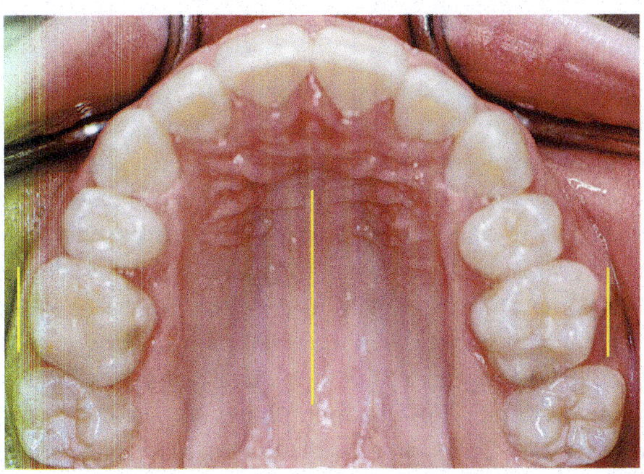

Figure 27-3 Occlusal view of a finished case where the buccal surface of the upper first molar is parallel to the midpalatal raphe.

angulation is important for good esthetics of the smile (Fig. 27-7).[1] Significant emphasis on the upper canine and first premolar third-order inclination has been proposed by some clinicians.[6] In general, the buccal surfaces of these teeth should be close to parallel to the midsagittal facial line in an ideal smile.

The final intra-arch objective is to achieve a gentle curve of Spee from the anterior teeth to the posterior buccal segments.[1] The magnitude of this curve will vary depending on the overbite (inter-arch relation) and incisor display (an extraoral objective, discussed below).

Inter-Arch Analysis

The first molars and canines are the most important teeth to evaluate regarding the interocclusal relationship. Traditionally, orthodontists have classified malocclusion in the anteroposterior dimension and thus the static analysis of the occlusion has primarily been based on the first molar relationship. Additionally, the canine is of primary importance if canine-guided functional occlusion is to be achieved. The main objective is to "seat" the canines in a Class I relationship and obtain good coupling with the antagonistic canines. This ideal interocclusal relationship is difficult to achieve when a significant tooth size discrepancy exists between the dental arches (i.e., a Bolton discrepancy).[7] The upper lateral incisors and lower second premolars are usually responsible for this inter-arch tooth size discrepancy,[8] as abnormal tooth morphology is more common in these teeth. This results in less than ideal occlusion, such as a Class II canine tendency on that side, that becomes apparent during finishing (Fig. 27-8).

Two types of occlusion have been considered ideal: cusp-to-fossa and cusp-to–interproximal space relationships. In the natural dentition, a cusp-to–interproximal space relationship is most characteristic.[3] The lingual cusps in the upper arch and the buccal cusps in the lower arch are primarily responsible for function. The buccal cusps of the upper premolars and the lingual cusps of the lower premolars should occlude in the interproximal space. In Class II

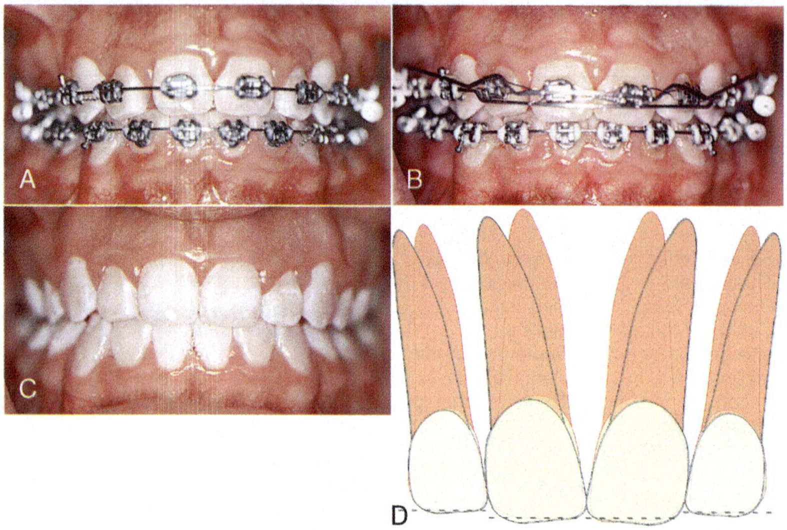

Figure 27-4 **A–C,** Patient shows no overjet but excess space between the incisors due to a Bolton discrepancy. These spaces can be closed or reduced by accentuating the distal root tip of the incisors, thereby increasing the interproximal contact distance. Incisal adjustments (enamoplasty) were done at the appliance removal visit. **D,** Diagram showing the distal tip and enamoplasty required.

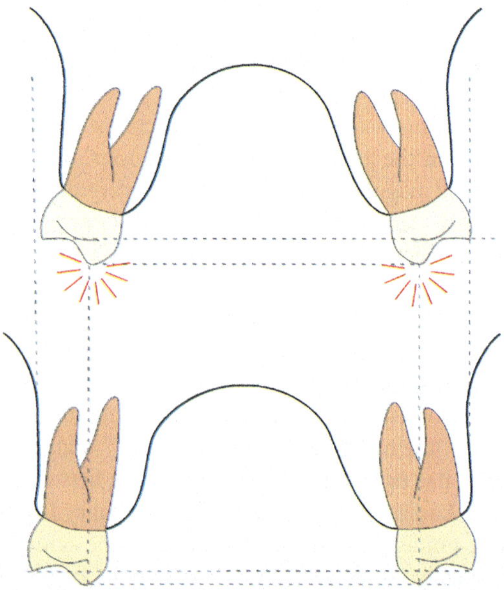

Figure 27-5 Proper third-order angulation needed in the posterior buccal segments may not be achieved in adults after arch width expansion without surgery. Occlusal balancing contacts may result from the dental third-order compensation. The lower diagram shows the difference in skeletal width and vertical cusp position that can be achieved with skeletal expansion.

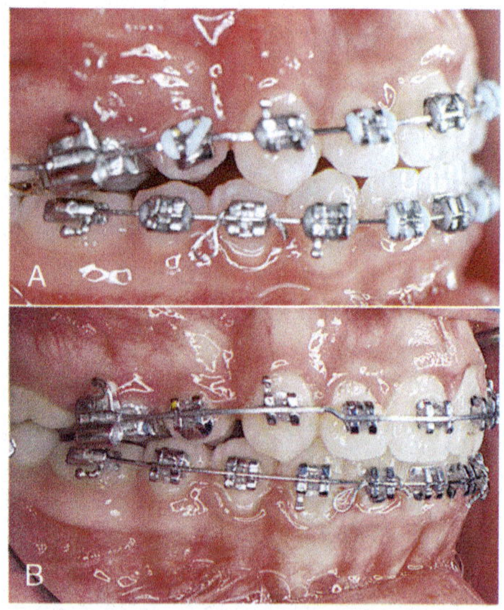

Figure 27-6 **A and B,** Patient showed an improvement in the occlusion after proper third-order angulation of the anterior teeth was obtained.

patients, some of the anteroposterior correction can be achieved by overrotation of the buccal cusps of the upper premolars distally to coincide with the lower interproximal spaces.[9,10] In the anterior segment, overbite and overjet are the most critical factors in achieving a proper interocclusal relationship. These two occlusal traits determine the disclusion of the posterior teeth during protrusive movements. More than 50% overbite may be excessive, as the contact of the lower incisors on the lingual surface of the upper incisors in these patients would not be on the cingulum (the most suitable portion to receive occlusal forces). Finally, it is important that the lingual surface of the upper incisors be properly inclined to allow the lower incisors to slide anteriorly in an angle that is in synchrony with the articular eminence.[11]

Arch coordination is also evaluated from the frontal view. This allows proper cusp seating to be visualized. The intercanine and inter-molar widths should be coordinated to prevent excessive buccal overjet or a buccal crossbite tendency. The premolar area is also inspected transversely for proper coordination between the upper and lower arches.

Midlines are also used to evaluate interocclusal relationships. During finishing, minor midline problems should be addressed. Any discrepancy >2-mm should have been addressed during the previous phases of treatment. A discrepancy of 1- to 2-mm or more between the midlines is usually due to a tooth size discrepancy and will probably result in an inadequate occlusal relationship, at least in one

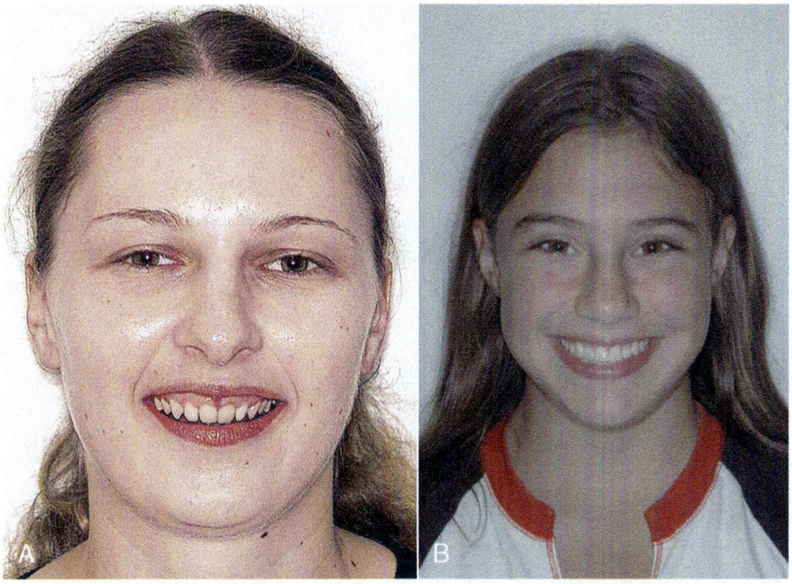

Figure 27-7 Depending on the upper anterior third-order angulation, light is reflected differently in the frontal view. **A,** Patient with retroclined incisors. Note the light reflected in the periodontal tissues. **B,** Patient with proper incisor inclination. Note the light reflected in the middle third of the incisors.

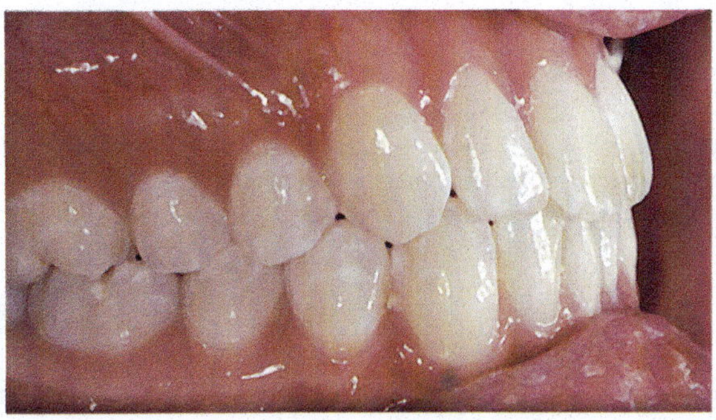

Figure 27-8 Bolton discrepancy reflected in the occlusion in the finishing stage. There is a tendency toward a Class II canine relationship due to the small upper laterals.

of the buccal segments (Class II or Class III on one side) (Fig. 27-9). The midline objectives in the finishing stage are evaluated in the extraoral finishing category as well, particularly in the upper arch.

EXTRAORAL OBJECTIVES

The extraoral objectives are based on esthetic concepts, with the majority of these concerning the smile. The key factors within the smile that must be addressed are smile arc, incisor display, gingival display, buccal corridors, incisal plane, midlines, upper incisor third-order inclination, and tooth morphology in the esthetic zone.

Smile Arc

The ideal smile arc is discussed in Chapter 1. In the finishing stage, little can be done to significantly affect the smile arc. Small finishing bends can differentially extrude or intrude the anterior teeth but that is about all that can be accomplished. The dilemma concerning these wire bends is the potential for antagonistic effects on the interocclusal finishing objectives. An example of this is seen when the overbite is perfect and the teeth need to be extruded to achieve an ideal smile arc. A choice between achieving an esthetic objective (ideal smile arc) and an occlusal objective (ideal overbite) is needed. A compromise might be the best decision. In such situations the initial objectives of the individual treatment plan must be reviewed. More importantly, a limit to the amount of compromise for each characteristic should be set (i.e., avoiding finishing with >50% overbite and a flat or reverse smile arc).

Incisor Display

On average, females show 2- to 3-mm of incisor at rest and 1-mm of gingiva when smiling.[12] Males show approximately 1-mm less incisor in each of these lip positions. During the diagnosis and treatment planning phases, an appropriate plan for correction of any deviation should be made. By the finishing phase of treatment the vertical incisor objectives should have already been accomplished. Detailing in this area should be limited to proper alignment and leveling of the incisal edges (provided no restorations are needed). Attempting to significantly intrude or extrude the incisors may complicate and prolong treatment.

Open-bite malocclusions with moderate to excessive incisor display present a challenge, as they are difficult to correct. It is not unusual to find an open-bite tendency still present at the finishing phase in this type of malocclusion. If no additional upper incisor display is desired, the overbite correction should be done by extruding the lower anterior teeth. This can be accomplished by accentuating the lower curve of Spee.

Gingival Display

The amount and characteristics of the gingival display (symmetry and height relationships of adjacent teeth) are

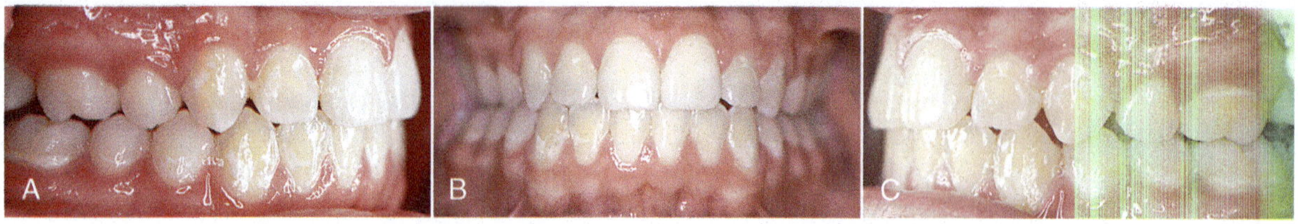

Figure 27-9 **A–C,** Midline discrepancy of approximately 2-mm to the right. A tendency toward a Class III canine occlusion is seen on the left side.

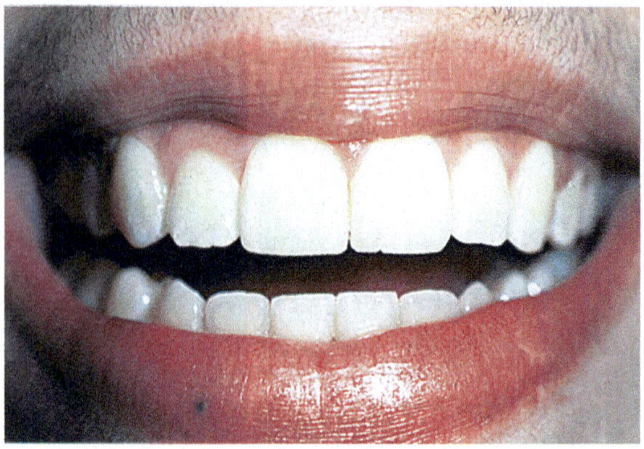

Figure 27-10 Finished treatment in a young female patient who displays the upper gingiva on smiling. An asymmetry in the gingival heights of the lateral incisors is evident.

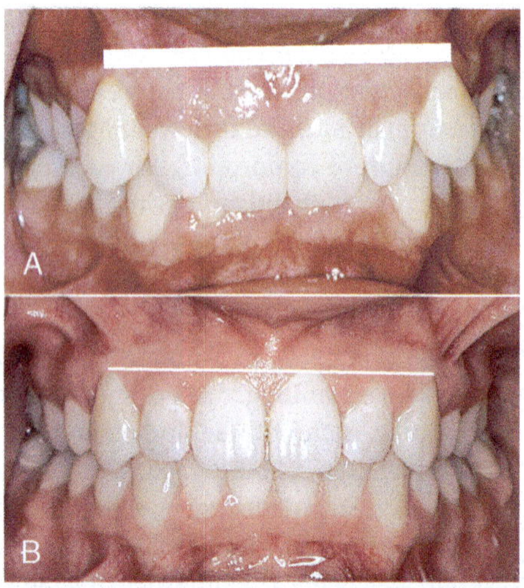

Figure 27-11 **A,** Incisal edges reflect the discrepancies in the gingival heights provided that no incisal wear is present. **B,** Correction of the incisal edges generally results in adequate gingival heights.

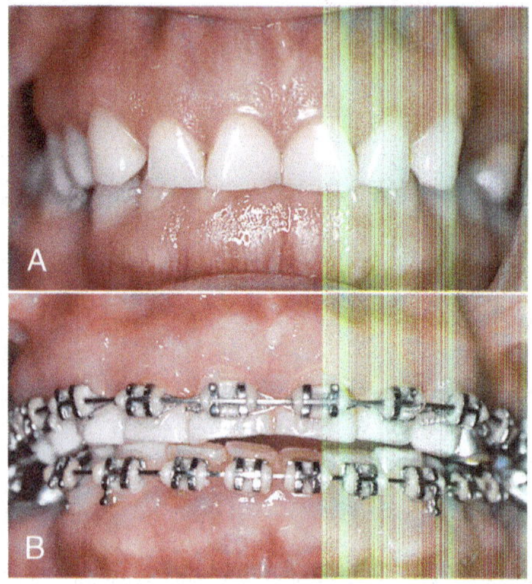

Figure 27-12 **A,** Inadequate gingival height in the upper anterior region with excessive overbite and worn incisors. **B,** Intrusion mechanics of the four upper anterior teeth to obtain proper gingival heights. Restoration of the incisors is needed to achieve adequate proportions and overbite.

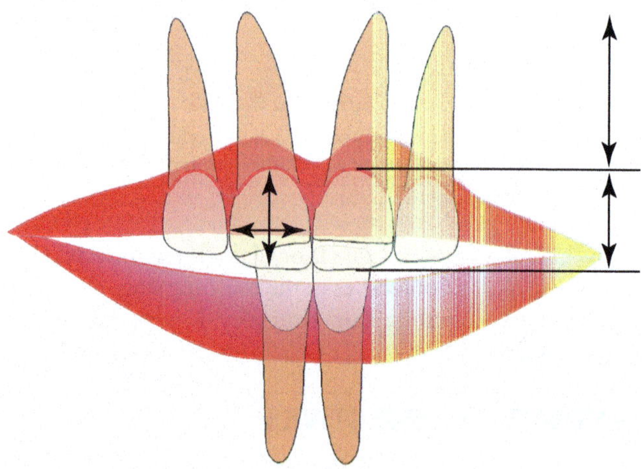

Figure 27-13 Factors involved in the final incisal edge position. The interrelationship of gingival height, tooth proportions, lip to tooth relationship, crown/root ratio, and overbite determines the position of the upper incisor in space.

important aspects to consider in a smile. Generally, males do not show any marginal gingiva when smiling. Females, on the other hand, display approximately 1-mm of gingiva on smiling.[13] Symmetry in the gingiva and proper gingival height relationships in the upper arch are important considerations during initial bracket positioning and final finishing repositions (Fig. 27-10).

During finishing, gingival display and symmetry can be altered within a narrow range of approximately 1-mm by selective intrusion or extrusion of any of the anterior teeth. Most frequently, the incisal edges will reflect gingival height asymmetries provided that incisal wear is not present (Fig. 27-11). The overbite will be the limiting factor of the magnitude of the finishing bends. However, if wear is present, the gingival height relationship will determine the finishing movements of the anterior teeth in the vertical dimension, instead of it being determined by the level of the incisal edges (Fig. 27-12).[14] The final incisal edge position, if there is significant incisal wear, is determined by proper tooth proportions, gingival heights, relationship to the upper lip, crown/root ratio, and overbite (Fig. 27-13).

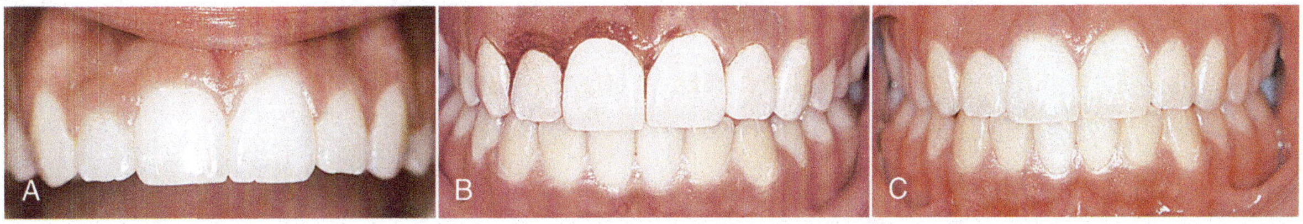

Figure 27-14 Asymmetrical gingival heights. **A,** Upper right lateral incisor has a more coronal gingival height. The upper right central incisor also has a slight coronal relationship of the gingival margin compared with its contralateral tooth. **B,** Gingivectomy performed on the upper right central and lateral incisors. **C,** Postsurgery.

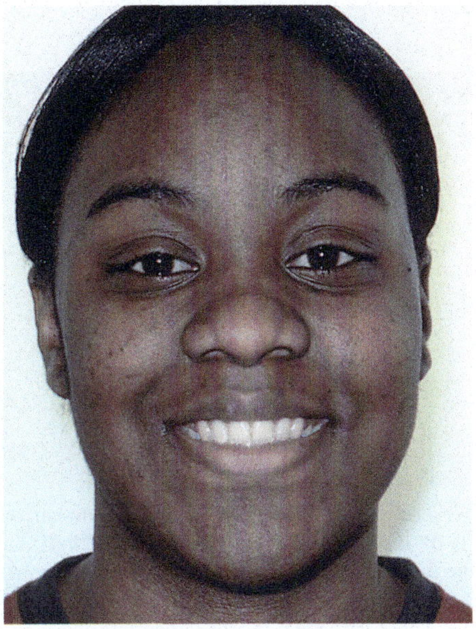

Figure 27-15 Excess gingival show on the upper buccal segments. Gingival heights are adequate from canine to canine. A smoother transition from the canine to the first premolar can be obtained through periodontal surgical procedures.

Periodontal procedures should be considered as an adjunct to the esthetic objectives after finishing in patients with an excessive gingival display or asymmetrical gingival heights. The periodontal procedures that can be considered are gingivectomy or crown lengthening (depending on the alveolar bone level) (Fig. 27-14). These procedures may also be combined with prosthetic alternatives in patients with worn incisal edges or abnormally shaped incisors (i.e., peg laterals).

A common unesthetic result after gingivectomies or crown lengthening (performed exclusively in the anterior segment) is seen in the transition area from the canine to the premolars. Ideally, there should be a 1-mm step down in gingival height between these teeth. When gingivectomies are not carried to the premolars, excess gingiva remains more pronounced in the corners of the smile (Fig. 27-15).[15]

In the literature little attention has been given to the gingival heights of the lower teeth. Symmetry and gingival height of the lower incisors in relation to the canines are important factors, especially in individuals over 30 years of age, as the lower gingival margin is more visible.[12] It is not uncommon to find a discrepancy in gingival heights between the lower incisors and the canines, particularly in deep bite patients (Fig. 27-16). In young patients, the gingival margin usually follows the incisal edges of the lower anterior teeth. This problem is corrected as the canines and central incisors are leveled during the initial phases of orthodontic treatment. In the adult, wear facets can complicate the determination of where proper gingival heights should be located. As the incisors supraerupt, a good incisal edge relationship with the canines will exist but a significant discrepancy in the gingival height will develop. To correct this discrepancy a decision must be made from the following choices: gingivectomy/crown lengthening to match gingival heights with no restorations, gingivectomy/crown lengthening and restorations (composites or veneers or crowns), intrusion of the four anterior teeth to level the gingival heights (no surgery), and restorations (composites, veneers, or crowns). A very important additional factor in deciding among these alternatives is the crown/root ratio. Any osseous resective periodontal procedure (crown lengthening) increases this ratio; therefore a good assessment of the eventual remaining root structure is required (Fig. 27-17).

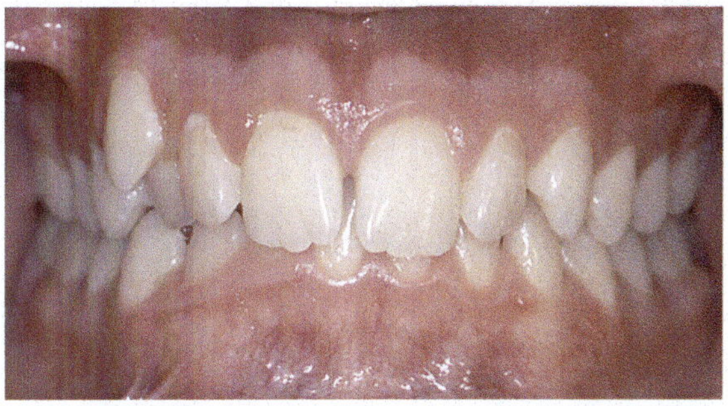

Figure 27-16 Discrepancy between the gingival heights of the lower incisors and the canines. Supraeruption of the lower incisors is evident at the incisal edges and is reflected on the overbite.

Buccal Corridors

The esthetic objective of widening the narrow buccal corridors, if indicated (see Chapter 1), should have been achieved long before the finishing stage. Any type of arch expansion during the finishing stage is difficult to achieve and unstable in the long-term.

Incisal Plane

In the frontal view, a cant in the upper incisor segment is sometimes found during finishing procedures. This cant may be limited to the incisor segment or involve the entire

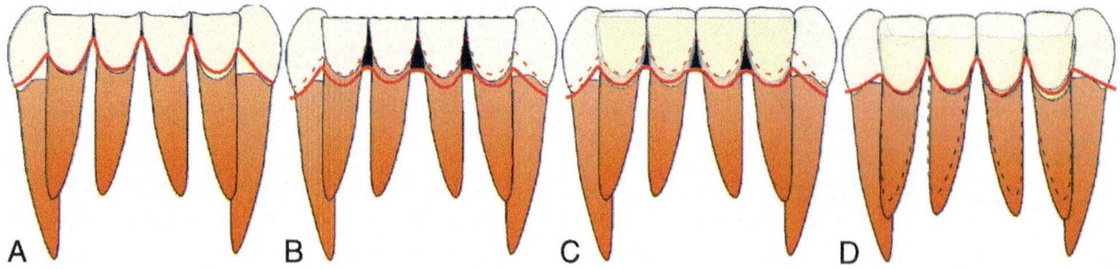

Figure 27-17 **A,** Significant attrition with supraeruption of the lower incisors. Different treatment modalities include the following. **B,** Gingivectomy/crown lengthening to match the gingival heights. As the gingival margin is brought down, a more tapered crown morphology is observed. Black triangles may result with this alternative. **C,** Gingivectomy/crown lengthening with additional restorations (crowns or veneers). The crown morphology is restored to normal tooth proportions and the crown/root ratio is increased. **D,** Orthodontic intrusion plus restorative procedures. The crown/root ratio is more favorable.

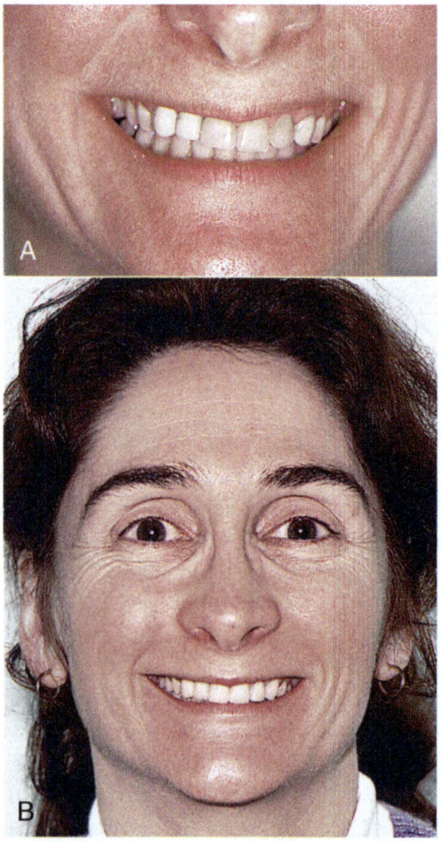

Figure 27-18 **A,** Occlusal cant of the maxilla evidenced on the left side. Gingiva is displayed only on the left side in relation to the labial commissure. **B,** Cant was camouflaged by prosthodontic work. Crowns were elongated on the right side and shortened on the left. Interproximal contacts were made more parallel to the facial midline.

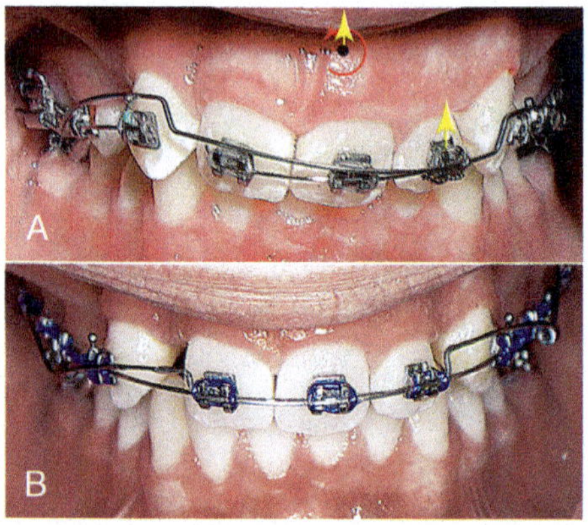

Figure 27-19 Asymmetrical intrusion arch placed to correct the incisal cant. **A,** A 0.017-inch × 0.025-inch nickel-titanium (Ni-Ti) intrusion arch is tied to the distal aspect of the upper left lateral incisor. A continuous 0.017-inch × 0.025-inch stainless steel segment from the upper right central incisor to the upper left lateral incisor is tied into the brackets of these teeth. The force system produces an intrusive force *(yellow arrows)* and a moment at the center of resistance *(red curved arrow)* of the anterior segment. **B,** Correction seen 1 month later. The cant was corrected and the midline discrepancy had improved.

maxillary arch. The incisal cant can be the result of incorrect bracket positioning, asymmetrical mechanics, or a true maxillary skeletal cant that was undetected during diagnosis due to dental compensations. Therefore a differential diagnosis between a dental and a skeletal incisal cant is important.

Patients who have an incisal cant due to a skeletally canted maxilla generally present with uneven heights between the labial commissure and the occlusal surfaces of the premolars (Fig. 27-18). This can also be identified by an uneven gingival display between the left and right sides when smiling. Care must be taken when developing a differential diagnosis between a true maxillary cant (skeletal etiology) and an asymmetrical smile (soft tissue etiology). A true maxillary cant is difficult to correct and, when the discrepancy is excessive, a maxillary Le Fort I osteotomy may be the best treatment. Other alternatives may involve periodontic and prosthodontic options to camouflage the cant (see Fig. 27-18, B).

In patients where the cant involves only the anterior teeth, corrections in the finishing stage are difficult but possible. An option is to place an intrusive force on the area that needs to be intruded (Fig. 27-19).[16,17] If the rotation of the anterior segment needs to be around the center of resistance, two cantilevers (with equal and opposite forces that produce a couple) may be placed to achieve intrusion of one side and extrusion of the opposite side (Fig. 27-20, A). A second method to achieve rotation around the center of resistance is to place a cantilever in an auxiliary tube of the anterior segment (Fig. 27-20, B).

Midlines

A discrepancy between the upper and lower dental midlines is generally most noticeable at the end of treatment. Coincidentally, it is also at this time that this problem is most difficult to correct. To achieve coincident midlines during

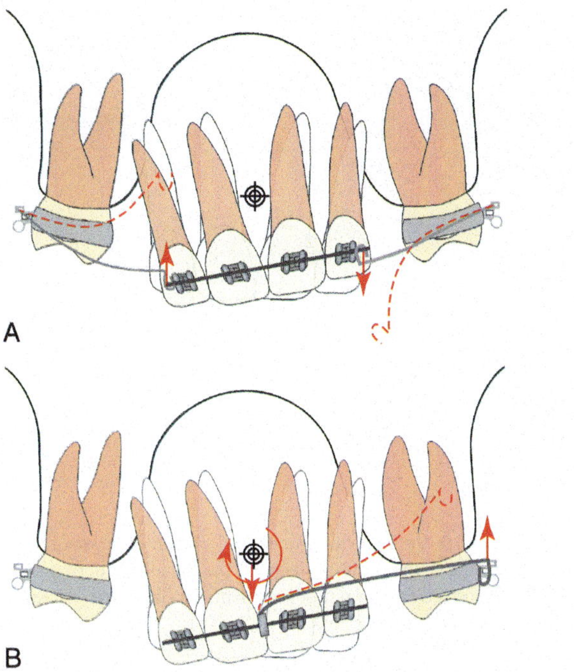

Figure 27-20 **A,** Moment produced by two cantilevers with the same amount of force in opposite directions. **B,** Moment produced by a cantilever with the single couple tied to an auxiliary tube in the anterior segment. A transpalatal arch is used in both situations as a solid anchor unit to minimize the side effects.

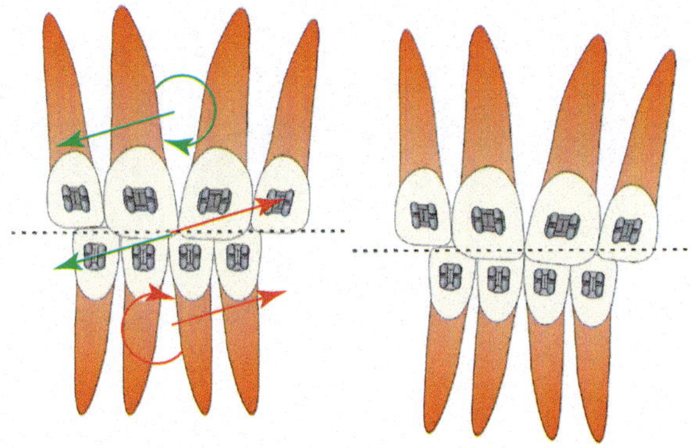

Figure 27-21 Vertical effects produced by an anterior cross elastic. The vertical component of the elastic force to correct midline discrepancy may produce canting of the incisal plane.

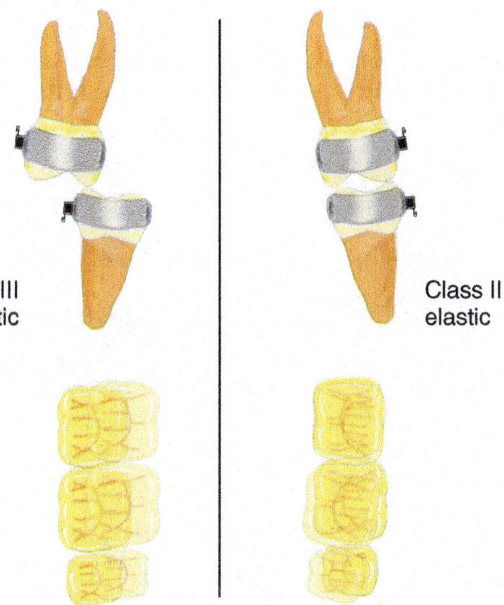

Figure 27-22 Class II and Class III elastics produce rotation around the y axis. Brodie bite tendency is seen on the Class III elastic side and a crossbite tendency is seen on the Class II elastic side.

finishing, the range of correction for each arch is approximately 1-mm to each side. Tipping is the major type of tooth movement that can be used to correct midlines at the finishing stage. It is important to stress that a slight discrepancy between the upper midline is esthetically acceptable[18–20] and generally does not have any functional implications.

On occasion there is a relationship between an incisal cant and a midline discrepancy. By correcting the incisal cant the midline problem may be improved (see Fig. 27-19), although in some instances the midline discrepancy might be accentuated. It is important to consider all smile characteristics together; correction of one characteristic should maintain, if not improve, the others.

The techniques used to correct midline problems during the finishing phase mainly rely on the use of anterior cross elastics. In some instances a combination of Class II elastics on one side and Class III elastics on the other side can be used. This method seems easy but can result in serious side effects if used indiscriminately. The orthodontist must watch for the side effects that may occur in the vertical and transverse planes with this method of long-term elastic use. In the vertical direction, canting of the occlusal plane as a result of the vertical component of the anterior cross elastic force may occur (Fig. 27-21). In the transverse plane, rotation of the dental arches around the y axis with the use of Class II or Class III elastics may result in a crossbite tendency on one buccal segment and a Brodie bite tendency on the other (Fig. 27-22).[21]

A final method to correct the dental midline in the finishing stage is the use of a cantilever with the active force along the x axis. The upper anteriors are treated as a segment and a force is applied at the bracket level of this segment. The anchor unit (posterior segment) is made up of the molars and premolars. A palatal arch is used to offset the rotational moment and lingual force on the anchor unit where the cantilever (couple side) is inserted (Fig. 27-23).

Upper Incisor Third-Order Inclination

Esthetic considerations of the upper incisal inclination are important not only from the profile view, but also from the frontal view. A common occurrence in the final stages of treatment, particularly in extraction cases, is excessive lingual crown torque. Although this is easily visualized in the lateral view, it can also be appreciated in the frontal view.[22] Third-order tooth corrections are difficult and time-consuming movements.

Extensive bone remodeling needs to occur as root correction is pursued and side effects such as upper molar mesial

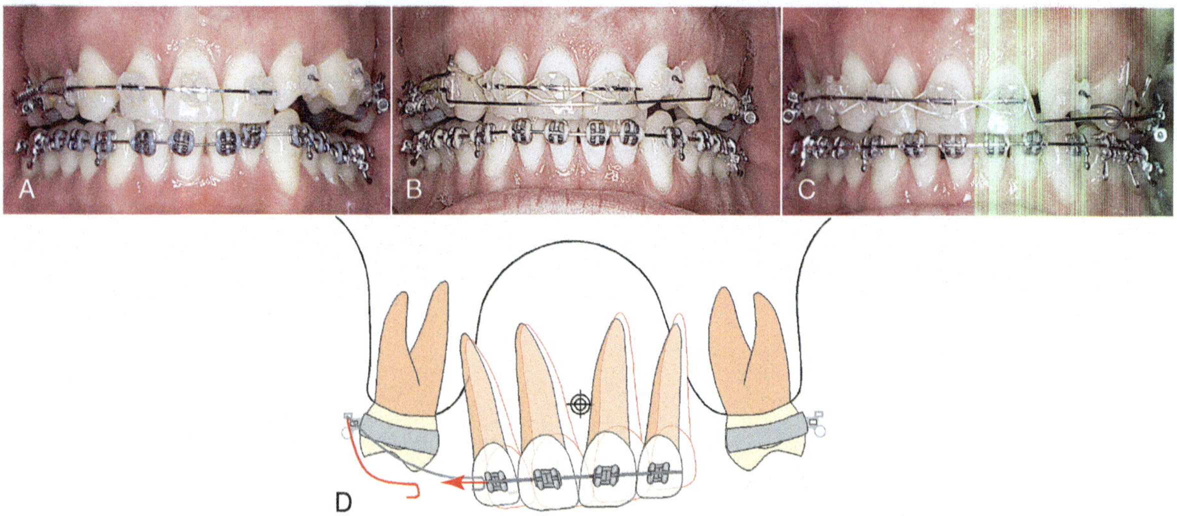

Figure 27-23 Method for correction of small midline deviations. **A,** Upper incisors tipped to the left with a midline deviation of approximately 2-mm. **B,** Force system in place (see **D** for detailed illustration.). A transpalatal arch offsets the moment on the posterior segment (mesial in). A continuous base arch bypassing the incisors aids in preventing their extrusion as they tip. The cantilever can be tied directly to the anterior segment. An elastic was placed for patient comfort. **C,** Force from the cantilever tips the teeth in the direction of the midline correction. **D,** Force system.

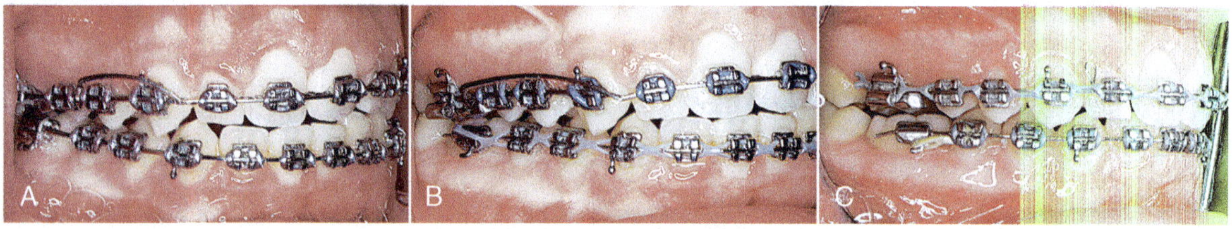

Figure 27-24 **A,** Upright upper incisors with anterior crossbite tendency. The torquing spring produces an anterior moment and an extrusive force needed in the anterior segment. The upper arch is laced together to prevent anterior spacing. **B,** Correction seen after 1 month. **C,** Final correction achieved in approximately 3 months.

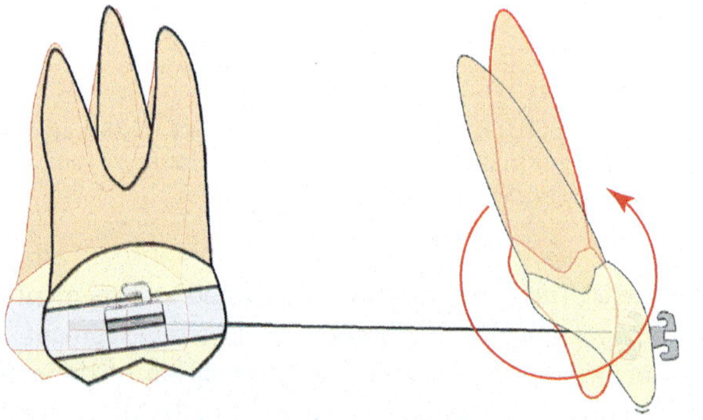

Figure 27-25 Rowboat effect produced by the lingual root correction moment (facial crown movement).

migration become common. Perhaps the best way to approach this objective is by maintaining a proper moment/force ratio during the retraction phase in extraction cases.[23] Some of the alternative mechanics in the finishing phase include auxiliary torquing springs (Fig. 27-24). Care must be taken to prevent the incisors from flaring if only root correction is needed. This can be achieved by cinching the archwires or lacing together the entire arch. The clinician must also be aware of the rowboat effect that is generated with root correction (Fig. 27-25).[24] Simultaneous use of Class II elastics is recommended to prevent this effect. Additionally, a mild bowing of the anterior segment with the torquing spring is expected due to the intrusive lateral forces on the posterior segment.

Tooth Morphology

Tooth morphology in the anterior or esthetic zone is of primary importance. The upper lateral incisors most often exhibit abnormal morphology in this zone. It is less common to find abnormally shaped central incisors. Preliminary planning regarding the space distribution for restoring teeth with abnormal morphology should be accomplished during the diagnosis and treatment planning phase. Involving a restorative dentist and a periodontist during the treatment planning phase is a good practice. In the finishing phase, communication within the team is crucial and will help to determine any precise finishing orthodontic tooth movements needed. Many of the restorative procedures should be done in conjunction with periodontal procedures to achieve the best tooth proportions.

Tooth proportions are influenced by the position of the gingival margin as well as the width and height of the tooth. These factors can be affected by the restorative dentist in conjunction with the periodontist. The shape of the incisor and the restorative option (composite buildup, veneers, or

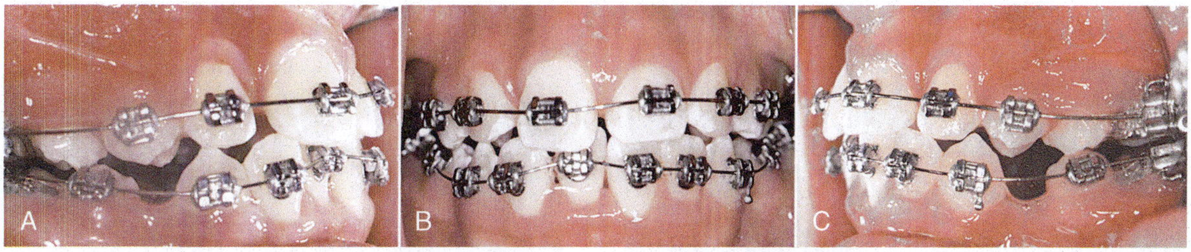

Figure 27-26 **A–C,** Early contouring of the canines to resemble lateral incisor morphology.

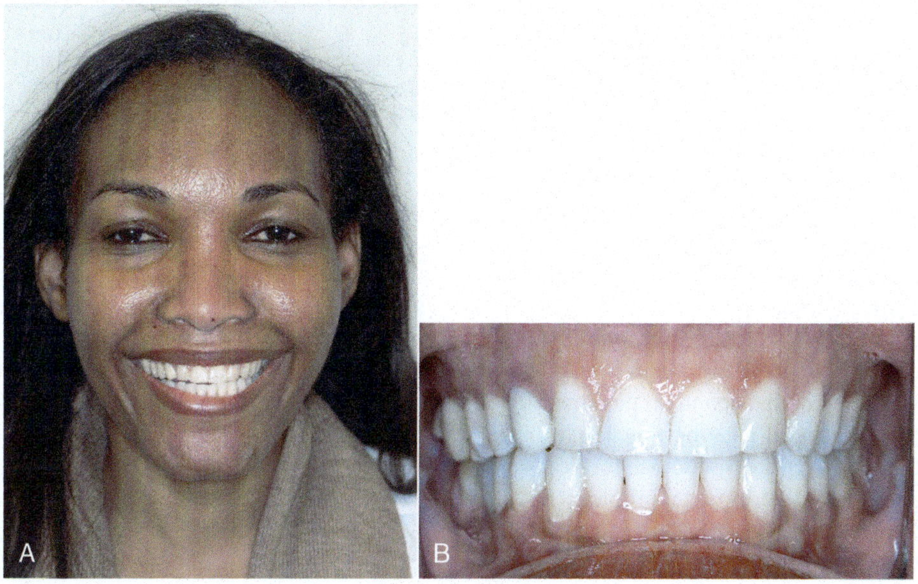

Figure 27-27 **A,** Patient with canine substitution showing good esthetic results. **B,** Note the reduced canine prominence and the similar emergence profile of a maxillary lateral incisor.

crowns) will determine the position of the abnormally shaped lateral incisor within the dental arch.[15]

It is of primary importance in achieving excellent esthetic results that good communication is maintained with the restorative dentist. Slight contouring of the incisal edges of the upper anterior teeth, especially the canines, has been recommended at the end of treatment for most patients.[25] The incisal edges of the anterior teeth with a small incisal edge fracture can also be contoured after previous extrusion. The gingival height relationship to the adjacent tooth may be altered with the extrusion of the incisor; thus an additional gingivectomy or crown lengthening procedure may be indicated if the patient displays gingiva on smiling. In patients with congenitally missing lateral incisors that have been treated by canine substitution, the alteration of canine morphology to mimic a lateral incisor is usually done in the early stages of treatment, with small detailing left for the finishing stages (Fig. 27-26). The premolars that substitute for canines also need to be contoured on the lingual cusps to avoid balancing interferences. One important consideration often overlooked in the esthetics of canine substitution is the emergence profile of the canine. To replicate the anatomy of the lateral incisor, significant lingual root torque is necessary in the canine. This small detail enhances the possibility of mimicking the lateral incisor and allows the restorative dentist to achieve a better esthetic result (Fig. 27-27).

The final situation in which abnormalities in tooth morphology are considered during finishing is the pronounced lingual fossae of the upper incisors. This abnormal crown morphology is found most frequently in Asian and African populations.[26] In these patients the mesial and distal ridges adjacent to the fossa are pronounced and prevent a good intercuspation in the buccal segments. It is recommended that the height of these ridges should be reduced to achieve better posterior occlusion.

RADIOGRAPHIC OBJECTIVES

Just before starting the finishing stage of treatment, it is always recommended that a panoramic radiograph be taken to evaluate root angulation and root parallelism. Problems in second-order angulation of the upper lateral incisors, lower premolars, and teeth adjacent to the extraction sites are commonly found (Fig. 27-28). Clinically, marginal ridge discrepancies are also a good method to detect possible root angulation discrepancies. However, the panoramic radiograph provides better evidence of root position, angulation, and parallelism.

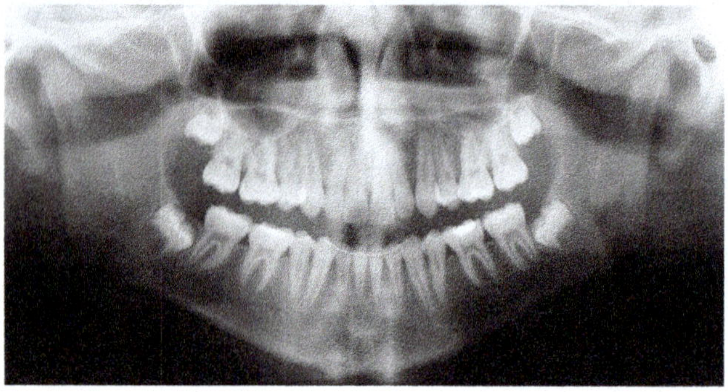

Figure 27-28 Finished four-premolar-extraction (upper first premolars and lower second premolars) patient with poor root alignment of the lower first premolars and upper laterals.

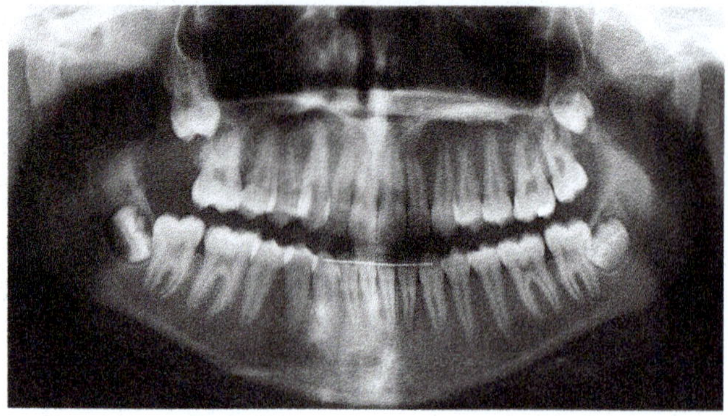

Figure 27-29 Panoramic x-ray should be taken before appliance removal to evaluate root apices, root parallelism, and status of unerupted teeth. This panoramic x-ray reveals an abnormally erupting second molar, which was noticed only after appliance removal.

Root angulation problems observed in the finishing panoramic radiograph might also be related to abnormal tooth morphology and/or bracketing errors. This is especially evident in the buccal segments, where it is difficult to gain access for bracket placement and premolars with abnormal crown morphology are common.

Root parallelism is important for three reasons. First, the occlusal load of the forces will be transmitted properly across the longitudinal axis of the tooth. Second, in patients where only the crown has been tipped and the root is not in its proper position, there is a greater potential for relapse.[27] Finally, there is a potential for periodontal problems due to root proximity. However, the rationale for this last statement is not well supported by the literature; no deleterious effects on the periodontium have been found in finished orthodontic cases with root proximity.[28]

The finishing panoramic radiograph is also helpful in evaluating root resorption. If external apical root resorption is observed, the orthodontist may want to decrease the length of time spent on the finishing stage. Although monitoring for root resorption has been recommended during the first 6 months of treatment,[29,30] usually it is noticed on the finishing panoramic radiograph.

Finally, two other important pieces of information can be obtained from a panoramic radiograph: evidence of any deterioration in periodontal health and the eruption angle of the third molars. If the eruption of the second molars is delayed or the orthodontic treatment is being finished before complete eruption of the second molars, it is important to evaluate their position and the eruption pattern (Fig. 27-29).

Periapical radiographs are usually indicated only in the finishing stage to obtain a more detailed view of any significant findings observed in the panoramic radiograph, such as extensive root resorption, root parallelism between adjacent teeth to an implant site, or evidence of periodontal bone loss.

FUNCTIONAL OBJECTIVES

A proper functional occlusion is the goal in every orthodontic treatment. However, as mentioned in Chapter 1, the definition of an ideal functional occlusion is not completely clear. In general, a mutually protected occlusion is considered the ideal goal.

To achieve this ideal occlusion during the finishing stage, it is important to have the maximum amount of normal occlusal contacts during maximum intercuspation. Although a coinciding centric relation with centric occlusion is the goal proposed by some clinicians, a small discrepancy between these two occlusal relationships is acceptable (long centric).[11]

With lateral movements of the jaw, a canine disclusion is the standard, although group function is acceptable. More importantly, no balancing contacts should be present. Canine disclusion is also a major protective factor in patients who receive any type of anterior esthetic restorations (veneers, composites, or porcelain crowns). Finally, the anterior teeth should disclude the posterior teeth during protrusive movements. All of these movements should be evaluated during the finishing stage and proper adjustments in crown angulations (relative to tip and torque) should be achieved. Small adjustments can be made after appliance removal (e.g., occlusal adjustments with rotary instruments); however, these should be minimal, as there is a limit to the amount of tooth structure that can be removed.

OVERCORRECTION

Rotational Correction

During finishing, the concept of overcorrection can be applied to the alignment (first-order corrections) and to certain malocclusions.[10,31–33] It is believed by some that overcorrection of rotated teeth, especially in the anteroinferior segment of teeth, may be necessary for stability. Since the amount of, and to a certain extent the direction of, rotational relapse is unpredictable,[34] this practice may not be indicated.

Vertical Correction

Overcorrection in some malocclusions, such as open-bite and deep bite cases, may be beneficial. This process ideally should begin during initial bracket placement but even

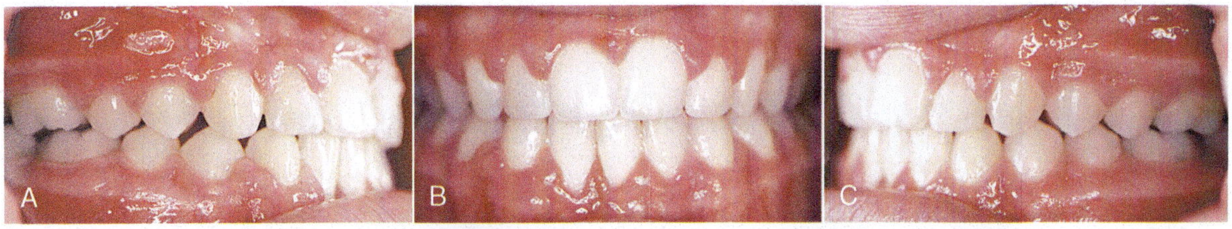

Figure 27-30 **A–C,** Patient with a lower incisor extraction finished with an ideal overjet but a Class III tendency on the right side and poor interdigitation. Gingival contours are not ideal, especially in the area of incisor extraction.

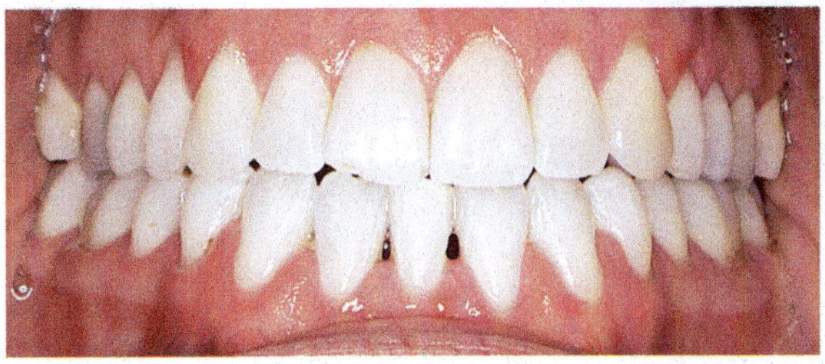

Figure 27-31 Black triangles are often seen in adult patients who have lower incisor extraction. The canine overjet is excessive.

during the finishing stage the clinician can fine-tune the process. Brackets on the anterior teeth could be placed 0.5-mm more gingival in cases with an open-bite tendency and 0.5-mm more incisal in deep bite cases.

UNIQUE FINISHING SITUATIONS

Lower Incisor Extraction

Lower incisor extraction treatment introduces a Bolton (tooth size) discrepancy that complicates orthodontic finishing. If no tooth size discrepancies are present (i.e., excessive tooth mass in the lower arch), the patient will generally finish with either a Class I canine relationship with excessive overjet or an ideal overjet and a Class III canine tendency relationship (Fig. 27-30).

Another problem frequently observed with incisor extractions is that the patient ends up with black interproximal triangles in the lower incisor segment (Fig. 27-31). To solve this problem, slight interproximal enamel reduction and/or root reapproximation on the lower teeth is done to move the contact more gingivally and to decrease the size of these black triangles. To some degree this procedure will accentuate the overjet because more tooth structure is removed from the lower anterior incisors, thus increasing the inter-arch tooth size discrepancy. Finally, major efforts should be made to coordinate the arches as the lower incisor extraction space is closed. Lower incisor extraction also results in a decrease in the intercanine distance[35] and thereby an excessive canine overjet could occur (see Figs. 27-30, B, and 27-31).

Finishing with Primary Teeth

Finishing can be challenging when a patient is missing permanent teeth (most commonly second premolars) and has overretained or ankylosed primary molars. Some advocate extraction of the primary molar and closure of the space while others believe that the primary molar should be kept for as long as possible and then be restored with an implant or bridge on its eventual loss.[36] The extent of finishing and detailing would depend on the initial treatment objectives of the individual case and any planned compromises in the buccal segment occlusion should be discussed with the patient and/or parent.

Bypassing Debilitated Teeth during Finishing

In certain clinical situations, after taking a finishing panoramic radiograph there may be evidence of localized root resorption. Two options are available: minimize the time spent on the finishing stage or bypass the affected tooth in order to avoid any force that will perpetuate the root resorption. Figure 27-32 illustrates the latter option during finishing. Sound biomechanical principles should be used to achieve the desired tooth movement with minimum side effects (the ideal objective during finishing).

Canine Substitution of Missing Lateral Incisors

When canines replace lateral incisors, it is difficult to adjust their morphology to resemble that of lateral incisors. Ideally, the majority of the canine contouring should have been accomplished in the early phases of treatment. During finishing, only minor contouring should be done in consultation with the restorative dentist.

One of the most challenging esthetic concerns for the restorative dentist in these situations is the gingival heights. In a patient with normal gingival architecture, the premolar that is replacing the canine usually has a gingival height that is 1- to 1.5-mm occlusal than that of the canine, and the canine's gingival height is usually at the same level of the central incisor. To achieve proper gingival heights, the canine substituting the lateral incisor morphology should be extruded slightly (approximately 0.5- to 1.0-mm) and for the premolar replacing the canine, the only option is a periodontal resective procedure.

However, this periodontal procedure must be done with caution, as the anatomic crown height of the premolar is much smaller than that of the canine and such a procedure may end up exposing the cementum on the facial aspect of the premolar.

Another challenge with canine substitution concerns lingual cusp contouring of the upper first premolar. This cusp should be reduced mainly for functional reasons to avoid balancing interferences during disocclusion. Care should be taken not to remove excessive amounts of tooth structure, in order to avoid postoperative sensitivity.

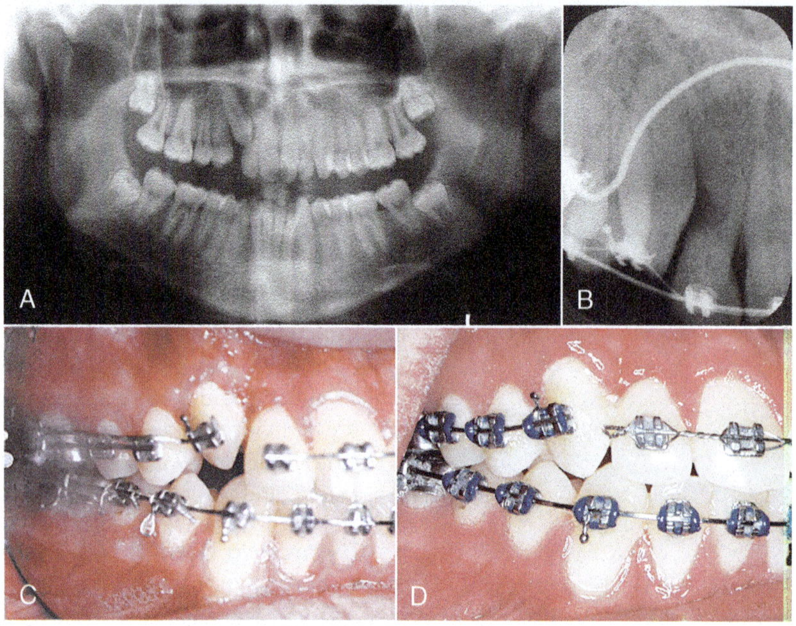

Figure 27-32 **A and B,** Patient with extensive root resorption on the upper right lateral tooth. **C,** This tooth was bypassed using segmental mechanics to position the canine in the arch. A 0.017-inch × 0.025-inch stainless steel segment was placed from the upper right first molar to the first premolar. A transpalatal arch *(not seen)* connected this segment to the other side of the arch. A 0.017-inch × 0.025-inch CNA beta-titanium segment was tied from the molar to the canine. The resultant geometry of the two-couple force system produced a distal crown tip and intrusive force on the canine in the second order. The intrusive force was counteracted by a vertical elastic. **D,** Canine correction in 4 weeks. Finishing detailing for the canine was done by sectioning the wire without engaging the upper right lateral incisor.

Edentulous Site for an Implant

One of the most common mistakes made when an edentulous space is prepared to receive an implant is to leave inadequate space. The minimum space that should be opened for an implant is approximately 6-mm. This measurement derives from the 3.5-mm mesiodistal width of the fixture and the 1-mm mesial and distal space to the fixture for a papilla in the interproximal space.[37]

The restorative dentist encounters not only a space problem at the coronal level, but also a root angulation problem of the teeth adjacent to the implant site at the apical level. Since the space is usually achieved by a push coil mechanism at the coronal level, the roots of the teeth tip into the implant space (Fig. 27-33). During finishing, adequate moments for root correction should be placed in these adjacent teeth to achieve the minimum 6-mm distance throughout the entire implant site. It is important to note that new developments in implant fixture shape (anatomically shaped implants) allow more leeway in this respect (Fig. 27-34). The key to success in such a multidisciplinary case scenario is coordination between the orthodontist, oral surgeon, and prosthodontist.

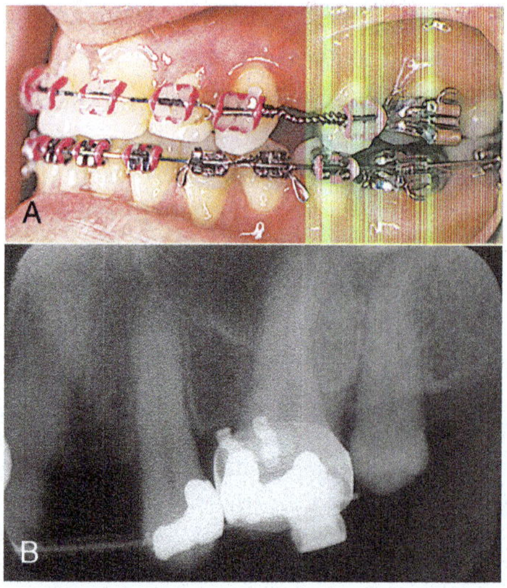

Figure 27-33 **A,** Push coil mechanism pushes the crown apart and the roots together. **B,** X-ray depicts the root convergence with no space in the apical portion to place an implant.

INTERPROXIMAL REDUCTION DURING FINISHING

Interproximal tooth reduction generally has been advocated where tooth size discrepancies exist and in some instances it has been recommended during finishing. This procedure is used to achieve a better occlusal relationship in the finishing stages.[25] Since the amount of interproximal enamel reduction is limited, it should be noted that tooth size discrepancies should be evaluated during the diagnosis phase to avoid last-minute quick-fix solutions in the finishing stage and to prevent long-term tooth sensitivity. Thus a slight interproximal reduction of certain teeth with abnormal morphology contributing to the discrepancy, usually between the upper lateral incisors and the lower second premolars,[8] can be done selectively instead of reducing teeth indiscriminately as a result of inappropriate diagnosis and treatment planning.

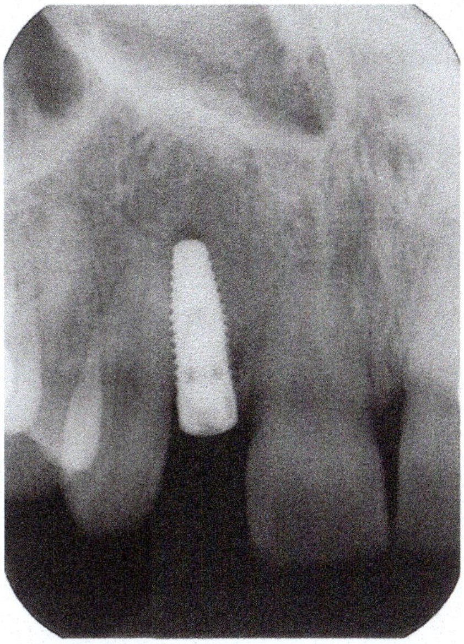

Figure 27-34 Anatomically shaped implants may allow fixture placement in sites where adjacent roots converge.

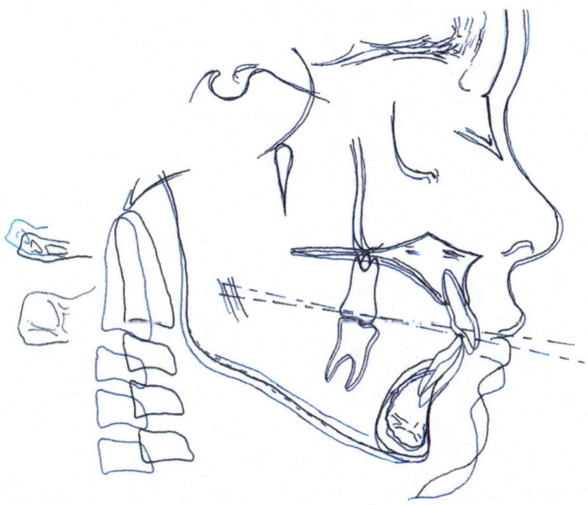

Figure 27-35 Treatment changes with Class II mechanics. Occlusal plane changes and retroclined and extruded upper incisors *(treatment changes in blue)* are seen.

FINISHING WITH CLASS II MECHANICS

Usually, in Class II mechanics using elastics or inter-arch Class II appliances, correction of the malocclusion is achieved by rotating the occlusal plane in a clockwise direction. As a result, the maxillary incisors finish with a retroclined angulation (Fig. 27-35). To address this problem, torque needs to be applied to the anterior teeth. This can be accomplished using a bracket prescription with an excessive amount of torque for the anteriors (i.e., 17 degrees or more) or by applying buccal crown torque to the archwire (via individual bends or adding a gentle curve of Spee). Another method involves using a torquing spring that adds a moment to the teeth that will correct the root angulation (see Fig. 27-24).

FINISHING SEQUENCE

Figure 27-1 provides a schematic outline and checklist that clinicians can use to address finishing in orthodontics. Third-order objectives during finishing should be addressed first since these usually take the most time to correct. The buccolingual inclination of the upper anterior segment is important in the finishing stage for occlusal and esthetic reasons. Proper incisor inclination is a key factor in achieving good buccal occlusion and an esthetic smile.

The major factors involved in achieving this proper anterosuperior incisor inclination are the bracket and wire coupling. Therefore, depending on the existing buccolingual inclination of the tooth and the relation of the bracket to the occlusal plane, a specific archwire with a medium-to-low load deflection rate (such as a 0.017-inch × 0.025-inch beta-titanium CNA archwire; Ortho Organizers Inc., San Marcos, CA.) can be selected. For example, if a patient has a lingual inclination of the crowns of the upper incisors, a counterclockwise moment given by the coupling between the wire and the bracket is needed to achieve a proper buccolingual inclination. Another option is to increase the dimension of the rectangular wire in a preadjusted bracket system (e.g., 0.021-inch × 0.025-inch in a 0.022-inch slot size bracket) while trying to maintain a medium load deflection (achieving the desired moment) or adding bends to the existing archwire to create the couple. Other options include selecting the proper prescription for patients in whom loss of third-order control in the incisors is anticipated or changing from a 0.022-inch slot to a 0.018-inch slot in the anterior segment. Torque is affected significantly by archwire dimension and edge shape as well as by bracket slot dimension.[38]

In the straight-wire appliance, proper third-order angulation can be achieved through rectangular archwires engaged into prescription brackets that can then express the torque of the appliance. For additional third-order correction on specific teeth, a 0.019-inch × 0.025-inch beta-titanium CNA (Ortho Organizers Inc.) is recommended. Third-order bends are placed in this archwire, which provides an adequate load-deflection rate[39] to achieve proper buccolingual inclination.

After the third-order objectives are met, second-order movements are addressed. Adjustments in this plane take a significant amount of time because they also involve root correction. To achieve second-order objectives, either with a 0.016-inch × 0.022-inch beta-titanium CNA (Ortho Organizers Inc.) or a 0.016-inch steel round archwire can be used, provided that all third-order objectives have been met. This allows marginal ridge discrepancies and root parallelism problems to be corrected.

The final step in finishing is the correction of first-order problems. Usually these problems are obvious clinically and can be corrected quickly. In many instances only small correction bends in the archwire are needed. Correction can also be achieved with auxiliary plastic rotation wedges on the brackets or by making small bends in either the 0.016-inch

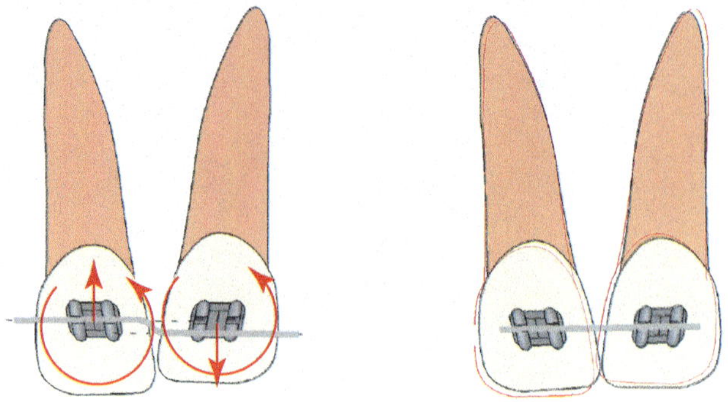

Figure 27-36 Step bends on the finishing wires can produce undesirable side effects.

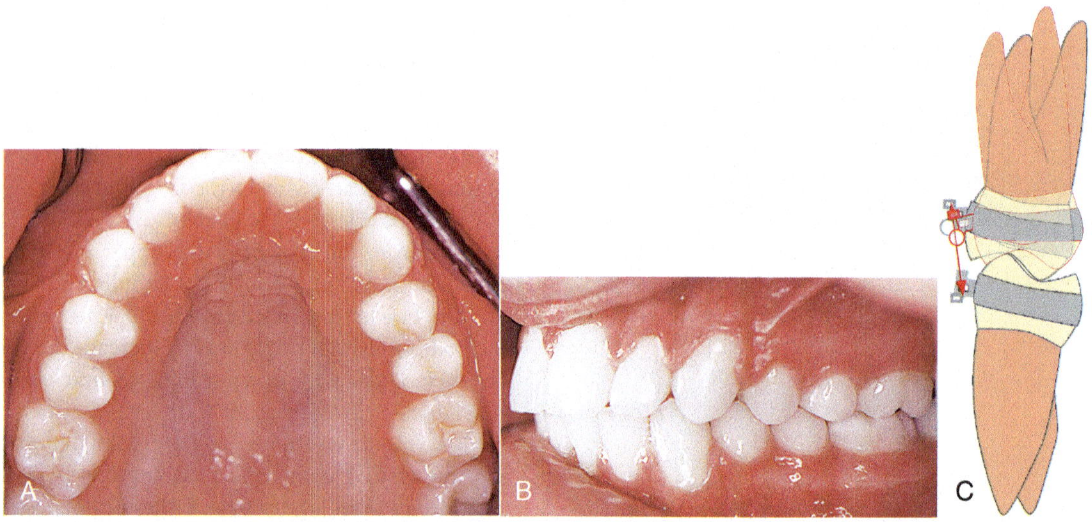

Figure 27-37 **A,** Long-term (6 weeks or more) vertical elastics with no or very light wires used to seat the occlusion may affect the upper arch form. **B,** Good buccal occlusion obtained at the expense of the arch form and **(C)** the third order of the upper left first premolar.

× 0.022-inch beta-titanium CNA (Ortho Organizers Inc.) or the 0.016-inch steel archwire.

All of the finishing bends placed in an archwire will result in either a V-bend or a step bend.[40] Care must be taken, as all of these bends will have vertical side effects and rotational tendencies on the adjacent teeth (Fig. 27-36).

Inter-arch objectives are the last to be addressed in the finishing stage. In many instances the intra-arch adjustments mentioned above will result in a good occlusion. To achieve good final intercuspation of the buccal segments, vertical elastics may be worn for a short period of time, usually 2 to 3 weeks.

It is important to note that although some orthodontists expect settling of the occlusion to occur during retention, the amount of settling is unpredictable[41] and in some patients it may not occur. Care must also be taken with the elastics in the finishing stages. Prolonged wear of vertical elastics with light or no archwires may result in deformation of the arch form and/or lingual inclination of the teeth (Fig. 27-37) as a result of the elastic force applied buccally to the center of resistance (see Fig. 27-37, C).

SUMMARY

The literature addressing the topic of orthodontic finishing is scarce. Most of the approaches and theories on finishing are anecdotal and subjective in nature. This supports the idea that orthodontic finishing is predominantly an art rather than a science. The common consensus on guidelines to evaluate finishing are described by the ABO standards. The evaluation is based on intraoral criteria and does not incorporate esthetic or functional objectives. This chapter provides an overview of the most important aspects of finishing using sound biomechanical principles. The goals for each of the four categories (intraoral objectives, extraoral objectives, radiographic objectives, and functional objectives) are described. The key to good orthodontics relies heavily on the diagnosis, treatment planning, and application of good mechanics. The key to excellence in orthodontics lies in the ability to identify and correct the small details needed for a perfect smile with an ideal occlusion.

REFERENCES

1. Andrews LF. The six keys to normal occlusion. *Am J Orthod.* 1972;62:296–309.
2. Casko JS, Vaden JL, Kokich VG, et al. Objective grading system for dental casts and panoramic radiographs. American Board of Orthodontics. *Am J Orthod Dentofacial Orthop.* 1998;114(5):589–599.
3. Bennett JC, McLaughlin RP. First molars. In: Bennett JC, McLaughlin RP, eds. *Orthodontic Management of the Dentition with Preadjusted Appliance.* St. Louis, MO: Mosby; 2002:281–310.
4. McNamara JA Jr. Transpalatal arches. In: McNamara JA Jr, Brudon WL. *Orthodontics and Dentofacial Orthopedics.* Ann Arbor, MI: Needham Press; 2001:199–209.

5. McNamara JA Jr. The transverse dimension. In: McNamara JA Jr, Brudon WL. *Orthodontics and Dentofacial Orthopedics*. Ann Arbor, MI: Needham Press; 2001:97–110.
6. Zachrisson BU. Making the premolar extraction smile full and radiant. *World J Orthod*. 2002;3:260–265.
7. Bolton WA. The clinical application of a toothsize analysis. *Am J Orthod*. 1962;48:504–529.
8. Smith SS, Buschang PH, Watanabe E. Interarch tooth size relationships of 3 populations: "does Bolton's analysis apply?" *Am J Orthod Dentofacial Orthop*. 2000;117:169–714.
9. Swartz M. Comprehensive fixed appliance therapy. In: McNamara JA Jr, Brudon WL, eds. *Orthodontics and Dentofacial Orthopedics*. Ann Arbor, MI: Needham Press; 2001:149–168.
10. JCO interviews Dr. Bjorn U. Zachrisson on excellence in finishing, part 1. *J Clin Orthod*. 1986:20(7):460–482.
11. Ash MM, Ramfjord S. *Occlusion*. 4th ed. Philadelphia, PA: WB Saunders; 1995.
12. Vig RG, Brundo GC. The kinetics of anterior tooth display. *J Prosthet Dent*. 1978;39:502–504.
13. Tjan AH, Miller GD, The JG. Some esthetic factors in a smile. *J Prosthet Dent*. 1984;51(1):24–28.
14. Kokich VG, Spear FM. Guidelines for managing the orthodontic-restorative patient. *Semin Orthod*. 1997;3(1):3–20.
15. Poling R. A method of finishing the occlusion. *Am J Orthod Dentofacial Orthop*. 1999;115:476–487.
16. van Steenbergen E, Nanda R. Biomechanics of orthodontic correction of dental asymmetries. *Am J Orthod Dentofacial Orthop*. 1995;107: 618–624.
17. Nanda R, Margolis MJ. Treatment strategies for midline discrepancies. *Semin Orthod*. 1996;2(2):84-89.
18. Johnston CD, Burden DJ, Stevenson MR. The influence of dental to facial midline discrepancies on dental attractiveness ratings. *Eur J Orthod*. 1999;21(5):517–522.
19. Kokich VO, Kiyak HA, Shapiro PA. Comparing the perception of dentists and lay people to altered dental esthetics. *J Esthet Dent*. 1999;11: 311–324.
20. Beyer JW, Lindauer SJ. Evaluation of dental midline position. *Semin Orthod*. 1998;4:146–152.
21. Burstone CJ. Diagnosis and treatment planning of patients with asymmetries. *Semin Orthod*. 1998;4:153–164.
22. Peluso C, Kuhlberg A. The axial inclination of central incisors and its effects on the perception of the facial profile. Paper presented at: Annual American Dental Association Meeting; October 2002; Memphis, TN.
23. Uribe F, Nanda R. Treatment of Class II, Division 2 malocclusion in adults: biomechanic considerations. *J Clin Orthod*. 2003;37:599–606.
24. Shroff B. Root correction during orthodontic therapy. *Semin Orthod*. 2001;7:50–58.
25. McNamara JA, Nolan PJ, West KS. Finishing and retention. In: McNamara JA Jr, Brudon WL. *Orthodontics and Dentofacial Orthopedics*. Ann Arbor, MI: Needham Press; 2001:453–474.
26. Kharat DU, Saini TS, Mokeem S. Shovel-shaped incisors and associated invagination in some Asian and African populations. *J Dent*. 1990;18: 216–220.
27. Hatasaka HH. A radiographic study of roots in extraction sites. *Angle Orthod*. 1976;46:64–68.
28. Artun J, Kokich VG, Osterberg SK. Long-term effect of root proximity on periodontal health after orthodontic treatment. *Am J Orthod Dentofacial Orthop*. 1987;91:125–130.
29. Levander E, Bajka R, Malmgren O. Early radiographic diagnosis of apical root resorption during orthodontic treatment: a study of maxillary incisors. *Eur J Orthod*. 1998;20:57–63.
30. O'Hea CM. A prospective investigation of maxillary central incisor root resorption incident to orthodontic therapy [Masters thesis]. Farmington, CT: Department of Orthodontics, University of Connecticut; 1999: 151.
31. Joondeph D. Retention and relapse. In: Graber TM, Vanarsdall RL, eds. *Orthodontics: Current Principles and Techniques*. 3rd ed. St. Louis, MO: Mosby; 2000:985–1012.
32. Proffit WR. The third stage of comprehensive treatment: finishing. In: Proffit WR, ed. *Contemporary Orthodontics*. 3rd ed. St. Louis, MO: Mosby; 2000:578–596.
33. McLaughlin R, Bennett J. Finishing with the preadjusted orthodontic appliance. *Semin Orthod*. 2003;9:165–183.
34. Little RM, Riedel RA, Artun J. An evaluation of changes in mandibular anterior alignment from 10 to 20 years postretention. *Am J Orthod Dentofacial Orthop*. 1988;93:423–428.
35. Faerovig E, Zachrisson BU. Effects of mandibular incisor extraction on anterior occlusion in adults with Class III malocclusion and reduced overbite. *Am J Orthod Dentofacial Orthop*. 1999;115:113–124.
36. Kokich VO Jr. Congenitally missing teeth: orthodontic management in the adolescent patient. *Am J Orthod Dentofacial Orthop*. 2002;121: 594–595.
37. Spear FM, Mathews DM, Kokich VG. Interdisciplinary management of single-tooth implants. *Semin Orthod*. 1997;3:45–72.
38. Archambault A, Lacoursiere R, Badawi H, Major PW, Carey J, Flores-Mir C. Torque expression in stainless steel orthodontic brackets: a systematic review. *Angle Orthod*. 2010;80(1):201–210.
39. Johnson E. Relative stiffness of beta titanium archwires. *Angle Orthod*. 2003;73:259–269.
40. Burstone CJ, Koenig HA. Creative wire bending: the force system from step and V bends. *Am J Orthod Dentofacial Orthop*. 1988;93(1):59–67.
41. Parkinson CE, Buschang PH, Behrents RG, Throckmorton GS, English JD. A new method of evaluating posterior occlusion and its relation to posttreatment occlusal changes. *Am J Orthod Dentofacial Orthop*. 2001; 120:503–512.

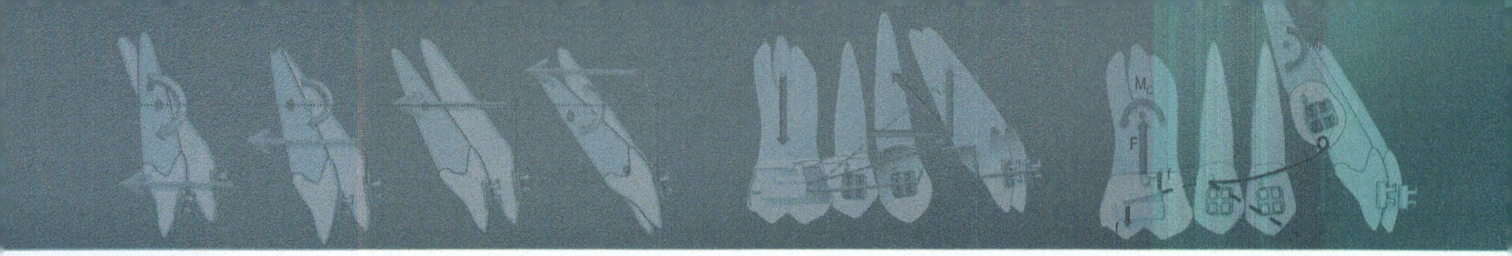

INDEX

Page numbers followed by "f" indicate figures, "t" indicate tables, and "b" indicate boxes.

D

Printed and bound by CPI Group (UK) Ltd, Croydon, CR0 4YY
14/09/2026
02216412-0001